Fifth Edition

BD Chaurasia's

Human Anatomy

for Dental Students

As per the syllabus prescribed by the Dental Council of India

Salient Features

- Regional and Applied Anatomy
- Dissection and Clinical Anatomy
- Facts to Remember
- Clinicoanatomical Problems
- Multiple Choice Questions
- Mnemonics
- General Anatomy
- Clinical Procedures
- Genetics
- Embryology
- Histology

New Topics

- Frequently Asked Questions
- Viva Voce
- Further Reading
- Molecular Basis of Development
- Flowcharts of Cranial Nerves
- Videos on Osteology and Soft Parts

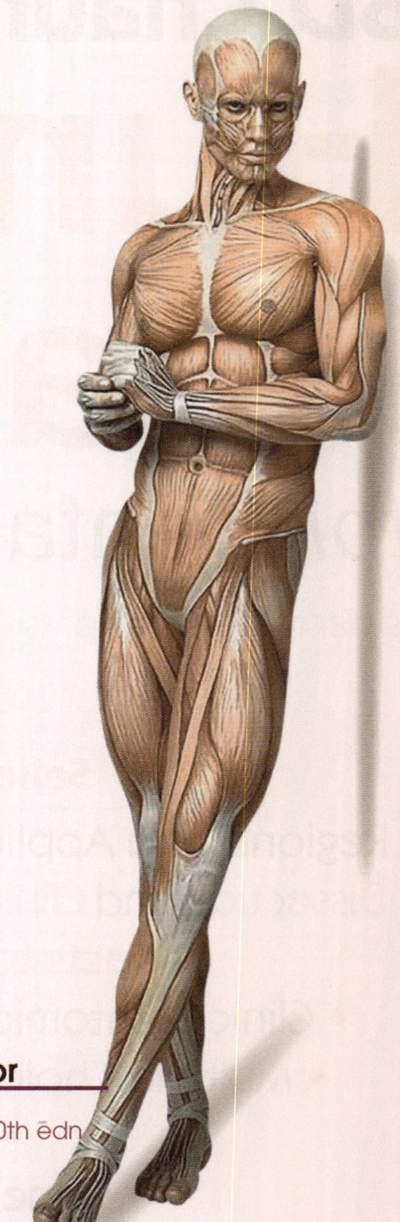

Other CBS Bestsellers in Human Anatomy by the Same Author

BD Chaurasia's **Human Anatomy: Regional and Applied | Dissection and Clinical** 10th edn
Volume **1: Upper Limb and Thorax**
Volume **2: Lower Limb, Abdomen and Pelvis**
Volume **3: Head and Neck**
Volume **4: Brain–Neuroanatomy**

BD Chaurasia's **Handbook of General Anatomy** 7th edn

BD Chaurasia's *dream* **Human Embryology** 2nd edn

Textbook of Histology 6th edn

Textbook of Neuroanatomy with Clinical Orientation 6th edn

Practical Anatomy Workbook revised 4th edn

Practical Histology Workbook revised 3rd edn

Practical Anatomy Workbook for Dental Students 2nd edn

Manual of Human Anatomy Dissection

Fifth Edition

BD Chaurasia's Human Anatomy *for* Dental Students

As per the syllabus prescribed by the Dental Council of India

Salient Features

- Regional and Applied Anatomy
- Dissection and Clinical Anatomy
- Facts to Remember
- Clinicoanatomical Problems
- Multiple Choice Questions
- Mnemonics
- General Anatomy
- Clinical Procedures
- Genetics
- Embryology
- Histology

New Topics

- Frequently Asked Questions
- Viva Voce
- Further Reading
- Molecular Basis of Development
- Flowcharts of Cranial Nerves
- Videos on Osteology and Soft Parts

Edited by

Krishna Garg

MBBS MS PhD FIMSA FIAMS FAMS FASI

Legend of Anatomy; Nation's Who's Who
Fellow, Anatomical Society of India
Lifetime Achievement Awardee
DMA Distinguished Service Awardee

Ex-Professor and Head, Department of Anatomy
Lady Hardinge Medical College, New Delhi

Visiting Faculty of Anatomy
Kalka Dental College, Meerut, UP

CBS Publishers & Distributors Pvt Ltd

New Delhi • Bengaluru • Chennai • Kochi • Kolkata • Lucknow • Mumbai
Gujarat • Hyderabad • Jharkhand • Nagpur • Patna • Pune • Uttarakhand

Disclaimer

Science and technology are constantly changing fields. New research and experience broaden the scope of information and knowledge. The editor has tried her best in giving information available to her while preparing the material for this book. Although all efforts have been made to ensure optimum accuracy of the material, yet it is quite possible some errors might have been left uncorrected. The publisher, the printer and the editor will not be held responsible for any inadvertent errors, omissions or inaccuracies.

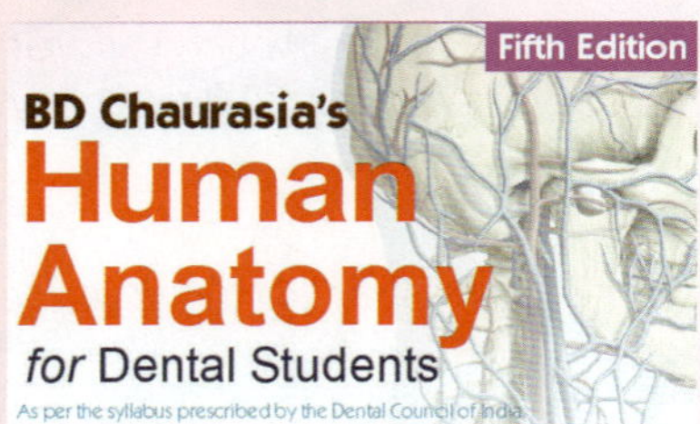

ISBN: 978-93-54666-08-7

Fifth Edition: 2024
Reprint: 2026
First Edition: 2007
Second Edition: 2012
Third Edition: 2016
Fourth Edition: 2020
Reprint: 2021, 2022

Published by Satish Kumar Jain and produced by Varun Jain for
CBS Publishers & Distributors Pvt Ltd
4819/XI Prahlad Street, 24 Ansari Road, Daryaganj, New Delhi 110 002, India.
Ph: 011-23289259, 23266838
Website: www.cbspd.com
e-mail: delhi@cbspd.com

Corporate Office: 204 FIE, Industrial Area, Patparganj, Delhi 110 092, India
Ph: 011-4934 4934 Fax: 4934 4935 e-mail: publishing@cbspd.com; publicity@cbspd.com

Branches

- **Bengaluru:** Seema House 2975, 17th Cross, K.R. Road, Banasankari 2nd Stage, Bengaluru 560 070, Karnataka, India
  Ph: +91-80-26771678/79 Fax: +91-80-26771680 e-mail: bangalore@cbspd.com
- **Chennai:** 18/8B, Subbarayan Street, Shenoy Nagar, Chennai 600 030, Tamil Nadu, India
  Ph: +91-44-42032115, 26681266 e-mail: chennai@cbspd.com
- **Kochi:** 42/1325, 1326, Power House Road, Opposite KSEB, Power House, Ernakulum 682 018, Kochi, Kerala, India
  Ph: +91-484-4059061-65 Fax: +91-484-4059065 e-mail: kochi@cbspd.com
- **Kolkata:** 147, Hind Ceramics Compound, 1st Floor, Nilgunj Road, Belghoria, Kolkata-700056, West Bengal, India
  Ph: +91-33-25330055/56 e-mail: kolkata@cbspd.com
- **Lucknow:** Basement, Khushnuma Complex, 7 Meerabai Marg (Behind Jawahar Bhawan), Lucknow-226001, UP, India
  Ph: +91-522-4000032 e-mail: tiwari.lucknow@cbspd.com
- **Mumbai:** PWD Shed, Gala No. 25/26, Ramchandra Bhatt Marg, Next to JJ Hospital Gate No. 2, Opp. Union Bank of India, Noorbaug, Mumbai-400009, Maharashtra, India
  Ph: +91-22-66661880/89 e-mail: mumbai@cbspd.com

Representatives

- **Gujarat** • **Hyderabad** • **Jharkhand** • **Nagpur** • **Patna** • **Pune** • **Uttarakhand**

For trade terms please contact customercare@cbspd.com
For general enquiries please contact info@cbspd.com

Printed at Goyal Offset Works Pvt. Ltd. Haryana, India

Preface to the Fifth Edition

Human Anatomy for Dental Students had a successful innings in its fourth edition. Since change for keeping in sync with the newer developments is necessary, the fifth edition is being published.

The text has been updated and diagrams have been corrected and improved.

Molecular basis of development of various organs has been initiated as most of the diseases have a genetic origin.

Some references as "Further Reading" are given at the end of all chapters of head, neck and brain for inquisitive students. Hallmark of this edition continues to be the inclusion of *Viva Voce* questions at the end of Head and Neck and Brain sections. Learning their answers will prepare the students for their numerous practical examinations. These would even give them confidence for their postgraduate medical entrance examinations and the interviews for their jobs.

Accordingly, the various sections in this book are as follows:

Section I General Anatomy contains 8 chapters.

Section II Head and Neck comprises the most important component of anatomy for BDS students. Numerous unique line diagrams, originally hand-drawn by late Dr BD Chaurasia and used in the first edition of the book, after thoughtful moderation, have now been incorporated in the present edition. Our criteria for the selection and manipulation of these drawings were clearly based on the simplicity and lucidity of the anatomic description. These simply structured illustrations can be easily reproduced by the students in multitudes of tests and examinations, including university examinations. Revision can be done by facts to remember, frequently asked questions, MCQ and *viva voce* at the end of all chapters. Indications for viewing videos from BD Chaurasia's *Human Anatomy* (Vol. 3) Head and Neck have been given in this section at relevant places.

Section III Brain highlights of this section are flowcharts of the cranial nerves.

Section IV Other Regions of Human Body covers upper limb, thorax, abdomen and pelvis and lower limb, very briefly, giving important clinical anatomy points.

Section V Topics of Importance in Human Anatomy contains clinical procedures, genetics, embryology and histology.

Chapter on embryology gives a bird's-eye view of the general embryology. Emphasis has been given on the molecular development and congenital anomalies of structures in head and neck, namely tongue, thyroid, parathyroid, pharyngeal arches, pouches, clefts, skull, face, teeth, eye, ear, etc. Some parts have been updated.

Chapter on histology is in two parts. General histology is given with relevant drawings. As far as systemic histology is concerned, only the parts necessary for BDS students are given, such as histology of salivary glands, trachea and general plan of gastrointestinal tract with diagrams of oesophagus, stomach, duodenum, jejunum, ileum, colon, vermiform appendix, liver, gallbladder, pancreas. The diagrams of kidney, ureter, urinary bladder, testis and ovary are also provided. All these diagrams have been complemented with three points of identification. In addition, the endocrine system and special senses are described to complete the organs studied by BDS students.

Obligations are due to Mr SK Jain, Chairman and Managing Director; Mr Varun Jain, Director; Mr YN Arjuna, Senior Vice President (Publishing, Editorial and Publicity); Ms Ritu Chawla, GM (Production); and the entire editorial and production teams at CBSPD. Thanks to Mr Tarun Rajput who has done the formatting part very efficiently, Mr Sanjay Chauhan for doing beautiful graphic work and Mr Prasenjit Paul who has proficiently done the proofreading.

I shall be obliged to the readers for any constructive criticism and suggestions for improvement of the book.

Krishna Garg
dr.krishnagarg@gmail.com

Preface to the First Edition

With an ever-increasing number of students pursing dentistry as a profession, an urgent need was felt for a comprehensive book on human anatomy for dental students. The books presently available for dental students have a large number of lacunae which require appropriate rectification. With this broad objective in mind, this book has been planned to provide gross anatomy of the whole body with detailed anatomy of the head and neck according to the syllabus prescribed by the Dental Council of India. I am grateful to the Almighty for providing me this unique opportunity.

The fourth edition of BD Chaurasia's Human Anatomy published in 2004 and edited by me has been widely accepted as the base-line book on the subject for dental students. In this book the text material of Volume 3 (Head and Neck section) has been revised and included. Dissection as per requirement of BDS students have been given in blue boxes. Multiple Choice Questions and Clinico-anatomical Problems of head and neck region have also been incorporated.

The other regions, namely, brain, upper limb, thorax, abdomen, pelvis and lower limb, have been condensed in description, however, without any compromise on the illustrations which have been revised and improved substantially. It is thus a continuous, well illustrated study of each region. Muscles of all the regions have been tabulated. Besides, at the end of each section the entire course of all the nerves with clinical terms has been incorporated from the viewpoint of revision and retention. Similarly, the brief course of arteries and their branches have been tabulcted to aid quick memorization.

The clinical anatomy has also been illustrated profusely with relevant photographs to provide a glimpse of the future to the first year students of BDS course.

I am obliged to Prof Ved Prakash, Prof Mohini Kaul, Prof Indira Bahl and Prof Kumkum Rana for providing help whenever required.

I am grateful to Dr Suvira Gupta, Ex-Director Professor and Head, Department of Radiology, GB Pant Hospital, New Delhi, for her expert guidance on various radiographs, CT, ultrasound and MRI scans in head and neck sections of the book. Thanks are due to Dr Neeta Agarwal and Dr Dalvinder Singh for constantly encouraging me.

Mr Ankur Mittal and Mr Ajit Kumar, students of BPT 2004 batch from Banarasidas Chandiwala Institute of Physiotherapy, New Delhi, have diligently read the entire text and helped me in correcting the errors of omission. Their help is gratefully acknowledged.

I am obliged to Mr YN Arjuna, Publishing Director of CBS Publishers & Distributors, for providing exemplary guidance and constructive critism for this book in spite of his extremely busy schedule. His team comprising Mr Karzan Lal Prasher, Mr. Mukesh Kumar Sharma, Ms Neelam, Mr Akhilesh Kumar Dubey and Ms Mehjabeen, has given the best technical support in getting the book in its present format which is attractive and appealing.

Mr SK Jain, Managing Director, CBS Publishers & Distributors, has been constantly monitoring the progress of the book so that it is released at the appropriate time.

I wish to thank all my family members for their cooperation. It is my fervent hope that prayer and the dedication put in this book proves to be useful for BDS and MDS students. I earnestly welcome the teachers and the students in all the colleges to provide suggestions that would help make further improvements in this book.

Krishna Garg

Contents

Section II HEAD AND NECK

45. Histology 690

Syllabus for Undergraduate (BDS)
as Prescribed by Dental Council of India

HUMAN ANATOMY, EMBRYOLOGY, HISTOLOGY AND MEDICAL GENETICS

1. Introduction

1. Anatomical terms.
2. Skin, superficial fascia and deep fascia.
3. Cardiovascular system, portal system collateral circulation and arteries.
4. Lymphatic system, regional lymph nodes.
5. Osteology—including ossification and growth of bones.
6. Myology—including types of muscle tissue and innervation.
7. Syndesmology—including classification of Joints.
8. Nervous system.

2. Head and Neck

1. Scalp, face and temple, lacrimal apparatus
2. Neck—deep fascia of neck, posterior triangle, suboccipital triangle, anterior triangle, anterior median region of the neck, deep structures in the neck.
3. Cranial cavity—meninges, parts of brain, ventricles of brain, dural venous sinuses, cranial nerves attached to the brain, pituitary gland.
4. Cranial nerves—III, IV, V, VI, VII, IX, XII in detail.
5. Orbital cavity—muscles of the eyeball, supports of the eyeball, nerves and vessels in the orbit.
6. Parotid gland.
7. Temporomandibular joint, muscles of mastication, infratemporal fossa, pterygo-palatine fossa.
8. Submandibular region
9. Walls of the nasal cavity, paranasal air sinuses
10. Palate
11. Oral cavity, tongue
12. Pharynx (palatine tonsil and the auditory tube) Larynx. Osteology—foetal skull, adult skull, individual bones of the skull, hyoid bone and cervical vertebrae.

3. Thorax

Demonstration on a dissected specimen of:

1. Thoracic wall
2. Heart chambers
3. Coronary arteries
4. Pericardium
5. Lungs—surfaces; pleural cavity
6. Diaphragm

4. Abdomen

Demonstration on a dissected specimen of:

1. Peritoneal cavity
2. Organs in the abdominal and pelvic cavity.

5. Clinical Procedures

a. *Intramuscular injections:* Demonstration on a dissected specimen and on a living person of the following sites of injection.
   1. Deltoid muscle and its relation to the axillary nerve and radial nerve.
   2. Gluteal region and the relation of the sciatic nerve.
   3. Vastus lateralis muscle.

b. *Intravenous injections and venesection:* Demonstration of veins in the dissected specimen and on a living person.
   1. Median cubital vein
   2. Cephalic vein
   3. Basilic vein
   4. Long saphenous vein

c. *Arterial pulsations:* Demonstration of arteries on a dissected specimen and feeling of pulsation of the following arteries on a living person.
   1. Superficial temporal
   2. Facial
   3. Carotid
   4. Axillary
   5. Brachial
   6. Radial
   7. Ulnar
   8. Femoral
   9. Popliteal
   10. Dorsalis pedis

d. *Lumbar puncture:* Demonstration on a dissected specimen of the spinal cord, cauda equina and epidural space and the inter vertebral space between L4 and L5.

6. Embryology

Oogenesis, spermatogenesis, fertilisation, placenta, primitive streak, neural crest, bilaminar and trilaminar embryonic disc, intra embryonic mesoderm—formation and fate, notochord formation and fate, pharyngeal arches, pouches and clefts, development of face, tongue, palate, thyroid gland, pituitary gland, salivary glands, and anomalies in their development, tooth development in brief.

7. Histology

The cell: Basic tissues—epithelium, connective tissue including cartilage and bone, muscle tissue.

Nervous tissue: Peripheral nerve, optic nerve, sensory ganglion, motor ganglion, skin.

Classification of glands: Salivary glands (serous, mucous and mixed gland), blood vessels, lymphoid tissue tooth, lip, tongue, hard palate, oesophagus, stomach, duodenum, ileum, colon, vermiform appendix, liver, pancreas, lung, trachea, epiglottis, thyroid gland, para thyroid gland, supra-renal gland and pituitary gland, kidney, ureter, urinary bladder, ovary and testis.

8. Medical Genetics

Mitosis, meiosis, chromosomes, gene structure, mendelism, modes of inheritance.

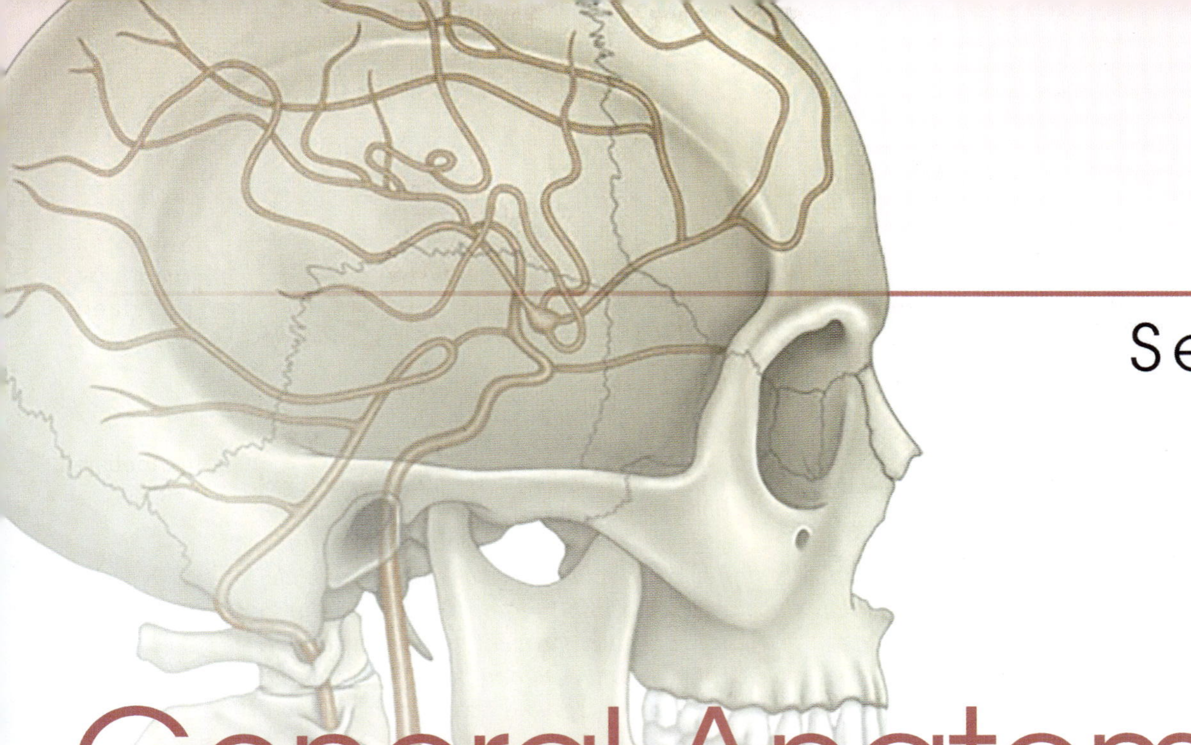

Section

I

General Anatomy

Anatomy Made Easy

Anatomical position is the position to learn Anatomy
Bone constitutes the strength of the body,
Muscles move the bones at the joints.
Blood vessels supply oxygen and take back carbon dioxide,
Nerves stimulate the muscles and inform brain about everything.
Skin is the outer garment and largest organ,
All these constitute General Anatomy, which is essential
to understand textbooks of Antomy

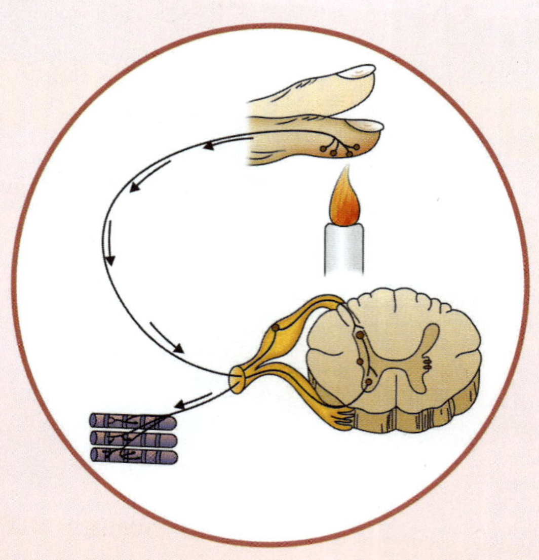

Chapter 1

Introduction

"Life is a book with three chapters. Two are already written by God—birth and death. The chapter in the middle is empty; fill it with smile, love and faith."
—Anonymous

Human anatomy is the science which deals with the structure of the human body.

The main subdivisions of anatomy are:

1 *Cadaveric anatomy* is studied on dead embalmed (preserved) bodies usually with the naked eye (macroscopic or gross anatomy).
Head and neck and brain are studied as regional anatomy (Fig. 1.1).
2 *Living anatomy* is studied by inspection (Fig. 1.2), palpation, percussion, auscultation, radiography, etc.
3 *Embryology (developmental anatomy)* is the study of the prenatal developmental changes in an individual (Fig. 1.3).

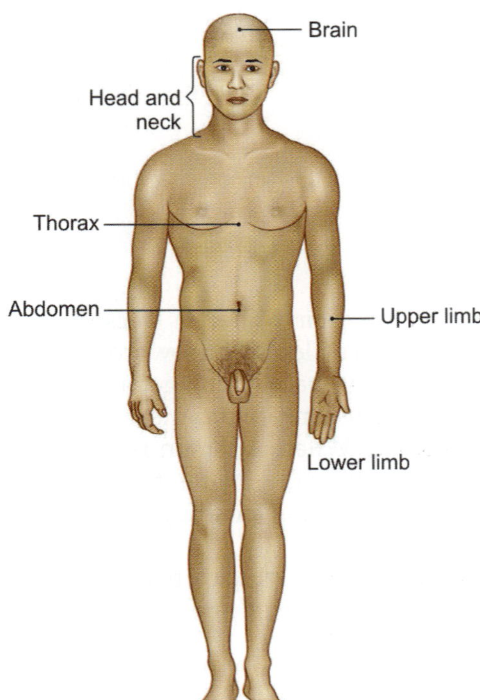

Fig. 1.1: Various regions of the body

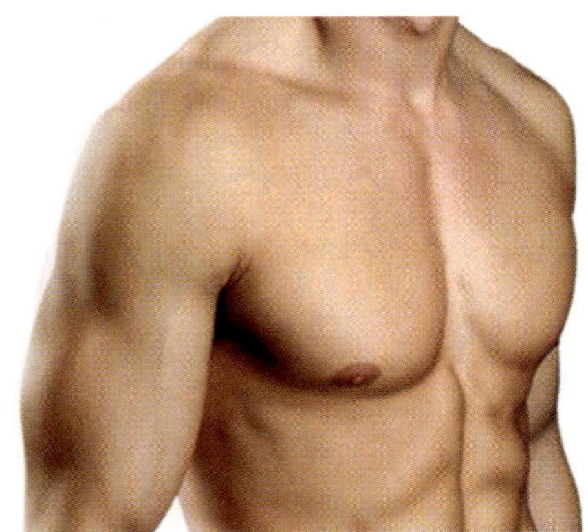
Fig. 1.2: Inspection of the chest

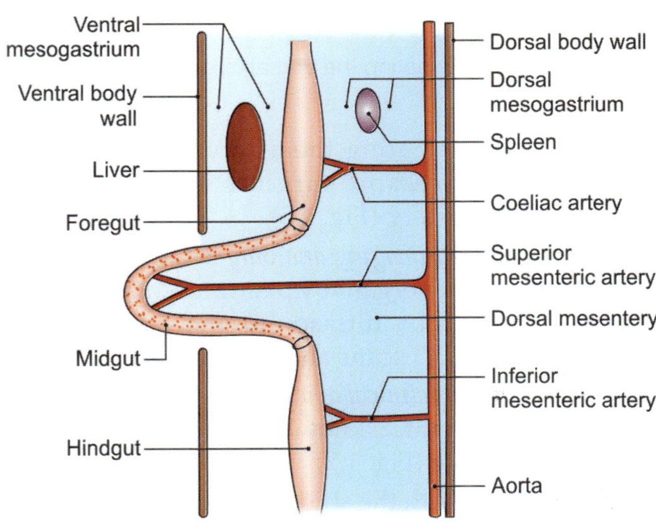

Fig. 1.3: Development of various parts of the gut

4 *Histology (microscopic anatomy)* is the study of structures with the aid of a microscope (Fig. 1.4).
5 *Surface anatomy (topographic anatomy)* is the study of deeper parts of the body in relation to the skin

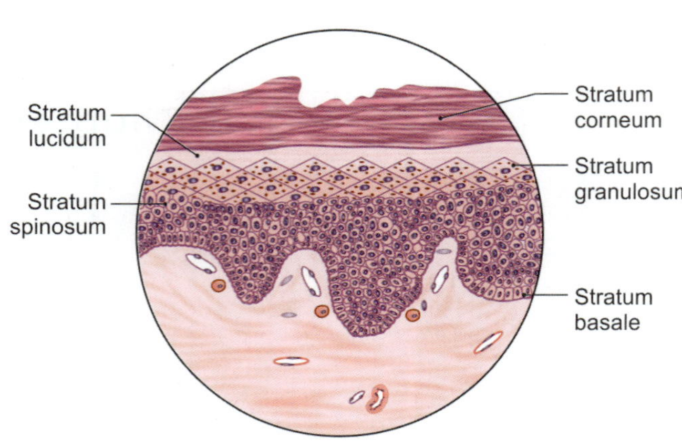

Fig. 1.4: Histology of the epidermis of thick skin

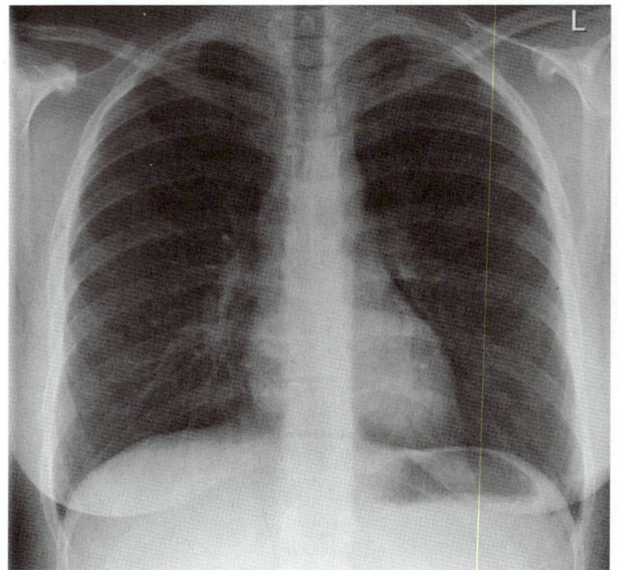

Fig. 1.6: X-ray chest: Posteroanterior view

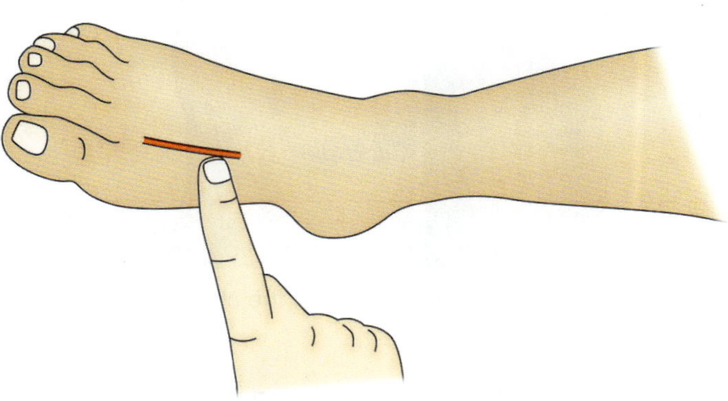

Fig. 1.5: Palpating the dorsalis pedis artery

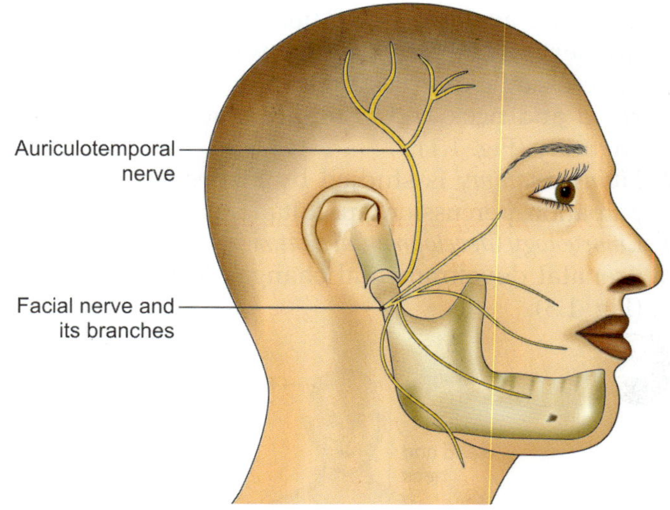

Fig. 1.7: Close relation of the two nerves to the temporomandibular joint

surface, e.g. palpating the artery. It is helpful in clinical practice and surgical operations, e.g. palpating the artery (Fig. 1.5).

6 *Radiographic and imaging anatomy* is the study of the bones and deeper organs by plain and contrast radiography (X-ray), by ultrasound and computerised tomographic (CT) scans and MRI scans (Fig. 1.6).
7 *Applied anatomy (clinical anatomy)* deals with application of the anatomical knowledge to the medical and surgical practice (Fig. 1.7).
8 *Genetics* deals with the study of information present in the chromosomes (*see* Chapter 43).

LANGUAGE OF ANATOMY

Various positions, planes, terms in relation to various regions specially head and neck and their movements are described.

Positions

- *Anatomical position:* When a person is standing straight with eyes looking forwards, both arms by the side of body, palms facing forwards, both feet together, the position is anatomical position (Fig. 1.8).
- *Supine position:* When a person is lying on her/his back, arms by the side, palms facing upwards and feet put together, the position is supine position (Fig. 1.9).
- *Prone position:* Person lying on his/her face, chest and abdomen is said to be in prone position (Fig. 1.10).

Planes

- A plane passing through the centre of the body dividing it into two equal right and left halves, is

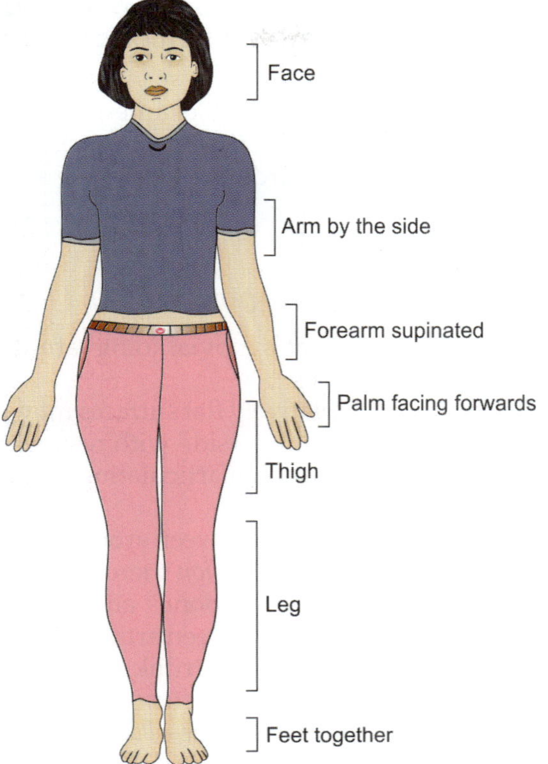

Fig. 1.8: Anatomical position

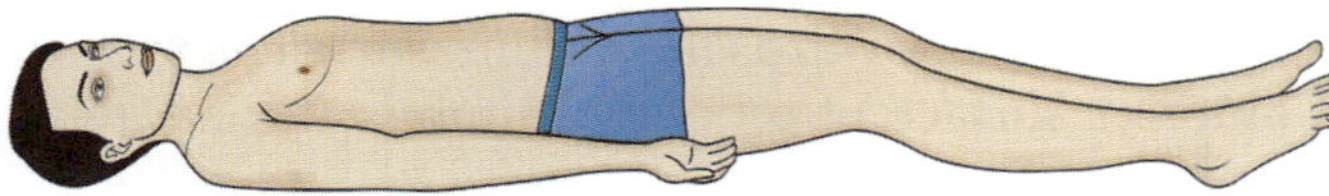
Fig. 1.9: Supine position

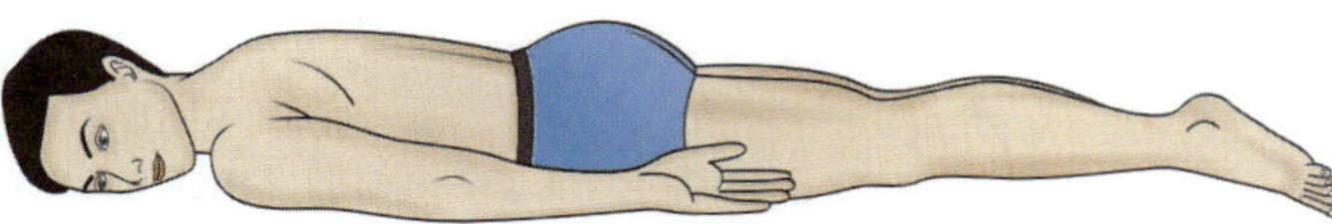
Fig. 1.10: Prone position

the median or midsagittal plane (Fig.1.11). Plane parallel to median or midsagittal plane is the sagittal plane.

- A plane at right angles to sagittal or median plane which divides the body into anterior and posterior halves is called a *coronal plane*.
- A plane at right angles to both sagittal and coronal planes which divides the body into upper and lower parts is called a *transverse—horizontal plane*.

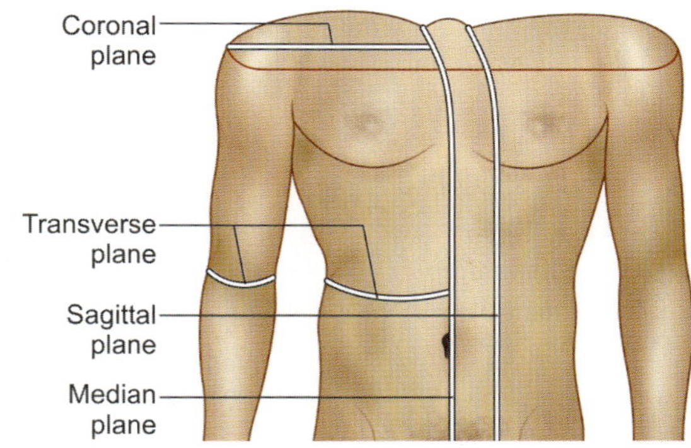

Fig. 1.11: Median, sagittal, coronal and horizontal planes

Terms Used in Relation to Trunk, Neck and Face

- *Ventral* or *anterior* is the front of trunk, neck and face.
- *Dorsal* or *posterior* is the back of trunk, neck and face.
- *Medial* is a plane close to the median plane.
- *Lateral* is plane away from the median plane.
- *Proximal/cranial/superior* is close to the head end of body (Figs 1.12 and 1.13).
- *Distal/caudal/inferior* is close to the lower end of the trunk.
- *Superficial* is close to skin/towards the surface of body.
- *Deep* is away from skin/away from the surface of body.
- *Ipsilateral* is on the same side of the body as another structure.
- *Contralateral* is on opposite side of the body from another structure.
- *Invagination* is projection inside.
- *Evagination* is projection outside.

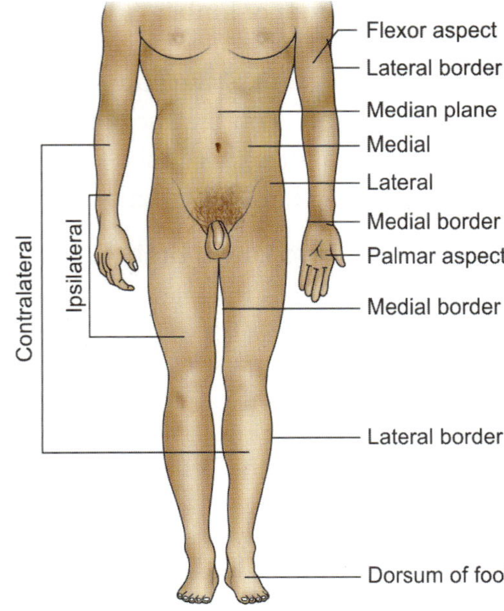

Fig. 1.12: Language of anatomy

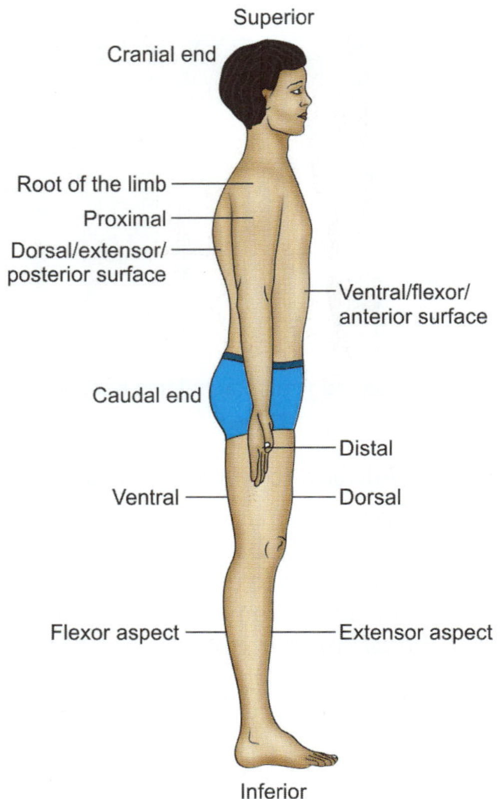

Fig. 1.13: Anatomical terms

Terms Used in Relation to Upper Limb

- *Ventral* or *anterior* is the front aspect.
- *Dorsal* or *posterior* is the back aspect.
- *Medial border* lies along the little finger, medial border of forearm and arm.
- *Lateral border* follows the thumb, lateral border of forearm and arm.
- *Proximal* is close to root of limb, while *distal* is away from the root (Fig. 1.13).
- *Palmar* aspect is the front of the palm (Fig. 1.12).
- *Dorsal* aspect of hand is on the back of palm.
- *Flexor* aspect is front of upper limb.
- *Extensor* aspect is back of upper limb.

Terms Used in Relation to Lower Limb

- *Posterior/ventral* aspect is the back of lower limb.
- *Anterior/dorsal* aspect is the front of lower limb (Fig. 1.13).
- *Medial border* lies along the big toe or hallux, medial border of leg and thigh (Fig. 1.12).
- *Lateral border* lies along the little toe, lateral border of leg and thigh.
- *Flexor* aspect is back of lower limb.
- *Extensor* aspect is front of lower limb (Fig. 1.13).
- *Proximal* is close to the root of limb, while *distal* is away from it (Fig. 1.13).

Terms of Relation Commonly Used in Embryology and Comparative Anatomy, but Sometimes in Gross Anatomy

a. *Ventral*—towards the belly (like anterior).
b. *Dorsal*—towards the back (like posterior).
c. *Cranial or rostral*—towards the head (like superior) (Fig. 1.13).
d. *Caudal*—towards the tail.

TERMS RELATED TO BODY MOVEMENTS

Movements in general at synovial joints are divided into four main categories.

1 *Gliding movement*: Relatively flat surfaces move back-and-forth and from side-to-side with respect to one another. The angle between articulating bones does not change significantly.
2 *Angular movements*: Angle between articulating bones decreases or increases. In *flexion* there is decrease in angle between articulating bones and in *extension* there is increase in angle between articulating bones. *Lateral flexion* is movement of trunk sideways to the right or left at the waist. *Adduction* is movement of bone toward midline, whereas *abduction* is movement of bone away from midline (Figs 1.14 and 1.15).
3 *Special movements*: These occur only at certain joints, e.g. pronation, supination at radioulnar joints, protraction and retraction at temporomandibular joint (Figs 1.21 to 1.23).
4 *Rotation*: A bone revolves around its own longitudinal axis. In *medial rotation* anterior surface of a bone of limb is turned towards the midline. In *lateral rotation* anterior surface of a bone of limb is turned away from midline.

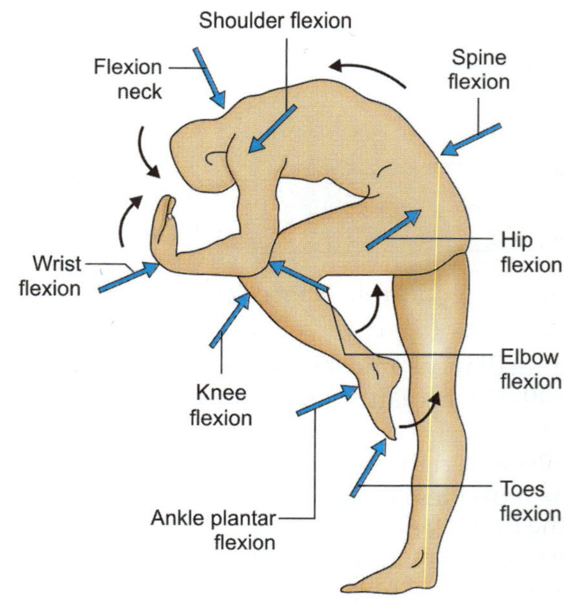

Fig. 1.14: Flexion

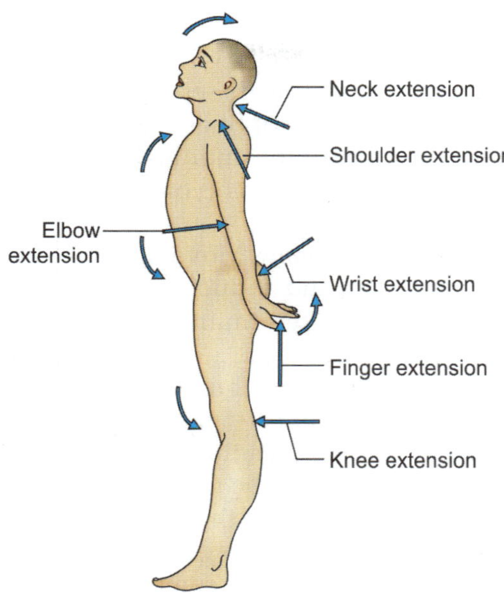

Fig. 1.15: Extension

In the Neck

- *Flexion*: When face comes closer to chest.
- *Extension*: When face is taken away from the chest (Fig. 1.16).
- *Lateral flexion*: When ear is brought close to shoulder (Fig. 1.17).
- *Rotation*: When neck rotates so that chin goes to opposite side.
- *Opening the mouth*: When lower jaw is lowered to open the mouth (Fig. 1.18).
- *Closure of the mouth*: When lower jaw is opposed to the upper jaw, closing the mouth (Fig. 1.19).
- *Protraction*: When lower jaw slides forwards in its socket in the temporal bone of skull (Fig. 1.20).
- *Retraction*: When lower jaw slides backwards in its socket in the temporal bone of skull (Fig. 1.21).

In Upper Limb

- *Flexion*: When two flexor surfaces are brought close to each other, e.g. in wrist joint when front of arm and palm move close to each other (Fig. 1.22).
- *Extension*: When extensor or dorsal surfaces are brought in as much approximation as possible, e.g. straighten the forearm at the elbow joint.
- *Abduction of shoulder*: When limb is taken away from the body.
- *Adduction of shoulder*: When limb is brought close to the body.
- *Flexion of shoulder*: If arm is taken towards the front of the chest wall.
- *Extension*: Arm is taken backwards and laterally.
- *Circumduction*: It is movement of distal end of a part of the body in a circle. A combination of extension,

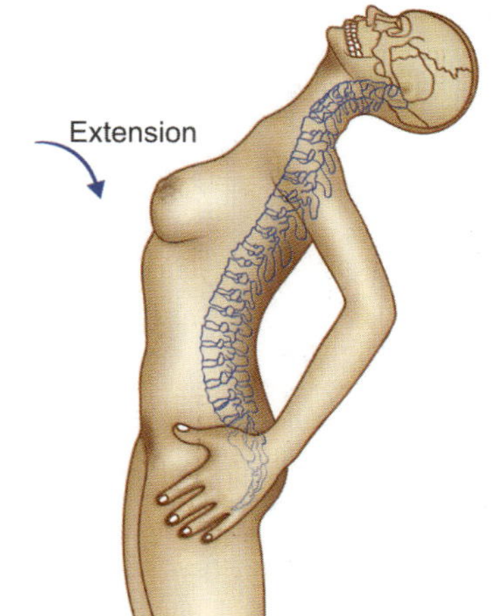

Fig. 1.16: Extension of neck and trunk

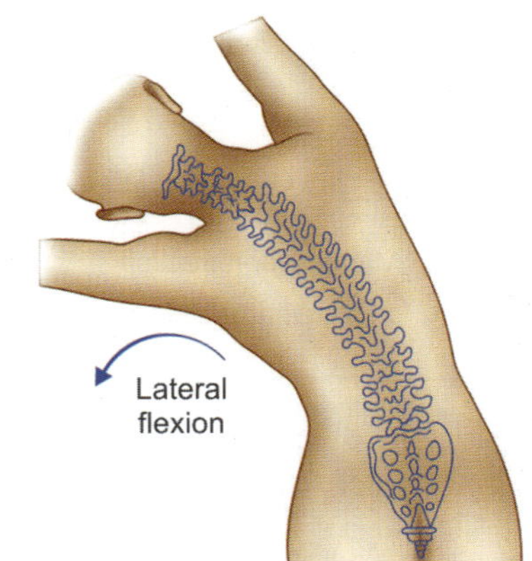

Fig. 1.17: Lateral flexion of neck and trunk

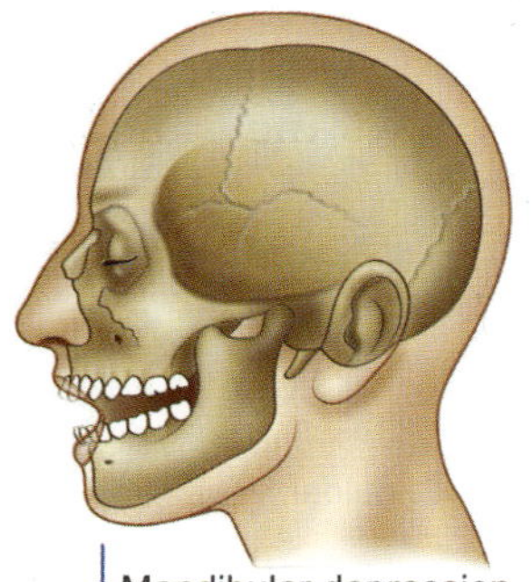

Fig. 1.18: Opening the mouth

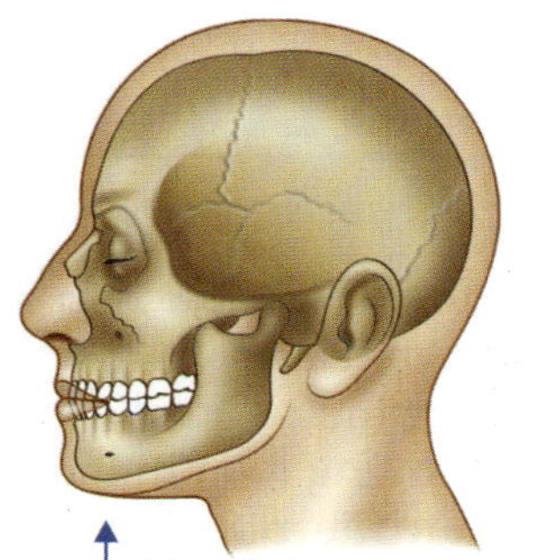

Fig. 1.19: Closure of the mouth

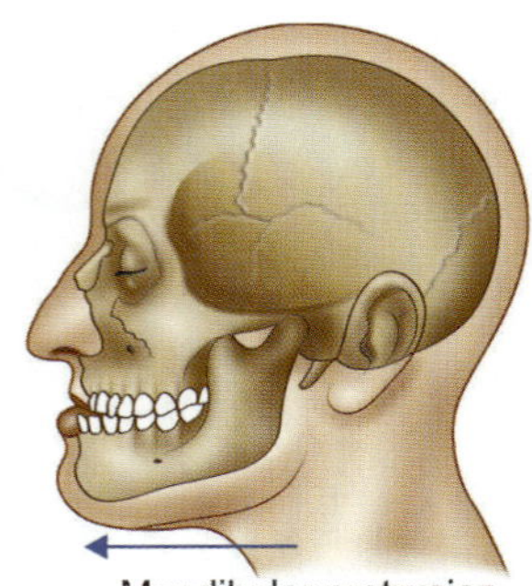

Fig. 1.20: Protraction of lower jaw

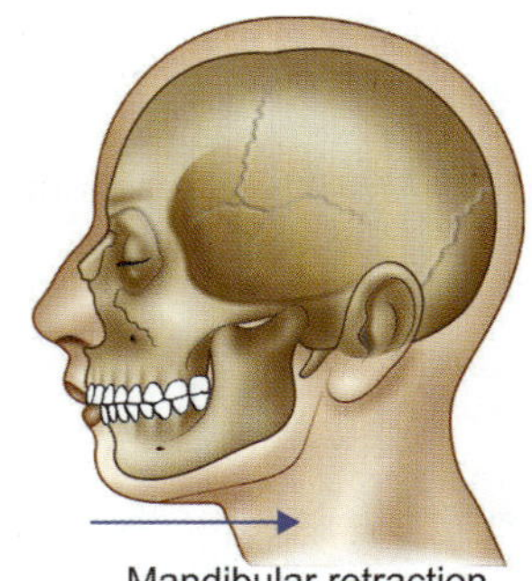

Fig. 1.21: Retraction of lower jaw

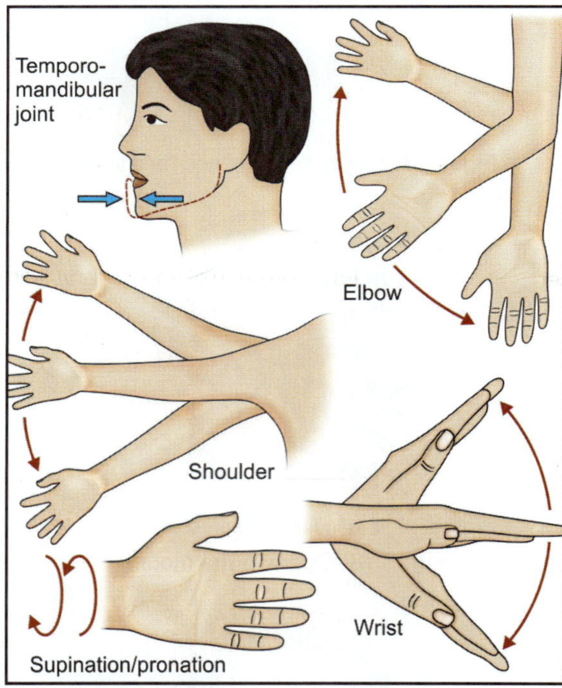

Fig. 1.22: Movements of some of the joints

abduction, flexion and adduction in a sequence is called circumduction as in bowling.

- *Supination*: When the palm is facing forwards or upwards, as in putting food in the mouth.
- *Pronation*: When the palm faces backwards or downwards, as in picking food with fingers from the plate (Fig. 1.22).
- *Adduction of digits/fingers*: When all the fingers get together.
- *Abduction*: When all fingers separate.
  The axis of movement of fingers is the line passing through the centre of the middle finger.
- *Opposition of thumb*: When tip of thumb touches the tips of any of the fingers.
- *Circumduction of thumb*: Movement of extension, abduction, flexion and adduction in sequence.
- *Flexion of thumb*: When thumb is taken across the palm.
- *Extension of thumb*: When thumb is taken backwards in the plane of the palm.
- *Abduction of thumb*: When thumb is put vertically at right angles to plane of the palm.
- *Adduction of thumb*: When thumb is in close contact with lateral side of index finger
- *Flexion of wrist*: When palm comes closer to front of forearm.
- *Extension of wrist*: When dorsum of hand comes closer to back of forearm.
- *Flexion of metacarpophalangeal and interphalangeal joints*: When attempting to make a fist.
- *Extension of metacarpophalangeal and interphalangeal joints*: When opening the fist.

In Lower Limb

- *Flexion of thigh*: When front of thigh comes close to or in contact with front of abdomen (Fig. 1.23).
- *Extension of thigh*: When person stands erect.

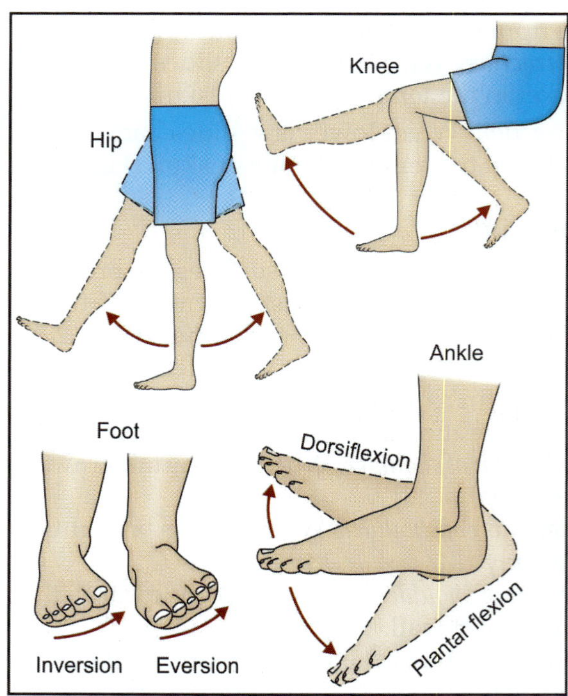

Fig. 1.23: Movements of joints of lower limb

- *Abduction*: When thigh is taken away from the median plane.
- *Adduction*: When thigh is brought close to median plane.
- *Medial rotation*: When thigh is turned medially. It is done by pointing the big toe medially.
- *Lateral rotation*: When thigh is turned laterally. It is done by pointing the big toe laterally.
- *Circumduction*: When flexion, adduction, extension and abduction are done in sequence
- *Flexion of knee*: When back of thigh and back of leg come close to or are in opposition.

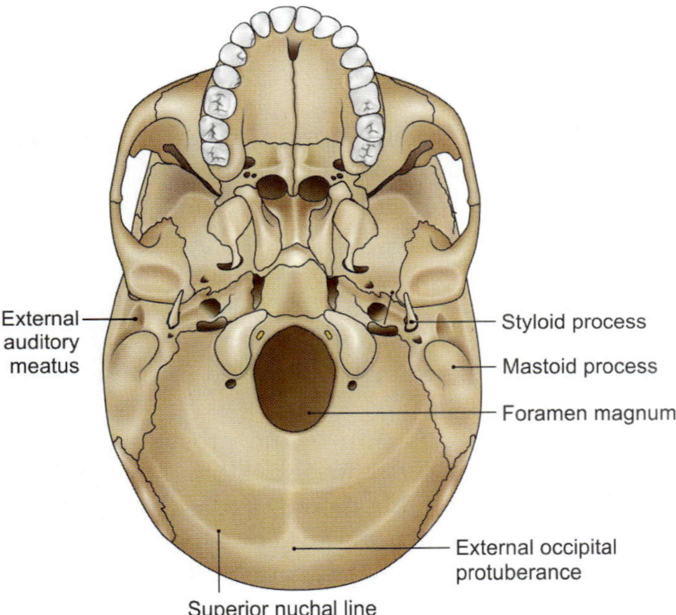

Fig. 1.24: Terms used for describing bone features

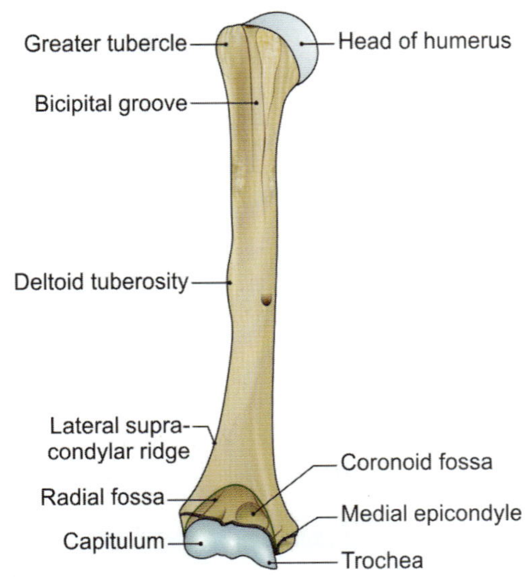

Fig. 1.25: Terms used for describing bone features

Terms Used for Describing Bone Features

Bone marking	*Example*
Linear elevation	
Line	Superior nuchal line and inferior nuchal line of the occipital bone (Fig. 1.24)
Crest	The illac crest of the hip bone of spine, of scapula
Ridge	The medial and lateral supracondylar ridges of the humerus (Fig. 1.25)
Rounded elevation	
Tubercle	Pubic tubercle, lesser and greater tubercles of humerus (Fig. 1.25)
Protuberance	External occipital protuberance
Tuberosity	Ischial tuberosity of the hip bone, deltoid tuberosity
Malleolus	Medial malleolus of the tibia, lateral malleolus of the fibula
Trochanter	Greater and lesser trochanters of the femur
Sharp elevation	
Spine or spinous process	Ischial spine, spine of vertebra, anterior superior iliac spine
Styloid process	Styloid process of temporal bone (Fig. 1.24)
Expanded ends for articulation	
Head	Head of humerus, head of femur, head of radius
Condyle	Medial and lateral condyles of femur
Epicondyle (a prominence situated just above condyle)	Medial and lateral epicondyles of femur, medial and lateral epicondyles of humerus
Small flat area for articulation	
Facet	Facet on head of rib for articulation with vertebral body
Depressions	
Notch	Greater sciatic notch and lesser sciatic notch of hip bone
Groove or sulcus	Bicipital groove of humerus
Fossa	Radial and coronoid fossae of humerus, acetabular fossa of hip bone
Openings	
Fissure	Superior orbital and inferior orbital fissures (Fig. 1.26)
Foramen	Infraorbital foramen of the maxilla
Canal	Carotid canal of temporal bone
Meatus	External acoustic meatus and internal acoustic meatus of temporal bone

- *Extension of knee*: When thigh and leg are in straight line as in standing (Fig. 1.23).
- *Dorsiflexion of foot*: When dorsum of foot is brought close to front of leg and sole faces forwards.
- *Plantar flexion of foot*: When sole of foot or plantar aspect of foot faces backwards (Fig. 1.23).

- *Inversion of foot*: When medial border of foot is raised from the ground.
- *Eversion of foot*: When lateral border of foot is raised from the ground (Fig. 1.23).

In the Trunk

- Backward bending is called *extension* (Fig. 1.16).
- Forward bending is *flexion*.
- Sideward movement is *lateral flexion* (Fig. 1.17).
- Sideward rotation is *lateral rotation*.

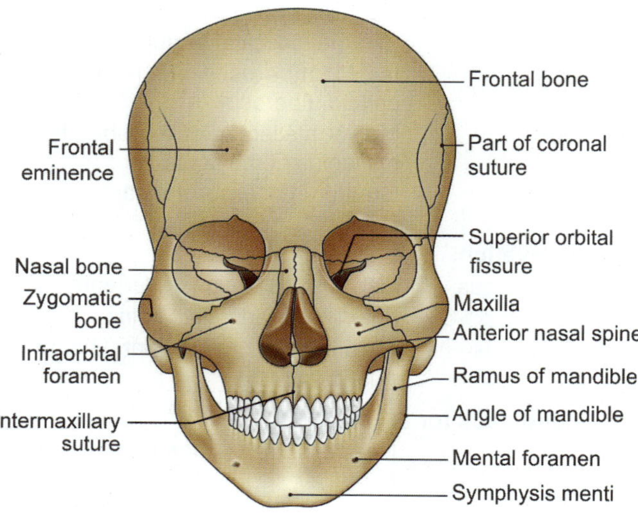

Fig. 1.26: Terms used for describing bone features

CLINICAL ANATOMY

1. ***Inflammation*** is the local reaction of the tissues to an injury or an abnormal stimulation caused by a physical, chemical, or biologic agent. It is characterized by:
   a. Swelling
   b. Pain
   c. Redness
   d. Warmth or heat
   e. Loss of function.
2. ***Paralysis***: Loss of motor power (movement) of a part of body due to denervation or primary disease of the muscles.
3. ***Hemiplegia***: Paralysis of one-half of the body.
4. ***Paraplegia***: Paralysis of both the lower limbs.
5. ***Monoplegia***: Paralysis of any one limb.
6. ***Anaesthesia***: Loss of sensation.
7. ***Tumour (neoplasm)***: A circumscribed, noninflammatory, abnormal growth arising from the body tissues.
8. ***Benign***: Mild illness or growth which does not endanger life.
9. ***Malignant***: Severe form of illness or growth, which may be resistant to treatment.

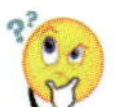

FACTS TO REMEMBER

- Hippocrates is the father of medicine.
- Dr Inderjit Dewan researched on osteology and anthropology.
- Anatomical position is the most important position for understanding anatomy.
- Pronation and supination of forearm are special movements which permit "picking up of food (pronation)" and "putting it in the mouth (supination)".
- Big toe being in the same plane as rest of the toes is unique to human.
- There are 12 systems in the body. Medical students learn anatomy as regional anatomy, whereas nursing students learn it as systemic anatomy.

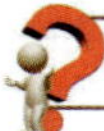

Multiple Choice Questions

1. Anatomical position has following features, *except*:
   a. Person standing erect
   b. Forearms are pronated
   c. Feet together
   d. Eyes looking forwards

2. What is the position of forearms in the anatomical position?
   a. Pronated
   b. Supinated
   c. Midprone
   d. None of the above

3. The term cranial means:
   a. Towards the head
   b. Towards the back
   c. Towards the tail
   d. Towards the front

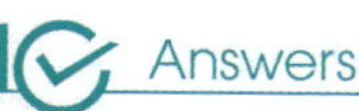

1. b **2.** b **3.** a

Chapter 2

Skeleton

"One quarter of what you eat keeps you alive; the three quarters keep doctors alive."
—Anonymous

Skeleton includes bones and cartilages. It forms the main supporting framework of the body, and is primarily designed for a more effective production of movements by the attached muscles.

BONES

Synonyms

1 Os (L)
2 Osteon (G).

Compare with the terms, osteology, ossification, osteomyelitis, osteomalacia, osteoma, osteotomy, etc.

Definition

Bone is one-third connective tissue. It is impregnated with calcium salts which constitute the remaining two-thirds part.

The inorganic calcium salts (mainly calcium phosphate, partly calcium carbonate, and traces of other salts) make it hard and rigid, which can afford resistance to compressive forces of weight-bearing and impact forces of jumping. The organic connective tissue (collagen fibres) makes it tough and resilient (flexible), which can afford resistance to tensile forces. In strength, bone is comparable to iron and steel.

The inorganic calcium salt is calcium hydroxyapatite $[Ca_{10}(PO_4)_6(OH)_2]$. If it is removed by putting the bone in acid, it becomes flexible and can be tied as a 'knot'. If organic tissue is removed by burning, the bone crumples into small pieces.

Despite its hardness and high calcium content, the bone is very much a living tissue. It is highly vascular, with a constant turnover of its calcium content. It shows a characteristic pattern of growth. It is subjected to disease and heals after a fracture. It has greater regenerative power than any other tissue of the body, except blood. It can mould itself according to changes in stress and strain it bears. It shows disuse atrophy and overuse hypertrophy.

Functions

1 Bones give shape and support to the body, and resist any forms of stress (Fig. 2.1).
2 These provide surface for the attachment of muscles, tendons, ligaments, etc.
3 These serve as levers for muscular actions.
4 The skull, vertebral column and thoracic cage protect brain, spinal cord and thoracic and some abdominal viscera, respectively.
5 Bone marrow manufactures blood cells.
6 Bones store 97% of the body calcium and phosphorus.
7 Bone marrow contains reticuloendothelial cells which are phagocytic in nature and take part in immune responses of the body.
8 The larger paranasal air sinuses, e.g. ethmoidal sinuses affect the timbre of the voice.

CLASSIFICATION OF BONES

A. According to Shape

1 *Long bones:* Each long bone has an elongated shaft (diaphysis) and two expanded ends (epiphyses) which are smooth and articular (Fig. 2.2). The shaft typically has 3 surfaces separated by 3 borders, a central medullary cavity, and a nutrient foramen directed away from the growing end. Examples: *Typical long bones:* These are humerus, radius, ulna, femur, tibia and fibula; with two secondary epiphyses.
2 *Short bones:* Their shape is usually cuboid (like a cube), or scaphoid (boat shaped). Examples: Tarsal and carpal bones (Fig. 2.1).
3 *Flat bones:* Resemble shallow plates and form boundaries of certain body cavities. Examples: Bones

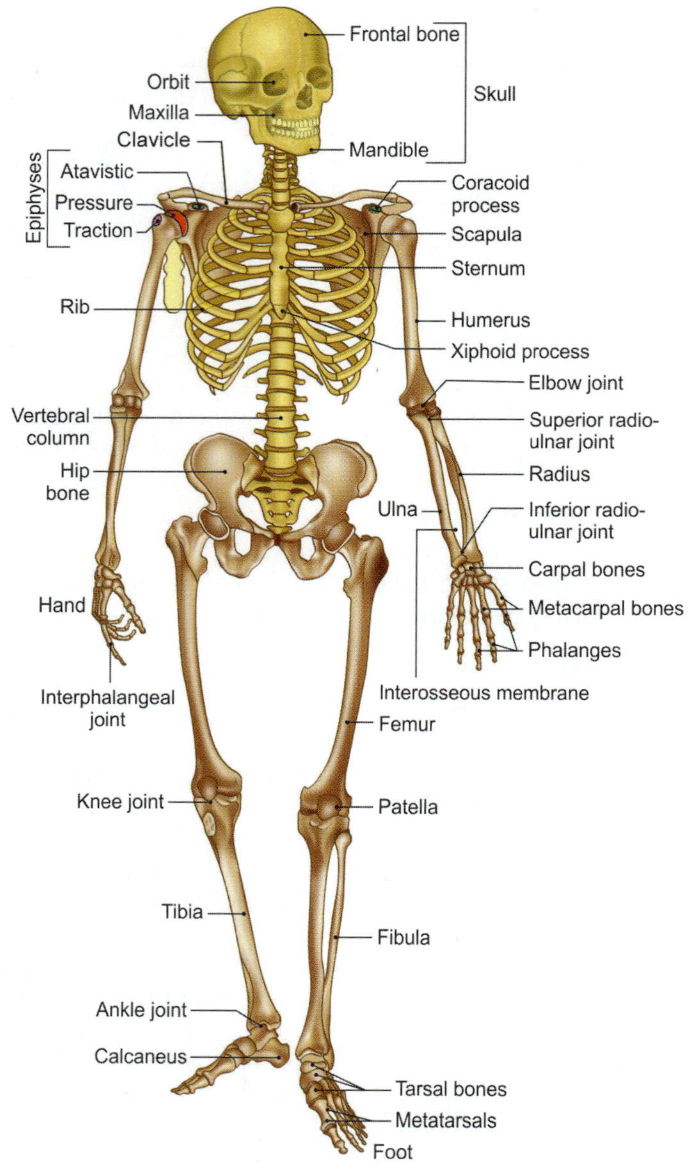

Fig. 2.1: Anterior view of skeleton. Axial skeleton is colored

in the vault of the skull, sternum, ribs, and scapula (Fig. 2.1).

4 *Irregular bones:* Examples: Hip bone (Fig. 2.1) and bones in the base of the skull, e.g. sphenoid and first and second cervical vertebrae.

5 *Pneumatic bones:* Certain irregular bones contain large air spaces lined by epithelium. Examples: Maxilla, sphenoid, ethmoid (Fig. 2.3), etc. They make the skull (a) light in weight, (b) help in resonance of voice, and (c) act as air conditioning chambers for the inspired air.

6 *Sesamoid bones:* These are bony nodules found embedded in the tendons or joint capsules. They have no periosteum and ossify after birth. Example: Patella in the tendon of quadriceps femoris (Fig. 2.1).

Divisions of the Skeletal System (Fig. 2.1)

Regions of the skeleton	*Number of bones*	*Cranial and facial bones (mnemonic is A–Z)*	
AXIAL SKELETON			
Skull			
Cranium	8	**A–D**	–
Face	14	Ethmoid	1
Hyoid	1	Frontal	1
Auditory ossicles (3 in each ear):	6	**G–H**	–
(Malleus, incus, stapes)		Inferior nasal	
Vertebral column	26	choncha	2
Thorax		**J–K**	–
Sternum	1	Lacrimal	2
Ribs	24	Maxilla	2
APPENDICULAR SKELETON		Mandible	1
Pectoral (shoulder) girdles		Nasal	2
Clavicle	2	Occipital	1
Scapula	2	Parietal	2
Upper extremities		Palatine	2
Humerus	2	**Q–R**	–
Ulna	2	Sphenoid	1
Radius	2	Temporal	2
Carpals	16	**U**	–
Metacarpals	10	Vomer	1
Phalanges	28	**W–Y**	–
Pelvic (hip) girdle		Zygomatic	2
Pelvic, or hip bone	2		
Lower extremities			
Femur	2		
Fibula	2		
Tibia	2		
Patella	2		
Tarsals	14		
Metatarsals	10		
Phalanges	28		
	—		
Total	**206**		

B. Developmental Classification

1 • *Membrane (dermal) bones:* Ossify in membrane (intramembranous or mesenchymal ossification), and are thus derived from mesenchymal condensations. Examples: Bones of the vault of skull like frontal, parietal and facial bones like maxilla (Fig. 2.1).

• *Cartilaginous bones:* Ossify in cartilage (intracartilaginous or endochondral ossification), and are thus derived from replacement of preformed cartilaginous models. Examples: Bones of limbs like humerus, femur, vertebral column and thoracic cage (Fig. 2.1).

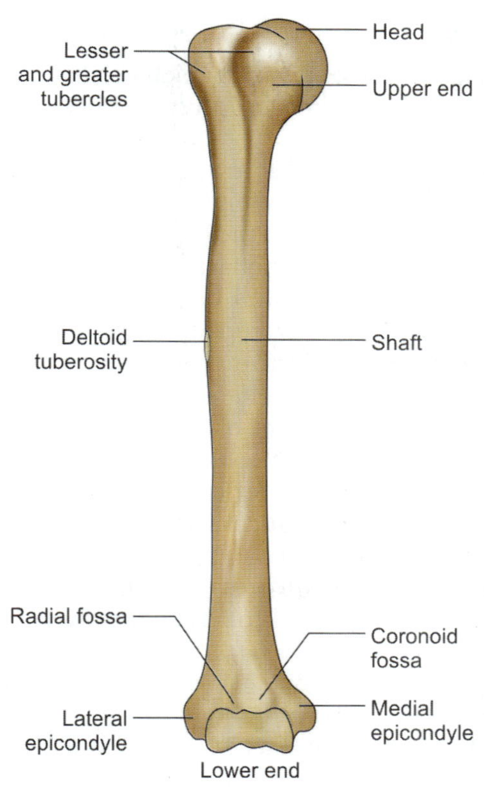

Fig. 2.2: Typical long bone

- *Membranocartilaginous bones:* Ossify partly in membrane and partly in cartilage. Examples: Clavicle (sternal end ossifies by endochondral ossification while the rest of the bone ossifies by intramembranous ossification) (Fig. 2.1); mandible, occipital, temporal, sphenoid.

2 • *Somatic bones:* Most of the bones are somatic.

- *Visceral bones:* These are a few and develop from pharyngeal arches. Examples are hyoid bone, part of mandible (Fig. 2.1) and ear ossicles.

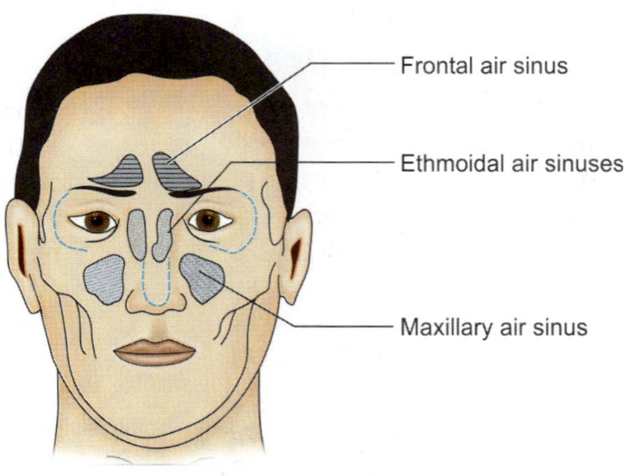

Fig. 2.3: Pneumatic bones

C. Regional Classification

1 *Axial skeleton:* Includes skull, vertebral column and thoracic cage (Fig. 2.1).

2 *Appendicular skeleton:* Includes bones of the limbs, e.g. pectoral girdle, free upper limb and pelvic girdle, free lower limb (Fig. 2.1).

D. Structural Classification

Macroscopically, the architecture of bone may be compact or cancellous.

1 Compact bone is dense in texture like ivory, but is extremely porous.

2 Cancellous or spongy or trabecular bone is open in texture, and is made up of a meshwork of trabeculae (rods and plates) between which are marrow containing spaces. Table 2.1 shows their comparison.

GROSS STRUCTURE OF AN ADULT LONG BONE

Naked eye examination of the longitudinal and transverse sections of a long bone shows the following features.

1 *Shaft:* From without inwards, it is composed of periosteum, cortex and medullary cavity.

a. Periosteum is a thick fibrous membrane covering the surface of the bone. It is made up of an outer fibrous layer, and an inner cellular layer which is osteogenic in nature. Periosteum is united to the underlying bone by Sharpey's fibres, and the union is particularly strong over the attachments of tendons, and ligaments. At the articular margin the periosteum is continuous with the capsule of the joint. The abundant periosteal arteries nourish the outer part of the underlying cortex also. Periosteum has a rich nerve supply which makes it the most sensitive part of the bone.

b. Cortex is made up of a compact bone which gives it the desired strength to withstand all possible mechanical strains (Fig. 2.4).

Table 2.1: Comparison of compact and cancellous bones

	Compact bone	*Cancellous (spongy) bone*
Location	In shaft (diaphysis) of long bone	In the epiphyses of long bone
Lamellae	Arranged to form Haversian system	Arranged in a mesh-work, so Haversian systems are not present
Bone marrow	Yellow which stores fat after puberty. It is red before puberty	Red, produce RBCs, granular series of WBC and platelets throughout life
Nature	Hard and ivory like	Spongy

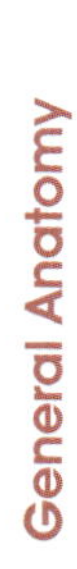

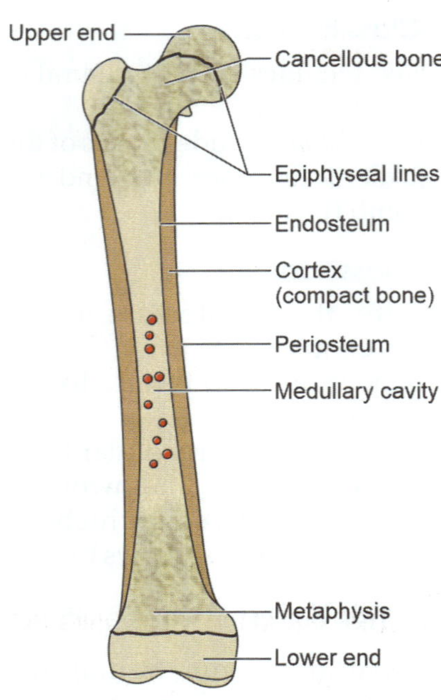

Fig. 2.4: Components of a long bone

c. Medullary cavity is lined by endosteum. The osteoblasts in endosteum help in bone repair and remodelling of bone.

The medullary cavity is filled with red or yellow bone marrow. At birth the marrow is red everywhere with widespread active hemopoiesis. As the age advances, the red marrow at many places atrophies and is replaced by yellow, fatty marrow, with no power of hemopoiesis. Red marrow persists in the cancellous ends of long bones, sternum, ribs, iliac crest, vertebrae and skull bones throughout life.

2 The two ends of a long bone are made up of cancellous bone covered with hyaline (articular) cartilage.

PARTS OF A YOUNG GROWING BONE

There are four parts of a young bone:

1. Epiphysis
2. Diaphysis
3. Metaphysis
4. Epiphysial plates

A typical long bone ossifies in three parts, the two ends from secondary centres (ossification centre appearing after birth), and the intervening shaft from a primary centre (ossification centre appearing before birth) (Fig. 3.2). Before ossification is complete the above mentioned parts of the bone can be defined.

1. Epiphysis

The ends and tips of a bone which ossify from secondary centres are called epiphyses. These are of the following types.

a. *Pressure epiphysis:* It is articular and takes part in transmission of the weight. Examples: Head of humerus; lower end of radius, etc. (Fig. 2.1)
b. *Traction epiphysis:* It is nonarticular and does not take part in the transmission of the weight. It always provides attachment to one or more tendons which exert a traction on the epiphysis. The traction epiphyses ossify later than the pressure epiphyses. Examples: Trochanters of femur and tubercles of humerus (Fig. 2.1).
c. *Atavistic epiphysis:* It is phylogenetically an independent bone which in human becomes fused to another bone.
   Examples: Coracoid process of scapula (Fig. 2.1) and os trigonum or lateral tubercle of posterior process of talus.

2. Diaphysis

It is the elongated shaft of a long bone which ossifies from a primary centre of ossification.

3. Metaphysis

The epiphysial ends of a diaphysis are called metaphyses.

Each metaphysis is the zone of active growth. Before epiphysial fusion, the metaphysis is richly supplied with blood through end arteries forming 'hair-pin' bends (Fig. 2.5).

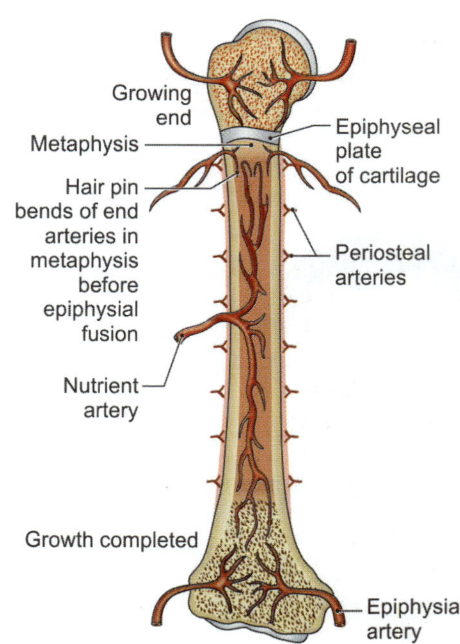

Fig. 2.5: Arterial supply of a young long growing bone

Thus metaphysis is the common site of osteomyelitis in children because the bacteria or emboli are easily trapped in the hair-pin bends, causing infarction.

After the epiphysial fusion, vascular communications are established between the metaphysial and epiphysial arteries. Now the metaphysis contains no more end-arteries and can no longer be subjected to osteomyelitis.

4. Epiphysial Plate of Cartilage

Epiphysial plate separates epiphysis from metaphysis.

Proliferation of cells in this cartilaginous plate is responsible for lengthwise growth of a long bone.

After the epiphysial fusion, the bone can no longer grow in length.

The growth cartilage is nourished by both the epiphysial and metaphysial arteries.

BLOOD SUPPLY OF BONES

Arterial Supply

Young Long Bones

The arterial supply of a long bone is derived from the following sources (Fig. 2.5).

a. *Nutrient artery*
- It enters the shaft through the nutrient foramen, runs through the cortex, and divides into ascending and descending branches in the medullary cavity.
- Each branch divides into a number of small parallel channels which terminate in the adult metaphysis by anastomosing with the epiphysial, metaphysial and periosteal arteries.
- The nutrient artery supplies medullary cavity, inner 2/3rd of cortex and metaphysis.
- The growing ends of bones in upper limb are upper end of humerus and lower ends of radius and ulna. In lower limb, the lower end of femur and upper end of tibia are the growing ends.
- The nutrient foramen is directed away from the growing end of the bone. Their directions are indicated by a jingle, 'To the elbow I go, from the knee I flee' (Fig. 2.6).

b. *Periosteal arteries*
- These are especially numerous beneath the muscular and ligamentous attachments.
- They ramify beneath the periosteum and enter the Volkmann's canals to supply the outer 1/3rd of the cortex.

c. *Epiphysial arteries*
- These are derived from periarticular vascular arcades (circulus vasculosus) found on the nonarticular bony surface.

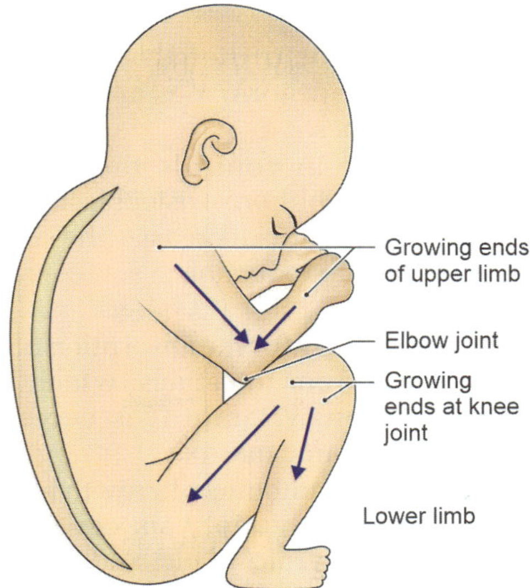

Fig. 2.6: Directions of nutrient foramina shown

- Out of the numerous vascular foramina in this region, only a few admit the arteries (epiphysial and metaphysial), and the rest are venous exits.

d. *Metaphysial arteries*
- These are derived from the neighbouring systemic vessels.

Venous Drainage

Veins are numerous and large in the cancellous red marrow containing bones (e.g., basivertebral veins). In the compact bone, they accompany arteries in the Volkmann's canals.

Lymphatic Drainage

Lymphatics accompany the periosteal blood vessels, which drain to the regional lymph nodes.

NERVE SUPPLY OF BONES

Nerves accompany the blood vessels. Most of them are sympathetic and vasomotor in function.

A few of them are sensory which are distributed to the articular ends and periosteum of the long bones.

GROWTH OF A LONG BONE

1. Bone grows in length by multiplication of cells in the epiphysial plate of cartilage (*see* Fig. 3.2).
2. Bone grows in thickness by multiplication of cells in the deeper layer of periosteum.
3. Bones grow by deposition of new bone on the surface and at the ends. This process of bone deposition by osteoblasts is called appositional growth or surface accretion. However, in order to maintain the shape the unwanted bone must be removed. This process of bone removal by osteoclasts is called remodelling. This is how marrow cavity increases in size.

Factors Affecting Growth

Adequate amounts of proteins, carbohydrates, minerals, vitamins and hormones are necessary for proper growth of bones.

1 *Vitamins:* Vitamin A controls the activity, co-ordination and distribution of osteoblasts and osteoclasts. Lack of vitamin decreases the activity of osteoclasts leading to reduction in size of cranial and spinal foramina.
   Vitamin D is necessary for the absorption of calcium and phosphorus from intestines, which helps in proper ossification. Vitamin C is necessary for maintenance of organic matrix.
2 *Hormonal:* Adequate amounts of growth hormone of anterior pituitary (hypophysis cerebri), parathormone of parathyroid gland and calcitonin of thyroid gland are also necessary.

CARTILAGE

Definition

Cartilage is a connective tissue composed of cells (chondrocytes) and fibres (collagen or yellow elastic) embedded in a firm, gel-like matrix which is rich in a mucopolysaccharide. It is much more elastic than bone. Table 2.2 shows comparison of bone and cartilage.

General Features of Cartilage

1 Cartilage has no blood vessels or lymphatics. The nutrition of cells diffuses through the matrix.
2 Cartilage has no nerves. It is, therefore, insensitive.
3 Cartilage is surrounded by a fibrous membrane, called perichondrium, which is similar to periosteum in structure and function. The articular cartilage has no perichondrium, so that its regeneration after injury is inadequate.

Table 2.2: Comparison between bone and cartilage

Bone	*Cartilage*
1. Bone is hard	Cartilage is firm
2. Matrix has inflexible material called ossein	It has chondroitin providing flexibility
3. Matrix possesses calcium salt	Calcium salts not present
4. Bone has rich nerve supply. It is vascular in nature	It does not have nerve supply. It is avascular in nature
5. Bone marrow is present	Bone marrow is absent
6. Growth is only by apposition (by surface deposition)	Growth is both appositional and interstitial (from within)

Types of Cartilage

There are three types of cartilages:

1 Hyaline cartilage (Fig. 2.7)
2 Fibrocartilage (Fig. 2.8)
3 Elastic cartilage (Fig. 2.7).

Table 2.3 reveals the comparison among three types of cartilages.

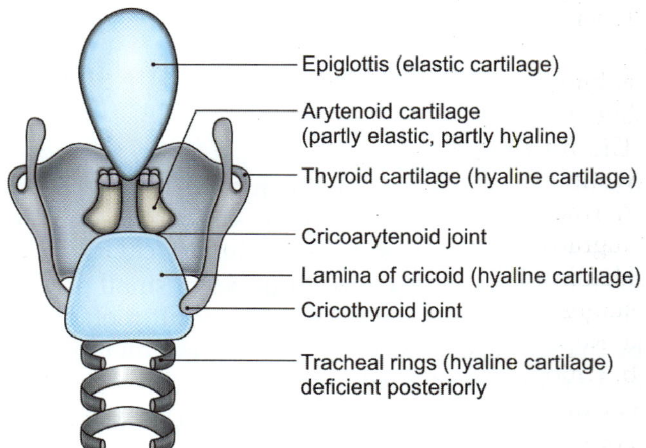

Fig. 2.7: Hyaline and elastic cartilages

Table 2.3: Comparison of three types of cartilages

	Hyaline cartilage	*Fibrocartilage*	*Elastic cartilage*
Location	In the articular cartilages of long bones, epiphysial plates, nasal cartilages, thyroid, cricoid, most of arytenoid, trachea, bronchi and costal cartilages (Fig. 2.7)	In the intervertebral disc, interpubic disc of symphysis pubis, articular discs of temporomandibular joints (TMJ), sternoclavicular joint and inferior radioulnar joint. Articular cartilages of TMJ and sternoclavicular joint (Fig. 2.8)	In the pinna, external auditory meatus, eustachian tubes, epiglottis, vocal process of arytenoid cartilage, corniculate and cuneiform cartilages (Fig. 2.7)
Colour	Bluish white	Glistening white	Yellowish
Appearance	Shiny or translucent	Opaque	Opaque
Fibres	Very thin, having same refractive index as matrix, so these are not seen	Numerous white fibres	Numerous yellow fibres
Elasticity	Flexible	More firm, strongest	Most flexible
Perichondrium	Present	Absent	Present
Cells	Maximum	Minimum, squeezed between fibres	Moderate

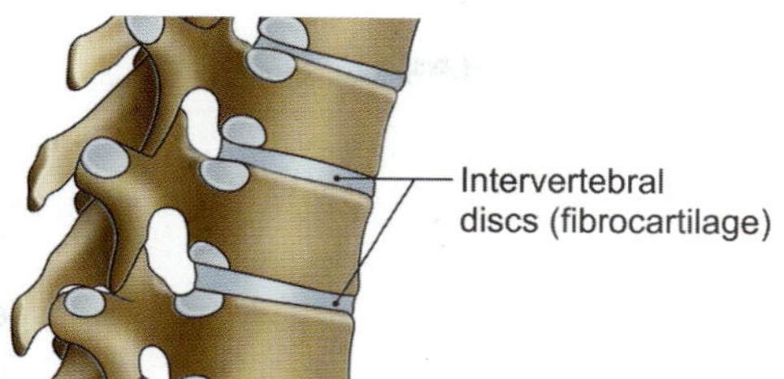

Fig. 2.8: Fibrocartilage in intervertebral disc

CLINICAL ANATOMY

- Periosteum is particularly sensitive to tearing or tension. Drilling into the compact bone without anaesthesia causes only mild pain or an aching sensation; drilling into spongy bone is much more painful. Fractures, tumours and infections of the bone are very painful.
- *Blood supply* of bone is so rich that it is very difficult to interrupt it sufficiently to kill the bone. Passing a metal pin into the medullary cavity hardly interferes with the blood supply of the bone.
- **Fracture** is a break in the continuity of a bone. The fracture which is not connected with the skin wound is known as simple (closed) fracture. The fracture line may be (a) spiral, (b) horizontal or (c) oblique. The fracture which communicates with the skin wound is known as (d) compound (open) fracture. A fracture requires "reduction" by which the alignment of the broken ends is restored.
  Healing (repair) of a fracture takes place in three stages:
  a. Repair by granulation tissue
  b. Union by callus
  c. Consolidation by mature bone.
- Axis or 2nd cervical vertebra may get fractured. If dens of axis gets separated from the body (as in hanging), it hits the vital centres in the medulla oblongata causing instantaneous death. Even fracture of laminae may cause death.
- Deficiency of calcium in bones in old age leads to *osteoporosis*, seen both in females and males. Due to osteoporosis, there is forward bending of the vertebral column, leading to kyphosis.
- Nerves are closely related to bones in some areas. Fracture of the bones of those areas may lead to injury to the nerve, leading to paralysis of muscles supplied, including the sensory loss.
- **Bone marrow biopsy:** Bone marrow can be taken either from manubrium sterni or iliac crest in various clinical conditions.

FACTS TO REMEMBER

- Inorganic calcium salt as calcium hydroxyapatite $[Ca_{10}(PO_4)_6(OH)_2]$ is present in the bone.
- Femur is the longest and strongest bone.
- Stapes of the middle ear is the shortest bone.
- Three bony ossicles of middle ear are fully developed at birth.
- Hyoid bone, mandible and 3 bony ossicles of middle ear develop from branchial cartilages.
- Clavicle is a long, horizontally placed bone with the medullary cavity in medial 2/3rd.
- Periosteum does not cover the sesamoid bones and the 3 bony ossicles of middle ear.
- Bone marrow puncture is done in iliac crest in children and in manubrium sterni in adult.
- Bone fractures are seen more often in persons without adequate protein, calcium and vitamin D.
- External ear or pinna is made of elastic cartilage. Its size does not increase even if it is pulled as part of punishment.
- Elastic cartilage is present in epiglottis and vocal process of arytenoid cartilage. This cartilage does not calcify/ossify.
- Fibrocartilage gives strength to the site of its presence. It is chiefly present in midline joints.
- Hyaline cartilage is maximum in the body. All the somatic bones initially were composed of hyaline cartilage.

Multiple Choice Questions

1. What percentage of calcium of the body is stored in the bones?
   a. 90% b. 80%
   c. 97% d. 75%
2. The cartilaginous model of bone arises from:
   a. Ectoderm
   b. Mesoderm
   c. Endoderm
   d. Neuroectoderm
3. Which cartilage has no periosteum?
   a. Hyaline
   b. Elastic
   c. White fibrocartilage
   d. All of the above

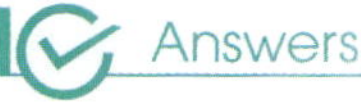

1. c **2.** b **3.** c

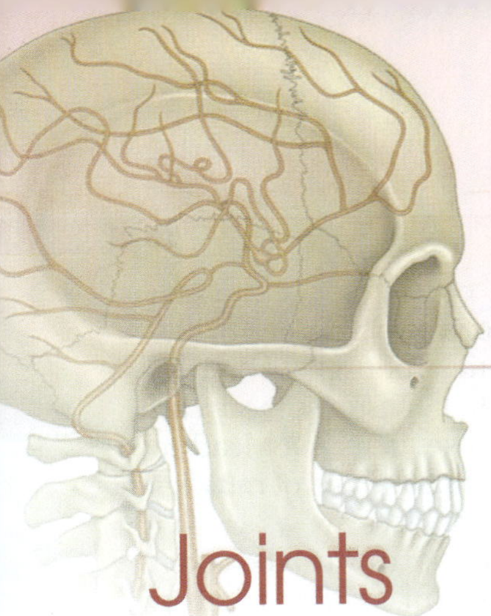

Chapter

3

Joints

"What I hear, I forget, What I see, I remember, What I do, I understand."
—Anonymous

Related Terms

1 Arthron (G a joint). Compare with the terms arthrology, synarthrosis, diarthrosis, arthritis, arthrodesis, etc.
2 Articulatio (L a joint); articulation (NA).
3 Junctura (L a joint).
4 Syndesmology (G syndesmosis = ligament) is the study of ligaments and related joints.

Definition

Joint is a junction between two or more bones or cartilages. It is a device to permit movements.

However, immovable joints are primarily meant for growth. Primary cartilaginous joints of long bones increase length of bone. A newborn baby is about 15″ long and length increases to 60–70″ in an adult due to growth at these joints. Fontanelles of skull may permit moulding during childbirth.

There are more joints in a child than in an adult because as growth proceeds some of the bones fuse together, e.g. the ilium, ischium and pubis to fuse form the pelvic bone. The two halves of the infant frontal bone, and of the infant mandible also fuse to form single frontal and mandible bone respectively. The five sacral vertebrae fuse to form sacrum at about 20 years and the four coccygeal vertebrae join to form coccyx.

Joints help to form cavities like cranial, thoracic, abdominal and pelvic cavities where the respective organs are safely kept. Joints of thoracic cage help in increasing transverse and anteroposterior diameters of the cage, helping in respiration. Joints of laryngeal cartilages help in speech.

CLASSIFICATION OF JOINTS

A. Structural Classification

1. *Fibrous Joints*

a. Sutures
b. Syndesmosis
c. Gomphosis

2. *Cartilaginous Joints*

a. Primary cartilaginous joints or synchondrosis
b. Secondary cartilaginous joints or symphysis or amphiarthrosis

3. *Synovial Joints*

a. Ball-and-socket or spheroidal joints
b. Sellar or saddle joints
c. Condylar or bicondylar joints
d. Ellipsoid joints
e. Hinge joints
f. Pivot or trochoid joints
g. Plane joints

B. Functional Classification (According to the Degree of Mobility)

1 Synarthroses (immovable), like sutures of the fibrous joints (Fig. 3.1), and epiphyseal plate of a young growing bone (Fig. 3.2).

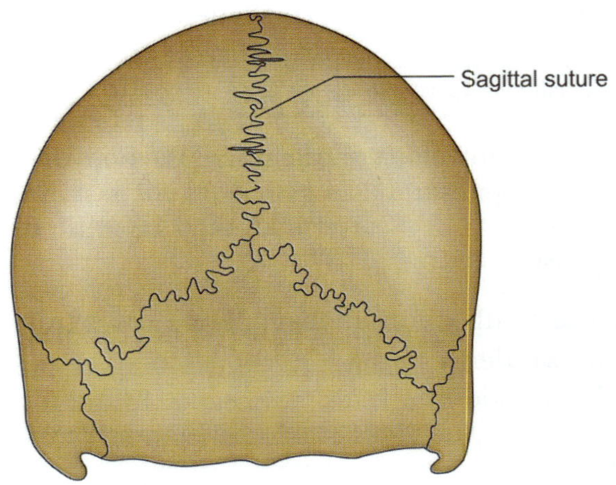

Fig. 3.1: Fibrous joint—sutures

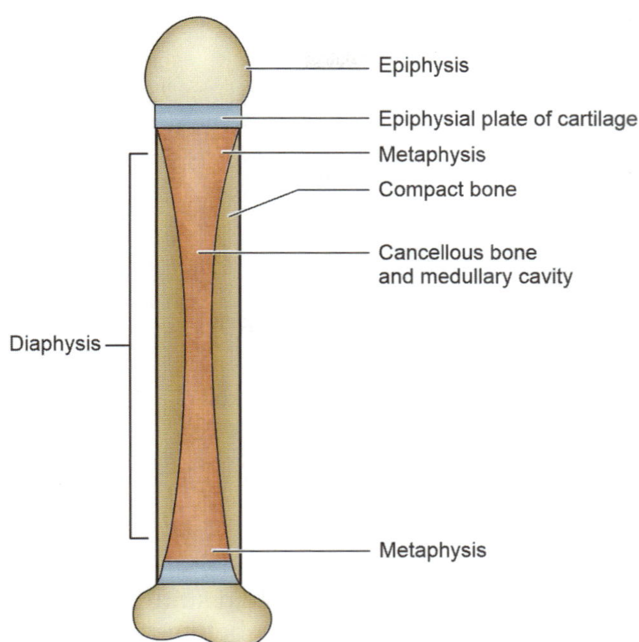

Fig. 3.2: Primary cartilaginous joint

2 Amphiarthroses (slightly movable), like secondary cartilaginous joints (Fig. 3.10).
3 Diarthroses (freely movable), like synovial joints (Fig. 3.3).

Synarthroses are fixed joints at which there is no movement. The articular surfaces are joined by tough fibrous tissue. Often the edges of the bones are dovetailed into one another as in the sutures of the skull.

Amphiarthroses are joints at which slight movement is possible. The articulating bones are covered by hyaline cartilage. A pad of fibrocartilage lies between the bone surfaces, and there are fibrous ligaments to hold the bones and cartilages in place. The cartilages of such joints also act as shock absorbers, e.g. the intervertebral discs between the bodies of the vertebrae.

Diarthroses or synovial joints are known as freely movable joints, though at some of them the movement is restricted by the shape of the articulating surfaces and by the ligaments which hold the bones together. These ligaments are of elastic connective tissue.

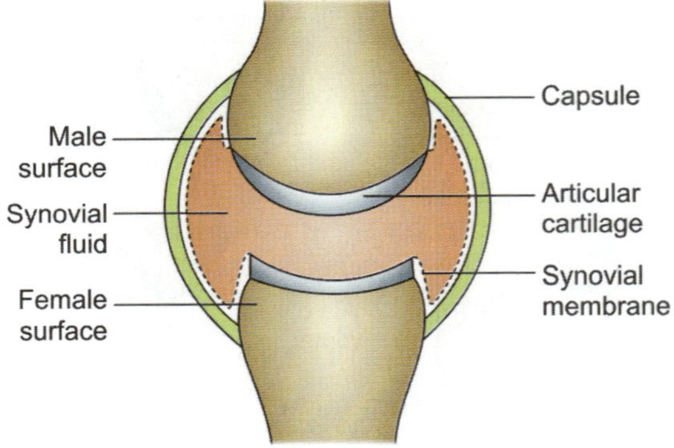

Fig. 3.3: Structure of simple synovial joint

A synovial joint has a fluid-filled cavity between articular surfaces which are covered by articular cartilage. The fluid, known as synovial fluid is produced by the synovial membrane. The synovial membrane lines the cavity except for the actual articular surfaces. It covers any ligaments or tendons which pass through the joint. Synovial fluid acts as a lubricant.

The form of the articulating surfaces controls the type of movement which takes place at any joint.

The movements possible at synovial joints are:

Angular—flexion: Decreasing the angle between two bones or two parts;

extension: Increasing the angle between two bones or two parts;

abduction: Moving the part away from the midline;

adduction: Bringing the part towards the midline

Rotatory—rotation: Rotating along the vertical axis

circumduction: Moving the extremity or the part round in a circle so that the whole part inscribes a cone. When flexion, abduction, extension and adduction occur in sequence, the movement is called the circumduction

Gliding: One part slides on another.

C. Regional Classification

1 *Skull type*: Immovable
2 *Vertebral type*: Slightly movable
3 *Limb type*: Freely movable

D. According to Number of Articulating Bones

1 *Simple joint*: When only two bones articulate, e.g. interphalangeal joints (Fig. 3.3).
2 *Compound joint*: More than two bones articulate within one capsule, e.g. elbow joint, radiocarpal joint (Fig. 3.4).
3 *Complex joint*: When joint cavity is divided by an intra-articular disc, e.g. temporomandibular joint (Fig. 3.5), sternoclavicular joint. Figure 3.6 is a diagrammatic representation of complex joint.

The *structural* classification is most commonly followed, and will be considered in detail in the following paragraphs.

FIBROUS JOINTS

In fibrous joints the bones are joined by fibrous tissue. These joints are either immovable or permit a slight degree of movement. These can be grouped in the following three subtypes.

1 *Sutures*: Sutures are present only in skull. Two bones are separated by connective tissue. The sutural side of each bone is covered by a layer of osteogenic cells/ cambial layer, covered by capsular layer which is continuous with the periosteum. The area between

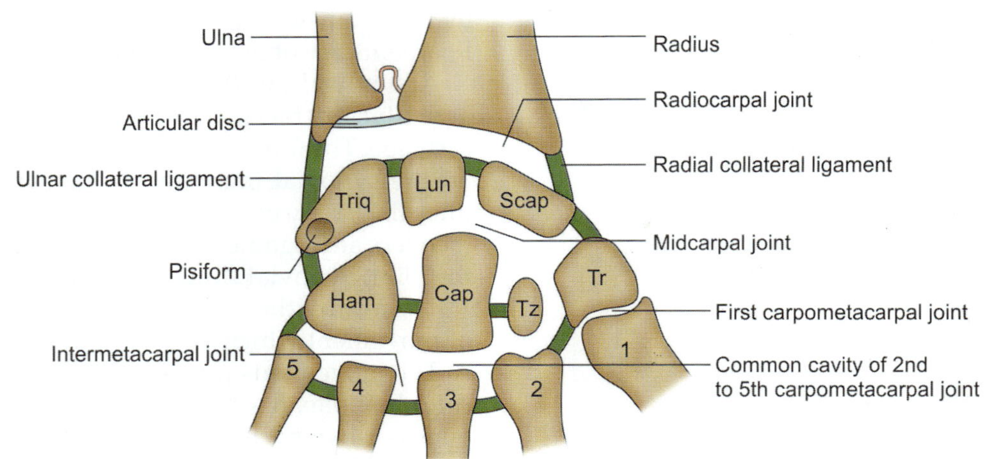

Fig. 3.4: Some simple and compound joints

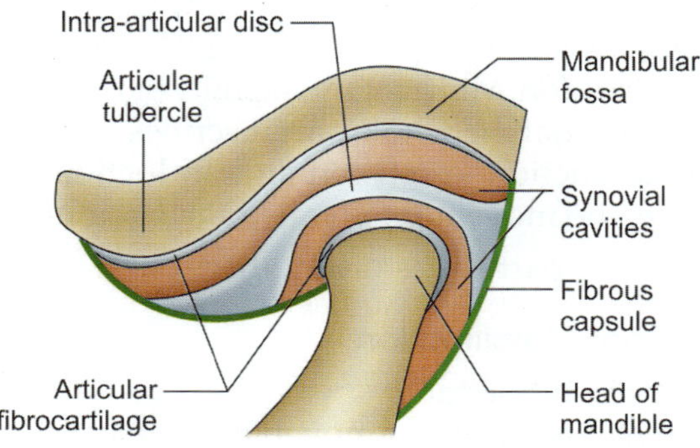

Fig. 3.5: Condylar joint—temporomandibular joint

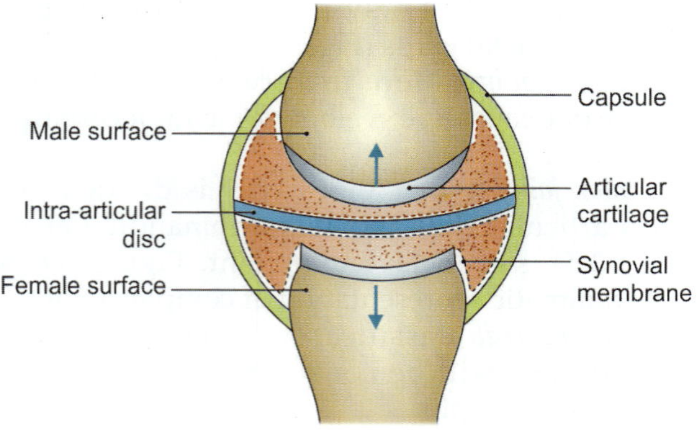

Fig. 3.6: Complex joint

the bones decreases with age, so that osteogenic surfaces become opposed. Sutures may synostose and get obliterated as age advances.

Sutures are peculiar to skull, and are immovable. According to the shape of bony margins, the sutures can be:

i. Plane, e.g. internasal suture (Fig. 3.7)
ii. Serrate, e.g. interparietal suture
iii. Squamous, e.g. temporoparietal suture
iv. Denticulate, e.g. lambdoid suture
v. Schindylesis type, e.g. between rostrum of sphenoid and upper border of vomer.

Neonatal skull reveals fontanelles which are temporary in nature permit moulding during normal childbirth. At six specific points on the sutures (in newborn skull) are membrane filled gaps called "fontanelles". These also allow the underlying brain to increase in size. Anterior fontanelle is used to judge the hydration of the infant. All these fontanelles become bone by 18 months (Fig. 3.8).

2 *Syndesmosis*: It is a fibrous union between bones. It may be represented as interosseous ligament as in inferior tibiofibular joint.

3 *Gomphosis*: It is a peg and socket junction between the tooth and its socket. The periodontal ligament connects the dental element to the alveolar bone (Fig. 3.9).

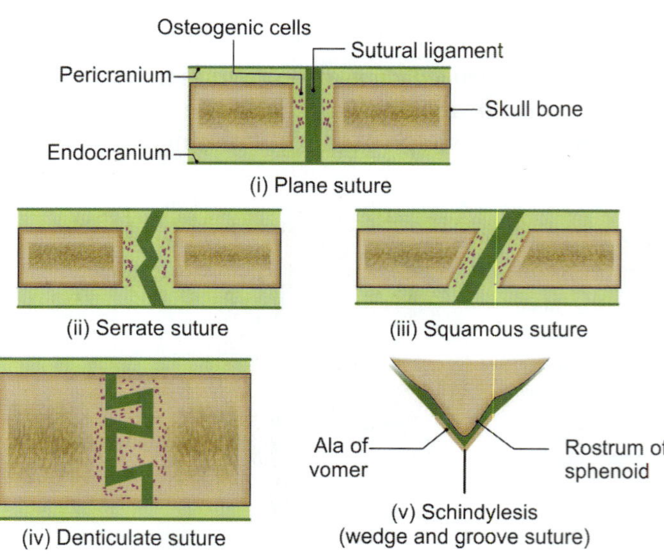

Fig. 3.7: Types of sutures

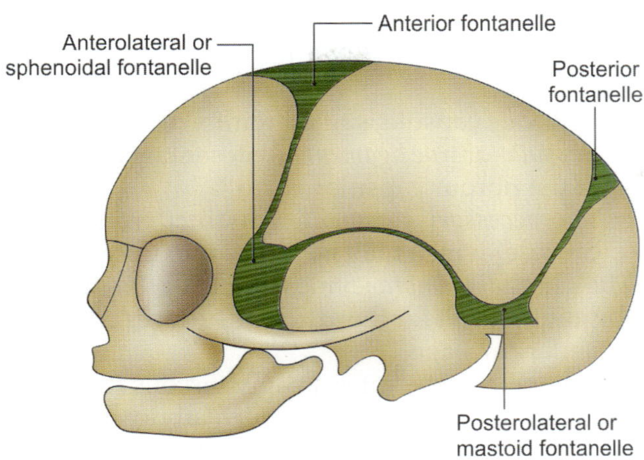

Fig. 3.8: Fontanelles of skull of a newborn baby

CARTILAGINOUS JOINTS

In this type of joints the bones are joined by cartilage. These are of the following two types:

1 *Primary cartilaginous joints* (synchondrosis, or hyaline cartilage joints): The bones are united by a plate of hyaline cartilage (epiphysial plate) so that the joint is immovable and strong.

These joints are temporary in nature because after a certain age the cartilaginous plate is replaced by bone (synostosis). These are seen in between epiphysis and diaphysis of long bone. These are associated with growth of epiphysial plates and increasing length of the bone. Primary cartilaginous joints or synchondrosis become synostosed after some age and are not identifiable.

Examples:

a. Joint between epiphysis and diaphysis of a growing long bone (Fig. 3.2)

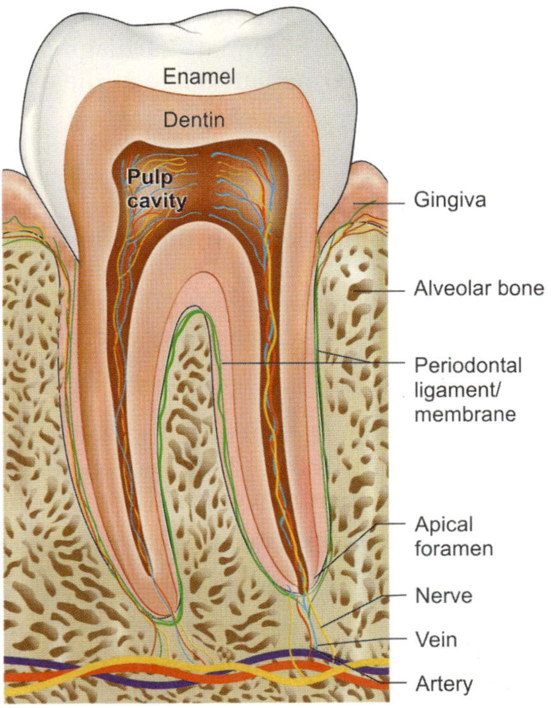

Fig. 3.9: Gomphosis

b. Spheno-occipital joint
c. First chondrosternal joint
d. Costochondral joints.

2 *Secondary cartilaginous joints* (symphyses or fibrocartilaginous joints): The articular surfaces are covered by a thin layer of hyaline cartilage, and united by a disc of fibrocartilage (Fig. 3.10).

These joints are permanent and persist throughout life. In this respect symphysis menti is a misnomer as it is a synostosis. Typically the secondary cartilaginous joints occur in the median plane of the body.

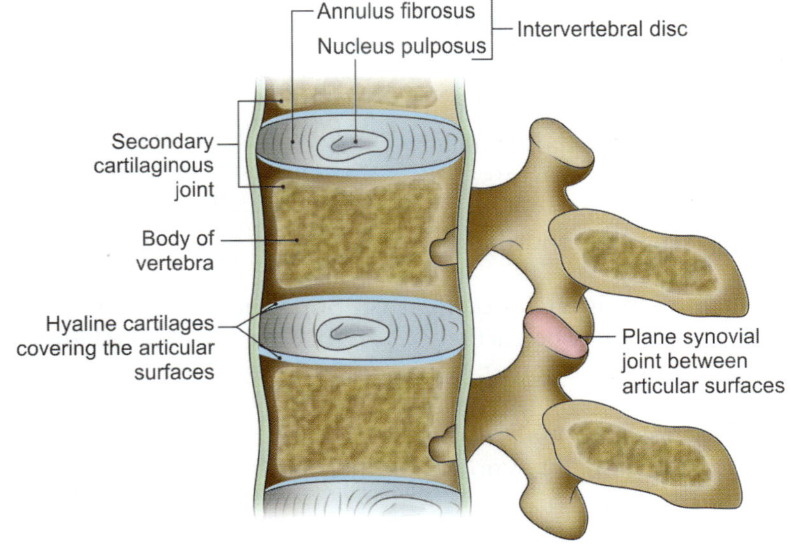

Fig. 3.10: Secondary cartilaginous joints with plane synovial joint

The thickness of fibrocartilage is directly related to the range of movement. Secondary cartilaginous joints may represent an intermediate stage in the evolution of synovial joints.

Examples:

a. Symphysis pubis
b. Manubriosternal joint
c. Intervertebral joints between the vertebral bodies (Fig. 3.10).

The disc varies from few mm to 10 mm and there is dense connective tissue with a few chondrocytes.

SYNOVIAL JOINTS

Synovial joints are most evolved, and, therefore, most mobile type of joints. Table 3.1 shows classification of synovial joints and their movements.

Table 3.1: Classification of synovial joints and their movements

Type of joint	*Movement*
A. Plane or gliding type	Gliding movement
B. Uniaxial joints	
1. Hinge joint	Flexion and extension
2. Pivot joint	Rotation only
C. Biaxial joints	
1. Condylar joint	Flexion, extension, and limited rotation
2. Ellipsoid joint	Flexion, extension, abduction, adduction, and circumduction
D. Multiaxial joints	
1. Saddle joint	Flexion and extension, abduction, adduction, and conjunct rotation
2. Ball-and-socket	Flexion and extension, abduction and adduction, (spheroidal) joint circumduction, medial and lateral rotation, i.e. adjunct rotation

Characters

1 The articular surfaces are covered with hyaline (articular) cartilage (fibrocartilage in certain membrane bones) like clavicle and mandible.
Articular cartilage is avascular, non-nervous and elastic. Lubricated with synovial fluid, the cartilage provides slippery surfaces for free movements, like 'ice on ice'.
The surface of the cartilage shows fine undulations filled with synovial fluid.

2 Between the articular surfaces there is a *joint cavity* filled with synovial fluid. The cavity may be partially or completely subdivided by an intra-articular disc or meniscus (Fig. 3.6).

3 The joint is surrounded by an *articular capsule* which is made up of a fibrous capsule lined by synovial membrane.
Because of its rich nerve supply, the *fibrous capsule* is sensitive to stretches imposed by movements. This sets up appropriate reflexes to protect the joint from any sprain. This is called the 'watchdog' action of the capsule.
The fibrous capsule is often reinforced by:
a. *Capsular* or *true ligaments* representing thickenings of the fibrous capsule.
b. The *accessory ligaments* (distinct from fibrous capsule) which may be intra- or extracapsular.
The *synovial membrane* lines whole of the interior of the joint, except for the articular surfaces covered by articular cartilage.
The membrane secretes a slimy viscous fluid called the synovia or *synovial fluid* which lubricates the joint and nourishes the articular cartilage. The viscosity of fluid is due to hyaluronic acid secreted by cells of the synovial membrane.

4 Varying degrees of movements are always permitted by the synovial joints.

Classification of Synovial Joints

1. *Plane Synovial Joints*

Articular surfaces are more or less flat (plane). They permit gliding movements (translations) in various directions.

Examples:

a. Intercarpal joints (Fig. 3.4)
b. Intertarsal joints
c. Joints between articular processes of vertebrae
d. Cricothyroid joint (*see* Fig. 2.7)
e. Cricoarytenoid joint (*see* Fig. 2.7)

2. *Hinge Joints (Ginglymi)*

Articular surfaces are pulley-shaped. There are strong collateral ligaments. Movements are permitted in one plane around a transverse axis.

Examples:

a. Elbow joint (*see* Fig. 2.1)
b. Ankle joint (*see* Fig. 2.1)
c. Interphalangeal joints (*see* Fig. 2.1)

3. *Pivot (Trochoid) Joints*

Articular surfaces comprise a central bony pivot (peg) surrounded by an osteoligamentous ring. Movements are permitted in one plane around a vertical axis.

Examples:

a. Superior and inferior radioulnar joints (*see* Fig. 2.1)
b. Median atlantoaxial joint (Fig. 3.11).

4. *Condylar (Bicondylar) Joints*

Articular surfaces include two distinct condyles (convex male surfaces) fitting into reciprocally concave female surfaces (which are also, sometimes, known as condyles, such as in tibia). These joints permit movements mainly in one plane around a transverse

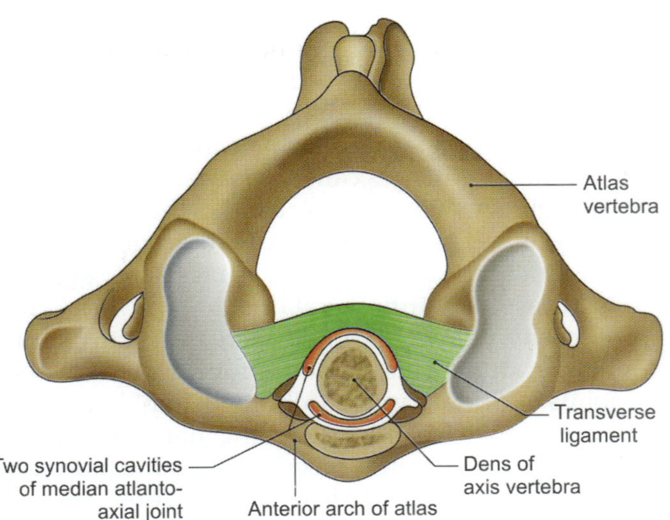

Fig. 3.11: Median atlantoaxial joint

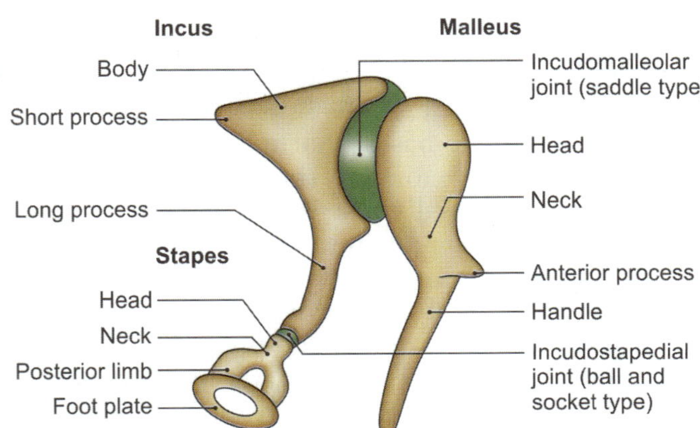

Fig. 3.12: Visceral bones, the ear ossicles with their joints

axis, but partly in another plane (rotation) around a vertical axis.

Examples:

a. Knee joint (*see* Fig. 2.1)
b. Right and left jaw joints or temporomandibular joint (Fig. 3.5).

5. *Ellipsoid Joints*

Articular surfaces include an oval, convex, male surface fitting into an elliptical, concave female surface. Free movements are permitted around both the axes; flexion and extension around the transverse axis, and abduction and adduction around the anteroposterior axis. Combination of movements produces circumduction. Typical rotation around a third (vertical) axis does not occur.

Examples:

a. Atlanto-occipital joints (*see* Fig. 17.6).
b. Wrist radiocarpal joint (Fig. 3.4)
c. Metacarpophalangeal joints

6. *Saddle (Sellar) Joints*

Articular surfaces are reciprocally concavoconvex. Movements are similar to those permitted by an ellipsoid joint, with addition of some rotation (conjunct rotation) around a third axis which, however, cannot occur independently.

Examples:

a. First carpometacarpal joint (Fig. 3.4)
b. Sternoclavicular joint
c. Calcaneocuboid joint
d. Incudomalleolar joint (Fig. 3.12)
e. Between femur and patella.

7. *Ball-and-Socket (Spheroidal) Joints*

Articular surfaces include a globular head (male surface) fitting into a cup-shaped socket (female surface). Movements occur around an indefinite number of axes which have one common centre. Flexion, extension, abduction, adduction, medial rotation, lateral rotation, and circumduction, all occur quite freely.

Examples:

a. Shoulder joint
b. Hip joint (*see* Fig. 2.1)
c. Talocalcaneonavicular joint
d. Incudostapedial joint (Fig. 3.12)

Mechanism of Lubrication of a Synovial Joint

1 Synovial fluid, secreted by synovial membrane, is sticky and viscous due to hyaluronic acid (a mucopolysaccharide). It serves the main function of lubrication of the joint. It also nourishes the articular cartilage.
2 *Hyaline cartilage*: Covering the articular surfaces possesses inherent slipperiness, like that of the ice.
3 *Intra-articular fibrocartilages, articular discs or menisci, complete or incomplete*: Help in spreading the synovial fluid throughout the joint cavity, but particularly between the articular surfaces, e.g. temporomandibular joint (Fig. 3.5). The disc divides the joint into two cavities for diverse movements in 2 cavities. The disc strengthens the joint.

Blood Supply

The articular and epiphysial branches given off by the neighbouring arteries form a periarticular arterial plexus. Numerous vessels from this plexus pierce the fibrous capsule and form a rich vascular plexus in the deeper parts of synovial membrane. The blood vessels of the synovial membrane terminate around the articular margins in a fringe of looped anastomoses termed the circulus vasculosus (*circulus articularis vasculosus*). It supplies capsule, synovial membrane and the epiphysis. The articular cartilage is avascular.

Nerve Supply

The *capsule* and *ligaments* possess a rich nerve supply, which makes them acutely sensitive to pain. The synovial membrane has a poor nerve supply and is relatively insensitive to pain. The articular cartilage is non-nervous and totally insensitive. Articular nerves contain sensory and autonomic fibres. Autonomic fibres are vasomotor or vasosensory. The joint pain is often diffuse, and may be associated with nausea, vomiting, slowing of pulse and fall in blood pressure.

The pain commonly causes reflex contraction of muscles which fix the joint in a position of maximum comfort. Like visceral pain, the joint pain is also referred to uninvolved joints.

Lymphatic Drainage

Lymphatics form a plexus in the subintima of the synovial membrane, and drain along the blood vessels to the regional deep nodes.

Stability

The various factors maintaining stability at a joint are described here in order of their importance.

1 *Muscles*: The tone of different groups of muscles acting on the joint is the most important and indispensable factor in maintaining the stability.
2 *Ligaments*: These are important in preventing any over-movement, and in guarding against sudden accidental stresses. However, they do not help against a continuous strain, because once stretched, they tend to remain elongated. In this respect, the elastic ligaments (ligamenta flava and ligaments of the joints of auditory ossicles) are superior to the common type of white fibrous ligaments.

CLINICAL ANATOMY

- Intervertebral disc forms secondary cartilaginous joint between the bodies of the vertebrae. If the nucleus pulposus part of the disc protrudes backwards, it may press on the spinal nerve leaving out from the intervertebral foramina. The condition is known as *herniation of the disc* or disc prolapse. If disc prolapse occurs in lumbar vertebrae there is radiating pain in the lower limb, and the condition is called **sciatica**.
- The joints may get dislocated, i.e. the end of one of the bones gets out of its socket. In subluxation, the end of the bone partially leaves its socket.
- Stiffness of joints is related to weather. The viscosity of synovial fluid increases with fall in temperature. This accounts for stiffness of the joints in cold weather. Mobility of joint in itself is an important factor in promoting lubrication. Thus the stiffness of joints experienced in the morning gradually passes off as the movements are resumed.

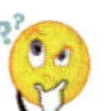

FACTS TO REMEMBER

- Joint is a junction between two or more bones or cartilages.
- Joints are classified as fibrous, cartilaginous and synovial types.
- There are more joints in a child than in an adult. The primary cartilaginous joints at the ends of long bones after fusion disappear in the adult, decreasing the number of joints.
- Joints help in increasing the length of bones, increasing the size of cranial, thoracic and pelvic cavities.
- Joints in thorax help in respiratory movements.
- Joints are vital for locomotion.
- The secondary cartilaginous joints are in midline of the body.
- Joints in ossicles of middle ear are synovial joints.
- Joints chiefly suffer in osteoarthritis and rheumatoid arthritis.
- Joints in the laryngeal cartilages help us in speech.

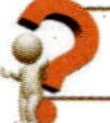

Multiple Choice Questions

1. Which of the following joints contains an intra-articular disc?
a. Ankle joint
b. Sternoclavicular joint
c. Elbow joint
d. Shoulder joint

2. Condylar joints are:
a. Uniaxial b. Biaxial
c. Multiaxial d. Symphysis

3. Which is not a fibrous joint?
a. Sutures b. Gomphosis
c. Xiphisternal d. Inferior tibiofibular

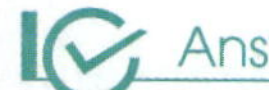

Answers

1. b **2.** b **3.** c

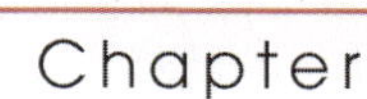

Chapter 4

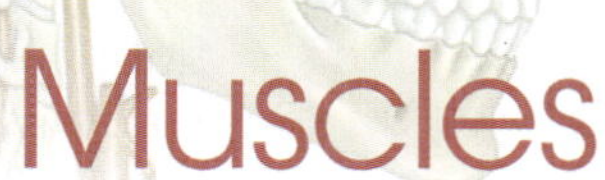

Muscles

"Smile does not cost anything, but it improves your 'face valve, much better than any cosmetics'."
—Anonymous

DERIVATION OF NAME

Muscles (L Mus = mouse) are so named because, many of them resemble a mouse, with their tendons representing the tail.

Definition

Muscle is a contractile tissue which brings about movements. Muscles can be regarded as motors of the body.

Types of Muscles

The muscles are of three types, skeletal, smooth and cardiac. The characters of each type are summarized in Table 4.1 and Figs 4.1 to 4.3.

SKELETAL MUSCLES

Synonyms

1 Striped muscles
2 Striated muscles
3 Somatic muscles
4 Voluntary muscles

Parts of a Muscle

A. *Two Ends*

1 *Origin* is one end of the muscle which mostly remains fixed during its contraction.
2 *Insertion* is the other end which mostly moves during its contraction. In the *limb* muscles, the origin is usually proximal to insertion.

However, the terms origin and insertion, are at times interchangeable, and at other times difficult to define, as in the intercostal muscles. Muscles of pharynx, oesophagus, and the diaphragm act as involuntary muscles.

Table 4.1: Types of muscles

Striated/skeletal	*Non-striated/smooth*	*Cardiac*
1. Striated muscles are present in the limbs, body wall, tongue, pharynx and beginning of oesophagus (Fig. 4.1)	Oesophagus (distal part), urogenital tract, urinary bladder, blood vessels, iris of eye, arrector pili muscle of hair (Fig. 4.2)	Wall of heart (Fig. 4.3)
2. Long and cylindrical	Spindle shaped	Short and cylindrical
3. Fibres unbranched	Fibres unbranched	Fibres branched
4. Multinucleated	Uninucleated	Uninucleated
5. Bounded by sarcolemma	Bounded by plasmalemma	Bounded by plasmalemma
6. Light and dark bands present	Light and dark bands absent	Faint light and dark bands present
7. No intercalated disc (junctional complex)	No intercalated discs	Intercalated disc present and a characteristic feature
8. Nerve supply from central nervous system	Nerve supply from autonomic nervous system	Nerve supply from autonomic nervous system
9. Blood supply is abundant	Blood supply is scanty	Blood supply is abundant
10. Very rapid contraction	Slow contraction	Rapid contractions
11. They soon get fatigued	They do not get fatigued	They never get fatigued
12. Voluntary	Involuntary	Involuntary

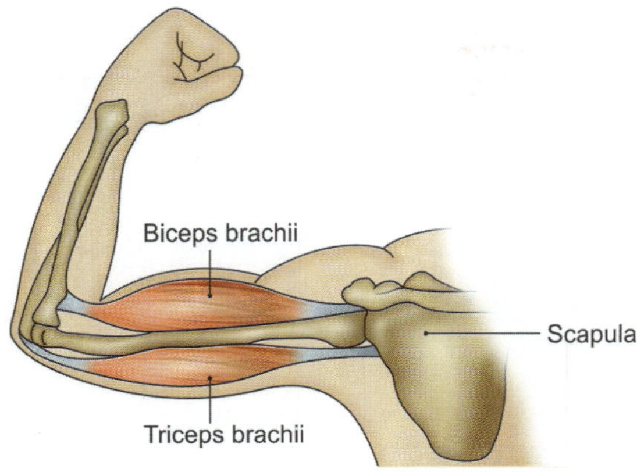

Fig. 4.1: Skeletal muscle

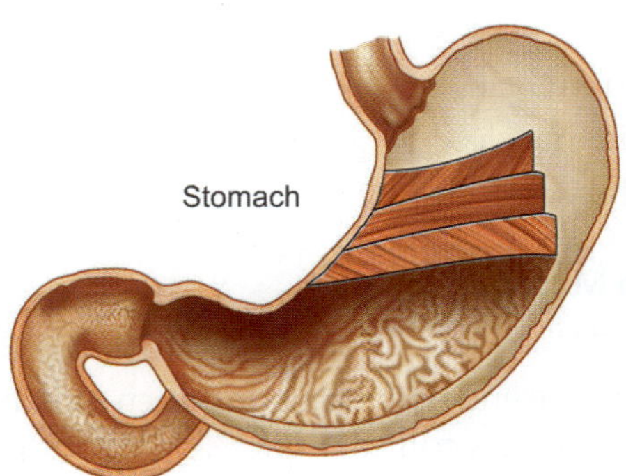

Fig. 4.2: Smooth muscle

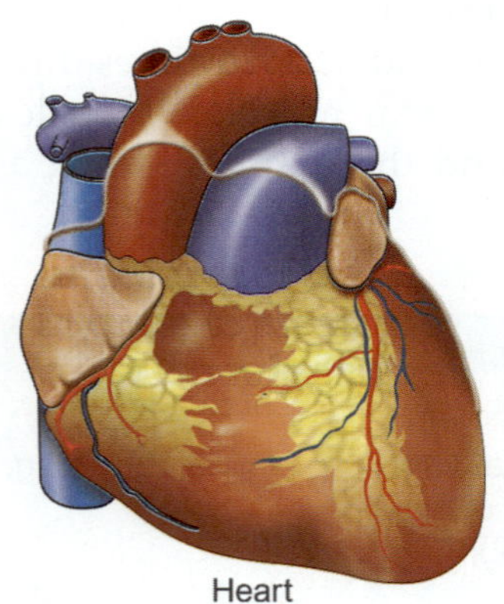

Fig. 4.3: Cardiac muscle

B. *Two Parts*

1 *Fleshy part* is contractile, and is called the 'belly'.
2 *Fibrous part* is noncontractile and inelastic. When cord-like or rope-like, it is called tendon (Fig. 4.4); when flattened, it is called aponeurosis. The tendon receives Golgi tendon nerve endings. It is supplied by capillaries extending from the fleshy part and also from the periosteal arteries of the bone where the tendon terminates or gets inserted.

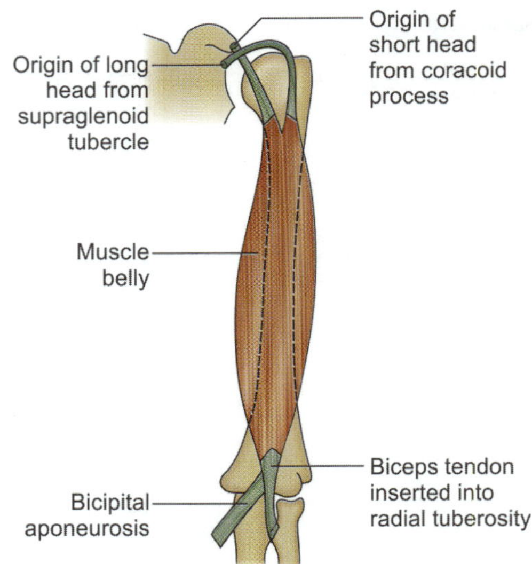

Fig. 4.4: Biceps brachii

STRUCTURE OF STRIATED MUSCLE

A. Contractile Tissue

Each muscle is composed of numerous muscle fibres. Each *muscle fibre* is a multinucleated, cross-striated cylindrical cell (myocyte) 1–300 mm long. It is made up of sarcolemma (cell membrane) enclosing sarcoplasm (cytoplasm).

Embedded in the sarcoplasm there are (a) several hundred nuclei arranged at the periphery beneath the sarcolemma and (b) a number of evenly distributed longitudinal threads called myofibrils. Each myofibril shows alternate dark and light bands. Dark bands are known as A bands (anistropic) and the light bands as I bands (isotropic). The bands of adjacent fibrils are aligned transversely so that the muscle fibre appears cross-striated. In the middle of dark band there is a light H band. In the middle of I band there is a dark Z line or Krause's membrane. The segment of myofibril between two Z lines is called sarcomere (Fig. 4.5).

Muscle → fasciculi → fibres → myofibril → myofilaments

B. Supporting Tissue

Supporting tissue helps in organization of the muscle. *Endomysium* surrounds each muscle fibre separately. *Perimysium* surrounds bundles (fasciculi or myonemes) of muscle fibres of various sizes. *Epimysium* surrounds the entire muscle. The connective tissue of the muscle becomes continuous with the tendon (Fig. 4.6).

Arterioles and motor nerves reach the muscle fibres along the supporting tissue. Venules, lymphatics and proprioceptive nerves leave the fibres along the same supporting tissues.

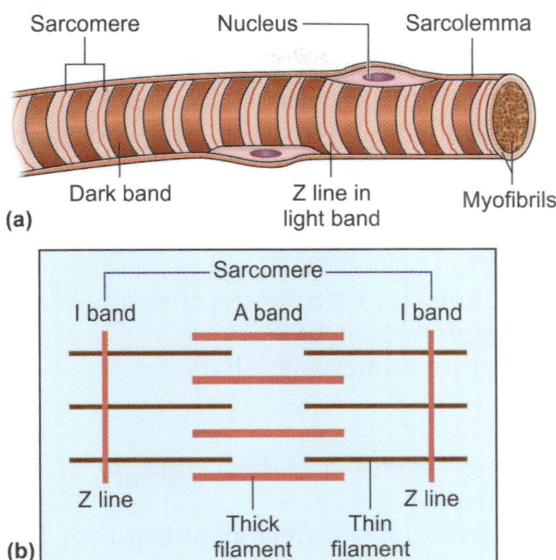

Figs 4.5a and b: Myofibrils in skeletal muscle

Fascicular Architecture of Muscles

The arrangement of muscle fibres varies according to the direction, force and range of habitual movement at a particular joint. The force of movement is directly proportional to the number and size of muscle fibres, and the range of movement is proportional to the length of fibres. The muscles can be classified according to the arrangement of their fasciculi into the following groups.

A. *Parallel Fasciculi*

When the fasciculi are parallel to the line of pull, the muscle may be:

1 *Quadrilateral* (thyrohyoid) (*see* Fig. 12.6).
2 *Strap-like* (sternohyoid and sartorius).

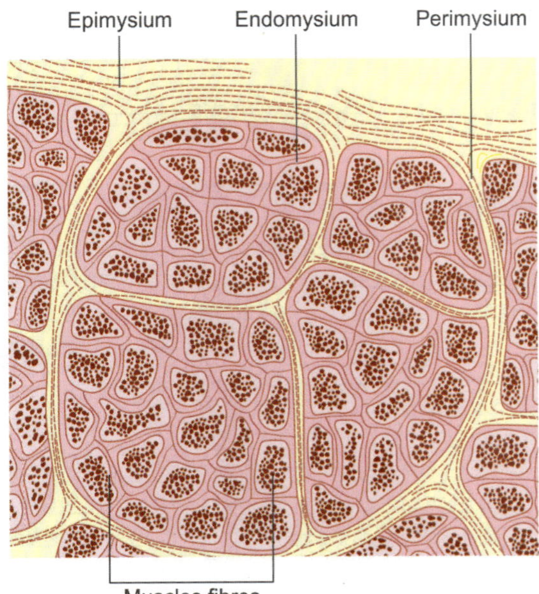

Fig. 4.6: Supporting tissue of skeletal muscle

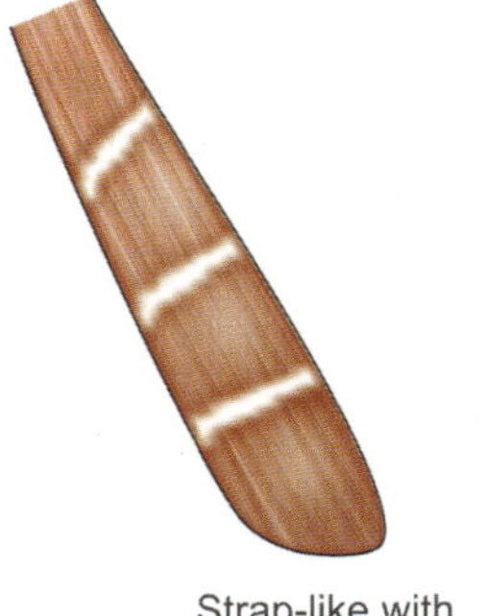

Fig. 4.7: Rectus abdominis

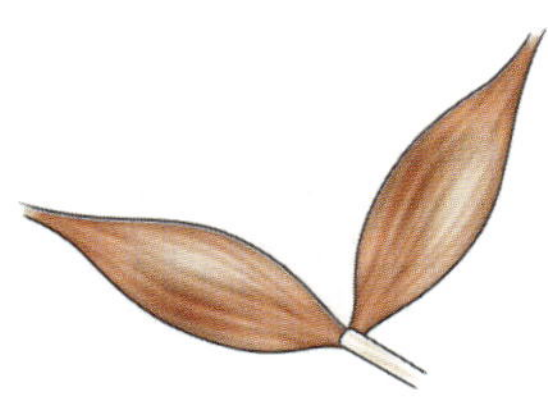

Fig. 4.8: Digastric muscle

3 *Strap-like with tendinous intersections* (rectus abdominis, Fig. 4.7).
4 *Fusiform* (biceps brachii, digastric, etc.). The range of movement in such muscles is maximum (Fig. 4.8).

B. *Oblique Fasciculi*

When the fasciculi are oblique to the line of pull, the muscle may be triangular, or pennate (feather-like) in its construction. This arrangement makes the muscle more powerful, although the range of movement is reduced. Oblique arrangements are of the following types:

1 *Triangular*, e.g. temporalis (Fig. 4.9).
2 *Bipennate*, e.g. rectus femoris (Fig. 4.12).
3 *Multipennate*, e.g. acromial fibres of deltoid (Fig. 4.11)

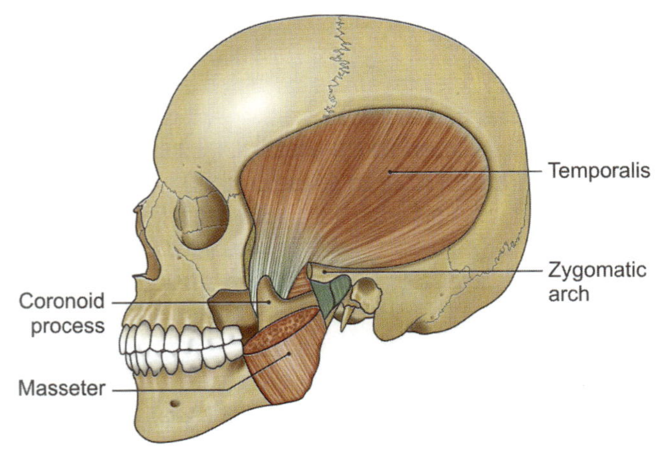

Fig. 4.9: Triangular muscle—temporalis

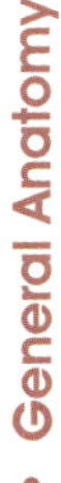

C. Spiral or Twisted Fasciculi

Spiral or twisted fibres are found in trapezius, pectoralis major, latissimus dorsi, supinator, etc. In certain muscles the fasciculi are crossed. These are called *cruciate* muscles, e.g. sternocleidomastoid (Fig. 4.10), masseter.

NAMING THE MUSCLES

Features Used in Naming Muscles

Following features are used for naming the muscles:

Shape

Deltoid (triangular, Fig. 4.11)
Rectus (straight)—rectus abdominis (Fig. 4.7)

Size

Major (big)—pectoralis major
Latissimus (broadest)—latissimus dorsi
Longissimus (longest)—longissimus thoracis

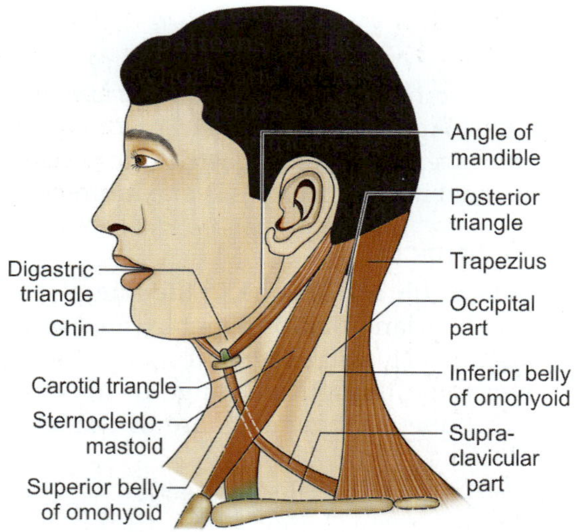

Fig. 4.10: Sternocleidomastoid muscle

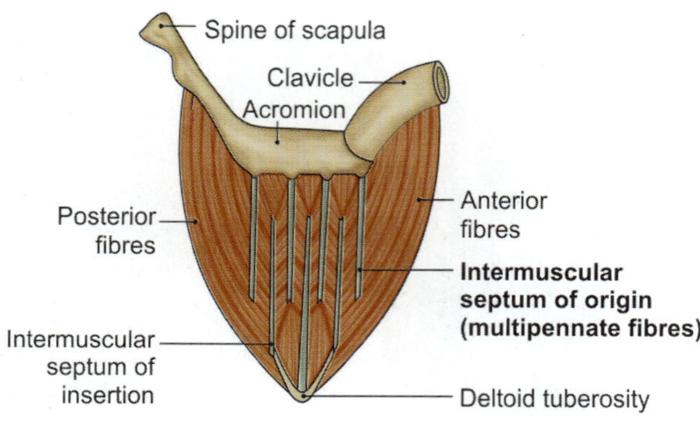

Fig. 4.11: Multipennate fibres—deltoid

Number of Heads

Biceps (two heads)—biceps brachii (Fig. 4.4)
Triceps (three heads)—triceps brachii
Quadriceps (four heads)—quadriceps femoris (Fig. 4.12)
Digastric (two bellies)—anterior and posterior bellies of digastric (Fig. 4.8).

Attachment

Sternocleidomastoid (from sternum and clavicle to mastoid process, Fig. 4.10)
Brachialis (from humerus to ulna).

Depth

Externus (external)—external oblique of anterior abdominal wall
Internus (internal)—internal oblique of anterior abdominal wall

Position

Anterior (front)—tibialis anterior
Posterior (back)—tibialis posterior
Lateralis (lateral side)—vastus lateralis (Fig. 4.12)
Medialis (medial side)—vastus medialis (Fig. 4.12)
Superior (upper side)—superior rectus of eyeball
Inferior (lower side)—inferior rectus of eyeball
Oris (of the mouth)—orbicularis oris (Fig. 4.13)
Oculi (of the eye)—orbicularis oculi (Fig. 4.13)

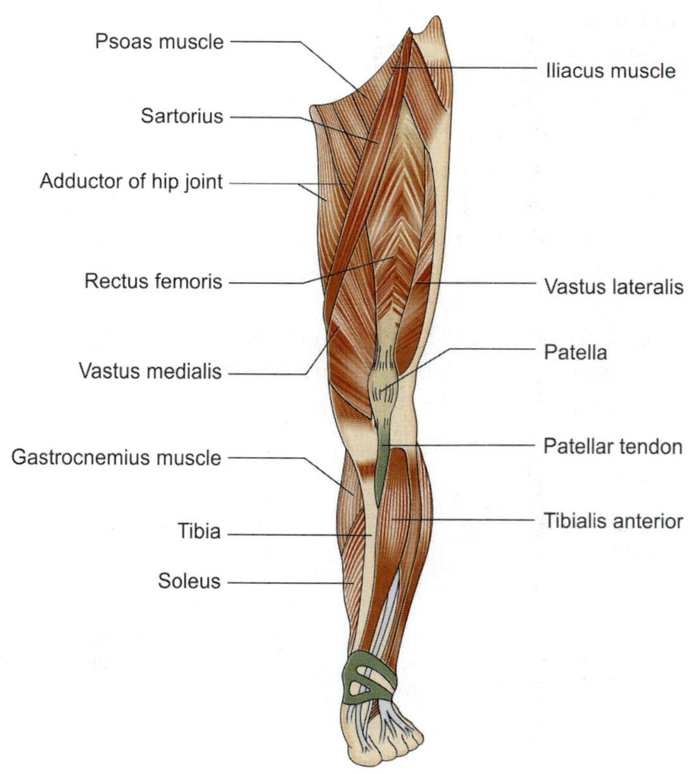

Fig. 4.12: Muscle of lower limb—anterior aspect

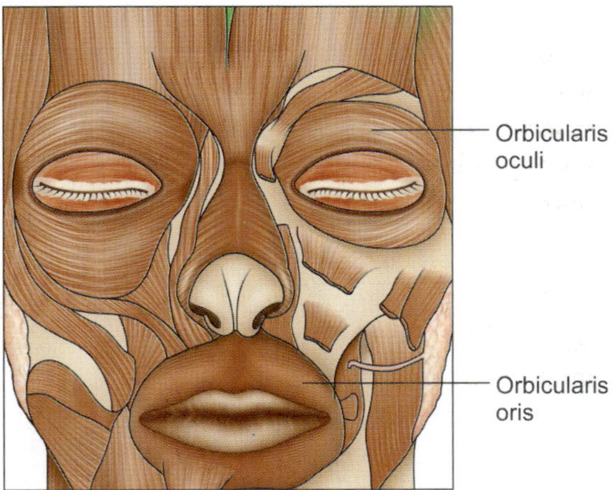

Fig. 4.13: Muscle of facial expression

Action

Extensor (increase the angle between forearm and palm)—extensor digitorum.
Levator (to elevate)—levator anguli oris
Depressor (to pull down)—depressor anguli oris
Supinator (turning palm anteriorly)—supinator
Pronator (turning palm posteriorly)—pronator teres
Constrictor (to narrow)—constrictor pupillae
Dilator (to dilate)—dilator pupillae

NERVE SUPPLY OF SKELETAL MUSCLE

The nerve supplying a muscle is called motor nerve. In fact it is a mixed nerve and consists of the following types of fibres.

1 *Motor fibres (60%) comprise:*
   a. Large myelinated alpha efferents which supply extrafusal muscle fibres. Fibre ends at motor end plate (Fig. 4.14)
   b. Smaller myelinated gamma efferents which supply intrafusal fibres of the muscle spindles which refine and control muscle contraction (Fig. 4.15).
   c. The fine non-myelinated autonomic efferents which supply smooth muscle fibres of the blood vessels.

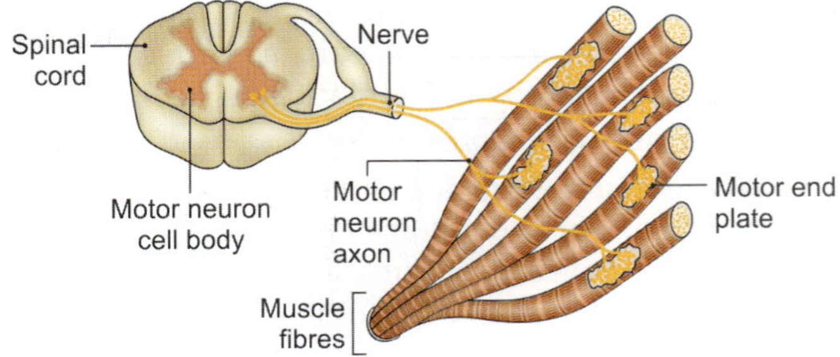

Fig. 4.14: Nerve supply to muscle fibres

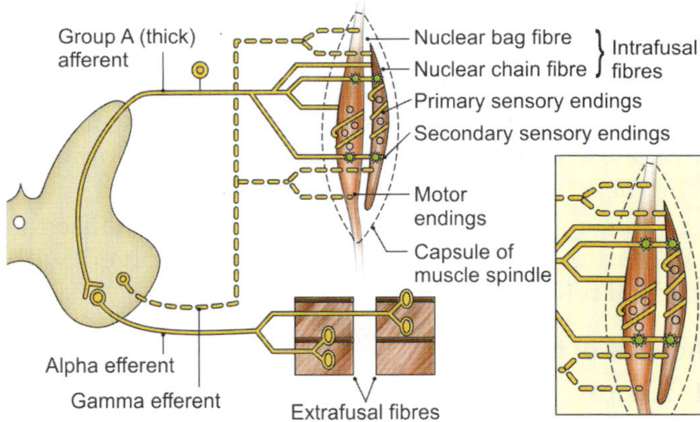

Fig. 4.15: Muscle spindle

2 *Sensory fibres (40%) comprise*: Myelinated fibres distributed to muscle spindles for proprioception, and also to tendons.

Motor point is the site where the motor nerve enters the muscle. It may be one or more than one. Electrical stimulation at the motor point is more effective.

Motor unit is defined as a single alpha motor neuron together with the muscle fibres supplied by it. The size of motor unit depends upon the precision of muscle control. Small motor units (5–10 muscle fibres) are found in muscles of fine movements (extraocular muscles). Large motor units (100–2000 muscle fibres) are found in muscles of gross movements (proximal limb muscles).

Composite/hybrid muscle: Muscle supplied by two different motor nerves with different root values is called a *composite* or *hybrid* muscle, e.g. adductor magnus, flexor digitorum profundus and pectoralis major.

Adductor magnus comprises an adductor part, supplied by obturator nerve (L2, 3, 4) and an hamstring part supplied by sciatic nerve (L4, 5, S1, 2, 3).

Flexor digitorum profundus comprises part destined for index and middle fingers is supplied by median nerve (C5, 6, 7, 8 T1). The part destined for ring and little fingers gets supplied by ulnar nerve (C7, 8, T1).

NERVE SUPPLY OF SMOOTH MUSCLE

According to nerve supply the smooth muscles are classified into:

Single-unit type: Seen in intestines. The nerve impulse reaches one muscle cell, is transmitted to other cells by the mechanical pull through the fused cell membrane. The nerve supply is sparse.

Multi-unit type: Seen in the muscles of the ductus deferens. Each muscle cell receives a separate nerve fibre. The contraction is simultaneous. The nerve supply is rich.

NERVE SUPPLY OF CARDIAC MUSCLE

Heart is supplied by sympathetic and parasympathetic nerve fibres. Sympathetic nerves stimulate both the heart rate and blood pressure and dilate the coronary arteries. The sensory fibres convey painful impulses from heart.

Parasympathetic fibres decrease and normalise the heart rate. Their sensory fibres are involved with visceral reflexes.

Actions of Muscles

1 Broadly, when a muscle contracts, it shortens by one-third (30%) of its belly-length, and brings about a movement. The range of movement depends on the length of fleshy fibres, and the power or force of movement on the number of fibres.

However, the actual behaviour of muscle contraction is more complex.

i. Length may remain unchanged (*isometric* contraction), e.g. holding the hand in outstretched position. Exercise without movement is isometric contraction.

ii. During contraction the length of the muscle may increase or decrease but the tension is constant (*isotonic* contraction). Exercise with movement is isotonic contraction.

iii. Length may increase, according to the functional demands of the body. It is called *eccentric* contraction, e.g. when the upper limb is lowered to the side of the body.

iv. *Concentric* contraction is when there is increasing tension in the muscle as it contracts and shortens. Most of contractions of muscle are concentric.

In each circumstance the tension generated at the ends may either increase, persist, or decrease, depending upon the number and state of its active motor units and the external conditions like loading. Daily activities involve use of both isotonic and isometric contractions.

2 Each movement at a joint is brought about by a coordinated activity of different groups of muscles. These muscle groups are classified and named according to their function.

a. *Prime movers (agonists)* bring about the desired movement. It is the chief/prime muscle for the movement, e.g. medial pterygoid is prime mover for closing the mouth.

b. *Antagonists (opponents)* oppose the prime movers. Lateral pterygoid opens the mouth and is antagonistic to medial pterygoid.

c. *Fixators* are the groups of muscles which stabilize the proximal joints of a limb, so that the desired movement at the distal joint may occur on a fixed base. Muscles acting on shoulder joint, e.g. trapezius, deltoid fix it for better movement of fingers.

d. *Synergists*: Two or more muscles causing one movement are synergist (Fig. 4.12). Masseter and temporalis are synergists to medial pterygoid muscle.

CLINICAL ANATOMY

- ***Paralysis***

Loss of motor power (power of movement) is called paralysis. This is due to inability of the muscles to contract, caused either by damage to the motor neural pathways (upper or lower motor neuron), or by the inherent disease of muscles (myopathy). Damage to the upper motor neuron causes *spastic paralysis* with exaggerated tendon jerks. Damage to the lower motor neuron causes *flaccid paralysis* with loss of tendon jerks, e.g. poliomyelitis (Fig. 4.16).

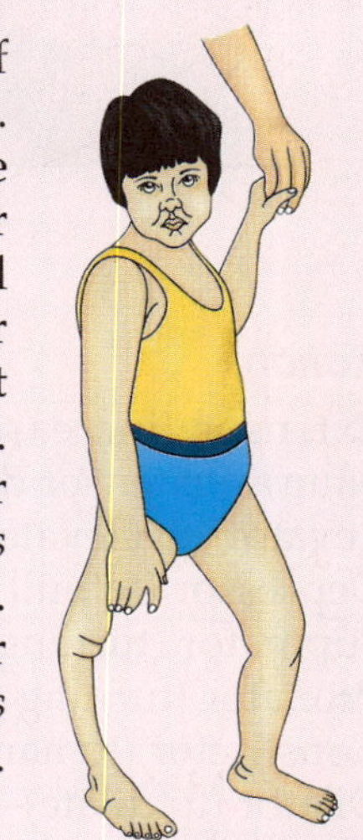

Fig. 4.16: Case of poliomyelitis

- ***Disuse atrophy and hypertrophy***

The muscles which are not used for long times become thin and weak. This is called *disuse atrophy*. Conversely, adequate or excessive use of particular muscles causes their better development, or even *hypertrophy*. Muscular 'wasting' (reduction in size) is a feature of lower motor neuron paralysis and generalized debility.

- ***Regeneration of skeletal muscle***

Skeletal muscle is capable of limited regeneration. If large regions are damaged, regeneration does not occur and the missing muscle is replaced by connective tissue.

- ***Hyperplasia***

Increase in number of smooth muscle fibres. It always occurs in uterus during pregnancy.

- ***Angina pectoris*** is episode of chest pain due to temporary ischaemia of cardiac muscle. It is usually relieved by rest and nitrites.

- ***Myocardial ischaemia***

Persistent ischaemia due to blockage of more than one arteries or a main artery results in necrosis (death) of the cardiac muscle. Pain, not relieved by rest, gets referred to left arm, chest, and neighbouring areas.

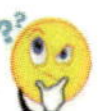

FACTS TO REMEMBER

- Cardiac muscles are least in amount, smooth muscles are intermediate and the skeletal muscles are maximum in amount and weight.
- Sartorius is the longest muscle with parallel fibres.
- The tendocalcaneus is the longest tendon.
- Soleus is called peripheral heart as it contains many venous sinuses.
- Gluteus maximus is the largest muscle.
- Red muscle fibres are used in marathons.
- Richest nerve supply is to extraocular muscles as these have small motor units. One nerve fibre supplies 5–10 muscle fibres.
- Smooth/visceral muscles have maximum regeneration capacity, skeletal muscles repair sparsely due to multiplication of satellite cells. Cardiac muscle does not regenerate.
- Muscles used for intramuscular injections are deltoid, gluteus medius and vastus lateralis.
- Hybrid/composite muscle is supplied by two different motor nerves with different root values, e.g. flexor digitorum profundus partly supplied by branch of median nerve and partly by ulnar nerve. Adductor magnus, pectineus and digastric are other hybrid muscles.

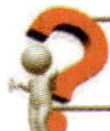

Multiple Choice Questions

1. Skeletal and smooth muscles are mixed in all *except* one muscle:
a. Anal sphincter
b. Upper eyelid
c. Middle region of oesophagus
d. Tongue

2. Connective tissue sheath around each muscle fibre of skeletal muscle is:
a. Epimysium b. Perimysium
c. Endomysium d. Sarcolemma

3. All the following are characteristics of cardiac muscle, *except*:
a. Striations b. Multinucleated
c. Intercalated disc d. Involuntary

4. Tendinous intersections are present in one of the following muscles:
a. Rectus femoris b. Rectus abdominis
c. Biceps brachii d. Biceps femoris

5. What is the role of triceps brachii during flexion of elbow joint?
a. Synergist b. Antagonist
c. Prime mover d. Fixator

6. Which fibres of deltoid are multipennate?
a. Clavicular
b. Acromial
c. Spine of scapula
d. All of the fibres

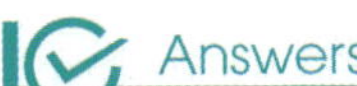

Answers

1. d **2.** c **3.** b **4.** b **5.** b **6.** b

Chapter 5

Circulatory System

"Health is the greatest possession, contentment is the greatest treasure, confidence is the greatest friend."
—Lao Tzu

Blood vessels form the transport system of the body, through which the nutrients are conveyed to places where these are utilized, and the metabolites (waste products) are conveyed to appropriate places from where these are expelled.

The conveying medium is a liquid tissue, the blood, which flows in tubular channels called blood vessels. The circulation is maintained by the central pumping organ called the heart.

COMPONENTS

1 *Heart:* It is a four-chambered muscular organ which pumps blood to various parts of the body (Fig. 5.1). Each half of the heart has a receiving chamber called atrium, and a pumping chamber called ventricle. It is the first organ of the body which starts functioning.

2 *Arteries:* These are distributing channels which carry blood away from the heart. Aorta is the largest artery (Fig. 5.1).

a. The arteries branch like trees on their way to different parts of the body. These contain oxygenated blood except pulmonary trunk and its two branches, the pulmonary arteries, which carry deoxygenated blood. During foetal life the umbilical arteries contain deoxygenated blood.

b. The large arteries are rich in elastic tissue, but as branching progresses there is an ever-increasing amount of smooth muscle in their walls.

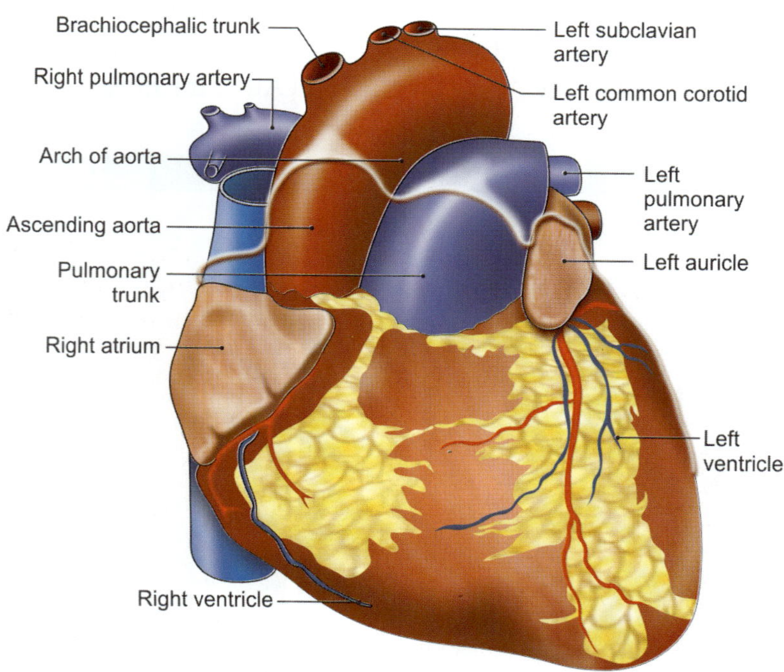

Fig. 5.1: Heart with main blood vessels

Table 5.1: Comparing the systemic circulation and pulmonary circulation

Systemic circulation	*Pulmonary circulation*
Left ventricle ↓	Right ventricle ↓
Aortic valve ↓	Pulmonary valve ↓
Aorta ↓	Pulmonary trunk and pulmonary arteries ↓
Oxygenated blood to all tissues except lungs ↓	Only to lungs ↓
Venous blood collected ↓	Deoxygenated blood gets oxygenated ↓
Superior vena cava and inferior vena cava ↓	4 pulmonary veins ↓
Right atrium	Left atrium

   c. The minute branches which are just visible to naked eye are called arterioles (Fig. 5.2). These give maximum peripheral resistance.

3 *Veins:* These are draining channels which carry deoxygenated blood from different parts of the body back to the heart.
   a. Like rivers, the veins are formed by tributaries.
   b. The small veins (venules) join together to form larger veins (Fig. 5.2). These in turn unite to form great veins called venae cavae. Inferior vena cava is the largest vein. The four pulmonary veins carry oxygenated blood. In foetal life the umbilical vein carries oxygenated blood.

Capillaries: These are networks of microscopic vessels which connect arterioles with the venules (Fig. 5.2).

- These come in intimate contact with the tissues for a free exchange of nutrients and metabolites across their walls between the blood and the tissue fluid.

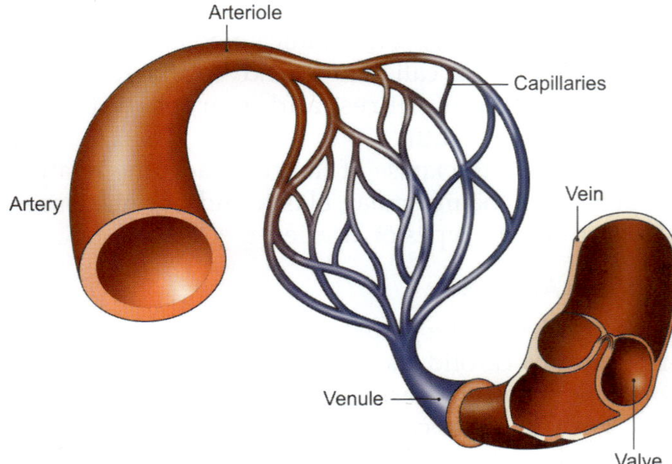

Fig. 5.2: Arteriole, capillaries and venule

- The metabolites are partly drained by the capillaries and partly by lymphatics.
- Capillaries are replaced by sinusoids in certain organs, like liver and spleen.

Functionally, the blood vessels can be classified into the following five groups.

a. Distributing vessels, including arteries (Fig. 5.2)
b. Resistance vessels, including arterioles and precapillary sphincters
c. Exchange vessels, including capillaries, sinusoids, and postcapillary venules
d. Reservoir (capacitance) vessels, including larger venules and veins; and
e. Shunts, including various types of anastomoses.

Types of Circulation of Blood

Total amount of blood in adult is 4.5–5 litres.

Systemic (greater) circulation: The blood flows from the left ventricle, through various parts of the body, to the right atrium, i.e. from the left to the right side of the heart (Fig. 5.3).

Pulmonary (lesser) circulation: The blood flows from the right ventricle, through the lungs, to the left atrium, i.e. from the right to the left side of the heart.

Table 5.1 shows the comparison between systemic circulation and pulmonary circulation.

Portal circulation: It is a part of systemic circulation, which has the following characteristics.

a. The blood passes through two sets of capillaries before draining into a systemic vein (Fig. 5.3).
b. The vein draining the first capillary network is known as portal vein which branches like an artery to form the second set of capillaries or sinusoids. Examples: Hepatic portal circulation, hypothalamo-hypophyseal portal circulation (Fig. 5.4) and renal portal circulation (Fig. 5.3).

ARTERIES

Characteristic Features

1 Arteries are thick-walled, being uniformly thicker than the accompanying veins, except for the arteries within the cranium and vertebral canal where these are thin (Fig. 5.5).
2 Their lumen is smaller than that of the accompanying veins.
3 Arteries have no valves.
4 An artery is usually accompanied by vein(s), nerve(s), and lymphatics and all of them together form the neurovascular bundle which is surrounded and supported by a fibroareolar sheath.

Types of Arteries and Structure

1 Large arteries of elastic type, e.g. aorta and its main branches [brachiocephalic, common carotid,

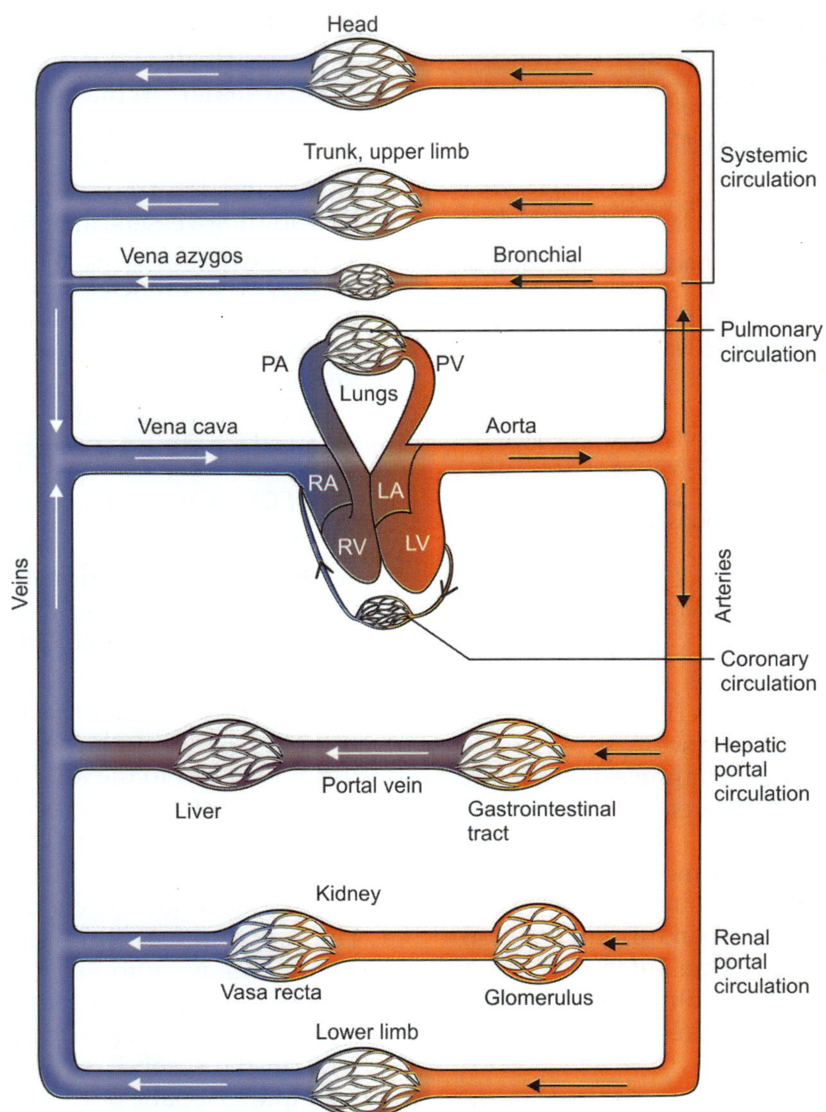

Fig. 5.3: Types of circulation

subclavian, common iliac and the pulmonary trunk (Fig. 5.1)].

2 Medium and small arteries of muscular type, e.g. ulnar, radial, femoral and popliteal, etc. (Fig. 5.6).

3 Smallest arteries of muscular type are called arterioles. They measure 50–100 micron in diameter. Arterioles divide into terminal arterioles with a diameter of 15–20 micron, and having one or two layers of smooth muscle in their walls. The side branches from terminal arterioles are called metarterioles which measure 10–15 micron at their origin and about 5 micron at their termination.

The terminal narrow end of metarteriole is surrounded by a precapillary sphincter which regulates blood flow into the capillary bed.

It is important to know that the muscular arterioles are responsible for generating peripheral resistance, and thereby for regulating the diastolic blood pressure.

Microscopically, all arteries are made up of three coats.

a. The inner coat is called tunica intima (Fig. 5.5).
b. The middle coat is called tunica media.
c. The outer coat is called tunica adventitia. It is made up of collagen fibres and merges with the perivascular sheath.

The relative thickness of the coats and the relative proportion of the muscular, elastic and fibrous tissues vary in different types of arteries.

Palpable Arteries

Some arteries can be palpated through the skin. These are: Common carotid, facial, brachial, radial, abdominal aorta, femoral, posterior tibial and dorsalis pedis (Fig. 5.6). The most commonly felt pulse is the radial pulse on the anterolateral aspect of wrist. Carotid pulse next to trachea is also easily felt.

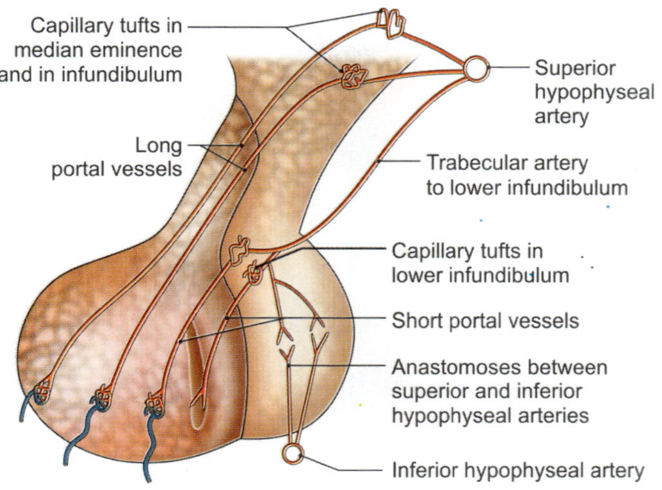

Fig. 5.4: Hypothalamo-hypophyseal circulation

VEINS

Characteristic Features

1. Veins are thin-walled, being thinner than the arteries (Fig. 5.7).
2. Their lumen is larger than that of the accompanying arteries.
3. Veins have valves which maintain the unidirectional flow of blood, even against gravity (Fig. 5.8).
4. The muscular and elastic tissue content of the venous walls is much less than that of the arteries. This is directly related to the low venous pressure.
5. Large veins have dead space around them for their dilatation during increased venous return. The dead space commonly contains the regional lymph nodes (Fig. 5.7).

Structure of Veins

Veins are made up of usual three coats which are found in the arteries. But the coats are ill-defined, and the muscle and elastic tissue content is poor (Fig. 5.5).

Table 5.2 shows the comparison of arteries and veins.

CAPILLARIES

Capillaries (capillus = hair) are networks of microscopic endothelial tubes interposed between the arterioles and venules (Fig. 5.2). The true capillaries (without any smooth muscle cell) begin after a transition zone of 50–100 micron beyond the precapillary sphincters.

The capillaries are replaced by cavernous (dilated) spaces in the sex organs, splenic pulp and placenta.

Size

The average diameter of a capillary is 6–8 micron, just sufficient to permit the red blood cells to pass through in 'single file'. But the size varies from organ to organ. It is smallest in the brain and intestines, and is largest (20 micron) in the skin and bone marrow.

Sinusoids

Sinusoids, replace capillaries in certain organs, like liver, spleen, bone marrow, suprarenal glands, parathyroid glands, carotid body, etc. Here the fenestrations are present both in the basement membrane and endothelial cells.

ANASTOMOSES

Definition

A precapillary or postcapillary communication between the neighbouring vessels is called anastomoses. Circulation through the anastomosis is called collateral circulation.

Types

A. Arterial anastomoses is the communication between the arteries, or branches of arteries. It may be actual or potential.
   1. In actual arterial anastomosis the arteries meet end to end. For example, palmar arches, plantar arch, circle of Willis (Fig. 5.9), intestinal arcades, labial branches of facial arteries.
   2. In potential arterial anastomoses the communication takes place between the terminal arterioles.

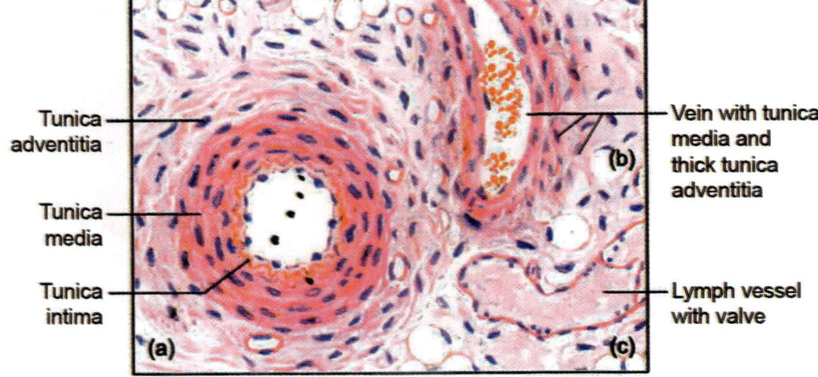

Fig. 5.5: Microscopic structure of (a) an artery; (b) vein and (c) lymph vessel

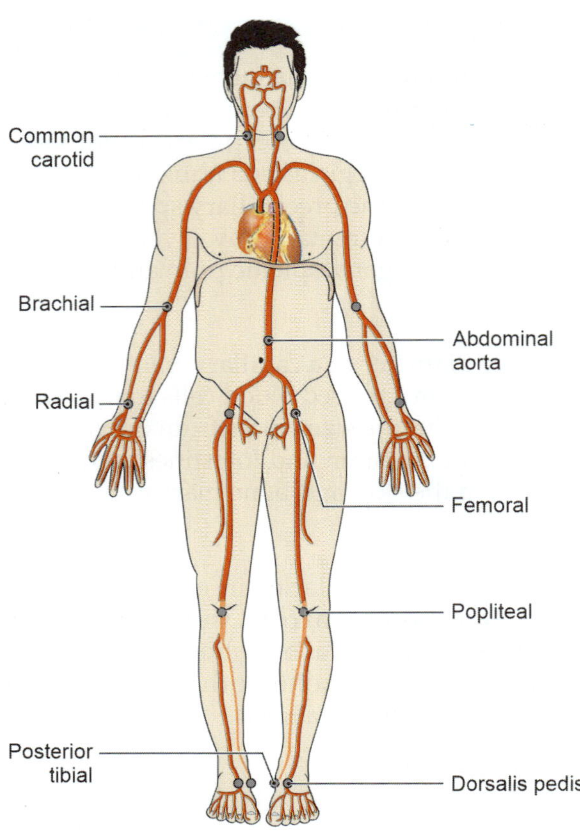

Fig. 5.6: Main arteries and various palpable arteries (with dots)

Such communications can dilate only gradually for collateral circulation. Therefore on sudden occlusion of a main artery, the anastomoses may fail to compensate the loss. The examples are seen in the coronary arteries (Fig. 5.10). The coronary arteries get filled during diastole of the heart.

B. Venous anastomoses is the communication between the veins or tributaries of veins. For example, the dorsal venous arches of the hand and foot.

C. Arteriovenous anastomosis (shunt) is the communication between an artery and a vein. It serves the function during phasic activity of the organ. When the organ is active, these shunts are closed and the blood circulates through the capillaries.

END ARTERIES

Definition

Arteries which do not anastomose with their neighbours are called end arteries. Examples:

1 Central artery of retina and labyrinthine artery of internal ear are the best examples of absolute end arteries.

2 Central branches of cerebral arteries and vasa recta of mesenteric arteries.

3. Arteries of spleen, kidney, lungs and metaphyses of long bones (*see* Fig. 2.5).

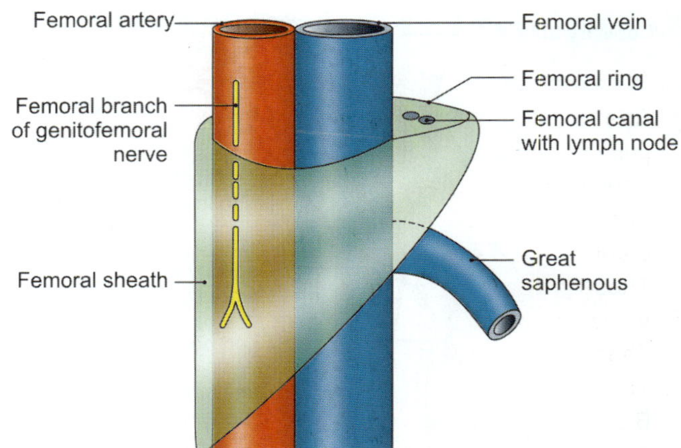

Fig. 5.7: Femoral sheath with its contents

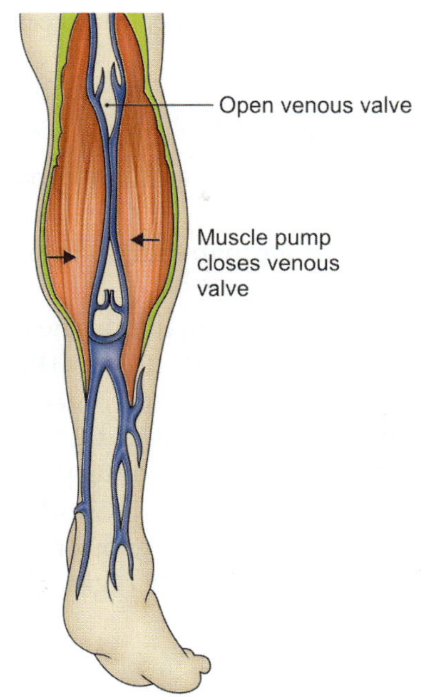

Fig. 5.8: Venous valves for unidirectional flow of venous blood

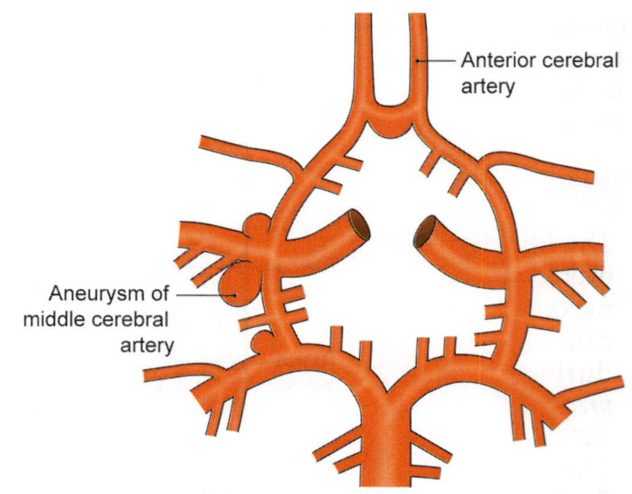

Fig. 5.9: Central branches of cerebral arteries. Aneurysms seen in the cerebral arteries

Table 5.2: Comparison of arteries and veins

	Arteries (Fig. 5.9)	*Veins* (Fig. 5.10)
1.	Arteries carry oxygenated blood, away from the heart except pulmonary trunk and pulmonary arteries	Veins carry deoxygenated blood, towards the heart except four pulmonary veins
2.	These are mostly deeply situated in the body	These are superficial and deep in location
3.	These are thick-walled, highly muscular except arteries of cranium and vertebral column	These are thin-walled
4.	These possess narrow lumen	These possess wide lumen
5.	Valves are absent	Valves are present which provide unidirectional flow of blood
6.	These are reddish in colour	These are bluish in colour
7.	These show spurty flow of blood giving pulse	These show sluggish flow of blood
8.	Blood in arteries moves with pressure	Blood in veins moves under very low pressure
9.	Arteries get empty up at the time of death	Veins get filled up at time of death
10.	If arterial wall is injured, the blood comes out like a 'fountain' in a large area all around the artery	If venous wall is injured, blood comes out, collects in a pool in a small area around vein

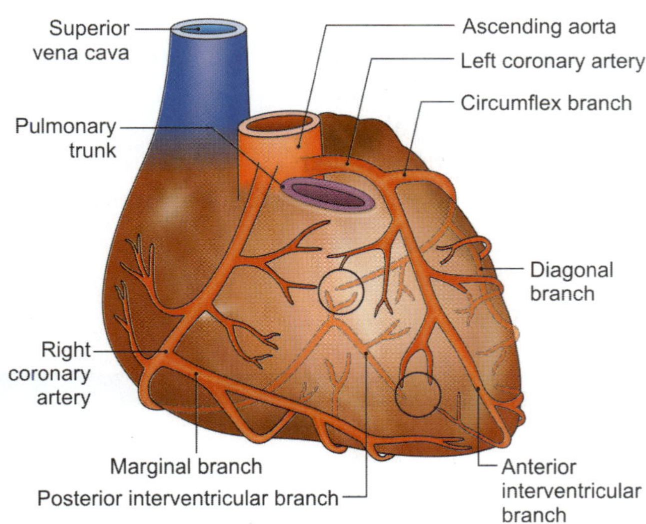

Fig. 5.10: Potential arterial anastomoses shown as circles

Importance

Occlusion of an end-artery causes serious nutritional disturbances resulting in death of the tissue supplied by it. For example, occlusion of central artery of retina results in blindness.

CLINICAL ANATOMY

- The ***blood pressure*** (BP) is the arterial pressure exerted by the blood on the arterial walls. The maximum pressure during ventricular systole is called *systolic pressure;* the minimum pressure during ventricular diastole is called *diastolic pressure.* Normally, the blood pressure is roughly 120/80 mm Hg, the systolic pressure ranging from 110–130, and the diastolic pressure from 70–80. BP is universally measured by auscultating the brachial artery at the elbow joint.
- ***Haemorrhage*** (bleeding) is the obvious result of rupture of the blood vessels. Arterial haemorrhage causes spurting of blood, venous haemorrhage results in pooling of blood.
- ***Coronary arteries blockage*:** These may be opened up by stents. Blocked coronary artery may be replaced by a graft. The graft is taken from the longest vein, the long or great saphenous vein of lower limb or anterior thoracic artery.
- ***Varicose veins*:** When the vein wall is subjected to increased pressure over long time, there is atrophy of muscle and elastic tissue with fibrous tissue replacement. This leads to stretching of the vein with tortuosity and localized bulging.

FACTS TO REMEMBER

- Systemic circulation starts from left ventricle, goes to most of the tissues of the body and returns to right atrium of heart.
- Pulmonary circulation starts from right ventricle, goes to lungs and returns to left atrium of heart.
- Portal circulation passes through two sets of capillaries. It starts like a vein, but ends like an artery. This circulation carries nutritive substances, hormone releasing factors, etc.
- Vessel wall comprises inner tunica intima, middle tunica media and outermost tunica adventitia. Arteries have thickest tunica media. Veins have thickest tunica adventitia.
- Veins have thinner walls, larger lumen and usually have blood cells in their lumen as compared to their parallel arteries.

- Some arteries in the body are superficial and are palpated to count heart rate. These are radial, common carotid, facial and superficial temporal, etc.
- Normal functioning valves of veins are responsible for unidirectional flow of blood especially in lower limb.
- End artery is an artery which does not anastomose with any other artery.
- Hypertension or high blood pressure must be controlled, or it may lead to haemorrhage, or aneurysm of the arteries.

Multiple Choice Questions

1. One of the following organs does not have sinusoids:
   a. Parotid gland b. Spleen
   c. Liver d. Bone marrow
2. Which vessels show valves?
   a. Capillaries b. Arteries
   c. Veins of neck d. Veins of lower limb
3. Which is the thickest layer in veins?
   a. Tunica intima
   b. Tunica media
   c. Tunica adventitia
   d. All tunicae are of the same thickness
4. Which is the thickest layer in the arteries?
   a. Tunica intima
   b. Tunica media
   c. Tunica adventitia
   d. All layers of equal thickness
5. All features of veins are correct, *except*:
   a. Their lumen is larger
   b. These have valves
   c. These are thin walled
   d. Muscle tissue and elastic tissue are more in veins
6. End arteries are present in:
   a. Skeletal muscle b. Bone
   c. Retina d. Middle ear

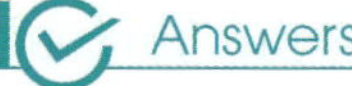

Answers

1. a **2.** d **3.** c **4.** b **5.** d **6.** c

Chapter

6

Lymphatic System

"Lives of great men all remind us, we can make our lives subline.
And departing leave behind us, foot prints on the sands of time."
—William Wordsworth

Lymphatic system is essentially a drainage system which is accessory to the venous system (Fig. 6.1).

Most of the tissue fluid formed at the arterial end of capillaries is absorbed back into the blood by the venous ends of the capillaries and the postcapillary venules. The rest of the tissue fluid (10–20%) is absorbed by the lymphatics which begin blindly in the tissue spaces.

It is important to know that the larger particles (proteins and particulate matter) can be removed from the tissue fluid only by the lymphatics. Therefore, the lymphatic system may be regarded as 'drainage system of coarse type' and the venous system as 'drainage system of fine type'.

Certain parts of the lymphatic system (lymphoreticular organs), however, are chiefly involved in phagocytosis, raising immune responses, and contributing to cell populations of the blood and lymph.

The tissue fluid flowing in the lymphatics is called lymph. It passes through filters (lymph nodes) placed in the course of lymphatics, and finally drains into the venous blood.

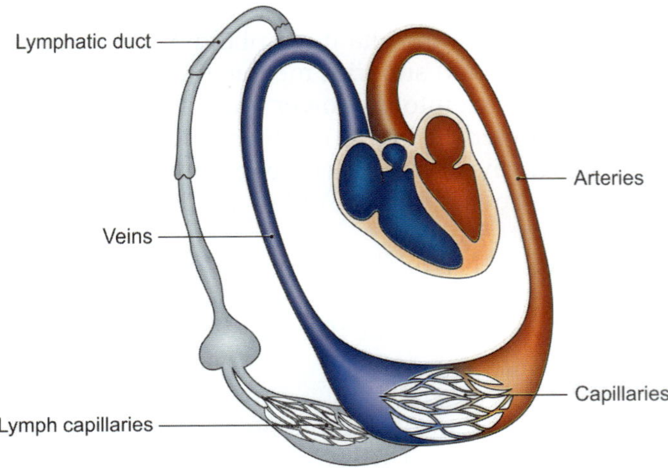

Fig. 6.1: Beginning and termination of lymph vessels

Lymph from most of the tissues is clear and colourless, but the lymph from small intestine is milky-white due to absorption of fat. The intestinal milky lymph is called *chyle,* and lymph vessels, the *lacteals*.

COMPONENTS

The lymphatic system comprises:

1 Lymph capillaries and lymph vessels
2 Central lymphoid tissues
3 Peripheral lymphoid organs
4 Circulating pool of lymphocytes

1. Lymph Capillaries and Lymph Vessels

The lymph capillaries begin blindly in the tissue spaces and form intricate networks. Their calibre is greater and less regular than that of blood capillaries, and their endothelial wall is permeable to substances of much greater molecular size.

Lymph capillaries are absent from the cellular structures like brain, spinal cord, splenic pulp, bone marrow, articular cartilage, epidermis, hair, nail and cornea.

The lymph capillaries join to form lymphatics, which are superficial and deep lymphatics. The superficial lymphatics accompany veins, while the deep lymphatics accompany arteries.

The lymph passes through filters or barriers of the regional lymph nodes which trap the particulate matter.

The filtered lymph passes through larger lymphatics and is eventually collected into two large trunks, the *thoracic duct* and *right lymphatic duct*, which pour their lymph into the brachiocephalic veins (Fig. 6.2). Thoracic duct drains *both* lower limbs, abdomen, left halves of thorax, head and neck and left upper limb. Right lymphatic duct only drains right halves of thorax, head and neck and right upper limb.

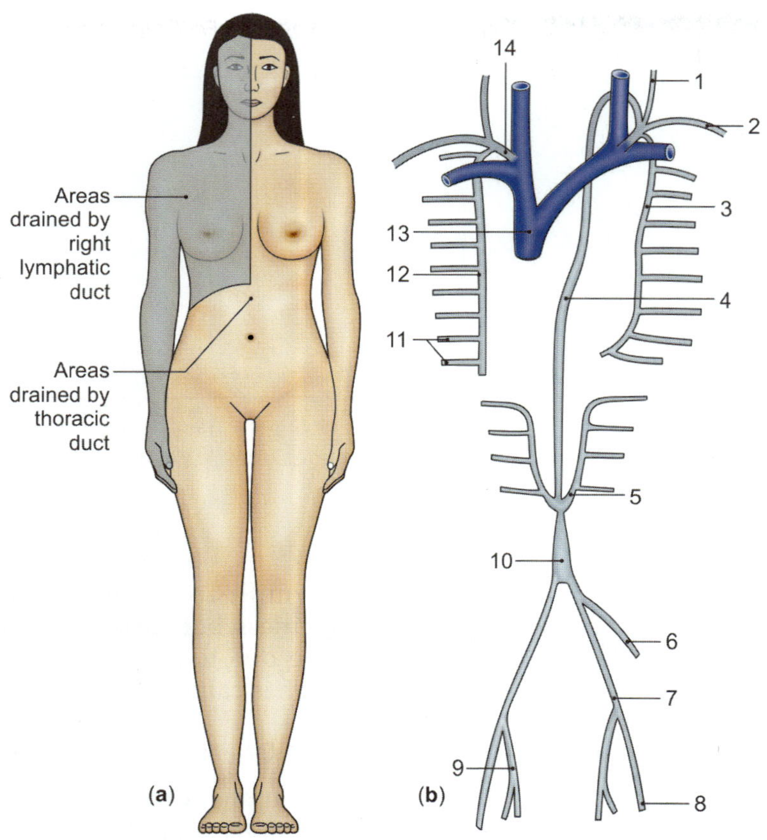

Figs 6.2a and b: (a) Areas drained by thoracic duct and (b) right lymphatic duct

1. Jugular lymph trunk
2. Left subclavian lymph trunk
3. Left broncho-mediastinal lymph trunk
4. Thoracic duct
5. Descending thoracic lymph trunk
6. Intestinal lymph trunk
7. Left lumbar lymph trunk
8. External iliac lymph trunk
9. Internal iliac lymph trunk
10. Cisterna chyli
11. Intercostal lymph vessels
12. Right broncho-mediastinal lymph trunk
13. Superior vena cava
14. Right lymphatic duct

The lymphatics anastomose freely with their neighbours of the same side as well as of the *opposite side*. Larger lymphatics are supplied with their *vasa vasorum* and are accompanied by a plexus of fine blood vessels which form red streaks seen in lymphangitis.

2. Central Lymphoid Tissues

Central lymphoid tissues comprise bone marrow and thymus.

Bone Marrow

All 'pluripotent' lymphoid stem cells are initially produced by bone marrow, except during early fetal life when these are produced by liver and spleen. The stem cells undergo differentiation in the central lymphoid tissues, so that the lymphocytes become competent defensive elements of the immune system.

Bone marrow helps differentiation of the (committed) B-lymphocytes which are capable of synthesizing antibodies after getting transformed into plasma cells.

Thymus

The thymus is an important lymphoid organ, situated in the anterior and superior mediastina of the thorax, extending above into the lower part of the neck. It is well developed at birth, continues to grow up to puberty, and thereafter undergoes gradual atrophy and replacement by fat. It is the only lymphoid organ well developed at birth.

The thymus is a bilobed structure, made up of two pyramidal lobes of unequal size which are connected together by areolar tissue (Fig. 6.3).

Functions

1 The thymus controls lymphopoiesis, and maintains an effective pool of circulating lymphocytes, competent to react to innumerable antigenic stimuli.

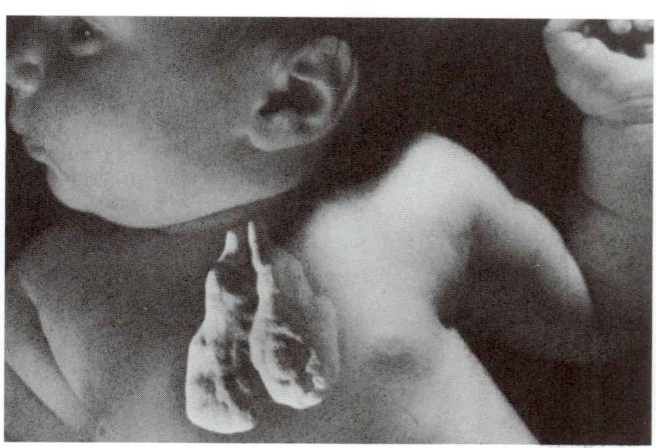

Fig. 6.3: Thymus in a child

2 It controls development of the peripheral lymphoid tissues of the body during the neonatal period. By puberty, the main lymphoid tissues are fully developed.

3 The cortical lymphocytes of the thymus arise from stem cells of bone marrow origin. Most (95%) of the lymphocytes (T lymphocytes) produced are autoallergic (act against the host or 'self antigens'), short-lived (3–5 days) and never move out of the organ. They are destroyed and their remnants are seen in Hassall's corpuscles. The remaining 5% of the T lymphocytes are longer living and join the circulating pool of lymphocytes where they act as immunologically competent but uncommitted cells. On the other hand, the other circulating lymphocytes (from lymph nodes, spleen, etc.) are committed only when exposed to a particular antigen. The process of involution are all intrinsically controlled.

4 The medullary epithelial cells of the thymus are thought to secrete:
   a. *Lymphopoietin,* which stimulates lymphocyte production, both in the cortex of the thymus and in peripheral lymphoid organs.
   b. The *competence-inducing factor,* which may be responsible for making new lymphocytes competent to react to antigenic stimuli.

5 Normally, there are no germinal centres in the thymic cortex. Such centres appear in autoimmune diseases. This may indicate a defect in the normal function of the thymus.

3. Peripheral Lymphoid Organs

Peripheral lymphoid organs comprise lymph nodes, and spleen. Any part of this may become overactive on appropriate stimulation.

The progenies of B- and T-lymphocytes reach these organs where the cells may proliferate and mature into competent cells. The mature lymphocytes join the circulating pool of lymphocytes.

Lymphatic Follicle (Nodule)

Collections of lymphocytes occur at many places in the body. Everywhere there is a basic pattern, the *lymphatic follicle.* The follicle is a spherical collection of lymphocytes with a pale centre known as *germinal centre,* where the lymphocytes are more loosely packed.

The central cells are larger in size, stain less deeply, and divide more rapidly, than the peripheral cells.

Lymph Nodes

Lymph nodes are small nodules of lymphoid tissue found in the course of smaller lymphatics.

The lymph passes through one or more lymph nodes before reaching the larger lymph trunks.

The nodes are oval or reniform in shape, 1–25 mm long, and light brown, black (pulmonary), or creamy white (intestinal) in colour.

Usually they occur in groups (cervical, axillary, inguinal, mesenteric, mediastinal, etc.), but at times there may be a solitary lymph node.

Superficial nodes are arranged along the veins, and the deep nodes along the arteries.

Cervical lymph nodes form a ring at the junction of head and neck and vertical chains in the neck (Fig. 6.4). These drain whole of head and neck. On right side jugular *lymph* trunk drains into right lymphatic duct, while on left side it drains into thoracic duct. Lymph vessels of abdominal wall above a line passing horizontally through umbilicus drain into respective sides of axillary lymph nodes. Lymph vessels below this line drain into inguinal group of lymph nodes. This line is called "watershed" (Fig. 6.5).

Each lymph node has a slight depression on one side, called hilum. The artery enters the node, and the vein with efferent lymphatic comes out of it, at the hilum.

The afferent lymphatics enter the node at different parts of its periphery.

Structurally, a lymph node is made up of the following parts (Fig. 6.6).

a. *Fibrous and reticular framework*: The lymph node is covered by a capsule. From the deep surface of the capsule a number of trabeculae extend radially into the interior of the node, where they are continuous with the fine reticulum which forms the supporting framework for the lymphoid tissue.
b. *Lymphatic channels*: The *subcapsular sinus* lies beneath the capsule and surrounds the node except at the hilum. Many afferent lymphatics of the node open into the subcapsular sinus. Lymph filters through reticulin fibres and leaves the node by only *one* efferent lymphatic vessel.
c. *Cortex*: It is the outer part of the lymph node situated beneath the subcapsular sinus, being absent at the hilum.

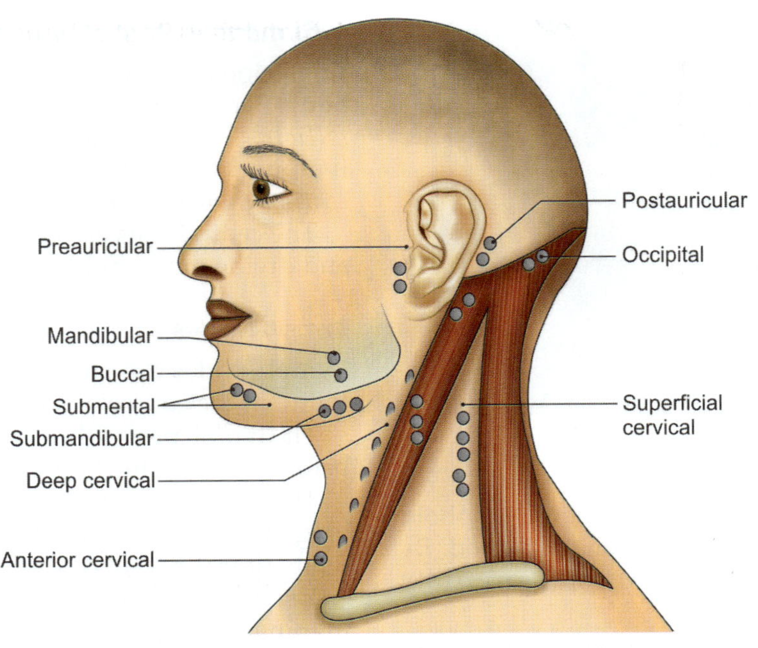

Fig. 6.4: Some lymph nodes of the neck

It is made up of lymphatic follicles and is traversed by fibrous trabeculae.

The cortex is far more densely cellular than the medulla.

According to the distribution of B- and T-lymphocytes, the cortex is divided into:

1 An outer part which contains immature B-lymphocytes.
2 An inner part, between the germinal centre and the medulla, which contains T-lymphocytes. This part is known as *paracortex* or *thymus dependent zone.*

The mature B-lymphocytes (plasma cells) are found in the medulla.

d. *Medulla*: It is the central part of the lymph node, containing loosely packed lymphocytes (forming irregular branching medullary cords), the plasma cells, and macrophages.

e. *Blood channels*: The artery enters at the hilum and divides into straight branches which run in the trabeculae. In the cortex the arteries further divide to form arcades of arterioles and capillaries with many anastomosing loops.

The capillaries give rise to venules and veins, which run back to the hilum. The capillaries are more profuse around the follicles, and the postcapillary venules are more abundant in the paracortical zones for lymphatic migration.

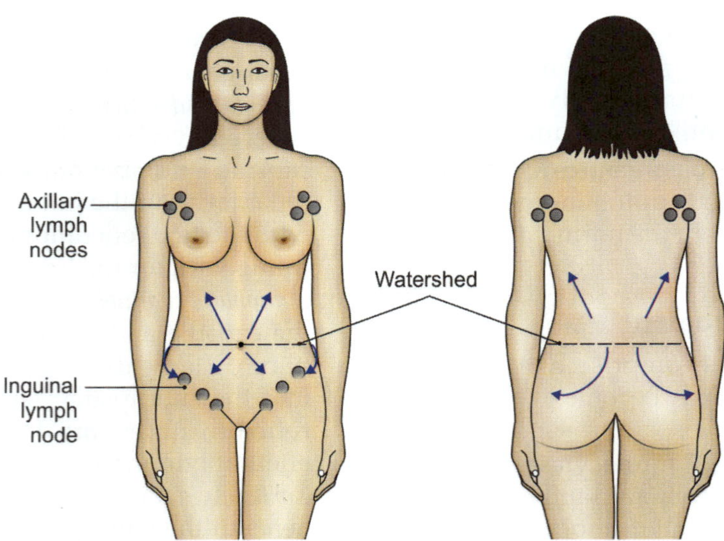

Fig. 6.5: Areas drained by axillary and inguinal lymph nodes

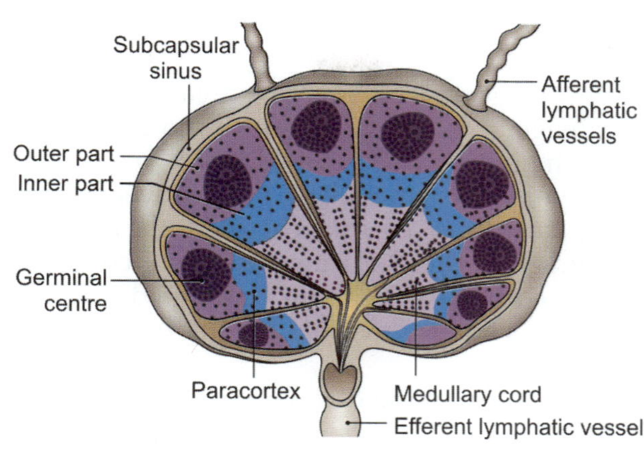

Fig. 6.6: Structure of a lymph node

Spleen

Spleen is the largest lymphoid organ and is covered by a dense connective tissue *capsule* (Fig. 6.7). *Trabeculae* extend inwards from capsule. Cellular material of spleen is divided into *white pulp* and *red pulp*. Red pulp consists of blood filled venous sinuses and white pulp comprises lymphatic tissue, consisting of lymphocytes and macrophages. Spleen is part of the lymphatic system and its functions are:

1 *Phagocytosis*: Leukocytes, platelets are phagocytosed in spleen. Old and abnormal RBCs are destroyed in spleen and break down products (bilirubin and iron) are passed to the liver.
2 *Storage of blood*: Spleen contains up to 350 ml blood. In shock, sympathetic stimulation can return a large part of this volume to circulation.
3 *Immunity*: Spleen contains B- and T-lymphocytes which are important in immune response to infections.
4 *Erythropoiesis*: RBC production occurs in spleen and liver in fetal life.
5 Storage of platelets.

4. Circulating Pool of Lymphocytes

The pool contains mature progenies of B- and T-lymphocytes which may be called upon during antigenic emergencies (Roitt, 1977). Table 6.1 shows the differences between T- and B-lymphocytes.

Table 6.2 shows the approximate percentage of lymphocytes in lymphoid organs.

Growth Pattern of Lymphoid Tissue

Lymphoid tissue of the body is prominent at birth, and grows rapidly during childhood. There are about 600–800 lymph nodes in an adult.

The growth ceases at about the time of puberty, and is followed by partial atrophy in the later years.

This growth pattern is shared by lymph nodes, thymus, tonsils, lymphoid tissue of the intestines, and the follicles of spleen.

However, the lymph nodes may enlarge again in response to inflammation (lymphadenitis) or tumour formation (Hodgkin's disease, lymphosarcoma, etc.).

Lymph nodes are commonly enlarged by metastases (spread) of malignant growths (carcinoma).

Functions of Lymphoid System

1 Lymph capillaries absorb and remove the large protein molecules and other particulate matter from the tissue spaces. Thus the cellular debris and foreign particles (dust particles inhaled into the lungs, bacteria and other micro-organisms) are conveyed to the regional lymph nodes. Lymphatics (lacteals) help in transportation of fat from the gut.
2 Lymph nodes serve a number of functions.
   a. They act as filters for the lymph which percolates slowly through the intricate network of its spaces. Thus the foreign particles are prevented from entering the blood stream.
   b. The foreign particles are engulfed by the macrophages in the sinuses.

Table 6.1: Differences between T- and B-lymphocytes

	T-lymphocytes	*B-lymphocytes*
Origin	Bone marrow →Thymus → Lymphoid tissue	Bone marrow → Bursa-equivalent → Lymphoid tissue
Life span	Months to years	Less than one month
Location		
Lymph nodes	Between germinal centre and medulla	Germinal centre and outer part
Spleen	Perifollicular	Germinal centre
Peyer's patches	Perifollicular	Central follicles
Number in blood	80%	20%
Function	i. Cell-mediated immunity via Tc cells (cytotoxic) ii. Immunoregulation of T- and B-lymphocytes via T_H cells (helper) iii. Memory T cells	i. Humoral immunity IgG (most abundant). It is via immunoglobulins produced by plasma cells Formed by enlargement and modification of B-lymphocytes Memory B cells

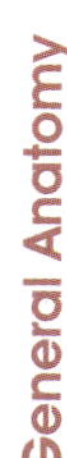

Table 6.2: Approximate percentage of lymphocytes in lymphoid organs

Lymphoid organ	*T-lymphocytes*	*B-lymphocytes*
Thymus	100%	0%
Lymph node	60%	40%
Spleen	45%	55%
Bone marrow	10%	90%
Blood	80%	20%

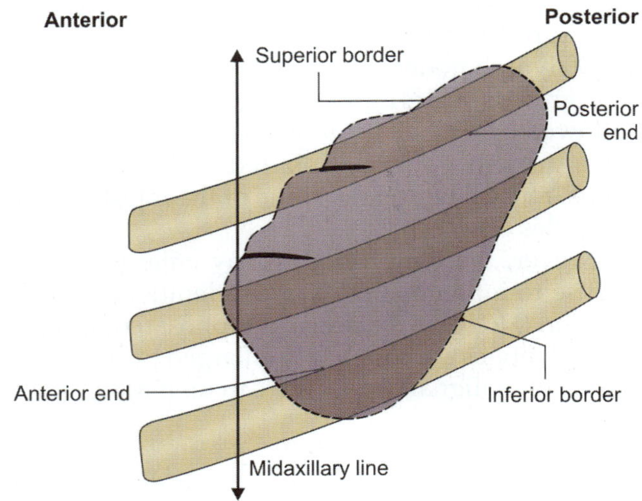

Fig. 6.7: Spleen with its ends and borders

c. Antigens are also trapped by the phagocytes.
d. The mature B-lymphocytes (plasma cells capable of producing antibodies) and mature T-lymphocytes are produced in the node.
e. Both the cellular and humoral immune responses are mounted against the antigen-laden phagocytes.
f. The circulating lymphocytes can pass back into the lymphatic channels within the node.
g. Humoral antibodies are freely produced by the lymph nodes.

3 Production (proliferation) and maturation of B- and T-lymphocytes is the main function of lymphoid tissue.

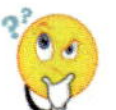

CLINICAL ANATOMY

- Lymphatics are primarily meant for coarse drainage, from the tissue spaces to the regional lymph nodes.
- The lymphatics provide the most convenient *route of spread of the cancer cells*. Therefore, the lymphatic drainage of those organs which are commonly involved in cancer should be studied in greater details. The reasons for detailed study are as follows:
  a. It is helpful in the diagnosis of the primary site of the cancer.
  b. It helps in predicting the prognosis and in classifying the stage of cancer.
  c. It helps the surgeon in doing the block dissections during operative removal of the cancer.
- Enlargement of thymus may cause **myasthenia gravis**, which produces extreme weakness of the skeletal muscles. It may be treated by removal of enlarged thymus, or by drug treatment.

FACTS TO REMEMBER

- Lymph mostly consists of macromolecules not able to course through the blood capillaries. Lymph carries absorbed products of fats to the blood circulation.
- Lymph vessels also carry cancer cells from the original site of disease to nearby or distant regions.
- Lymph nodes/palatine tonsil/thymus, etc. are maximum in size till puberty. Then these start involuting/decreasing in size.
- Lymph nodes increase in size (lymphadenitis) during chronic infections like tuberculosis, syphilis, lymphomas.
- Lymphatic system forms the first line of defence of the body.

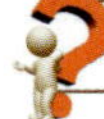

Multiple Choice Questions

1. Components of lymphatic system are all, *except*:
a. Lymph vessels
b. Central lymphoid tissues
c. Peripheral lymphoid organs
d. Circulating red blood cells

2. Splenomegaly commonly occurs in:
a. Malaria b. Cirrhosis of liver
c. Anaemia d. Elephantiasis

3. Thoracic duct drains the following areas, *except*:
a. Left upper limb b. Left lower limb
c. Right lower limb d. Right upper limb

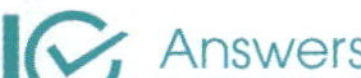

Answers

1. d **2.** a **3.** d

Chapter

7

Nervous System

"We only use 5% of our intelligence, while Albert Einstein used up to 15–20%. There is such a gap between what we do and what we can do."

—William James

Nervous system is the chief controlling and coordinating system of the body. It controls and regulates all activities of the body, whether voluntary or involuntary, and adjusts the individual (organism) to the given surroundings.

This is based on the special properties of sensitivity, conductivity and responsiveness of the nervous system.

The protoplasmic extensions of the nerve cells form the neural pathways called nerves. The nerves resemble the electricity wires. Like the electric current flowing through the wires, the impulses (sensory and motor) are conducted through the nerves.

The sensory impulses are transmitted by the sensory (afferent) nerves from the periphery (skin, mucous membranes, muscles, tendons, joints, and special sense organs) to the central nervous system (CNS).

The motor impulses are transmitted by the motor (efferent) nerves from the central nervous system to the periphery (muscles and glands) (Fig. 7.1).

Thus the CNS is kept continuously informed about the surroundings (environment) through various sensory impulses, both general and special.

The CNS in turn brings about necessary adjustment of the body by sending appropriate orders which are passed on as motor impulses to the muscles, vessels, viscera and glands. The adjustment of the organism to the given surroundings is the most important function of the nervous system, without which it will not be possible for the organism to survive.

PARTS OF NERVOUS SYSTEM

The nervous system is broadly divided into central and peripheral parts which are continuous with each other. Further subdivisions of each part are given below.

A. *Central nervous system (CNS) includes:*
   1. Brain or encephalon, which occupies cranial cavity, and contains the higher governing centres (Fig. 7.2).
   2. Spinal cord or spinal medulla, which occupies upper two-thirds of the vertebral canal, and contains many reflex centres.

B. *Peripheral nervous system (PNS)* is subdivided into the following two components.

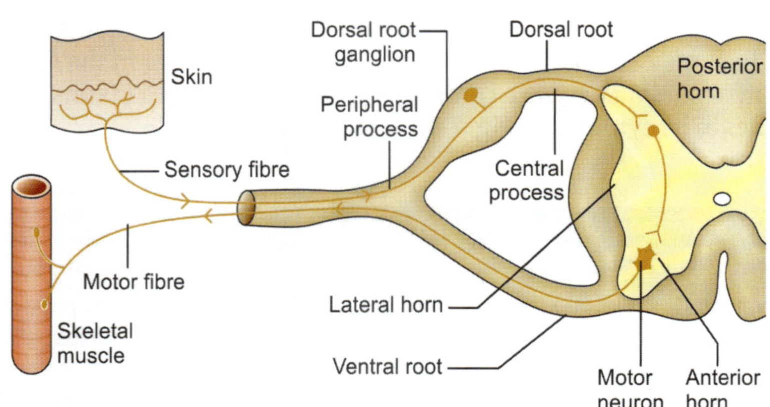

Fig. 7.1: Afferent and efferent pathways through the spinal cord

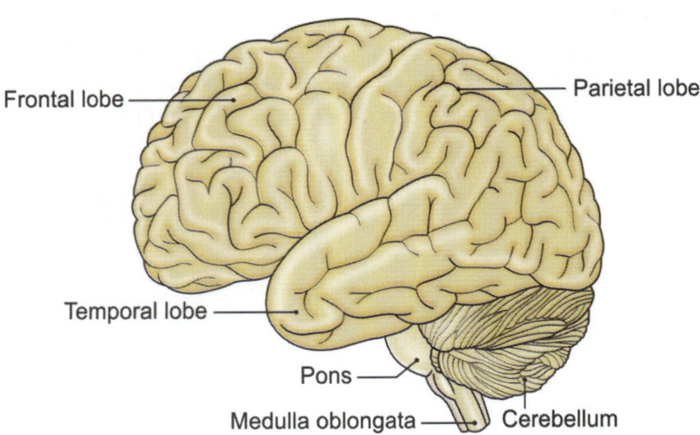

Fig. 7.2: Superolateral surface of cerebral hemisphere, pons, medulla oblongata and cerebellum

1. Cerebrospinal nervous system is the somatic component of the peripheral nervous system, which includes 12 pairs of cranial nerves and 31 pairs of spinal nerves (Fig. 7.3). It innervates the somatic structures of the head and neck, limbs and body wall, and mediates somatic sensory and motor functions.
2. Peripheral autonomic nervous system is the visceral component of the peripheral nervous system, which includes the visceral or splanchnic nerves that are connected to the CNS through the somatic nerves. It innervates the viscera, glands, blood vessels and nonstriated muscles, and mediates the visceral functions.

The cerebrospinal and autonomic nervous systems differ from each other in their efferent pathways. Table 7.1 shows comparison of the above two systems.

CELL TYPES OF NERVOUS SYSTEM

The nervous tissue is composed of two distinct types of cells:

a. The excitable cells are the nerve cells or neurons; and
b. The non-excitable cells constitute neuroglia and ependyma in the CNS, and Schwann cells in the PNS.

1. Neuron

Each nerve cell or neuron has:

a. A cell body or perikaryon or somata having a central nucleus and Nissl granules in its cytoplasm (Fig. 7.4).

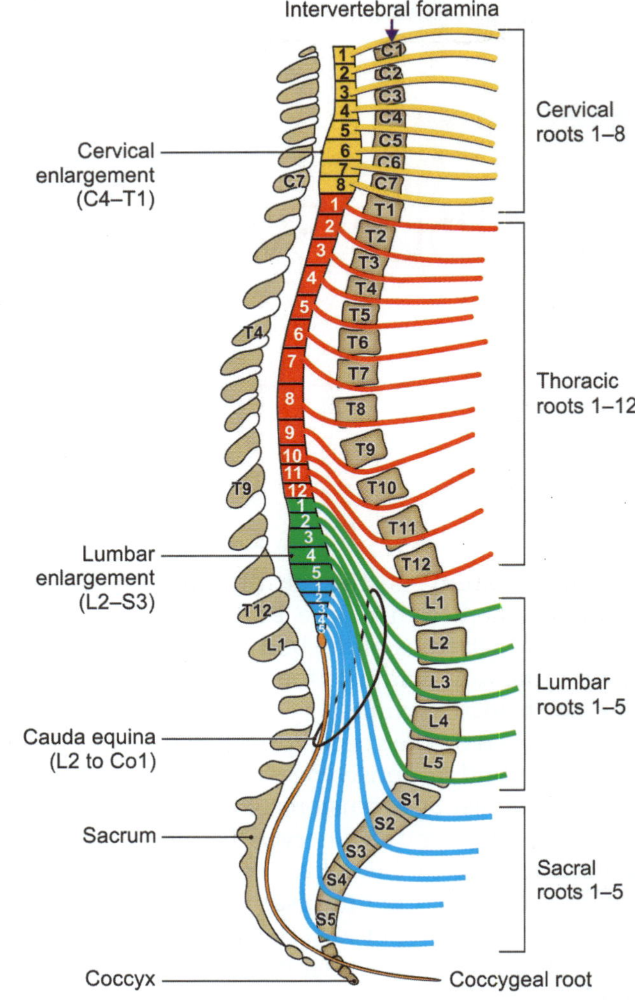

Fig. 7.3: Segments of spinal cord with 31 pairs of spinal nerves

b. Cell processes called neurites, which are of two types.

Many short afferent processes, which are freely branching and varicose, are called dendrites.

A single long efferent process called axon, arising from axon hillock. It may give off occasional branches (collaterals) and is of uniform diameter.

The terminal branches of the axon are called axon terminals or telodendria.

The cell bodies (somata) of the neurons form grey matter and nuclei in the CNS, and ganglia in the PNS. The cell processes (axons) form tracts in the CNS, and nerves in the PNS.

Table 7.1: Comparison of cerebrospinal and peripheral autonomic nervous systems

Cerebrospinal nervous system	*Peripheral autonomic nervous system*
The somatic efferent pathway is made up of one neuron which passes directly to the effector organ (skeletal muscles) Neuron ↓ axon Skeletal muscle	The autonomic efferent pathway is made up of two neurons (preganglionic and postganglionic) with an intervening ganglion for the relay of the preganglionic fibre. The effector organ (viscera) is supplied by the postganglionic fibre

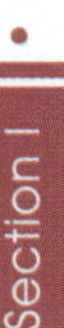

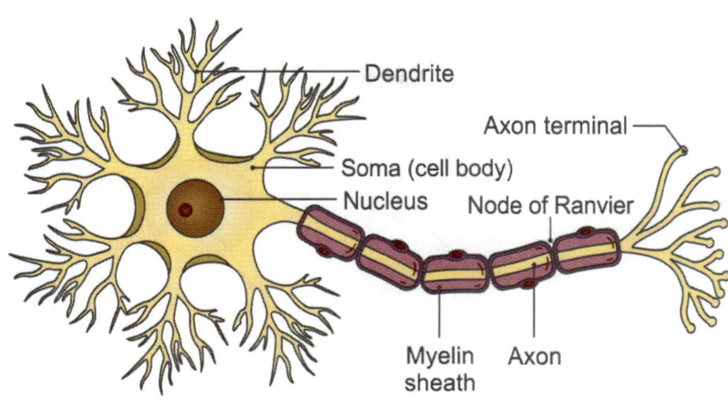

Fig. 7.4: Components of a neuron with a peripheral nerve

Table 7.2 shows the differences between axon and dendrite.

Types of neurons: Neurons can be classified in several ways.

I. According to the number of their processes (neurites) they may be:
   a. Unipolar, e.g. mesencephalic nucleus
   b. Pseudounipolar, e.g. sensory ganglia or spinal ganglia (Fig. 7.5)
   c. Bipolar, e.g. spiral and vestibular ganglia and bipolar neurons of retina.
   d. Multipolar, neurons in cerebrum and cerebellum.

II. According to the length of axon, the neurons are classified as
   a. Golgi type I neurons, with a long axon; and
   b. Golgi type II neurons (microneurons), with a short or no axon.

Dynamic polarity: The neurons show dynamic polarity in their processes. The impulse flows towards the soma in the dendrites, and away from the soma in the axon. However, in certain microneurons, where the axon is absent, the impulse can flow in either direction through their dendrites.

Synapse: The neurons form long chains along which the impulses are conducted in different directions. Each junction between the neurons is called a synapse (Fig. 7.6). It is important to know that the contact between the neurons is by contiguity and not by continuity. This is neuron theory of Waldeyer (1891). The impulse is transmitted across a synapse by specific neurotransmitters, like acetylcholine, catecholamines (noradrenalin and dopamine), serotonin, histamine, glycine, GABA and certain polypeptides.

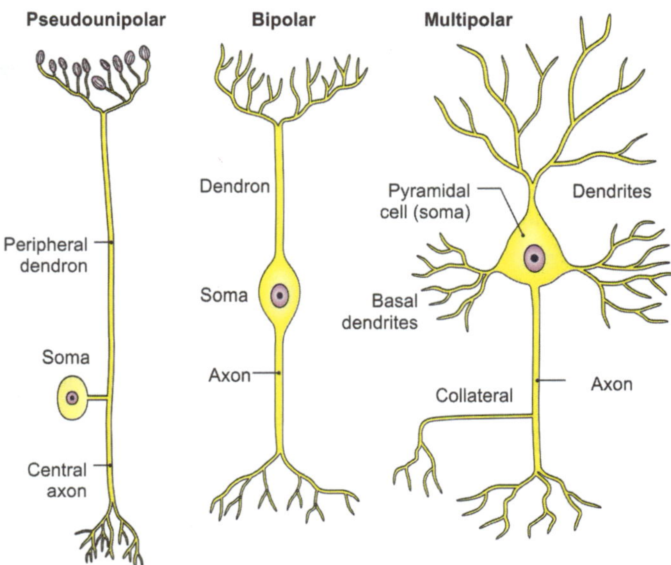

Fig. 7.5: Types of neurons

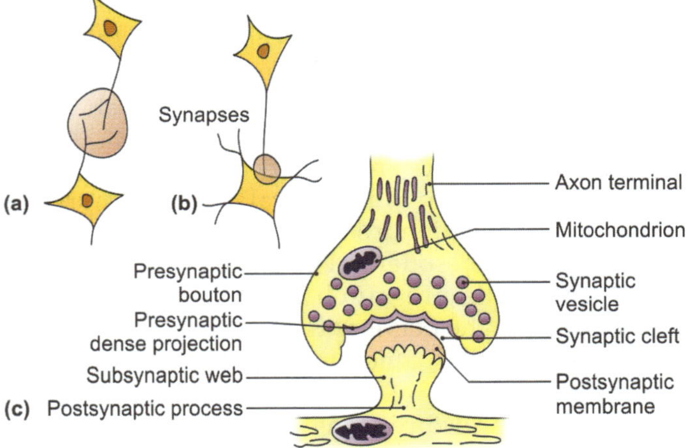

Figs 7.6a to c: Types of synapses: (a) Axodendritic, (b) axosomatic and (c) structure of a synapse

Table 7.2: Comparison of axon and dendrite

Axon	*Dendrite*
1. Only one axon is present in a neuron.	Usually multiple in a neuron.
2. Thin long process of uniform thickness and smooth surface.	These are short multiple processes. Their thickness diminishes as these divide repeatedly. The branches are studded with spiny projections.
3. The branches of axon are fewer and at right angles to the axon.	The dendrites branch profusely and are given off at acute angles.
4. Axon contains neurofibrils and no Nissl granules.	Dendrites contain both neurofibrils and Nissl granules.
5. Forms the efferent component of the impulse.	Forms the afferent component of the impulse.

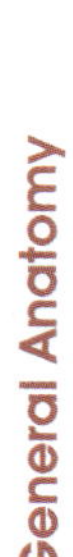

The most common types of the synapse are axo-dendritic, axo-somatic, (Figs 7.6a and b). In synaptic glomeruli, groups of axons make contact with the dendrites of one or more neurons for complex interactions. Figure 7.6c shows the ultrastructure of a synapse.

Functionally, a synapse may either be inhibitory or excitatory.

2. Neuroglia

The non-excitable supporting cells of the nervous system form a major component of the nervous tissue. These cells include the following:

1 Neuroglial cells, found in the parenchyma of brain and spinal cord.
2 Ependymal cells lining the internal cavities or ventricles.
3 Capsular or satellite cells, surrounding neurons of the sensory and autonomic ganglia.
4 Schwann cells, forming sheaths for axons of peripheral nerves.
5 Several types of supporting cells, ensheathing the motor and sensory nerve terminals, and supporting the sensory epithelia.

The neuroglial cells, found in the parenchyma of brain and spinal cord, are broadly classified as:

A. Macroglia, of ectodermal (neural) origin, comprising astrocytes, oligodendrocytes, and glioblasts.
B. Microglia, of mesodermal origin.

All glial cells are much smaller but far more numerous than the nerve cells.

a. *Astrocytes:* As the name suggests, these cells are star-shaped because of their numerous processes radiating in all directions. Astrocytes are of two types.
   Protoplasmic astrocytes, with thick and symmetrical processes are found in the grey matter.
   Fibrous astrocytes, with thin and asymmetrical processes, are found in the white matter.
   The processes of astrocytes often end in plate-like expansions on the blood vessels, ependyma, and pial surface of the CNS (Fig. 7.7).
b. *Oligodendrocytes:* As the name suggests these cells have fewer cell processes. According to their distribution, the oligodendrocytes may be intrafascicular or perineuronal. The intrafascicular cells are found in the myelinated tracts.
   The perineuronal cells are seen on the surface of the somata of neurons.
c. *Glioblast:* These are stem cells which can differentiate into macroglial cells. They are particularly numerous beneath the ependyma.
d. *Microglia:* These are the smallest of the glial cells which have a flattened cell body with a few short, fine processes.

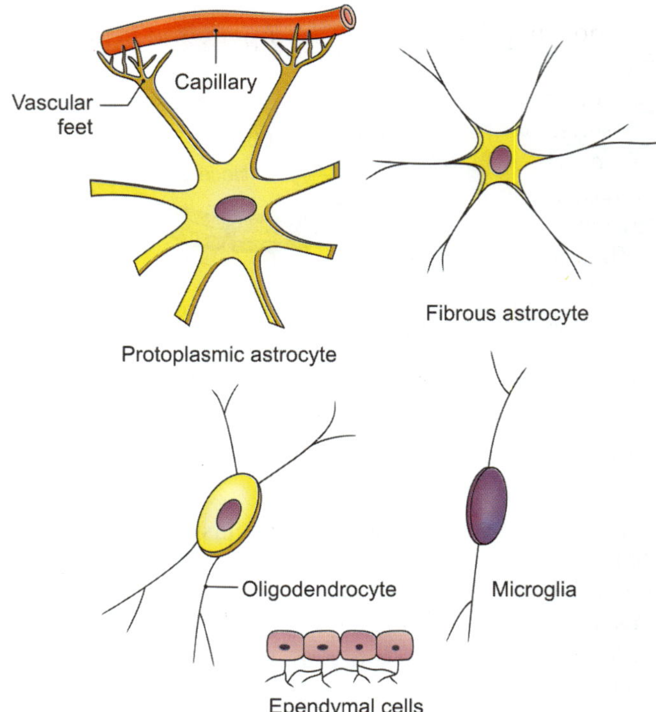

Fig. 7.7: Types of neuroglia

They are often related to capillaries, and are said to be phagocytic in nature.

Microglial cells are possibly derived from the circulating monocytes which migrate into the CNS during the late foetal and early postnatal life.

Functions of Glial and Ependymal Cells

1 They provide mechanical support to neurons.
2 Because of their non-conducting nature, the glial cells act as insulators between the neurons and prevent neuronal impulses from spreading in unwanted directions.
3 They can remove the foreign material and cell debris by phagocytosis.
4 They can repair the damaged areas of nervous tissue. By proliferation (gliosis) they form glial scar tissue, and fill the gaps left by degenerated neurons.
5 Glial cells can take up and store neurotransmitters released by the neighbouring synapses. These can either be metabolized or released again from the glial cells.
6 They help in neuronal functions by maintaining a suitable metabolic and ionic environment for the neurons.
7 Oligodendrocytes myelinate tracts.
8 Ependymal cells secrete cerebro-spinal fluid.

REFLEX ARC

A reflex arc is the basic functional unit of the nervous system which can perform an integrated neural activity.

A monosynaptic reflex arc, is simplest and is made up of:

a. A receptor, e.g. skin;
b. A sensory or afferent neuron;
c. A motor or efferent neuron; and
d. An effector, e.g. muscle.

An involuntary motor response of the body is called a reflex action. The stretch reflexes (tendon jerks) are the examples of monosynaptic reflexes (Fig. 7.8).

The complex forms of reflex arc are polysynaptic due to addition of one or more internuncial neurons (interneurons) in between the afferent and efferent neurons (Fig. 7.9). Withdrawal reflex response to a painful stimulation is polysynaptic reflex.

PERIPHERAL NERVES

The nerves are solid white cords composed of bundles (fasciculi) of nerve fibres.

Each motor nerve fibre is an axon with its coverings.

The nerve fibres are supported and bound together by connective tissue sheaths at different levels of organization of the nerve. The whole nerve trunk is ensheathed by epineurium, each fasciculus by perineurium, and each nerve fibre by a delicate endoneurium. The toughness of a nerve is due to its fibrous sheaths, otherwise the nerve tissue itself is very delicate and friable (Fig. 7.10).

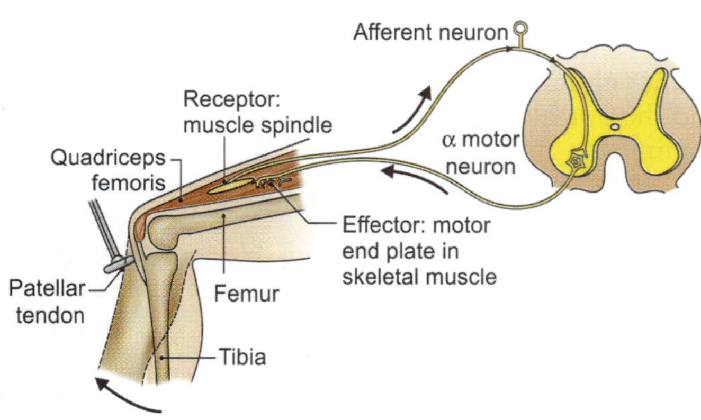

Fig. 7.8: Monosynaptic reflex arc

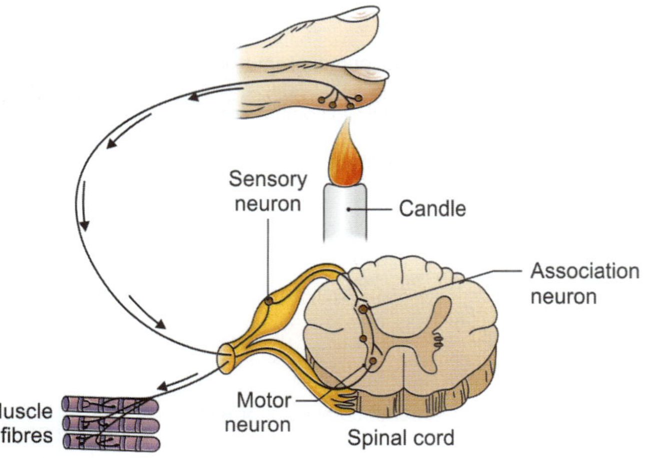

Fig. 7.9: Polysynaptic reflex arc

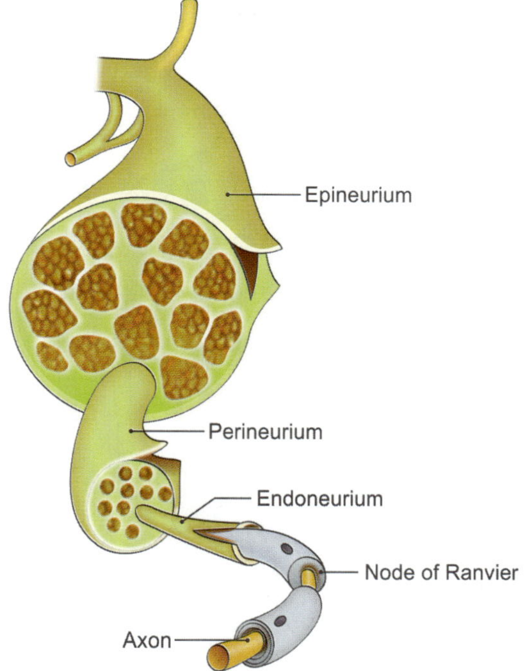

Fig. 7.10: Fibrous support of the nerve fibres

SPINAL NERVES

There are 31 pairs of spinal nerves, including 8 cervical, 12 thoracic, 5 lumbar, 5 sacral and 1 coccygeal.

Area of skin supplied by a single segment of spinal cord giving origin to one pair of spinal nerves is called a **dermatome**.

The distribution of dermatomes to the skin is shown in Fig. 7.11. Each spinal nerve is connected with the spinal cord by two roots, a ventral root which is motor, and a dorsal root which is sensory (Fig. 7.12).

The dorsal root is characterized by the presence of a spinal ganglion. In the majority of nerves the ganglion lies in the intervertebral foramen.

The ventral and dorsal nerve roots unite together within the intervertebral foramen to form the spinal nerve.

The nerve emerges through the intervertebral foramen, gives off recurrent meningeal branches, and then divides immediately into a dorsal and a ventral ramus.

The dorsal ramus passes backwards and supplies the intrinsic muscles of the back, and the skin covering them.

The ventral ramus is connected with the sympathetic ganglion, and is distributed to the limb or the anterolateral body wall.

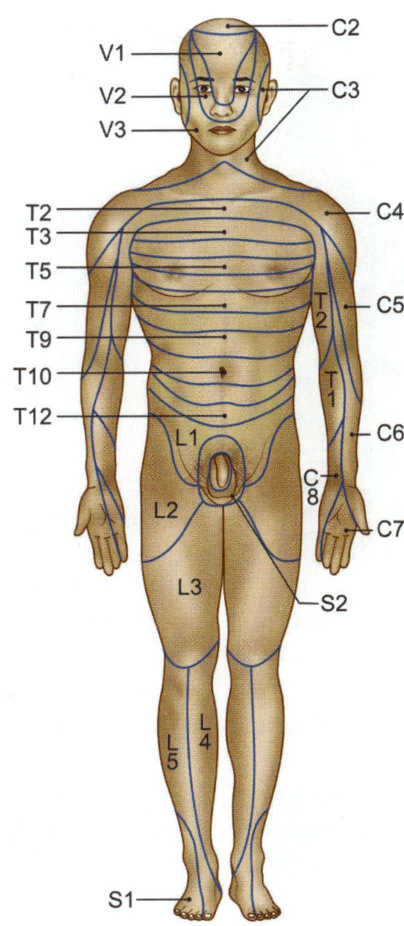

Fig. 7.11: Dermatome—anterior aspect

In case of a typical (thoracic) spinal nerve, the ventral ramus does not mix with neighbouring rami, and gives off several muscular branches, a lateral cutaneous branch, and an anterior cutaneous branch. However, the ventral rami of other spinal nerves are plaited to form the nerve plexuses for the limbs, like the brachial plexus, lumbar plexus, etc.

Nerve Plexuses for Limbs

All nerve plexuses are formed only by the ventral rami, and never by the dorsal rami.

These supply the limbs.

Against each plexus the spinal cord is enlarged, e.g. 'cervical enlargement' for the brachial plexus, and 'lumbar enlargement' for the lumbosacral plexus. Plexus formation resembles a tree (Fig. 7.13).

Various nerve plexuses are:

Cervical: Formed by C1, C2, C3 and C4 ventral primary rami.

Brachial: Formed by C5, C6, C7, C8 and T1 ventral primary rami.

Lumbar: Formed by L2, L3 and part of L4 ventral primary rami.

Sacral plexus: Formed by part of L4, L5, S1, S2 and S3 ventral primary rami.

Each nerve root of the plexus (ventral ramus) divides into a ventral and a dorsal division.

The ventral division supplies the flexor compartment, and the dorsal division, the extensor compartment, of the limb.

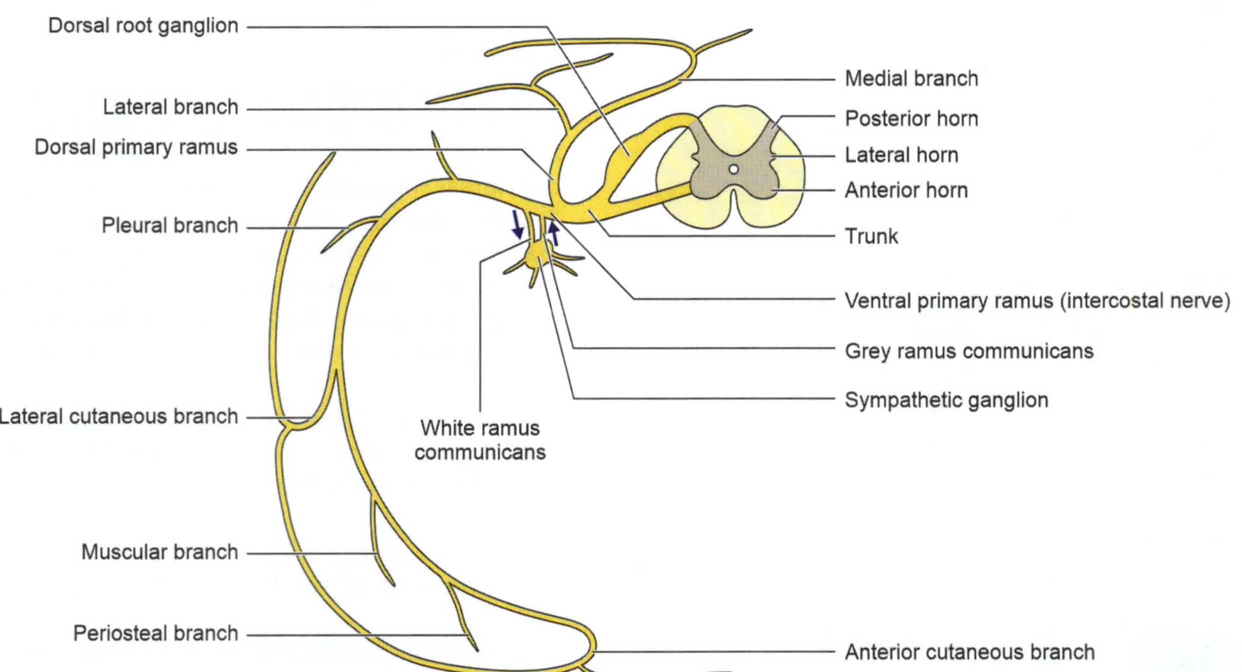

Fig. 7.12: Course of typical thoracic nerve

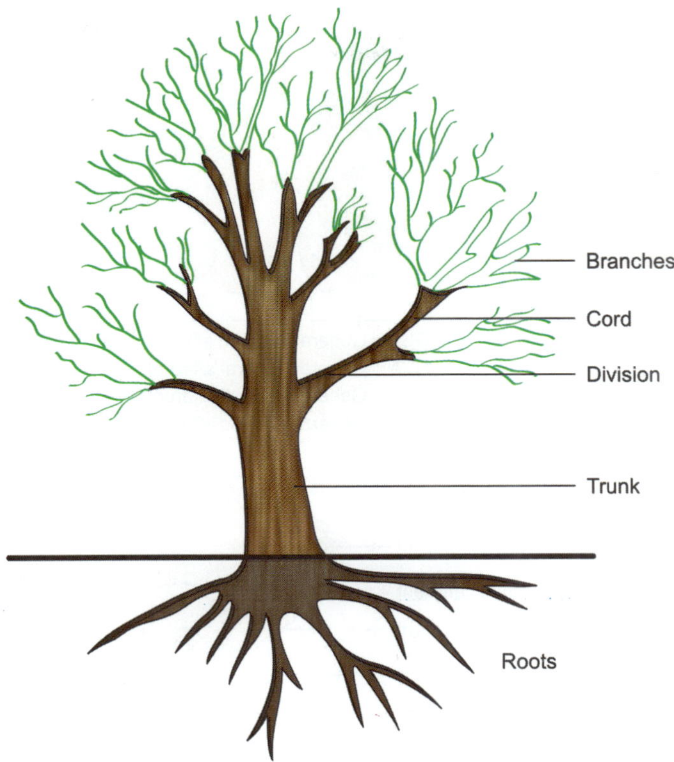

Fig. 7.13: Nerve plexuses likened to a tree

The flexor compartment has a richer nerve supply than the extensor compartment. The flexor skin is more sensitive than the extensor skin, and the flexor muscles (antigravity, bulkier muscles) are more efficient and are under a more precise control than the coarse extensor muscles.

The plexus formation is a physiological or functional adaptation, and is perhaps the result of the following special features in the limbs.

1 Overlapping of dermatomes
2 Overlapping of myotomes
3 Composite nature of muscles
4 Possible migration of muscles from the trunk to the limbs
5 Linkage of the opposite groups of muscles in the spinal cord for reciprocal innervation.

Blood and Nerve Supply of Peripheral Nerves

The peripheral nerves are supplied by vessels, called vasa vasorum, which form longitudinal anastomoses on the surface of the nerves. The nerves distributed to the sheaths of the nerve trunks are called nervi nervorum.

NERVE FIBRES

Each motor nerve fibre is an axon with its coverings.

Larger axons are covered by a myelin sheath and are termed myelinated or medullated fibres (Fig. 7.14a).

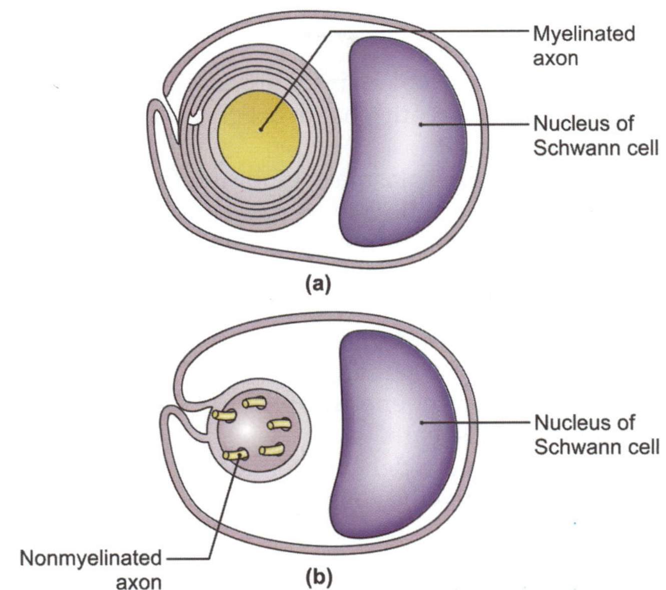

Figs 7.14a and b: (a) Myelinated, and (b) nonmyelinated axon

The fatty nature of myelin is responsible for the glistening whiteness of the peripheral nerve trunks and white matter of the CNS.

Thinner axons, of less than one micron diameter, have thin layers myelin sheath and are therefore termed nonmyelinated or non-medullated (Fig. 7.14b).

However, all the fibres whether myelinated or nonmyelinated have a neurolemmal sheath, which is uniformly absent in the tracts. In peripheral nerves, both the myelin and neurolemmal sheaths are derived from Schwann cells.

Myelinated Fibres

Myelinated fibres form the bulk of the somatic nerves. Structurally, they are made up of following parts from within outwards:

1 Axis cylinder axon forms the central core of the fibre. It consists of axoplasm covered by axolemma (Fig. 7.4).
2 Myelin sheath, derived from Schwann cells, surrounds the axis cylinder. It is made up of alternate concentric layers of lipids and proteins formed by spiralization of the mesaxon; the lipids include cholesterol, glycolipids and phospholipids.
   Myelin sheath is interrupted at regular intervals called the nodes of Ranvier where the adjacent Schwann cells meet (Fig. 7.4).
   Collateral branches of the axon arise at the nodes of Ranvier.
   Thicker axons possess a thicker coat of myelin and longer internodes.
   Each internode is myelinated by one Schwann cell. Oblique clefts in the myelin, called incisures of Schmidt Lantermann, provide conduction channels

for metabolites into the depth of the myelin and to the subjacent axon.

Myelin sheath acts as an insulator for the nerve fibres.

3 Neurolemmal sheath (sheath of Schwann) surrounds the myelin sheath.

It represents the plasma membrane (basal lamina) of the Schwann cell.

Beneath the membrane there lies a thin layer of cytoplasm with the nucleus of the Schwann cell.

The sheaths of two cells interdigitate at the nodes of Ranvier. Neurolemmal sheath is necessary for regeneration of a damaged nerve.

Tracts do not regenerate because of absence of neurolemmal sheath.

4 Endoneurium is a delicate connective tissue sheath which surrounds the neurolemmal sheath (Fig. 7.10).

Nonmyelinated Fibres

Nonmyelinated fibres comprise the smaller axons of the CNS, in addition to peripheral postganglionic autonomic fibres, several types of fine sensory fibres (C fibres of skin, muscle and viscera), olfactory nerves, etc. Structurally, a 'nonmyelinated fibre' consists of a group of small axons (0.12–2 micron diameter) that have invaginated separately a single Schwann cell (in series) without any spiralling of the mesaxon (Fig. 7.14). The endoneurium, instead of ensheathing individual axons, surrounds all the neurolemmal sheath by virtue of which the non-myelinated fibres, like the myelinated fibres, can regenerate after damage.

Classification of Peripheral Nerve Fibres

A. According to their function, the cranial nerves have following nuclear columns.

1 General somatic efferent, to supply striated muscles of somatic origin, e.g. III, IV, VI, XII cranial nerves (Fig. 7.15).

2 Special visceral efferent (branchial efferent) to supply striated muscles of branchial origin, e.g. V, VII, IX, X, XI cranial nerves.

3 General visceral efferent to supply smooth muscles and glands, e.g. III, VII, IX, X cranial nerves.

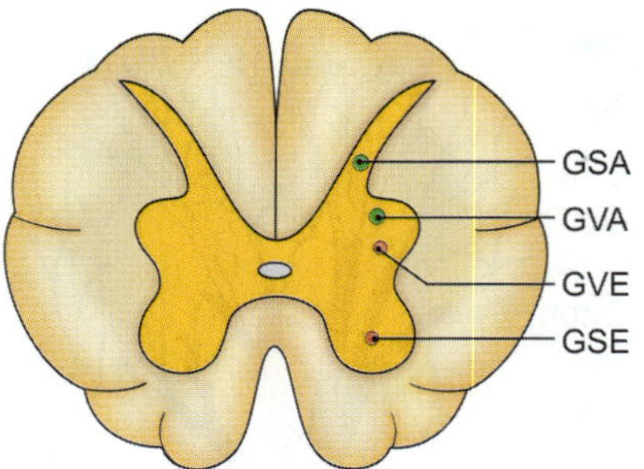

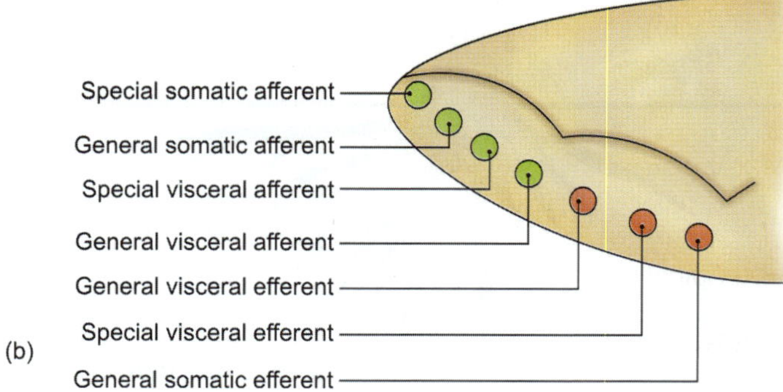

Figs 7.15a and b: Nuclear columns of (a) spinal cord, and (b) medulla oblongata

4 General visceral afferent, to carry visceroceptive impulses (like pain) from the viscera, e.g. X cranial nerve.

5 Special visceral afferent, to carry the sensation of taste, e.g. VII, IX, X cranial nerves.

6 General somatic afferent, to carry exteroceptive impulses from the skin of face and proprioceptive impulses from the muscles, tendons and joints (Figs 7.15a and b), e.g. V cranial nerve.

7 Special somatic afferent to carry the sensations of hearing and equilibrium, e.g. VIII cranial nerve.

B. According to their size and speed of conduction, the nerve fibres are divided into three categories, namely A, B and C. These have been compared in Table 7.3. Table 7.4 shows the summary of cranial nerves.

Table 7.3: Comparison of types of nerve fibres

Group A fibre	Group B fibre	Group C fibre
1. Thickest and fastest	Medium size	Thinnest and slowest
2. Myelinated	Myelinated	Non-myelinated
3. Diameter: 1.5–22 micron	Diameter: 1.5–3.4 micron	Diameter: 0.1–2 micron
4. Speed: 4–120 metres/sec, e.g. skeletomotor fibre, fusimotor fibre afferent to skin, muscles and tendons	Speed: 3–15 metres/sec, e.g. preganglionic autonomic efferents	Speed: 0.5–4 metres/sec, e.g. postganglionic autonomic efferents, afferent fibre to skin, muscle and viscera
5. Fast conduction	Slow conduction	Very slow conduction

Table 7.4: Summary of the cranial nerves

Nerve	Function	Details
I Olfactory	Smell	20 rootless, pass through root of nose to reach temporal lobe of brain
II Optic	Vision	From the retina via optic chiasma and lateral geniculate body to the occipital lobe of brain
III Oculomotor	Motor + para sympathetic	Supplies 4½ extraocular muscles. Also two sets of muscles which help in accomodation
IV Trochlear	Motor	One muscle of eyeball (superior oblique)
V Trigeminal	Sensory + motor	Most of the skin of face, nasal mucous membrane, conjunctiva; motor to muscles of mastication
VI Abducent	Motor	Motor to one muscle of eye (lateral rectus)
VII Facial	Motor + special sense + parasympathetic	Motor to muscles of the face those around eyes and mouth; taste from anterior 2/3rd of tongue; secretomotor to submandibular, lacrimal, nasal glands, etc.
VIII Vestibulocochlear	Hearing and balance	Vestibular part for balancing the body and maintenance of posture; cochlear part for hearing, appreciated in temporal lobe
IX Glossopharyngeal	Special sense + motor + parasympathetic	Taste from posterior 1/3rd of tongue, motor to one muscle of pharynx and secretory to parotid gland
X Vagus + Cranial root of accessory	Motor + special sense + parasympathetic	Taste from posterior most part of tongue, motor to muscles of soft palate, pharynx, larynx, stomach and intestines and secretory to glands of respiratory and most part of digestive system
XI Spinal root of accessory	Motor	Motor to two important muscles of neck, i.e. sternocleidomastoid and trapezius
XII Hypoglossal	Motor	To seven out of eight muscles of each half of tongue

AUTONOMIC NERVOUS SYSTEM

Autonomic nervous system controls involuntary activities of the body, like sweating, salivation, peristalsis, etc. It differs fundamentally from the somatic nervous system in having:

a. Preganglionic fibres arising from the CNS
b. Ganglia for relay of the preganglionic fibres
c. Postganglionic fibres arising from the ganglia which supply the effectors (smooth muscles and glands).

In contrast, the somatic nerves after arising from the CNS reach their destination without any interruption (Fig. 7.1).

Autonomic nervous system is divided into two more or less complementary parts, the sympathetic and parasympathetic systems.

The sympathetic activities are widespread and diffuse, and combat the acute emergencies.

The parasympathetic activities are usually discrete and isolated, and provide a comfortable environment.

Both systems function in absolute coordination and adjust the body involuntarily to the given surroundings.

SYMPATHETIC NERVOUS SYSTEM

1 It is also known as 'thoracolumbar' outflow because it arises from Tl to L2 segments of the spinal cord (Fig. 7.16).
2 The medullated preganglionic fibres (white rami communicantes) arise from the lateral column of the spinal cord, emerge through the ventral rami where the white rami are connected to the ganglia of the sympathetic chain (Fig. 7.16).
3 Preganglionic fibres relay either in the lateral ganglia (sympathetic chain) or in the collateral ganglia, e.g. the coeliac ganglion. The nonmedullated postganglionic fibres (grey rami communicantes) run for some distance before reaching the organ of supply. **The adrenal medulla is a unique exception in the body; it is supplied by the preganglionic fibres** (Fig. 7.16).
4 Sympathetic nerve endings are adrenergic in nature, meaning thereby that noradrenalin is produced for neurotransmission. The only exception to this general rule is the cholinergic sympathetic nerves supplying the sweat glands and skeletal muscle vessels for vasodilatation.
5 Functionally, sympathetic nerves are vasomotor (vasoconstrictor), sudomotor (secretomotor to sweat glands), and pilomotor (contract the arrector pili and cause erection of hair) in the skin of limbs and body wall (Fig. 7.16). In addition, sympathetic activity causes dilation of pupil, pale face, dry mouth, tachycardia, rise in blood pressure, inhibition of hollow viscera, and closure of the perineal sphincters.

The blood supply to the skeletal muscles, heart and brain is markedly increased (Fig. 7.17).

Thus, sympathetic reactions tend to be 'mass reactions', widely diffused in their effect and that they are directed towards mobilization of the resources of the body for expenditure of energy in dealing with the emergencies or emotional crises (fright, fight, flight).

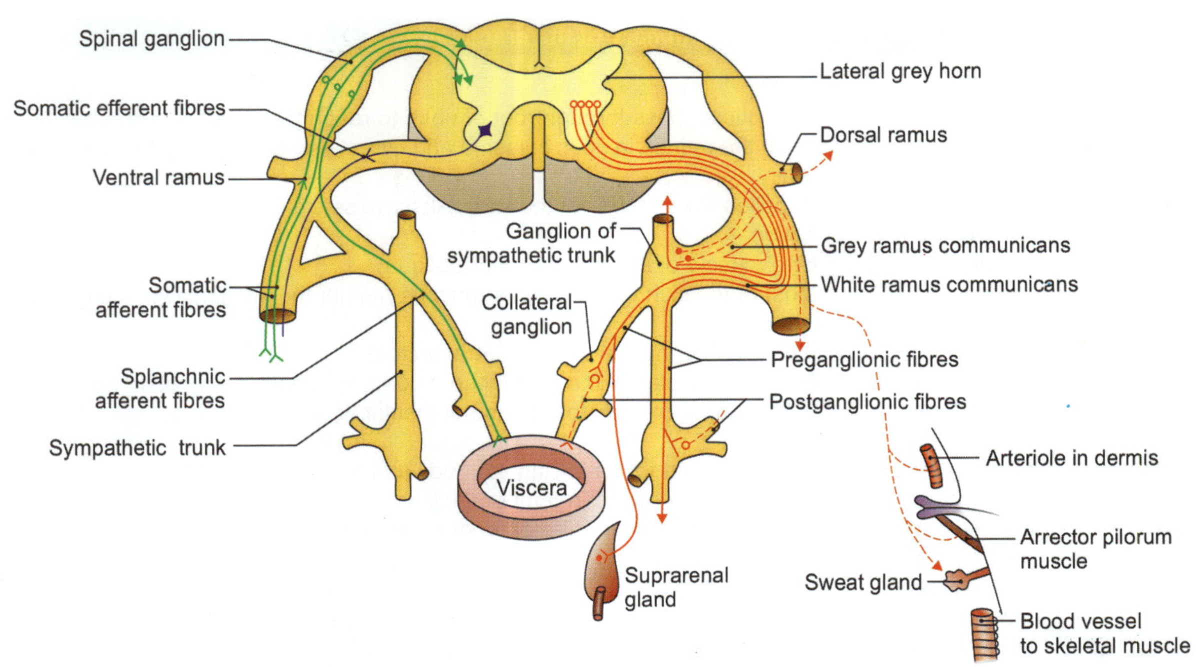

Fig. 7.16: Course of sympathetic fibres

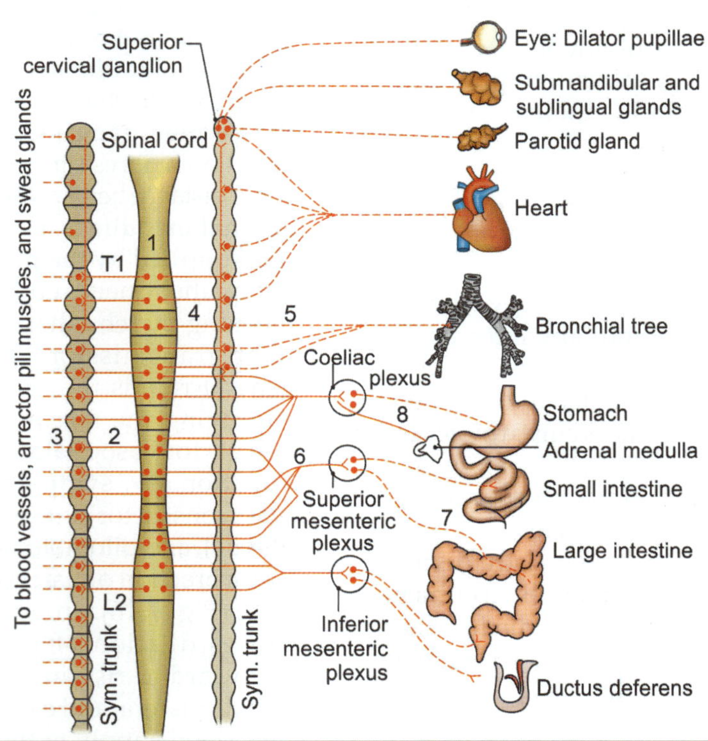

1. Spinal cord, T1 to L2 segments of spinal cord; 2. White ramus communicans to sympathetic ganglia; 3. Grey ramus communicans to structures in skin; 4. Preganglionic fibres for thoracic viscera; 5. Postganglionic fibres for thoracic viscera; 6. Preganglionic fibres for abdominal and pelvic viscera; 7. Long post-ganglionic fibres for abdominal and pelvic viscera and 8. Preganglionic fibres for adrenal medulla

Fig. 7.17: Distribution of sympathetic nervous system

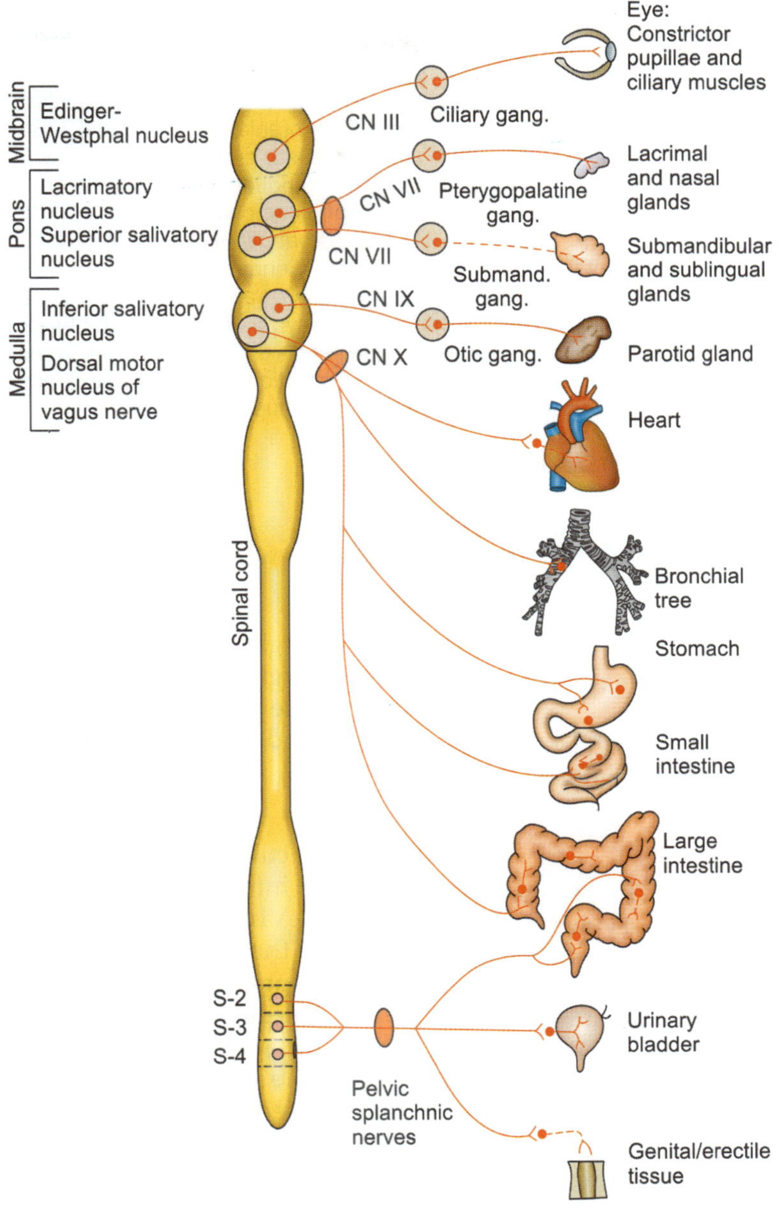

Fig. 7.18: Distribution of parasympathetic nervous system

PARASYMPATHETIC NERVOUS SYSTEM

1 It is also known as craniosacral outflow because it arises from the brain (mixed with III, VII, IX and X cranial nerves) and sacral 2–4 segments of the spinal cord. Thus it has a cranial and a sacral part (Fig. 7.18).

2 The preganglionic fibres are very long, reaching right up to the viscera of supply. The ganglia, called terminal ganglia, are situated mostly on the viscera and, therefore, the postganglionic fibres are very short.

3 Parasympathetic nerve endings are cholinergic in nature, similar to the somatic nerves.

4 Functionally, parasympathetic activity is seen when the subject is fully relaxed. His pupils are constricted, lenses accommodated, face flushed, mouth moist, pulse slow, blood pressure low, bladder and gut contracting, and the perineal sphincters relaxed.

In general the effects of parasympathetic activity are usually discrete and isolated, and directed towards conservation and restoration of the resources of energy in the body.

Table 7.5 shows the comparison between the two divisions of autonomic nervous system.

Table 7.5: Comparison of sympathetic and parasympathetic nervous systems

Sympathetic nervous system	*Parasympathetic nervous system*
All neurons forming this system originate from T_1 to L_2 segment of spinal cord. So it is called "thoracolumbar outflow"	All neurons forming this system originate from brain (III, VII, IX, X cranial nerves) and S2–S4 segment of spinal cord. So it is called "craniosacral outflow"
Preganglionic fibres are short, relay either in lateral ganglia or collateral ganglia	Preganglionic fibres are very long reaching up to terminal ganglia mostly on viscera
Postganglionic fibres are long	Postganglionic fibres are short
Nerve endings are adrenergic in nature except in sweat gland	Nerve endings are cholinergic in nature
Functionally, sympathetic nerves are vasomotor, sudomotor and pilomotor to skin. It is seen when subject is in fear, fight and flight position. It dilates skeletal muscle blood vessels	Functionally, it is seen when subject is fully relaxed. Parasympathetic system has no effect on skin
Effect is widely diffused and directed towards mobilization of resources and expenditure of energy during emergency and emotional crisis	Effect is discrete, isolated, directed towards conservation and restoration of the resources of energy in the body
It supplies visceral blood vessels and skin. Afferents from viscera and specific area of skin reach the same spinal segment to go to the cerebrum. Since pain is better appreciated from the skin, it appears to be coming from skin rather than the viscera. This is the basis of *referred pain.*	It only supplies viscera

Neurotransmitters

Following neurotransmitters are released at various autonomic nerve endings:

- Preganglionic parasympathetic: Acetylcholine
- Preganglionic sympathetic: Acetylcholine
- Postganglionic parasympathetic: Acetylcholine
- Postganglionic sympathetic: Norepinephrine except those supplying skeletal muscle vessles and sweat glands which release acetylcholine.

CLINICAL ANATOMY

- ***Irritation*** of a motor nerve causes muscular spasm. Mild irritation of a sensory nerve causes tingling and numbness, but when severe it causes pain along the distribution of the nerve. Irritation of a mixed nerve causes combined effects.
- ***Bell's palsy*** is the compression of a facial nerve in or just outside stylomastoid foramen due to inflammation and oedema of the nerve. This causes paralysis of facial muscles and loss of facial expression on the affected side.
- ***Ageing***: Usually after 60–70 years or so there are changes in the brain. These are:
  a. Prominence of sulci due to cortical shrinkage.
  b. The gyri get narrow and sulci get broad.
  c. The subarachnoid space becomes wider.
  d. There is enlargement of the ventricles.
- ***Dementia***: In this condition, there is slow and progressive loss of memory, intellect and personality. The consciousness of the subject is normal. Dementia usually occurs due to Alzheimer's disease.
- ***Infections of brain***: (a) Bacterial, (b) viral, (c) miscellaneous types.
  a. **Bacterial** (through blood) may cause meningitis or brain abscess. Otitis media may cause meningitis or temporal lobe abscess. Tuberculosis: TB meningitis is due to blood-borne infection.
  b. **Viral infections:** Most viruses enter the body through blood. Viruses may cause meningitis or encephalitis.

Herpes simplex virus and encephalitis: This virus usually causes vesicles at angles of the mouth and alae of the nose, following cold or any other disease. In some cases it may cause encephalitis.

Herpes zoster: It presents as a vesicular rash affecting one or more dermatomes. This condition is very painful.

Poliomyelitis: The virus has attraction for anterior (motor) horn cells, especially of the spinal cord which get damaged. The nerves arising from these neurons get affected resulting in paresis or paralysis. There may be partial or complete recovery. Under Polio Eradication Programme, India has been declared "polio free" in March 2014—a great achievement.

c. **Miscellaneous types:**

Parkinson's disease: The extrapyramidal system which connects the higher centers and the anterior horn cells get affected in this disease. There is usually deficiency of neurotransmitter dopamine in the affected nuclei of the extrapyramidal system, including depigmentation of substantia nigra.

The face is mask like and expressionless, the posture is bent forwards with stiff pill-rolling movements and tremors of the hands.

Upper motor neuron damage: When the fibres are interrupted from their cortical origin till these synapse with anterior horn cells of the spinal cord, it is called upper motor neuron damage. The tendon jerks are exaggerated and the plantar reflex is of the extensor type.

Lower motor neuron damage: When the anterior horn cells (motor neurons) are affected, usually by poliomyelitis virus, there is paresis or paralysis of the muscles supplied by the nerves arising from the affected neurons. The affected muscles atrophy, and reflexes are absent.

FACTS TO REMEMBER

- Neuron is the unit of nervous tissue.
- Neuron has only one axon while the dendrites are variable.
- At synapse there is only contiguity of cell membrances. There is no continuity of cytoplasm at the synapse.
- Astrocytes form part of "blood–brain barrier."
- Cervical (spinal) nerves are 8 while cervical vertebrae are 7 only.
- Coccygeal nerve is one while coccygeal vertebrae are 4.
- Limbs are mostly supplied by ventral primary rami of the spinal nerves.
- Endoneurium surrounds each nerve fibre, perineurium is around the nerve fascicle, epineurium is around the entire nerve.
- Nerve plexuses are only formed by ventral primary rami of the spinal nerves.
- Plexuses are cervical, brachial, lumbosacral and coccygeal.
- Sympathetic nervous system is thoracolumbar outflow.
- Parasymphathetic nervous system is craniosacral outflow.
- Sympathetic nervous system supplies the whole body from head to toes, while parasympathetic nerves only supply the viscera.
- Sympathetic is sudomotor, vasomotor and pilomotor to skin.
- Sympathetic is unsympathetic to the digestive system.
- Sympathetic nerves are mostly responsible for the referred pain.

Multiple Choice Questions

1. Number of spinal nerves in cervical region is:
a. 7 nerves
b. 8 nerves
c. 6 nerves
d. 9 nerves

2. Bipolar neurons are absent in:
a. Spiral ganglia
b. Vestibular ganglia
c. Olfactory cells
d. Neurons in posterior horn of spinal cord

3. Supporting tissue around nerve fibres are following, *except*:
a. Endoneurium
b. Perineurium
c. Epineurium
d. Epimysium

4. Nerve plexuses are only formed by:
a. Dorsal rami
b. Ventral rami
c. Dorsal roots
d. Ventral roots

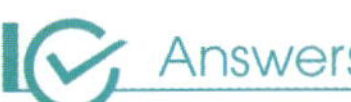

Answers

1. b **2.** d **3.** d **4.** b

Chapter 8

Skin, Fasciae and Ligaments

"Give a man a fish, and you feed him for a day. Teach a man to fish, and you feed him for a lifetime."
—Lao Tzu

SKIN

Synonyms

1. Cutis (L); 2. Derma (G); 3. Integument. Compare with the terms cutaneous, dermatology and dermatomes.

Definition

Skin is the general covering of the entire external surface of the body, including the external auditory meatus and the outer surface of tympanic membrane.

It is continuous with the mucous membrane at the orifices of the body.

Because of a large number of its functions, the skin is regarded as an important organ of the body. Figure 8.1 shows the histological structure of thin skin.

SURFACE AREA

In an adult the surface area of the skin is 1.5–2 (average 1.7) sq. metres. In order to assess the area involved in burns, one can follow the rule of nines: Head and neck 9%; each upper limb 9%; the front of the trunk 18%; the back of the trunk (including buttocks) 18%; each lower limb 18%; and perineum 1% (Fig. 8.2a). The percentage of area in a child is shown in Fig. 8.2b.

The surface area of an individual can be calculated by Du Bois formula. Thus, A = W × H × 71.84, where A = surface area in sq. cm, W = weight in kg, and H = height in cm.

PIGMENTATION OF SKIN

The colour of the skin is determined by at least five pigments present at different levels and places of the skin. These are:

1 Melanin (brown), present in the germinative zone of the epidermis.
2 Melanoid, (resembles melanin), present diffusely throughout the epidermis.
3 Carotene (yellow to orange), present in stratum corneum and the fat cells of dermis and superficial fascia.

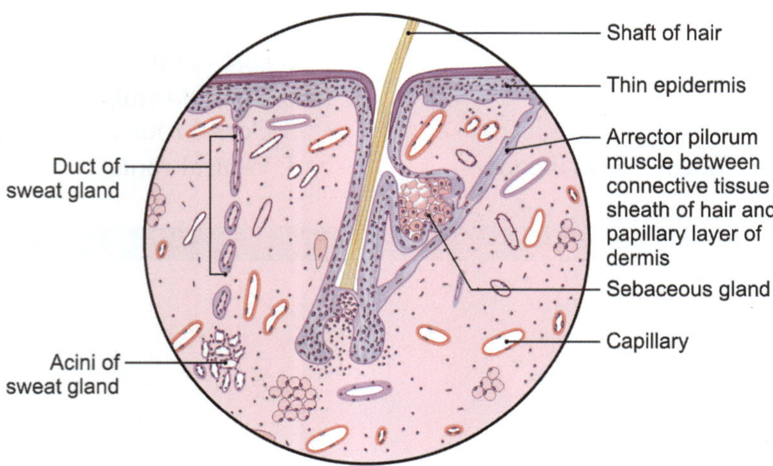

Fig. 8.1: Histological structure of thin skin

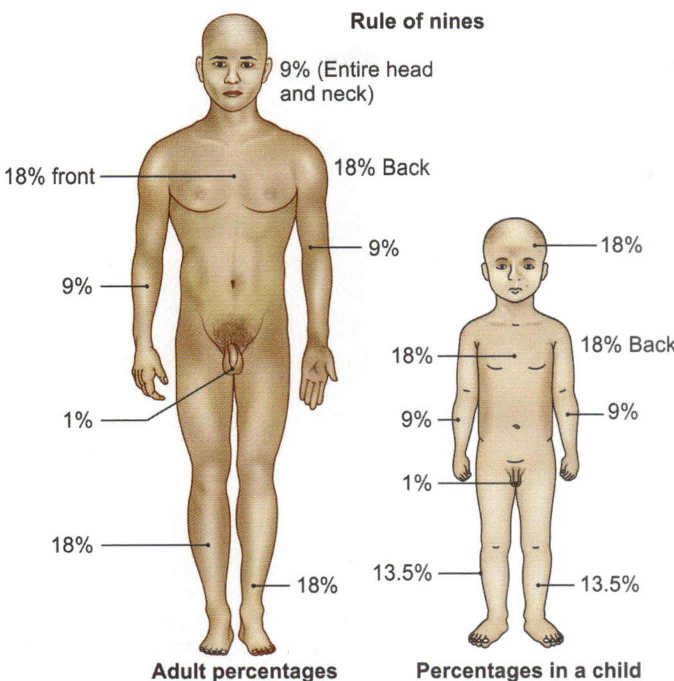

Fig. 8.2: Percentages of area in burn: (a) Adult, and (b) child

4 Haemoglobin (purple).
5 Oxyhaemoglobin (red), present in the cutaneous vessels.

The amounts of first three pigments vary with the race, age, and part of the body. In white races, the colour of the skin depends chiefly on the vascularity of the dermis and thickness (translucency) of the keratin. The colour is red where keratin is thin (lips), and it is white where keratin is thick (palms and soles).

Thickness

The thickness of the skin varies from about 0.5 to 3 mm.

STRUCTURE OF SKIN

The skin is composed of two distinct layers, epidermis and dermis.

A. Epidermis

It is the superficial, avascular layer of stratified squamous epithelium. It is ectodermal in origin and gives rise to the appendages of the skin, namely hair, nails, sweat glands and sebaceous glands.

Structurally, the epidermis is made up of a deep germinative zone, comprising (i) stratum basale, (ii) stratum spinosum, (iii) stratum granulosum and a superficial cornified zone, (iv) stratum lucidum, and (v) a stratum corneum (*see Textbook of Histology*, 6th edition by K Garg, G Rath and M Chandra).

The cells of the deepest layer proliferate and pass towards the surface to replace the cornified cells lost due to wear and tear. As the cells migrate superficially, they become more and more flattened, and lose their nuclei to form the flattened dead cells of the stratum corneum.

In the germinative zone, there are (i) 'dopa' positive melanocytes (melanoblasts, dendritic cells, or clear cells) of neural crest origin, which synthesize melanin. (ii) Langerhans cells which are phagocytic in nature. (iii) Merkel's cells which are sensory receptor cells in stratum basale.

B. Dermis or Corium

Dermis or corium is the deep, vascular layer of the skin, derived from mesoderm.

It is made up of connective tissue (with variable elastic fibres) mixed with blood vessels, lymphatics and nerves. The connective tissue is arranged into a superficial papillary layer and a deep reticular layer.

The papillary layer forms conical, blunt projections (dermal papillae) which fit into reciprocal depressions on the undersurface of the epidermis. The reticular layer is composed chiefly of the white fibrous tissue arranged mostly in parallel bundles.

The direction of the bundles, constituting flexor or cleavage lines (Langer's lines), is longitudinal in the limbs and horizontal in the trunk and neck (Fig. 8.3).

In old age the elastic fibres atrophy and the skin becomes wrinkled. Overstretching of the skin may lead to rupture of the fibres, followed by scar formation. These scars appear as white streaks on the skin (e.g. linea gravidarum).

At the flexure lines of the joints, the skin is firmly adherent to the underlying deep fascia. Dermis is the real skin, because, when dried it makes green hide, and when tanned it makes leather. Its deep surface is continuous with the superficial fascia.

SURFACE IRREGULARITIES OF THE SKIN

The skin is marked by three types of surface irregularities, the tension lines, flexure lines and papillary ridges.

1 *Tension lines:* Form a network of linear furrows which divide the surface into polygonal or lozenge-shaped areas. These lines to some extent correspond to variations in the pattern of fibres in the dermis. These are seen clearly on dorsum of hand.
2 *Flexure lines* (skin creases or skin joints): Are certain permanent lines along which the skin folds during habitual movements (chiefly flexion) of the joints. The skin along these lines is thin and firmly bound to the deep fascia.
   The lines are prominent opposite the flexure of the joints, particularly on the palms, soles digits and neck (Fig. 8.3).
3 *Papillary ridges* (friction ridges): Are confined to palms and soles and their digits. They form narrow

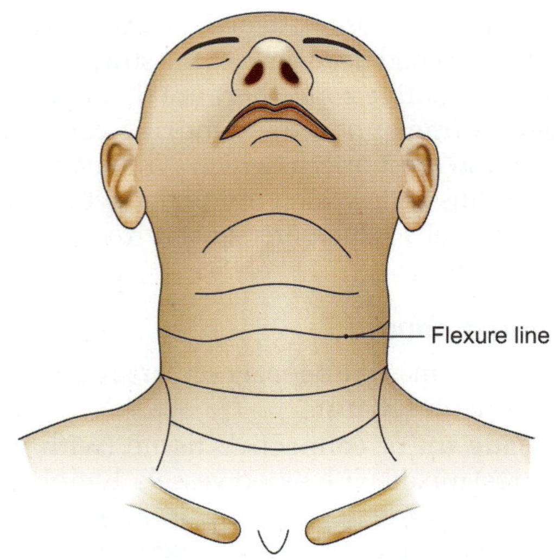

Fig. 8.3: Flexure/Langer's lines

ridges separated by fine parallel grooves, arranged in curved arrays. They correspond to patterns of dermal papillae. Their study constitutes a branch of science, called dermatoglyphics.

Three major patterns in the human fingerprints include loops, whorls and arches. These patterns and many other minor features are determined genetically by multifactorial inheritance (Fig. 8.4). These do not change throughout life, except to enlarge. This serves as a basis for identification through fingerprints or footprints.

Skin of palm and sole is thick, rest of the body has thin skin. Table 8.1 compares the two types of skin.

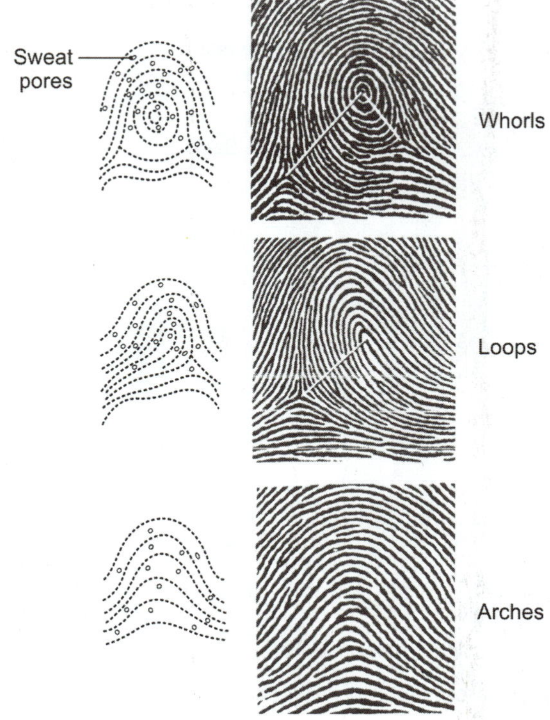

Fig. 8.4: Types of papillary ridges

APPENDAGES OF SKIN

1. Nails

Synonyms. (a) Onych or onycho (G); and (b) ungues (L). Compare with the terms paronychia, koilonychia and onychomycosis.

Nails are hardened keratin plates (cornified zone) on the dorsal surface of the tips of fingers and toes, acting as a rigid support for the digital pads of terminal phalanges. Each nail has the following parts.

a. Root is the proximal hidden part which is burried into the nail groove and is overlapped by the nail fold of the skin (Fig. 8.5).
b. Body is the exposed part of the nail which is adherent to the underlying skin; a and b together form nail plate.
c. Free border is the distal part free from the skin. It is attached to the under surface by hyponychium.

Table 8.1: Comparison of thick and thin skin

Features	*Thick skin*	*Thin skin*
Epidermal layers	Comprises 5 layers stratum basale stratum spinosum stratum granulosum stratum lucidum stratum corneum	Comprises 4 layers stratum basale stratum spinosum stratum granulosum — stratum corneum thin
Epidermal ridges	Present	Absent
Sebaceous gland hair follicle and arrector pili muscle	Absent	Present
Sweat gland	Many	Few
Sensory receptors	Many	Few
Location	Palm and sole and palmar aspects of digits	All parts of body except palm, sole and palmar aspects of digits

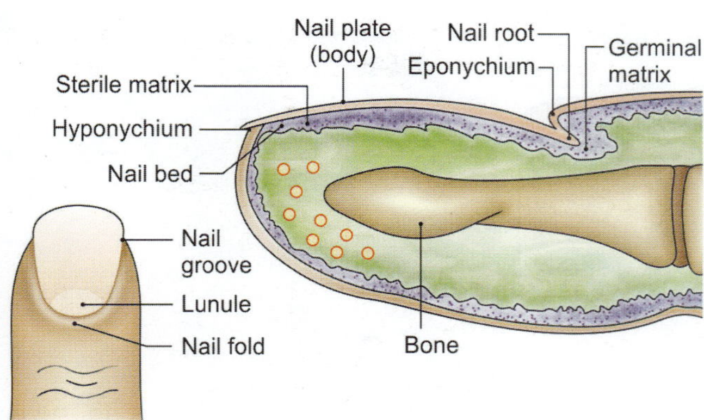

Fig. 8.5: Parts of a nail

The proximal part of the body presents a white opaque crescent called lunule. It is overlapped by a fold of skin, the eponychium.

Each lateral border of the nail body is overlapped by a fold of a skin, termed the nail fold and the groove between nail body and nail fold is called nail groove.

The skin (germinative zone + corium) beneath the root and body of the nail is called nail bed. The germinative zone of the nail bed beneath the root and lunule is thick and proliferative (germinal matrix), and is responsible for the growth of the nail.

The rest of the nail bed is thin (sterile matrix) over which the growing nail glides.

Under the translucent body (except lunule) of the nail, the corium is very vascular. This accounts for their pink colour.

Nail of middle finger grows the fastest.

2. Hair

Hair are keratinous filaments derived from invaginations of the germinative layer of epidermis into the dermis.

These are peculiar to mammals (like feathers to the birds), and help in conservation of their body heat.

However, in man the heat loss is prevented by the cutaneous sensation of touch.

Hair are distributed all over the body, except for the palms, soles, dorsal surface of distal phalanges, umbilicus, glans penis, inner surface of prepuce, the labia minora, and inner surface of labia majora. The length, thickness and colour of the hair vary in different parts of the body and in different individuals.

Structure of Hair

Each hair has an implanted part called the root, a bulb and a projecting part, called the shaft.

Layers of Shaft

Innermost is:

i. The medulla, comprising of cells with eleidin granules and air spaces.
ii. The cortex is the middle part made of elongated cells with melanin pigment.
iii. Cuticle is a single layer of flat keratinised cells.

The root is surrounded by a hair follicle (a sheath of epidermis and dermis), and is expanded at its proximal end to form the hair bulb. Each hair bulb is invaginated at its end by hair papilla (vascular connective tissue) which forms the neurovascular hilum of the hair and its sheath.

Hair follicle surrounds the hair. Wall of the follicle comprises (i) inner root sheath, (ii) outer root sheath and (iii) connective tissue sheath (Fig. 8.6).

i. Inner root sheath surrounds the beginning of the shaft. Its cells degenerate above the sebaceous gland.
ii. Outer root sheath is continuous with epidermal cells and it shows all the layers of epidermis.
iii. Connective tissue sheath is derived from the dermis.

Hair grows at the hair bulb, by proliferation of its cells capping the papilla.

The hair follicles, enclosing hair roots lie obliquely to the surface of the skin, which is responsible for the characteristic hair streams in different parts of the body.

The arrectores pilorum muscles (smooth muscles supplied by sympathetic nerve) connect the undersurface of the follicles to the superficial part of the dermis. Arrector pili muscles are absent in a few regions like hair of face, axilla, eyelashes, eyebrows, hair of anterior nares and of external auditory meatus.

Colour of Hair

Colour of hair depends upon the amount and type of melanin pigment and the air inside the hair.

3. Sweat Glands

Sudoriferous or sweat glands are distributed all over the skin, except for the lips, glans penis, and nail bed. These glands are of two types, eccrine and apocrine.

Eccrine Glands

The eccrine glands are much more abundant and distributed in almost every part of the skin.

Each gland is a single tube, the deep part of which is coiled into a ball. The coiled part, called the body of the gland, lies in the deeper part of corium or in the subcutaneous tissue. The straight part, called the duct, traverses the dermis and epidermis and opens on the surface of the skin.

Location: The glands are a few in the axilla and groin, most numerous in the palms and soles, and least numerous in the neck and back.

The eccrine glands are merocrine in nature, i.e. produce the thin watery secretion without any disintegration of the epithelial cells.

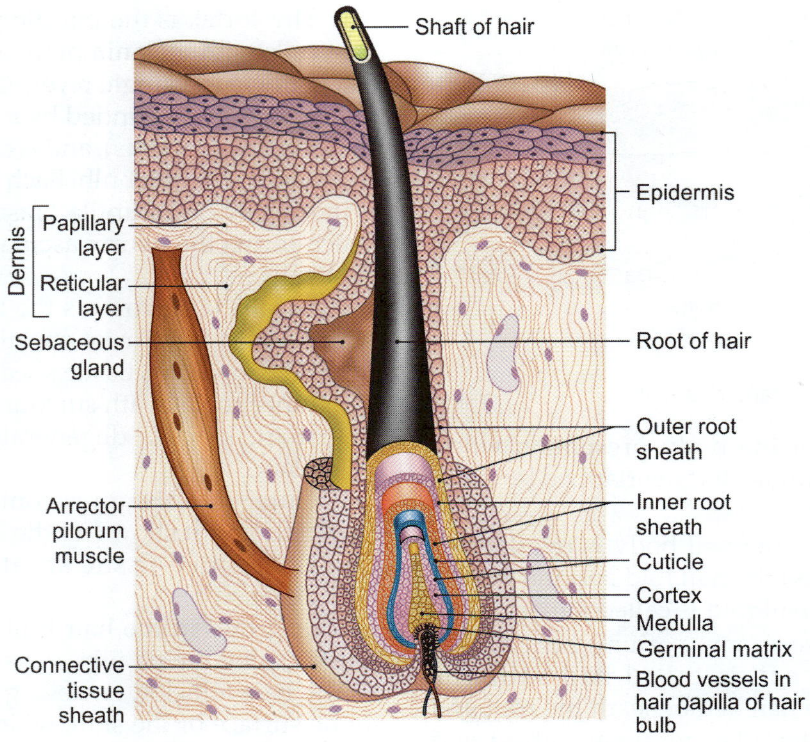

Fig. 8.6: Hair follice with arrector pilorum muscle

Control: They are supplied and controlled by cholinergic sympathetic nerves.

Functions: The glands help in regulation of the body temperature by evaporation of sweat, and also help in excreting the body salts. In dogs, sweat glands are confined to foot pads. Therefore, dogs do not sweat, they pant.

Apocrine Glands

Apocrine glands are confined to axilla, eyelids (Moll's glands), nipple and areola of the breast, perianal region, and the external genitalia.

Structure: They are larger than eccrine glands and produce a thicker secretion having a characteristic odour. They develop in close association with hair and their ducts typically open into the distal ends of the hair follicles. Ceruminous glands of the external auditory meatus are modified apocrine sweat glands.

Nervous control: The apocrine glands also are merocrine in nature, but are regulated by a dual autonomic control. Some workers are not inclined to call them as sweat glands at all because they do not respond sufficiently to temperature changes.

Functions: In animals they produce chemical signals or pheromones, which are important in courtship and social behaviour.

On an average one litre of sweat is secreted per day; another 400 ml of water is lost through the lungs, and 100 ml through the faeces.

This makes a total of about 1500 ml, a rough estimate of the invisible loss of water per day.

However, in hot climates the secretion of sweat may amount to 3–10 litres per day, with a maximum of 1–2 litres per hour.

So long as the sweat glands are intact, the skin can regenerate. If the sweat glands are lost, skin grafting becomes necessary.

4. Sebaceous Glands

Location: Sebaceous glands, producing an oily secretion, are widely distributed all over the dermis of the skin (Figs 8.1 and 8.6), except for the palms and soles. They are especially abundant in the scalp and face, and are also numerous around the apertures of the ear, nose, mouth and anus.

Structure: Sebaceous glands are small and sacculated in appearance, made up of a cluster of about 2–5 piriform alveoli.

Most of their ducts open into the hair follicles. But the ducts of sebaceous glands of lips, glans penis, inner surface of prepuce, labia minora, nipple and areola of the breast, and tarsal glands of the eyelids, open on the surface of the skin.

Sebaceous glands are holocrine in nature, i.e. they produce their secretion by complete fatty degeneration of the central cells of the alveolus, which are then replaced by the proliferating peripheral cells.

Nervous control: The secretion is under hormonal control, especially the androgens.

The oily secretion of sebaceous glands is called sebum.

Functions: It lubricates skin and protects it from moisture, desiccation, and the harmful sun rays. Sebum also lubricates hair and prevents them from becoming brittle.

In addition, sebum also has some bactericidal action.

Sebum makes the skin waterproof. Water evaporates from the skin, but the fats and oils are absorbed by it.

FUNCTIONS OF SKIN

1. *Protection:* Skin protects the body from mechanical injuries.
   i. *Physical barrier.* Due to stratum corneum, skin acts as a barrier against bacterial infections, heat and cold, wet and drought, acid and alkali.
   ii. *Immune properties.* Langerhans cells phagocytose antigen and take it to T lymphocytes.
   iii. *Reflex action.* Sensory nerve endings start reflex action against painful stimuli and prevent it from damage.
   iv. The actinic rays of the sun are absorbed by melanocytes.
2. *Sensory.* Skin is sensory to touch, pain and temperature.
3. *Regulation of body temperature.* Heat is lost through evaporation of sweat. It is conserved by the fat and hair.
4. *Absorption.* Oily substances are freely absorbed by the skin.
5. *Secretion.* Skin secretes sweat and sebum.
6. *Excretion.* The excess of water, salts and waste products are excreted through the sweat.
7. *Regulation of pH.* A good amount of acid is excreted through the sweat.
8. *Synthesis.* In the skin, vitamin D is synthesized from ergosterol by the action of ultraviolet rays of the sun.
9. *Storage.* Skin stores chlorides.
10. *Reparative.* The cuts and wounds of the skin are quickly healed.
11. *Water balance.* Skin does not permit water to pass in and out of skin. Thus it maintains the water balance of the body.

Blood Supply

The dermis is vascular while epidermis is avascular. Epidermal cells especially those of stratum basale are supplied nourishment by diffusion.

Nerve Supply

There are motor and sensory nerves. The motor nerve fibres are autonomic nerve fibres which are sudomotor (increase the sweat) and vasomotor. The sensory nerves endings in the skin are of the following types:

i. Free nerve endings in the epidermis for perception of pain.
ii. Merkel's disc end on Merkel's cells situated in stratum basale, acting as mechanoreceptors.
iii. Meissner's corpuscles are present in dermal papillae, acting as mechanoreceptors.
iv. Pacinian corpuscles are sensitive to deep pressure.
v. Ruffini's endings are sensitive to heat.
vi. Krause's bulbs in dermis detects cold. The plexuses around hair follicles detect pain and movement.

FASCIAE

Fasciae are of two types: Superficial fascia and deep fascia.

SUPERFICIAL FASCIA

Definition

Superficial fascia is a general coating of the body beneath the skin, made up of loose areolar tissue with varying amounts of fat.

Distribution of Fat in this Fascia

1 Fat is abundant in the gluteal region (buttocks), lumbar region (flanks), front of the thighs, anterior abdominal wall below the umbilicus, mammary gland (Fig. 8.7), postdeltoid region, and the cervicothoracic region.
2 In females, fat is more abundant and is more evenly distributed than in males.
3 Fat is absent from the eyelids, external ear, penis, and scrotum.
4 The subcutaneous layer of fat is called the panniculus adiposus.

In females fat is in the superficial fascia of the lower abdomen, upper thigh, whereas in males it is inside the abdominal cavity.

In general, in women fat forms a thicker and more even layer than in men.

Fat (adipose tissue) fills the hollow spaces like axilla, orbits and ischiorectal fossa.

Fat present around the kidneys in abdomen, supports these organs.

Types of Fats

There are two types of fat, i.e. yellow and brown fat.

Most of the body fat is yellow, only in hibernating animals it is brown. The cells of brown fat are smaller with several small droplets, and multiple mitochondria.

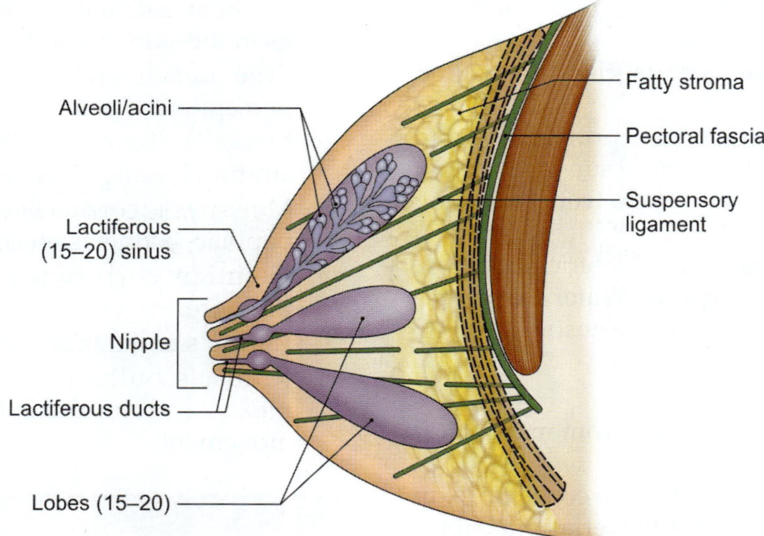

Fig. 8.7: Fat in mammary gland

Fat cells are specialised cells, and the size of fat cells increases during accumulation of fat, rather than the number of cells.

Any attempt to reduce excessive fat (obesity) must be slow and steady and not drastic, as the latter may cause harm to the body.

Important Features

1 Superficial fascia is most distinct in the lower part of the anterior abdominal wall, perineum, and the limbs.
2 It is very thin on the dorsal aspect of the hands and feet, sides of the neck, face, and around the anus.
3 It is very dense in the scalp, palms, and soles.
4 Superficial fascia shows stratification (into two layers) in the lower part of anterior abdominal wall, perineum, and uppermost part of the thighs.
5 It contains:
   a. Subcutaneous muscles in the face (muscles of facial expression), neck (platysma) and scrotum (dartos).
   b. Mammary gland
   c. Deeply situated sweat glands
   d. Localized groups of lymph nodes
   e. Cutaneous nerves and vessels.

Functions

1 Superficial fascia facilitates movements of the skin.
2 It serves as a soft medium for the passage of the vessels and nerves to the skin.
3 It conserves body heat because fat is a bad conductor of heat.

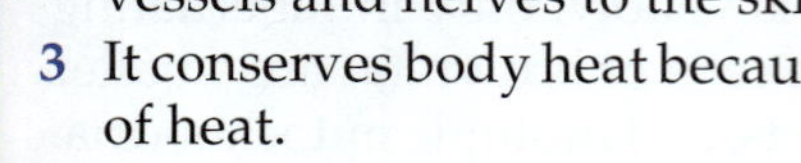

DEEP FASCIA

Definition

Deep fascia is a tough inelastic fibrous sheet which invests the body beneath the superficial fascia. It is devoid of fat.

Distribution

1 Deep fascia is best defined in the limbs where it forms tough and tight sleeves, and in the neck where it forms a collar.
2 It is absent on the trunk and face. On the trunk its absence permits expansion of organs. On the face its absence allows movements of facial expression and of mastication.

Important Features

1 Extensions (prolongations) of the deep fascia form:
   a. The intermuscular septa which divide the limb into compartments (Fig. 8.8).
   b. The fibroareolar sheaths for the muscles, vessels and nerves.
2 Thickenings of the deep fascia form:
   a. Retinacula (retention bands) around certain joints like wrist (Fig. 8.9) and ankle.
   b. The palmar and plantar aponeuroses, for protection of nerves and blood vessels.
3 Interruptions in the deep fascia on the subcutaneous bones.

Deep fascia never crosses a subcutaneous bone. Instead it blends with its periosteum and is bound down to the bone.

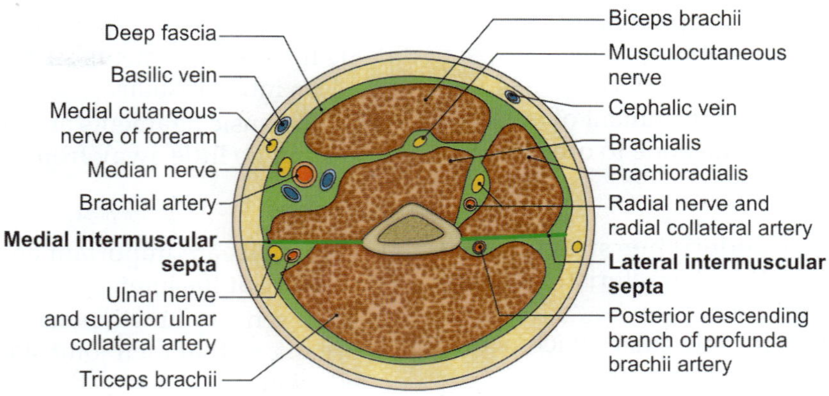

Fig. 8.8: Fascial compartments

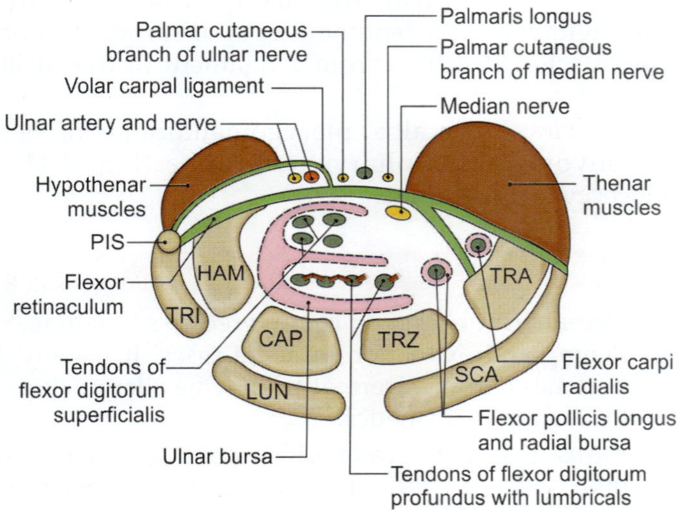

Fig. 8.9: Flexor retinaculum of wrist. Sca: Scaphoid, Lun: Lunate, Tri: Triquetral, Pi: Pisiform, Tra: Trapezium, Trz: Trapezoid, cap: Capitate, Ham: Hamate

MODIFICATIONS OF DEEP FASCIA

1 Forms the intermuscular septa separating functionally different groups of muscles into separate compartments (Fig. 8.8).
2 Covers each muscle as epimysium which sends in the septa to enclose each muscle fasciculus known as perimysium. From the perimysium septa pass to enclose each muscle fibre. These fine septa are the endomysium. Through all these connective tissue septa, e.g. epimysium, perimysium and endomysium, arterioles, capillaries, venules, lymphatics and nerves traverse to reach each muscle fibre (*see* Fig. 4.6).
3 Deep fascia covers each nerve as epineurium, each nerve fascicle as perineurium and individual nerve fibre as endoneurium. These connective tissue coverings support the nerve fibres and carry capillaries and lymphatics (*see* Fig. 7.10).
4 Forms sheaths around large arteries, e.g. femoral sheath. The deep fascia is dense around the artery and rather loose around the vein to give an allowance for the vein to distend.
5 Modified to form the capsule, synovial membrane and bursae in relation to the joints.
6 Forms tendon sheaths wherever tendons cross over a joint like radial/ulnar bursa. This mechanism prevents wear and tear of the tendon.
7 In the region of palm and sole it is modified to form aponeuroses, e.g. palmar and plantar aponeuroses which afford protection to the underlying structures (Fig. 8.10). It also forms septa between various muscles. These septa are specially well developed in the calf muscles of lower limb. The contraction of calf muscles in the tight sleeve of deep fascia helps in pushing the venous blood and lymph towards the heart.

Thus the deep fascia helps in venous and lymphatic return from the lower limb.

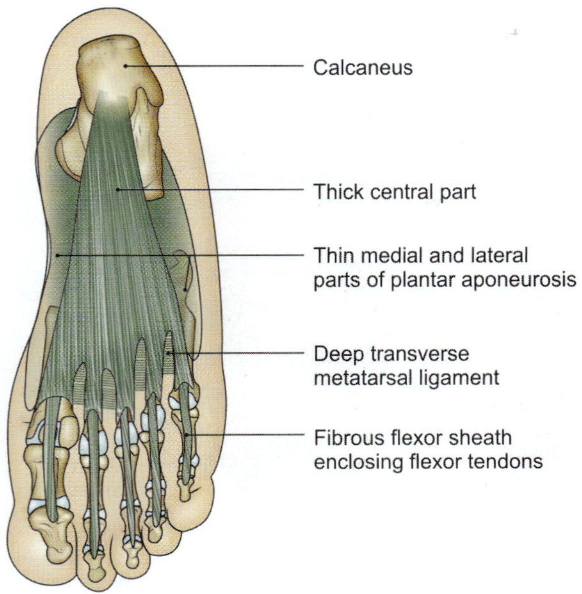

Fig. 8.10: Plantar aponeurosis

8 In the forearm and leg, the deep fascia is modified to form the interosseous membrane, which keeps:
   a. The two bones at optimum distance.
   b. Increases surface area for attachment of muscles.
   c. Transmits weight from one bone to other.

Functions

1 Deep fascia keeps the underlying structures in position and preserves the characteristic surface contour of the limbs and neck.
2 It provides extra surface for muscular attachments.
3 It helps in venous and lymphatic return.
4 It assists muscles in their action by the degree of tension and pressure it exerts upon their surfaces.
5 The retinacula act as pulleys and serve to prevent the loss of power. In such situations the friction is minimized by the synovial sheaths of the tendons also called radial and ulnar bursa (Fig. 8.9).

LIGAMENTS

DEFINITION

Ligaments are fibrous bands which connect the adjacent bones, forming integral parts of the joints. They are tough and unyielding, but at the same time are flexible and pliant, so that the normal movements can occur without any resistance, but the abnormal movements are prevented.

Types of Ligaments

A. According to their composition
   1. Most of the ligaments are made up of collagen fibres. These are inelastic and unstretchable.
   2. A few ligaments, like the ligamenta flava and ligaments of auditory ossicles, are made up of elastic fibres (predominantly). These are elastic and stretchable.

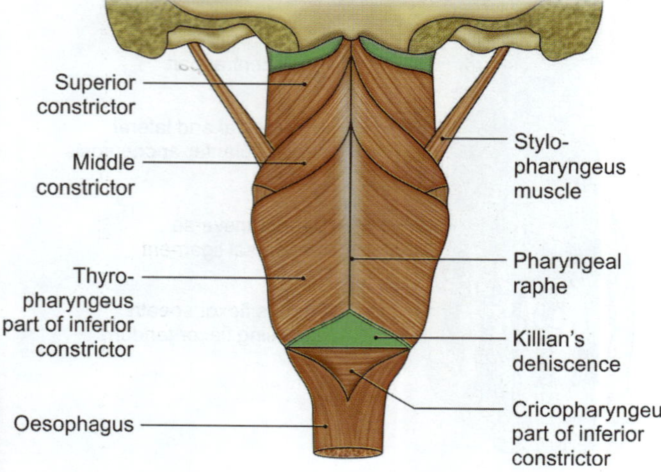

Fig. 8.11: Pharyngeal raphe

B. According to their relation to the joint
   1. Intrinsic ligaments surround the joint, and may be intracapsular.
   2. Extrinsic ligaments are independent of the joint; and lie little away from it.

Functions

1 Ligaments are important agents in maintaining the stability at the joint.
2 Their sensory function makes them important reflex organs, so that their joint stabilizing role is far more efficient.

RAPHE

A raphe is a linear fibrous band formed by interdigitation of the tendinous or aponeurotic ends of the muscles. It differs from a ligament in that it is *stretchable.*

Examples: Linea alba, pterygomandibular raphe, mylohyoid raphe, pharyngeal raphe (Fig. 8.11), anococcygeal raphe, etc.

CLINICAL ANATOMY

- ***Dermatitis or eczema***: There is redness, swelling, itching and exudation in acute cases. It usually becomes chronic. Dermatitis may be allergic due to soaps and cosmetics.
- ***Burns***: It is a condition which occurs due to too much heat or cold, acids, alkalies and electricity, etc. If only epidermis is affected, the burn is called *superficial*. If both dermis and epidermis are affected, the burn is called *deep*. Burn results in dehydration, shock and contractures.
- ***Sebaceous cyst*** is common in the scalp. It is due to obstruction of the duct of a sebaceous gland, caused either by trauma or infection. If the duct of sebaceous gland of cheek is blocked, it leads to closed comedones or acne. If the condition gets severe, the condition is acne vulgaris.
- ***Scabies*** is a mite infection. It is commonly seen in genital region and in interdigital cleft.
- ***Keloid*** is overgrowth of connective tissue at site of injury or burn.
- ***Fungal infection of nail*** is common. It may occur in between the toes also.
- ***Vitiligo*** is an autoimmune disease leading to white patches on skin.
- ***Baldness*** is related to hormones. Alopecia areata is an autoimmune disease.
- ***Retinacula*** keep the tendons and nerves in position. Sometimes the delicate nerve may get

compressed as it traverses under the retinacula. Median nerve may get compressed deep to the flexor retinaculum, leading to the *carpal tunnel syndrome* (Fig. 8.9).

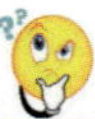

FACTS TO REMEMBER

- "Rule of Nines" is taken for counting percentages of burn.
- Dermis is processed/tanned to make leather.
- Epidermis contains mainly free nerve endings.
- Skin is the largest organ of the body in terms of surface area and sensory nerve endings.
- Nails take nearly 4 months to grow fully.
- Hair of face, axilla, eyelashes, eyebrows, external auditory meatus and anterior nares lack arrector pilorum muscles.
- Grey hair with lack of melanin and more of air after a certain age make a person graceful.
- Grey hair are lighter and float on the scalp like "clouds in the sky." Dyes are chemicals which do harm the body.
- Grey hair shows the experience of the person. Cosmetics should be occasionally used.
- Finger prints are unique to each and every person.
- Acne occurs due to blockage of the duct of sebaceous gland.
- Hair contain sulphur and emits peculiar smell on burning.
- Long hair are present on the scalp while short hair are situated on the eyelids.
- Sweat glands are maximum in palm/sole. These are supplied by sympathetic fibres. Sympathetic stimulation makes the palm wet.
- Superficial fascia is very thin on dorsum of hands, feet, face and neck, while it is very dense in scalp, palms and soles.
- Mammary gland is situated in the superficial fascia and is largest modified gland.
- Deep fascia helps in venous and lymphatic return.
- It is modified to form numerous structures around the joints.
- Deep fascia in temporal region is the toughest. It is absent on face and anterior abdominal wall.

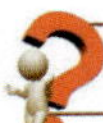

Multiple Choice Questions

1. Appendages of skin are all, *except*:
a. Hair
b. Nail
c. Sebaceous glands
d. Arrector pilorum muscles

2. Arrector pilorum is a:
a. Skeletal muscle
b. Smooth muscle
c. Cardiac muscle
d. Mixture of skeletal and smooth muscles

3. Following except one are subcutaneous muscles:
a. Dartos
b. Muscles of facial expression
c. Palmaris brevis
d. Palmaris longus

4. Carotid sheath is thin:
a. Around artery
b. Around vein
c. Around nerve
d. Around all structures

5. Deep fascia in the leg helps in:
a. Making compartments in the leg
b. Forms an effective mechanisms of venous return
c. Forms sheath around blood vessels
d. Forms aponeurosis

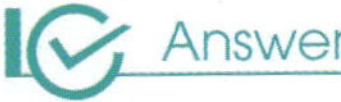

Answers

1. d **2.** b **3.** d **4.** b **5.** d

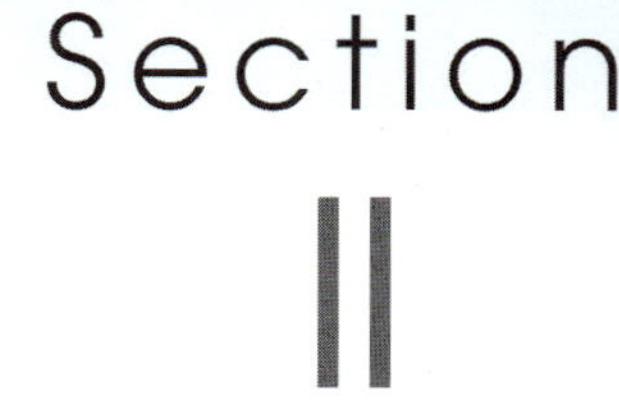

Section

II

Head and Neck

Anatomy Made Easy

Ichchak dana, bichchak dana, dane upar dana
Hands naache, feet naache, brain hai khushnama Ichhak dana
Teen inch lambi hai, pink aur khurdari hai,
chat pakori, pizza hut chalte iske bal se
Soch vichar express hote hai iske dum se,
achha bolna, thoda bolna, sukh se reh jana
Kehna hai aasan, magar mushkil hai nibhana
Ichhak dana
Bolo kya—tongue, bolo kya—tongue

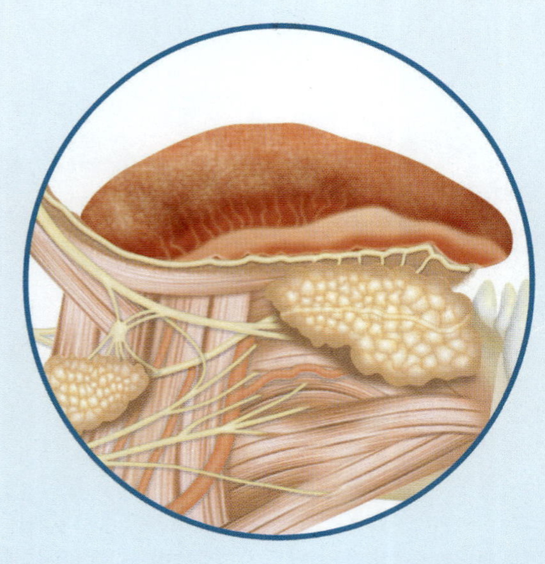

Chapter 9

Introduction and Osteology

"Uneasy lies the head that wears the crown."
—Shakespeare

INTRODUCTION

Face is the anterior aspect of head and the muscles present here express facial movements. Scalp overlies the lateral, posterior and superior aspects of skull.

Compartments of Neck

1 Posterior or vertebral compartment contains 7 cervical vertebrae with their muscles.
2 Anterior/visceral compartment contains glands like thyroid, parathyroid, thymus and parts of digestive and respiratory tracts.
3 Two lateral vascular compartments, one on each side, containing major arteries, veins, lymph vessels and lymph nodes.

Neck also contains pharynx and larynx. Pharynx is a musculofascial tube with openings in anterior wall, two posterior nasal openings, one opening of mouth and lowest is opening of inlet of larynx. These parts are called nasopharynx, oropharynx and laryngopharynx, respectively.

Larynx or voice box is a part of respiratory system. It lies between hyoid bone and trachea. A number of cartilages and membranes form the skeleton of larynx. There are two lateral vocal folds projecting towards each other from sides of laryngeal cavity. Muscles of larynx move the vocal folds. Function of larynx is to give passage to air and produce speech.

FUNCTIONS OF HEAD AND NECK

1 Protection to brain, endocrine glands and special senses.
2 Gives passage to food and air and connects their upper parts to respective lower parts.
3 Produces voice for communication.

Head and neck is the uppermost part of the body. Head comprises skull and lodges the brain covered by meninges, hypophysis cerebri, special senses, teeth and blood vessels. Brain is the highest seat of intelligence. Human is the most evolved animal so far, as there is maximum nervous tissue. To accommodate the increased volume of nervous tissue, the cranial cavity had to enlarge. Correspondingly, the lower jaw or mandible had to retract. The eyes also had come more anteriorly, on each side of the nose. The external nose also got prominent. During the course of evolution, external ear becomes vestigeal and chin is pushed forwards to accommodate the broad tongue. Tongue, the organ for speech, is securely placed in the oral cavity for articulation of words, i.e. speech. In human, the vocalisation centre is quite big to articulate various words and speak distinctly. Speech is a special and chief characteristic of the human.

Skull comprises a number of bones, and their respective regions are:

Frontal region: Lies in front of skull.

Parietal region: Lies on top of skull, formed chiefly by the parietal bones. It is seen from the top.

Occipital region: Forms back of skull.

Temporal region: It is the area above the ears. The sense of hearing and balance is appreciated and understood in the temporal lobe of brain situated on its inner aspect.

Ocular region: It is the region around the large orbital openings, containing the precious eyeball, muscles to move the eyeball, nerves and blood vessels to supply those muscles. There are accessory structures like the lacrimal apparatus and protective eyelids.

Auricular region: The region of the external ear with external auditory meatus comprises the auricular region. Air waves enter the ear through the meatus which change into fluid waves and finally into nerve impulses to be received in the temporal lobe of the cerebrum.

Nasal region: The region of the external nose, its muscles and the associated cavity comprise the nasal region. Sense of smell is perceived from this region.

Oral region: Comprises upper and lower lips and the angle of the mouth, where the lips join on each side. Numerous muscles are present here, to express the feelings and emotions. These are parts of the muscles of facial expression. They show the feelings, without words.

Oral cavity: It houses the organ of speech and taste. Tongue is not swallowed, though everything put on the tongue passes downwards. It is held in position by extrinsic muscles arising from surrounding bones. It says so much and manages to hide inside the oral cavity to be protected by 32 teeth in an adult.

Parotid region: Lies on the side of the face. It contains the biggest serous parotid salivary gland, which lies around the external auditory meatus.

Head is followed by the tubular neck which continues downwards with chest or thorax.

Each half of the neck comprises two triangles between anterior median line and posterior median line.

Posterior triangle: Lies between sternocleidomastoid, the *neck and chin turning muscle*; trapezius, *the shrugging muscle* and middle one-third of the clavicle. It contains proximal parts of the important brachial plexus, subclavian vessels with its branches and tributaries. Its apex is above and base is below.

Anterior triangle: Lies between the anterior median line and the anterior border of sternocleidomastoid muscle. Its apex is in lower part of neck, close to sternum and base above. It contains the carotid arteries and their branches. Isthmus of thyroid gland lies in the lower part of the triangle.

Bones of head and neck include the skull, i.e. cranium with mandible, seven cervical vertebrae, the hyoid, and six ossicles of the ear.

The skull cap is formed by frontal, parietal, squamous temporal and a part of occipital bones. These develop by intramembranous ossification, being a quicker one-stage process.

The base of the skull in contrast ossifies by intra-cartilaginous ossification which is a two-stage process (membrane–cartilage–bone).

Skull lodges the brain, teeth and also special senses like cochlear and vestibular apparatus, retina, olfactory mucous membrane, and taste buds.

The weight of the brain is not felt as it is floating in the cerebrospinal fluid. Our personality, power of speech, attention, concentration, judgement, and intellect are because of the brain that we possess and its proper use.

SKULL

Terms

The skeleton of the head is called the *skull*. It consists of several bones that are joined together to form the *cranium*. The term skull also includes the mandible or lower jaw which is a separate bone. However, the two terms, skull and cranium, are often used synonymously.

The skull can be divided into two main parts:

a. The *calvaria* or *brain box/neurocranium* is the upper part of the cranium which encloses the brain. It consists of a skull cap/vault (upper part) and a base (lower part).
b. The facial skeleton/viscerocranium constitutes the rest of the skull and includes the mandible.

Bones of the Skull

The skull consists of 22 bones which are named as follows.

a. The calvaria or brain case is composed of 8 bones.

Paired	Unpaired
1. Parietal (2)	1. Frontal (1)
2. Temporal (2)	2. Occipital (1)

b. The *facial skeleton* is composed of 14 bones.

Paired	Unpaired
1. Maxilla (2)	1. Mandible (1)
2. Zygomatic (2)	2. Vomer (1)
3. Nasal (2)	
4. Lacrimal (2)	
5. Palatine (2)	
6. Inferior nasal concha (2)	

Skull Joints

The joints in the skull are mostly sutures, a few primary cartilaginous joints and three pairs of synovial joints. Two pairs of synovial joints are present between the ossicles of middle ear. One pair is the largest temporo-mandibular joint. This mobile joint permits us to speak, eat, drink and laugh.

Sutures are:

Plane	– internasal suture
Serrate	– coronal suture
Denticulate	– lambdoid suture
Squamous	– parietotemporal suture

Anatomical Position of Skull

The skull can be placed in proper orientation by considering any one of the two planes.

1 Reid's base line is a horizontal line obtained by joining the infraorbital margin to the centre of external acoustic meatus, i.e. auricular point.
2 The Frankfurt's horizontal plane of orientation is obtained by joining the infraorbital margin to the upper margin of the external acoustic meatus (Fig. 9.1).

Methods of Study of the Skull

The skull can be studied as a whole.

The whole skull can be studied from the outside or externally in different views:

a. Superior view or norma verticalis
b. Posterior view or norma occipitalis
c. Anterior view or norma frontalis
d. Lateral view or norma lateralis
e. Inferior view or norma basalis

The whole skull can be studied from the inside or internally after removing the roof of the calvaria or skull cap:

a. Internal surface of the cranial vault.
b. Internal surface of the cranial base which shows a natural subdivision into anterior, middle and posterior cranial fossae.

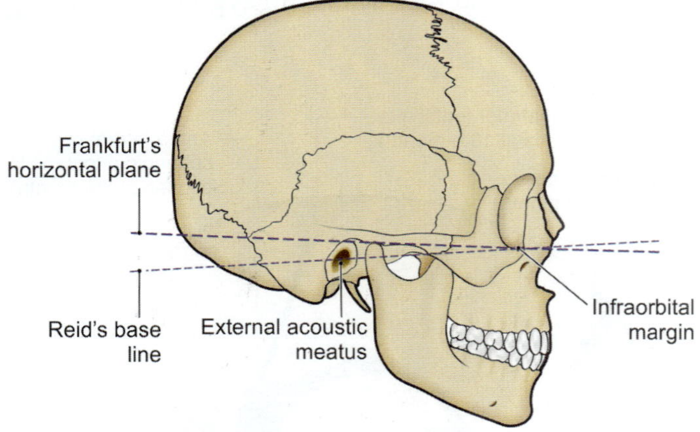

Fig. 9.1: Anatomical position of skull

The skull can also be studied as individual bones. Mandible, maxilla, ethmoid and zygomatic, etc. have been described.

Peculiarities of Skull Bones

1 Base of skull ossifies in cartilage, while the skull cap ossifies in membrane.
2 At birth, skull comprises one table only. By 4 years or so, two tables are formed. Between the two tables, there are *diploes* (Greek double), i.e. spaces containing red bone marrow forming RBCs, granular series of WBCs and platelets. Four diploic veins drain the formed blood cells into neighbouring veins.
3 At birth, the 4 angles of parietal bone have membranous gaps or fontanelles. These allow overlapping of bones during vaginal delivery, if required. These also allow skull bones to increase in size after birth, for housing the delicate brain.
4 Some skull bones have air cells in them and are called pneumatic bones, e.g. frontal, maxilla.
   a. They reduce the weight of skull.
   b. They maintain humidity of inspired air.
   c. They give resonance to voice.
   d. These may get infected resulting in sinusitis.
5 Skull bones are united mostly by sutures.
6 Skull has foramina for 'emissary veins' which connect intracranial venous sinuses with extracranial veins. These try to relieve raised intracranial pressure. Infection may reach through the emissary veins into cranial venous sinuses as these veins are valveless (Table 9.1).
7 Petrous temporal is the densest bone of the body. It lodges internal ear, middle ear including three ossicles, i.e. malleus, incus and stapes. Ossicles are 'bones within the bone' and are fully formed at birth.
8 Skull lodges brain, meninges, CSF, glands like hypophysis cerebri and pineal, venous sinuses, teeth, special senses like retina of eyeball, taste buds of tongue, olfactory epithelium, cochlear and vestibular nerve endings.

Table 9.1: The emissary veins of the skull

Name	*Foramen of skull*	*Veins outside skull*	*Venous sinus*
1. Parietal emissary vein	Parietal foramen	Veins of scalp	Superior sagittal sinus
2. Mastoid emissary vein	Mastoid foramen	Veins of scalp (posterior auricular vein)	Sigmoid sinus
3. Emissary vein	Hypoglossal canal	Internal jugular vein	Sigmoid sinus
4. Condylar emissary vein	Posterior condylar foramen	Suboccipital venous plexus	Sigmoid sinus
5. 2–3 emissary veins	Foramen lacerum	Pharyngeal venous plexus	Cavernous sinus
6. Emissary vein	Foramen ovale	Pterygoid venous plexus	Cavernous sinus
7. Emissary vein	Foramen caecum	Veins from upper part of nose	Superior sagittal sinus

EXTERIOR OF THE SKULL

NORMA VERTICALIS

Shape

When viewed from above, the skull is usually oval in shape. It is wider posteriorly than anteriorly. The shape may be more nearly circular.

Bones

1 Upper part of frontal bone—anteriorly.
2 Uppermost part of occipital bone—posteriorly.
3 A parietal bone—on each side.

Sutures

1 *Coronal suture:* This is placed between the frontal and the two parietal bones. The suture crosses the cranial vault from side-to-side and runs downwards and forwards (Fig. 9.2).
2 *Sagittal suture:* It is placed in the median plane between the two parietal bones.
3 *Lambdoid suture:* It lies posteriorly between the occipital and the two parietal bones, and it runs downwards and forwards across the cranial vault.
4 *Metopic* (Latin forehead) *suture:* This is occasionally present in about 3 to 8% individuals. It lies in the median plane and separates the two halves of the frontal bone. Normally, it fuses at 6 years of age.

Some other Named Features

1 *Vertex* is the highest point on sagittal suture.
2 *Vault* of skull is the arched roof for the dome of skull.
3 *Bregma* is the meeting point between the coronal and sagittal sutures. In the foetal skull, this is the site of a membranous gap, called the anterior fontanelle, which closes at 18 to 24 months of age. It allows growth of brain (Fig. 9.3).
4 The *lambda* is the meeting point between the sagittal and lambdoid sutures. In the foetal skull, this is the site of the posterior fontanelle which closes at birth—2 to 3 months of age.
5 The *parietal tuber (eminence)* is the area of maximum convexity of the parietal bone. This is a common site of fracture of the skull.
6 The *parietal foramen,* one on each side, pierces the parietal bone near its upper border, 2.5 to 4 cm in front of the lambda. The parietal foramen transmits an emissary vein from the veins of scalp to superior sagittal sinus (Fig. 9.2).
7 The *obelion* is the point on the sagittal suture between the two parietal foramina.
8 The *temporal lines* begin at the zygomatic process of the frontal bone, arch backwards and upwards, and cross the frontal bone, the coronal suture and the parietal bone. Over the parietal bone, there are two lines—superior and inferior. Traced anteriorly, they fuse to form a single line. Traced posteriorly, the superior line fades out over the posterior part of the parietal bone, but the inferior temporal line continues downwards and forwards with zygomatic arch.

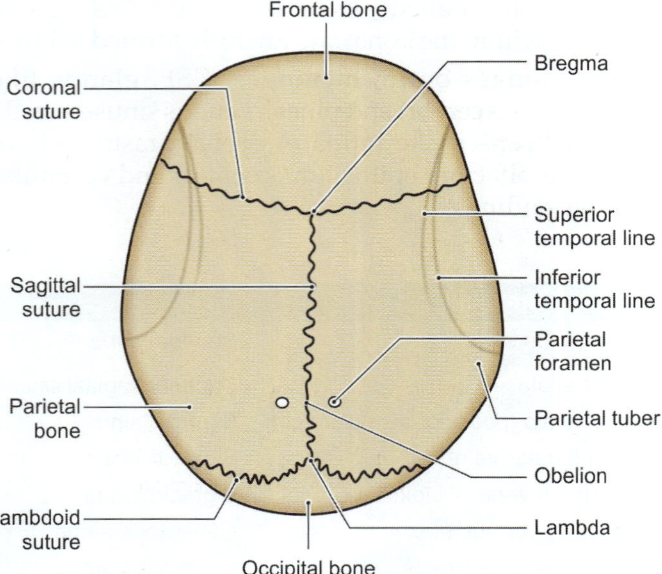

Fig. 9.2: Norma verticalis

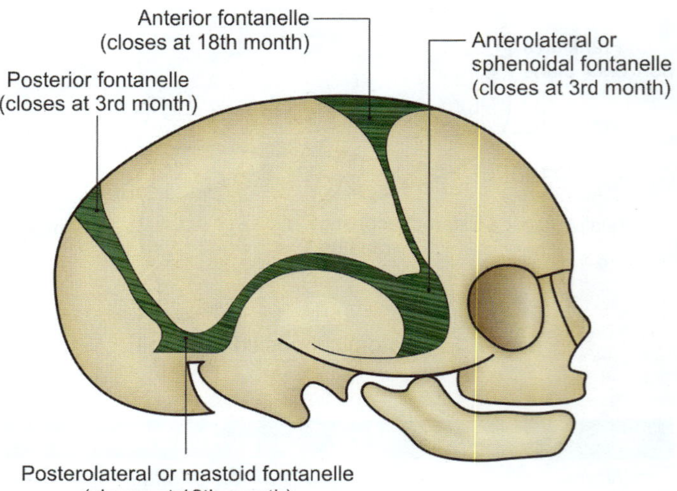

Fig. 9.3: Fontanelles of skull

CLINICAL ANATOMY

- Fontanelles are sites of growth of skull, permitting growth of brain and help to determine age.

- If fontanelles fuse early, brain growth is stunted; such children are less intelligent.
- If anterior fontanelle is bulging, there is raised intracranial pressure. If anterior fontanelle is depressed, it shows decreased intracranial pressure, mostly due to dehydration.
- Bones override at the fontanelle helping to decrease size of head during vaginal delivery.
- *Caput succedaneum* is soft tissue swelling on any part of skull due to rupture of capillaries during delivery. Skull becomes normal within a few days in postnatal life (Fig. 9.4).

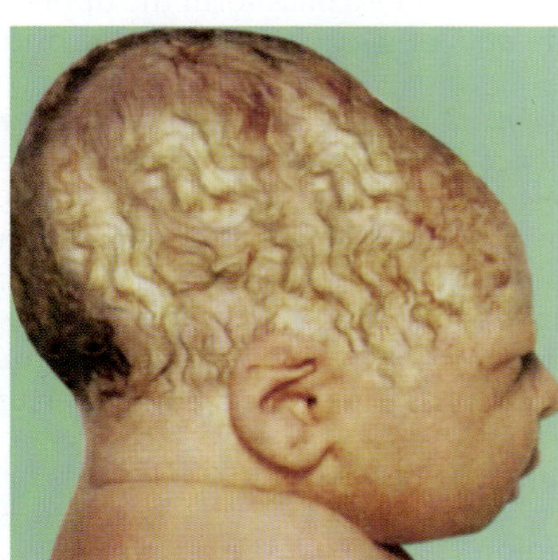

Fig. 9.4: Caput succedaneum

NORMA OCCIPITALIS

Norma occipitalis is convex upwards and on each side, and is flattened below.

Bones

1 Posterior parts of the parietal bones—above.
2 Upper part of the squamous part of the occipital bone—below (Fig. 9.5).
3 Mastoid part of the temporal bone—on each side.

Sutures

1 The *lambdoid suture* lies between the occipital bone and the two parietal bones. Sutural or wormian bones are common along this suture.
2 The *occipitomastoid suture* lies between the occipital bone and mastoid part of the temporal bone.
3 The *parietomastoid suture* lies between the parietal bone and mastoid part of the temporal bone.
4 The posterior part of the *sagittal suture* is also seen.

Other Features

1 *Lambda, parietal foramina* and *obelion* have been examined in the norma verticalis.
2 The *external occipital protuberance* is a median prominence in the lower part of this norma. It marks the junction of the head and the neck. The most prominent point on this protuberance is called the *inion*.

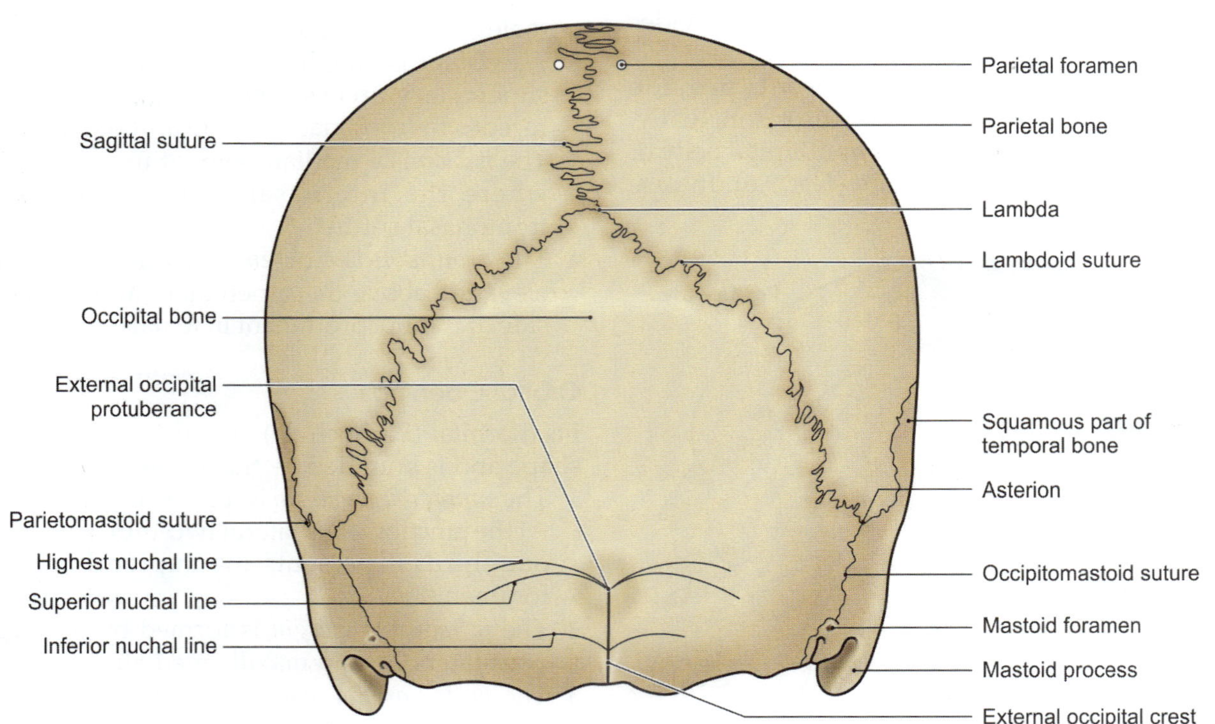

Fig. 9.5: Norma occipitalis

3 The *superior nuchal lines* are curved bony ridges passing laterally from the protuberance. These also mark the junction of the head and the neck. The area below the superior nuchal lines will be studied with the norma basalis.
4 The *highest nuchal lines* are not always present. They are curved bony ridges situated about 1 cm above the superior nuchal lines. They begin from the upper part of the external occipital protuberance and are more arched than the superior nuchal lines.
5 The *occipital point* is a median point, a little above the inion. It is the point farthest from the glabella.
6 The *mastoid* (Greek breast) *foramen* is located on the mastoid part of the temporal bone at or near the occipitomastoid suture. Internally, it opens at the sigmoid sulcus. The mastoid foramen transmits an emissary vein (Table 9.1) and the meningeal branch of the occipital artery.
7 The *interparietal bone* (inca bone) is occasionally present. It is a large triangular bone located at the apex of the squamous occipital. This is not a sutural or accessory bone, but represents the membranous part of the occipital bone which has failed to fuse with the rest of the bone.

Attachments

1 The upper part of the external occipital protuberance gives origin to the trapezius, and the lower part gives attachment to the upper end of the ligamentum nuchae (Fig. 9.14).
2 The medial one-third of the superior nuchal line gives origin to the trapezius, and the lateral part provides insertion to the sternocleidomastoid.
3 The highest nuchal lines, if present, provide attachment to the epicranial aponeurosis medially, and give origin to the occipitalis or occipital belly of occipitofrontalis muscle laterally (Fig. 9.6). In case of absence of highest nuchal lines, these structures are attached to superior nuchal lines.

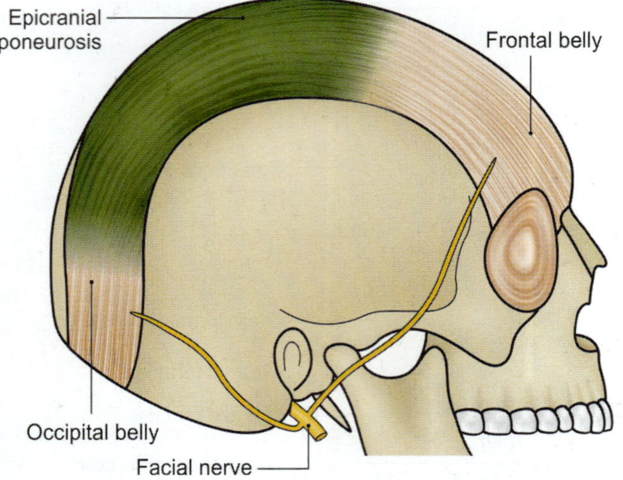

Fig. 9.6: Attachments of the occipitofrontalis muscle

NORMA FRONTALIS

The norma frontalis is roughly oval in outline, being wider above than below.

Bones

1 *Frontal* bone forms the forehead. Its upper part is smooth and convex, but the lower part is irregular and is interrupted by the orbits and by the anterior bony aperture of nose (Fig. 9.7).
2 The right and left *maxillae* form the upper jaw.
3 The right and left *nasal* bones form the bridge of the nose.
4 The *zygomatic* (Greek yoke) bones form the bony prominence of the superolateral part of the cheeks.
5 The *mandible* forms the lower jaw.

The *norma frontalis* can be studied under the following heads.

a. Frontal region
b. Orbital openings
c. Anterior piriform-shaped bony aperture of the nose
d. Lower part of the face.

Frontal Region

The frontal region presents the following features:

1 The *superciliary arch* is a rounded, curved elevation situated just above the medial part of each orbit. It overlies the frontal sinus and is better marked in males than in females.
2 *The glabella* is a median elevation connecting the two superciliary arches. Below the glabella, the skull recedes to frontonasal suture at root of the nose.
3 The *nasion* is a median point at the root of the nose where the internasal suture meets with the frontonasal suture.
4 The *frontal tuber* or *eminence* is a low rounded elevation above the superciliary arch—one on each side. It is more prominent in females and in children.

Orbital Openings

Each orbital (Latin circle) opening is quadrangular in shape and is bounded by the following four margins.

1 The *supraorbital margin* is formed by the frontal bone. At the junction of its lateral two-thirds and its medial one-third, it presents the supraorbital notch or foramen (Fig. 9.7).
2 The *infraorbital margin* is formed by the zygomatic bone laterally, and maxilla medially.
3 The *medial orbital margin* is ill-defined. It is formed by the frontal bone above, and by the lacrimal crest of the frontal process of the maxilla below.

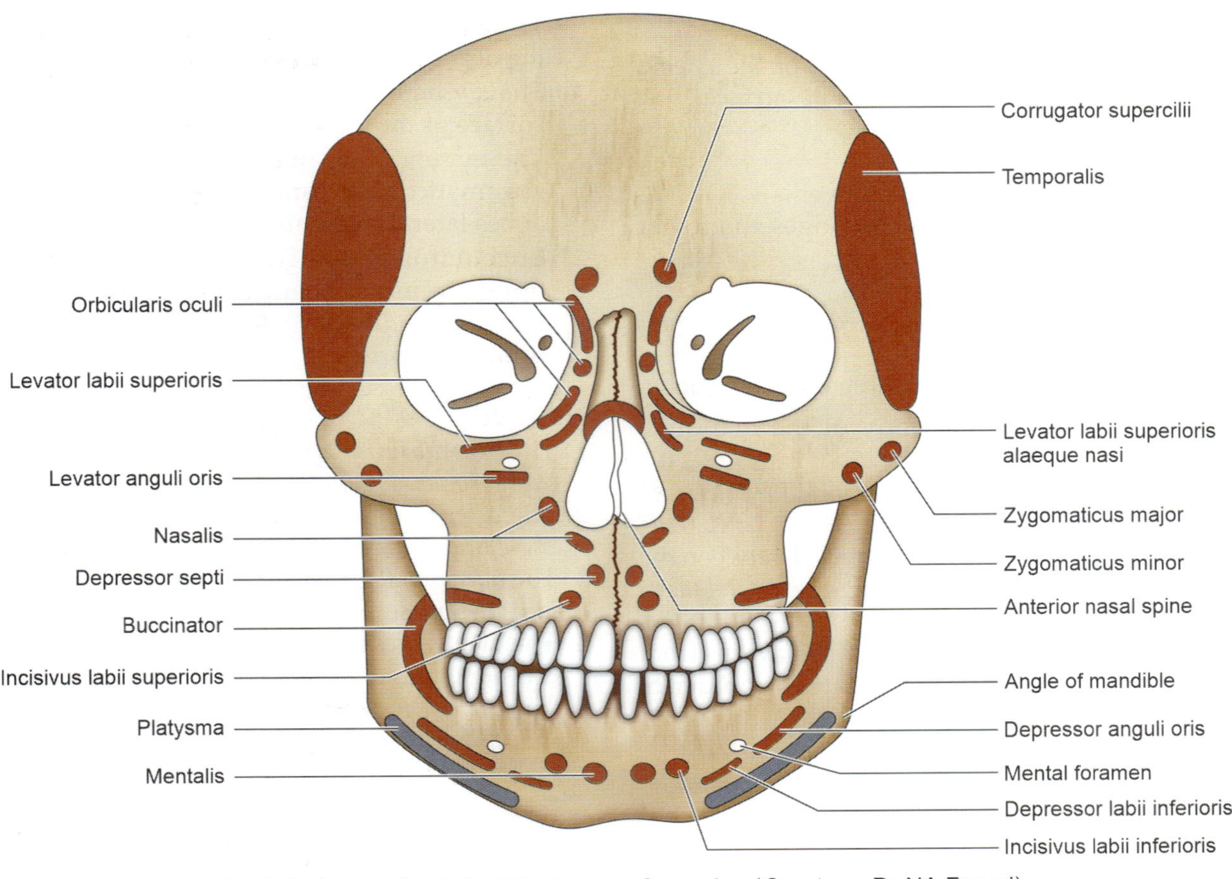

Fig. 9.7: Norma frontalis: Attachment of muscles (*Courtsey:* Dr NA Faruqi)

4 The *lateral orbital margin* is formed mostly by the frontal process of zygomatic bone, but is completed above by the zygomatic process of frontal bone. *Frontozygomatic suture* lies at their union.

Anterior Bony Aperture of the Nose

The anterior bony aperture is pear-shaped, being wide below and narrow above.

Boundaries

Above: By the lower border of the nasal bones.

Below: By the nasal notch of the body of maxilla on each side.

Features: Note the following:

1 *Articulations of the nasal bone:*
   a. *Anteriorly*, with the opposite bone at the internasal suture.
   b. *Posteriorly*, with the frontal process of the maxilla.
   c. *Superiorly*, with the frontal bone at the frontonasal suture.
   d. *Inferiorly*, the upper nasal cartilage is attached to it.
2 The *anterior nasal spine* is a sharp projection in the median plane in the lower boundary of the piriform aperture (Fig. 9.7).
3 Rhinion is the lowermost point of the internasal suture.

Lower Part of the Face

Maxilla

Maxilla contributes a large share in the formation of the facial skeleton. The anterior surface of the body of the maxilla presents:

a. The *nasal notch* medially;
b. The *anterior nasal spine;*
c. The *infraorbital foramen,* 1 cm below the infraorbital margin;
d. The *incisive fossa* above the incisor teeth, and
e. The *canine fossa* lateral to the canine eminence.

In addition, three out of four processes of the maxilla are also seen in this norma.

a. The *frontal process of the maxilla* is directed upwards. It articulates anteriorly with the nasal bone, posteriorly with the lacrimal bone, and superiorly with the frontal bone (Fig. 9.7).
b. The *zygomatic process of the maxilla* is short but stout and articulates with the zygomatic bone.
c. The *alveolar process of the maxilla* bears sockets for the upper teeth.

Zygomatic Bone (Malar Bone)

Zygomatic bone forms the prominence of the cheek. The *zygomaticofacial foramen* is seen on its surface.

Mandible (Lower Jaw Bone)

Mandible (Latin to chew) forms the lower jaw.

The *upper border* or *alveolar arch* lodges the lower teeth.

The *lower border* or *base* is rounded.

The middle point of the base is called the *mental point or gnathion.*

The point on the angle of mandible is called *gonion*.

The *anterior surface* of the body of the mandible presents:

a. The *symphysis menti*, the *mental protuberance* and *mental tubercles*, anteriorly (Fig. 9.7).
b. The *mental foramen* below the interval between the two premolar teeth, transmitting the *mental nerve and vessels*.
c. The *oblique line* runs upwards and backwards from the mental prominence to the anterior border of *ramus* (Latin branch) of the mandible.

Sutures of the Norma Frontalis

- Internasal (Fig. 9.7)
- Frontonasal
- Nasomaxillary
- Lacrimomaxillary
- Frontomaxillary
- Intermaxillary
- Zygomaticomaxillary
- Zygomaticofrontal

Attachments

1 The medial part of the superciliary arch gives origin to the corrugator supercilii muscle (*see* Fig. 10.9).
2 The procerus muscle arises from the nasal bone near the median plane (*see* Fig. 10.9).
3 The orbital part of the orbicularis oculi arises from the frontal process of the maxilla and from the nasal part of the frontal bone (*see* Fig. 10.9).
4 The medial palpebral ligament is attached to the frontal process of the maxilla between the frontal and maxillary origins of the orbicularis oculi.
5 The levator labii superioris alaeque nasi arises from the frontal process of the maxilla in front of the orbicularis oculi (Fig. 9.7).
6 The levator labii superioris arises from the maxilla between the infraorbital margin and the infraorbital foramen (Fig. 9.7).
7 The levator anguli oris arises from the canine fossa.
8 The nasalis and the depressor septi arise from the surface of the maxilla bordering the nasal notch.
9 The incisivus muscle arises from an area just below the depressor septi. It forms part of orbicularis oris.
10 The zygomaticus major and minor arise from the surface of the zygomatic bone (Fig. 9.7).
The zygomaticus minor muscle arises below the zygomaticofacial foramen. The zygomaticus major arises lateral to the minor muscle (Fig. 9.7).
11 Buccinator arises from maxilla and mandible opposite molar teeth (*see* Fig. 10.10) and from *pterygomandibular raphe*. It also forms part of orbicularis oris.

Structures Passing through Foramina

1 The *supraorbital notch or foramen* transmits the *supraorbital nerves and vessels* (*see* Fig. 10.5).
2 The *external nasal nerve* emerges between the nasal bone and upper nasal cartilage (*see* Fig. 10.16).
3 The *infraorbital foramen* transmits the *infraorbital nerve* and *vessels* (*see* Fig. 10.16).
4 The *zygomaticofacial foramen* transmits the nerve of the same name, a branch of *maxillary nerve.*
5 The *mental foramen* on the mandible transmits the mental nerve and vessels (*see* Fig. 10.16).

CLINICAL ANATOMY

The *nasal bone is one of the most commonly fractured bones of the face*. Mandible and parietal eminence are the next bones to be fractured (Fig. 9.8).

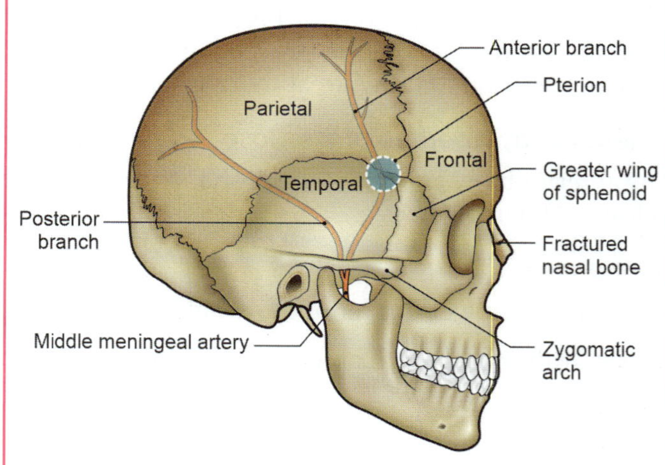

Fig. 9.8: Fractured nasal bone and position of anterior division of middle meningeal artery against the pterion

NORMA LATERALIS

Bones

1 Frontal
2 Parietal (Fig. 9.9a)
3 Occipital
4 Temporal (Figs 9.9b and c)

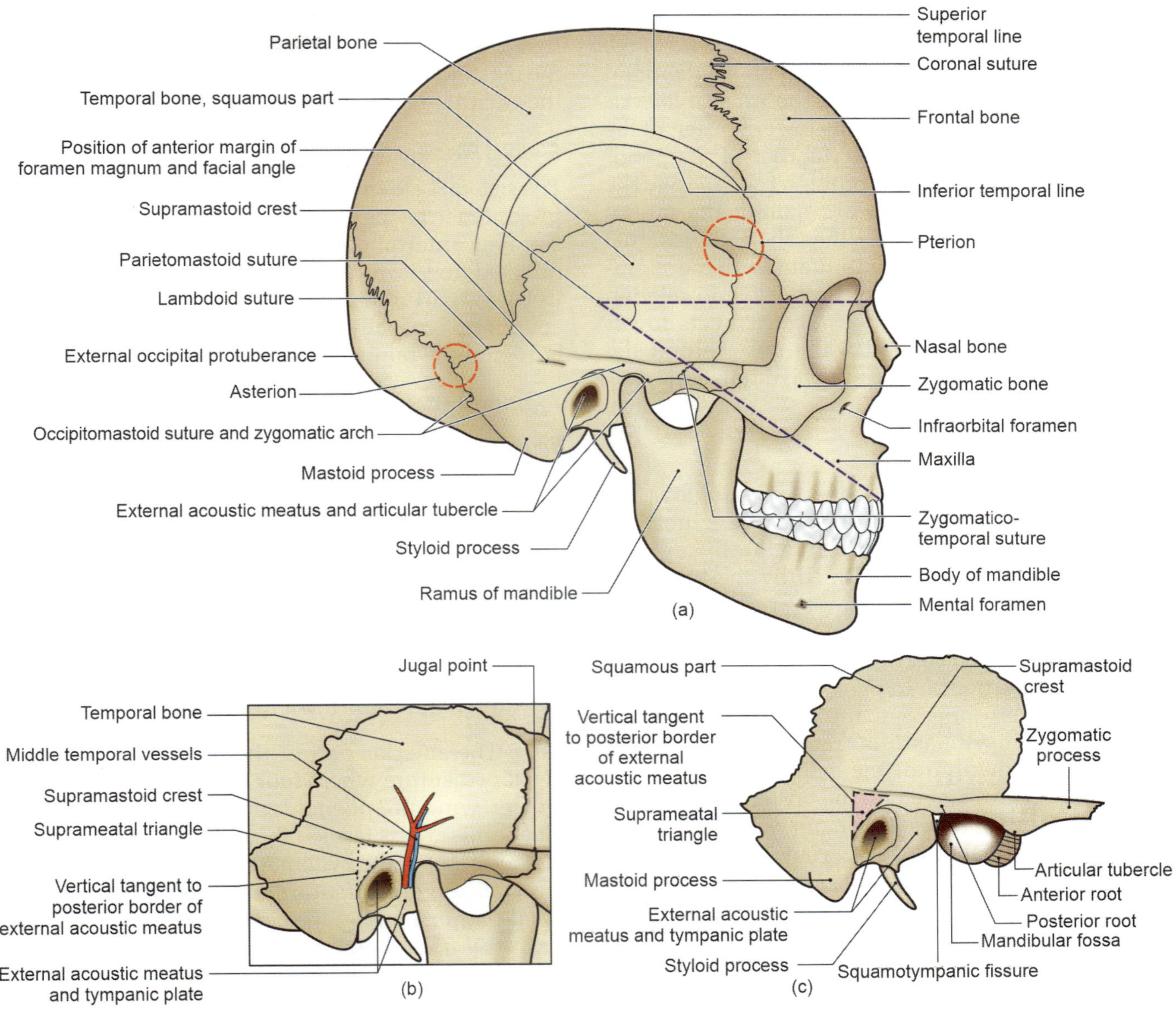

Figs 9.9a to c: (a) Norma lateralis with facial angle; (b) Bones forming norma lateralis; (c) Tympanic plate forming margins of external acoustic meatus

5 Sphenoid
6 Zygomatic
7 Mandible
8 Maxilla
9 Nasal

Features

Temporal Lines

The *temporal lines* have been studied in the norma verticalis. The inferior temporal line, in its posterior part, turns downwards and forwards and becomes continuous with the *supramastoid crest* on the squamous temporal bone near its junction with the mastoid temporal. This crest is continuous anteriorly with the posterior root of the zygomatic arch (Fig. 9.9b).

Zygomatic Arch or Zygoma

The *zygomatic arch* is a horizontal bar on the side of the head, in front of the ear, a little above the tragus. It is formed by the temporal process of the zygomatic bone in anterior one-third and the zygomatic process of the temporal bone in posterior two-thirds. The *zygomatico-temporal suture* crosses the arch obliquely downwards and backwards.

Above the zygomatic arch is temporal fossa, which is filled by temporalis muscle. Attached to lower margin of zygomatic arch is masseter muscle; contraction of both temporalis and masseter may be felt by clenching the teeth.

The arch is separated from the side of the skull by a gap which is deeper in front than behind. Its *lateral surface* is subcutaneous. The anterior end of the upper border is called the *jugal point*. The posterior end of the zygomatic arch is attached to the squamous temporal bone by *anterior* and *posterior roots*. The *articular tubercle of the root* of the zygoma lies on its lower border, at the junction of the anterior and posterior roots. The anterior root passes medially in front of the *articular fossa*. The posterior root passes backwards along the lateral margin of the mandibular fossa, then above the external acoustic meatus to become continuous with the supramastoid crest. Two projections are visible in relation to these roots. One is *articular tubercle* at its lower border. Another tubercle is visible just behind the mandibular or articular fossa and is known as *postglenoid tubercle*.

External Acoustic Meatus

The *external acoustic meatus* opens just below the posterior part of the posterior root of zygoma. Its anterior and inferior margins and the lower part of the posterior margin are formed by the tympanic plate, and the posterosuperior margin is formed by the squamous temporal bone. The margins are roughened for the attachment of auricular cartilage.

The *suprameatal triangle (trianlge of McEwen)* is a small depression posterosuperior to the meatus. It is *bounded* above by the supramastoid crest, in front by the posterosuperior margin of the external meatus, and behind by a vertical tangent to the posterior margin of the meatus. The *suprameatal spine* may be present on the anteroinferior margin of the triangle. The triangle forms the lateral wall of the tympanic or mastoid antrum (Fig. 9.9c).

Mastoid Part of the Temporal Bone

The *mastoid part of the temporal bone* lies just behind the external acoustic meatus. It is continuous anterosuperiorly with the squamous temporal bone (Fig. 9.9c). A partially obliterated squamomastoid suture may be visible in front of and parallel to the roughened area for muscular insertion.

The mastoid temporal bone articulates posterosuperiorly with the posteroinferior part of the parietal bone at the horizontal *parietomastoid suture*, and posteriorly with the squamous occipital bone at the *occipitomastoid suture*. These two sutures meet at the lateral end of the lambdoid suture. The *asterion* is the point where the parietomastoid, occipitomastoid and lambdoid sutures meet. In infants, the asterion is the site of the *posterolateral* or *mastoid fontanelle*, which closes by 12 months (Fig. 9.3).

The *mastoid process* is a breast-like projection from the lower part of the mastoid temporal bone, posteroinferior to the external acoustic meatus. It appears during the second year of life. The *tympanomastoid fissure* is placed on the anterior aspect of the base of the mastoid process. The *mastoid foramen* lies at or near the occipitomastoid suture (Fig. 9.5).

Styloid Process

The *styloid* (Latin pen) *process* is a needle-like thin, long projection from the temporal bone seen in norma basalis situated anteromedial to the mastoid process. It is directed downwards, forwards and slightly medially. Its base is partly ensheathed by the tympanic plate. The apex or tip is usually hidden from view by the posterior border of the ramus of the mandible.

Temporal Fossa

Boundaries

1. *Above*, by the superior temporal line.
2. *Below*, by the upper border of the zygomatic arch laterally, and by the infratemporal crest of the greater wing of the sphenoid bone medially. Through the gap deep to the zygomatic arch, temporal fossa communicates with the infratemporal fossa.
3. The *anterior wall* is formed by the zygomatic bone and by parts of the frontal and sphenoid bones. This wall separates the fossa from the orbit.

Floor: The anterior part of the floor is crossed by an H-shaped suture where four bones—frontal, parietal, greater wing of sphenoid and temporal adjoin each other. This area is termed the *pterion*. It lies 4 cm above the midpoint of the zygomatic arch and 2.5 cm behind the frontozygomatic suture. Deep to the pterion lie, the *middle meningeal vein*, the *anterior division of the middle meningeal artery*, and the *stem of the lateral sulcus of brain (Sylvian point)* (Fig. 9.8).

On the temporal surface of the zygomatic bone forming the anterior wall of the fossa, there is the *zygomaticotemporal foramen*.

Attachments

1. The temporal fascia is attached to the superior temporal line and to the area between the two temporal lines. Inferiorly, it is attached to the outer and inner lips of the upper border of the zygomatic arch.
2. The temporalis muscle arises from the whole of the temporal fossa, except the part formed by the zygomatic bone (*see* Fig. 14.4). Beneath the muscle, there lie the *deep temporal vessels* and *nerves*. The *middle temporal vessels* produce vascular markings on the temporal bone just above the external acoustic meatus (Fig. 9.9b).
3. The medial surface and lower border of the zygomatic arch give origin to the masseter (*see* Fig. 14.3).

4 The lateral ligament of the temporomandibular joint is attached to the tubercle of the root of the zygoma (*see* Chapter 14).
5 The sternocleidomastoid, splenius capitis and longissimus capitis are inserted from before backwards on the posterior part of the lateral surface of the mastoid process (Fig. 9.14). Posterior belly of digastric arises from mastoid notch. The groove obliquely placed behind mastoid notch is due to occipital artery (*see* Fig. 15.3).
6 The *gap* between the zygomatic arch and the side of the skull transmits:
   a. Tendon of the temporalis muscle
   b. Deep temporal vessels
   c. Deep temporal nerves.

Infratemporal Fossa

Boundaries and the contents are described in Chapter 14.

Pterygopalatine Fossa

Pterygopalatine fossa is described in Chapter 23.

Structures Passing through Foramina

1 The *tympanomastoid fissure* on the anterior aspect of the base of the mastoid process transmits the *auricular branch* of *vagus nerve.*
2 The mastoid foramen transmits:
   a. An *emissary vein* connecting the *sigmoid sinus* with the *posterior auricular vein* (Table 9.1).
   b. A meningeal branch of the occipital artery.
3 The *zygomaticotemporal foramen* transmits the nerve of the same name and a minute artery (*see* Fig. 10.16).

CLINICAL ANATOMY

Pterion site of anterolateral fontanelle is the thin part of skull. In roadside accidents, the anterior division of middle meningeal artery at pterion (Fig. 9.8) may be ruptured, leading to clot formation between the skull bone and dura mater or extradural haemorrhage. The clot compresses the motor area of brain, leading to paralysis of the opposite side. The clot must be sucked out at the earliest by trephining (Fig. 9.10). The head must be protected by a helmet during driving a two-wheeler.

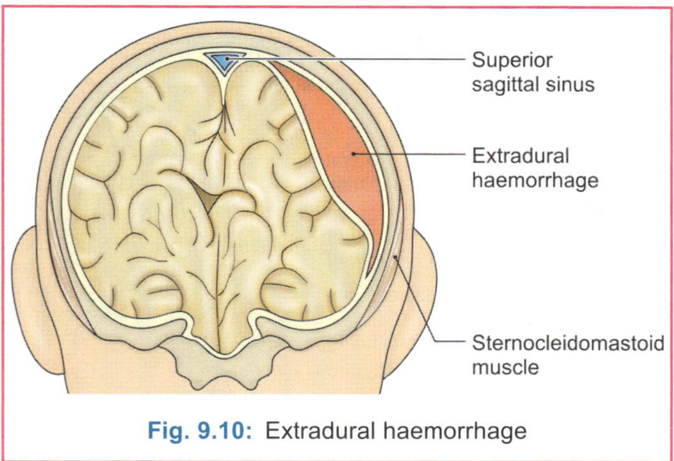

Fig. 9.10: Extradural haemorrhage

NORMA BASALIS

For convenience of study, the norma basalis is divided arbitrarily into anterior, middle and posterior parts. The *anterior part* is formed by the hard palate and the alveolar arches. The *middle and posterior parts* are separated by an imaginary transverse line passing through the anterior margin of the foramen magnum (Figs 9.11a–c).

Anterior Part of Norma Basalis

Alveolar Arch

Alveolar arch bears sockets for the roots of the upper teeth.

Hard Palate

1 *Formation:*
   a. Anterior two-thirds, by the palatine processes of the maxillae.
   b. Posterior one-third, by the horizontal plates of the palatine.
2 *Sutures:* The palate is crossed by a cruciform suture made up of intermaxillary, interpalatine and palatomaxillary sutures.
3 *Dome:*
   a. It is arched in all directions.
   b. Shows pits for the palatine glands.
4 The *incisive foramen* is a deep fossa situated anteriorly in the median plane (Fig. 9.12).

   Two *incisive* canals, right and left, pierce the walls of the incisive foramen, usually one on each side, but occasionally in the median plane, the left being anterior and the right, posterior.
5 The *greater palatine foramen,* one on each side, is situated just behind the lateral part of the palatomaxillary suture. A groove leads from the foramen towards the incisive fossa (Fig. 9.11a).
6 The *lesser palatine foramina,* two or three in number on each side, lie behind the greater palatine foramen, and perforate the pyramidal process of the palatine bone (Fig. 9.11a).
7 The *posterior border* of the hard palate is free and presents the *posterior nasal spine* in the median plane.
8 The *palatine crest* is a curved ridge near the posterior border. It begins behind the greater palatine foramen and runs medially (Fig. 9.12).

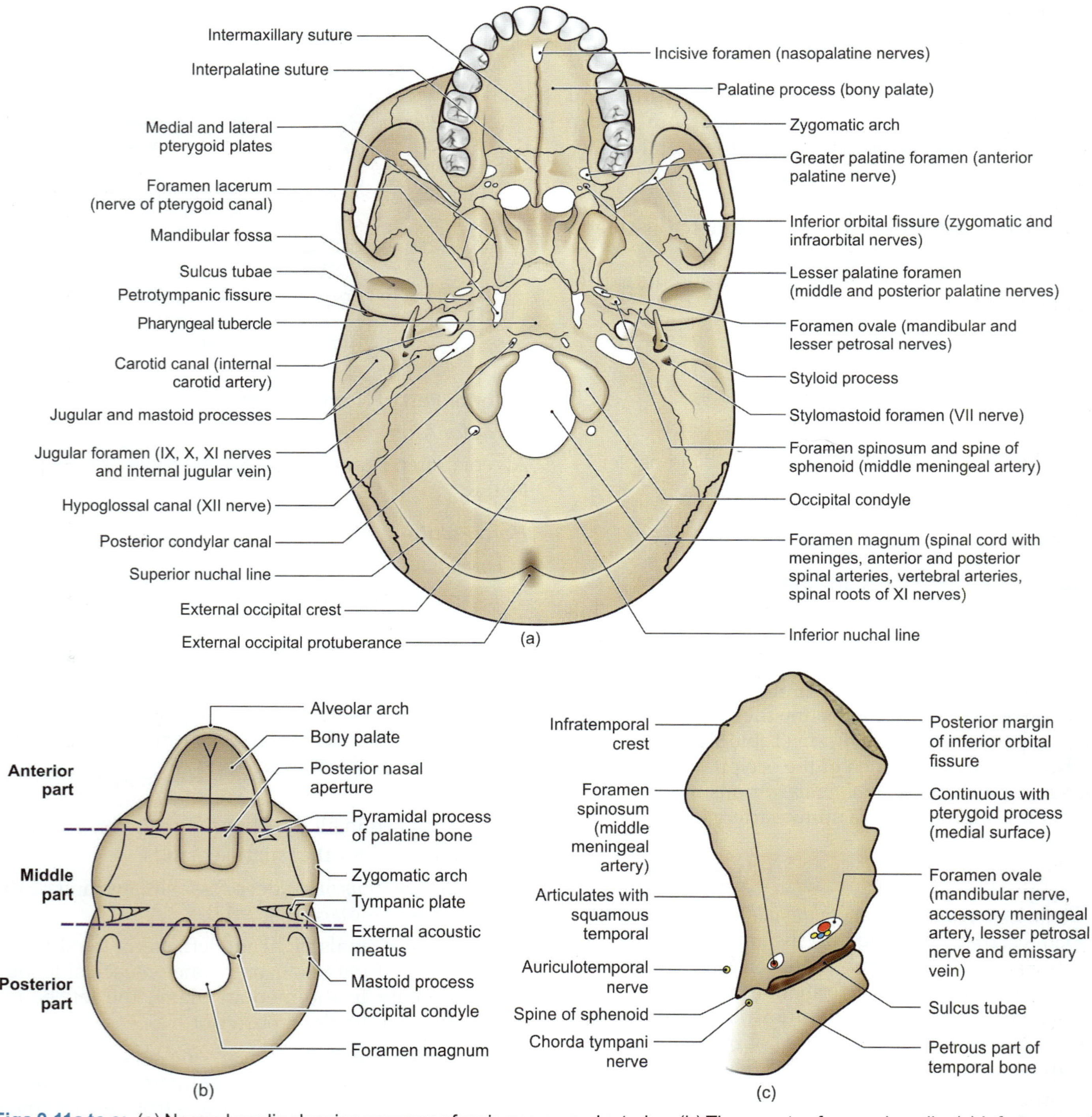

Figs 9.11a to c: (a) Norma basalis showing passage of main nerves and arteries; (b) Three parts of norma basalis; (c) Infratemporal surface of greater wing of sphenoid

Middle Part of Norma Basalis

The middle part extends from the posterior border of the hard palate to the arbitrary transverse line passing through the anterior margin of the foramen magnum.

Median Area

1 The median area shows:
   a. The posterior border of the *vomer*.
   b. A *broad bar of bone* formed by fusion of the posterior part of the body of sphenoid and the basilar part of occipital bone (Fig. 9.13).

2 The vomer separates the two posterior nasal apertures. Its inferior border articulates with the bony palate. The superior border splits into two *alae* and articulates with the *rostrum* of the *sphenoid bone* (Fig. 9.13).

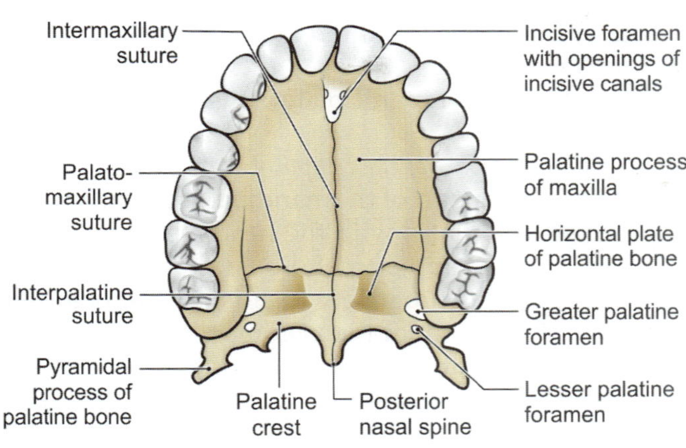

Fig. 9.12: Anterior part of the norma basalis

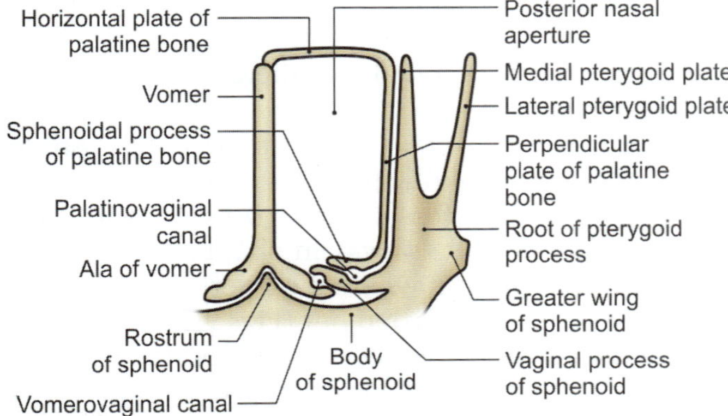

Fig. 9.13: Posterior view of a coronal section through the posterior nasal aperture showing the formation of the palatinovaginal and vomerovaginal canals

3 *Palatinovaginal canal*: The inferior surface of the vaginal process of the medial pterygoid plate is marked by an anteroposterior groove which is converted into the palatinovaginal canal by the upper surface of the sphenoidal process of the palatine bone. The canal opens anteriorly into the posterior wall of the pterygopalatine fossa (*see* Fig. 23.16).

4 *Vomerovaginal canal:* The lateral border of each ala of the vomer comes into relationship with the vaginal process of the medial pterygoid plate, and may overlap it from above to enclose the vomerovaginal canal (Fig. 9.13).

5 The broad bar of the bone is marked in the median plane by the *pharyngeal tubercle*, a little in front of the foramen magnum (Fig. 9.11a).

Lateral Area

1 The lateral area shows two parts of the sphenoid bone—pterygoid process and greater wing. Also seen are three parts of the temporal bone, i.e. petrous temporal, tympanic plate and squamous temporal.

2 The *pterygoid process* projects downwards from the junction of greater wing and the body of sphenoid behind the third molar tooth.
Inferiorly, it divides into the *medial and lateral pterygoid plates* which are fused together anteriorly, but are separated posteriorly by the V-shaped *pterygoid fossa.*
The fused anterior borders of the two plates articulate medially with the perpendicular plate of the palatine bone, and are separated laterally from the posterior surface of the body of the maxilla by the pterygo-maxillary fissure.
The *medial pterygoid plate* is directed backwards. It has medial and lateral surfaces and a free posterior border.
The upper end of posterior border divides to enclose a triangular depression called the *scaphoid fossa.* The lower end of the posterior border is prolonged downwards and laterally to form the *pterygoid hamulus.*
The *lateral pterygoid plate* is directed backwards and laterally. It has medial and lateral surfaces and a free posterior border. The lateral surface forms the medial wall of the infratemporal fossa. Its lateral and medial surfaces give origin to muscles.
The posterior border sometimes has a projection at its middle called the pterygospinous process which projects towards the spine of the sphenoid.

3 The *infratemporal surface of the greater wing of the sphenoid* is pentagonal.
   a. Its *anterior margin* forms the posterior border of the inferior orbital fissure (Fig. 9.11c).
   b. Its *anterolateral margin* forms the infratemporal crest.
   c. Its *posterolateral margin* articulates with the squamous temporal.
   d. Its *posteromedial margin* articulates with petrous temporal.
   e. *Anteromedially*, it is continuous with the pterygoid process and with the body of the sphenoid bone.

The posteriormost point between the posterolateral and posteromedial margins projects downwards to form the *spine* of the sphenoid.

Along the posteromedial margin, the surface is pierced by the following foramina.
   a. The *foramen ovale* is large and oval in shape. It is situated posterolateral to the upper end of the posterior border of lateral pterygoid plate (Figs 9.11a and c).
   b. The *foramen spinosum* is small and circular in shape. It is situated posterolateral to the foramen ovale, and is limited posterolaterally by the spine of sphenoid (Figs 9.11a and c).

c. Sometimes, there is the *emissary sphenoidal foramen or foramen of Vesalius.* It is situated between the foramen ovale and the scaphoid fossa. Internally, it opens between the foramen ovale and the foramen rotundum.

d. At times, there is a *canaliculus innominatus* situated between the foramen ovale and the foramen spinosum.

The *spine* of the sphenoid may be sharply pointed or blunt (Figs 9.11a and c).

The *sulcus tubae* is the groove between the posteromedial margin of the greater wing of the sphenoid and the petrous temporal bone. It lodges the *cartilaginous part of the auditory tube*. Posteriorly, the groove leads to the bony part of the auditory tube which lies within the petrous temporal bone (Figs 9.11a and c).

4 The inferior surface of the *petrous* (Greek rock) part of the temporal bone is triangular in shape with its apex directed forwards and medially.

It lies between the greater wing of the sphenoid and the basiocciput. Its *apex* is perforated by the upper end of the carotid canal, and is separated from the sphenoid by the foramen lacerum. The *inferior surface* is perforated by the lower end of the *carotid canal* posteriorly.

The *carotid canal* runs forwards and medially within the petrous temporal bone.

The *foramen lacerum* is a short, wide canal, 1 cm long. Its lower end is bounded posterolaterally by the apex of the petrous temporal, medially by the basiocciput and the body of the sphenoid, and anteriorly by the root of the pterygoid process and the greater wing of the sphenoid bone.

A part of the petrous temporal bone, called the *tegmen tympani*, is present in the middle cranial fossa. It has a down turned edge which is seen in the *squamotympanic fissure* and divides it into the posterior *petrotympanic* and anterior *petrosquamous* fissures (Fig. 9.11a).

5 *The tympanic part of the temporal bone, also called the tympanic plate,* is a triangular curved plate which lies in the angle between the petrous and squamous parts. Its apex is directed medially and lies close to the spine of the sphenoid.

The *base or lateral border* is curved, free and roughened. Its *anterior surface* forms the posterior wall of the mandibular fossa. The *posterior surface* is concave and forms the anterior wall, floor, and lower part of the posterior wall of the bony external acoustic meatus (Fig. 9.9c).

Its *upper border* bounds the petrotympanic fissure. The *lower border* is sharp and free.

Medially: It passes along the anterolateral margin of the lower end of the carotid canal.

Laterally: It forms the anterolateral part of the *sheath of the styloid process*.

Internally: The tympanic plate is fused to the petrous temporal bone.

6 *The squamous part of the temporal bone* forms:

a. The anterior part of the mandibular articular fossa which articulates with the head of the mandible to form the temporomandibular joint.

b. The articular tubercle which is continuous with the anterior root of the zygoma.

c. A small posterolateral part of the roof of the infratemporal fossa.

Posterior Part of Norma Basalis

Median Area

The median area shows from before backwards:

a. The foramen magnum
b. The external occipital crest
c. The external occipital protuberance
d. Nuchal lines.

a. The *foramen magnum* (Latin great) is the largest foramen of the skull. It opens upwards into the posterior cranial fossa, and downwards into the vertebral canal. It is oval in shape, being wider behind than in front where it is overlapped on each side by the occipital condyles (Figs 9.11b and 9.14).

b. The *external occipital crest* begins at the posterior margin of the foramen magnum and ends posteriorly and above at the external occipital protuberance (Fig. 9.11).

c. The *external occipital protuberance* is a projection located at the posterior end of the crest. It is easily felt in the living, in the midline, at the point where the back of the neck becomes continuous with the scalp (Fig. 9.11a).

d. *Nuchal lines:* The superior nuchal lines begin at the external occipital protuberance and the inferior nuchal lines at the middle of the crest. Both of them curve laterally and backwards and then laterally and forwards. Highest nuchal line is faded and seen above superior nuchal line (occasionally).

Lateral Area

The *lateral area* shows:

- The condylar part of the occipital bone.
- The squamous part of the occipital bone.
- The jugular foramen between the occipital and petrous temporal bones.
- The styloid process of the temporal bone.
- The mastoid part of the temporal bone.

a. The *condylar or lateral part of the occipital bone* presents the following.

i. The *occipital condyles* are oval in shape and are situated on each side of the anterior part of the foramen magnum. Their long axis is directed forwards and medially (Fig. 9.11a).

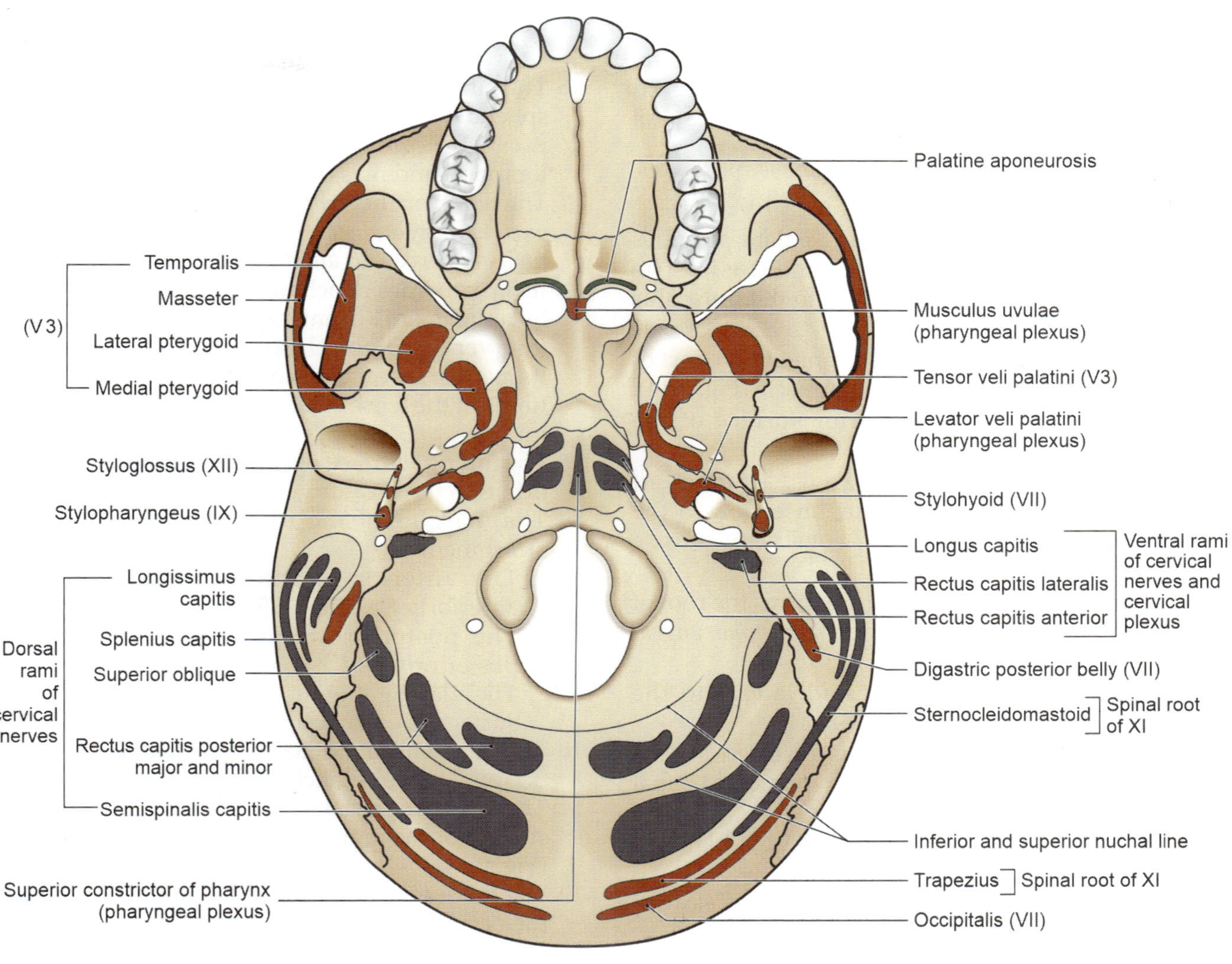

Fig. 9.14: Muscles attached to the base of skull with their nerve supply

They articulate with the superior articular facets of the atlas vertebra to form the atlanto-occipital joints.

ii. The *hypoglossal* or *anterior condylar canal* pierces the bone anterosuperior to the occipital condyle, and is directed laterally and slightly forwards.

iii. The *condylar* or *posterior condylar canal* is occasionally present in the floor of a condylar fossa present behind the occipital condyle. Superiorly, it opens into the sigmoid sulcus.

iv. The *jugular process of the occipital bone* lies lateral to the occipital condyle and forms the posterior boundary of jugular foramen (Fig. 9.11a).

b. *Squamous part of occipital bone* is marked by the superior and inferior nuchal lines mentioned above (Fig. 9.5).

c. The *jugular foramen* is large and elongated, with its long axis directed forwards and medially. It is placed at the posterior end of the petro-occipital suture (Fig. 9.11a).

At the posterior end of the foramen, its anterior wall (petrous temporal) is hollowed out to form *jugular fossa* which lodges the superior bulb of the internal jugular vein. The fossa is larger on the right side than on the left.

The lateral wall of the jugular fossa is pierced by a minute canal, the *mastoid canaliculus*.

Near the medial end of the jugular foramen, there is the *jugular notch*. At the apex of the notch, there is an opening that leads into the *cochlear canaliculus*.

The *tympanic canaliculus* opens on or near the thin edge of bone between the jugular fossa and the lower end of the carotid canal.

d. *Styloid process* is described in Chapter 16.

The *stylomastoid foramen* is situated posterior to the root of the styloid process, at the anterior end of the mastoid notch.

e. The *mastoid process*, a component of mastoid part, is a large conical projection located posterolateral to the stylomastoid foramen. It is directed downwards and forwards. It forms the lateral wall of the *mastoid notch* (Fig. 9.5).

Attachments on Exterior of Skull

1 The posterior border of the hard palate provides attachment to the palatine aponeurosis. The posterior nasal spine gives origin to the musculus uvulae (Fig. 9.14).

2 The palatine crest provides attachment to a part of the tendon of tensor veli palatini muscle (Fig. 9.14).

3 The attachments on the inferior surface of the basiocciput are as follows:
   a. The *pharyngeal tubercle* gives attachment to the raphe which provides insertion to the upper fibres of the superior constrictor muscle of the pharynx (Fig. 9.14).
   b. The area in front of the tubercle forms the roof of the *nasopharynx* and supports the *pharyngeal tonsil*.
   c. The longus capitis is inserted lateral to the pharyngeal tubercle (Fig. 9.14).
   d. The rectus capitis anterior is inserted a little posterior and medial to the hypoglossal canal (Fig. 9.14).

4 The attachments on the medial pterygoid plate are as follows:
   a. The pharyngobasilar fascia is attached below to the processus tuberis.
   Processus tuberis/pterygospinous process is a triangular projection which is present at the middle of the posterior border of medial pterygoid plate. It supports the medial end of cartilaginous part of auditory tube.
   b. The lower part of the posterior border and the pterygoid hamulus give origin to the superior constrictor of the pharynx.
   c. The upper part of the posterior border is notched by the *auditory* tube.
   d. The pterygomandibular raphe is attached to the tip of the *pterygoid hamulus* at one end and to the mandible behind 3rd molar tooth at the other end.
   e. The pterygospinous process which is present at the middle of medial pterygoid plate gives attachment to the ligament of same name.

5 The attachments on the lateral pterygoid plate are as follows.
   a. Its lateral surface gives origin to the larger lower head of lateral pterygoid muscle (Fig. 9.14).
   b. Its medial surface gives origin to the deep head of the medial pterygoid. The small, superficial head of this muscle arises from the *maxillary tuberosity* and the adjoining part of the pyramidal process of the palatine bone (Fig. 9.14).

6 The infratemporal surface of the greater wing of the sphenoid gives origin to the upper head of the lateral pterygoid muscle, and is crossed by the deep temporal and masseteric nerves.

7 The *spine* of the *sphenoid is related laterally* to the *auriculotemporal nerve*, and *medially to the chorda tympani nerve* and *auditory tube* (Fig. 9.11c).
   Its *tip* provides attachment to the (i) sphenomandibular ligament, (ii) anterior ligament of malleus, and (iii) pterygospinous ligament.
   Its *anterior aspect* gives origin to the most posterior fibres of the tensor veli palatini and tensor tympani muscles.

8 The inferior surface of petrous temporal bone gives origin to the levator veli palatini (Fig. 9.14).

9 The margins of the foramen magnum provide attachment to:
   a. The anterior atlanto-occipital membrane, anteriorly (*see* Fig. 17.5d).
   b. The posterior atlanto-occipital membrane, posteriorly.
   c. The alar ligaments on the roughened medial surface of each occipital condyle (*see* Fig. 17.6).

10 The ligamentum nuchae is attached to the external occipital protuberance and crest.

11 The rectus capitis lateralis is inserted into the inferior surface of the jugular process of the occipital bone (Fig. 9.14).

12 The following are attached to the squamous part of the occipital bone (Fig. 9.14).
   - The area between the superior and inferior nuchal lines provides insertion medially to the semispinalis capitis, and laterally to the superior oblique muscle.
   - The area below the inferior nuchal line provides insertion medially to the rectus capitis posterior minor, and laterally to the rectus capitis posterior major (Fig. 9.14).

13 The mastoid notch gives origin to the posterior belly of digastric muscle (Fig. 9.14).

Structures Passing through Foramina

1 Each *incisive foramen* transmits:
   a. The terminal parts of the *greater palatine vessels* from the palate to the nose.
   b. The terminal part of the *nasopalatine nerve* from the nose to the palate (Fig. 9.11a).

2 The *greater palatine foramen* transmits:
   a. The *greater palatine vessels* (Fig. 9.12).
   b. The *anterior palatine nerve*, both of which run forwards in the groove that passes forwards from the foramen.

3 The *lesser palatine foramina* transmit the *middle* and *posterior palatine nerves*.

4 The *palatinovaginal canal* transmits:
   a. A *pharyngeal branch* from the *pterygopalatine ganglion* (see Fig. 23.16a).
   b. A small *pharyngeal branch* of the *maxillary artery.*
5 The *vomerovaginal canal* (if patent) transmits branches of the *pharyngeal branch* from pterygopalatine ganglion and vessels.
6 The *foramen ovale* transmits (mnemonic—**MALE**)
   a. The ***m**andibular nerve* (Fig. 9.11a)
   b. The ***a**ccessory meningeal artery*
   c. The ***l**esser petrosal nerve*
   d. An ***e**missary vein* connecting the cavernous sinus with the pterygoid plexus of veins.
   e. Anterior trunk of middle meningeal vein (occasionally).
7 The *foramen spinosum* transmits the *middle* meningeal artery (Fig. 9.11a), the meningeal branch of the mandibular nerve or nervus spinosus, and the posterior trunk of the middle meningeal vein.
8 The *emissary sphenoidal foramen* (foramen of Vesalius) transmits an *emissary vein* connecting the cavernous sinus with the pterygoid plexus of veins.
9 When present the *canaliculus innominatus* transmits the lesser petrosal nerve (in place of foramen ovale).
10 The *carotid canal* transmits the *internal carotid artery,* and the *venous* and *sympathetic plexuses* around the artery (Fig. 9.11a).
11 The structures passing through the *foramen lacerum:* During life, the lower part of the foramen is filled with cartilage, and no significant structure passes through the whole length of the canal, except for the meningeal branch of the ascending pharyngeal artery and an emissary vein from the cavernous sinus.
   However, the upper part of the foramen is traversed by the internal carotid artery with venous and sympathetic plexuses around it. In the anterior part of the foramen, the *greater petrosal nerve* unites with *the deep petrosal nerve* to form the *nerve of the pterygoid canal* (Vidian's nerve) which leaves the foramen by entering the pterygoid canal in the anterior wall of the foramen lacerum (Figs 9.15a and b).
12 The medial end of the *petrotympanic fissure* (Fig. 9.11a) transmits the chorda tympani nerve, anterior ligament of malleus and the anterior tympanic artery.
13 The *foramen magnum* (Fig. 9.16a) transmits the following.
   Through the narrow anterior part:
   a. Apical ligament of dens
   b. Vertical band of cruciate ligament
   c. Membrana tectoria
   Through wider posterior part:
   a. Lowest part of medulla oblongata
   b Three meninges.
   Through the subarachnoid space pass:
   a. Spinal accessory nerves
   b. Vertebral arteries
   c. Sympathetic plexus around the vertebral arteries
   d. Posterior spinal arteries
   e. Anterior spinal artery.
14 The *hypoglossal* or *anterior condylar* canal transmits the *hypoglossal nerve,* the *meningeal branch* of the hypoglossal nerve (These are the sensory fibres of first cervical spinal nerve supplying the dura mater of posterior cranial fossa.), the *meningeal branch* of the ascending pharyngeal artery, and an *emissary vein* connecting the sigmoid sinus with the internal jugular vein (Table 9.1).
15 The *posterior condylar canal* transmits an emissary vein connecting the sigmoid sinus with suboccipital venous plexus (Table 9.1).

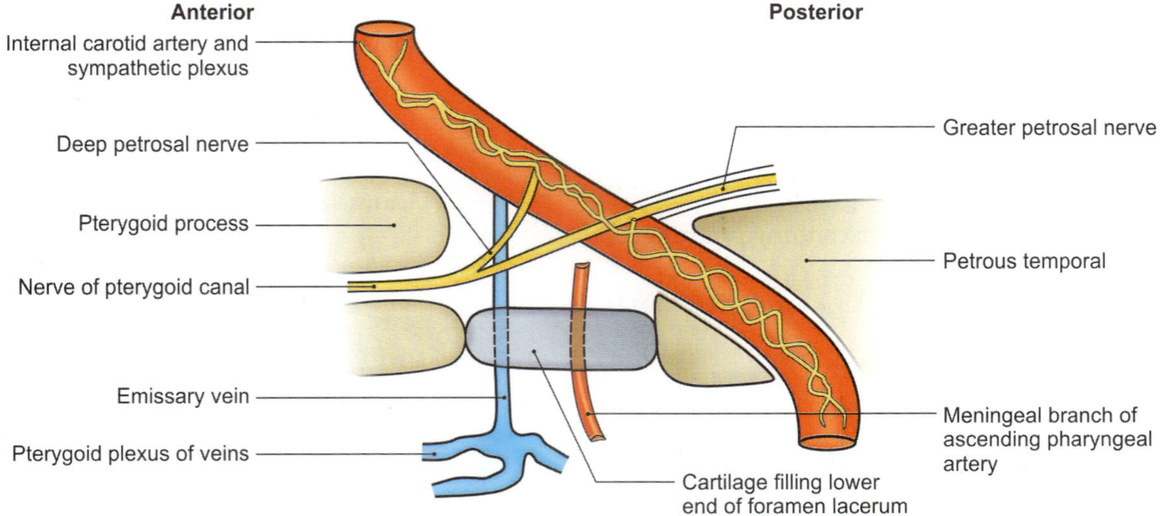

Fig. 9.15a: Structures related to the foramen lacerum

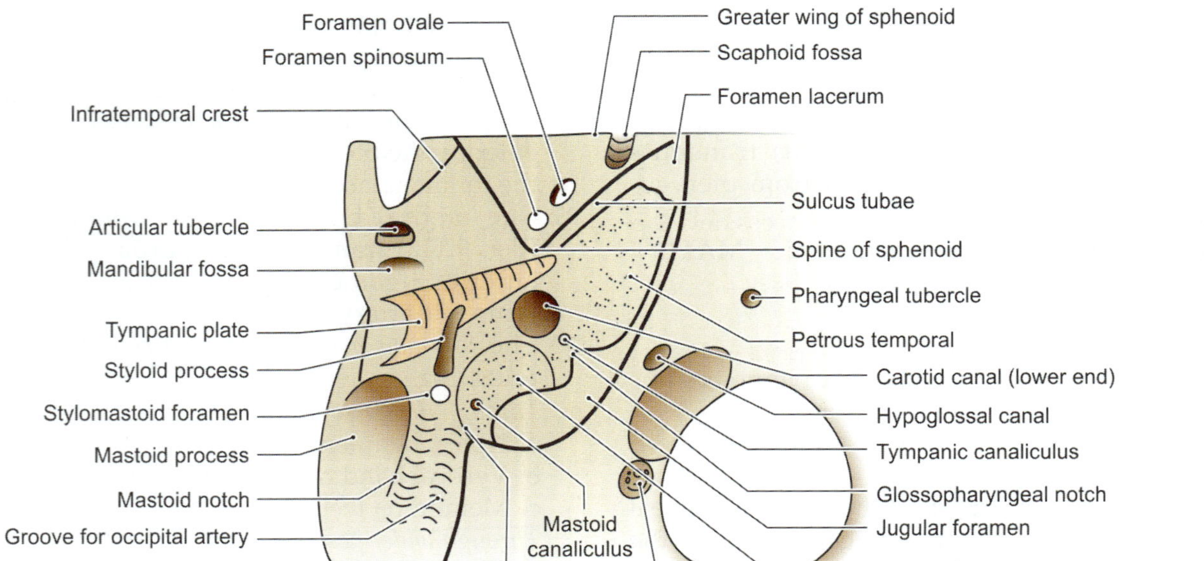

Fig. 9.15b: Portion of right norma basalis showing foramina of middle and posterior parts

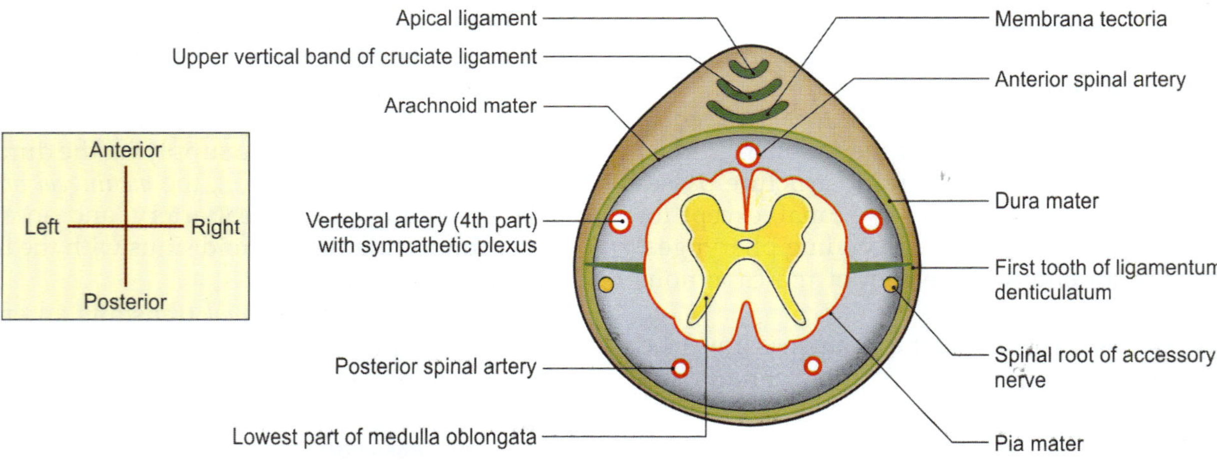

Fig. 9.16a: Structures passing through foramen magnum

16 The *jugular foramen* transmits the following structures:

i. *Through the anterior part:*
   a. Inferior petrosal sinus (Fig. 9.16b).
   b. Meningeal branch of the ascending pharyngeal artery.

ii. *Through the middle part*: IX, X and XI cranial nerves.

iii. *Through the posterior part:*
   a. Internal jugular vein (Fig. 9.11a).
   b. Meningeal branch of the occipital artery.

The glossopharyngeal notch near the medial end of the jugular foramen lodges the inferior ganglion of glossopharyngeal nerve.

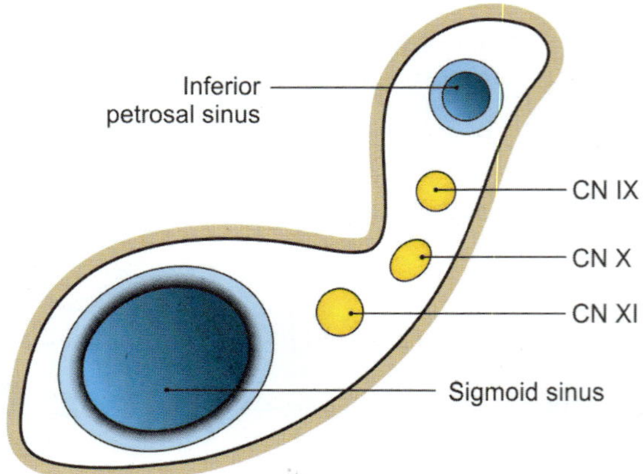

Fig. 9.16b: Jugular foramen (CN, cranial nerve)

17 The mastoid canaliculus (Arnold's canal) in the lateral wall of the jugular fossa transmits the auricular branch of the vagus (Arnold's nerve). The nerve passes laterally through the bone, crosses the facial canal, and emerges at the tympanomastoid fissure. The nerve is extracranial at birth, but becomes surrounded by bone as the tympanic plate and mastoid process develop (also called Alderman's nerve).
18 The *tympanic canaliculus* on the thin edge of partition between the jugular fossa and carotid canal transmits the tympanic branch of glossopharyngeal nerve (Jacobson's nerve) to the middle ear cavity.
19 The *stylomastoid foramen* transmits the facial nerve and the stylomastoid branch of the posterior auricular artery.

INTERIOR OF THE SKULL

Before beginning a systematic study of the interior, the following general points may be noted.

1 The cranium is lined internally by *endocranium* which is continuous with the pericranium through the foramina and sutures.
2 The *thickness* of the cranial vault is variable. The bones covered with muscles, i.e. temporal and posterior cranial fossae, are thinner than those covered with scalp. Further, the bones are thinner in females than in males, and in children than in adults.
3 Most of the cranial bones consist of:
   a. An *outer table* of compact bone which is thick, resilient and tough (Fig. 9.17b).
   b. An *inner table* of compact bone which is thin and brittle.
   c. The *diploe* which consists of spongy bone filled with red marrow, in between the two tables.

The skull bones derive their blood supply mostly from the meningeal arteries from inside and very little from the arteries of the scalp. Blood supply from the outside is rich in those areas where muscles are attached, e.g. the temporal fossa and the suboccipital region. The blood from the diploes is drained by four diploic veins on each side draining into venous sinuses (Table 9.2 and Fig. 9.17a).

Many bones, like *vomer* (Latin plowshare), pterygoid plates, do not have any diploe.

Table 9.2: Diploic veins

Vein	*Foramen*	*Drainage*
1. Frontal diploic vein	Supraorbital foramen	Drain into supraorbital vein
2. Anterior temporal or parietal diploic vein	In the greater wing of sphenoid	Sphenoparietal sinus or in anterior deep temporal vein
3. Posterior temporal or parietal diploic vein	Mastoid foramen	Transverse sinus
4. Occipital diploic vein (largest)	Foramen in occipital bone	Occipital vein or confluence of sinuses
5. Small unnamed diploic veins	Pierce inner table of skull close to the margins of superior sagittal sinus	Venous lacunae

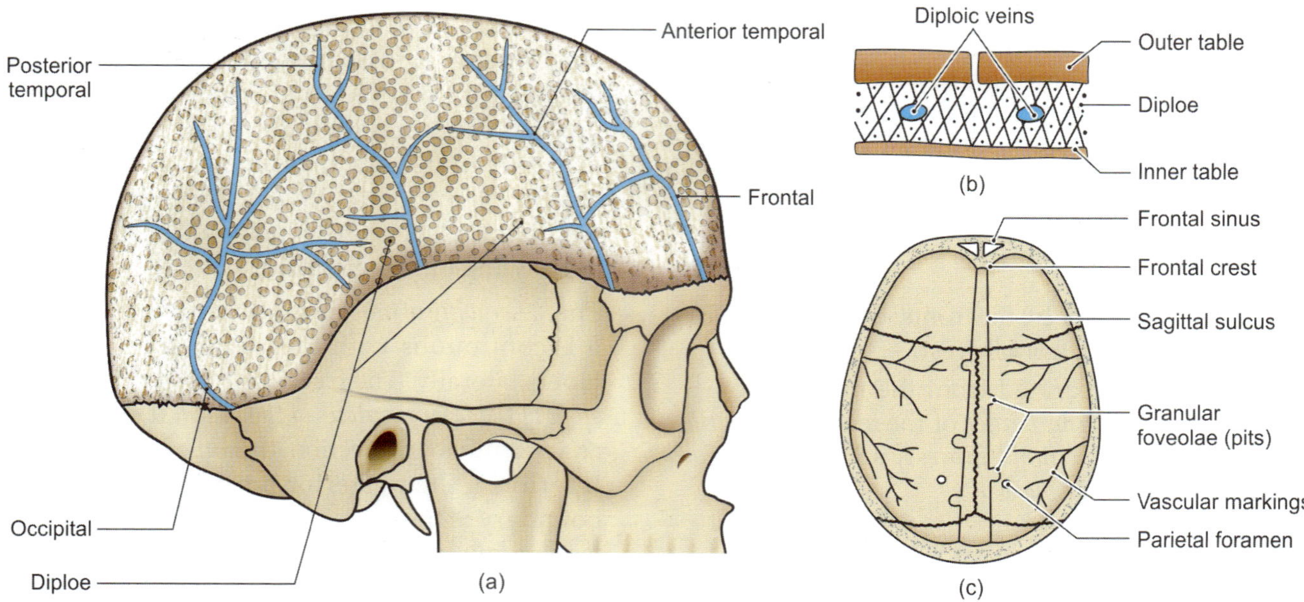

Figs 9.17a to c: (a) Diploic veins in an adult; (b) Section of cranial bone showing its structure; (c) Internal surface of the skull cap

INTERNAL SURFACE OF CRANIAL VAULT

The shape, the bones present, and the sutures uniting them have been described with the norma verticalis.

The following features may be noted.

a. The *inner table* is thin and brittle. It presents *markings* produced by meningeal vessels, venous sinuses, arachnoid granulations, and to some extent by cerebral gyri. It also presents raised ridges formed by the attachments of the dural folds.
b. The *frontal crest* lies anteriorly in the median plane. It projects backwards.
c. The *sagittal sulcus* runs from before backwards in the median plane. It becomes progressively wider posteriorly. It lodges the superior sagittal sinus.
d. The *granular foveolae* are deep, irregular, large, pits situated on each side of the sagittal sulcus. They are formed by arachnoid granulations. They are larger and more numerous in aged persons.
e. *Vascular markings:* The groove for the anterior branch of the middle meningeal artery, and the accompanying vein runs upwards 1 cm behind the coronal suture. Smaller grooves for the branches from the anterior and posterior branches of the middle meningeal vessels run upwards and backwards over the parietal bone (Fig. 9.17c).
f. The *parietal foramina* open near the sagittal sulcus 2.5 to 3.75 cm in front of the lambdoid suture (Fig. 9.2).
g. The *impressions for cerebral gyri* are less distinct. These become very prominent in cases of raised intracranial tension.

INTERNAL SURFACE OF THE BASE OF SKULL

The interior of the base of skull presents natural subdivisions into the anterior, middle and posterior cranial fossae. The dura mater is firmly adherent to the floor of fossae and is continuous with pericranium through the foramina and fissures (Fig. 9.18a).

Anterior Cranial Fossa (refer to BDC App)

Boundaries

Anteriorly and on the sides, by the frontal bone (Fig. 9.18b). In the median plane is frontal crest.

Posteriorly, it is separated from the middle cranial fossa by the free *posterior border* of the *lesser wing of the sphenoid,* the *anterior clinoid process,* and the *anterior margin of the sulcus chiasmaticus.*

Floor

In the median plane, it is formed anteriorly by the *cribriform plate of the ethmoid bone,* and posteriorly by the superior surface of the anterior part of the body of the sphenoid or *jugum sphenoidale.*

On each side, the floor is formed mostly by the *orbital plate of the frontal bone,* and is completed posteriorly by the lesser wing of the sphenoid.

Other Features

1 The *cribriform plate of the ethmoid bone* separates the anterior cranial fossa from the nasal cavity. It is quadrilateral in shape (Fig. 9.18a).

   a. *Anterior* margin articulates with the frontal bone at the *frontoethmoidal suture* which is marked in the median plane by the *foramen caecum.* This foramen is usually blind, but is occasionally patent.
   b. *Posterior margin* articulates with the jugum sphenoidale. At the posterolateral corners, we see the *posterior ethmoidal canals.*
   c. Its *lateral margins* articulate with the orbital plate of the frontal bone: The suture between them presents the *anterior ethmoidal canal* placed behind the crista galli (Fig. 9.18a).

   Anteriorly, the cribriform plate has a midline projection called the *crista galli* (Latin *cock's comb).* On each side of the crista galli, there are foramina through which the *anterior ethmoidal nerve and vessels* pass to the nasal cavity. The plate is also perforated by *numerous foramina* for the passage of olfactory nerve rootlets.

2 The *jugum sphenoidale* separates the anterior cranial fossa from the sphenoidal sinuses.

3 The *orbital plate of the frontal bone* separates the anterior cranial fossa from the orbit. It supports the orbital surface of the frontal lobe of the brain, and presents reciprocal impressions. The *frontal air sinus* may extend into its anteromedial part. The *medial margin* of the plate covers the labyrinth of the ethmoid; and the *posterior margin* articulates with the lesser wing of the sphenoid.

4 The *lesser wing of the sphenoid* is broad medially where it is continuous with the jugum sphenoidale and tapers laterally. The free *posterior border* fits into the *stem of the lateral sulcus of the brain.* It ends medially as a prominent projection, the *anterior clinoid process.* Inferiorly, the posterior border forms the upper boundary of the *superior orbital fissure.* Medially, the lesser wing is connected to the body of the sphenoid by *anterior and posterior roots,* which enclose the *optic canal.*

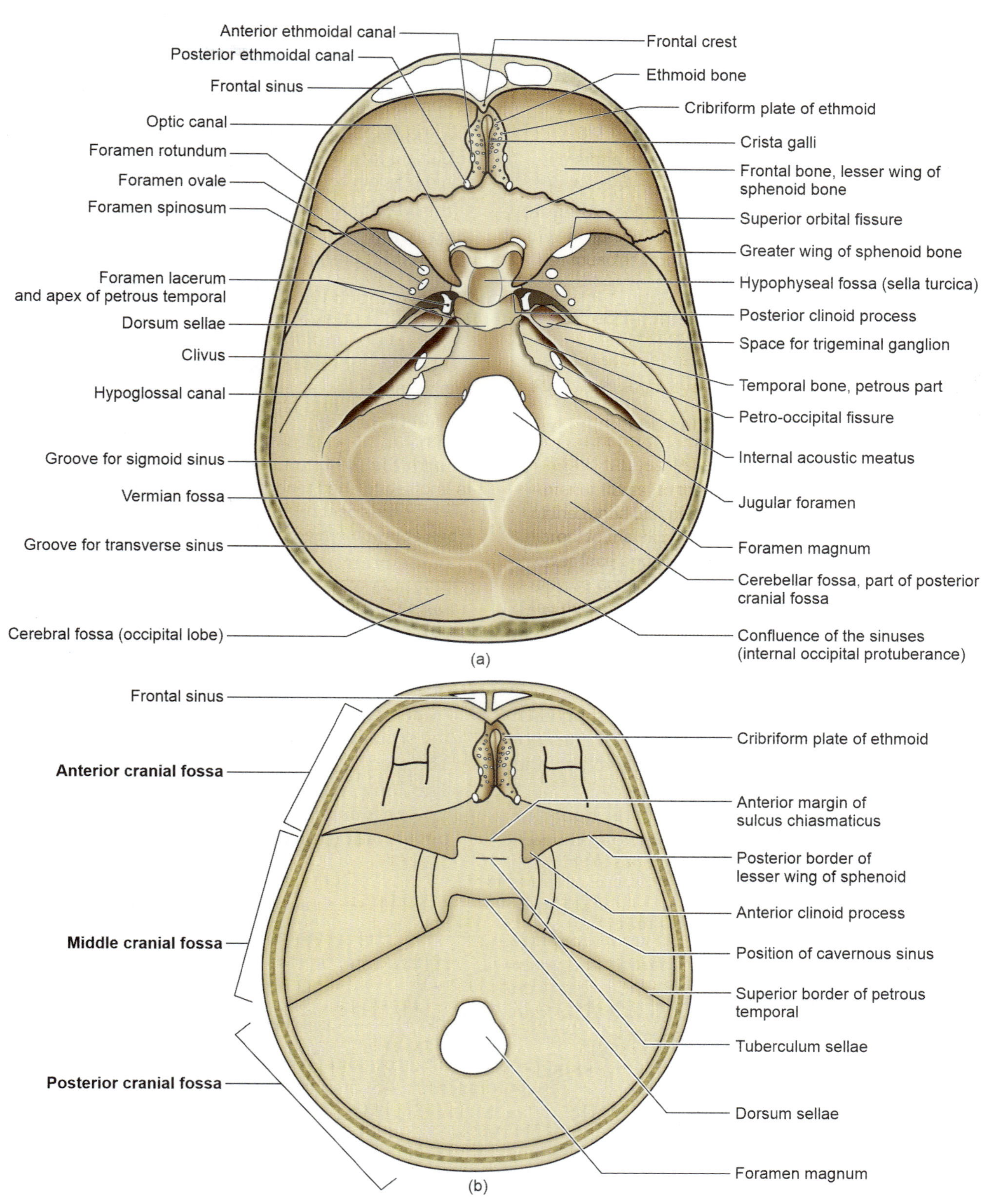

Figs 9.18a and b: (a) All three cranial fossae; (b) Divisions of skull into three fossae

CLINICAL ANATOMY

Fracture of the anterior cranial fossa may cause bleeding and discharge of cerebrospinal fluid through the nose. It may also cause a condition called *black eye* which is produced by seepage of blood into the eyelid, as frontalis muscle has no bony origin (*see* Fig. 10.8).

Middle Cranial Fossa (refer to BDC App)

It is deeper than the anterior cranial fossa, and is shaped like a butterfly, being narrow and shallow in the middle; and wide and deep on each side.

Boundaries

Anterior

1 Posterior border of the lesser wing of the sphenoid
2 Anterior clinoid process
3 Anterior margin of the sulcus chiasmaticus

Posterior

1 Superior border of the petrous temporal bone
2 The dorsum sellae of the sphenoid

Lateral

1 Greater wing of the sphenoid
2 Anteroinferior angle of the parietal bone
3 The squamous temporal bone

Floor

Floor is formed by body of sphenoid in the median region and by greater wing of sphenoid, squamous temporal and anterior surface of petrous temporal on each side.

Other Features

Median area: The body of the sphenoid presents the following features.

1 The *sulcus chiasmaticus* or *optic groove* leads, on each side, to the optic canal. The optic chiasma does not occupy the sulcus, it lies at a higher level well behind the sulcus.
2 The *optic canal* leads to the orbit. It is bounded laterally by the lesser wing of the sphenoid, in front and behind by the two roots of the lesser wing, and medially by the body of sphenoid.
3 *Sella turcica* (pituitary fossa or hypophyseal fossa): The upper surface of the body of the sphenoid is hollowed out in the form of a Turkish saddle, and is known as the *sella turcica*. It consists of the *tuberculum sellae* in front, the *hypophyseal fossa* in the middle and the *dorsum sellae* behind (Fig. 9.19).

The *tuberculum sellae* separates the optic groove from the *hypophyseal fossa*. Its lateral ends form the *middle clinoid process* which may join the anterior clinoid process.

The *hypophyseal fossa* lodges the hypophysis cerebri. Beneath the floor of fossa lie the sphenoidal air sinuses.

The *dorsum sellae* is a transverse plate of bone projecting upwards; it forms the back of the saddle. The superolateral angles of the dorsum sellae are expanded to form the *posterior clinoid processes.*

Lateral area

1 The lateral area is deep and lodges the temporal lobe of the brain.
2 It is related anteriorly to the orbit, laterally to the temporal fossa, and inferiorly to the infratemporal fossa.
3 The *superior orbital fissure* opens anteriorly into the orbit. It is *bounded* above by the lesser wing, below by the greater wing, and medially by the body of the sphenoid (*see* Fig. 21.4).
The medial end is wider than the lateral.
The long axis of the fissure is directed laterally, upwards and forwards. The lower border is marked by a small projection, which provides attachment

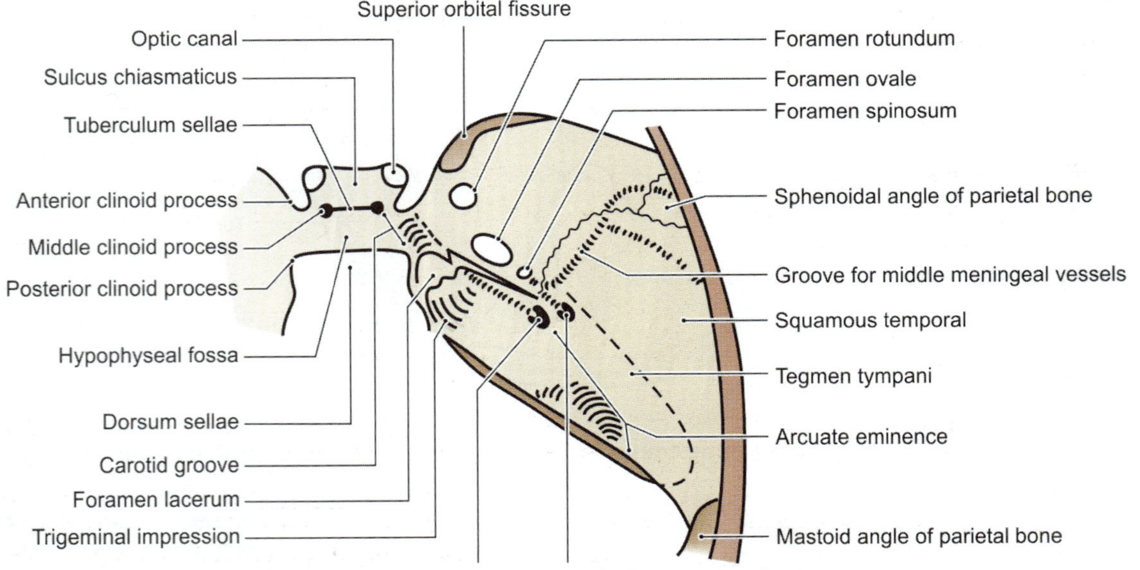

Fig. 9.19: Features of the middle cranial fossa

to the *common tendinous ring of Zinn*. The ring divides the fissure into three parts.

4 The *greater wing of the sphenoid* presents the following features.
   a. The *foramen rotundum* leads anteriorly to the pterygopalatine fossa containing pterygopalatine ganglia (*see* Fig. 23.15).
   b. The *foramen ovale* lies posterolateral to the foramen rotundum and lateral to the lingula. It leads inferiorly to the infratemporal fossa (Figs 9.18a and 9.19).
   c. The *foramen spinosum* lies posterolateral to the foramen ovale. It also leads, inferiorly, to the infratemporal fossa (Figs 9.18a and 9.19).
   d. The *emissary sphenoidal foramen* or foramen of Vesalius carries an emissary vein.

5 The *foramen lacerum* lies at the posterior end of the carotid groove, posteromedial to the foramen ovale.

6 The *anterior surface of the petrous temporal bone* presents the following features.
   a. The *trigeminal impression* lies near the apex, behind the foramen lacerum. It lodges the trigeminal ganglion within its dural cave (*see* Fig. 20.4).
   b. The *hiatus and groove for the greater petrosal nerve* are present lateral to the trigeminal impression. They lead to the foramen lacerum (Fig. 9.36).
   c. The *hiatus* and *groove for the lesser petrosal nerve* lie lateral to the hiatus for the greater petrosal nerve. They lead to the foramen ovale or to canaliculus innominatus to relay in otic ganglion (Fig. 9.36).
   d. Still more laterally there is the *arcuate eminence* produced by the superior semicircular canal.
   e. The *tegmen tympani* is a thin plate of bone anterolateral to the arcuate eminence. It forms a continuous sloping roof for the tympanic antrum, for the tympanic cavity and for the canal for the tensor tympani.

   The lateral margin of the tegmen tympani is turned downwards, it forms the lateral wall of the bony auditory tube.

   Its lower edge is seen in the squamotympanic fissure and divides it into the petrosquamous and petrotympanic fissures.

7 The *cerebral surface of the squamous temporal bone* is concave. It shows impressions for the temporal lobe and grooves for branches of the middle meningeal vessels.

CLINICAL ANATOMY

Fracture of the middle cranial fossa produces:
a. Bleeding and discharge of CSF through the ear.
b. Bleeding through the nose or mouth may occur due to involvement of the sphenoid bone.
c. The seventh and eighth cranial nerves may be damaged, if the fracture also passes through the internal acoustic meatus. If a semicircular canal is damaged, vertigo may occur.

Posterior Cranial Fossa (refer to BDC App)

This is the largest and deepest of the three cranial fossae. The posterior cranial fossa contains the *hindbrain* which consists of the *cerebellum behind and the pons and medulla in front*.

Boundaries

Anterior

1 The superior border of the petrous temporal bone
2 The dorsum sellae of the sphenoid bone (Fig. 9.18a)

Posterior: Squamous part of the occipital bone.

On each side

1 Mastoid part of the temporal bone
2 The mastoid angle of the parietal bone

Floor

Median area

1 Sloping area behind the dorsum sellae or clivus in front
2 The foramen magnum in the middle
3 The squamous occipital behind

Lateral area

1 Condylar or lateral part of occipital bone
2 Posterior surface of the petrous temporal bone
3 Mastoid temporal bone
4 Mastoid angle of the parietal bone

Other Features

Median area

1 The *clivus* is the sloping surface in front of the foramen magnum. It is formed by fusion of the posterior part of the body of the sphenoid including the dorsum sellae with the basilar part of the occipital bone or basiocciput. It is related to the *basilar plexus of veins*, and supports the pons and medulla (Fig. 9.18a).

   On each side, the clivus is separated from the petrous temporal bone by the *petro-occipital fissure* which is grooved by the inferior petrosal sinus, and is continuous behind with the jugular foramen.

2 The *foramen magnum* lies in the floor of the fossa. The anterior part of the foramen is narrow because it is *overlapped* by the medial surfaces of the occipital condyles.

3 The *squamous part of the occipital bone* shows the following features.

a. The *internal occipital protuberance* lies opposite the external occipital protuberance. It is related to the confluence of sinuses, and is grooved on each side by the beginning of transverse sinuses.
b. The *internal occipital crest* runs in the median plane from the internal occipital protuberance to the foramen magnum where it forms a shallow depression, the *vermian fossa* (Fig. 9.20).
c. The *transverse sulcus* is quite wide and runs laterally from the internal occipital protuberance to the mastoid angle of the parietal bone where it becomes continuous with the sigmoid sulcus. The transverse sulcus lodges the *transverse sinus.* The right transverse sulcus is usually wider than the left and is continuous medially with the superior sagittal sulcus (Fig. 9.20).
d. On each side of the internal occipital crest, there are *deep fossae* which lodge the cerebellar hemispheres (Fig. 9.20).

Lateral area

1 The *condylar part of the occipital bone* is marked by the following.
   a. The *jugular tubercle* lies over the occipital condyle.
   b. The *hypoglossal canal* (anterior condylar canal) pierces the bone posteroanterior to the jugular tubercle and runs obliquely forwards and laterally along the line of fusion between the basilar and the condylar parts of the occipital bone.
   c. The *condylar canal* (posterior condylar canal) opens in the lower part of the sigmoid sulcus which indents the jugular process of occipital bone.
2 The *posterior surface of the petrous part of the temporal bone* forms the anterolateral wall of the posterior cranial fossa. The following features may be noted.
   a. The *internal acoustic meatus* opens above the anterior part of the jugular foramen. It is about 1 cm long and runs transversely in a lateral direction. It is closed laterally by a perforated plate of bone known as *lamina cribrosa* which separates it from the internal ear (Figs 9.18a and 9.20).
   b. The orifice of the *aqueduct of the vestibule* is a narrow slit lying behind the internal acoustic meatus.
   c. The *subarcuate fossa* lies below the arcuate eminence, lateral to the internal acoustic meatus.
3 The *jugular foramen* lies at the posterior end of the petro-occipital fissure. The upper margin is sharp and irregular, and presents the *glossopharyngeal notch.* The lower margin is smooth and regular.
4 The *mastoid part of the temporal bone* forms the lateral wall of the posterior cranial fossa just behind the petrous part of the bone. Anteriorly, it is marked by the *sigmoid sulcus* which begins as a downward continuation of the transverse sulcus at the mastoid angle of the parietal bone, and ends at the jugular foramen. The sigmoid sulcus lodges the *sigmoid sinus* which become the internal jugular vein at the jugular foramen (Figs 9.18a and 9.20). The sulcus is related anteriorly to the *tympanic antrum.* The *mastoid foramen* opens into the upper part of the sulcus.

CLINICAL ANATOMY

Fracture of the posterior cranial fossa causes bruising over the mastoid region extending down over the sternocleidomastoid muscle.

ATTACHMENTS AND RELATIONS: INTERIOR OF THE SKULL

Attachment on Vault

1 The frontal crest gives attachment to the falx cerebri (*see* Fig. 20.2).
2 The lips of the sagittal sulcus give attachment to the falx cerebri (*see* Fig. 20.2).

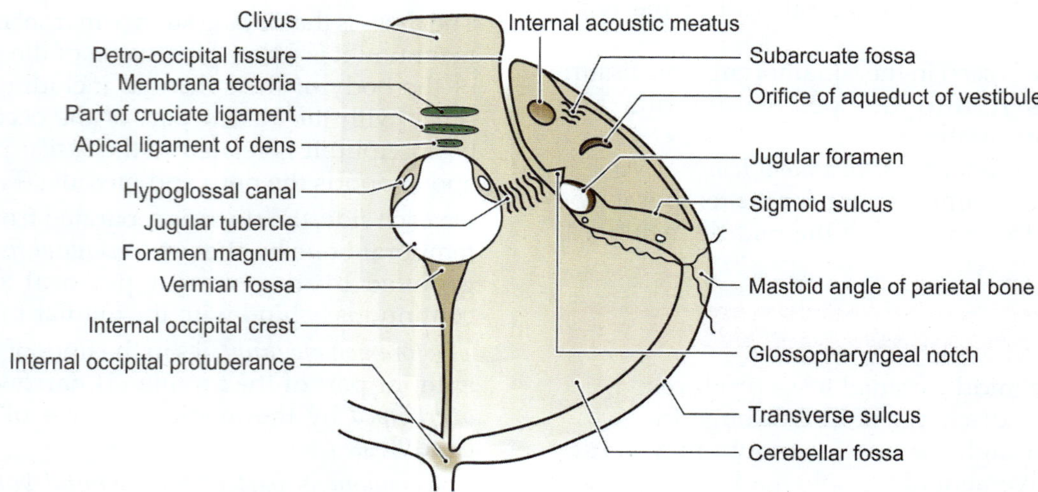

Fig. 9.20: Features of the posterior cranial fossa

Anterior Cranial Fossa

1 The crista galli gives attachment to the falx cerebri.
2 The orbital surface of the frontal bone supports the frontal lobe of the brain.
3 The anterior clinoid processes give attachment to the free margin of the tentorium cerebelli (*see* Fig. 20.3).

Middle Cranial Fossa

1 The middle cranial fossa lodges the *temporal lobe of the cerebral hemisphere.*
2 The tuberculum sellae provides attachment to the *diaphragma sellae* (*see* Fig. 20.5).
3 The hypophyseal fossa lodges the *hypophysis cerebri.*
4 Upper margin of the dorsum sellae provides attachment to the diaphragma sellae, and the posterior clinoid process to anterior end of the attached margin of tentorium cerebelli and to the petrosphenoidal ligament (*see* Fig. 20.3).
5 One *cavernous sinus* lies on each side of the body of the sphenoid. The internal carotid artery passes through the cavernous sinus (*see* Fig. 20.6).
6 The superior border of the petrous temporal bone is grooved by the *superior petrosal sinus* and provides attachment to the *attached margin of the tentorium cerebelli*. It is grooved in its medial part by the *trigeminal nerve* (trigeminal impression).

Posterior Cranial Fossa

1 The posterior cranial fossa contains the hindbrain which consists of the cerebellum behind, and the pons and medulla in front.
2 The lower part of the clivus provides attachment to the apical ligament of the dens near the foramen magnum, upper vertical band of cruciate ligament and to the *membrana tectoria* just above the apical ligament (Fig. 9.16a).
3 The internal occipital crest gives attachment to the falx cerebelli.
4 The jugular tubercle is grooved by the *ninth, tenth and eleventh cranial nerves* as they pass to the jugular foramen.
5 The subarcuate fossa on the posterior surface of petrous temporal bone lodges the *flocculus of the cerebellum.*

Structures Passing through Foramina

The following foramina seen in the cranial fossae have been dealt with under the norma basalis: Foramen ovale, foramen spinosum, emissary sphenoidal foramen, foramen lacerum, foramen magnum, jugular foramen, hypoglossal canal, and posterior condylar canal. Additional foramina seen in the cranial fossae are as follows.

1 The *foramen caecum* in the anterior cranial fossa is usually blind, but occasionally it transmits a vein from the upper part of nose to the superior sagittal sinus.
2 The *posterior ethmoidal canal* transmits the vessels of the same name. Note that the posterior ethmoidal nerve *does not pass* through the canal as it terminates earlier.
3 The *anterior ethmoidal canal* transmits the corresponding nerve and vessels.
4 The *optic canal* transmits the optic nerve and the ophthalmic artery.
5 The three parts of the *superior orbital fissure* (*see* Fig. 21.4) transmit the following structures.

   Lateral part
   a. Lacrimal nerve (Fig. 9.22a)
   b. Frontal nerve
   c. Trochlear nerve
   d. Superior ophthalmic vein

   Middle part
   e1 and e2. Upper and lower divisions of the oculomotor nerve (Table 9.4)
   f. Nasociliary nerve in between the two divisions of the oculomotor (Fig. 9.22a)
   g. The abducent nerve, inferolateral to the foregoing nerves (Fig. 9.22a)

   Medial part
   h. Inferior ophthalmic vein
   i. Sympathetic nerves from the plexus around the internal carotid artery
6 The *foramen rotundum* transmits the maxillary nerve (*see* Fig. 23.15).
7 The *internal acoustic meatus* transmits the *seventh and eighth cranial nerves* and the *labyrinthine vessels.*

PRINCIPLES GOVERNING FRACTURES OF THE SKULL

1 Fractures of the skull are prevented by:
   a. Its elasticity
   b. Rounded shape
   c. Construction from a number of secondary elastic arches, each made up of a single bone
   d. The muscles covering the thin areas.
2 Since the skull is an elastic sphere filled with the semifluid brain, a violent blow on the skull produces a *splitting effect* commencing at the site of the blow and tending to pass along the lines of least resistance.
3 The *base of the skull is more fragile* than the vault, and is more commonly involved in such fractures, particularly along the foramina.

4 The *inner table is more brittle* than the outer table. Therefore, fractures are more extensive on the inner table. Occasionally, only the inner table is fractured and the outer table remains intact.

5 The *common sites* of fracture in the skull are:

a. The *parietal area* of the vault

b. The *middle cranial fossa* of the base. This fossa is weakened by numerous foramina and canals.

The facial bones commonly fractured are:

a. The *nasal bone*

b. The *mandible*.

THE ORBIT

The orbits are pyramidal bony cavities, situated one on each side of the root of the nose. They provide sockets for rotatory movements of the eyeballs. They also protect the eyeballs (*refer to BDC App*).

Shape and Disposition

Each orbit resembles a four-sided pyramid. Thus, it has:

- *An apex* situated at the posterior end of orbit at the medial end of superior orbital fissure.
- *A base* seen as the orbital opening on the face.
- *Four walls*: Roof, floor, lateral and medial walls.

The long axis of the orbit passes backwards and medially. The medial walls of the two orbits are parallel and the lateral walls are set at right angles to each other (Fig. 9.21).

Roof

It is concave from side-to-side. It is formed:

1 Mainly by the orbital plate of the frontal bone.

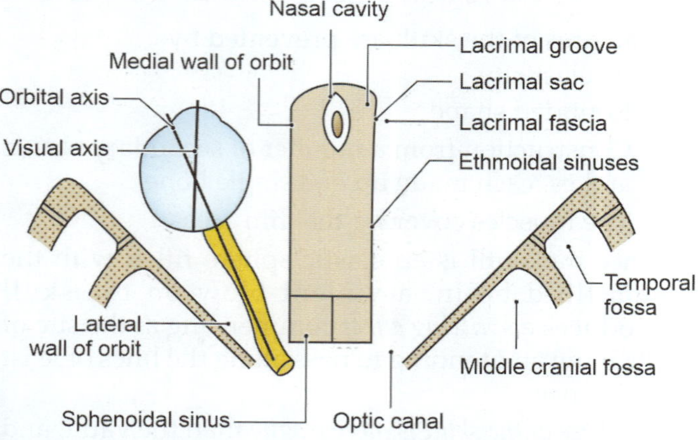

Fig. 9.21: Diagram comparing the orientation of the orbital axis and the visual axis

2 It is completed posteriorly by the lesser wing of the sphenoid (Fig. 9.22a).

Relations

1 It separates the orbit from the anterior cranial fossa.

2 The frontal air sinus may extend into its anteromedial part.

Named Features

1 The *lacrimal fossa,* placed anterolaterally, lodges the lacrimal gland (Fig. 9.22a).

2 The *optic canal* lies posteriorly, at the junction of the roof and medial wall (Figs 9.22a and b).

3 The *trochlear fossa* lies anteromedially. It provides attachment to the fibrous pulley or trochlea for the tendon of the *superior oblique muscle* (Fig. 9.22a).

Lateral Wall

This is the thickest and strongest of all the walls of the orbit. It is formed:

1 By the anterior surface of the greater wing of the sphenoid bone, posteriorly (Fig. 9.22b).

2 By the orbital surface of the frontal process of the zygomatic bone, anteriorly.

Relations

1 The greater wing of the sphenoid separates the orbit from the middle cranial fossa.

2 The zygomatic bone separates it from the temporal fossa.

Named Features

1 The *superior orbital fissure* occupies the posterior part of the junction between the roof and lateral wall.

2 The *foramen for the zygomatic nerve* is seen in the zygomatic bone.

3 *Whitnall's* or *zygomatic tubercle* is a palpable elevation on the zygomatic bone just within the orbital margin. It provides attachment to the lateral check ligament of eyeball (Fig. 9.22a).

Floor

It slopes upwards and medially to join the medial wall. It is formed:

1 Mainly by the orbital surface of the maxilla (Fig. 9.22b).

2 By the lower part of the orbital surface of the zygomatic bone, anterolaterally.

3 The orbital process of the palatine bone, at the posterior angle.

Relation

It separates the orbit from the maxillary sinus.

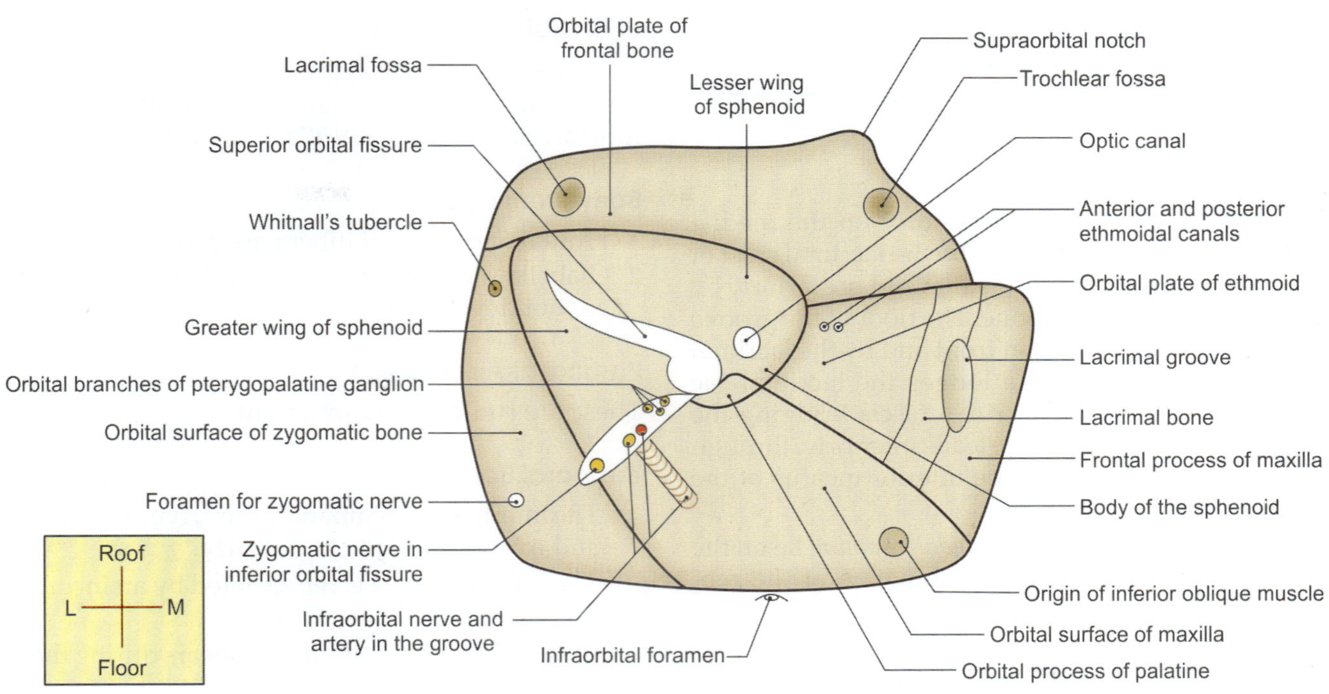

Fig. 9.22a: The orbit seen from the front (schematic)

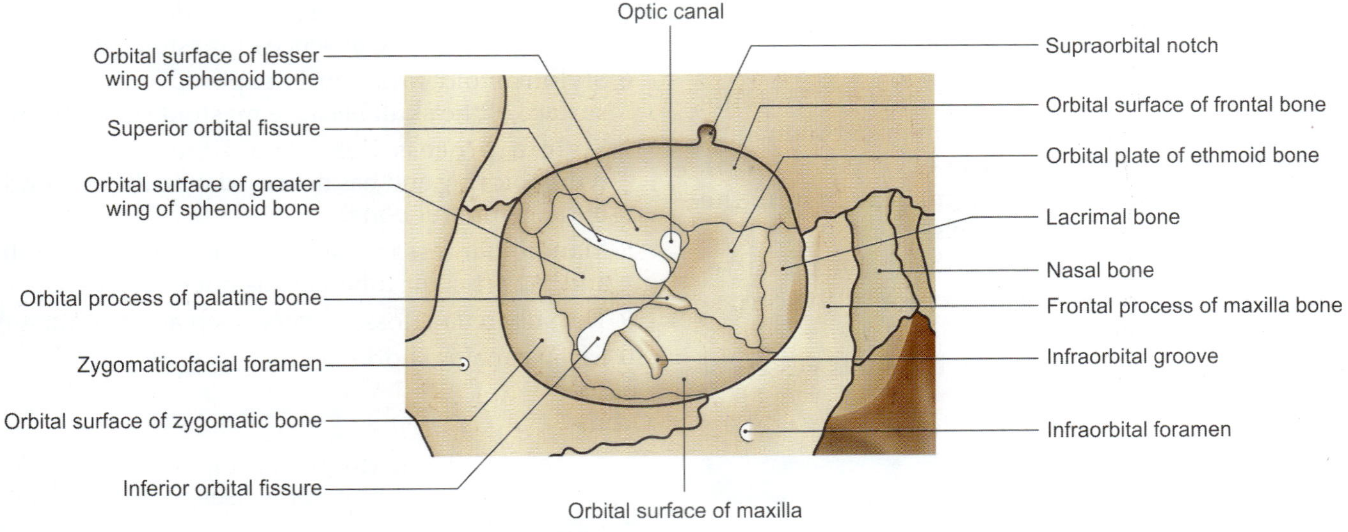

Fig. 9.22b: The orbit seen from the front

Named Features

1. The *inferior orbital fissure* occupies the posterior part of the junction between the lateral wall and floor. Through this fissure, the orbit communicates with the infratemporal fossa anteriorly and with the pterygopalatine fossa posteriorly (Figs 9.22a and b).
2. The *infraorbital groove* runs forwards in relation to the floor.
3. A small depression on anteromedial part of the floor gives origin to *inferior oblique muscle*.

Medial Wall

It is very thin. From before backwards, it is formed by:

1. The frontal process of the maxilla
2. The lacrimal bone (Fig. 9.22a)
3. The orbital plate of the ethmoid
4. The body of the sphenoid bone.

Relations

1. The *lacrimal groove*, formed by the maxilla and the lacrimal bone, separates the orbit from the nasal cavity.

2 The orbital plate of the ethmoid separates the orbit from the ethmoidal air sinuses.
3 The sphenoidal sinuses are separated from the orbit only by a thin layer of bone.

Named Features

1 The lacrimal groove lies anteriorly on the medial wall. It is bounded anteriorly by the lacrimal crest of the frontal process of the maxilla, and posteriorly by the crest of the lacrimal bone. The floor of the groove is formed by the maxilla in front and by the lacrimal bone behind. The groove lodges the lacrimal sac which lies deep to the lacrimal fascia bridging the lacrimal groove. The groove leads inferiorly, through the nasolacrimal duct, to the inferior meatus of the nose (*see* Fig. 10.22).
2 The *anterior and posterior ethmoidal foramina* lie on the frontoethmoidal suture, at the junction of the roof and medial wall.

Foramina in Relation to the Orbit

1 The structures passing through the optic canal and through the superior orbital fissure have been described in cranial fossae (*see* Fig. 21.4).
2 The *inferior orbital fissure* transmits:
   a. The *zygomatic nerve*,
   b. The *orbital branches of the pterygopalatine ganglion*,
   c. The *infraorbital nerve and vessels*, and the communication between the inferior ophthalmic vein and the pterygoid plexus of veins (Fig. 9.22a).
3 The *infraorbital groove and canal* transmit the corresponding nerve and vessels.
4 The *zygomatic foramen* transmits the zygomatic nerve.
5 The *anterior ethmoidal foramen* transmits the corresponding nerve and vessels.
6 *Posterior ethmoidal foramen* only transmits vessels of same name (Fig. 9.22a).

FOETAL SKULL/NEONATAL SKULL

DIMENSIONS

1 *Skull* is large in proportion to the other parts of skeleton.
2 *Facial skeleton* is small as compared to calvaria. In foetal skull, the facial skeleton is 1/7th of calvaria; in adults, it is half of calvaria. The facial skeleton is small due to rudimentary mandible and maxillae, non-eruption of teeth, and small size of maxillary sinus and nasal cavity. The large size of calvaria is due to precocious growth of brain.
3 *Base of the skull* is short and narrow, though internal ear is almost of adult size, the petrous temporal has not reached the adult length.

STRUCTURE OF BONES

The bones of cranial vault are smooth and unilamellar; there is no diploe. The tables and diploes appear by fourth year of age (Fig. 9.17a and Table 9.2).

Bony Prominences

1 Frontal and parietal tubera are prominent.
2 Glabella, superciliary arches and mastoid processes are not developed.

Paranasal Air Sinuses

These are rudimentary or absent.

Temporal Bone

1 The internal ear, tympanic cavity, tympanic antrum, and ear ossicles are of adult size.
2 The tympanic part is represented by an incomplete tympanic ring.
3 Mastoid process is absent, it appears during the later part of second year.
4 External acoustic meatus is short and straight. Its bony part is unossified and represented by a fibrocartilaginous plate.
5 Tympanic membrane faces more downwards than laterally due to the absence of mastoid process.
6 Stylomastoid foramen is exposed on the lateral surface of the skull because mastoid portion is flat.
7 Styloid process lies immediately behind the tympanic ring and has not fused with the remainder of the temporal bone.
8 Mandibular fossa is flat and placed more laterally, and the articular tubercle has not developed.
9 The subarcuate fossa is very deep and prominent.
10 Facial canal is short.

Orbits

These are large. The germs of developing teeth lies close to the orbital floor. Orbit comprises base or an outer opening with upper, lower, medial and lateral walls. Its apex lies at the optic foramen/canal. It also has superior and inferior orbital fissures.

OSSIFICATION

- Two halves of frontal bone are separated by metopic suture.
- The mandible is also present in two halves. It is a derivative of first branchial arch.
- Occipital bone is in four parts (squamous one, condylar two, and basilar one).

- The four bony elements of temporal bone are separate, except for the commencing union of the tympanic part with the squamous and petrous parts. The second centre for styloid process has not appeared.
- Unossified membranous gaps, a total of 6 fontanelles at the angles of the parietal bones are present (Fig. 9.3).
- Squamous suture between parietal and squamous temporal bones is present.

POSTNATAL GROWTH OF SKULL

The growth of calvaria and facial skeleton proceeds at different rates and over different periods. Growth of calvaria is related to growth of brain, whereas that of the facial skeleton is related to the development of dentition, muscles of mastication, and of the tongue. The rates of growth of the base and vault are also different.

Growth of the Vault

1 *Rate:* Rapid during the first year, and then it slows up to the seventh year when it is almost of adult size.

2 *Growth in breadth:* This growth occurs at the sagittal suture, sutures bordering greater wings, occipitomastoid suture, and the petro-occipital suture at the base.

3 *Growth in height*: This growth occurs at the frontozygomatic suture, pterion, squamosal suture, and asterion.

4 *Growth in anteroposterior diameter:* This growth occurs at the coronal and lambdoid sutures.

Growth of the Base

The base grows in anteroposterior diameter at three cartilaginous plates situated between the occipital and sphenoid bones, between the pre- and post-sphenoids, and between the sphenoid and ethmoid.

Growth of the Face

1 Growth of orbits and ethmoid is completed by seventh year.

2 In the face, the growth occurs mostly during first year, although it continues till puberty and even later.

Closure of Fontanelles

Anterior fontanelle (bregma) closes by 18 months, mastoid fontanelle by 12 months, posterior fontanelle (lambda) by 2–3 months and sphenoidal fontanelle also by 2–3 months (Fig. 9.3).

CLINICAL ANATOMY

- Fontanelles help to determine the age in 1–2 years of child.
- Help to know the intracranial pressure. In case of increased pressure, bulging is seen and in case of dehydration, depression is seen at the site of fontanelles.

Thickening of Bones

1 Two tables and diploe appear by fourth year. Differentiation reaches maximum by about 35 years, when the diploic veins produce characteristic marking in the radiographs.

2 Mastoid process appears during second year, and the mastoid air cells during sixth year.

Obliteration of Sutures of the Vault

1 Obliteration begins on the inner surface between 30 and 40 years, and on the outer surface between 40 and 50 years.

2 The timings are variable, but it usually takes place first in the lower part of the coronal suture, next in the posterior part of the sagittal suture, and then in the lambdoid suture.

In Old Age

The skull generally becomes thinner and lighter but in small proportion of cases, it increases in thickness and weight. The most striking feature is reduction in the size of mandible and maxillae due to loss of teeth and absorption of alveolar processes. This causes decrease in the vertical height of the face and a change in the angles of the mandible which become more obtuse.

SEX DIFFERENCES IN THE SKULL

There are no sex differences until puberty. The postpubertal differences are listed in Table 9.3.

Wormian or Sutural Bones

These are small irregular bones found in the region of the fontanelles, and are formed by additional ossification centres.

They are most common at the lambda and at the asterion; common at the pterion (epipteric bone); and rare at the bregma (Os Kerckring). Wormian bones are common in hydrocephalic skulls.

CRANIOMETRY

Cephalic Index

It expresses the shape of the head, and is the proportion of breadth to length of the skull. Thus:

Table 9.3: Sex differences in the skull

Features	Males	Females
1. Weight	Heavier	Lighter
2. Size	Larger	Smaller
3. Capacity	Greater in males	10% less than males
4. Walls	Thicker	Thinner
5. Muscular ridges, glabella, superciliary arches, temporal lines, mastoid processes, superior nuchal lines, and external occipital protuberance	More marked	Less marked
6. Tympanic plate	Larger and margins are more roughened	Smaller and margins are less roughened
7. Supraorbital margin	More rounded	Sharp
8. Forehead	Sloping (receding)	Vertical
9. Frontal and parietal tubera	Less prominent	More prominent
10. Vault	Rounded	Somewhat flattened
11. Contour of face	Longer due to greater depth of the jaws. Chin is bigger and projects more forwards. In general, the skull is more rugged due to muscular markings and processes; and zygomatic bones are more massive	Rounded, facial bones are smoother, and mandible and maxillae are smaller.

$$\text{Cephalic index} = \frac{\text{Breadth}}{\text{Length}} \times 100$$

The length or longest diameter is measured from the glabella to the occipital point, the breadth or widest diameter is measured usually a little below the parietal tubera.

Human races may be:

a. *Dolichocephalic* or long-headed when the index is 75 or less.
b. *Mesaticephalic* when the index is between 75 and 80.
c. *Brachycephalic* or short-headed or round-headed when the index is above 80.
d. Dolichocephaly is a feature of primitive races, like Eskimos, Negroes, etc.
e. Brachycephaly through mesaticephaly has been a continuous change in the advanced races, like the Europeans.

Facial Angle

This is the angle between two lines drawn from the nasion to the basion or anterior margin of foramen magnum and a line drawn from basion to the prosthion or central point on upper incisor alveolus (Fig. 9.9).

Facial angle is a rough index of the degree of development of the brain because it is the angle between facial skeleton, i.e. viscerocranium, and the calvaria, i.e. neurocranium, which are inversely proportional to each other. The angle is the smallest in the most evolved races of man, it is larger in lower races, and still larger in anthropoids.

Abnormal Crania

Oxycephaly or acrocephaly, tower-skull, or steeple-skull is an abnormally tall skull. It is due to premature closure of the suture between presphenoid and postsphenoid in the base, and the coronal suture in skull cap, so that the skull is very short anteroposteriorly. Compensation is done by the upward growth of skull for the enlarging brain.

Scaphocephaly or boat-shaped skull is due to premature synostosis in the sagittal suture, as a result the skull is very narrow from side-to-side but greatly elongated.

MANDIBLE

The *mandible*, or the lower jaw, is the largest and the strongest bone of the face. It develops from the *first pharyngeal arch*. It has a horseshoe-shaped body which lodges the teeth, and a *pair of rami* which project upwards from the posterior ends of the *body*. The rami provide attachment to the muscles of mastication (*refer to BDC App*).

BODY

Each half of the body has outer and inner surfaces, and upper and lower borders.

The *outer surface* presents the following features.

a. The *symphysis menti* is the line at which the right and left halves of the bone meet each other. It is marked by a faint ridge (Fig. 9.23a).
b. The *mental protuberance* (*mentum* = chin) is a median triangular projecting area in the lower part of the midline. The inferolateral angles of the protuberance form the *mental tubercles*.
c. The *mental foramen* lies below the interval between the premolar teeth (Table 9.4).
d. The *oblique line* is the continuation of the sharp anterior border of the ramus of the mandible. It runs downwards and forwards towards the mental tubercle.
e. The *incisive fossa* is a depression that lies just below the incisor teeth.

The *inner surface* presents the following features.

a. The *mylohyoid line* is a prominent ridge that runs obliquely downwards and forwards from below the third molar tooth to the median area below the genial tubercles (*see* below) (Fig. 9.23b).
b. Below the mylohyoid line, the surface is slightly hollowed out to form the *submandibular fossa*, which lodges the submandibular gland.
c. Above the mylohyoid line, there is the *sublingual fossa* in which the sublingual gland lies.
d. The posterior surface of the symphysis menti is marked by four small elevations called the *superior and inferior genial tubercles*.
e. The mylohyoid groove (present on the ramus) extends onto the body below the posterior end of the mylohyoid line.

The *upper or alveolar border* bears sockets for the teeth.

The *lower border* of the mandible is also called the *base*. Near the midline, the base shows an oval depression called the *digastric fossa*.

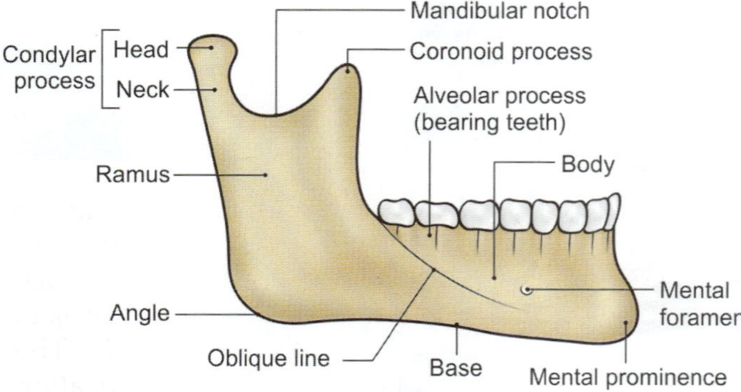

Fig. 9.23a: Outer surface of right half of the mandible

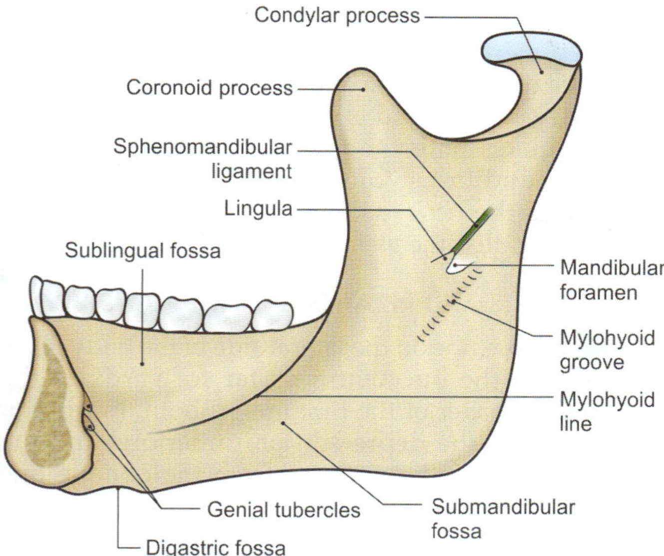

Fig. 9.23b: Inner surface of right half of the mandible

RAMUS

The ramus is quadrilateral in shape and has:

- Two surfaces—lateral and medial
- Four borders—upper, lower, anterior and posterior
- Two processes—coronoid and condyloid.

The *lateral surface* is flat and bears a number of oblique ridges.

The *medial surface* presents the following.

1. The *mandibular foramen* lies a little above the centre of ramus at the level of occlusal surfaces of the teeth. It leads into the *mandibular canal* which descends into the body of the mandible and opens at the *mental foramen* (Fig. 9.23b).
2. The anterior margin of the mandibular foramen is marked by a sharp tongue-shaped projection called the *lingula*. The lingula is directed towards the head or condyloid process of the mandible.
3. The *mylohyoid groove* begins just below the mandibular foramen, and runs downwards and forwards to be gradually lost over the submandibular fossa.

The *upper border* of the ramus is thin and is curved downwards forming the *mandibular notch*.

The *lower border* is the backward continuation of the base of the mandible. Posteriorly, it ends by becoming continuous with the posterior border at the *angle* of the mandible.

The *anterior border* is thin, while the *posterior border* is thick.

The *coronoid* (Greek crow's beak) *process* is a flattened triangular upward projection from the anterosuperior part of the ramus. Its anterior border is continuous with the anterior border of the ramus. The posterior border bounds the mandibular notch.

The *condyloid* (Latin knuckle like) *process* is a strong upward projection from the posterosuperior part of the ramus. Its upper end is expanded from side-to-side to form the *head*. The head is covered with fibrocartilage and articulates with the temporal bone to form the temporomandibular joint. The constriction below the head is the *neck*. Its anterior surface presents a depression called the *pterygoid fovea*.

ATTACHMENTS AND RELATIONS OF THE MANDIBLE

1 The oblique line on the lateral side of the body gives origin to the buccinator as far forwards as the anterior border of the first molar tooth. In front of this origin, the depressor labii inferioris and the depressor anguli oris arise from the oblique line below the mental foramen (Fig. 9.24).
2 The incisive fossa gives origin to the mentalis and mental slips of the orbicularis oris.
3 The parts of both the inner and outer surfaces just below the alveolar margin are covered by the mucous membrane of the mouth.
4 Mylohyoid line gives origin to the mylohyoid muscle (Fig. 9.23b).
5 Superior constrictor muscle of the pharynx arises from an area above the posterior end of the mylohyoid line.
6 Pterygomandibular raphe is attached immediately behind the third molar tooth in continuation with the origin of superior constrictor.
7 *Upper genial tubercle* gives origin to the genioglossus, and the *lower tubercle* to geniohyoid (Fig. 9.25).
8 Anterior belly of the digastric muscle arises from the digastric fossa (Fig. 9.25).
9 Deep cervical fascia (investing layer) is attached to the whole length of lower border.
10 The platysma is inserted into the lower border (Fig. 9.24).
11 Whole of the lateral surface of ramus except the posterosuperior part provides insertion to the masseter muscle (Fig. 9.24).
12 Posterosuperior part of the lateral surface is covered by the *parotid gland.*
13 Sphenomandibular ligament is attached to the lingula (Fig. 9.23b).
14 The medial pterygoid muscle is inserted on the medial surface of the ramus, on the roughened area below and behind the mylohyoid groove (Fig. 9.25).
15 The temporalis is inserted into the apex and medial surface of the coronoid process. The insertion extends downwards on the anterior border of the ramus (Fig. 9.24).
16 The lateral pterygoid muscle is inserted into the pterygoid fovea on the anterior aspect of the neck (Fig. 9.24).
17 The lateral surface of neck provides attachment to the lateral ligament of the temporomandibular joint (*see* Fig. 14.9).

FORAMINA AND RELATIONS TO NERVES AND VESSELS

1 The mental foramen transmits the *mental nerve and vessels* (Fig. 9.24).
2 The *inferior alveolar nerve and vessels* enter the *mandibular canal through the mandibular foramen*, and run forwards within the canal.
3 The *mylohyoid nerve and vessels* lie in the *mylohyoid groove* (Fig. 9.25).
4 The *lingual nerve* is related to the medial surface of the ramus in front of the mylohyoid groove (Fig. 9.25).
5 The area above and behind the mandibular foramen is related to the *inferior alveolar nerve and vessels* and to the *maxillary artery* (Fig. 9.25).

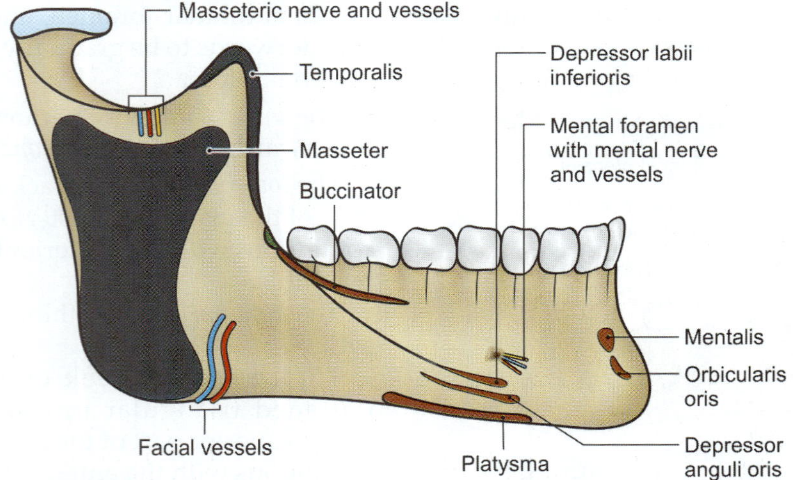

Fig. 9.24: Muscle attachments and relations of outer surface of the mandible

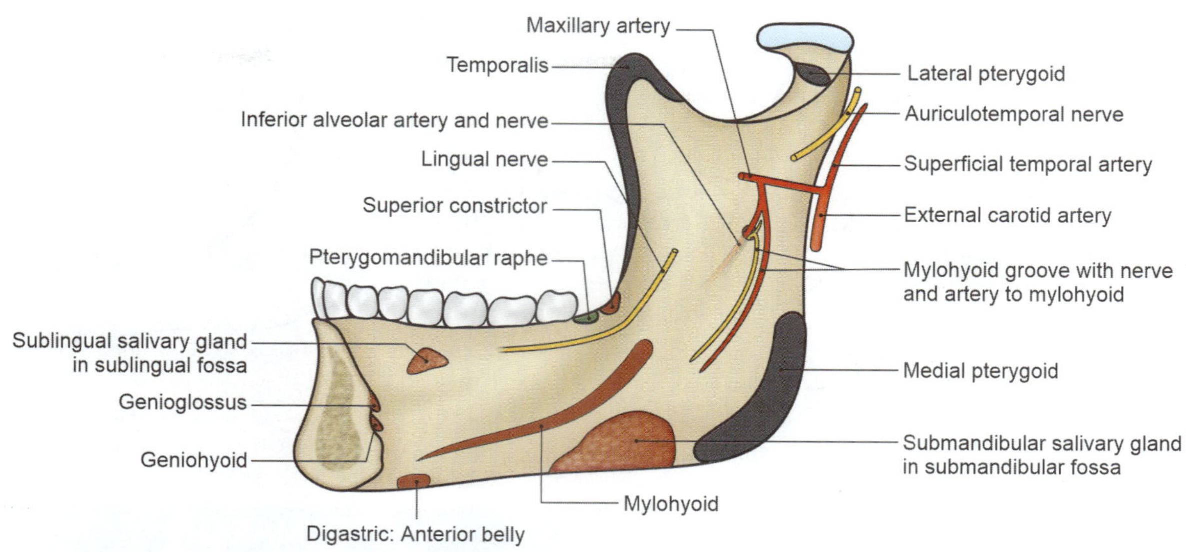

Fig. 9.25: Muscle attachments and relations of inner surface of the mandible

6 The *masseteric nerve and vessels* pass through the mandibular notch (Fig. 9.24).
7 The *auriculotemporal nerve* and *superficial temporal artery* are related to the medial side of the neck of mandible (Fig. 9.25).
8 Facial artery is palpable on the lower border of mandible at anteroinferior angle of masseter (Fig. 9.24).
9 Facial and maxillary arteries are not accompanied by respective nerves. The lingual nerve does not get company of its artery.

OSSIFICATION

The mandible is the *second bone, next to the clavicle, to ossify* in the body. Its greater part ossifies *in membrane*. The parts ossifying in *cartilage* include the *incisive part* below the incisor teeth, the *coronoid and condyloid processes*, and the *upper half of the ramus* above the level of the mandibular foramen.

Each half of the mandible ossifies from only one *centre* which appears at about the *sixth week* of intrauterine life in the mesenchymal *sheath of Meckel's cartilage* near the future mental foramen. Meckel's cartilage is the skeletal element of *first pharyngeal arch*.

At birth, the mandible consists of two halves connected at the *symphysis menti* by fibrous tissue. Bony union takes place during the first year of life.

AGE CHANGES IN THE MANDIBLE

In Infants and Children

1 The two halves of the mandible fuse during the first year of life (Fig. 9.26a).
2 At birth, the *mental foramen* opens below the sockets for the two deciduous molar teeth *near the lower border*. This is so because the bone is made up only of the alveolar part with teeth sockets. The *mandibular canal* runs near the lower border. The foramen and canal gradually shift upwards.
3 The angle is *obtuse*. It is 140° or more because the head is in line with the body. The coronoid process is large and projects upwards above the level of the condyle.

In Adults

1 The *mental foramen* opens midway between the upper and lower borders because the alveolar and sub-alveolar parts of the bone are equally developed. The mandibular canal runs parallel with the mylohyoid line.
2 The *angle* reduces to about 110° or 120° because the ramus becomes almost vertical (Fig. 9.26b).

In Old Age

1 Teeth fall out and the alveolar border is absorbed, so that the height of body is markedly reduced (Fig. 9.26c).
2 The *mental foramen* and the *mandibular canal* are close to the alveolar border.
3 The *angle* again becomes obtuse about 140° because the ramus is oblique.

STRUCTURES RELATED TO MANDIBLE

Salivary glands: Parotid, submandibular and sublingual (Figs 9.23a and b).

Lymph nodes: Parotid, submandibular and submental.

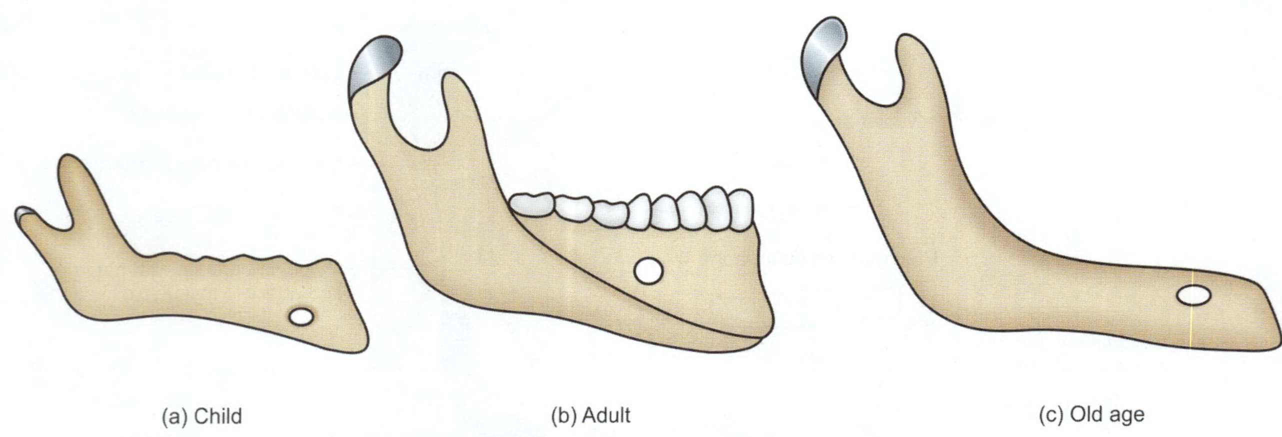

Figs 9.26a to c: Age changes in the mandible

Arteries: Maxillary, superficial temporal, masseteric, inferior alveolar, mylohyoid, mental and facial (Figs 9.24 and 9.25).

Nerves: Lingual, auriculotemporal, masseteric, inferior alveolar, mylohyoid and mental (Fig. 9.25).

Muscles of mastication: Insertions of temporalis, masseter, medial pterygoid and lateral pterygoid.

Ligaments: Lateral ligament of temporomandibular joint, stylomandibular ligament, sphenomandibular and pterygomandibular raphe.

CLINICAL ANATOMY

- The mandible is commonly fractured at the canine socket where it is weak (Fig. 9.27). Involvement of the inferior alveolar nerve in the callus may cause neuralgic pain, which may be referred to the areas of distribution of the buccal and auriculotemporal nerves. If the nerve is paralysed, the areas supplied by these nerves become insensitive.
- The next common fracture of the mandible occurs at the angle and neck of mandible (Fig. 9.27).

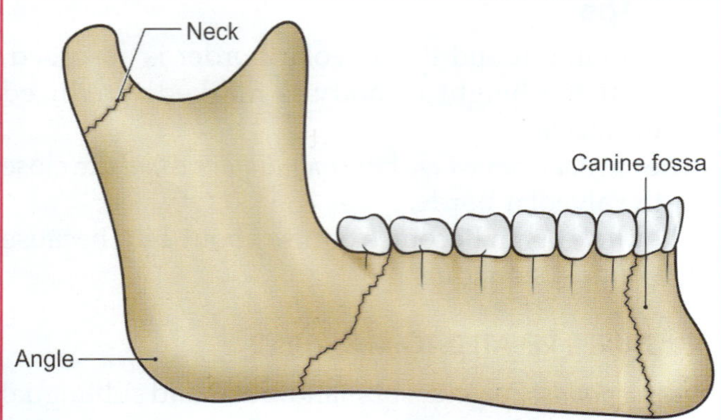

Fig. 9.27: Fracture of the mandible at the neck, at the angle and at canine fossa

MAXILLA

Maxilla (cheek) is the second largest bone of the face, the first being the mandible. The two maxillae form the whole of the upper jaw, and each maxilla forms a part each in the formation of face, nose, mouth, orbit, the infratemporal and pterygopalatine fossae.

SIDE DETERMINATION

1 Anterior surface ends medially into a deeply concave border, called the *nasal notch*. Posterior surface is convex (Fig. 9.28).
2 Alveolar border with sockets for upper teeth faces downwards with its convexity directed outwards. Frontal process is the longest process which is directed upwards.
3 Medial surface is marked by a large irregular opening, the *maxillary hiatus*/antrum of Highmore for maxillary air sinus.

FEATURES

Each maxilla has a body and four processes—the frontal, zygomatic, alveolar and palatine.

Body

The body of maxilla is pyramidal in shape, with its base directed medially at the nasal surface, and the apex pointing laterally at the zygomatic process. It has four surfaces and encloses a large cavity, the *maxillary sinus* described in Chapter 23.

The surfaces are:
- Anterior or facial,
- Posterior or infratemporal,
- Superior or orbital, and
- Medial or nasal.

Anterior or Facial Surface

1 Anterior surface is directed forwards and laterally.

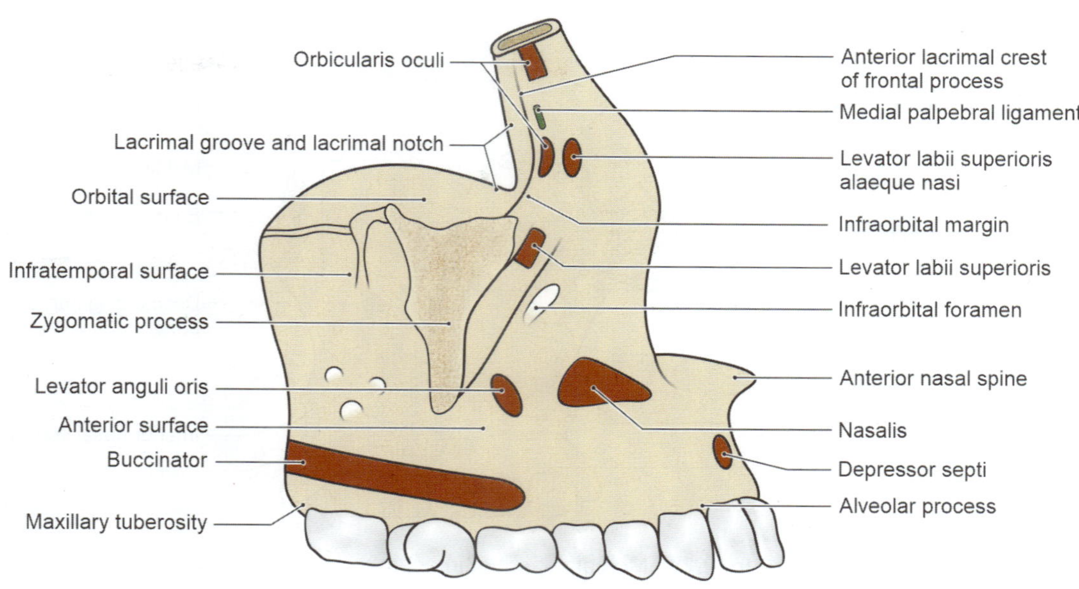

Fig. 9.28: Lateral aspect of maxilla with muscular attachments

2 Above the incisor teeth, there is a slight depression, the *incisive fossa,* which gives origin to depressor septi. Incisivus arises from the alveolar margin below the fossa, and the *nasalis* superolateral to the fossa along the nasal notch.

3 Lateral to canine eminence, there is a larger and deeper depression, the *canine fossa,* which gives origin to levator anguli oris.

4 Above the canine fossa, there is *infraorbital foramen,* which transmits *infraorbital nerve and vessels* (Fig. 9.28).

5 Levator labii superioris arises between the infraorbital margin and infraorbital foramen.

6 Medially, the anterior surface ends in a deeply concave border, the *nasal notch,* which terminates below into process which with the corresponding process of opposite maxilla forms the anterior nasal spine. Anterior surface bordering the nasal notch gives origin to nasalis and depressor septi.

Posterior or Infratemporal Surface

1 Posterior surface is convex and directed backwards and laterally.

2 It forms the anterior wall of *infratemporal fossa,* and is separated from anterior surface by the zygomatic process and a rounded ridge which descends from the process to the first molar tooth.

3 Near the centre of the surface open two or three *alveolar canals* for *posterior superior alveolar nerve and vessels.*

4 Posteroinferiorly, there is a rounded eminence, the *maxillary tuberosity,* which articulates superomedially with pyramidal process of palatine bone, and gives origin laterally to the superficial head of medial pterygoid muscle.

5 Above the maxillary tuberosity, the smooth surface forms anterior wall of *pterygopalatine fossa,* and is grooved by *maxillary nerve.*

Superior or Orbital Surface

1 Superior surface is smooth, triangular and slightly concave, and forms the greater part of the *floor of orbit.*

2 *Anterior border* forms a part of infraorbital margin. Medially, it is continuous with the lacrimal crest of the frontal process.

3 *Posterior border* is smooth and rounded, it forms most of the anterior margin of inferior orbital fissure. In the middle, it is notched by the infraorbital groove.

4 *Medial border* presents anteriorly the lacrimal notch which is converted into *nasolacrimal canal* by the descending process of lacrimal bone. Behind the notch, the border articulates from before backwards with the *lacrimal, labyrinth of ethmoid, and the orbital process of palatine bone* (Fig. 9.29).

5 The surface presents *infraorbital groove* leading forwards to *infraorbital canal* which opens on the anterior surface as *infraorbital foramen.* The groove, canal and foramen transmit the *infraorbital nerve and vessels.* Near the midpoint, the canal gives off laterally a branch, the *canalis sinuous,* for the passage of *anterior superior alveolar nerve and vessels.*

6 Inferior oblique muscle of eyeball arises from a depression just lateral to lacrimal notch at the anteromedial angle of the surface.

Medial or Nasal Surface

1 Medial surface forms a part of the *lateral wall of nose.*

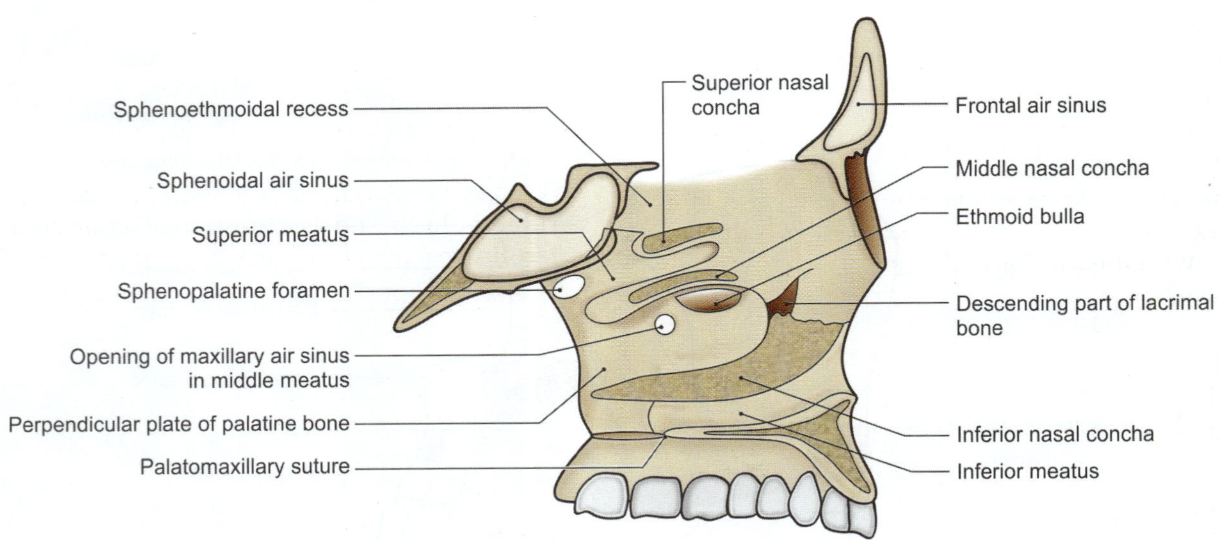

Fig. 9.29: Medial aspect of intact maxilla

2 *Posterosuperiorly*, it displays a large irregular opening of the maxillary sinus, the *maxillary hiatus* (Fig. 9.30).
3 Above the hiatus, there are *parts of air sinuses* which are completed by the ethmoid and lacrimal bones.
4 Below the hiatus, the smooth concave surface forms a part of *inferior meatus of nose*.
5 Behind the hiatus, the surface articulates with perpendicular plate of palatine bone, enclosing the *greater palatine canal* which runs downwards and forwards, and transmits *greater palatine vessels and the anterior, middle and posterior palatine nerves* (Fig. 9.12).
6 In front of the hiatus, there is *nasolacrimal groove*, which is converted into the nasolacrimal canal by articulation with the *descending process of lacrimal bone* and the *lacrimal process of inferior nasal concha*. The canal transmits *nasolacrimal duct to the inferior meatus of nose*.
7 More anteriorly, an oblique ridge forms the *conchal crest* for articulation with the inferior nasal concha.
8 Above the conchal crest, the shallow depression forms a part of the *atrium of middle meatus* of nose.

Processes of Maxilla

Zygomatic Process

The zygomatic process is a pyramidal lateral projection on which the anterior, posterior, and superior surfaces of maxilla converge. In front and behind, it is continuous with the corresponding surfaces of the body, but superiorly it is rough for articulation with the zygomatic bone.

Frontal Process

1 The frontal process projects upwards and backwards to *articulate* above with the nasal margin of frontal

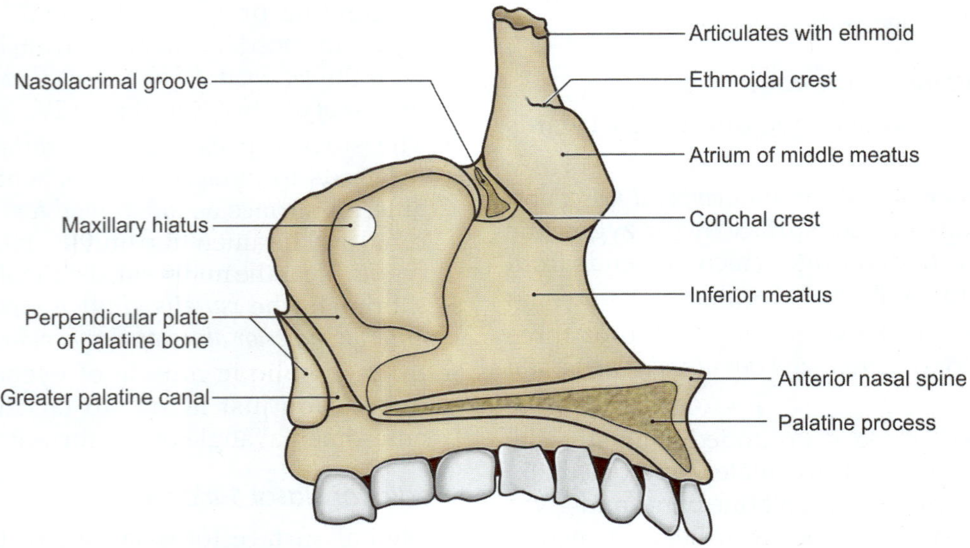

Fig. 9.30: Medial aspect of disarticulated left maxilla

bone, in front with nasal bone, and behind with lacrimal bone.

2 *Lateral surface* is divided by a vertical ridge, the *anterior lacrimal crest*, into a smooth anterior part and a grooved posterior part.

The lacrimal crest gives attachment to lacrimal fascia and the medial palpebral ligament, and is continuous below with the infraorbital margin.

The anterior smooth area gives origin to the orbital part of orbicularis oculi and levator labii superioris alaeque nasi. The posterior grooved area forms the anterior half of the floor of *lacrimal groove* (Fig. 9.45).

3 *Medial surface* forms a part of the lateral wall of nose. The surface presents following features:

a. Uppermost area is rough for articulation with ethmoid to close the anterior ethmoidal sinuses.

b. *Ethmoidal crest* is a horizontal ridge about the middle of the process. Posterior part of the crest articulates with middle nasal concha, and the anterior part lies beneath the agger nasi (*see* Fig. 23.8).

c. The area below the ethmoidal crest is hollowed out to form the atrium of the middle meatus.

d. Below the atrium is the *conchal crest* which articulates with inferior nasal concha.

e. Below the conchal crest, there lies the inferior meatus of the nose with nasolacrimal groove ending just behind the crest (*see* Fig. 23.8).

Alveolar Process

1 The alveolar process forms half of the alveolar arch, and bears sockets for the roots of upper 8 teeth. In adults, there are eight *sockets*: *Canine socket* is deepest; *molar sockets* are widest and divided into three minor sockets by septa; the *incisor and second premolar sockets* are single; and the *first premolar socket* is sometimes divided into two.

2 Buccinator arises from the posterior part of its outer surface up to the first molar tooth (Fig. 9.28).

3 A rough ridge, the *maxillary torus*, is sometimes present on the inner surface opposite the molar sockets.

Palatine Process

1 Palatine process is a thick horizontal plate projecting medially from the lowest part of the nasal surface. It forms a large part of the roof of mouth and the floor of nasal cavity (Fig. 9.30).

2 *Inferior surface* is concave, and the two palatine processes form anterior three-fourths of the bony palate. It presents numerous vascular foramina and pits for palatine glands.

Posterolaterally, it is marked by two anteroposterior grooves for the greater palatine vessels and anterior palatine nerves.

3 *Superior surface* is concave from side-to-side, and forms greater part of the floor of nasal cavity.

4 *Medial border* is thicker in front than behind. It is raised superiorly into the nasal crest.

Groove between the nasal crests of two maxillae receives lower border of vomer; anterior part of the ridge is high and is known as *incisor crest* which terminates anteriorly into the anterior nasal spine (Fig. 9.28).

Incisive canal traverses near the anterior part of the medial border.

5 *Posterior border* articulates with horizontal plate of palatine bone.

6 *Lateral border* is continuous with the alveolar process.

ARTICULATIONS OF MAXILLA

1 Superiorly, it articulates with three bones—the nasal, frontal and lacrimal.

2 Medially, it articulates with five bones—the ethmoid, inferior nasal concha, vomer, palatine and opposite maxilla.

3 Laterally, it articulates with one bone—the zygomatic.

OSSIFICATION

Maxilla ossifies in membrane from three centres, one for the maxilla proper, and two for os incisivum or *premaxilla*. The centre for maxilla proper appears above the canine fossa during sixth week of intrauterine life.

Of the two premaxillary centres, the main centre appears above the incisive fossa during seventh week of intrauterine life. The second centre (paraseptal or prevomerine) appears at the ventral margin of nasal septum during tenth week and soon fuses with the palatal process of maxilla. Though premaxilla begins to fuse with alveolar process almost immediately after the ossification begins, the evidence of premaxilla as a separate bone may persist until the middle decades.

AGE CHANGES

1 *At birth*:

a. The transverse and anteroposterior diameters are each more than the vertical diameter.

b. Frontal process is well marked.

c. Body consists of a little more than the alveolar process, the tooth sockets reaching to the floor of orbit.

d. Maxillary sinus is a mere furrow on the lateral wall of the nose.

2 *In the adult:* Vertical diameter is greatest due to development of the alveolar process and increase in the size of the sinus.

3 *In the old:* The bone reverts to infantile condition. Its height is reduced as a result of absorption of the alveolar process.

PARIETAL BONE

Two parietal bones form a large part of the roof and sides of vault of skull. Each bone is roughly quadrilateral in shape with its convexity directed outwards (Fig. 9.31).

SIDE DETERMINATION

Outer surface is convex and smooth, inner surface is concave and depicts vascular markings.

Anteroinferior angle is pointed and shows a groove for anterior division of middle meningeal artery.

FEATURES

Parietal bone has two surfaces, four borders, and four angles.

Surfaces

1 Outer convex
2 Inner concave (Fig. 9.32)

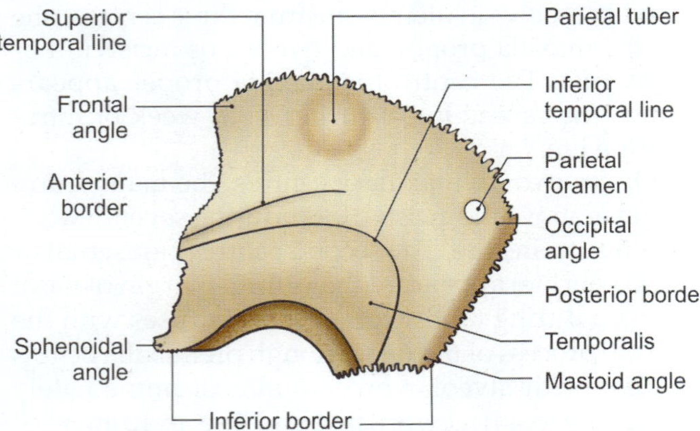

Fig. 9.31: Outer surface of left parietal bone

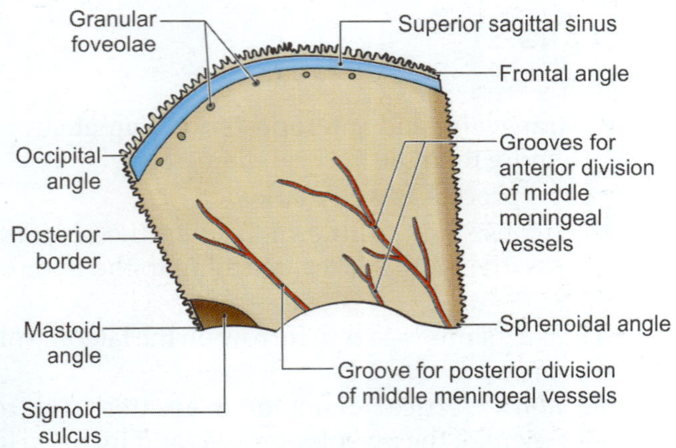

Fig. 9.32: Inner surface of left parietal bone

Borders

1 Superior or sagittal
2 Inferior or squamosal
3 Anterior or frontal
4 Posterior or occipital

Angles

1 Anterosuperior or frontal
2 Anteroinferior or sphenoidal
3 Posterosuperior or occipital
4 Posteroinferior or mastoid

At each of the four angles, are four fontanelles. These are:

1 One anterior fontanelle—closes at 18 months.
2 One posterior fontanelle—closes at 3 months
3 Two anterolateral or sphenoidal fontanelles—close at 3 months.
4 Two posterolateral or mastoid fontanelles—close at about 12 months of life.

Details can be studied from *norma verticalis* and *norma lateralis* and *inner aspect of skull cap*.

OCCIPITAL BONE

Single occipital bone occupies posterior and inferior parts of the skull (Fig. 9.33).

ANATOMICAL POSITION

It is concave forwards and encloses the largest foramen of skull, foramen magnum, through which cranial cavity communicates with the vertebral canal.

On each side of foramen magnum is the occipital condyle which articulates with atlas vertebra.

FEATURES

Occipital bone is divided into three parts:

1 Squamous part—above, below and behind foramen magnum.
2 Basilar part—lies in front of foramen magnum.
3 Condylar or lateral part—on each side of foramen magnum.

Squamous Part

Comprises two surfaces, three angles and four borders.

Surfaces: External convex surface and internal concave surface.

Angles: One superior angle and two lateral angles.

Borders: Two lambdoid borders in upper part and two mastoid borders in lower part.

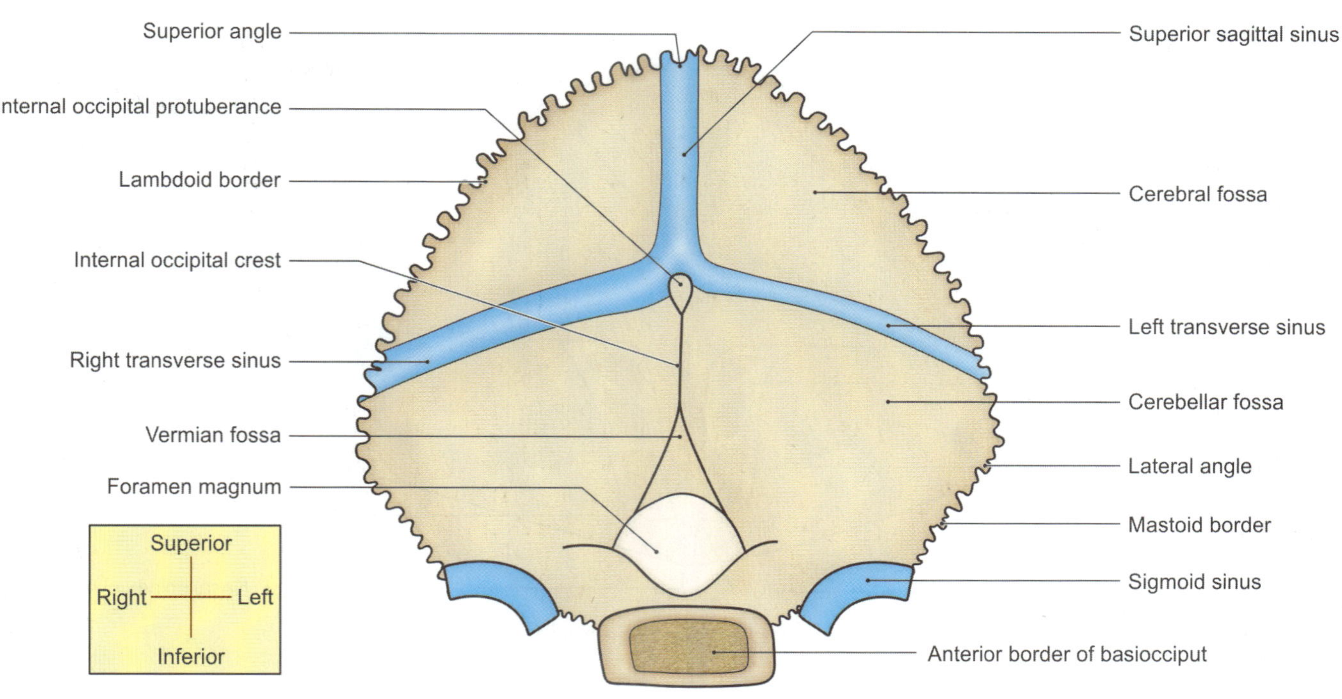

Fig. 9.33: Inner surface of occipital bone

Basilar Part

The basilar part of occipital bone is called basiocciput. It articulates with basisphenoid to form the base of skull. It is quadrilateral in shape and comprises two surfaces and four borders.

Surfaces are superior and inferior.

Borders are anterior, posterior and lateral, on each side.

Condylar Part

It comprises:
- Superior surface
- Inferior surface which shows occipital condyles and hypoglossal canal.

The details can be read from descriptions of *norma occipitalis* and *posterior cranial fossa*.

FRONTAL BONE

Frontal bone forms the forehead, most of the roof of orbit, and most of the floor of anterior cranial fossa. Its parts are squamous, orbital and nasal bones (Fig. 9.34).

ANATOMICAL POSITION

Squamous part is vertical and is convex forwards.

Two orbital plates are horizontal thin plates projecting backwards.

Nasal part is directed forwards and downwards.

Squamous Part

The squamous part presents two surfaces, two borders and encloses a pair of frontal air sinuses.

Outer Surface

It is smooth and shows:
1. Frontal tuberosity
2. Superciliary arches
3. Glabella
4. Frontal air sinus is a cavity within outer and inner tables of frontal bone, divided by a bony septum into two parts
5. Metopic suture
6. Upper or parietal border: Articulates with parietal bone
7. Lower or orbital border: Free, presents supra-orbital notch foramen
8. Zygomatic process
9. Temporal line and temporal surfaces

Inner Surface

It is concave and presents:
1. Sagittal sulcus
2. Frontal crest

Orbital Parts (Plates)

Orbital plates are separated from each other by a wide gap—the ethmoidal notch.

Orbital or inferior surface of the plate is smooth and presents lacrimal fossa, anterolaterally and trochlear spine, anteromedially.

Ethmoidal notch is occupied by cribriform plate of ethmoid bone. On each side of notch are small air spaces which articulates with the labyrinth of ethmoid to

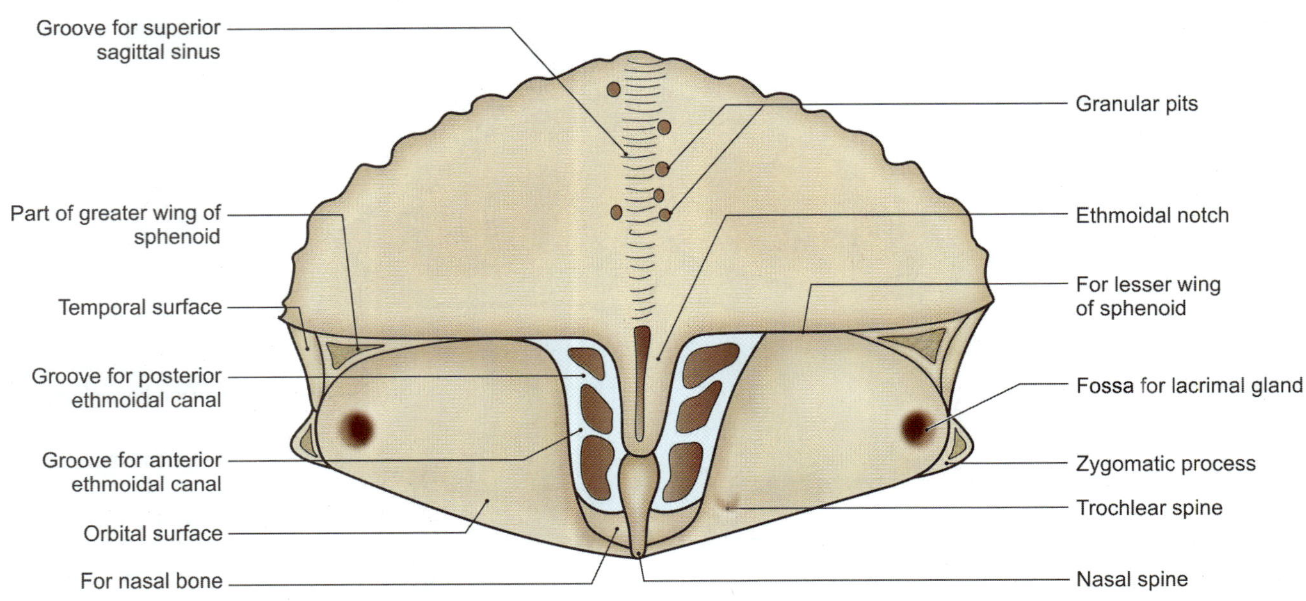

Fig. 9.34: Frontal bone from below

complete ethmoidal air sinuses. At the margins are anterior and posterior ethmoidal canals.

Nasal Part

Lies between two supraorbital margins.

The margins of the nasal notch on each side articulate with nasal, frontal process of maxilla and lacrimal bones.

Details can be studied from descriptions of *norma frontalis, norma lateralis, inner aspect of skull cap and anterior cranial fossa.*

TEMPORAL BONE

Temporal bones are situated at the sides and base of skull.

SIDE DETERMINATION

- Plate-like squamous part is directed upwards and laterally.
- Strong zygomatic process is directed forwards.
- Petrous part, triangular in shape, is directed medially.
- External acoustic meatus, enclosed between squamous and tympanic parts, is directed laterally.

FEATURES

It comprises following parts:

a. Squamous part (Fig. 9.35)
b. Petromastoid part
c. Tympanic part
d. Styloid process

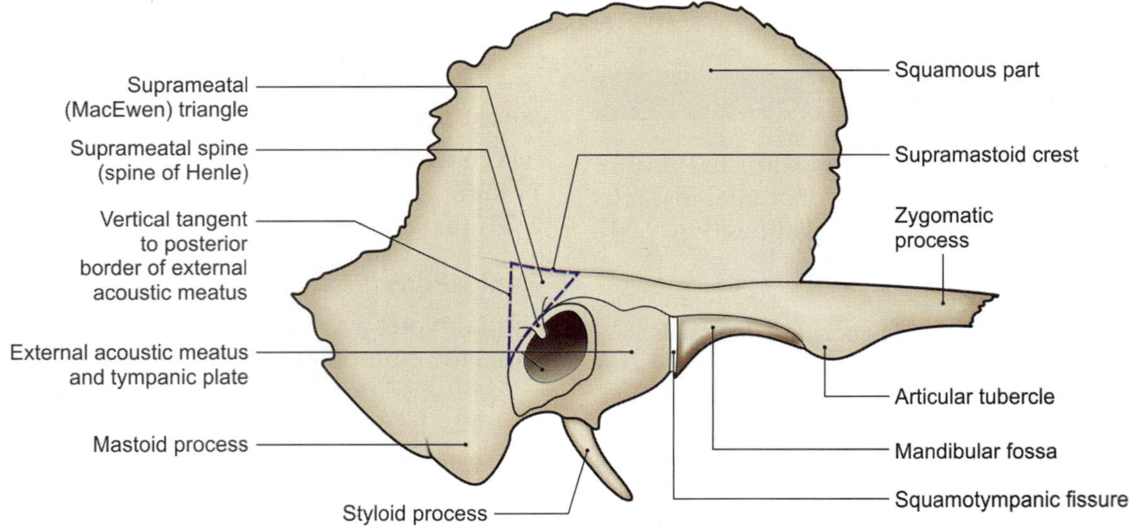

Fig. 9.35: Outer aspect of left temporal bone

Squamous Part

Two surfaces: Outer and inner

Two borders: Superior and anteroinferior

Surfaces

Outer or temporal

It is smooth and forms a part of temporal fossa.

Above external acoustic meatus, there is a groove for middle temporal artery.

Its posterior part presents supramastoid crest.

Below the anterior end of supramastoid crest and posterosuperior to external acoustic meatus, there is suprameatal triangle.

Zygomatic process springs forwards from the outer surface of squamous part. Its posterior part comprises superior and inferior surfaces. The inferior surface is bounded by two roots which converge at the tubercle of root of the zygoma. Anterior root projects as the articular tubercle in front of mandibular fossa.

Posterior root begins above the external acoustic meatus.

Mandibular fossa lies behind articular tubercle and consists of anterior articular part formed by squamous part of temporal bone and a posterior non-articular portion formed by tympanic plate.

Inner or cerebral

It is concave and shows grooves for the middle meningeal vessels. Its superior border articulates with the lower border of parietal bone. Its anteroinferior border articulates with the greater wing of sphenoid.

Borders

Superior border: Articulates with parietal bone.

Anteroinferior border: Articulates with greater wing of sphenoid bone.

Petromastoid Part

Mastoid Part

Mastoid (Greek breast) part forms posterior part of temporal bone. It has:

- Two surfaces—outer and inner
- Two borders—superior and posterior, and enclose the mastoid air cells. (The outer surface forms a downwards projecting conical process, the mastoid process.)

Surfaces

Outer: The outer surface gives attachment to occipitalis muscle. Mastoid foramen opens near its posterior border and transmits an emissary vein and a branch of occipital artery.

Mastoid process appears at the end of 2nd year. Lateral surface gives attachment to sternocleidomastoid, splenius capitis, and longissimus capitis (Fig. 9.14).

Medial surface of the process shows a deep mastoid notch for the origin of posterior belly of digastric. Medial to this notch is a groove for the occipital artery.

Inner: The inner surface is marked by a deep sigmoid sulcus (Fig. 9.36).

Borders

Superior border: Articulates with parietal bone at asterion.

Posterior border: Articulates with occipital bone at occipitomastoid suture.

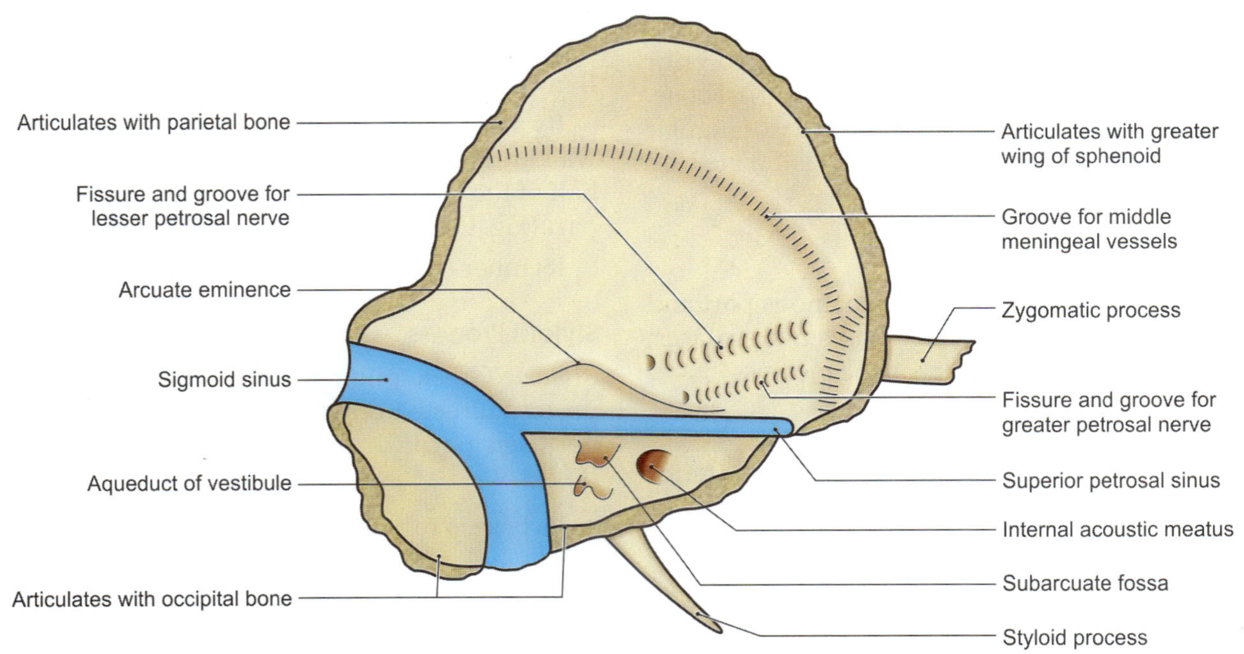

Fig. 9.36: Inner aspect of the left temporal bone

Petrous Part

Petrous (Latin rock) part is triangular in shape. It has a base, an apex, three surfaces—anterior, posterior and inferior; and three borders—superior, anterior and posterior.

Base is fused with squamous and mastoid parts.

Apex is irregular and forms posterolateral boundary of foramen lacerum.

Surfaces

Anterior:

- Trigeminal impression
- Part forming roof of anterior part of carotid canal.
- Arcuate eminence
- Tegmen tympani lying most laterally. In the anterior part of tegmen tympani are hiatus and groove for greater petrosal nerve and a smaller hiatus and groove for the lesser petrosal nerve.

Posterior: Internal acoustic meatus is present here.

Aqueduct of vestibule lies behind internal acoustic meatus.

Inferior: Forms part of norma basalis. It shows lower opening of carotid canal (refer to *norma basalis* for details). Jugular fossa lies behind carotid canal (Fig. 9.37).

Borders

a. *Superior:* It is grooved by superior petrosal sinus. Margins of the groove provide attachment to tentorium cerebelli.
b. *Anterior:* Medial part articulates with greater wing of sphenoid. Lateral part joins squamous part of petrosquamosal suture.
c. *Posterior:* Medial part forms a sulcus for inferior petrosal sinus with a similar sulcus on occipital bone. The lateral part forms anterior boundary of jugular foramen whose posterior boundary is formed by jugular notch of occipital bone.

Tympanic Part

It is a curved plate of bone below squamous part and in front of mastoid process. It comprises two surfaces, three borders and an external acoustic meatus.

Surfaces

Anterior and posterior concave part forming anterior wall, floor and lower part of the posterior wall of external acoustic meatus.

Borders

Lateral border forms the margin of external acoustic meatus.

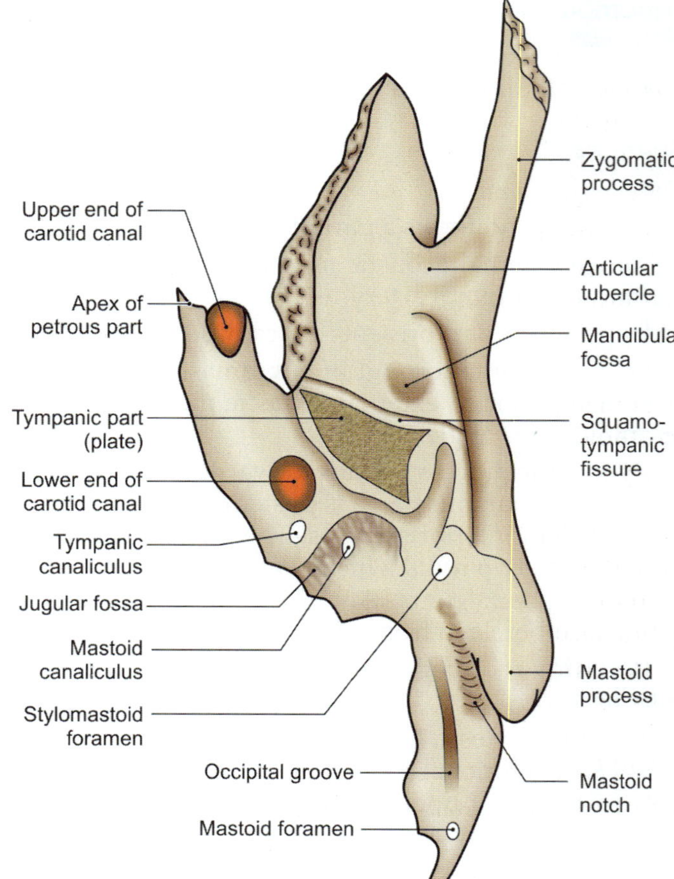

Fig. 9.37: Inferior view of the temporal bone

Upper and lower borders, which in its lateral part, split to enclose the root of styloid process.

External Acoustic Meatus

Bony part of meatus is about 16 mm long.

Its anterior wall, floor and lower part of posterior wall are formed by tympanic part. Its roof and upper half of the posterior wall are formed by the squamous part (Fig. 9.35).

Its inner end is closed by tympanic membrane.

Styloid Process

Styloid (Greek pillar form) process is long pointed process directed downwards, forwards and medially between parotid gland and internal jugular vein (Fig. 9.36).

- Its base is related to facial nerve
- Its apex is crossed by external carotid artery.
- It gives attachment to three muscles and two ligaments (*see* Chapter 16) (*refer* to *norma lateralis* for details).

SPHENOID BONE

Sphenoid (Greek wedge) bone resembles a bat with outstretched wings. It comprises:

- A body in the centre (Fig. 9.38).
- Two lesser wings from the anterior part of body.
- Two greater wings from the lateral part of body.
- Two pterygoid (wing-like) processes, directed downwards from the junction of body and greater wings.

BODY OF SPHENOID

It comprises six surfaces and enclose a pair of sphenoidal air sinuses.

Superior or Cerebral Surface

It articulates with ethmoid bone anteriorly and basilar part of occipital bone posteriorly. It shows:

1 Jugum sphenoidale
2 Sulcus chiasmaticus
3 Tuberculum sellae
4 Sella turcica
5 Dorsum sellae
6 Clivus

Refer to *middle cranial fossa* for details.

Inferior Surface

1 Rostrum of sphenoid (Fig. 9.39a)
2 Sphenoid conchae (Fig. 9.39b)
3 Vaginal processes of medial pterygoid plate

Refer to *norma basalis* for details.

Anterior Surface

Sphenoidal crest articulates with perpendicular plate of ethmoid to form a small part of septum of nose.

Opening of sphenoidal air sinus is seen (Fig. 9.39b).

Sphenoidal conchae close the sphenoid air sinuses leaving the openings. Each half of anterior surface has two parts—superolateral and inferomedial.

The superolateral depression articulates with labyrinth of ethmoid to complete the posterior ethmoidal air sinuses. The inferomedial smooth triangular area forms the posterior part of the root of the nose.

Posterior Surface

It articulates with basilar part of occipital bone.

Lateral Surfaces

Carotid sulcus, a broad groove curved like letter 'f' for lodging cavernous sinus and internal carotid artery. Below the sulcus, it articulates with greater wing of sphenoid laterally and with pterygoid process which is directed downwards.

Sphenoidal Air Sinuses

These are asymmetrical air sinuses in the body of sphenoid, and are closed by sphenoidal conchae. The sinus opens into the lateral wall of nose in the sphenoethmoidal recess above the superior concha.

GREATER WINGS

These are two strong processes which curve laterally and upwards from the sides of the body. It has three surfaces.

Superior or Cerebral Surface

It forms the floor of middle cranial fossa and presents from before backwards:

1 Foramen rotundum (Fig. 9.39a)
2 Foramen ovale

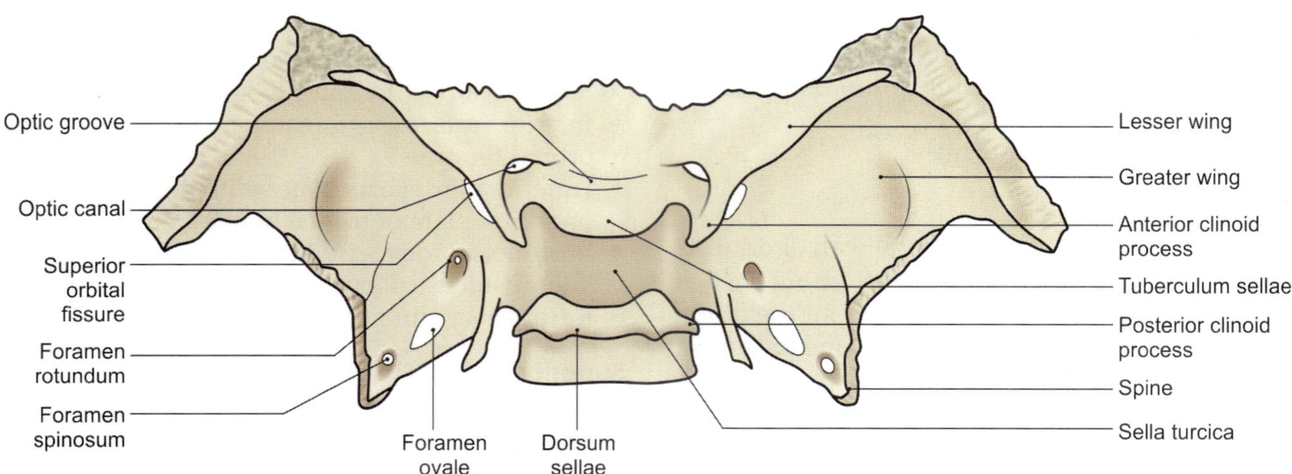

Fig. 9.38: Superior view of the sphenoid bone

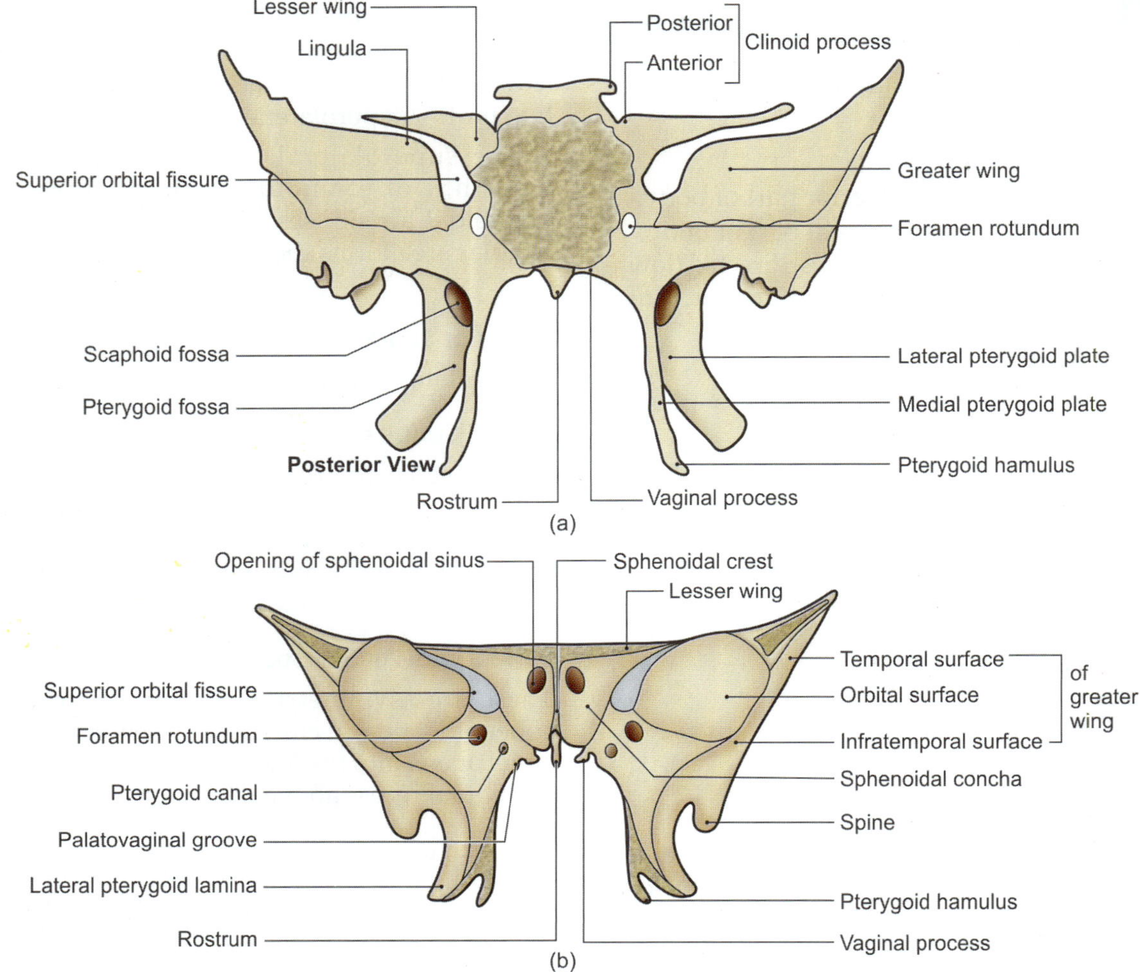

Figs 9.39a and b: (a) Posterior view of sphenoid; (b) Greater and lesser wings of sphenoid

3 Emissary sphenoidale foramen
4 Foramen spinosum

Lateral Surface

A horizontal ridge, the infratemporal crest divides this surface into upper or temporal surface and a lower or infratemporal surface. It is pierced by foramen ovale and foramen spinosum. Its posterior part presents spine of sphenoid.

Refer to *norma basalis* for details.

Orbital Surface

Forms the posterior wall of the lateral wall of orbit.

Its medial border bears a small tubercle for attachment of a common tendinous ring for the origin of recti muscles of the eyeball. Below the medial end of superior orbital fissure, the grooved area forms the posterior wall of the pterygopalatine fossa and is pierced by foramen rotundum (Fig. 9.39b).

Borders are surrounding the greater wing of sphenoid.

LESSER WINGS

Lesser wings are two triangular plates projecting laterally from the anterosuperior part of the body. It comprises:

- A base forming medial end of the wing. It is connected to the body by two roots which enclose the optic canal.
- Tip forms the lateral end of the wing.
- Superior surface forming floor of anterior cranial fossa.
- Inferior surface forming upper boundary of superior orbital fissure.
- Anterior border articulates with the posterior border of orbital plate of frontal bone.
- Posterior border is free and projects into the stem of lateral sulcus of brain. Medially, it terminates into the anterior clinoid process.

Superior Orbital Fissure

It is a triangular gap through which middle cranial fossa communicates with the orbit. The structures passing through it are put in list of foramina and nerves passing through them seen in Fig. 9.22a.

PTERYGOID PROCESSES

One *pterygoid* (Greek wing) process on each side projects downwards from the junction of the body with the greater wing of sphenoid (Fig. 9.38).

Each pterygoid process divides inferiorly into the medial and lateral pterygoid plates. The plates are fused together in their upper parts, but are separated in their lower parts by the pterygoid fissure. Posteriorly, the pterygoid plates enclose a 'V-shaped interval', the pterygoid fossa. The medial pterygoid plate in its upper part presents a scaphoid fossa.

Refer to *norma basalis* for medial and lateral pterygoid plates.

ETHMOID BONE

Ethmoid (Greek sieve) is a very light cuboidal bone situated in the anterior of base of cranial cavity between the two orbits. It forms:

1 Part of medial orbital walls
2 Part of nasal septum (Fig. 9.40a)
3 Part of medial wall of orbit
4 Lateral walls of the nasal cavity

Ethmoid bone comprises:

1 Cribriform plate (Fig. 9.40b)
2 Perpendicular plate
3 A pair of labyrinth

CRIBRIFORM PLATE

It is a horizontal perforated bony lamina, occupying ethmoidal notch of frontal bone. It contains foramina for olfactory nerve rootlets.

Crista Galli

Crista galli is a median, tooth-like upward projection in the floor of anterior cranial fossa. Foramen transmitting anterior ethmoidal nerve to nasal cavity is situated by the side of crista galli.

PERPENDICULAR PLATE

It is a thin lamina projecting downwards from the undersurface of the cribriform plate, forming upper part of nasal septum.

LABYRINTHS

These are two light cubical masses situated on each side of the perpendicular plate, suspended from the undersurface of the cribriform plate (Fig. 9.40c).

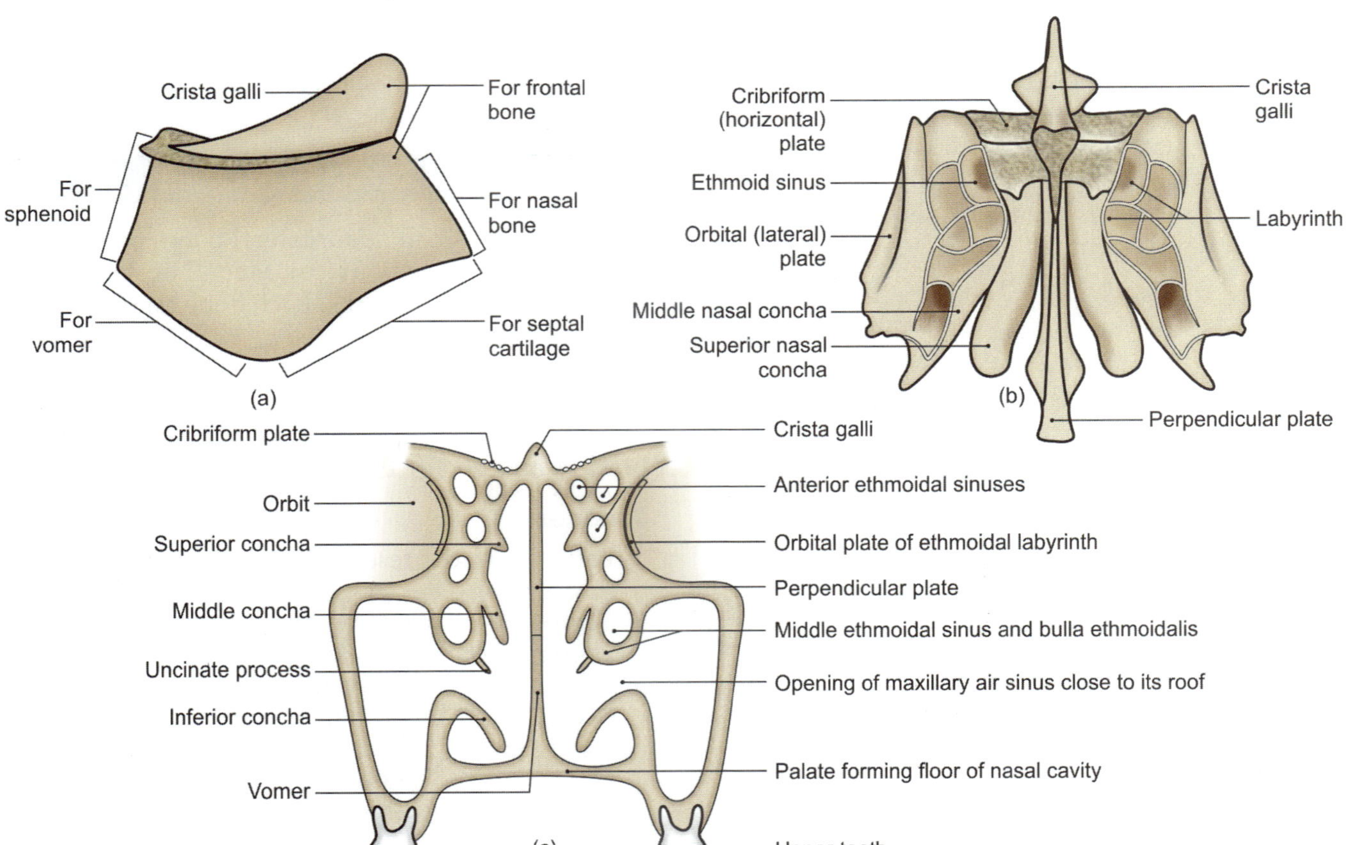

Figs 9.40a to c: (a) Articulations of perpendicular plate of ethmoid bone; (b) Posterior view of the ethmoid bone; (c) Ethmoid bone articulating with neighbouring bones

Each labyrinth also encloses large number of 'air cells' arranged in three groups—the anterior, middle and posterior ethmoidal air sinuses. Its surfaces are:

- Anterior surface articulates with frontal process of maxilla to complete anterior ethmoidal air cells.
- Posterior surface articulates with sphenoidal concha to complete posterior ethmoidal air cells.
- Superior surface articulates with orbital plate of frontal bone.
- Inferior surface articulates with nasal surface of maxilla.
- Lateral surface forms medial wall of orbit.
- Medial surface presents small superior nasal concha, middle nasal concha, superior meatus below superior concha, and middle meatus below middle concha.

VOMER

Vomer (Latin plough share) is a single thin, flat bone forming posteroinferior part of the nasal septum. It comprises:

- Right and left surfaces marked by nasopalatine nerves which course downwards and forwards.
- Superior border splits into two alae with a groove is occupied by rostrum of sphenoid (Fig. 9.13).
- Inferior border articulates with nasal crests of maxillae and palatine bones (Fig. 9.41).
- Anterior, longest border, articulates with perpendicular plate of ethmoid above and with septal cartilage below.
- Posterior border is free and separates the two posterior nasal openings.

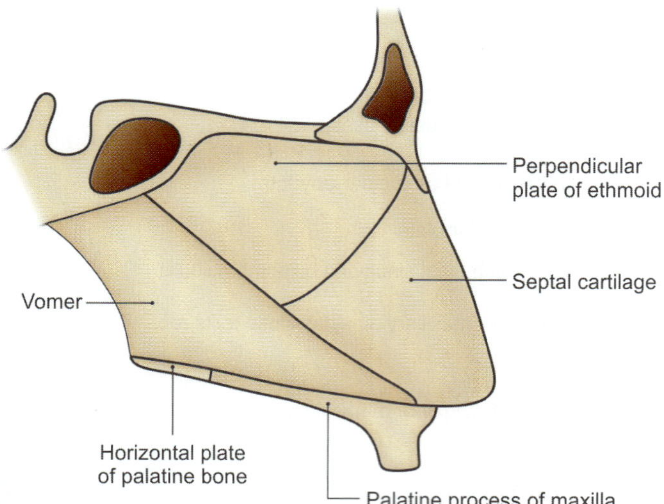

Fig. 9.41: Vomer forming posteroinferior part of the nasal septum with its various borders

INFERIOR NASAL CONCHAE

The inferior nasal conchae are two curved bony laminae, these are horizontally placed in the lower part of lateral walls of the nose. Between this concha and floor of the nose lies the inferior meatus of the nose. It comprises two surfaces, two borders and two ends.

- Medial convex surface is marked by vascular grooves.
- Lateral concave surface forms the medial wall of inferior meatus of the nerve.
- Superior border is irregular and articulates with lacrimal, maxilla, ethmoid and palatine bones (Fig. 9.42).
- Inferior border is free, thick and spongy.
- Posterior end is more pointed than the anterior end.

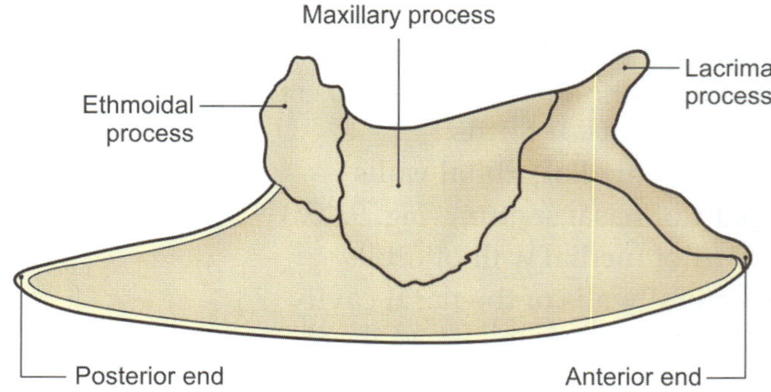

Fig. 9.42: Lateral view of the left inferior nasal concha

ZYGOMATIC BONES

These are two small quadrilateral bones present in the upper and lateral part of face. The bone forms prominence of the cheeks. Each bone takes part in the formation of:

- Floor and lateral wall of the orbit
- Walls of temporal and infraorbital fossae.

Zygomatic bone comprises three surfaces, five borders and two processes.

Surfaces

1. Lateral surface presenting zygomaticofacial foramen (Fig. 9.43a).
2. Temporal surface is smooth and concave and presents zygomaticotemporal foramen (Fig. 9.43b).
3. Orbital surface is also smooth and concave one or two zygomatico-orbital foramen on this surface and this leads to zygomaticofacial and zygomaticotemporal foramina (Fig. 9.22a).

Borders

1. Anterosuperior or orbital
2. Anteroinferior or maxillary
3. Posteroinferior or temporal border

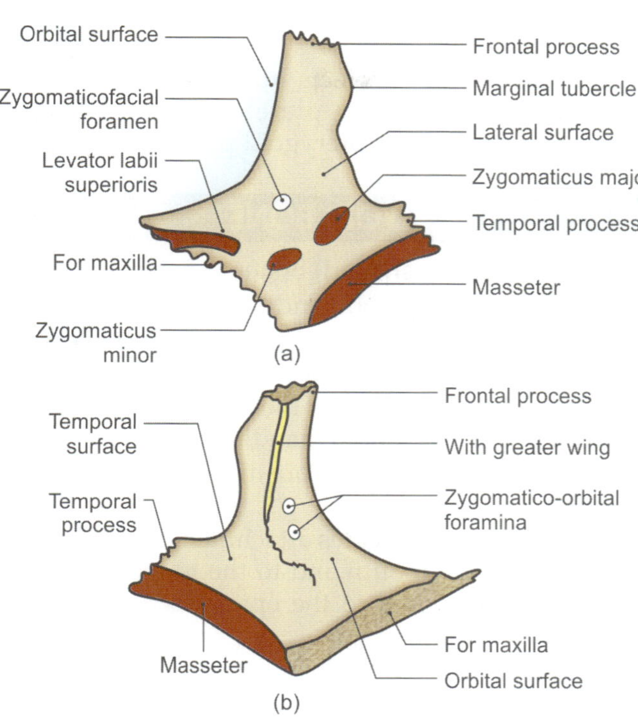

Figs 9.43a and b: Features of the left zygomatic bone: (a) Outer view; (b) Inner view

4 Posteroinferior border
5 Posteromedial border

Processes

1 Frontal process, which is directed upwards.
2 Temporal process, which is directed backwards.

NASAL BONES

Nasal bones are two small oblong bones, which form the bridge of the nerve.

Each nasal bone has two surfaces and four borders (Fig. 9.44).

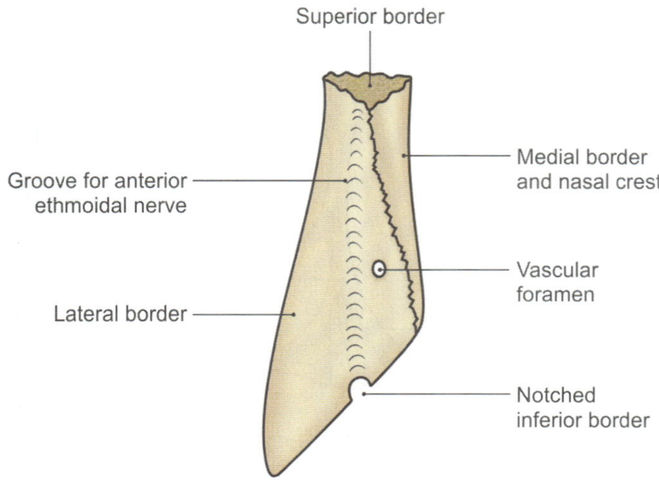

Fig. 9.44: Inner view of the left nasal bone

Surfaces

1 The outer surface is convex from side-to-side.
2 The inner surface is concave from side-to-side and is traversed by a vertical groove for anterior ethmoidal nerve.

Borders

1 Superior border is thick and serrated and articulates with nasal part of frontal bone.
2 Inferior border is thin and notched and articulates with lateral nasal cartilage.
3 Medial border articulates with opposite nasal bone.
4 Lateral border articulates with frontal process of maxilla.

LACRIMAL BONES

Lacrimal bones are extremely delicate and smallest of the skull bones. These form the anterior part of the medial part of the orbit. Each lacrimal bone comprises two surfaces and four borders.

Surfaces

1 Lateral or orbital surface is divided by posterior lacrimal crest into anterior and posterior parts. The anterior grooved part forms posterior half of the floor of lacrimal groove for lacrimal sac. The posterior smooth part forms part of medial wall of orbit (Fig. 9.22).
2 Medial or nasal surface forms a part of middle meatus of the nose (Fig. 9.45). It ends below in lacrimal hamulus which together with maxilla completes the upper opening of nasolacrimal canal. Descending process articulates with nasolacrimal groove of maxilla and lacrimal process of inferior concha to complete nasolacrimal duct.

Borders

1 Anterior border articulates with frontal process of maxilla.

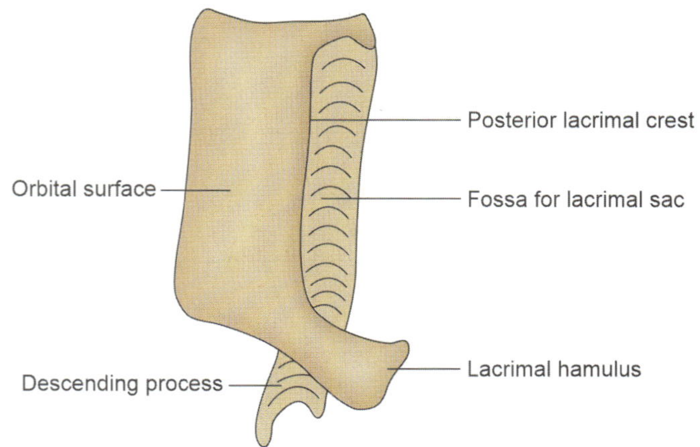

Fig. 9.45: Lateral surface of the left lacrimal bone

2 Posterior border with orbital plate of ethmoid.
3 Superior border with frontal bone.
4 Inferior border with orbital surface of maxilla.

PALATINE BONES

Palatine bones are two L-shaped bones present in the posterior part of nasal cavity. Each bone forms:

- Lateral wall and floor of nasal cavity (Fig. 9.46a)
- Roof of mouth cavity (Fig. 9.29)
- Floor of the orbit
- Parts of pterygopalatine fossa

Each palatine bone has two plates and three processes.

Plates

1 Horizontal plate forms posterior one-fourth part of bony palate. It has two surfaces and four borders (Fig. 9.46b).
2 Perpendicular plate of palatine bone is vertical in shape and comprises two surfaces and four borders *(refer* to *norma basalis)*. It is fixed to posterior part of medial surface of maxilla.

Processes

Pyramidal

Pyramidal process projects downwards from the junction of two plates. Its inferior surface is pierced by lesser palatine foramina.

Orbital

Orbital process projects upwards and laterally from the perpendicular plate. Its orbital surface is triangular and forms the posterior part of the floor of the orbit (Fig. 9.46b).

Sphenoidal

Sphenoidal process projects upwards and medially from the perpendicular plate. Its lateral surface articulates with medial pterygoid plate.

HYOID BONE

The *hyoid* (Greek U-shaped) bone is U-shaped.

It develops from second and third branchial arches.

It is situated in the anterior midline of the neck between the chin and the thyroid cartilage (*refer to BDC App*).

At rest, it lies at the level of the third cervical vertebra behind and the base of the mandible in front.

It is kept suspended in position by muscles and ligaments.

The hyoid bone provides attachment to the muscles of the floor of the mouth and to the tongue above, to the larynx below, and to the epiglottis and pharynx behind (Fig. 9.47).

The bone consists of the central part, called the body, and of two pairs of cornua—greater and lesser.

Body

It has two surfaces—anterior and posterior, and two borders—upper and lower.

The *anterior surface* is convex and is directed forwards and upwards. It is often divided by a median ridge into two lateral halves.

The *posterior surface* is concave and is directed backwards and downwards.

Each lateral end of the body is continuous posteriorly with the greater horn or cornua. However, till middle life, the connection between the body and greater cornua is fibrous.

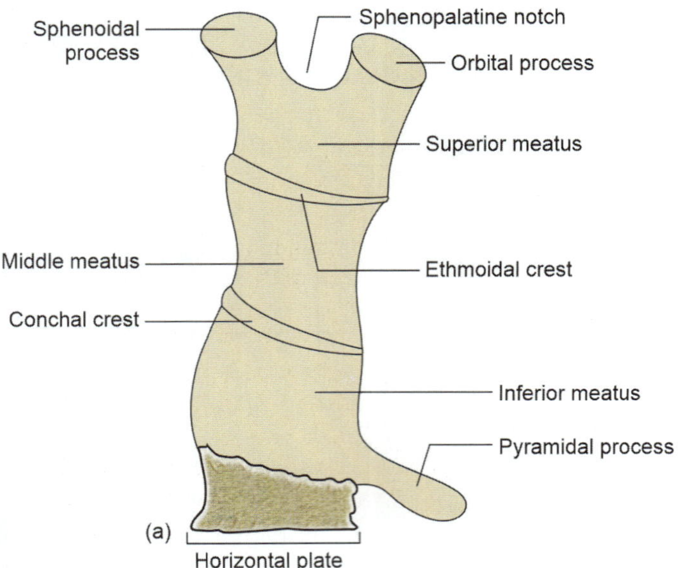

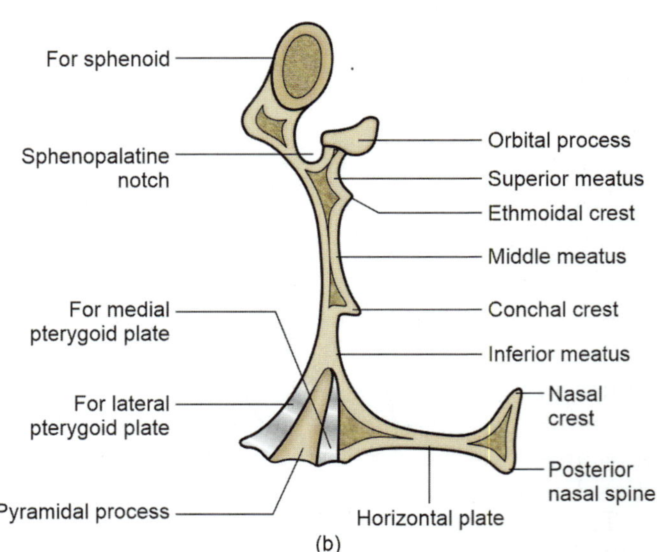

Figs 9.46a and b: (a) Medial view of the left palatine bone; (b) Various processes of palatine bone

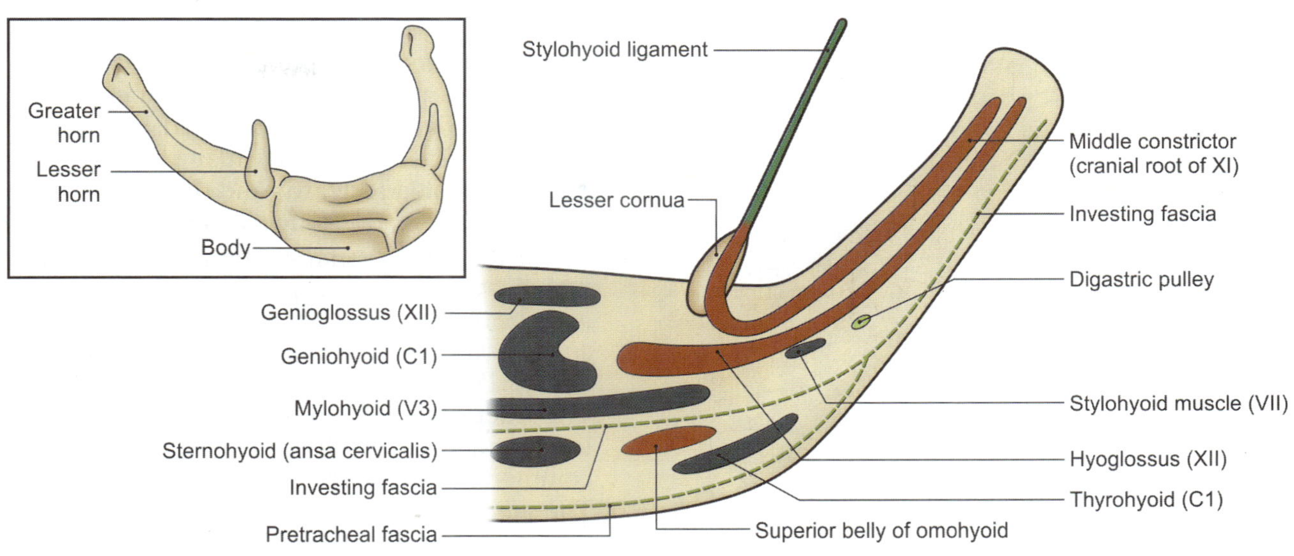

Fig. 9.47: Anterosuperior view of the left half of hyoid bone showing its attachments (Inset: Hyoid bone)

Greater Cornua/Horn

These are flattened from above downwards. Each cornua tapers posteriorly, but ends in a tubercle. It has two surfaces—upper and lower, two borders—medial and lateral and a tubercle.

Lesser Cornua/Horn

These are small conical pieces of bone which project upwards from the junction of the body and greater cornua. The lesser cornua are connected to the body by fibrous tissue. Occasionally, they are connected to the greater cornua by synovial joints which usually persist throughout life, but may get ankylosed.

ATTACHMENTS ON THE HYOID BONE

The anterior surface of the body provides insertion to the geniohyoid and mylohyoid muscles and gives origin to a part of the hyoglossus which extends to the greater cornua (Fig. 9.47).

The *upper border* of the body provides insertion to the lower fibres of the genioglossi and attachment to the thyrohyoid membrane.

The *lower border* of the body provides attachment to the pretracheal fascia. In front of the fascia, the *sternohyoid* is inserted medially and the superior belly of omohyoid laterally.

Below the omohyoid, there is the linear attachment of the thyrohyoid, extending back to the lower border of the greater cornua.

The *medial border* of the greater cornua provides attachment to the thyrohyoid membrane, stylohyoid muscle and digastric pulley.

The *lateral border* of the greater cornua provides insertion to the thyrohyoid muscle anteriorly. The investing fascia is attached throughout its length.

The lesser cornua provides attachment to the stylohyoid ligament at its tip. The middle constrictor muscle arises from its posterolateral aspect extending onto the greater cornua (*see* Fig. 22.21).

DEVELOPMENT

Upper part of body and lesser cornua develop from second branchial arch, while lower part of body and greater cornua develop from the third arch.

CLINICAL ANATOMY

In a suspected case of murder, fracture of the hyoid bone strongly indicates throttling or strangulation.

CERVICAL VERTEBRAE

IDENTIFICATION

The cervical vertebrae are identified by the presence of foramina transversaria.

There are seven cervical vertebrae, out of which the third to sixth are typical, while the first, second and seventh are atypical (Figs 9.48a and b) (*refer to BDC App*).

TYPICAL CERVICAL VERTEBRAE

Body

1. The body is *small* and *broader* from side-to-side than from before backwards.
2. Its *superior surface* is concave transversely with upward projecting lips on each side. The anterior border of this surface may be bevelled.

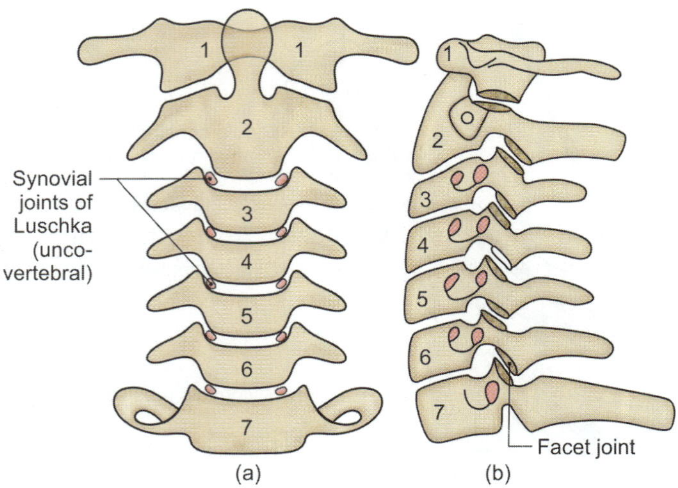

Figs 9.48a and b: Cervical vertebrae: (a) Anterior view; (b) Lateral view

3 The *inferior surface* is saddle-shaped, being convex from side-to-side and concave from before backwards. The lateral borders are bevelled and form synovial joints with the projecting lips of the next lower vertebra. The anterior border projects downwards and may hide the intervertebral disc.

4 The *anterior and posterior surfaces* resemble those of other vertebrae (Fig. 9.49).

Vertebral Foramen

Vertebral foramen is larger than the body. It is triangular in shape because the pedicles are directed backwards and laterally.

Vertebral Arch

1 The *pedicles* are directed backwards and laterally. The superior and inferior vertebral notches are of equal size.

2 The *laminae* are relatively long and narrow, being thinner above than below.

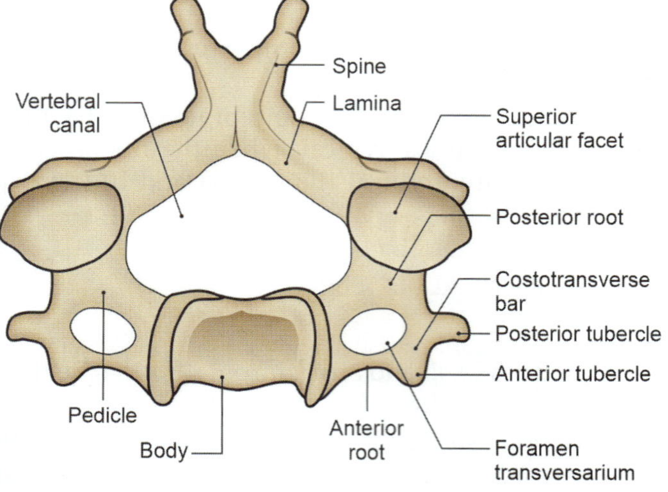

Fig. 9.49: Typical cervical vertebra seen from above

3 The *superior and inferior articular processes* form articular pillars which project laterally at the junction of pedicle and the lamina. The superior articular facets are flat. They are directed backwards and upwards. The inferior articular facets are also flat but are directed forwards and downwards.

4 The *transverse processes* are pierced by foramina transversaria. Each process has *anterior* and *posterior roots* which end in tubercles joined by the *costotransverse bar*. The *costal element is represented by the anterior root, anterior tubercle, the costotransverse bar and the posterior tubercle*. Posterior root represents the transverse process. The anterior tubercle of the sixth cervical vertebra is large and is called the *carotid tubercle* because the common carotid artery can be compressed against it.

5 The *spine* is short and bifid. The notch is filled up by the ligamentum nuchae (Fig. 9.49).

Attachments and Relations

1 The anterior and posterior longitudinal ligaments are attached to the upper and lower borders of the body in front and behind, respectively. On each side of the anterior longitudinal ligament, the vertical part of the longus colli is attached to the anterior surface. The posterior surface has two or more foramina for passage of *basivertebral veins*.

2 The upper borders and lower parts of the anterior surfaces of the laminae provide attachment to the ligamenta flava.

3 The *foramen transversarium* transmits the *vertebral artery*, the *vertebral veins* and a *branch from the inferior cervical ganglion*. The *anterior tubercles* give origin to the scalenus anterior, the longus capitis, and the oblique part of the longus colli.

4 The *costotransverse bars* are grooved by the *anterior primary rami* of the corresponding cervical nerves.

5 The *posterior tubercles* give origin to the scalenus medius, scalenus posterior, the levator scapulae and insertion to the splenius cervicis, the longissimus cervicis, and the iliocostalis cervicis (*see* Fig. 18.3).

6 The spine gives origin to the deep muscles of the back of the neck—interspinales, spinalis cervicis, and insertion to semispinalis thoracis, cervicis and multifidus (*see* Figs 18.2 and 18.4).

OSSIFICATION

A typical cervical vertebra ossifies from three primary and six secondary centres. There is one *primary centre* for each half of the neural arch during 9 to 10 weeks of foetal life and one for the *centrum* in 3 to 4 months of foetal life. The two halves of the neural arch fuse posteriorly with each other during the first year. Synostosis at the neurocentral synchondrosis occurs during the third year.

The *secondary centres, two* for the annular epiphyseal discs for the peripheral parts of the upper and lower surfaces of the body, *two* for the tips of the transverse processes, and *two* for the bifid spine, appear during puberty, and fuse with the rest of the vertebrae by 25 years.

FIRST CERVICAL VERTEBRA

It is called the *atlas* (Tiltan, who supported the heaven). It can be identified by the following features.

1 It is ring-shaped. It has neither a body nor a spine (Fig. 9.50).
2 The atlas has a short anterior arch, a long posterior arch, right and left lateral masses, and transverse processes.
3 The *anterior arch* is marked by a median *anterior tubercle* on its anterior aspect. Its posterior surface bears an *oval facet* which articulates with the *dens* (Fig. 9.50).
4 The *posterior arch* forms about two-fifths of the ring and is much longer than the anterior arch. Its posterior surface is marked by a median posterior tubercle. The upper surface of the arch is marked behind the lateral mass by a *groove*.

Each *lateral mass* shows the following important features.

a. Its upper surface bears the *superior articular facet.* This facet is elongated (forwards and medially), concave, and is directed upwards and medially. It articulates with the corresponding condyle to form an atlanto-occipital joint.
b. The lower surface is marked by the *inferior articular facet*. This facet is nearly circular, more or less flat, and is directed downwards, medially and backwards. It articulates with the corresponding facet on the axis vertebra to form an atlantoaxial joint.
c. The medial surface of the lateral mass is marked by a small roughened tubercle.
d. The *transverse process* projects laterally from the lateral mass. It is unusually long and can be felt on the surface of the neck between the angle of mandible and the mastoid process. Its long length allows it to act as an effective lever for rotatory movements of the head. The transverse process is pierced by the foramen transversarium.

Attachments and Relations

1 The anterior tubercle provides attachment (in the median plane) to the anterior longitudinal ligament, and provides insertion on each side to the upper oblique part of longus colli.
2 The upper border of the anterior arch gives attachment to the anterior atlanto-occipital membrane.
3 The lower border of the anterior arch gives attachment to the lateral fibres of the anterior longitudinal ligament.
4 The posterior tubercle provides attachment to the ligamentum nuchae in the median plane and gives origin to the rectus capitis posterior minor on each side (Fig. 9.50).
5 The groove on the upper surface of the posterior arch is occupied by the *vertebral artery* and by the *first cervical nerve*. Behind the groove, the upper border of the posterior arch gives attachment to the posterior atlanto-occipital membrane (*see* Fig. 18.5).
6 The lower border of the posterior arch gives attachment to the highest pair of ligamenta flava.
7 The tubercle on the medial side of the lateral mass gives attachment to the transverse ligament of the atlas.

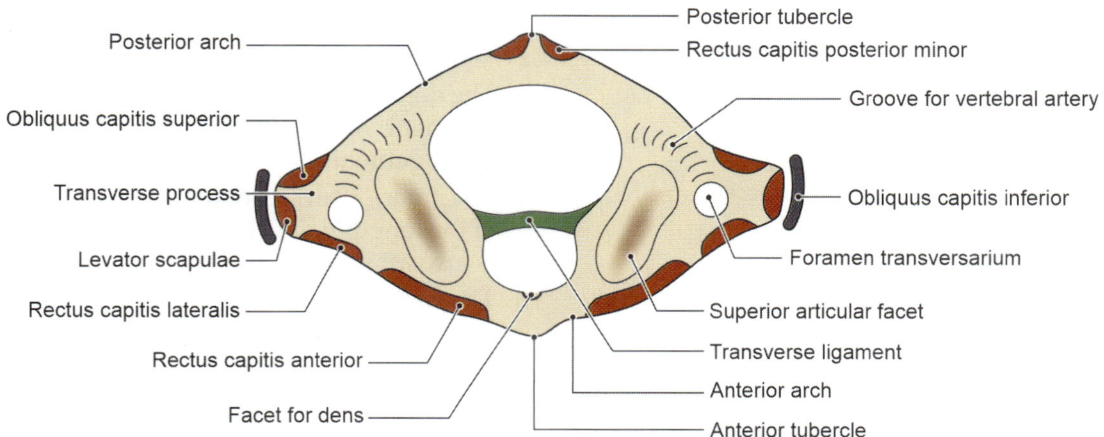

Fig. 9.50: Atlas vertebra seen from above

8 The anterior surface of the lateral mass gives origin to the rectus capitis anterior.
9 The transverse process gives origin to the rectus capitis lateralis from its upper surface anteriorly, the obliquus capitis superior from its upper surface posteriorly, the levator scapulae from its lateral margin and lower border, scalenus medius from its lower surface of the tip and insertion to obliquus capitis inferior and splenius cervicis from the posterior tubercle of transverse process.

OSSIFICATION

Atlas ossifies from three centres, one for each lateral mass with half of the posterior arch, one for the anterior arch. The centres for the lateral masses appear during seventh week of intrauterine life and unite posteriorly at about 3 years. The centre for anterior arch appears at about first year and unites with the lateral mass at about 7 years.

SECOND CERVICAL VERTEBRA

This is called the *axis* (Latin *axile*). It is identified by the presence of the dens or *odontoid* (Greek tooth) process which is a strong, tooth-like process projecting upwards from the body. The dens is usually believed to represent the centrum or body of the atlas which has fused with the centrum of the axis (Figs 9.51a and b).

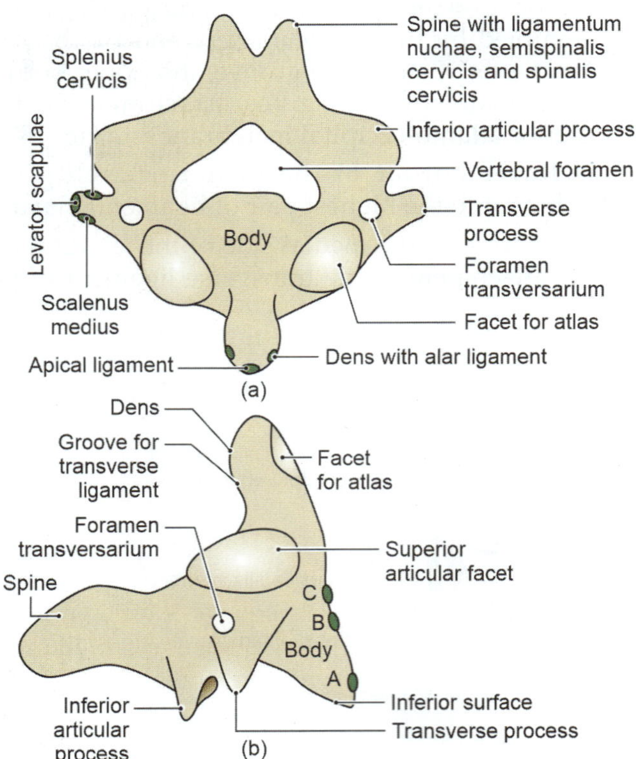

Figs 9.51a and b: The axis vertebra: (a) Posterosuperior view; (b) Lateral view. A–posterior longitudinal ligament; B–membrana tectoria; C–vertical limb of cruciate ligament

Body and Dens

1 The *superior surface* of the body is fused with the dens, and is encroached upon on each side by the superior articular facets. The dens articulates anteriorly with oval fact on posterior surface of the anterior arch of the atlas, and posteriorly with the transverse ligament of the atlas.
2 The *inferior surface* has a prominent anterior margin which projects downwards.
3 The *anterior surface* presents a median ridge on each side of which there are hollowed out impressions.

Vertebral Arch

1 The *pedicles* are concealed superiorly by the superior articular processes. The inferior surface presents a deep and wide *inferior vertebral notch*, placed in front of the inferior articular process. The superior vertebral notch is very shallow and is placed on the upper border of the lamina, behind the superior articular process.
2 The *laminae* are thick and strong.
3 Articular facets: Each *superior articular facet* occupies the upper surfaces of the body and of the massive pedicle. Laterally, it overhangs the foramen transversarium. It is a large, flat, circular facet which is directed upwards and laterally. It articulates with the inferior facet of the atlas vertebra to form the atlantoaxial joint. Each *inferior articular facet* lies posterior to the transverse process and is directed downwards and forwards to articulate with the third cervical vertebra.
4 The *transverse processes* are very small and represent the true posterior tubercles only. The foramen transversarium is directed upwards and laterally (Figs 9.51a and b).
5 The *spine* is large, thick and very strong. It is deeply grooved inferiorly. Its tip is bifid, terminating in two rough tubercles.

Attachments

1 The dens provides attachment at its apex to the apical ligament, and on each side, below the apex to the alar ligaments (Fig. 9.51a).
2 The anterior surface of the body receives the insertion of the longus colli. The anterior longitudinal ligament is also attached to the anterior surface.
3 The posterior surface of the body provides attachment, from below upwards, to the posterior longitudinal ligament, the membrana tectoria and the vertical limb of the cruciate ligament.
4 The laminae provide attachment to the ligamentum flava.

5 The transverse process gives origin by its tip to the levator scapulae, the scalenus medius anteriorly and insertion to the splenius cervicis posteriorly. The *intertransverse muscles* are attached to the upper and lower surfaces of the process.

6 The spine gives attachment to the ligamentum nuchae, insertion to semispinalis cervicis, the spinalis cervicis, the interspinalis and the multifidus and origin to rectus capitis posterior major and obliquus capitis inferior (*see* Chapter 18).

SEVENTH CERVICAL VERTEBRA

It is also known as the *vertebra prominens* because of its long spinous process, the tip of which can be felt through the skin at the lower end of the nuchal furrow.

Its spine is thick, long and nearly horizontal. It is not bifid, but ends in a tubercle (Fig. 9.52).

The transverse processes are comparatively large in size, the posterior root is larger than the anterior. The anterior tubercle is absent. The foramen transversarium is relatively small, sometimes double, or may be entirely absent. It does not transmit the vertebral artery.

Attachments

1 The tip of the *spine* provides attachment to the ligamentum nuchae, origin to trapezius, rhomboid minor, serratus posterior superior, splenius capitis, and insertion to semispinalis thoracis, interspinales, and the multifidus (*see* Fig. 18.3).

2 *Transverse process:* The *foramen transversarium* usually transmits only an accessory vertebral vein. The *posterior tubercle* provides attachment to the supra-pleural membrane. The lower *border* provides attachment to the levator costarum.

The anterior root of the transverse process may sometimes be separate. It then forms a *cervical rib* of variable size.

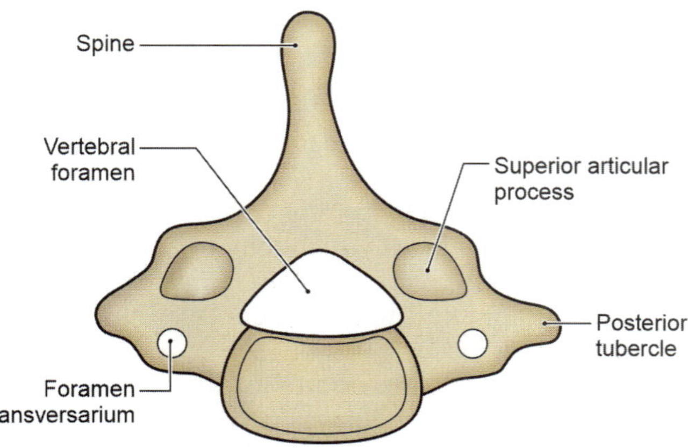

Fig. 9.52: Seventh cervical vertebra seen from above

OSSIFICATION

Its ossification is similar to that of a typical cervical vertebra. In addition, separate centre for each costal process appears during sixth month of intrauterine life and fuses with the body and transverse process during fifth to sixth years of life.

CLINICAL ANATOMY

- The costal element of seventh cervical vertebra may get enlarged to form a cervical rib (Fig. 9.53).
- A cervical rib is an additional rib arising from the C7 vertebra and usually gets attached to the 1st rib near the insertion of scalenus anterior. If the rib is more than 5 cm long, it usually displaces the brachial plexus and the subclavian artery upwards (Fig. 9.54).

  The symptoms are tingling pain along the inner border of the forearm and hand including weakness and even paralysis of the muscles of the palm.
- The intervertebral foramina of the cervical vertebrae lie anterior to the joints between the articular processes. Arthritic changes in these joints, if occur, cause tiny projections or osteophytes.

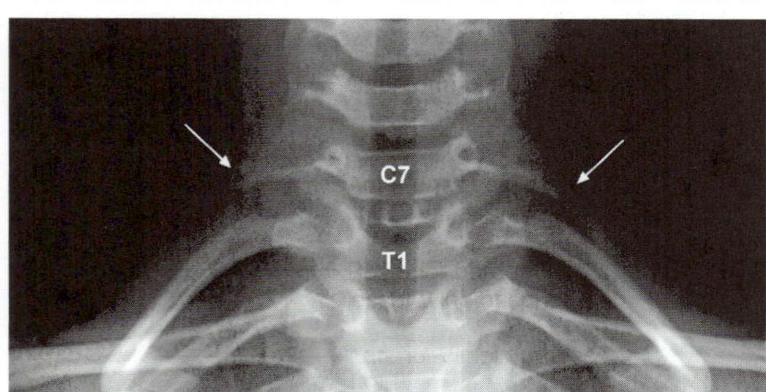

Fig. 9.53: Bilateral cervical ribs

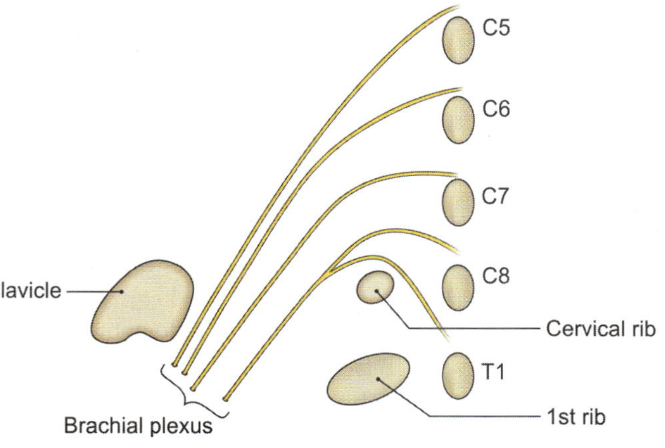

Fig. 9.54: Cervical rib causing pressure on the lower trunk of the brachial plexus

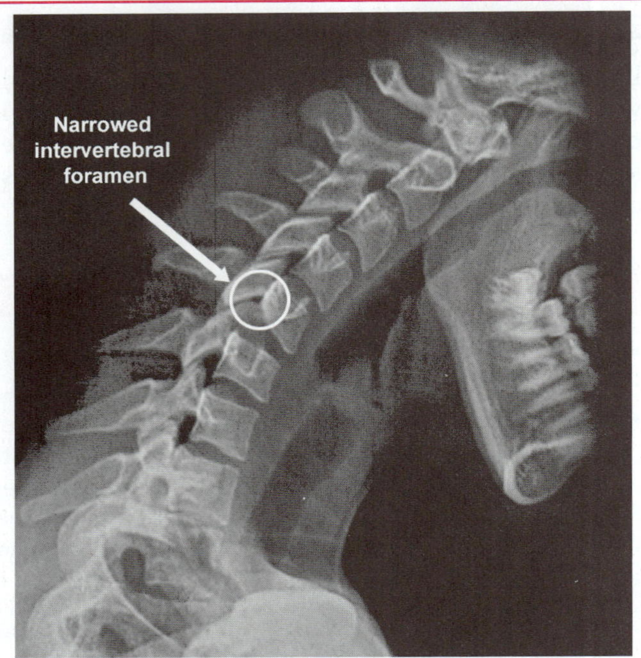

Fig. 9.55: Pressure on the cervical nerve due to bony changes

These osteophytes may press on the anteriorly placed cervical spinal nerves in the foramina causing pain along the course and distribution of these nerves (Fig. 9.55).

- The joints in the lateral parts of adjacent bodies of cervical vertebrae are called Luschka's joints. The osteophytes commonly occur in these joints. The cervical nerve roots lying posterolateral to these joints may get pressed causing pain along their distribution (Fig. 9.55).
- The vertebral artery coursing through the foramen transversarium lies lateral to Luschka's joints. The osteophytes of Luschka's joints may cause distortion of the vertebral artery leading to vertebrobasilar insufficiency. This may cause vertigo, dizziness, etc.
- Prolapse of the intervertebral disc occurs at the junction of different curvatures. So, the common site is lower cervical and upper lumbar vertebral regions. In the cervical region, the disc involved is above or below 6th cervical vertebra. The nerve roots affected are C6 and C7. There is pain and numbness along the lateral side of forearm and hand. There may be wasting of muscles of thenar eminence.
- During judicial hanging, the odontoid process usually breaks to hit upon the vital centres in the medulla oblongata (Fig. 9.56).
- Atlas may fuse with the occipital bone. This is called *occipitalization of atlas* and this may at times compress the spinal cord which requires surgical decompression.
- The pharyngeal and retropharyngeal inflammations may cause decalcification of atlas vertebra.

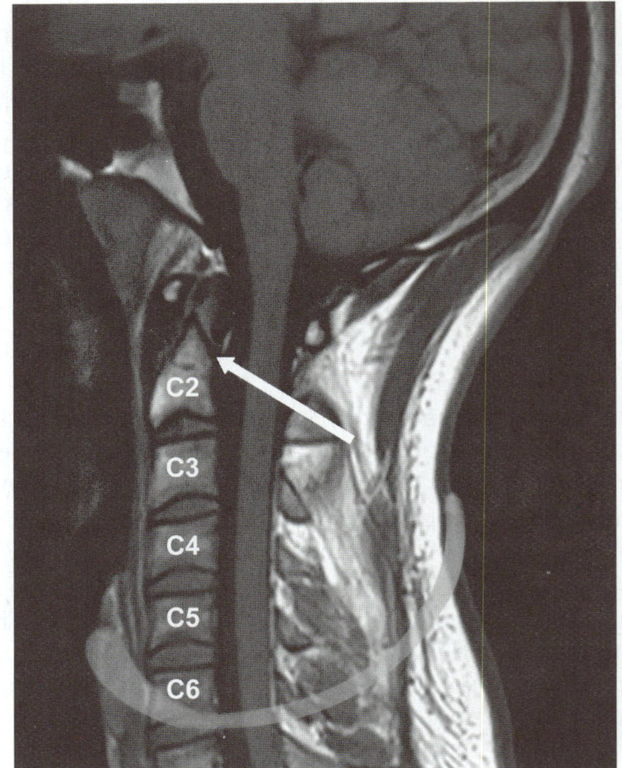

Fig. 9.56: Fracture of the odontoid process during hanging

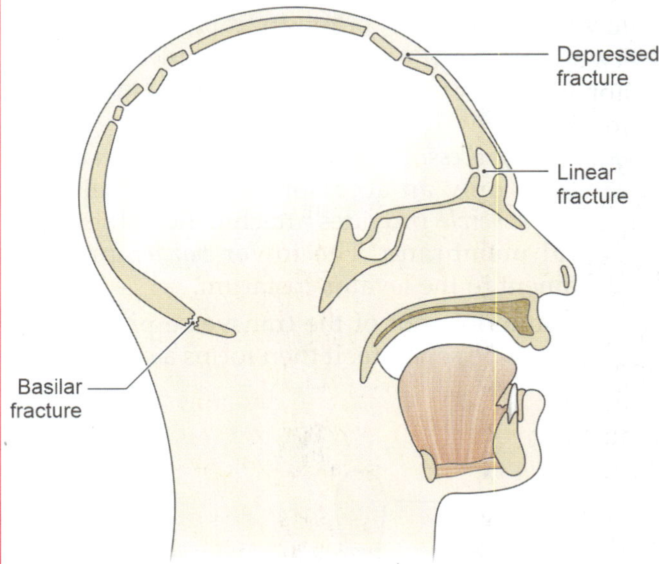

Fig. 9.57: Types of the fractures of the skull

This may lead to loosening of the attachments of transverse ligament which may eventually yield, causing *sudden death* from *dislocation of dens*.

- Fractures of skull may be depressed, linear and basilar (Fig. 9.57).
- Hangman's fracture occurs due to fracture of the pedicles of axis vertebra. As the vertebral canal gets enlarged, the spinal cord does not get pressed.

OSSIFICATION OF CRANIAL BONES

Intramembranous ossification of skull bones is one stage quicker process of ossification. Bones forming cap of skull, i.e. frontal, parietal, squamous temporal and upper part of occipital ossify in membrane as these cover and protect the vital brain.

Frontal: It ossifies in membrane. Two primary centres appear during eighth week near frontal eminences. At birth, the bone is in two halves, separated by a suture, which soon start to fuse. But remains of metopic suture may be seen in about 3–8% of adult skulls.

Parietal: It also ossifies in membrane. Two centres appear during seventh week near the parietal eminence and soon fuse with each other.

Occipital: It ossifies partly in membrane and partly in cartilage. The part of the bone above highest nuchal line ossifies in membrane by two centres which appear during second month of foetal life, it may remain separate as interparietal bone.

The following centres appear in cartilage:

- Two centres for squamous part below highest nuchal line appear during seventh week. One Kerckring centre appears for posterior margin of foramen magnum during sixteenth week.
- Two centres, one for each of the lateral parts, appear during eighth week. One centre appears for the basilar part during sixth week.

Temporal: *Squamous* and *tympanic* parts ossify in membrane. *Squamous part* by one centre which appears during seventh week. *Tympanic part* from one centre which appears during third month.

Petromastoid and *styloid* parts ossify in cartilage. *Petromastoid part* is ossified by several centres which appear in cartilaginous ear capsule during fifth month. *Styloid process* develops from cranial end of second branchial arch cartilage. Two centres appear in it. Tympanohyal before birth and stylohyal after birth.

Sphenoid: It ossifies in two parts:

- *Presphenoidal part* which lies in front of tuberculum sellae and lesser wings ossifies from six centres in cartilage: Two for body of sphenoid during ninth week; two for the two lesser wings during ninth week; two for the two sphenoidal conchae during fifth month.
- *Postsphenoidal part* consisting of posterior part of body, greater wings and pterygoid processes ossifies from eight centres: Two centres for two greater wings during eighth week forming the root only; two for postsphenoidal part of body during fourth month; two centres appear for the two pterygoid hamulus during third month of foetal life. These six centres appear in cartilage. Two centres for medial pterygoid plates appear during ninth week and the remaining portion of the greater wings and lateral plates ossify in membrane from the centres for the root of greater wing only.

Ethmoid: It ossifies in cartilage. Three centres appear in cartilaginous nasal capsule. One centre appears in perpendicular plate during first year of life. Two centres, one for each labyrinth, appear between fourth and fifth months of intra-uterine life.

Mandible: Each half of the body is ossified in membrane by one centre which appears during sixth week near the mental foramen. The upper half of ramus ossifies in cartilage. Ossification spreads in condylar and coronoid processes above the level of the mandibular foramen.

Inferior nasal concha: It ossifies in cartilage. One centre appears during fifth month in the lower border of the cartilaginous nasal capsule.

Palatine: One centre appears during eighth week in perpendicular plate. It ossifies in membrane.

Lacrimal: It ossifies in membrane. One centre appears during twelfth week.

Nasal: It also ossifies in membrane from one centre which appears during third month of intra-uterine life.

Vomer: It ossifies in membrane. Two centres appear during eighth week on either side of midline. These fuse by twelfth week.

Zygomatic: It ossifies in membrane by one centre which appears during eighth week.

Maxilla: It also ossifies in membrane by three centres. One for main body which appears during sixth week above canine fossa.

Two centres appear for premaxilla during seventh week and fuse soon.

Various foramina of anterior, middle and posterior cranial fossae and other foramina with their contents are shown in Table 9.4.

DEVELOPMENT OF NEUROCRANIUM

1 Membranous part: From mesenchyme around developing brain. Mesenchyme is derived from:
   i. Neural crest cells forming roof and sides of cranial vault.
   ii. Para-axial mesoderm forming small part in occipital region. Ossification is membranous ossification.

Table 9.4: Foramina of skull bones and their contents (*refer to BDC App*)

Foramina/apertures	*Contents*
ANTERIOR CRANIAL FOSSA	
Groove for superior sagittal sinus	Superior sagittal sinus
Foramen caecum	Emissary vein to superior sagittal sinus from upper part of nose
Anterior ethmoidal foramen	Anterior ethmoidal nerve and vessels
Foramina of cribiform plate	Olfactory nerve rootlets
Posterior ethmoidal foramen	Posterior ethmoidal vessels
MIDDLE CRANIAL FOSSA	
Optic canal	Optic nerve and ophthalmic artery
Superior orbital fissure:	
• Lateral part	*Lacrimal and frontal nerves* (branches of ophthalmic nerve); *trochlear nerve*; superior ophthalmic vein; meningeal branch of lacrimal artery; anastomotic branch of middle meningeal artery, which anastomoses with recurrent branch of lacrimal artery.
• Middle part	*Upper division of oculomotor nerve* (CN III), *nasociliary nerve, lower division of CN III, abducent nerve* (CN VI)
• Medial part	Inferior ophthalmic vein; sympathetic nerve from plexus around internal carotid artery.
Foramen rotundum	Maxillary nerve (CN V2)
Foramen ovale	Mandibular nerve (CN V3); accessory meningeal artery; lesser petrosal nerve; emissary vein connecting cavernous sinus with pterygoid plexus (MALE)
Foramen spinosum	Middle meningeal artery and vein, meningeal branch of mandibular nerve (CN V3)
Emissary sphenoidal foramen	Emissary vein connecting cavernous sinus with pterygoid plexus of veins
Foramen lacerum (Fig. 9.15)	During life, the foramen is filled with cartilage No significant structure passes through it; internal carotid artery and nerve plexus pass across its superior end; nerve to pterygoid canal passes through its anterior wall; meningeal branch of ascending pharyngeal artery and emissary vein pass through it.
Carotid canal	Internal carotid artery and nerve plexus (sympathetic)
Groove for lesser petrosal nerve	Lesser petrosal nerve
Groove for greater petrosal nerve	Greater petrosal nerve
POSTERIOR CRANIAL FOSSA	
Foramen magnum (Fig. 9.16)	Lowest part of medulla oblongata and three meninges; vertebral arteries; spinal roots of CN XI; anterior and posterior spinal arteries; apical ligament; vertical band of cruciate ligament and membrana tectoria.
Jugular foramen	CN IX; X; XI; inferior petrosal and sigmoid sinuses; meningeal branches of ascending pharyngeal and occipital arteries.
Hypoglossal canal/anterior condylar canal	CN XII
Internal acoustic meatus	CN VII; VIII and labyrinthine vessels
External opening of vestibular aqueduct	Endolymphatic duct
Posterior condylar canal	Emissary vein connecting sigmoid sinus with the suboccipital venous plexus
Mastoid foramen	Mastoid emissary vein and meningeal branch of occipital artery
OTHER FORAMINA	
External acoustic meatus	Air waves
External nasal foramen	External nasal nerve
Greater palatine foramen	Greater palatine vessels; anterior palatine nerve

(Contd...)

Table 9.4: Foramina of skull bones and their contents (*Contd...*)

Foramina/apertures	*Contents*
Incisive canal	Greater palatine vessels; terminal part of nasopalatine nerve
Inferior orbital fissure	Zygomatic nerve; orbital branches of pterygopalatine ganglion; infraorbital nerve and vessels
Infraorbital foramen	Infraorbital nerve and vessels
Lesser palatine foramen	Middle and posterior palatine nerves
Mandibular foramen/canal	Inferior alveolar nerve and vessels
Mandibular notch	Masseteric nerve and vessels
Mastoid canaliculus	Auricular branch of vagus nerve
Mental foramen	Mental nerve and vessels
Palatinovaginal canal	Pharyngeal branch from pterygopalatine ganglion; pharyngeal branch of maxillary artery
Parietal foramen	Emissary vein from scalp to superior sagittal sinus
Petrotympanic fissure	Chorda tympanic nerve and anterior tympanic artery
Pterygoid canal	Nerve to pterygoid canal and vessels
Pterygomaxillary fissure	Maxillary nerve
Pterygopalatine fossa	Pterygopalatine ganglion
Stylomastoid foramen	Facial nerve; stylomastoid branch of posterior auricular artery.
Supraorbital foramen	Supraorbital nerve and vessels
Tympanic canaliculus	Tympanic branch of glossopharyngeal nerve
Tympanomastoid fissure	Auricular branch of vagus nerve
Vomerovaginal canal	Branch of pharyngeal nerve and vessels
Zygomatic foramen	Zygomatic nerve
Zygomaticofacial foramen	Zygomaticofacial nerve
Zygomaticotemporal foramen	Zygomaticotemporal nerve

2 Mesenchyme formed directly into bone. Membranous bones are: Frontal, parietal, squamous temporal and interparietal part of occipital bones. These bones are united by sutures and fontanelles.

DEVELOPMENT OF SKULL BONES

Bones formed in membrane: Frontal and parietal develop in relation to mesenchyme covering developing brain.

Maxilla (excluding premaxilla), zygomatic, palatine parts of temporal bone are formed by mesenchyme of maxillary process.

Nasal, lacrimal and vomer are formed by membrane covering nasal capsule.

Bones formed in cartilage: Inferior nasal concha and ethmoid are formed from cartilage of nasal capsule.

Bones formed in cartilage and membrane

Sphenoid—only lateral part of greater wing and pterygoid laminae are formed in membrane, rest is formed in cartilage.

Occipital—only interparietal part is membranous, rest is cartilaginous.

Temporal—squamous and tympanic parts are formed in membrane. The other parts, i.e. petrous and mastoid are formed in cartilage. Styloid process is fromed in cartilage from 2nd branchial arch.

Mandible—most of the bone is formed in membrane in the mesenchyme of Meckel's cartilage. *Ventral part of Meckel's cartilage gets embedded in the bone*. Condylar and coronoid process are ossified from secondary cartilages.

Hyoid bone—develops from the 2nd and 3rd pharyngeal arches.

Cartilaginous part: Neural crest cells form mesenchyme which form cartilaginous models; these get replaced by bone. Bones thus formed are: Ethmoid, most of sphenoid, base of occipital, petrous temporal.

Development of viscerocranium: Viscerocranium includes bones of face. Some bones have membranous ossification while others have cartilaginous. These are formed by first pharynegeal arch cartilage—maxillary process → Maxilla, zygomatic, part of temporal. Mandibular process—mandible, malleus, incus.

Second arch <Dorsal end—stapes, styloid process, lesser cornua and upper part of body of hyoid bone.

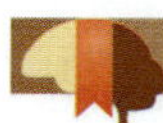

Mnemonics

Nerves related to mandible M3LIA

M3—masseteric nerve, mental nerve, nerve to mylohyoid
L—lingual nerve
I—inferior alveolar nerve
A—auriculotemporal nerve

Arteries related to mandible—M4IFS

M4—masseteric artery, maxillary, mental and artery to mylohyoid
I—inferior alveolar artery
F—facial artery
S—superficial temporal artery

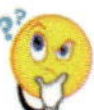

FACTS TO REMEMBER

- Eight bones in the calvaria and 14 facial bones make up the skull.
- Most of the joints are 'suture' type of joints. The joint between teeth and gums is gomphosis. There is a pair of temporomandibular joints, which is of synovial variety.
- The bony ossicles are malleus, incus and stapes and are 'bone within bone', as these are present in the petrous temporal bone. Between these three ossicles are two synovial joints.
- Diploe veins contain manufactured RBCs, granulocytes and platelets. These drain into the neighbouring veins.
- Paranasal sinuses give resonance to the voice, besides humidifying and warming up the inspired air.

CLINICOANATOMICAL PROBLEM

A young woman complains of pain and numbness along the lateral side of forearm and hand, with wasting of the muscles of thenar eminence.

- Why is there pain in forearm and hand with no injury to the affected area?
- Why are thenar muscles getting weaker?

Ans: There is no obvious injury in the hand or forearm. These symptoms are nervous in nature. One has to look for the nerve root which supplies this area. The nerve root is C6. Feel the cervical spine for any pain. An X-ray/CT scan may reveal prolapse of the intervertebral disc between C5 and C6 vertebrae compressing the C6 nerve root. These roots form part of lateral cutaneous nerve of forearm, and median nerves. Since median nerve (C6) supplies thenar muscles, there is wasting/weakness of these muscles. As lateral cutaneous nerve of forearm is pressed, there is numbness on lateral side of forearm and hand.

FURTHER READING

- Lahr MM. The Evolution of Modern Human Diversity: A study of Cranial Variation. Cambridge: Cambridge University Press. 1996.
- Tuli A, Choudhry R, Choudhry S, Raheja S, Agarwal S. Variation in shape of the lingula in the adult human mandible. J Anat 2000;197:313–17.
- Tubbs RS, Salter EG, Oakes WJ. Artificial deformation of the human skull: A review Clin Anat 2006;19:372–77.
  An excellent text when considering the extent of human variation and diversity.
  An excellent review article that highlights the incredible plasticity of the human skull.

Frequently Asked Questions

1. Enumerate the muscles attached to the hyoid bone. Give their nerve supply.
2. Name the structures traversing foramen magnum. Depict these with the help of a diagram.
3. Write short notes/enumerate:
   a. Structures passing though superior orbital fissure.
   b. Pterion bones meeting at this point and its clinical importance.
   c. Attachments of muscles on mastoid process with their nerve supply.
   d. Ligaments/membranes attached to atlas vertebra.
   e. Structure passing through jugular foramen.
4. Name paired bones of cranium and face.

Multiple Choice Questions

1. Which of the following structures does not pass through foramen magnum?
   a. Accessory pharyngeal artery
   b. Vertebral artery
   c. Spinal accessory nerve
   d. Vertical band of cruciate ligament
2. Which of the following nerves does not pass through jugular foramen?
   a. Vagus b. Hypoglossal
   c. Glossopharyngeal d. Accessory
3. Which is the thickest boundary of the orbit?
   a. Lateral b. Medial
   c. Roof d. Floor
4. Which bone is not a 'bone within the bone' in petrous temporal bone?
   a. Malleus b. Hyoid
   c. Incus d. Stapes
5. Which of the parasympathetic ganglia does not have a secretomotor root?
   a. Submandibular b. Pterygopalatine
   c. Otic d. Ciliary

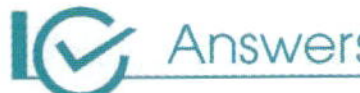

Answers

1. a **2.** b **3.** a **4.** b **5.** d

VIVA VOCE

- Name the paired and unpaired (brain case) bones of cranium.
- Name the paired and unpaired bones of facial skeleton.
- Name the fontanelles of the skull. When do these close?
- Name the 'bones within the bone'.
- Which is the last fontanelle to be closed and at what age does it close? What are the functions of fontanelle?
- Name the diploic veins.
- Name the emissary veins. What are their functions and clinical anatomy?
- What is pterion? Give its importance.
- Name the structures passing through foramen magnum.
- Name the structures traversing inferior orbital fissure.
- Name the structures passing through superior orbital fissure in order.
- Enumerate the nerves related to mandible.
- Enumerate the arteries related to mandible.
- What is type of atlantoccipital joint?
- What is type of median atlantoaxial joint?
- Name the muscles attached to styloid process including their nerve supply.

Bones of skull: Introduction, bones of skull, anterior cranial fossa, middle cranial fossa, posterior cranial fossa, orbit, mandible, foramina, norma frontalis, hyoid bone, cervical vertebrae.

Chapter

10

Scalp, Temple and Face

"Kiss is the anatomical juxtaposition of the orbicularis oris in a state of contraction."
—Anonymous

INTRODUCTION

Face is the most prominent part of the body. Facial muscles, being the muscles of facial expression, express a variety of emotions like happiness, joy, sadness, anger, frowning, grinning, etc. The face, therefore, is an *index of mind*. One's innerself is expressed by the face itself as it is controlled by the higher centres.

SURFACE LANDMARKS

1 The *forehead* is the part of the face between the hairline of adolescent's scalp and the eyebrows. The superolateral prominence of the forehead is known as the *frontal eminence*.

2 Identify the following in relation to the nose: The prominent ridge separating the right and left halves of the nose is called the *dorsum*. The upper narrow end of the nose, just below the forehead, is the *root of* the nose. The lower end of the dorsum is in the form of a somewhat rounded *tip*. At the lower end of the nose, we see the right and left *nostrils* or *anterior nares*. The two nostrils are separated by a soft median partition called the *columella*. This is continuous with the *nasal septum* which separates the two nasal cavities. Each nostril is bounded laterally by the *ala*.

3 The *palpebral fissure* is an elliptical opening between the two eyelids. The lids are joined to each other at the medial and lateral angles or *canthi* of the eye. The free margin of each eyelid has eyelashes or cilia arranged along its outer edge (Fig. 10.1a).

Through the palpebral fissure following are seen.

a. The opaque sclera or white of the eye

b. The transparent circular *cornea* through which the coloured iris and the dark circular *pupil* can be seen.

The eyeballs are lodged in bony sockets, called the *orbits*.

The *conjunctiva* is a moist, transparent membrane. The part which covers the anterior surface of the eyeball is the *bulbar conjunctiva*, and the part lining the inner surfaces of the lids is the *palpebral conjunctiva*. The space between the two is the *conjunctival* sac. The line along which the bulbar conjunctiva becomes the palpebral conjunctiva is known as the *conjunctival fornix*.

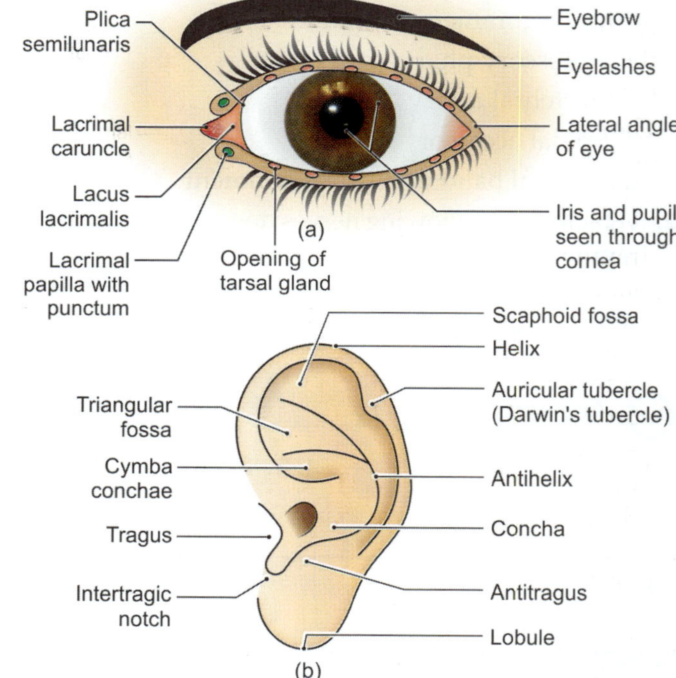

Figs 10.1a and b: (a) Some features to be seen on the face around the left eye; (b) Parts of the pinna

4 The *oral fissure* or mouth is the opening between the upper and lower *lips*. It lies opposite the cutting edges of the upper incisor teeth. The angle of the mouth usually lies just in front of first upper premolar tooth. Each lip has a *red margin* at mucocutaneous junction and a *dark margin*, with a non-hairy thin skin intervening between the two margins. The lips normally close the mouth along their red margins. The *philtrum* is the median vertical groove on the upper lip.

5 The *external ear* is made up of two parts: A superficial projecting part, called the *auricle or pinna;* and a deep canal, called the *external acoustic meatus*. The mobile auricle helps in catching the sound waves, and is a characteristic feature of mammals (Fig. 10.1b). Lobule is the lower, smaller soft part of the auricle. The upper larger stiff part shows: (a) Helix, the outer rolled margin; (b) A Y-shaped antihelix which is surrounded, except inferiorly, by the arched helix. The upper forked end of the antihelix encloses the triangular fossa. Antihelix is separated from the helix posterosuperiorly by the scaphoid fossa and anteroinferiorly by the cymba conchae. (c) Concha leads into external acoustic meatus. It is bounded anteriorly by tragus, inferiorly by the intertragic notch and the antitragus, posteriorly by the curved anterior end of the helix. The auricle is situated at the level of the eyebrow above and the nostrils below and is nearer the occiput than the face.

6 The *supraorbital margin* lies beneath the upper margin of the eyebrow. The supraorbital notch is palpable at the junction of the medial one-third with the lateral two-thirds of the supraorbital margin. A vertical line drawn from the supraorbital notch to the base of the mandible, passing midway between the lower two premolar teeth, crosses the infraorbital foramen 5 mm below the infraorbital margin, and the mental foramen midway between the upper and lower borders of the mandible.

7 The *superciliary* arch is a curved bony ridge situated immediately above the medial part of each supra-orbital margin. The *glabella* is the median elevation connecting the two superciliary arches, and corresponds to elevation between the two eyebrows.

SCALP AND SUPERFICIAL TEMPORAL REGION

SCALP

The soft tissues covering the cranial vault form the scalp (Fig. 10.2b).

Extent of Scalp

Anteriorly, supraorbital margins; posteriorly, external occipital protuberance and superior nuchal lines; and on each side, the superior temporal lines (Fig. 10.2b) or upto zygomatic arch and external auditory meatus (42nd, ed, Gray's Anatomy).

Structure

Conventionally, the superficial temporal region is studied with the scalp, and the following description, therefore, will cover both the regions.

DISSECTION

Place 2–3 wooden blocks under the head to raise it about 10–12 cm from the table. Figure 10.2a shows a median incision in the skin of scalp extending from root of the nose (i), to the prominent external occipital protuberance (ii). Give a coronal incision across the previous incision from root of one auricle to the other (iii). Extend the incision from the auricles to the mastoid process posteriorly (iv), and to root of zygoma anteriorly (v). Reflect the skin in four flaps. Usually, the skin is so adherent to the subjacent connective tissue and aponeurotic layers that these all come off together. Dissect the layers, including the nerves, vessels, lymphatics and identify these structures in the cadaver (*refer to BDC App*).

The scalp is made up of five layers (mnemonic **SCALP**)

a. **S**kin

b. Superficial fascia (**C**onnective tissue)

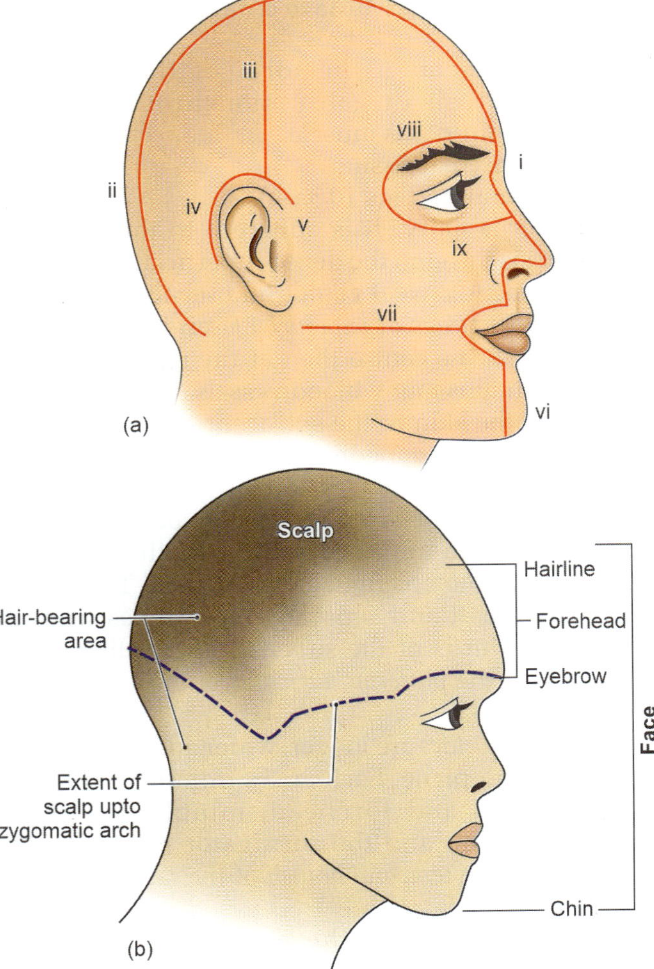

Figs 10.2a and b: (a) Lines of dissection for scalp, face and eyelids, (b) Extent of scalp

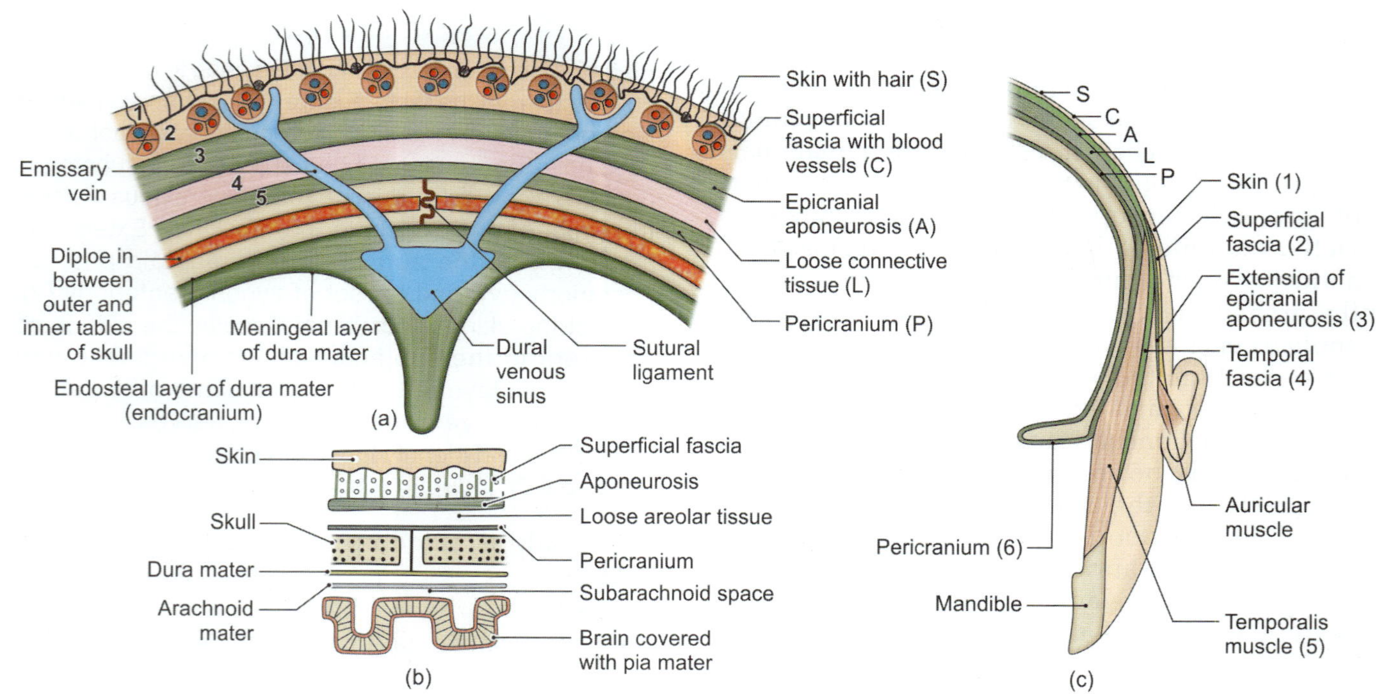

Figs 10.3a to c: (a) and (b) Layers of the scalp; (c) Layers of superficial temporal region

c. Deep fascia in the form of the epicranial **a**poneurosis or galea aponeurotica with the occipitofrontalis muscle
d. **L**oose areolar tissue
e. **P**ericranium (Figs 10.3a–c).

The *skin* is hairy. It is adherent to the epicranial aponeurosis through the dense superficial fascia. It has more number of sweat glands and sebaceous glands.

The *subcutaneous* or *superficial fascia* is more fibrous and dense in the centre than at the periphery of the head. It contains many blood vessels.

It binds the skin to the subjacent aponeurosis, and provides the proper medium for passage of vessels and nerves to the skin.

The *occipitofrontalis muscle* has two bellies, occipital or occipitalis and frontal or frontalis, both of which are inserted into the epicranial aponeurosis. The *occipital bellies* are small and separate. Each arises from the lateral two-thirds of the superior nuchal line, and is supplied by the *posterior auricular* branch of the *facial nerve* (Fig. 10.4a).

The *frontal bellies* are longer, wider and partly united in the median plane. Each arises from the skin of the upper eyelid and forehead, mingling with the orbicularis oculi and the corrugator supercilii. It is supplied by the *temporal branch* of the facial nerve (*see* Fig. 9.6).

The muscle raises the eyebrows and causes horizontal wrinkles in the skin of the forehead.

The *epicranial aponeurosis,* or galea aponeurotica is freely movable on the pericranium along with the

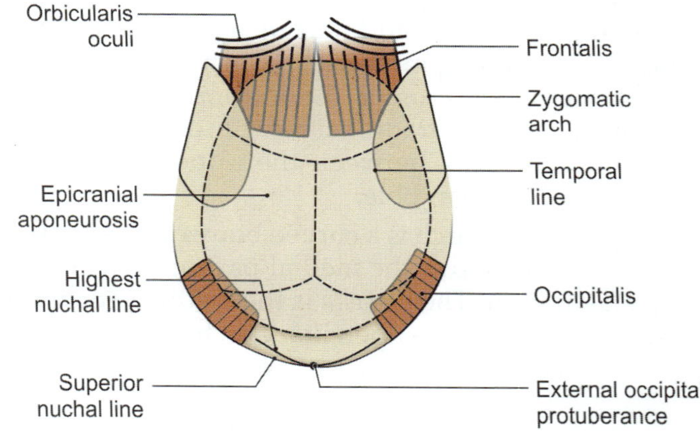

Fig. 10.4a: Bellies of the occipitofrontalis muscle

overlying and adherent skin and fascia (Figs 10.3a and 10.9). Anteriorly, it receives the insertion of the frontalis, posteriorly, it receives the insertion of the occipitalis and is attached to the external occipital protuberance, and to the highest/superior nuchal lines in between the occipital bellies. On each side, the aponeurosis is attached to the superior temporal line, but sends down a thin expansion which passes over the temporal fascia and is attached to the zygomatic arch (Fig. 10.3c).

First three layers of scalp are called *surgical layers of the scalp*. These are called scalp proper also.

The fourth layer of the scalp is made up of *loose areolar tissue*. It extends anteriorly into the eyelids (Fig. 10.4b), because the frontalis muscle has no bony attachment; posteriorly to the highest and superior nuchal lines; and on each side to the superior temporal

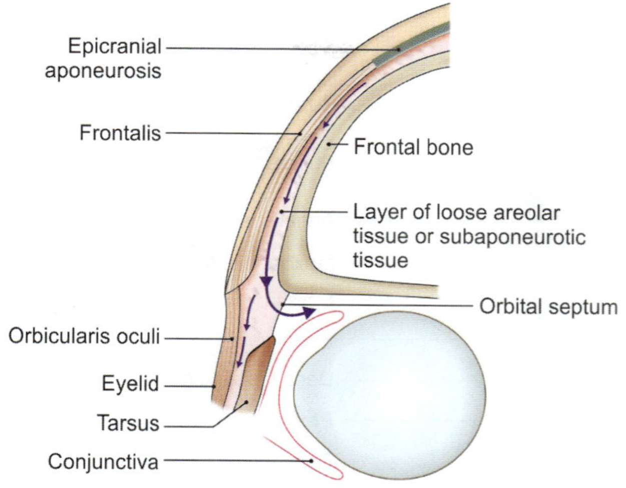

Fig. 10.4b: Schematic section through the scalp and upper eyelid to show how fluids can pass from the subaponeurotic space or layer of loose areolar tissue of the scalp into the eyelid, and into the subconjunctival area. Note that this is possible because the frontalis muscle has no bony attachment

lines. It gives passage to the emissary veins which connect extracranial veins to intracranial venous sinuses (Fig. 10.3a).

The fifth layer of the scalp, called the *pericranium*, is loosely attached to the surface of the bones, but is firmly adherent to their sutures where the sutural ligaments bind the pericranium to the endocranium (Fig. 10.3a).

SUPERFICIAL TEMPORAL REGION

It is the area between the superior temporal line and the zygomatic arch. It is considered as a part of scalp (42nd ed., Gray's Anatomy). This area contains the following 6 layers (Fig. 10.3c):

1. Skin
2. Superficial fascia
3. Thin extension of epicranial aponeurosis which gives origin to extrinsic muscles of the auricle
4. Temporal fascia
5. Temporalis muscle
6. Pericranium.

Tempus means time. Greying of hair first starts here.

Arterial Supply of Scalp and Superficial Temporal Region

In front of the auricle, the scalp is supplied from before backwards by the:

- *Supratrochlear*
- *Supraorbital*
- *Superficial temporal* arteries (Fig. 10.5).

The first two are branches of the ophthalmic artery which in turn is a branch of the internal carotid artery. The superficial temporal is a branch of the external carotid artery.

Behind the auricle, the scalp is supplied from before backwards by the:

- *Posterior auricular*
- *Occipital* (tortuous) arteries, both of which are branches of the external carotid artery.

Thus, the scalp has a *rich blood supply* derived from both the internal and the external carotid arteries, the two systems anastomosing over the temple.

Venous Drainage

The veins of the scalp accompany the arteries and have similar names. The *supratrochlear* and *supraorbital* veins

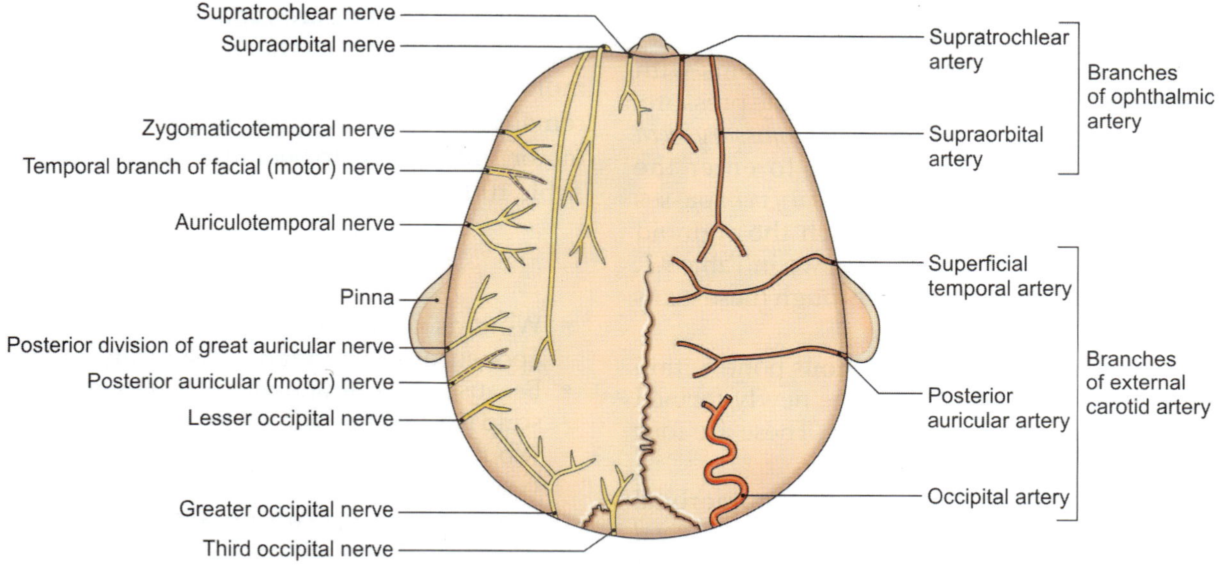

Fig. 10.5: Arterial and nerve supply of scalp and superficial temporal region

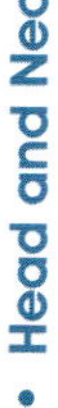

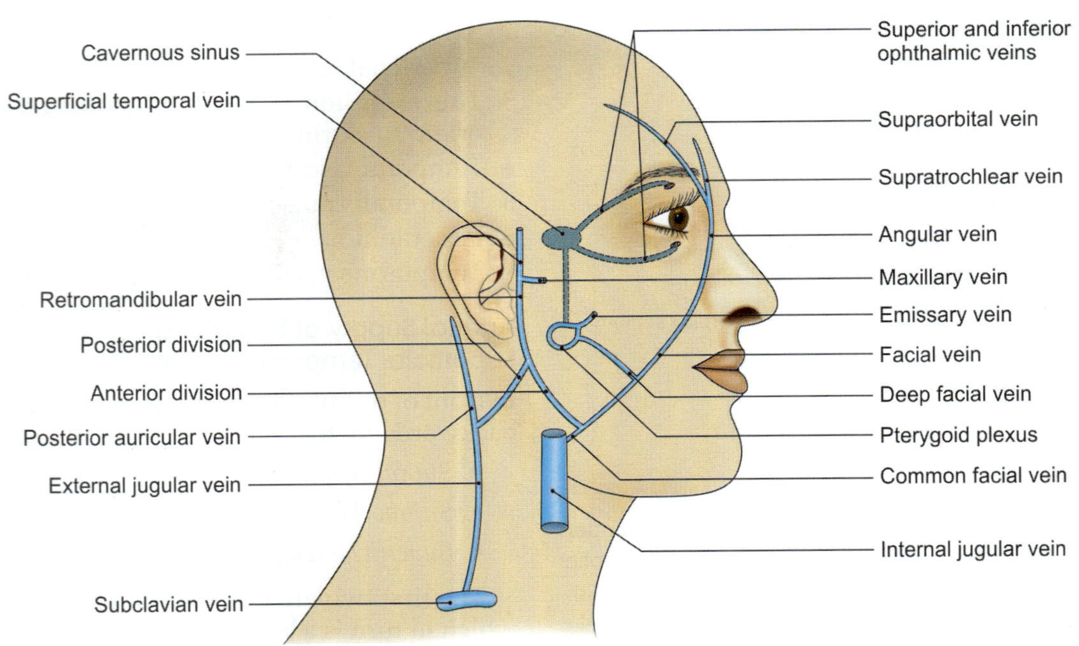

Fig. 10.6: The veins of the scalp, face and their deep connections with the cavernous sinus and the pterygoid plexus of veins

unite at the medial angle of the eye forming the *angular* vein which continues down as the *facial* vein.

The *superficial temporal vein* descends in front of the tragus, enters the parotid gland, and joins the maxillary vein to form the *retromandibular* vein. This vein divides into two divisions.

The anterior division of the retromandibular vein unites with the facial vein to form the common facial vein which drains into the internal jugular vein.

The posterior division of the retromandibular vein unites with the *posterior auricular vein* to form the *external jugular vein* which ultimately drains into the *subclavian vein*. The occipital veins terminate in the suboccipital venous plexus (Fig. 10.6).

Emissary veins connect the extracranial veins with the intracranial venous sinuses to equalise the pressure. These veins are valveless. The *parietal emissary vein* passes through the parietal foramen to enter the superior sagittal sinus. The *mastoid emissary vein* passes through the mastoid foramen to reach the sigmoid sinus. Remaining emissary veins are shown in Table 9.1. Extracranial infections may spread through these veins to intracranial venous sinuses.

Diploic veins start from the cancellous bone within the two tables of skull. These carry the newly formed blood cells into the general circulation. These are four veins on each side (*see* Fig. 9.17a).

The *frontal diploic vein* emerges at the supraorbital notch open into the supraorbital vein. *Anterior temporal diploic vein* ends in anterior deep temporal vein or sphenoparietal sinus. *Posterior temporal diploic vein* ends in the transverse sinus. The *occipital diploic vein* opens either into the occipital vein, or into the transverse sinus near the median plane (*see* Table 9.2).

Lymphatic Drainage

The anterior part of the scalp drains into the pre-auricular or parotid lymph nodes, situated on the surface of the parotid gland. The posterior part of the scalp drains into the posterior auricular or mastoid and occipital lymph nodes.

Nerve Supply

The scalp and temple are supplied by 10 nerves on each side. Out of these, five nerves (four sensory and one motor) enter the scalp in front of the auricle. The remaining five nerves (again four sensory and one motor) enter the scalp behind the auricle (Fig. 10.5 and Table 10.1).

CLINICAL ANATOMY

- Wounds of the scalp gape when the epicranial aponeurosis is divided transversely.
- Because of the abundance of sebaceous glands, the scalp is a common site for sebaceous cysts (Fig. 10.7).
- Wounds of the scalp bleed profusely because the vessels are prevented from retracting by the fibrous fascia. Bleeding can be arrested by applying pressure at the site of injury by a tight cotton bandage against the bone.

Table 10.1: Nerves of the scalp and superficial temporal region

In front of auricle	*Behind the auricle*
Sensory nerves	*Sensory nerves*
• Supratrochlear, branch of the frontal nerve (ophthalmic division of trigeminal nerve)	• Posterior division of great auricular nerve (C2, C3) from cervical plexus
• Supraorbital, branch of frontal nerve (ophthalmic division of trigeminal nerve)	• Lesser occipital nerve (C2), from cervical plexus
• Zygomaticotemporal, branch of zygomatic nerve (maxillary division of trigeminal nerve)	• Greater occipital nerve (C2, dorsal ramus)
• Auriculotemporal branch of mandibular division of trigeminal nerve	• Third occipital nerve (C3, dorsal ramus)
Motor nerve	*Motor nerve*
• Temporal branch of facial nerve	• Posterior auricular branch of facial nerve

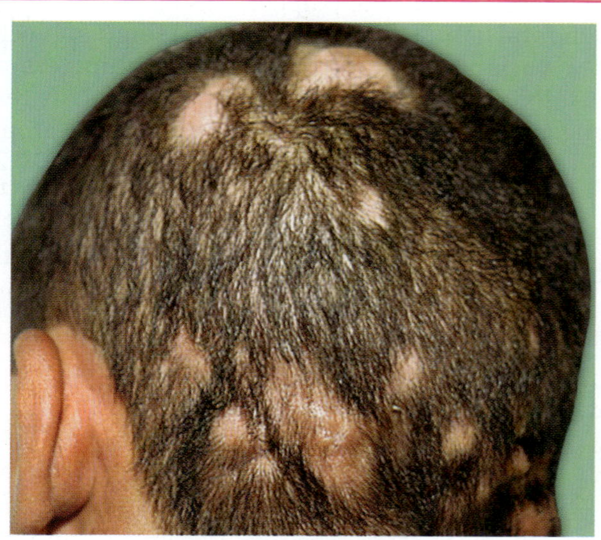

Fig. 10.7: Bilateral sebaceous cysts

- Because of the density of fascia, subcutaneous haemorrhages are never extensive, and the inflammations in this layer cause little swelling but much pain.
- Because the pericranium is adherent to sutures, collections of fluid deep to the pericranium known as *cephalhaematoma* take the shape of the bone concerned when there is fracture of particular bone.
- The layer of loose areolar tissue is known as the *dangerous area of the scalp* because the emissary veins, which course here, may transmit infection from the scalp to the cranial venous sinuses (Fig. 10.3a).

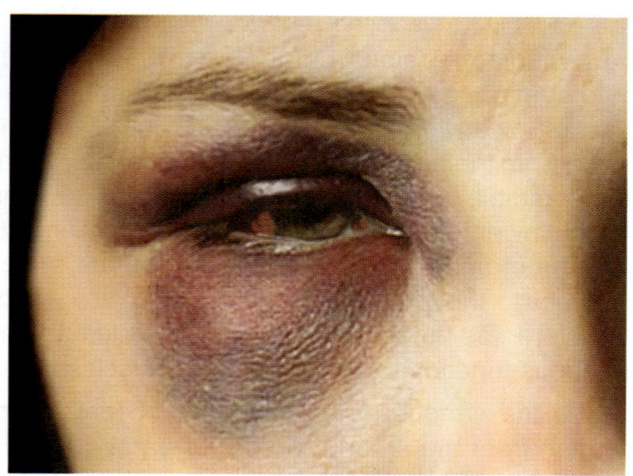

Fig. 10.8: Right eye—black eye due to injury to the scalp

- Collection of blood in the layer of loose connective tissue causes generalised swelling of the scalp. The blood may extend anteriorly into the root of the nose and into the eyelids (as frontalis muscle has no bony origin) resulting in black eye. The posterior limit of such haemorrhage is not seen (Fig. 10.8). If bleeding is due to local injury, the posterior limit of haemorrhage is seen.
- Because of the spread of blood, compression of brain is not seen and so this layer is also called safety layer.
- Since the blood supply of scalp and superficial temporal region is very rich; avulsed portions need not be cut away. They can be replaced in position and stitched: They usually take up and heal well.

FACE

Features

The face, or countenance, extends superiorly from the adolescent position of hairline, inferiorly to the chin and the base of the mandible, and on each side to the auricle. The forehead is, therefore, common to both the face and the scalp.

SKIN

1. The facial skin is *very vascular*. Rich vascularity makes the face blush and blanch. Wounds of the face bleed profusely but heal rapidly. The results of plastic surgery on the face are excellent for the same reason.
2. The facial skin is *rich in sebaceous and sweat glands*. Sebaceous glands keep the face oily, but also cause *acne* in young adults. Sweat glands help in regulation of the body temperature.
3. *Laxity* of the greater part of the skin facilitates rapid spread of oedema. Renal oedema appears first in the

DISSECTION

Give a median incision from the root of nose, across the dorsum of nose, centre of philtrum of upper lip, to centre of lower lip to the chin (vi). Give a horizontal incision from the angle of the mouth to posterior border of the mandible (vii). Reflect the lower flap towards and up to the lower border of mandible (Fig. 10.2a; line with dots). Direct and reflect the upper flap till the auricle. Subjacent to the skin, the facial muscles are directly encountered as these are inserted in the skin. Identify the various functional groups of facial muscles.

Trace the various motor branches of facial nerve emerging from the anterior border of parotid gland to supply these muscles. Amongst these motor branches on the face are the sensory branches of the three divisions of the trigeminal nerve. Try to identify all these with the help of their course given in the text (Fig. 10.16) (*refer to BDC App*).

eyelids and face before spreading to other parts of the body.

4 Boils in the nose and ear are acutely painful due to the *fixity* of the skin to the underlying cartilages.

5 Facial skin is very *elastic and thick* because the facial muscles are inserted into it. The wounds of the face, therefore, tend to gape.

SUPERFICIAL FASCIA

It contains: (i) The facial muscles, all of which are inserted into the skin, (ii) the vessels and nerves, to the muscles and to the skin, and (iii) a variable amount of fat. Fat is absent from the eyelids, but is well developed in the cheeks, forming the buccal pads that are very prominent in infants in whom they help in sucking.

The *deep fascia is absent* from the face, except over the parotid gland where it forms the parotid fascia, and over the buccinator where it forms the *buccopharyngeal fascia*.

FACIAL MUSCLES

The facial muscles are subcutaneous muscles. Since these muscles are inserted into skin, these bring out various facial expressions. So, these are secondarily known as muscles of facial expression. These have small motor units.

Embryologically, they develop from the mesoderm of the second branchial arch, and are, therefore, supplied by the facial nerve.

Morphologically, they represent the best remnants of the *panniculus carnosus*, a continuous subcutaneous muscle sheet seen in some animals. All of them are inserted into the skin.

Topographically, the muscles are grouped under the following six heads.

Functionally, most of these muscles may be regarded primarily as regulators of the three openings situated on the face, namely the palpebral fissures, the nostrils and the oral fissure. Each opening has a single sphincter, and a variable number of dilators. Sphincters are naturally circular and the dilators radial in their arrangement. These muscles are better developed around the eyes and mouth than around the nose (Table 10.2).

Table 10.2: Functional groups of facial muscles

Opening	*Sphincter*	*Dilators*
A. Palpebral fissure	Orbicularis oculi	1. Levator palpebrae superioris 2. Frontalis part of occipitofrontalis
B. Oral fissure	Orbicularis oris	All the muscles around the mouth, except the orbicularis oris, the sphincter, and the mentalis which does not mingle with orbicularis oris
C. Nostrils	Compressor naris	1. Dilator naris 2. Depressor septi 3. Medial slip of levator labii superioris alaeque nasi

Muscle of the Scalp

Occipitofrontalis—described in scalp.

Muscles of the Auricle

Situated around the ear:

1 Auricularis anterior
2 Auricularis superior
3 Auricularis posterior

These are vestigeal muscles.

Muscles of the Eyelids/Orbital Openings

1 Orbicularis oculi (Fig. 10.9 and Table 10.3)
2 *Corrugator* (Latin to wrinkle) supercilii (Fig. 10.9 and Table 10.3)
3 Levator palpebrae superioris (an extraocular muscle, supplied by sympathetic fibres and the third cranial nerve) is described in Chapter 21, *see* Fig. 10.21 as well.

Muscles of the Nose

1 Procerus (Fig. 10.9)
2 Compressor naris
3 Dilator naris
4 Depressor septi

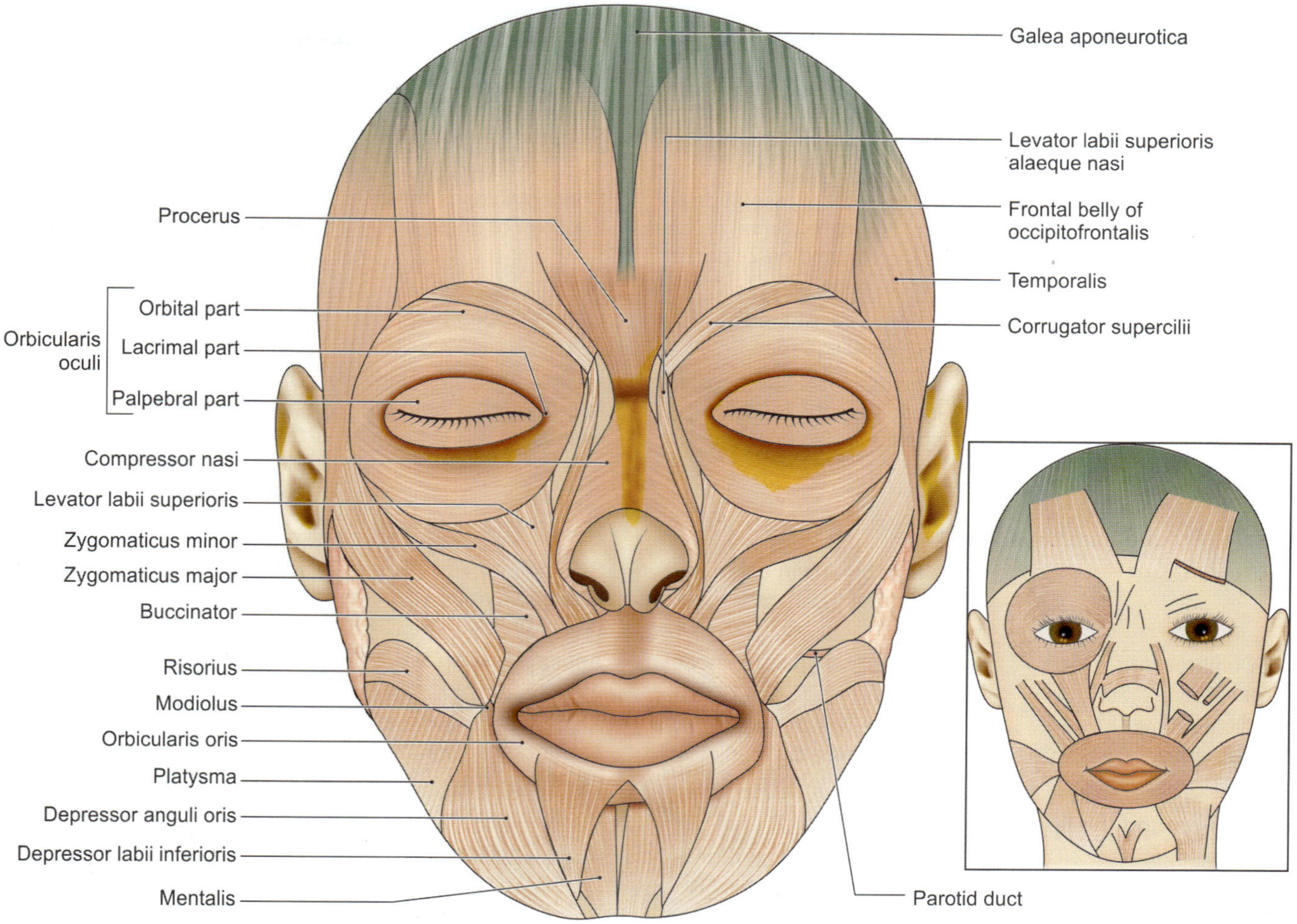

Fig. 10.9: The facial muscles

Muscles around the Mouth

1 Orbicularis oris (Fig. 10.9)
2 *Buccinator* (Latin cheek) (Fig. 10.10)
3 Levator labii superioris alaeque nasi (Fig. 10.10)
4 Zygomaticus major (Fig. 10.9)
5 Levator labii superioris (Fig. 10.9)

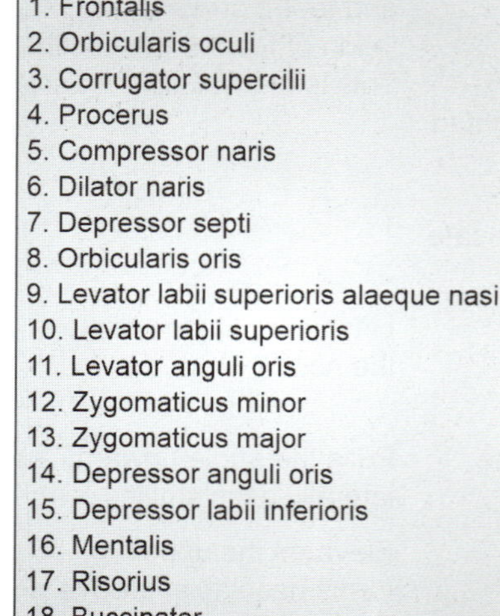

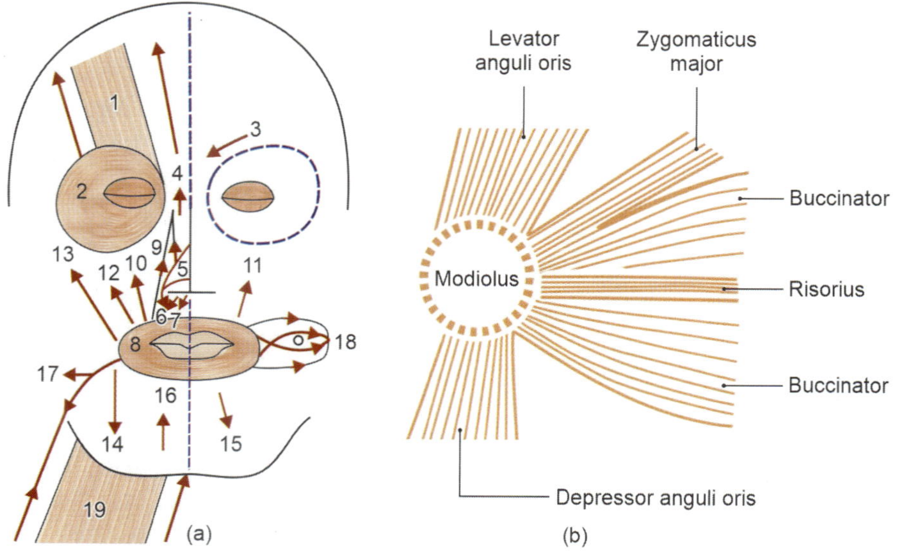

Fig. 10.10: Some facial muscles

Table 10.3: The facial muscles			
Name	*Origin*	*Insertion*	*Actions*
Muscles of eyelid/orbital opening			
1. Corrugator supercilii (Fig. 10.9)	Medial end of superciliary arch	Skin of mid-eyebrow	Vertical lines in forehead, as in frowning
2. Orbicularis oculi (Fig. 10.9) a. Orbital part, on and around the orbital margin	Medial part of medial palpebral ligament, frontal process of maxilla and nasal part of frontal bone	Concentric rings return to the point of origin	Protects eye from bright light, wind and rain. Cause forceful closure of eyelids
b. Palpebral part, in the lids	Lateral part of medial palpebral ligament	Lateral palpebral raphe	Closes lids gently as in blinking and sleeping
c. Lacrimal part, lateral and deep to the lacrimal sac	Lacrimal fascia and posterior lacrimal crest, forms sheath for lacrimal sac	Pass laterally in front of tarsal plates of both the eyelids	Dilates lacrimal sac for sucking of lacrimal fluid into the sac, directs lacrimal puncta into lacus lacrimalis; supports the lower lid
Muscles around nasal opening			
3. Procerus	Nasal bone and upper part of lateral nasal cartilage	Skin of forehead between eyebrows and on bridge of the nose	Causes transverse wrinkles
4. Compressor naris	Maxilla just lateral to nose	Aponeurosis across dorsum of nose	Nasal aperture compressed
5. Dilator naris	Maxilla over the lateral incisor	Alar cartilage of nose	Nasal aperture dilated
6. Depressor septi	Maxilla over the medial incisor	Lower mobile part of nasal septum	Nose pulled inferiorly
Muscles around the lips			
7. Orbicularis oris a. Intrinsic part, deep stratum, very thin sheet	Superior incisivus, from maxilla; inferior incisivus, from mandible	Angle of mouth	Closes lips and protrudes lips, numerous extrinsic muscles make it most versatile for various types of grimaces
b. Extrinsic part, two strata, formed by converging muscles (Fig. 10.9)	Thickest middle stratum, derived from buccinator; thick superficial stratum, derived from elevators and depressors of lips and their angles	Lips and the angle of the mouth	For detail, *see* p. 150
8. Buccinator, the muscle of the cheek (Fig. 10.10) Pierced by a. Parotid duct and b. Buccal branch of mandibular nerve	1. Upper fibres, from maxilla opposite molar teeth 2. Lower fibres, from mandible, opposite molar teeth 3. Middle fibres, from pterygomandibular raphe	1. Upper fibres, straight to the upper lip 2. Lower fibres, straight to the lower lip 3. Middle fibres decussate	Flattens cheek against gums and teeth; prevents accumulation of food in the vestibule. This is the *whistling muscle*
9. Levator labii superioris alaeque nasi	Frontal process of maxilla	Upper lip and alar cartilage of nose	Lifts upper lip and dilates the nostril
10. Zygomaticus major	Posterior aspect of lateral surface of zygomatic bone	Skin at the angle of the mouth	Pulls the angle upwards and laterally as in smiling
11. Levator labii superioris (Fig. 10.10)	Infraorbital margin of maxilla	Skin of upper lateral half of the upper lip	Elevates the upper lip, forms nasolabial groove
12. Levator anguli oris	Maxilla just below infraorbital foramen	Skin of angle of the mouth	Elevates angle of mouth, forms nasolabial groove

(Contd...)

Table 10.3: The facial muscles *(Contd...)*

Name	*Origin*	*Insertion*	*Actions*
13. Zygomaticus minor	Anterior aspect of lateral surface of zygomatic bone	Upper lip medial to its angle	Elevates the upper lip
14. Depressor anguli oris	Oblique line of mandible below first molar, premolar and canine teeth	Skin at the angle of mouth and fuses with orbicularis oris	Draws angle of mouth downwards and laterally
15. Depressor labii inferioris	Anterior part of oblique line of mandible	Lower lip at midline, fuses with muscles from opposite side	Draws lower lip downward
16. Mentalis	Mandible inferior to incisor teeth	Skin of chin	Elevates and protrudes lower lip as it wrinkles skin on chin
17. Risorius	Fascia on the masseter muscle	Skin at the angle of the mouth	Retracts angle of mouth
Muscles of the neck			
18. Platysma (Fig. 10.9)	Upper parts of pectoral and deltoid fasciae Fibres run upwards and medially	Anterior fibres, to the base of the mandible; posterior fibres, to the skin of the lower face and lip, and may be continuous with the risorius	Releases pressure of skin on the subjacent veins; depresses mandible; pulls the angle of the mouth downwards as in horror or fright

Modiolus: It is a compact, mobile fibromuscular structure present at about 1.25 cm lateral to the angle of the mouth opposite the upper second premolar tooth. The five muscles interlacing to form the modiolus are: zygomaticus major, buccinator, levator anguli oris, risorius and depressor anguli oris.

6 Levator anguli oris
7 Zygomaticus minor
8 Depressor anguli oris (Fig. 10.10)
9 Depressor labii inferioris
10 *Mentalis* (Latin chin)
11 *Risorius* (Latin laughter)

Muscle of the Neck

Platysma (Greek broad)

Details of these muscles are given in Table 10.3.

A few of the *common facial expressions* and the muscles producing them are given below (Fig. 10.11).

1 *Surprise:* Frontalis
2 *Dislike:* Corrugator supercilii and procerus
3 *Anger:* Dilator naris and depressor septi
4 *Smiling and laughing:* Zygomaticus major
5 *Grinning:* Risorius
6 *Sadness:* Levator labii superioris
7 *Grief:* Depressor anguli oris
8 *Closing the mouth:* Orbicularis oris
9 *Whistling/kissing:* Buccinator, and orbicularis oris
10 *Doubt:* Mentalis
11 *Horror, terror and fright:* Platysma

NERVE SUPPLY OF FACE

Motor Nerve Supply

The *facial nerve* is the motor nerve of the face. Its five terminal branches, temporal, zygomatic, buccal, marginal mandibular and cervical emerge from the parotid gland and diverge to supply the various facial muscles as follows.

Temporal—frontalis, auricular muscles, orbicularis oculi (Fig. 10.12a).

Zygomatic—orbicularis oculi (lower eyelid part).

Buccal—muscles of the cheek and upper lip.

Marginal mandibular—muscles of lower lip.

Cervical—platysma.

Branches of facial nerve can be simulated by putting your right wrist on the right ear and spreading five digits: The thumb over the temporal region, the index finger on the zygomatic bone, middle finger on the upper lip, the ring finger on the lower lip and the little finger over the neck (Fig. 10.12b).

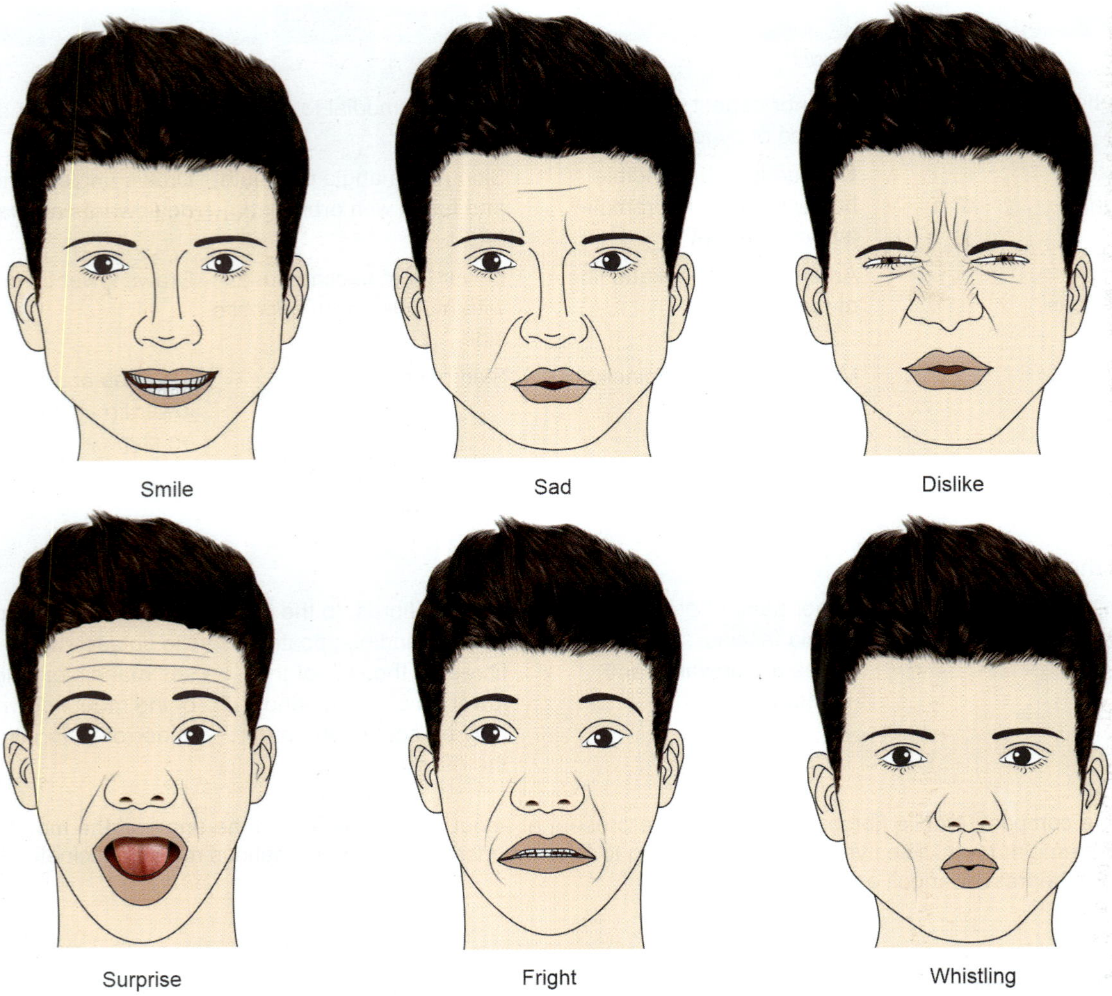

Smile

Sad

Dislike

Surprise

Fright

Whistling

Fig. 10.11: Some common facial expressions

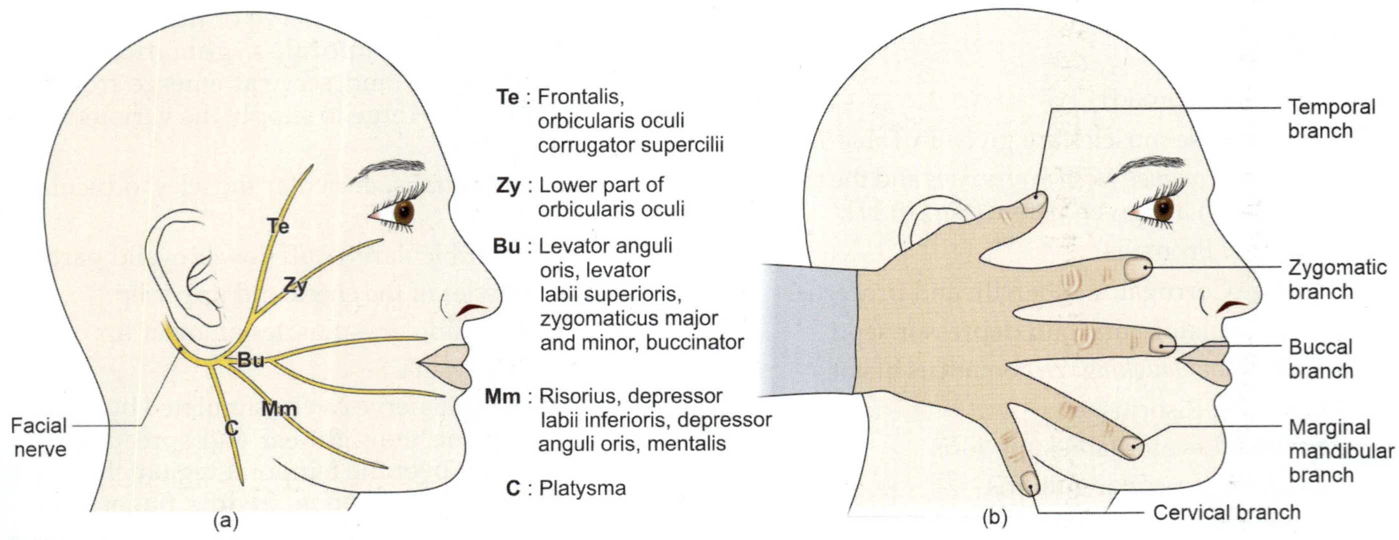

Figs 10.12a and b: Terminal branches of the facial nerve

CLINICAL ANATOMY

- The facial nerve is examined by testing the following facial muscles (Fig. 10.13).
  a. *Frontalis:* Ask the patient to look upwards without moving his head, and look for the normal horizontal wrinkles on the forehead (Fig. 10.13a).
  b. *Dilators of mouth:* Showing the teeth (Fig. 10.13b).
  c. *Orbicularis oculi:* Tight closure of the eyes (Fig. 10.13c).
  d. *Buccinator:* Puffing the mouth and then blowing forcibly as in whistling (Fig. 10.13d).
- Infranuclear lesion (Fig. 10.14) of the facial nerve, at the stylomastoid foramen is known as Bell's palsy, upper and lower quarters of the face on the same side get paralysed with atrophy of the facial muscles. It also causes loss of taste in anterior 2/3rds of tongue on same side.
  The face becomes asymmetrical and is drawn up to the normal side. The affected side is motionless. Wrinkles disappear from the forehead. The eye cannot be closed leading to keratitis. Any attempt to smile draws the mouth to the normal side. During mastication, food accumulates between the teeth and the cheek. Articulation of labials is impaired. Tears flow out from the eye. Saliva flows down from the angle of mouth.
- In supranuclear lesions of the facial nerve; usually a part of hemiplegia, with injury of corticonuclear fibres, only the lower quarter of the opposite side of face is paralysed. The upper quarter with the frontalis and orbicularis oculi escapes due to its bilateral representation in the cerebral cortex (Fig. 10.15). Only voluntary movements are affected and emotional expressions remain normal as there are separate pathways for voluntary and emotional movements. There is no atrophy of facial muscles.

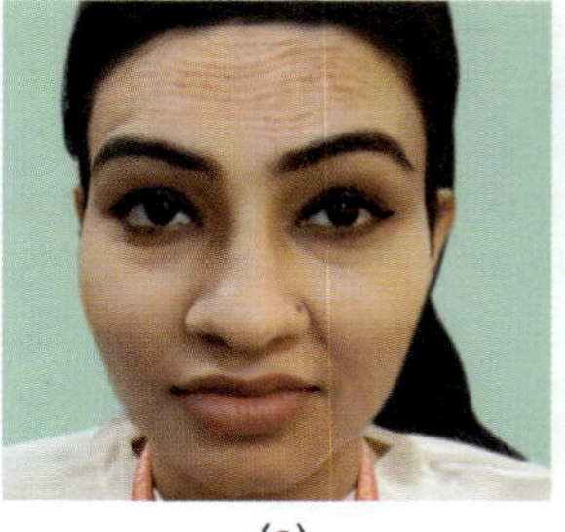
(a)
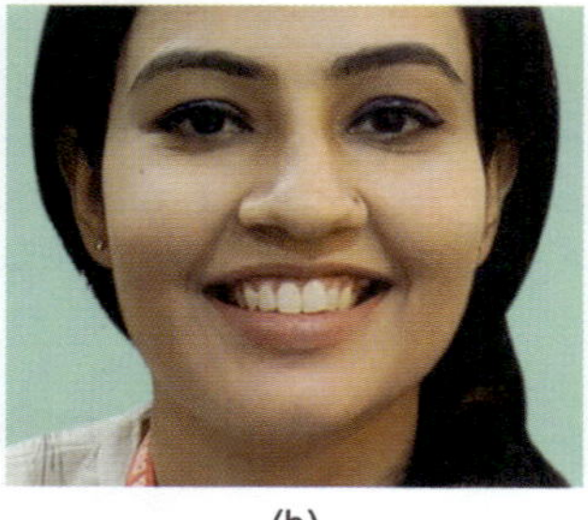
(b)
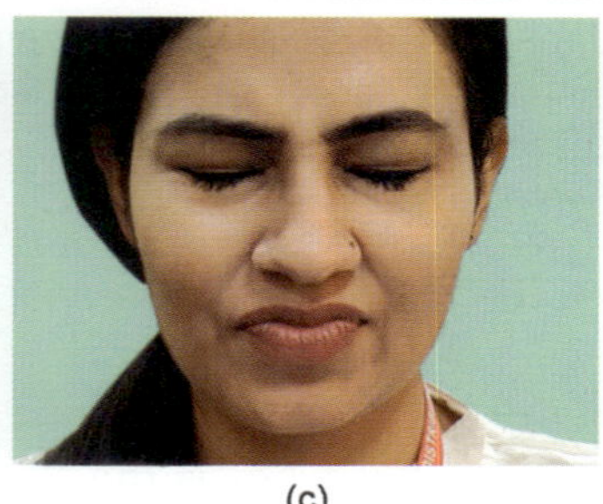
(c)
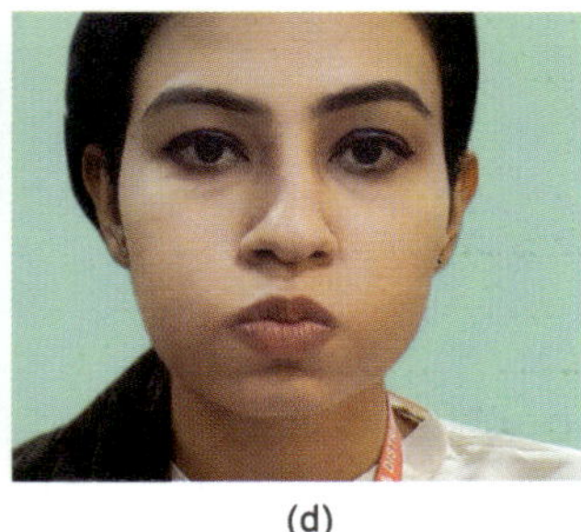
(d)

Figs 10.13a to d: (a) Test for frontalis; (b) Test for dilators of mouth; (c) Test for orbicularis oculi; (d) Test for buccinator

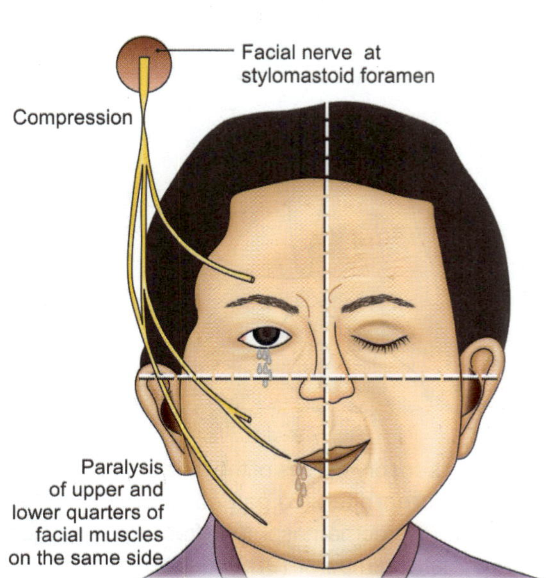

Fig. 10.14: Infranuclear lesion of right facial nerve or Bell's palsy

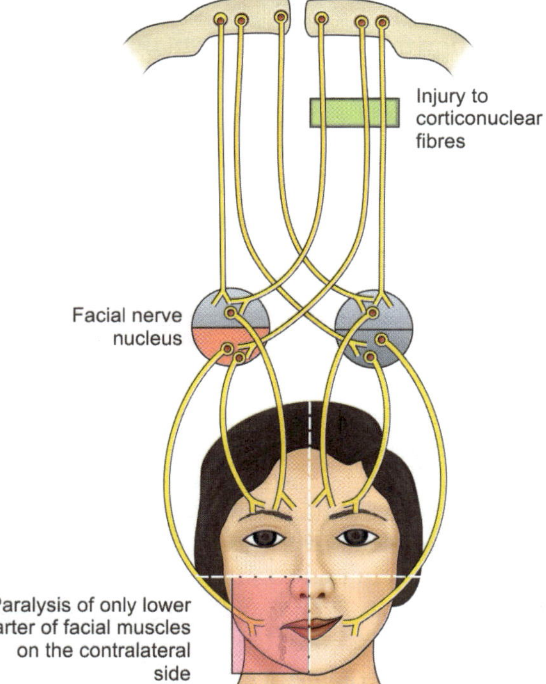

Fig. 10.15: Supranuclear lesion of left facial nerve

Table 10.4: Cutaneous nerves of the face

Source	*Cutaneous nerve*	*Area of distribution*
a. Ophthalmic division of trigeminal nerve	1. Supratrochlear nerve 2. Supraorbital nerve 3. Lacrimal nerve 4. Infratrochlear nerve 5. External nasal nerve	1. Upper eyelid and forehead 2. Upper eyelid, frontal air sinus, scalp 3. Lateral part of upper eyelid 4. Medial parts of both eyelids 5. Lower part of dorsum and tip of nose
b. Maxillary division of trigeminal nerve	6. Infraorbital nerve 7. Zygomaticofacial nerve 8. Zygomaticotemporal nerve	6. Lower eyelid, side of nose and upper lip 7. Upper part of cheek 8. Anterior part of temporal region
c. Mandibular division of trigeminal nerve	9. Auriculotemporal nerve 10. Buccal nerve 11. Mental nerve	9. Upper two-thirds of lateral side of auricle, temporal region 10. Skin of lower part of cheek 11. Skin over chin
d. Cervical plexus	12. Anterior division of great auricular nerve (C2, C3) 13. Upper and lower divisions of transverse (anterior) cutaneous nerve of neck (C2, C3) 14. Lesser occipital 15. Supraclavicular	12. Skin over angle of the jaw and over the parotid gland 13. Lower margin of the lower jaw and upper part of neck 14. Back of auricle 15. Front of thorax till 2nd costal cartilage and skin over upper ½ of deltoid muscle

Sensory Nerve Supply

The *trigeminal nerve* through its three branches is the chief sensory nerve of the face (Fig. 10.16 and Table 10.4). The skin over the angle of the jaw and over the parotid gland is supplied by the great auricular nerve (C2, C3).

In addition to most of the skin of the face, the sensory distribution of the trigeminal nerve is also to the nasal cavity, the paranasal air sinuses, the eyeball, the mouth cavity, palate, cheeks, gums, teeth and anterior two-thirds of tongue and the supratentorial part of the dura mater, including that lining the anterior and middle cranial fossae (Fig. 10.16).

CLINICAL ANATOMY

- The sensory distribution of the trigeminal nerve explains why headache is a uniformly common symptom in involvements of the nose (common cold, boils), the paranasal air sinuses (sinusitis), infections and inflammations of teeth and gums, refractive errors of the eyes, and infection of the meninges as in meningitis.
- Trigeminal neuralgia may involve one or more of the three divisions of the trigeminal nerve. It causes attacks of very severe burning and scalding pain along the distribution of the affected nerve.

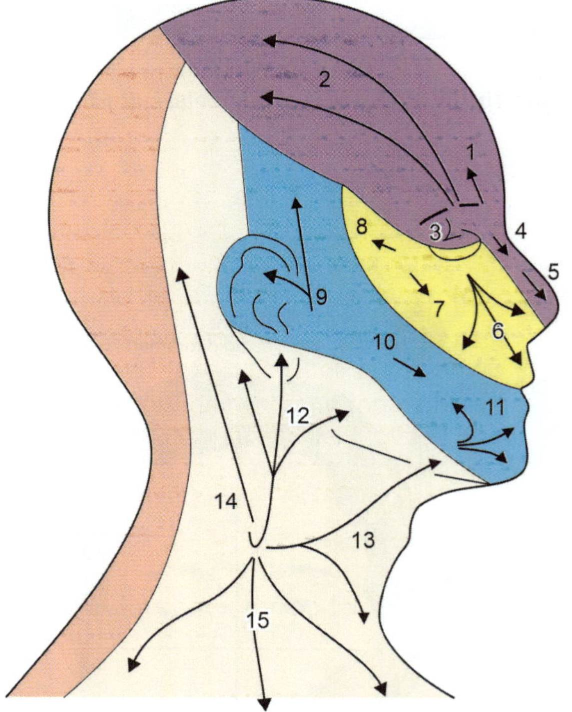

Fig. 10.16: The sensory nerves of the face and neck. (1) Supratrochlear, (2) supraorbital, (3) palpebral branch of lacrimal, (4) infratrochlear, (5) external nasal, (6) infraorbital, (7) zygomaticofacial, (8) zygomaticotemporal, (9) auriculotemporal, (10) buccal, (11) mental, (12) great auricular, (13) transverse cutaneous nerve of neck, (14) lesser occipital, and (15) supraclavicular

Pain is relieved either: (a) By injecting 90% alcohol into the affected division of the trigeminal ganglion, or (b) by sectioning the affected nerve, the main sensory root, or the spinal tract of the trigeminal nerve which is situated superficially in the medulla. The procedure is called medullary tractotomy.

ARTERIES OF THE FACE

Features

The face is richly vascular. It is supplied by:

1 The facial artery,
2 The transverse facial artery, and
3 Arteries that accompany the cutaneous nerves, which are small branches of ophthalmic, maxillary and superficial temporal arteries.

DISSECTION

Tortuous facial artery enters the face at the lower border of mandible. Dissect its course from the anteroinferior angle of masseter muscle running to the angle of mouth till the medial angle of eye, reflecting off some of the facial muscles, if necessary (Fig. 10.17).

Straight facial vein runs on a posterior plane than the artery.

Identify buccopharyngeal fascia on the external surface of buccinator muscle. Clean the deeply placed buccinator muscle situated lateral to the angle of mouth.

Identify parotid duct, running across the cheek 2 cm below the zygomatic arch. The duct pierces buccal pad of fat, buccopharyngeal fascia, buccinator muscle, mucous membrane of the mouth to open into its vestibule opposite second upper molar tooth (Fig. 10.20).

Facial Artery (Facial Part)

The facial artery is the chief artery of the face (Fig. 10.17). It is a branch of the external carotid artery given off in the carotid triangle just above the level of the tip of the greater cornua of the hyoid bone. In its cervical course, it passes through the submandibular region, and finally enters the face.

Course

1 It enters the face by winding around the base of the mandible, and by piercing the deep cervical fascia, at the anteroinferior angle of the masseter muscle. It can be palpated here and is called 'anaesthetist's artery'.
2 First it runs upwards and forwards to a point 1.25 cm lateral to the angle of the mouth. Then it ascends by the side of the nose up to the medial angle of the eye, where it terminates by supplying the lacrimal sac; and by anastomosing with the dorsal nasal branch of the ophthalmic artery.
3 The facial artery is very tortuous. The tortuosity of the artery prevents its walls from being unduly

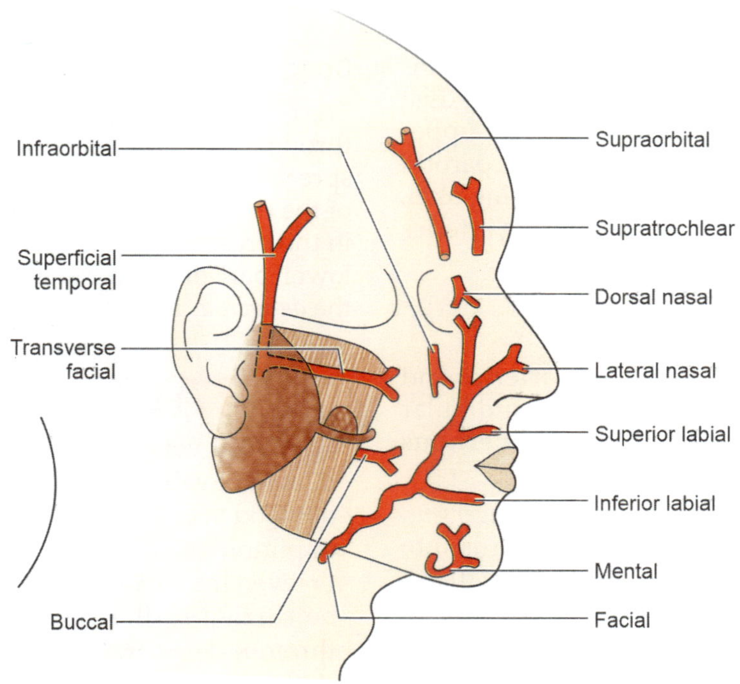

Fig. 10.17: Arteries of the face

stretched during movements of the mandible, the lips and the cheeks.

4 It lies between the superficial and deep muscles of the face.

The course of the artery in the neck is described in submandibular region.

Branches

The anterior branches on the face are large and named. They are:

1 *Inferior labial*, to the lower lip.
2 *Superior labial*, to the upper lip and the anteroinferior part of the nasal septum.
3 *Lateral nasal*, to the ala and dorsum of the nose.

The posterior branches are *small* and unnamed.

Anastomoses

1 The large anterior branches anastomose with similar branches of the opposite side and with the mental artery. In the lips, anastomoses are large, so that cut arteries spurt from both ends.
2 Small posterior branches anastomose with the transverse facial and infraorbital arteries.
3 At the medial angle of the eye, terminal branches of the facial artery anastomose with branches of the ophthalmic artery. This is, therefore, a site for anastomoses between the branches of the external and internal carotid arteries.

Transverse Facial Artery

This small artery is a branch of the superficial temporal artery. After emerging from the parotid gland, it runs forwards over the masseter between the parotid duct and the zygomatic arch, accompanied by the upper buccal branch of the facial nerve. It supplies the parotid gland and its duct, masseter and the overlying skin, and ends by anastomosing with neighbouring arteries (Fig. 10.17).

VEINS OF THE FACE

1 The veins of the face accompany the arteries and drain into the common facial and retromandibular veins. They communicate with the cavernous sinus.
2 The veins on each side form a *'W-shaped' arrangement*. Each corner of the 'W' is prolonged upwards into the scalp and downwards into the neck (Fig. 10.6).
3 The *facial vein* is the largest vein of the face with no valves. It begins as the angular vein at the medial angle of the eye. It is formed by the union of the supratrochlear and supraorbital veins. The angular vein continues as the facial vein, running downwards and backwards behind the facial artery, but with a straighter course. It crosses the anteroinferior angle of the masseter, pierces the deep fascia, crosses the submandibular gland, and joins the anterior division of the retromandibular vein below the angle of the mandible to form the common facial vein. It latter drains into the internal jugular vein. It is represented by a line drawn just behind the facial artery. The other veins drain into neighbouring veins.
4 *Deep connections* of the facial vein include:
   a. A communication between the supraorbital and superior ophthalmic veins.
   b. Another connection with the pterygoid plexus through the *deep facial* vein which passes backwards over the buccinator. The connection between facial vein and cavernous sinus is shown in Flowchart 10.1.

Flowchart 10.1: Connection between facial vein and cavernous sinus

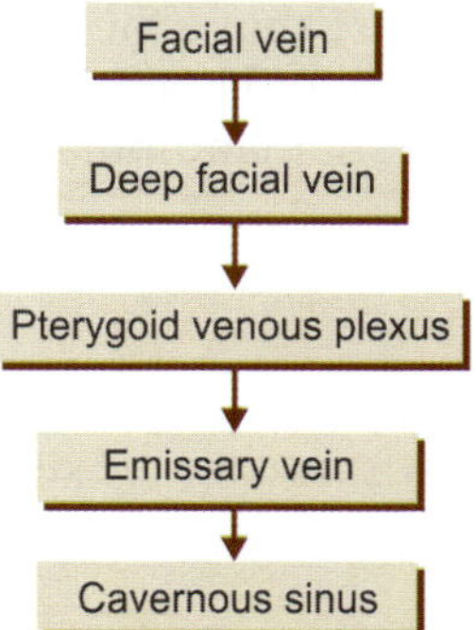

Dangerous Area of Face

The facial vein communicates with the cavernous sinus through emissary veins. Infections from the face can spread in a retrograde direction and cause *thrombosis* of the cavernous sinus. This is specially likely to occur in the presence of infection in the upper lip and in the lower part of the nose. This area is, therefore, called the *dangerous area of the face* (Fig. 10.18).

CLINICAL ANATOMY

The facial veins and its deep connecting veins are devoid of valves, making an uninterrupted passage of blood to cavernous sinus. Squeezing the pustules or pimples in the area of the upper lip or side of nose or even the cheeks may cause infection which may be carried to the cavernous sinus leading to its thrombosis. So the cheek area may also be included as the dangerous area (Fig. 10.18).

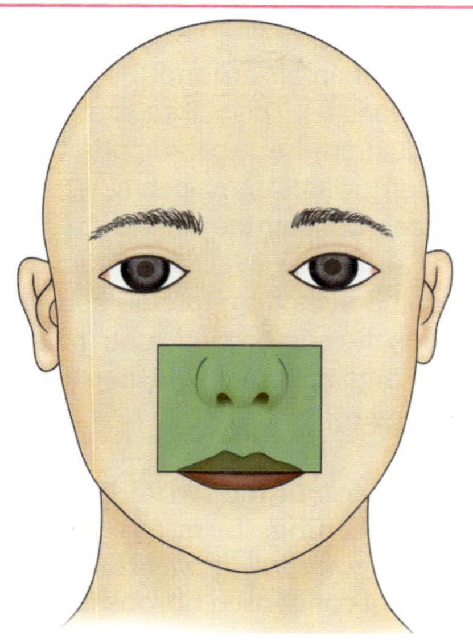

Fig. 10.18: Dangerous area of the face (stippled). Spread of infection from this area can cause thrombosis of the cavernous sinus

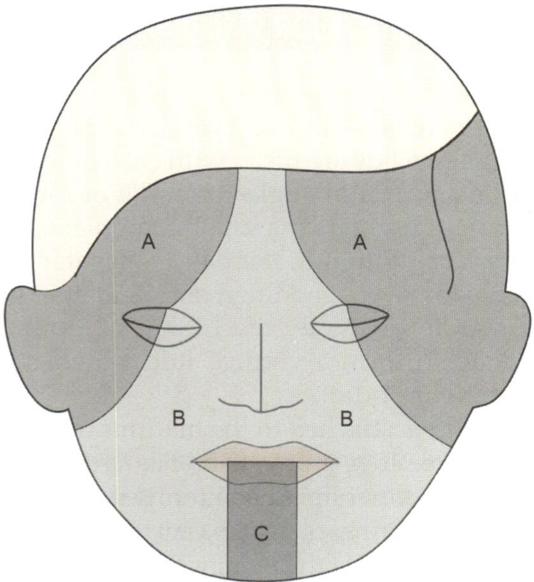

Fig. 10.19: The lymphatic territories of the face. Area A drains into the preauricular nodes, area B drains into the submandibular nodes, and area C drains into the submental nodes

LYMPHATIC DRAINAGE OF THE FACE

The face has three lymphatic territories:

1. *Upper territory*, including the greater part of the forehead, lateral halves of eyelids, conjunctiva, lateral part of the cheek and parotid area, drains into the *preauricular parotid nodes*.
2. *Middle territory*, including a strip over the median part of the forehead, external nose, upper lip, lateral part of the lower lip, medial halves of the eyelids, medial part of the cheek, and the greater part of lower jaw, drains into the *submandibular nodes*.
3. *Lower territory*, including the central part of the lower lip and the chin, drains into the *submental nodes* (Fig. 10.19).

Labial, Buccal and Molar Mucous Glands

The labial and buccal mucous glands are numerous. They lie in the submucosa of the lips and cheeks. The molar mucous glands, four or five, lie on the buccopharyngeal fascia around the parotid duct. All these glands open into the vestibule of the mouth (Fig. 10.20).

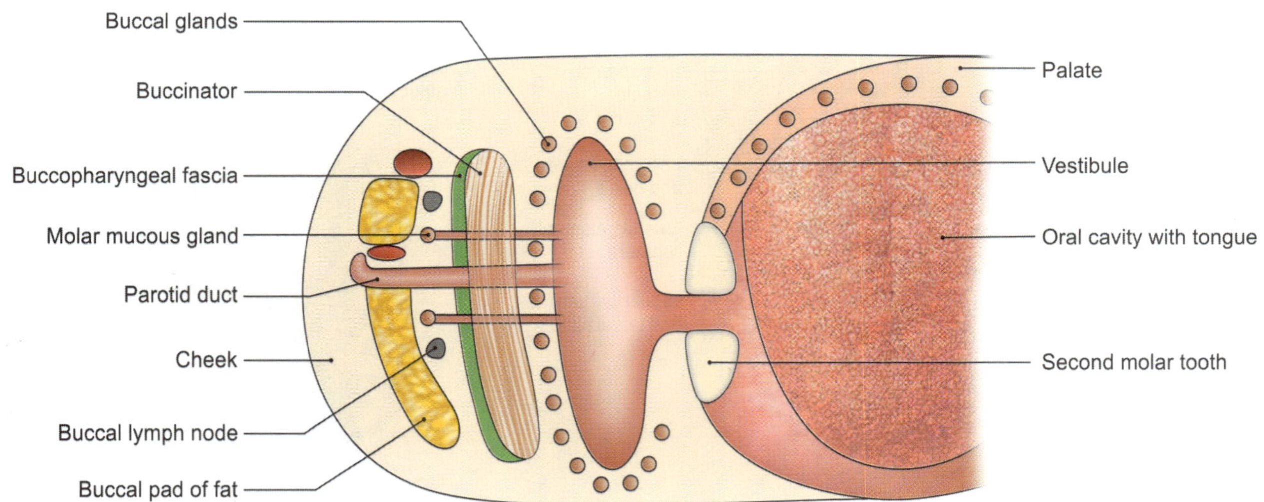

Fig. 10.20: Scheme of coronal section showing structures in the cheek. The parotid duct pierces buccal pad of fat, buccopharyngeal fascia, buccinator muscle and the mucous membrane to open into the vestibule of mouth opposite the crown of the upper second molar tooth

EYELIDS OR PALPEBRAE

Features

The space between the two eyelids is the palpebral fissure. The two lids are fused with each other to form the medial and lateral angles or *canthi* of the eye. At the inner canthus, there is a small triangular space, the *lacus lacrimalis*. Within it, there is an elevated *lacrimal caruncle*, made up of modified skin and skin glands. Lateral to the caruncle, the bulbar conjunctiva is pinched up to form a vertical fold called the *plica semilunaris* (Fig. 10.1a).

Each eyelid is attached to the margins of the orbital opening. Its free edge is broad and has a rounded outer lip and a sharp inner lip. The outer lip presents two or more rows of eyelashes or cilia, except in the boundary of the lacus lacrimalis. At the point where eyelashes cease, there is a *lacrimal papilla* on the summit of which there is the *lacrimal punctum* (Fig. 10.1a). Near the inner lip of the free edge, there is a row of openings of the tarsal glands.

The free margin of both the eyelids is subdivided into: Lateral 5/6th, the ciliary part with eyelashes and medial 1/6th, the lacrimal part, which lacks cilia.

Structure

Each lid is made up of the following layers from without inwards:

1 The *skin* is thin, loose and easily distensible by oedema fluid or blood.
2 The *superficial fascia* is without any fat. It contains the palpebral part of the orbicularis oculi. Deep to the muscle is loose areolar tissue which is continuous with loose areolar tissue of the scalp.

DISSECTION

Give a circular incision around the roots of eyelids (Fig. 10.2a—viii and ix). This will separate the orbital part of orbicularis oculi from the palpebral parts. Carefully reflect the palpebral part towards the palpebral fissure. Identify the structures present beneath the muscle as given in the text.

The upper and lower eyelids are movable curtains which protect the eyes from foreign bodies and bright light. They keep the cornea clean and moist. The upper eyelid is larger and more movable than the lower eyelid (Figs 10.21a and b).

3 The *palpebral fascia* of the two lids forms the *orbital septum*. Its thickenings form *tarsal plates* or *tarsi* in the lids and the *palpebral ligaments* at the angles. Tarsi are thin plates of condensed fibrous tissue located near the lid margins. They give stiffness to the lids (Müller's muscles) (Fig. 10.21a).
The palpebral fascia (orbital septum) is pierced by: (a) Palpebral part of lacrimal gland, (b) fibres of levator palpebral superioris, (c) vessels and nerves entering the face from the orbit.
The upper tarsus receives two tendinous slips from the *levator palpebrae superioris*, one from voluntary part and another from involuntary part or Müller's muscle (Fig. 10.21b). *Tarsal glands* or meibomian glands are embedded in the posterior surface of the tarsi; their ducts open in a row behind the cilia.
4 The *conjunctiva* lines the posterior surface of the tarsus.

Apart from the usual glands of the skin, and mucous glands in the conjunctiva, the larger glands found in the lids are:

a. Large sebaceous glands also called *Zeis glands* at the lid margin associated with cilia.

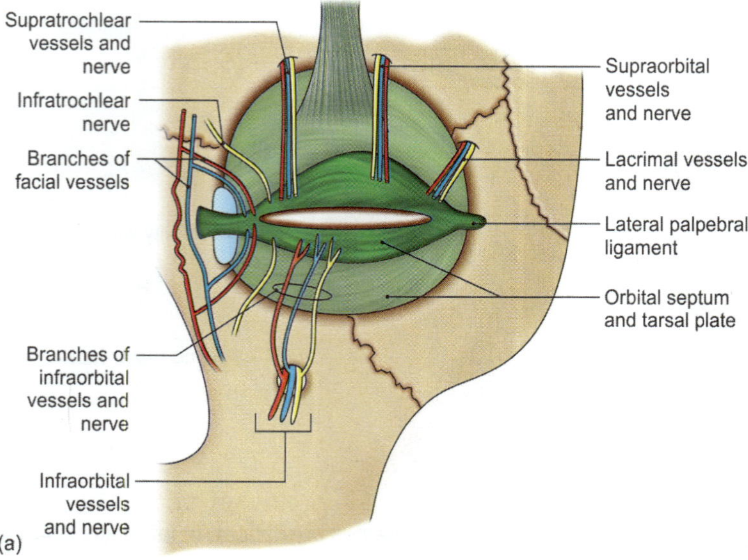

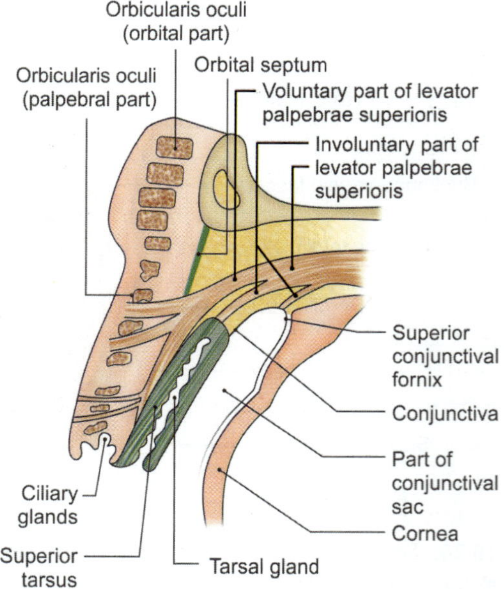

Figs 10.21a and b: (a) Orbital septum; (b) Sagittal section of the upper eyelid

b. Modified sweat glands or *Moll's glands* at the lid margin closely associated with Zeis glands and cilia.
c. Sebaceous or *tarsal glands* are also known as *meibomian glands*.

Blood Supply

The eyelids are supplied by:

1 The superior palpebral branches of lacrimal, supraorbital, supratrochlear arteries which are branches the ophthalmic artery (Fig. 10.21a).
2 The inferior palpebral branches of infraorbital and facial arteries. They form an arcade in each lid.

The veins drain into the ophthalmic and facial veins.

Nerve Supply

The upper eyelid is supplied by the lacrimal, supraorbital, supratrochlear and infratrochlear nerves from lateral to medial side.

The lower eyelid is supplied by the infraorbital and infratrochlear nerves (Fig. 10.21a).

Lymphatic Drainage

The medial halves of the lids drain into the submandibular nodes, and the lateral halves into the preauricular nodes (Fig. 10.19).

CLINICAL ANATOMY

- The Müller's muscle or involuntary part of levator palpebrae superioris is supplied by sympathetic fibres from the superior cervical ganglion. Paralysis of this muscle leads to partial ptosis. This is part of the Horner's syndrome.
- The palpebral conjunctiva is examined for anaemia and for conjunctivitis; the bulbar conjunctiva for jaundice.
- Conjunctivitis is one of the commonest diseases of the eye. It may be caused by infection or by allergy.
- Foreign bodies are often lodged in a groove situated 2 mm from the edge of each eyelid.
- Chalazion is inflammation of a tarsal gland, causing a localised swelling pointing inwards.
- Ectropion is due to eversion of the lower lacrimal punctum. It usually occurs in old age due to laxity of skin.
- Trachoma is a contagious granular conjunctivitis caused by the trachoma virus. It is regarded as the commonest cause of blindness.
- Stye or hordeolum is a suppurative inflammation of one of the glands of Zeis. The gland is swollen, hard and painful, and the whole of the lid is oedematous. The pus points near the base of one of the cilia.
- Blepharitis is inflammation of the eyelids, specially of the lid margin.

LACRIMAL APPARATUS

COMPONENTS

The structures concerned with secretion and drainage of the lacrimal or tear fluid constitute the lacrimal apparatus. It is made up of the following parts:

1 Lacrimal gland and its ducts (Fig. 10.22).
2 Conjunctival sac
3 Lacrimal puncta and lacrimal canaliculi
4 Lacrimal sac
5 Nasolacrimal duct.

Lacrimal Gland

It is a *serous gland* situated chiefly in the lacrimal fossa on the anterolateral part of the roof of the bony orbit and partly on the upper eyelid. Small *accessory lacrimal glands* are found in the conjunctival fornices. These are also called Krause's gland.

DISSECTION

On the lateral side of the upper lid, cut the palpebral fascia. This will show the presence of the lacrimal gland deep in this area. Its palpebral part is to be traced in the upper eyelid. On the medial ends of both the eyelids, look for lacrimal papilla. Palpate and dissect the medial palpebral ligament binding the medial ends of the eyelids. Try to locate the small lacrimal sac behind this ligament.

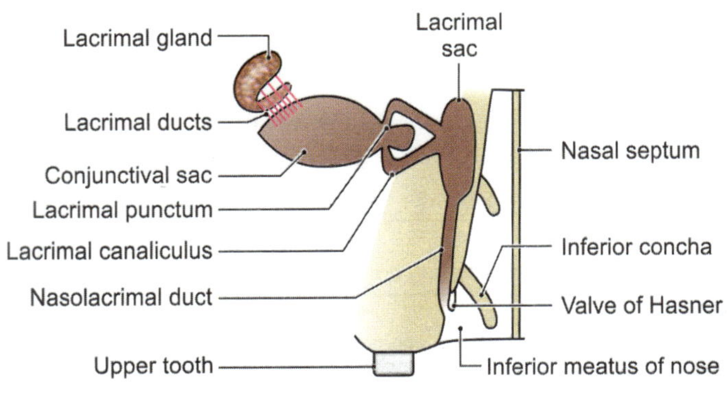

Fig. 10.22: Components of lacrimal apparatus

The gland is 'J' shaped, being indented by the tendon of the *levator palpebrae superioris* muscle. It has:

a. An *orbital part* which is larger and deeper, and
b. A *palpebral part* smaller and superficial, lying within the eyelid (Fig. 10.22).

About a dozen of its *ducts* pierce the conjunctiva of the upper lid and open into the conjunctival sac near the superior fornix. Most of the ducts of the orbital part pass through the palpebral part. Removal of the latter is functionally equivalent to removal of the entire gland. After removal, the conjunctiva and cornea are moistened by accessory lacrimal glands.

The gland is supplied by the lacrimal branch of the ophthalmic artery and by the *lacrimal nerve*. The nerve has both sensory and secretomotor fibres. Flowchart 10.2 shows the secretomotor fibres for lacrimal gland.

Flowchart 10.2: Secretomotor fibres for lacrimal gland

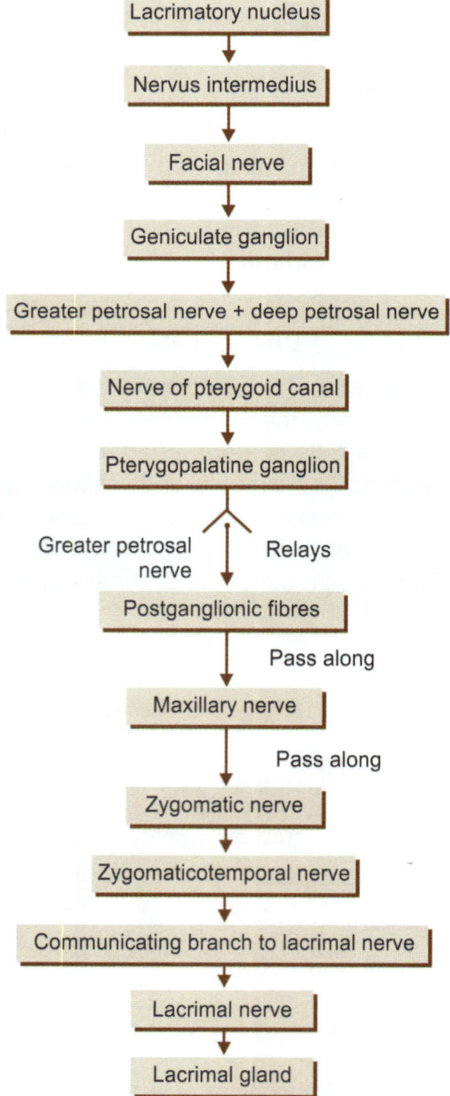

The lacrimal fluid (1.0–1.5 ml/24 hrs) secreted by the lacrimal gland flows into the conjunctival sac where it lubricates the front of the eye and the deep surface of the lids. Periodic blinking helps to spread the fluid over the eye. Most of the fluid evaporates. The rest is drained by the lacrimal canaliculi. When excessive, it overflows as *tears*.

Conjunctival Sac

The conjunctiva lining the deep surfaces of the eyelids is called palpebral conjunctiva and that lining the front of the eyeball is called bulbar conjunctiva. The potential space between the palpebral and bulbar parts is the *conjunctival sac*. The lines along which the palpebral conjunctiva of the upper and lower eyelids is reflected onto the eyeball are called the superior and inferior *conjunctival fornices*.

The *palpebral conjunctiva* is thick, opaque, highly vascular, and adherent to the tarsal plate. The *bulbar conjunctiva* covers the sclera. It is thin, transparent, and loosely attached to the eyeball. Over the cornea, it is represented by the anterior epithelium of the cornea.

Lacrimal Puncta and Canaliculi

Each lacrimal canaliculus begins at the *lacrimal punctum*, and is 10 mm long. It has a vertical part which is 2 mm long and a horizontal part which is 8 mm long. There is a dilated ampulla at the bend. Both canaliculi open close to each other in the lateral wall of the lacrimal sac behind the medial palpebral ligament.

Lacrimal Sac

It is a membranous sac, 12 mm long and 5 mm wide, situated in the lacrimal groove behind the medial palpebral ligament. Its upper end is blind. The lower end is continuous with the nasolacrimal duct.

The sac is related anteriorly to the medial palpebral ligament and to the orbicularis oculi. Medially, the lacrimal groove separates it from the nose. Laterally, it is related to the lacrimal fascia and the lacrimal part of the orbicularis oculi.

Nasolacrimal Duct

It is a membranous passage, 18 mm long. It begins at the lower end of the lacrimal sac, runs downwards, backwards and laterally, and opens into the inferior meatus of the nose. A fold of mucous membrane, called the *valve of Hasner*, forms an imperfect valve at the lower end of the duct.

CLINICAL ANATOMY

- Inflammation of the lacrimal sac is called *dacrocystitis*.
- The ducts of lacrimal gland open through its palpebral part into the conjunctival sac. Because

of this arrangement, the removal of palpebral part necessitates the removal of the orbital part as well.

- Excessive secretion of the lacrimal fluid overflowing on the cheeks is called epiphora. Epiphora may result due to obstruction in the lacrimal fluid pathway, either at the level of punctum or canaliculi or nasolacrimal duct.

DEVELOPMENT OF FACE

Five processes of face, one frontonasal, two maxillary and two mandibular processes form the face. Frontonasal process forms the forehead, the nasal septum, philtrum of upper lip and premaxilla bearing upper four incisor teeth.

Maxillary process forms whole of upper lip except the philtrum and most of the hard and soft palate except the part formed by the premaxilla.

Mandibular process forms the whole lower lip.

Cord of ectoderm gets buried at the junction of frontonasal and maxillary processes. Canalisation of ectodermal cord of cells gives rise to nasolacrimal duct.

Molecular Regulation

Face develops from pharyngeal arches. Facial skeleton develops from neural crest cells which migrate into the pharyngeal arches. In hindbrain, the segments are rhombomeres. From the rhombomeres, crest cells migrate to pharyngeal region. Genes responsible are:

First arch is HOX negative. It expresses OTX2, a homeodomain containing transcription factor.

Second arch expresses HOX-A2.

Third to sixth arches express HOX-A3, HOX-B3 and HOX-D3.

Following signaling molecules play an important part in development of face.

- BMP7—Bone morphogenetic protein
- FGF8—Fibroblast growth factor 8
- SHH—Sonic hedgehog proteins

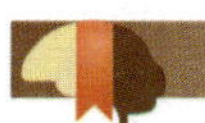

Mnemonics

Bell's palsy

Blink reflex abnormal
Ear ache
Lacrimation (deficient)
Loss of taste in anterior two-thirds of tongue
Sudden onset
Palsy of muscles of facial expression (unilateral)

Five branches of the facial nerve (VII)

(**T**en **Z**ebras **B**it **M**y **C**at)
Temporal
Zygomatic
Buccal
Marginal mandibular
Cervical

SCALP

From superficial to deep:
Skin
Connective tissue
Aponeurosis
Loose areolar tissue
Pericranium

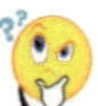

FACTS TO REMEMBER

- Forehead is common to both the scalp and the face.
- There are 5 layers in scalp and 6 layers in the superficial temporal region.
- Impulses from skin of the face reach the three branches of trigeminal nerve, whereas the muscles of facial expression are supplied by the facial nerve. To establish the reflex arc, nucleus of VII nerve comes closer to the spinal nucleus of V nerve at the level of lower pons. This is called 'neurobiotaxis'.
- Facial nerve though courses through the parotid gland, does not give any branch to the largest salivary gland.
- Buccinator is an accessory muscle of mastication, as it prevents food entering the vestibule of mouth.
- Part of the face between anterior nares and upper lip is called 'dangerous area of face' as the facial vein communicates with cavernous venous sinus situated in the cranial cavity. Any infection from this part of face can infect the intracranial venous sinus, i.e. cavernous sinus.
- Levator palpebrae superioris is supplied partly by oculomotor nerve and partly by sympathetic fibres.
- The facial muscles are subcutaneous in position and represent morphologically remnants of panniculus carnosus.

CLINICOANATOMICAL PROBLEMS

Case 1

A man of about 30 years comes to OPD with inability to close his left eye, tears overflowing on the left cheek and saliva dribbling from his left angle of the mouth.

- What is the reason for his sad condition?
- What is the nerve damaged and how is the integrity of the nerve tested?

Ans: The reason for the patient's sad condition is paralysis of his left facial nerve at the stylomastoid foramen. It is called Bell's palsy. It is treated by physiotherapy and medicines.

Facial nerve is tested by:

Asking the patient:

i. To look upwards without moving his head, and look for the normal horizontal wrinkles on the forehead.
ii. To show the teeth
iii. Tightly close the eyes to test the orbicularis oculi muscle.
iv. Puffing the mouth and then blowing out air forcibly to test the buccinator muscle.

Case 2

A teenage girl with infected acne tried to drain the pustules on her upper lip with her bare hands. After a few days, she noticed severe weakness in her eye muscles.

- How are the pustules connected to nerves supplying eye muscles?

Ans: Infection from pustules travels via facial vein, deep facial vein, pterygoid venous plexus, emissary vein to cavernous venous sinus and III, IV and VI cranial nerves related in its lateral wall. Since the nerves are infected, the extraocular muscles get weak and may get paralysed.

Orbicularis oris muscle (42nd ed., Gray's Anatomy) consists of 4 quadrants: Upper, lower on right side and upper, lower on left side. Each quadrant comprises pars peripheralis and pars marginalis.

1. Pars peripheralis is attached to modiolus. These are derived from elevators and depressors of lips and their angles. These fibres diverge and form muscular sheet which is triangular in shape. These pass across the midline to decussate with fibres of opposite side. These fibres press lips against teeth.
2. Pars marginalis arises from modiolus and comprises one band of fibres, which decussate with fibres of opposite side at vermiform zone of lips. These fibres are associated with speech and with production of musical notes (vermilion zone is the dark margin of the lips).

FURTHER READING

- Choudhry R, Raheja S, Gaur U, Choudhry S, Anand C. Mastoid canals in adult human skulls. J Anat 1996;188: 217–19.
- Wilkinson C, Rynn C. Craniofacial Identification. Cambridge: Cambridge University press. 2012.
  Forensic facial reconstruction is an area that requires an equal amount of scientific and artistic talent. This text addresses this complex subject in an approachable manner.

Frequently Asked Questions

1. Describe the arterial supply and venous drainage of the face, add a note on its clinical importance.
2. Enumerate the layers of the scalp. Give its blood supply, nerve supply and clinical importance.
3. Write short notes/enumerate:
   a. Buccinator muscle
   b. Sensory nerve supply of face
   c. Components of lacrimal apparatus
   d. Features of Bell's palsy
   e. Emissary veins

Multiple Choice Questions

1. Nasolacrimal duct opens into:
   a. Anterior part of inferior meatus
   b. Vestibule of nose
   c. Middle meatus
   d. Superior meatus
2. Dangerous area of face is named because of connection of cavernous sinus with facial vein through which vein?
   a. Maxillary
   b. Anterior ethmoidal
   c. Posterior ethmoidal
   d. Deep facial
3. Which of the following muscles separates the orbital and palpebral parts of the lacrimal gland?
   a. Superior oblique
   b. Superior rectus
   c. Inferior oblique
   d. Levator palpabrae superioris
4. Infection in dangerous area of face usually leads to:
   a. Superior sagittal sinus thrombosis
   b. Transverse sinus thrombosis
   c. Cavernous sinus thrombosis
   d. Brain abscess
5. Supraorbital artery is a branch of:
   a. Maxillary b. External carotid
   c. Ophthalmic d. Internal carotid
6. Which of the following nerves ascends along with occipital artery in the scalp?
   a. Greater occipital b. Lesser occipital
   c. Third occipital d. Suboccipital

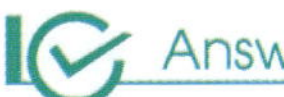

Answers

1. a **2.** d **3.** d **4.** c **5.** c **6.** a

VIVA VOCE

- Name the sensory and motor nerves supplying the scalp.
- How is the external jugular vein formed?
- What is air-embolism?
- Name the parts of orbicularis oculi muscle.
- Name the muscles attached to the modiolus.
- What is the effect of supranuclear lesion of left facial nerve?
- Which is the dangerous area of face?
- Why is this area of face called dangerous?
- Name the nerves supplying levator palpebrae superioris muscle.
- Enumerate the parts of lacrimal apparatus.
- Why is buccinator muscle an accessory muscle of mastication?
- Name the branches of facial nerve given on the face.
- What is the sensory nerve supply of the face?
- What are the structures piercing the buccinator muscle?
- Name the layers of upper eyelid.
- What are the effects of left Bell's palsy on the face?
- Which arteries are called 'an anaesthetist's arteries' and why?

Scalp and face

Chapter

11

Side of the Neck

"Life is a continuous process of adjustment."
—Indira Gandhi

INTRODUCTION

The beauty of the neck lies in its deep or cervical fascia (Fig. 11.1a). The sternocleidomastoid is an important landmark between the anterior and posterior triangles. The posterior triangle contains the spinal root of accessory nerve deep to its fascial roof and the roots and trunks of brachial plexus deep to its fascial floor. It also contains a part of the subclavian artery, which continues as the axillary artery for the upper limb. Arteries, like the rivers, are named according to the regions they pass through. Congestive cardiac failure can be seen at a glance by the raised jugular venous pressure. This external jugular vein lies in the superficial fascia and if cut, leads to air embolism, unless the deep fascia pierced by the vein is also cut to collapse the vein.

LANDMARKS

1 The *sternocleidomastoid* muscle is seen prominently when the neck and chin are turned to the opposite side. The ridge raised by the muscle extends from the clavicle and sternum to the mastoid process (Fig. 11.1b).
2 The *external jugular vein* crosses the sternocleidomastoid obliquely, running downwards and backwards from near the auricle to the clavicle. It is better seen in old age.
3 The *greater supraclavicular fossa* lies above and behind the middle one-third of the clavicle. It overlies the cervical part of the brachial plexus and the third part of the subclavian artery.
4 The *lesser supraclavicular fossa* is a small depression between the sternal and clavicular parts of the sternocleidomastoid. It overlies the internal jugular vein.
5 The *mastoid process* is a large bony projection behind the auricle.
6 The *transverse process of the atlas vertebra* can be felt on deep pressure midway between the angle of the mandible and the mastoid process, immediately anteroinferior to the tip of the mastoid process.
7 The *fourth cervical transverse process* is just palpable at the level of the upper border of the thyroid cartilage; and the *sixth cervical transverse process* at the level of the cricoid cartilage.
8 The anterior tubercle of the *transverse process of the sixth cervical vertebra* is the largest of all such processes and is called the *carotid tubercle* of Chassaignac. The common carotid artery can be best pressed against this tubercle, deep to the anterior border of the sternocleidomastoid muscle.
9 The *anterior border of the trapezius muscle* becomes prominent on elevation of the shoulder against resistance.

BOUNDARIES

The side of the neck is roughly quadrilateral in outline. It is *bounded* anteriorly, by the anterior median line; posteriorly, by the anterior border of trapezius; superiorly, by the base of mandible, a line joining angle of the mandible to mastoid process, and superior nuchal line; and inferiorly, by the clavicle.

This quadrilateral space is divided obliquely by the sternocleidomastoid muscle into the *anterior and posterior triangles* (Fig. 11.1b).

SKIN

The skin of the neck is supplied by the second, third and fourth cervical nerves. The anterolateral part is supplied by anterior primary rami through the (i) anterior cutaneous, (ii) great auricular, (iii) lesser occipital, and (iv) supraclavicular nerves. A broadband of skin over the posterior part is supplied by dorsal or posterior primary rami (*see* Fig. 10.16).

First cervical spinal nerve has no cutaneous distribution. Cervical fifth, sixth, seventh, eighth and thoracic first nerves supply the upper limb through the brachial plexus; and, therefore, do not supply the neck. The territory of fourth cervical nerve extends into the pectoral region through the supraclavicular nerves and meets second thoracic dermatome at the level of the second costal cartilage.

SUPERFICIAL FASCIA

Superficial fascia contains areolar tissue with platysma (*see* Table 10.3). Lying deep to platysma are cutaneous nerves (Fig. 11.6), superficial veins (*see* Fig. 10.6), *lymph vessels, lymph nodes* and small arteries.

DISSECTION

Give a median incision from the chin downwards towards the suprasternal notch situated above the manubrium of sternum.

Make one incision in the skin of base of mandible. Continue it by oblique incision along posterior border of ramus of mandible up to mastoid process and further along the superior nuchal line till the external occipital protuberance.

One incision is given along the upper border of clavicle (Fig. 11.1a). Reflect only the skin up towards the anterior border of trapezius muscle.

Platysma, a part of the subcutaneous muscle, is visible. Reflect the platysma towards the mandible. Identify the anterior or transverse cutaneous nerve of the neck in the upper part of superficial fascia. Anterior jugular vein running vertically close to the median plane is also encountered. Remove the superficial fascia till the deep fascia of neck is seen (Fig. 11.1a).

External jugular vein is seen above the clavicle.

To open up the suprasternal space, make a horizontal incision just above the sternum. Extend this incision along the anterior border of sternocleidomastoid muscle for 3–4 cm. Reflect the superficial lamina to expose the suprasternal space and identify its contents.

Define the attachments of investing layer, pretracheal layer, prevertebral layer and carotid sheath.

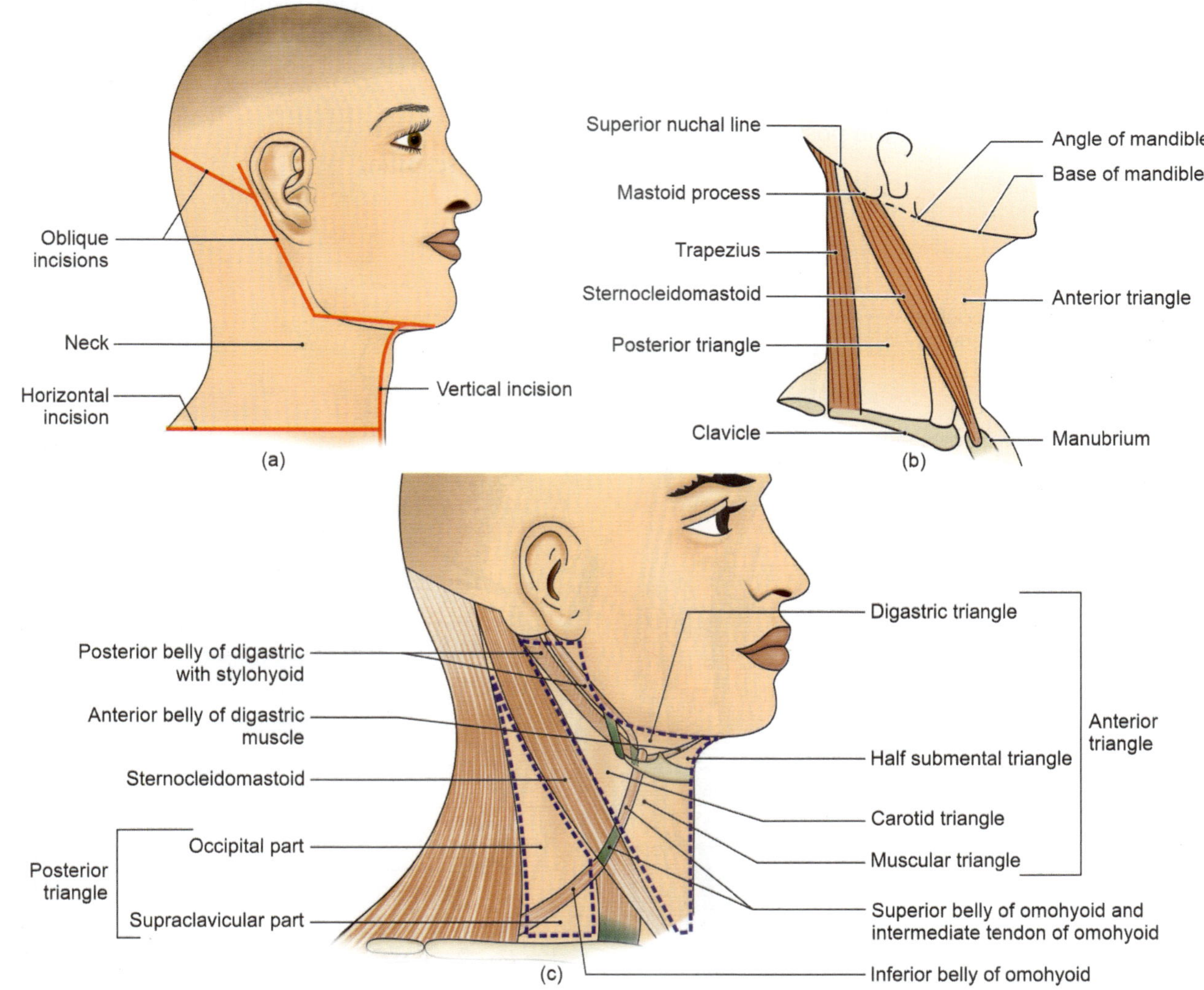

Figs 11.1a to c: (a) Lines of dissection; (b) Side of neck divided into anterior and posterior triangles; (c) Parts of posterior and anterior triangles

CLINICAL ANATOMY

The surgeon has to stitch platysma muscle separately so that skin does not adhere to deeper neck muscles, otherwise the skin will get an ugly scar.

DEEP CERVICAL FASCIA (FASCIA COLLI)

The deep fascia of the neck is condensed to form the following layers:

1 Investing layer (Fig. 11.2)
2 Pretracheal fascia
3 Prevertebral fascia
4 Carotid sheath
5 Buccopharyngeal fascia
6 Pharyngobasilar fascia.

INVESTING LAYER

It lies deep to the platysma, and surrounds the neck like a collar. It forms the roof of the posterior triangle of the neck (Fig. 11.3).

Attachments

Superiorly

a. External occipital protuberance
b. Superior nuchal line
c. Mastoid process, styloid process
d. External acoustic meatus, tympanic plate
e. Base of the mandible.

Between the angle of the mandible and the mastoid process, the fascia splits to enclose the parotid gland (Fig. 11.4a).

The superficial lamina, named *parotid fascia,* is thick and dense, and is attached to the zygomatic arch. The deep lamina is thin and is attached to the styloid process, the tympanic plate and the mandible. Between the styloid process and the angle of the mandible, the deep lamina is thick and forms the *stylomandibular ligament* which separates the parotid gland from the submandibular gland, and is pierced by the external carotid artery.

At the base of mandible, it encloses submandibular gland. The superficial lamina is attached to lower border of body of mandible and deep lamina to the mylohyoid line (Fig. 11.4b).

Inferiorly

a. Spine of scapula,

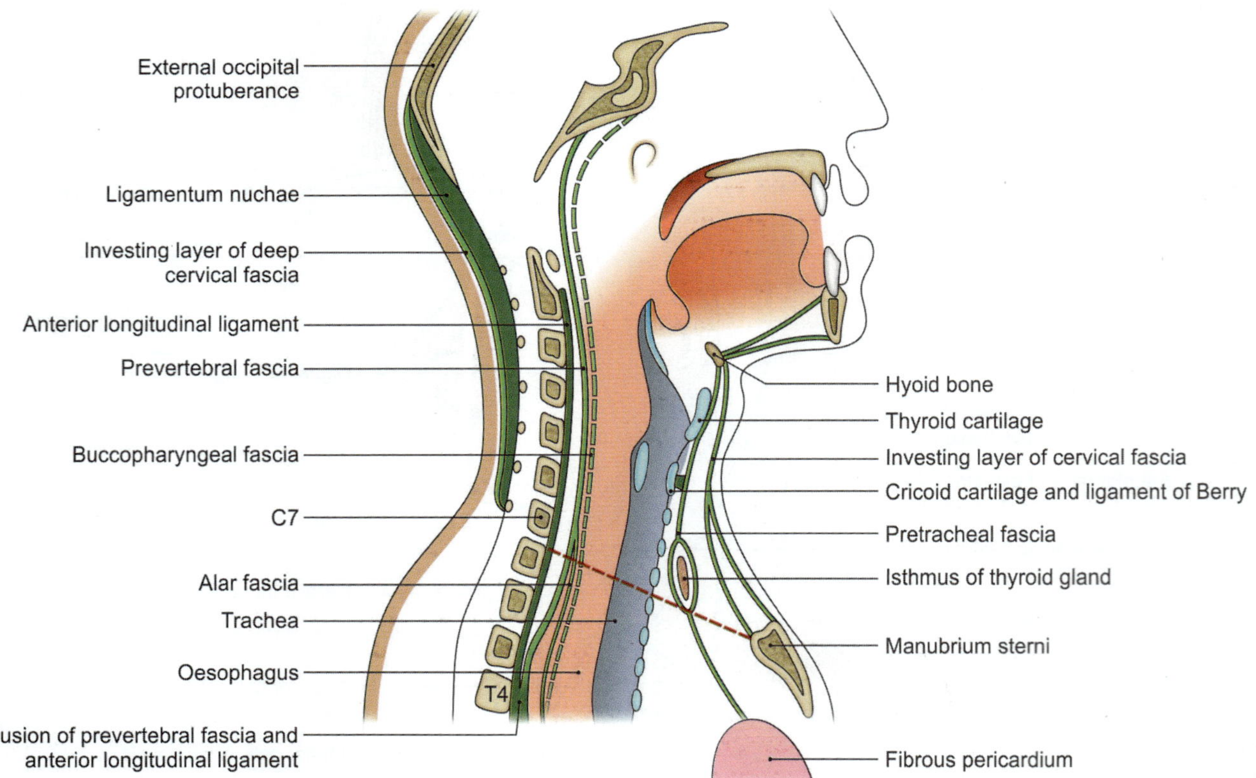

Fig. 11.2: Vertical extent of the first three layers of the deep cervical fascia

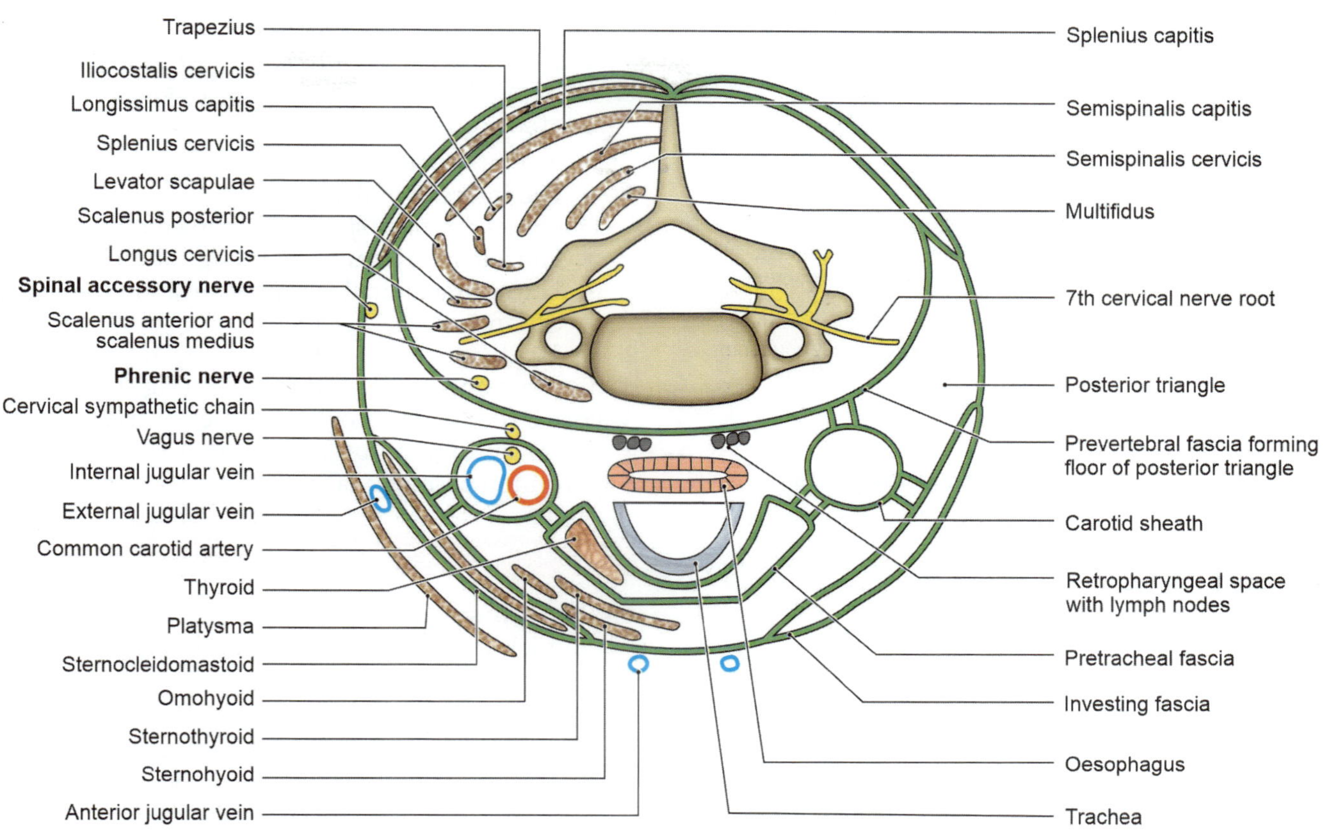

Fig. 11.3: Transverse section through the neck at the level of the seventh cervical vertebra

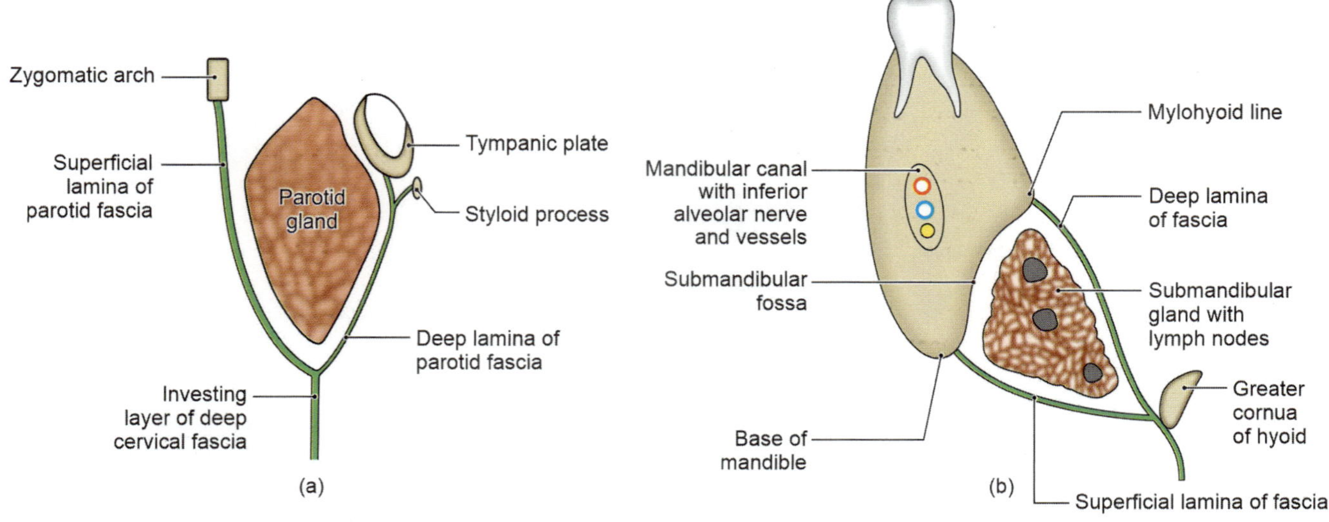

Figs 11.4a and b: Investing layer enclosing: (a) Parotid gland; (b) Submandibular gland

b. Acromion process,
c. Clavicle, and
d. Manubrium.

The fascia splits to enclose the suprasternal and supraclavicular spaces (Fig. 11.5), both of which are described as follows.

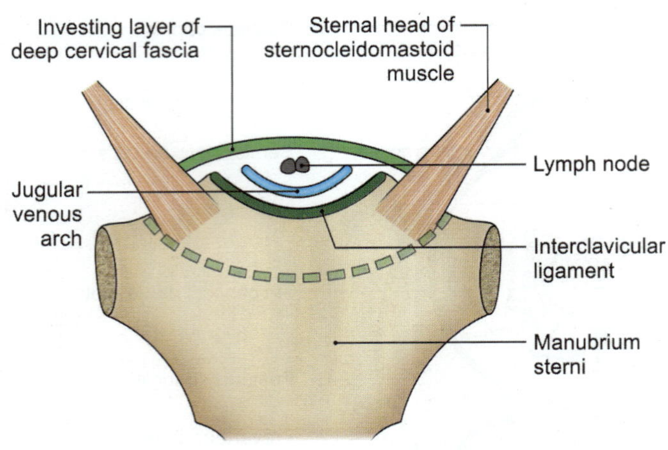

Fig. 11.5: Contents of suprasternal space

Posteriorly

a. Ligamentum nuchae, and
b. Spine of seventh cervical vertebra.

Anteriorly

a. Symphysis menti
b. Hyoid bone.

Both above and below the hyoid bone, it is continuous with the fascia of the opposite side.

Other Features

1 The investing layer of deep cervical fascia *splits* to enclose:
   a. *Muscles*: Trapezius and sternocleidomastoid (Fig. 11.3).
   b. *Salivary glands*: Parotid and submandibular (Fig. 11.4).
   c. *Spaces*: Suprasternal and supraclavicular.

   The *suprasternal space* or space of Burns contains:
   - The sternal heads of the right and left sternocleidomastoid muscles (Fig. 11.5),
   - The jugular venous arch,
   - A lymph node, and
   - The interclavicular ligament.

   The *supraclavicular space* is traversed by:
   - The external jugular vein (Fig. 11.6),
   - The supraclavicular nerves, and
   - Cutaneous vessels, including lymphatics.

2 It also forms *pulleys* to bind the tendons of the digastric and omohyoid muscles (Fig. 11.1c).
3 Forms roof of anterior and posterior triangles.
4 Forms stylomandibular ligament (Fig. 11.4a) and parotidomasseteric fascia.

CLINICAL ANATOMY

- Parotid swellings are very painful due to the unyielding nature of parotid fascia.
- While excising the submandibular salivary gland, the external carotid artery should be secured before dividing it, otherwise it may retract through the stylomandibular ligament and cause serious bleeding (Fig. 11.4a). This figure also shows the superior attachment of investing layer of deep cervical fascia to tympanic plate and styloid process.
- Division of the external jugular vein in the supraclavicular space may cause air embolism and consequent death because the cut ends of the vein are prevented from retraction and closure by the fascia, attached firmly to the vein (Fig. 11.6 and inset).

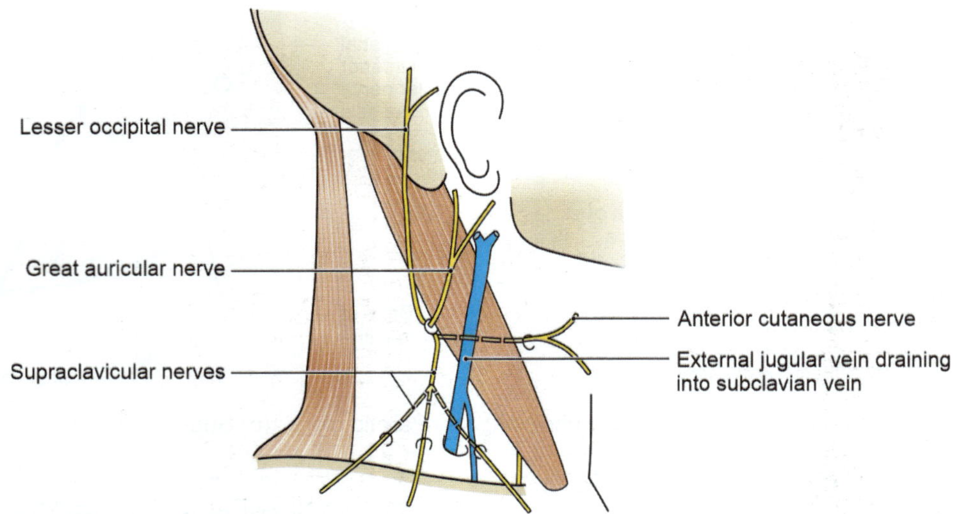

Fig. 11.6: Structures seen in relation to the fascial roof of the posterior triangle and structures seen in supraclavicular space

PRETRACHEAL FASCIA

The importance of this fascia is that it encloses and suspends the thyroid gland and forms its false capsule (Fig. 11.2). It is continuous with buccopharyngeal fascia.

Attachments

Superiorly

1 Hyoid bone in the median plane
2 Oblique line of thyroid cartilage—laterally
3 Cricoid cartilage—more laterally

Inferiorly

Below the thyroid gland, it encloses the inferior thyroid veins, passes behind the brachiocephalic veins, and finally blends with the arch of the aorta and fibrous pericardium.

On Either Side

It forms the front of the carotid sheath, and fuses with the fascia deep to the sternocleidomastoid (Fig. 11.3).

Other Features

1 The posterior layer of the thyroid capsule is thick. On either side, it forms a *suspensory ligament* for the thyroid gland known as *ligament of Berry* (*see* Fig. 16.4). The ligaments are attached chiefly to the cricoid cartilage, and may extend to the thyroid cartilage. They support the thyroid gland, and do not let it sink into the mediastinum. The capsule of the thyroid is very weak along the posterior borders of the lateral lobes.
2 The fascia provides a slippery surface for free movements of the trachea during swallowing.

CLINICAL ANATOMY

- Neck infections in front of the pretracheal fascia may bulge in the suprasternal area or extend down into the anterior mediastinum.
- The thyroid gland and all thyroid swellings move with deglutition because the thyroid is attached to cartilages of the larynx by the suspensory ligaments of Berry.

PREVERTEBRAL FASCIA

It lies in front of the prevertebral muscles, and forms the floor of the posterior triangle of the neck (Fig. 11.2).

Attachments and Relations

Superiorly

It is attached to the base of the skull (Fig. 11.2).

Inferiorly

It extends into the superior mediastinum where it splits into anterior and posterior layers. Anterior layer/alar fascia blends with buccopharyngeal fascia and posterior layer is attached to the anterior longitudinal ligament and to the body of the fourth thoracic vertebra.

Anteriorly

It is separated from the pharynx and buccopharyngeal fascia by the retropharyngeal space containing loose areolar tissue. In the lower part of neck, prevertebral and buccopharyngeal fasciae fuse (Fig. 11.3 and *see* Fig. 16.4). Lymph nodes lie in the retropharyngeal space.

Laterally

It lies deep to the trapezius and is attached to fascia of sternocleidomastoid muscle.

Other Features

1 The cervical and brachial plexuses lie behind the prevertebral fascia. The fascia is pierced by the four cutaneous branches of the cervical plexus (Fig. 11.6).
2 As the trunks of the brachial plexus and the subclavian artery pass laterally through the interval between the scalenus anterior and the scalenus medius, they carry with them a covering of the prevertebral fascia known as the *axillary sheath* which extends into the axilla (Fig. 11.7). The subclavian and axillary veins lie outside the sheath and as a result they can dilate during increased venous return from the limb.
3 Fascia provides a fixed base for the movements of the pharynx, the oesophagus and the carotid sheaths during movements of the neck and during swallowing.

CLINICAL ANATOMY

- Neck infections behind the prevertebral fascia arise usually from tuberculosis of the cervical vertebrae or cervical caries. Pus produced as a result may extend in various directions. It may pass forwards forming a chronic retropharyngeal abscess which may form a bulging in the posterior wall of the pharynx, in the median plane (Fig. 11.7). The pus may extend laterally through the axillary sheath and point in the posterior triangle, or in the lateral wall of the axilla. It may extend downwards into the superior mediastinum, where its descent is limited by fusion of the prevertebral fascia to the fourth thoracic vertebra.
- Neck infections in front of the prevertebral fascia in the retropharyngeal space usually arise from suppuration, i.e. formation of pus in the retropharyngeal lymph nodes. The pus forms an acute retropharyngeal abscess which bulges forwards in the paramedian position due to fusion of the buccopharyngeal fascia to the prevertebral fascia in the median plane. The infection may extend down through the superior mediastinum into the posterior mediastinum (Fig. 11.3).

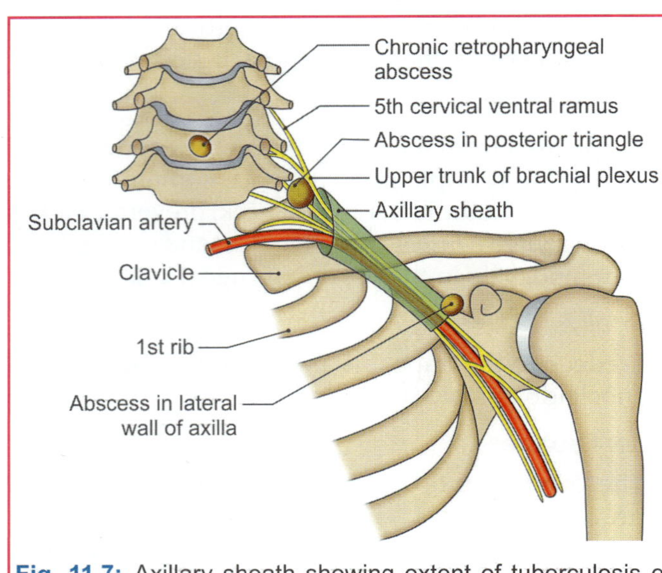

Fig. 11.7: Axillary sheath showing extent of tuberculosis of cervical vertebrae

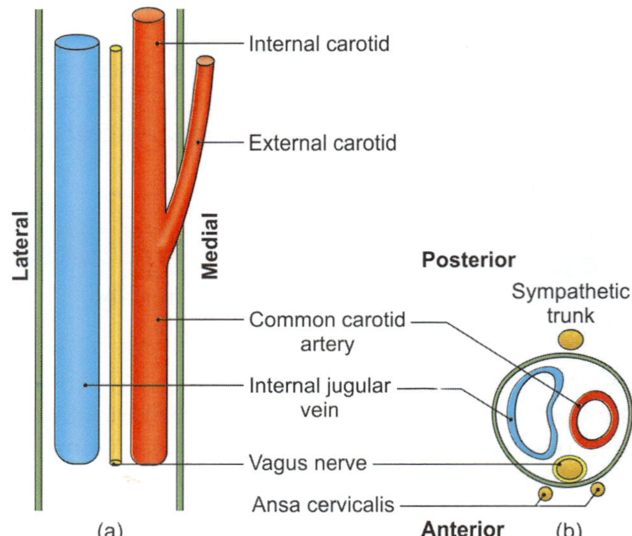

Figs 11.8a and b: Right carotid sheath with its contents: (a) Surface view; (b) Sectional view

CAROTID SHEATH

It is a condensation of the fibroareolar tissue around the main vessels of the neck.

***Formation*:** It is formed on anterior aspect by pretracheal fascia and on posterior aspect by prevertebral fascia.

***Contents*:** The contents are the common or internal carotid arteries, internal jugular vein and the vagus nerve. It is thin over the vein (Figs 11.8a and b). In the upper part of sheath, there are IX, XI, XII nerves also. These nerves pierce the sheet at different points.

***Relations*:**

1. The ansa cervicalis lies embedded in the anterior wall of the carotid sheath (Fig. 11.8b).
2. The cervical sympathetic chain lies behind the sheath, plastered to the prevertebral fascia.
3. The sheath is overlapped by the anterior border of the sternocleidomastoid, and is fused to the layers of the deep cervical fascia.

BUCCOPHARYNGEAL FASCIA

This fascia covers all the constrictor muscles externally and extends onto the superficial aspect of the buccinator muscle (Fig. 11.2) and is attached to pharyngeal tubercle. Retropharyngeal space lies posterior to buccopharyngeal fascia. Alar fascia is an ancillary layer of deep cervical fascia which divides retropharyngeal space into two parts. The posterior space between alar and prevertebral fasciae is the 'dangerous space in neck'.

PHARYNGOBASILAR FASCIA

This fascia is especially thickened between the upper border of superior constrictor muscle and the base of the skull. It lies deep to the pharyngeal muscles (*see* Figs 22.14 and 22.21).

PHARYNGEAL SPACES

RETROPHARYNGEAL SPACE

Situation:	Dead space behind pharynx.
Function:	Acts as a bursa for expansion of pharynx during deglutition
Boundaries:	Anterior: Buccopharyngeal fascia Posterior: Prevertebral fascia. The two get fused. Sides: Carotid sheath (Fig. 11.3)
Superior:	Base of skull
Inferior:	Open and continuous with superior mediastinum.
Contents:	Retropharyngeal lymph nodes, pharyngeal plexus of vessels and nerves, loose areolar tissue.
Clinical anatomy:	Pus collection due to lymph node abscess which lies in paramedian postion. It should be differentiated from cold abscess of spine of cervical vertebrae which is seen in median plane.

LATERAL PHARYNGEAL SPACE

Situation:	Side of pharynx
Boundaries:	Medial: Pharynx Posterolateral: Parotid gland Anterolateral: Medial pterygoid Posterior: Carotid sheath

Contents: Branches of maxillary artery
Fibrofatty tissue
Clinical anatomy: Pus collection/Ludwig's angina.

STERNOCLEIDOMASTOID MUSCLE (STERNOMASTOID)

The sternocleidomastoid and trapezius are large superficial muscles of the neck. Both of them are supplied by the spinal root of the accessory nerve. The trapezius, is described in Chapter 18. The sternocleidomastoid is described below.

Origin

1 The *sternal head* is tendinous and arises from the superolateral part of the front of the manubrium sterni (Fig. 11.1c).
2 The *clavicular head* is musculotendinous and arises from the medial one-third of the superior surface of the clavicle. It passes deep to the sternal head, and the two heads blend below the middle of the neck. Between the two heads, there is a small triangular depression of the lesser supraclavicular fossa, overlying the internal jugular vein.

Insertion

It is inserted:

1 By a thick tendon into the lateral surface of *mastoid process,* from its tip to superior border.
2 By a thin aponeurosis into the lateral half of the *superior nuchal line* of the occipital bone.

Nerve Supply

1 The spinal accessory nerve provides the motor supply. It passes through the muscle (Fig. 11.10).
2 Branches from the ventral rami of C2 and C3 are proprioceptive.

Blood Supply

Arterial supply—one branch each from superior thyroid artery and suprascapular artery and, two branches from the occipital artery supply the big muscle (*see* Fig. 12.16). Veins follow the arteries.

Actions

1 When one muscle contracts:
   a. It turns the chin to the opposite side.
   b. It can also tilt the head towards the shoulder of same side.
2 When both muscles contract together:
   a. They draw the head forwards, as in eating and in lifting the head from a pillow.
   b. With the longus colli, they flex the neck against resistance.
   c. It also helps in forced inspiration.

Relations

The sternocleidomastoid is enclosed in the investing layer of deep cervical fascia, and is pierced by the accessory nerve and by the four sternocleidomastoid arteries. It has the following relations.

Superficial

1 Skin
2 a. Superficial fascia
   b. Superficial lamina of the deep cervical fascia (Fig. 11.3)
3 Platysma
4 External jugular vein, and superficial cervical lymph nodes lying along the vein (Fig. 11.6).
5 a. Great auricular
   b. Transverse or anterior cutaneous
   c. Medial supraclavicular nerves (Fig. 11.6)
   d. Lesser occipital nerve
6 The parotid gland overlaps the muscle.

Deep

1 Bones and joints:
   a. Mastoid process—above (Fig. 11.1c)
   b. Sternoclavicular joint—below.
2 Carotid sheath (Fig. 11.8)
3 Muscles:
   a. Sternohyoid (Fig. 11.3)
   b. Sternothyroid
   c. Omohyoid
   d. Three scaleni
   e. Levator scapulae (Fig. 11.9b)
   f. Splenius capitis (Fig. 11.10)
   g. Longissimus capitis (*see* Fig. 19.3)
   h. Posterior belly of digastric (*see* Fig. 12.10).
4 Arteries:
   a. Common carotid (Fig. 11.8)
   b. Internal carotid
   c. External carotid
   d. Sternocleidomastoid arteries, two from the occipital artery, one from the superior thyroid, one from the suprascapular
   e. Occipital
   f. Subclavian
   g. Suprascapular
   h. Transverse cervical (Fig. 11.9)

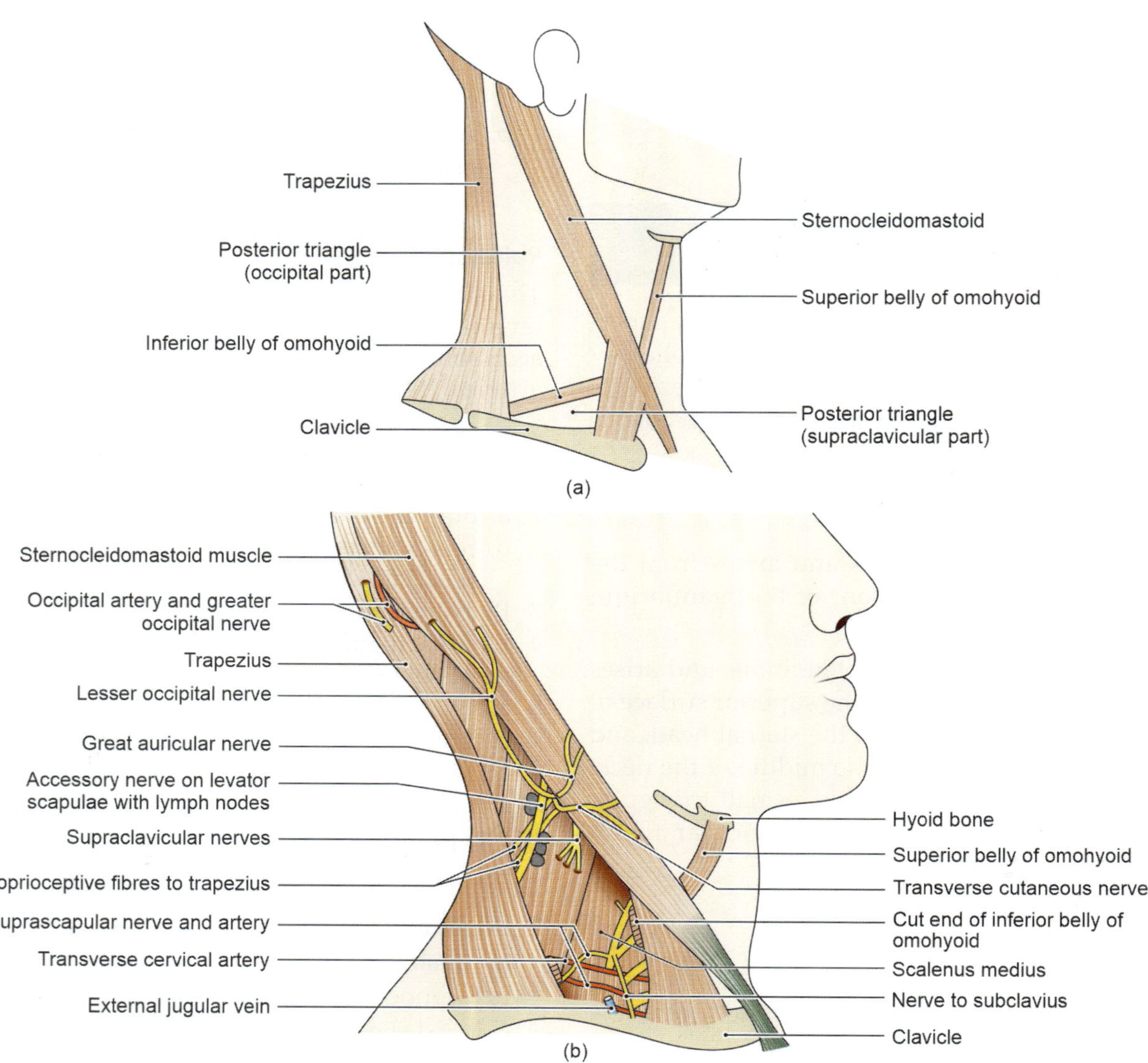

Figs 11.9a and b: (a) Boundaries; (b) Contents of posterior triangle

5 Veins:
   a. Internal jugular (Fig. 11.8)
   b. Anterior jugular
   c. Facial
   d. Lingual

6 Nerves:
   a. Vagus
   b. Parts of IX, XI, XII. Spinal root of XI leaves the SCM at middle of its posterior border to lie in posterior triangle (Figs 11.8 and 11.10)
   c. Cervical plexus
   d. Upper part of brachial plexus (Fig. 11.10)
   e. Phrenic (Fig. 11.10)
   f. Ansa cervicalis

7 Lymph nodes, superficial and deep cervical (*see* Figs 16.30 and 16.31).

CLINICAL ANATOMY

- Figure 11.5 shows inferior attachment of investing layer of deep cervical fascia. Fascia of supraclavicular space is pierced by external jugular vein to drain into subclavian vein (Fig. 11.6).
- Torticollis is a deformity in which the head is bent to one side and the chin points to the other side. This is a result of spasm or contracture of the muscles supplied by the spinal accessory nerve, these being the sternocleidomastoid and trapezius. Although there are many varieties of torticollis depending on the causes, the common types are:
   a. Rheumatic torticollis due to exposure to cold or draught.
   b. Reflex torticollis due to inflamed or suppurating cervical lymph nodes which irritate the spinal accessory nerve.

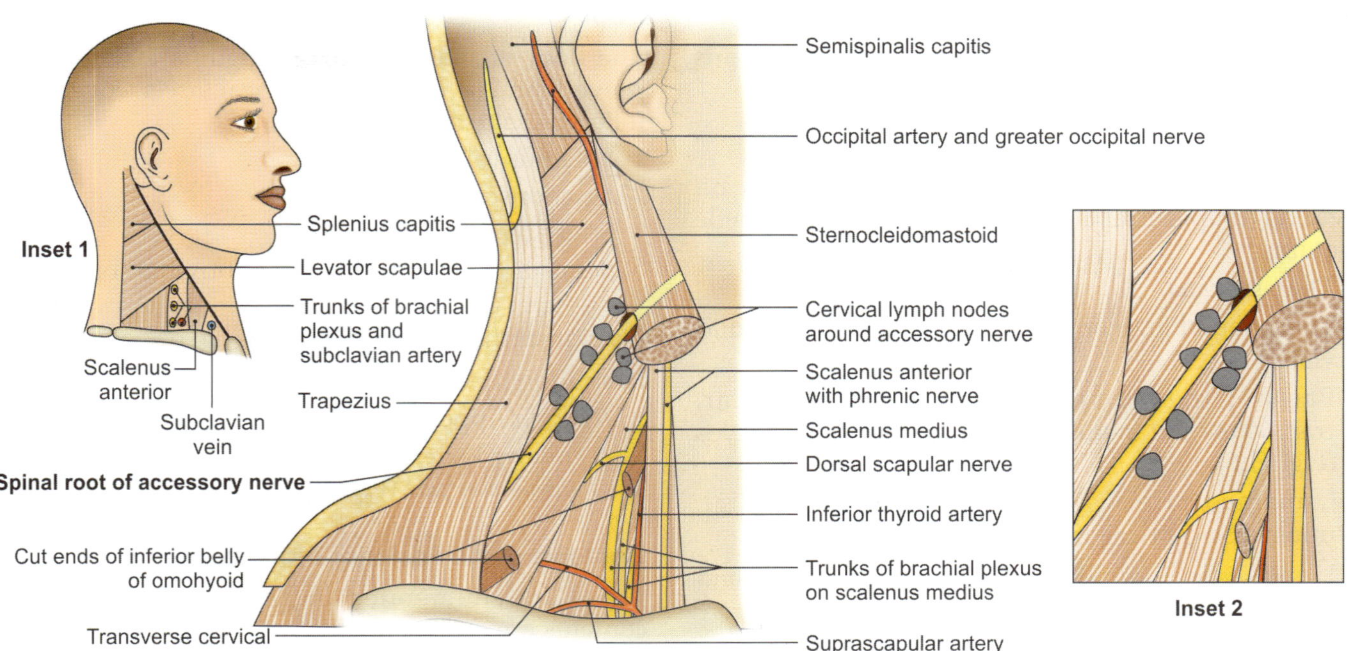

Fig. 11.10: The boundaries of posterior triangle of neck with its contents

c. Congenital torticollis due to birth injury.

Wry neck: Shortening of the muscle fibres due to intravascular clotting of veins within the muscle. It usually occurs during difficult delivery of the baby.

POSTERIOR TRIANGLE

Features

The posterior triangle is a space on the side of the neck situated behind the sternocleidomastoid muscle.

DISSECTION

Try to dissect and clean the cutaneous nerves (Fig. 11.6) which pierce the investing layer of fascia at the middle of posterior border of sternocleidomastoid muscle. Demarcate the course of external jugular vein. Cut carefully the deep fascia of posterior border of sterno-cleidomastoid muscle and reflect it towards trapezius muscle. Identify the accessory nerve lying just deep to the investing layer seen at the middle of the posterior border of sternocleidomastoid muscle and across the posterior triangle to reach the anterior border of trapezius which it supplies (Fig. 11.10).

Define the boundaries, roof, floor, divisions and contents of the posterior triangle (Fig. 11.1c).

Identify and clean the inferior belly of omohyoid. Find the transverse cervical artery along the upper border of this muscle. Trace it both ways. Deep to this muscle is the upper or supraclavicular part of brachial plexus. Identify the roots, trunks and their branches carefully. The branches are suprascapular nerve, dorsal scapular nerve, long thoracic nerve, nerve to subclavius (Fig. 11.10). Medial to the brachial plexus locate the third part of subclavian artery (*refer to BDC App*).

Follow the terminal part of external jugular vein through the deep fascia into the deeply placed subclavian vein (Fig. 11.6). Identify suprascapular artery running just above the clavicle (Fig. 11.9b).

Define the attachments and relations of sternocleido-mastoid muscle. To expose scalenus anterior muscle, cut across the clavicular head of sternocleidomastoid muscle and push it medially. Scalenus anterior muscle covered by well-defined prevertebral fascia can be identified. Clean the subclavian artery and upper part of brachial plexus deep to the scalenus anterior muscle.

Boundaries

Anterior

Posterior border of sternocleidomastoid (Figs 11.1b and c).

Posterior

Anterior border of trapezius.

Inferior or Base

Middle one-third of clavicle.

Apex

Lies on the superior nuchal line where the trapezius and sternocleidomastoid meet.

Roof

The roof is formed by the *investing layer of deep cervical fascia*. The superficial fascia over the posterior triangle contains:

1 The platysma
2 The external jugular and posterior external jugular veins
3 Parts of the supraclavicular, great auricular, transverse cutaneous and lesser occipital nerves (Fig. 11.6)
4 Unnamed arteries derived from the occipital, transverse cervical and suprascapular arteries.
5 Lymph vessels which pierce the deep fascia to end in the supraclavicular nodes.

External jugular vein: It lies deep to the platysma (Fig. 11.6). It is formed by union of the posterior auricular vein with the posterior division of the retromandibular vein. It begins within the lower part of the parotid gland, crosses the sternocleidomastoid obliquely, pierces the anteroinferior angle of the roof of the posterior triangle, and opens into the subclavian vein (*see* Fig. 10.6).

Its tributaries are:

a. The posterior external jugular vein
b. The transverse cervical vein
c. The suprascapular vein
d. The anterior jugular vein.

The oblique jugular vein connects the external jugular vein with the internal jugular vein across the middle one-third of the anterior border of the sternocleidomastoid.

CLINICAL ANATOMY

- The right external jugular vein is *examined to assess the venous pressure;* the right atrial pressure is reflected in it because there are no valves in the entire course of this vein and it is straight.
- As external jugular vein pierces the fascia, the margins of the vein get adherent to the fascia. So if the vein gets cut, it cannot close and air is sucked in due to negative intrathoracic pressure. That causes air embolism. To prevent this, the deep fascia has to be cut.

Floor

The floor of the posterior triangle is formed by the prevertebral layer of deep cervical fascia, covering the following muscles:

1 Splenius capitis
2 Levator scapulae
3 Scalenus medius (Fig. 11.9)

Semispinalis capitis may also form part of the floor.

Division of the Posterior Triangle

It is subdivided by the inferior belly of omohyoid into:

1 A larger upper part, called the *occipital part.*
2 A smaller lower part, called the *supraclavicular part* or *subclavian part* (Fig. 11.9a).

Contents of the Posterior Triangle

These are enumerated in Table 11.1. Some of the contents are considered below.

Relevant Features of the Contents of Posterior Triangle

1 The *spinal root of accessory nerve* emerges a little above the middle of the posterior border of the sternocleidomastoid. It runs through a tunnel in the fascia forming the roof of the triangle, passing downwards and laterally, and disappears under the anterior border of the trapezius about 5 cm above the clavicle (Figs 11.9 and 11.10). It is the only structure beneath the roof of triangle. It supplies both sternocleidomastoid and trapezius muscles.
2 The four *cutaneous branches of the cervical plexus* pierce the fascia covering the floor of the triangle, pass through the triangle and pierce the deep fascia at different points to become cutaneous (Fig. 11.6).
   a. *Transverse cutaneous nerve:* Arises from ventral rami of C2 and C3 nerves runs transversely across the sternocleidomastoid to supply skin of neck, till the sternum.
   b. *Supraclavicular nerves:* Formed from ventral rami of C3 and C4 nerves. Emerges at posterior border of sternocleidomastoid. It descends downwards and diverges into three branches. Medial one supplies the skin over the manubrium till manubriosternal joint. Intermediate nerve crosses the clavicle to supply skin of first intercostal space till the second rib. Lateral nerve runs across the lateral side of clavicle and acromion to supply skin over the upper half of the deltoid muscle.
   c. *Great auricular nerve:* It is the largest ascending branch of cervical plexus. Arises from ventral rami of C2 and C3 nerves. Ascends on the

Table 11.1: Contents of the posterior triangle

Contents	*Occipital triangle*	*Subclavian triangle*
A. Nerves	1. Spinal accessory nerve (Figs 11.9 and 11.10) 2. Four cutaneous branches of cervical plexus (Fig. 11.6): a. Lesser occipital (C2) b. Great auricular (C2, C3) c. Anterior cutaneous nerve of neck (C2, C3) d. Supraclavicular nerves (C3, C4) 3. Muscular branches: a. Two small branches to the levator scapulae (C3, C4) b. Two small branches to the trapezius (C3, C4) c. Nerve to rhomboids (proprioceptive) (C5)	1. Roots and trunks of brachial plexus 2. Nerve to serratus anterior (long thoracic, C5–C7) 3. Nerve to subclavius (C5, C6) 4. Suprascapular nerve (C5, C6)
B. Vessels	1. Transverse cervical artery and vein 2. Occipital artery	1. Third part of subclavian artery and subclavian vein 2. Suprascapular artery and vein 3. Commencement of transverse cervical artery and termination of the corresponding vein 4. Lower part of external jugular vein
C. Lymph nodes	Along the posterior border of the sternocleidomastoid, more in the lower part—the supraclavicular nodes and a few at the upper angle—the occipital nodes	A few members of the supraclavicular chain

sternocleidomastoid muscle to reach parotid gland, where it divides into anterior and posterior branches. Anterior branch supplies lower one-third of skin on lateral surface of pinna and skin over the parotid gland and connects the gland to the auriculotemporal nerve. This cross-connection is the anatomical basis for Frey's syndrome. Posterior branch supplies lower one-third of skin on medial surface of the pinna.

d. *Lesser occipital:* Arises from ventral ramus of C2 segment of spinal cord. Seen at the posterior border of sternocleidomastoid muscle. It then winds around and ascends on or along its posterior border to supply skin of upper two-thirds of medial surface of pinna adjoining part of the scalp.

3 *Branches to the levator scapulae and to the trapezius* (C3, C4) appear about the middle of the sternocleidomastoid. Those to the levator scapulae soon end in it; those to the trapezius run below and parallel to the accessory nerve across the middle of the triangle. Both nerves lie deep to the fascia of the floor.

4 Three trunks of the *brachial plexus* emerge between the scalenus anterior and medius, and carry the axillary sheath around them. The sheath contains the brachial plexus and the subclavian artery. These structures *lie deep* to *the floor* of posterior triangle. If prevertebral *fascia is left intact, all these structures are safe* (Fig. 11.9).

5 The *nerve to the rhomboid* or *dorsal scapular nerve* is from C5 root, pierces the scalenus medius and passes deep to the levator scapulae to reach the back where it lies deep or anterior to the rhomboid muscles (Fig. 11.10) and supplies these muscles.

6 The *nerve to the serratus anterior* (C5–C7) arises by three roots. The roots from C5 and C6 pierce the scalenus medius and join the root from C7 over the first digitation of the serratus anterior. The nerve passes behind the brachial plexus. It descends over the serratus anterior in the medial wall of the axilla and gives branches to the digitations of the muscle (Fig. 11.11).

7 The *nerve to the subclavius* (C5, C6) (Fig. 11.9b) descends in front of the brachial plexus and the subclavian vessels, but behind the omohyoid, the transverse cervical and suprascapular vessels and the clavicle to reach the deep surface of the subclavius muscle. As it runs near the lateral margin of the scalenus anterior, it sometimes gives off the *accessory phrenic nerve* which joins the phrenic nerve in front of the scalenus anterior.

8 The *suprascapular nerve* (C5, C6) arises from the upper trunk of the brachial plexus and crosses the lower part of the posterior triangle just above and lateral to the brachial plexus, deep to the transverse cervical vessels and the omohyoid. It passes backwards over the shoulder to reach the scapula. It supplies the supraspinatus and infraspinatus muscles (Fig. 11.9b).

9 The *subclavian artery* passes behind the tendon of the scalenus anterior, over the first rib (Fig. 11.12).

10 The *transverse cervical artery* is a branch of the thyrocervical trunk. It crosses the scalenus anterior, the phrenic nerve, the upper trunks of the brachial

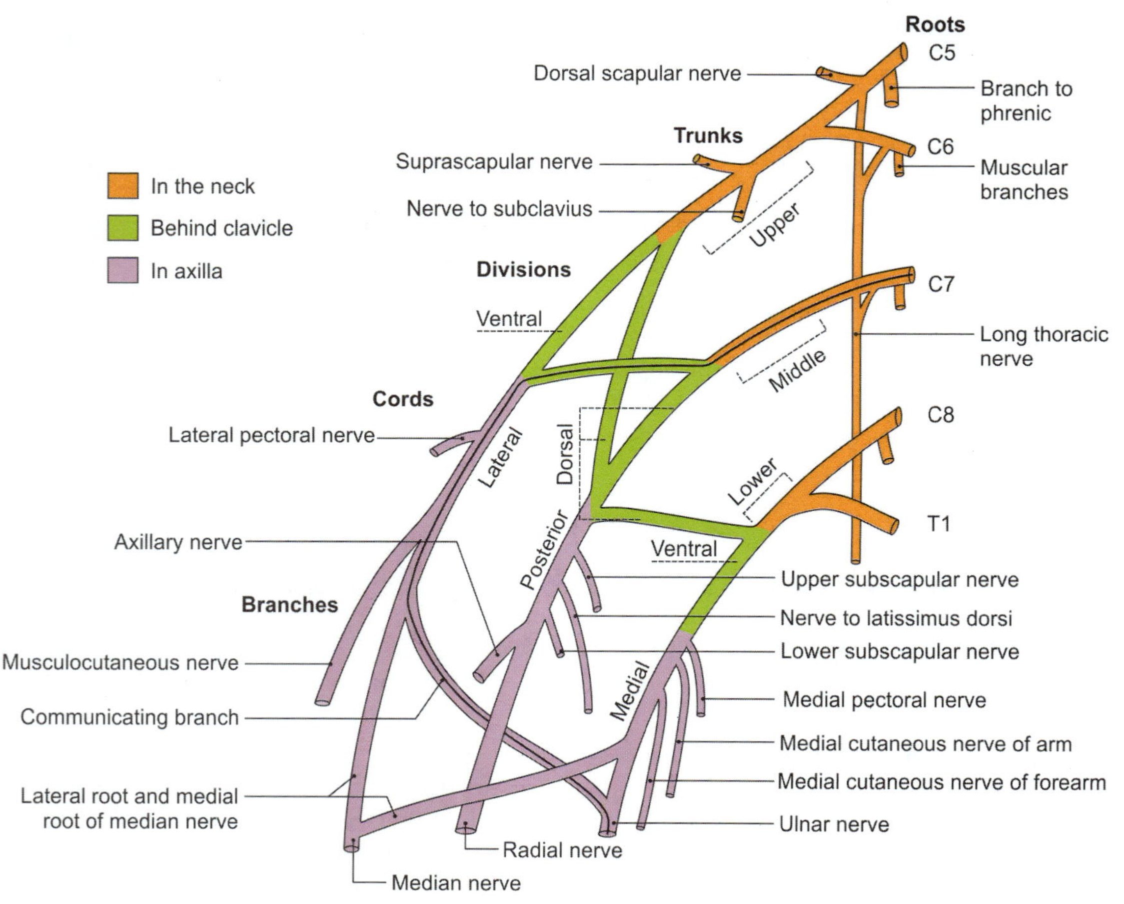

Fig. 11.11: Brachial plexus

plexus, the nerve to the subclavius, the suprascapular nerve, and the scalenus medius. At the anterior border of the levator scapulae, it divides into superficial and deep branches. The inferior belly of the omohyoid crosses the artery (Fig. 11.10).

11 The *suprascapular artery* is also a branch of the thyrocervical trunk. It passes laterally and backwards behind the clavicle (Fig. 11.10).

12 The *occipital artery* crosses the apex of the posterior triangle superficial to the splenius capitis (Fig. 11.9).

13 The subclavian vein passes in front of the tendon of scalenus anterior muscle.

14 Inferior belly of omohyoid arises from upper border of scapula near suprascapular notch, passes deep to trapezius and appears on its upper border in the posterior triangle. It courses through posterior triangle, dividing it in two parts, lies deep to sternocleidomastoid and continues as superior belly till hyoid bone.

CLINICAL ANATOMY

- The most common swelling in the posterior triangle is due to enlargement of the supraclavicular lymph nodes. While doing biopsy of the lymph node, one must be careful in preserving the accessory nerve which may get entangled amongst enlarged lymph nodes (Fig. 11.10).
- Supraclavicular lymph nodes are commonly enlarged in tuberculosis, Hodgkin's disease, and in malignant growths of the breast, arm or chest.
- Block dissection of the neck for malignant diseases is the removal of cervical lymph nodes along with other structures involved in the growth. This procedure does not endanger those nerves of the posterior triangle which lie deep to the prevertebral fascia, i.e. the brachial and cervical plexuses and their muscular branches.
- A cervical rib may compress the second part of subclavian artery. In these cases, blood supply to upper limb reaches via anastomoses around the scapula.
- Dysphagia caused by compression of the oesophagus by an abnormal subclavian artery is called *dysphagia lusoria*.
- Elective arterial surgery of the common carotid artery is done for aneurysms, AV fistulae or arteriosclerotic occlusions. It is better to expose the common carotid artery in its upper part where it is superficial. While ligating the artery, care

should be taken not to include the vagus nerve or the sympathetic chain.

- Second part of the subclavian artery may get pressed by the scalenus anterior muscle, resulting in decreased blood supply to the upper limb. If the muscle is divided, the effects are abolished (Fig. 11.12).

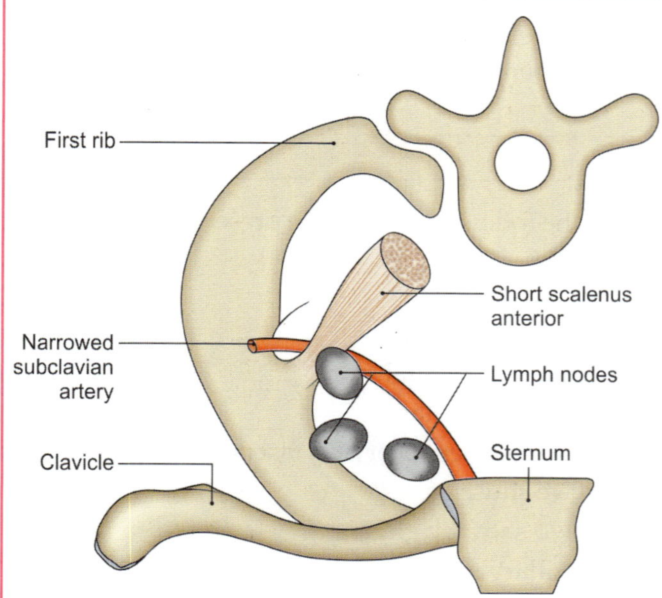

Fig. 11.12: Second part of subclavian artery narrowed by the short scalenus anterior

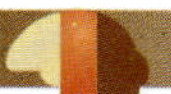

Mnemonics

Arrangement of the important nerves "GLAST":

Great auricular
Lesser occipital
Accessory nerve pops out between L and S
Supraclavicular
Transverse cervical

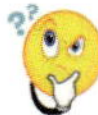

FACTS TO REMEMBER

Investing layer of deep cervical fascia encloses two muscles, two salivary glands; forms two pulleys; encloses two spaces and forms roof of posterior triangle.

- Prevertebral fascia forms the axillary sheath.
- Pretracheal fascia suspends the thyroid gland.
- Cold abscess of caries spine, can track down to the posterior triangle or axilla.
- Occipital part of posterior triangle contains the spinal root of accessory nerve as the most important constituent.
- Supraclavicular part of posterior triangle contains roots, trunks, branches of brachial plexus and third part of subclavian artery.
- Sternocleidomastoid divides the side of neck into anterior and posterior triangles.

CLINICOANATOMICAL PROBLEM

A middle-aged woman had a deep cut in the middle of her right posterior triangle of neck. The bleeding was arrested and wound was sutured. The patient later felt difficulty in combing her hair.

- What is the blood vessel severed?
- Why did the patient have difficulty in combing her hair?

Ans: The external jugular vein was severed. It passes across the sternocleidomastoid muscle to join the subclavian vein above the clavicle. Her accessory nerve is also injured as it crosses the posterior triangle close to its roof, causing paralysis of trapezius muscle. The trapezius with serratus anterior causes overhead abduction required for combing the hair. Due to paralysis of trapezius, she felt difficulty in combing her hair.

FURTHER READING

- Berkoviz BKB, Moxham BJ. Color Atlas of the Skull, London: Mosby-Wolfe. 1994.
  An excellent atlas that gives a clear illustration of the different components of the skull.
- Guidera, AK Daws PJD, Stringer MD. Cervical fascia: A terminological pain the neck. ANZ Surg 2012;82:786–91.
  A review that provides a critical appraisal of the terms used to describe the cervical fascia in order to achieve consensus and uniformitiy.
- Guidera AK, Dawes PJD, Fong A, et al. Head and neck fascia and compartments: No space for spaces. Head Neck 2014; 36:1058–68.
  A comprehensive review of the fascia of the head and neck and its associated compartments aiding the understanding of the variable and, at times, misleading terminology.

Frequently Asked Questions

1. Describe the cervical fascia under following headings:
   a. Attachments and structures enclosed by investing layer of cervical fascia
   b. Clinical importance of pretracheal fascia
   c. Contents of carotid sheath
2. Enumerate the boundaries and contents of posterior triangle of neck. How is external jugular vein formed and what is its clinical importance?
3. Write short notes/enumerate:
   a. Sternocleidomastoid muscle
   b. Contents of suprasternal space
   c. Suspensary ligament of Berry

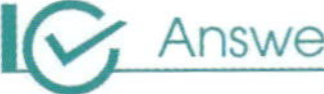

Multiple Choice Questions

1. All of the following structures are seen in the posterior triangle of neck, *except*:
   a. Spinal accessory nerve
   b. Transverse cervical artery
   c. Middle trunk of brachial plexus
   d. Superior belly of omohyoid
2. Spinal root of accessory nerve innervates:
   a. Serratus anterior
   b. Stylohyoid
   c. Styloglossus
   d. Sternocleidomastoid
3. Suprasternal space contains all, *except*:
   a. Sternal heads of right and left sternocleido-mastoid muscles
   b. Jugular venous arch
   c. Interclavicular ligament
   d. Sternohyoid muscles
4. All the following nerves are present in the posterior triangle, *except*:
   a. Spinal accessory
   b. Lesser occipital
   c. Greater occipital
   d. Great auricular
5. Investing layer of cervical fascia encloses all, *except*:
   a. Two muscles
   b. Two salivary glands
   c. Axillary vessels
   d. Two spaces
6. Ligament of Berry is formed by:
   a. Investing layer of cervical fascia
   b. Pretracheal layer
   c. Prevertebral layer
   d. Buccopharyngeal fascia

Answers

1. d **2.** d **3.** d **4.** c **5.** c **6.** b

VIVA VOCE

- Enumerate the contents of suprasternal space.
- Name the structures enclosed by investing layer of cervical fascia.
- What is the function of ligament of Berry.
- Name the contents of carotid sheath.
- Which layer of cervical fascia forms the axillary sheath?
- What are the boundaries of posterior triangle of neck?
- Which are the muscles supplied by spinal root of XI nerve?
- Name the arteries supplying the sternocleidomastoid muscle.
- Traction of which muscle may result in narrowing of the subclavian artery?
- Name the nerves arising from upper trunk of brachial plexus.
- What is the root value of 'nerve to serratus anterior'?

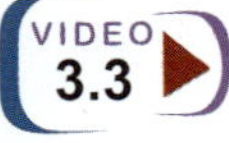

Side of the neck: Posterior triangle

Chapter 12

Anterior Triangle of the Neck

"One picture is worth more than thousand words."
—Anonymous

INTRODUCTION

The anterior triangle of the neck lies between midline of the neck and sternocleidomastoid muscle. It is subdivided into smaller triangles.

SURFACE LANDMARKS

1 The *mandible* forms the lower jaw (Fig. 12.1). The lower border of its horseshoe-shaped body is known as the *base of the mandible.* Anteriorly, this base forms the *chin*, and posteriorly it can be traced to the *angle of the mandible.*

2 The body of the U-shaped *hyoid bone* can be felt in the median plane just below and behind the chin, at the junction of the neck with the floor of the mouth. On each side, the body of hyoid bone is continuous posteriorly with the *greater cornua* which is overlapped in its posterior part by the sternocleidomastoid muscle.

3 The *thyroid cartilage* of the larynx forms a sharp protuberance in the median plane just below the hyoid bone. This protuberance is called the *laryngeal prominence or Adam's apple.* It is more prominent in males.

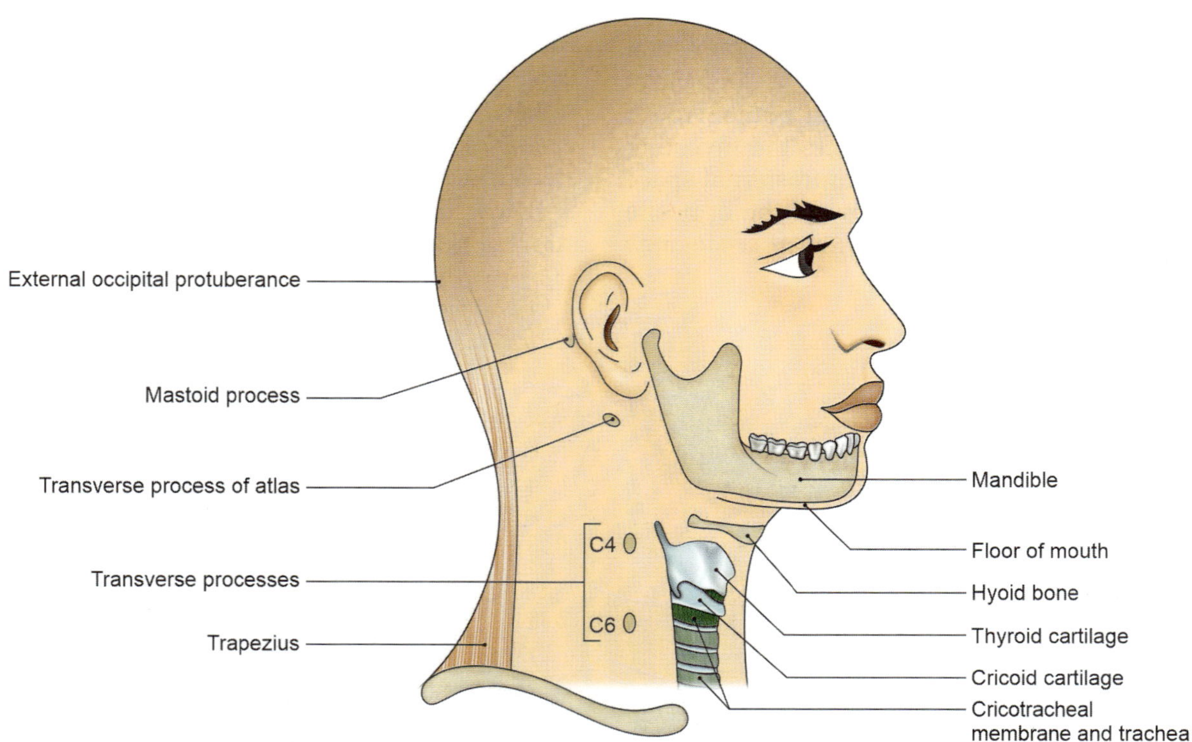

Fig. 12.1: Surface landmarks of neck

4 The rounded arch of the *cricoid cartilage* lies below the thyroid cartilage at the upper end of the trachea.
5 The trachea runs downwards and backwards from the cricoid cartilage. It is identified by its cartilaginous rings. However, it is partially masked by the *isthmus of the thyroid gland* which lies against second to fourth tracheal rings. The trachea is commonly palpated in the *suprasternal notch* which lies between the tendinous heads of origin of the right and left sternocleidomastoid muscles. In certain diseases, the trachea may shift to one side from the median plane. This indicates a shift in the mediastinum.

STRUCTURES IN THE ANTERIOR MEDIAN REGION OF THE NECK

Features

This region includes a strip 2 to 3 cm wide extending from the chin to the sternum. The structures encountered are listed below from superficial to deep.

Skin

It is freely movable over the deeper structures due to the looseness of the superficial fascia.

Superficial Fascia

It contains:

1 The upper decussating fibres of the *platysma* for 1 to 2 cm below the chin.
2 The *anterior jugular veins* beginning in the submental region below the chin. It descends in the superficial fascia about 1 cm from the median plane. About 2.5 cm above the sternum, it pierces the investing layer of deep fascia to enter the suprasternal space where it is connected to its fellow of the opposite side by a transverse channel, the *jugular venous arch*

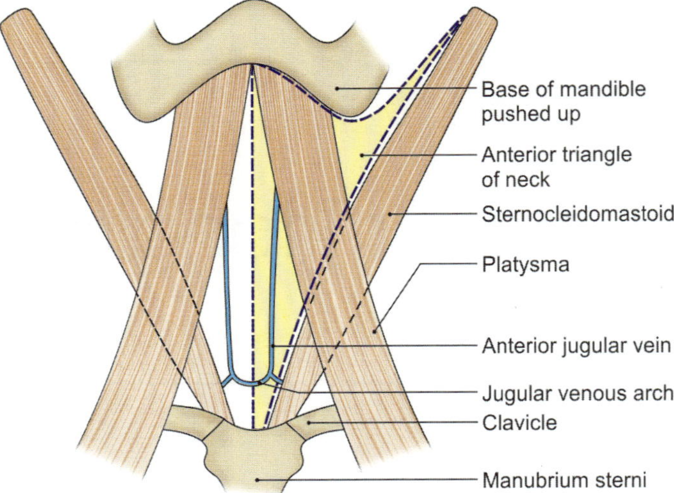

Fig. 12.2: Anterior triangles of the neck showing the platysma and the anterior jugular veins in the superficial fascia

(Fig. 12.2). The vein then turns laterally, runs deep to the sternocleidomastoid just above the clavicle, and *ends in the external jugular vein* at the posterior border of the sternocleidomastoid.
3 A few small *submental lymph nodes* lie on the deep fascia below the chin (Fig. 12.3).
4 The terminal filaments of the *transverse or anterior cutaneous nerve* of the neck may be present in it.

Deep Fascia

Above the hyoid bone, the investing layer of deep fascia is a single layer in the median plane, but splits on each side to enclose the submandibular salivary gland (*see* Fig. 11.4).

Between the hyoid bone and the cricoid cartilage, it is a single layer extending between the right and left sternocleidomastoid muscles.

Below the cricoid, the fascia splits to enclose the suprasternal space (*see* Fig. 11.5).

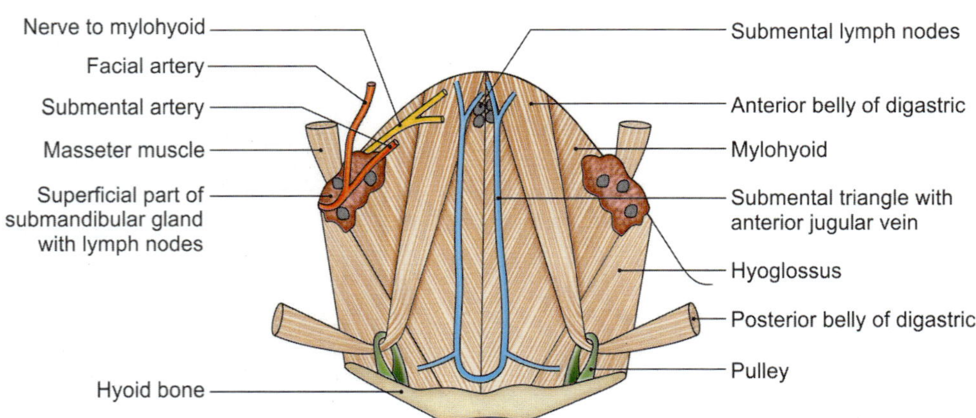

Fig. 12.3: Suprahyoid region, contents of submental and digastric triangles also shown

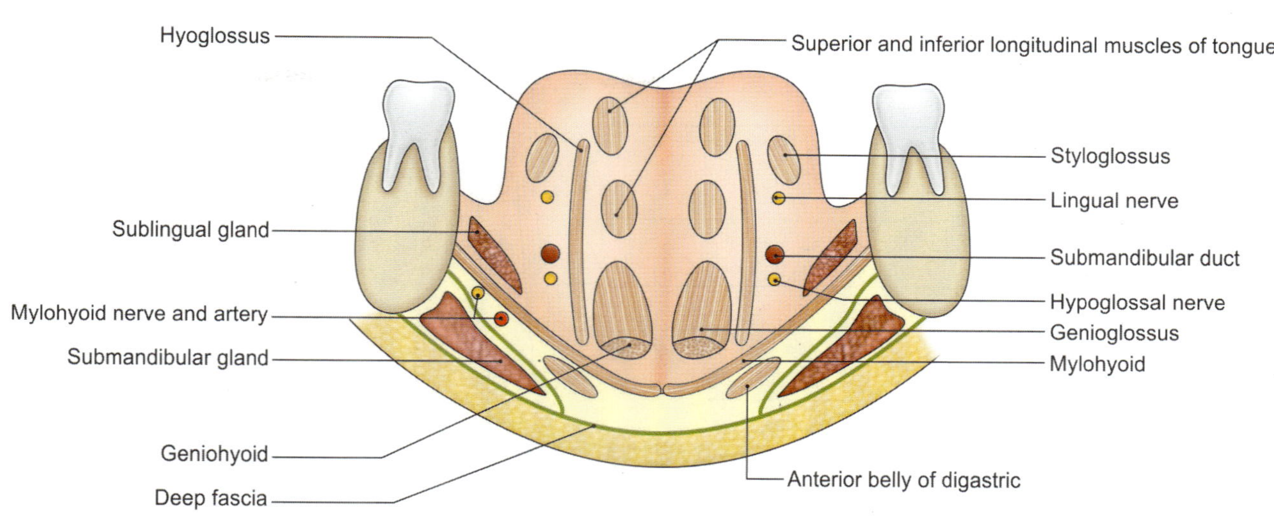

Fig. 12.4: Coronal section through the floor of the mouth

Deep Structures Lying above the Hyoid Bone

The *mylohyoid muscle* is overlapped by:

a. Anterior belly of *digastric* above the hyoid bone.
b. Superficial part of the *submandibular salivary gland* (Figs 12.3 and 12.4).
c. *Mylohyoid nerve and vessels.*
d. *Submental branch of the facial artery.*

The anteroinferior part of the *hyoglossus muscle* with its superficial relations may also be exposed during dissection. Structures lying in this corner are:

a. The intermediate tendon of the *digastric* muscle with its fibrous pulley (Fig. 12.3).
b. The bifurcated tendon of the *stylohyoid* muscle embracing the digastric tendon (Fig. 12.10).

The *subhyoid bursa* lies between the posterior surface of the body of the hyoid bone and the thyrohyoid membrane. It lessens friction between these two structures during the movements of swallowing (Fig. 12.5).

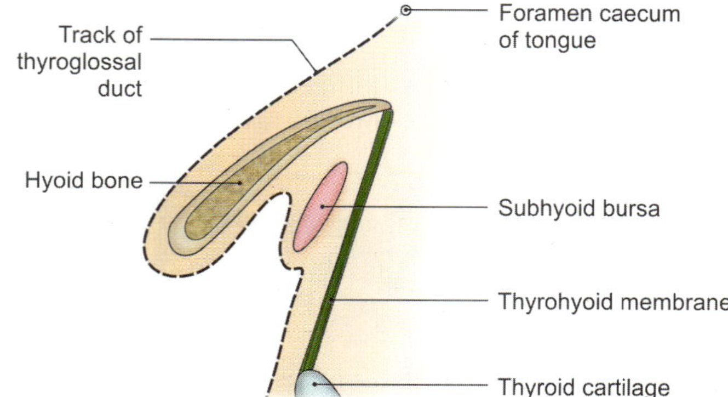

Fig. 12.5: Sagittal section through the hyoid region of the neck showing the subhyoid bursa and its relations

Structures Lying below the Hyoid Bone

These structures may be grouped into three planes: (1) Superficial plane containing the infrahyoid muscles, (2) a middle plane consisting of the pretracheal fascia and the thyroid gland, and (3) a deep plane containing the larynx, trachea and structures associated with them.

1 *Infrahyoid muscles:*
   a. Sternohyoid
   b. Sternothyroid
   c. Thyrohyoid
   d. Superior belly of omohyoid.
   These are described in Table 12.1 and shown in Fig. 12.6.
2 *Pretracheal fascia:* It forms the *false capsule of the thyroid gland* and the *suspensory ligaments of Berry* which attach the thyroid gland to the cricoid cartilage (*see* Fig. 16.4).
3 Deep to the pretracheal fascia, there are:
   a. The *thyrohyoid membrane* deep to the thyrohyoid muscle: It is pierced by the internal laryngeal nerve and the superior laryngeal vessels (Fig. 12.7).
   b. *Thyroid cartilage.*
   c. *Cricothyroid membrane* with the anastomosis of the cricothyroid arteries on its surface.
   d. Arch of the *cricoid cartilage.*
   e. *Cricothyroid muscle* supplied by the external laryngeal nerve.
   f. *Trachea,* partly covered by the isthmus of the thyroid gland from the second to fourth rings.
   g. *Carotid sheaths* lie on each side of the trachea (*see* Fig. 11.8).

DISSECTION

The skin over the anterior triangle has already been reflected following dissection in Chapter 11. Platysma is also reflected upwards. Identify the structures present in the superficial fascia and structures present in the anterior median region of neck.

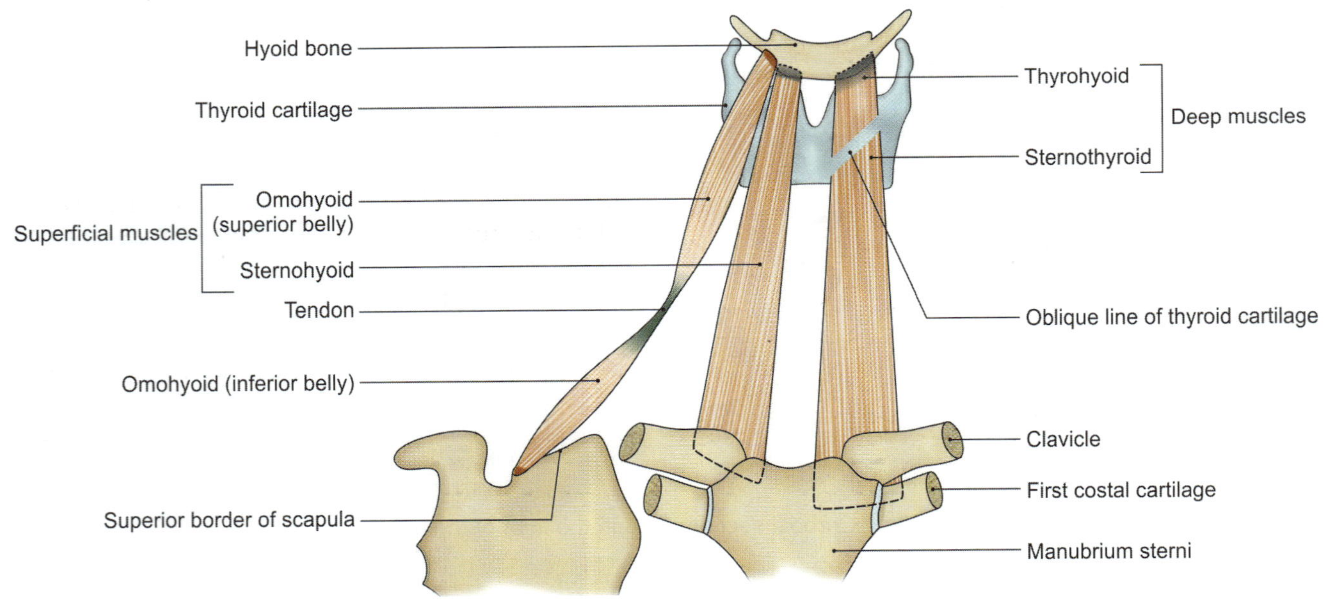

Fig. 12.6: The infrahyoid muscles

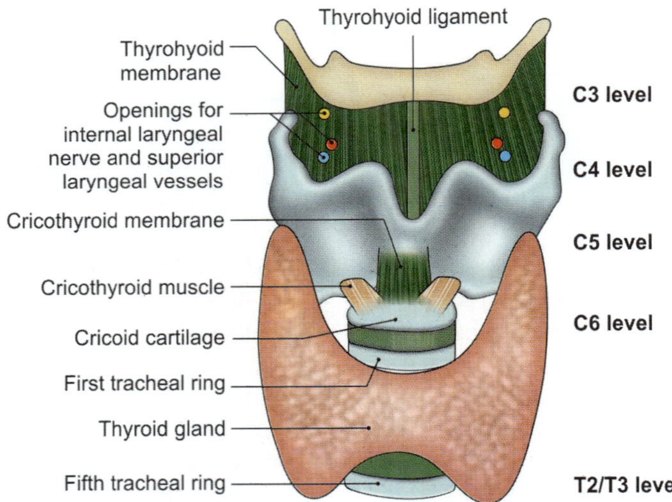

Fig. 12.7: The thyroid gland, the larynx and the trachea seen from the front

CLINICAL ANATOMY

- The common anterior midline swellings of the neck are:
  a. Enlarged submental lymph nodes and sublingual dermoid in the submental region.
  b. Thyroglossal cyst and inflamed subhyoid bursa just below the hyoid bone (Fig. 12.5).
  c. Goitre, carcinoma of larynx and enlarged lymph nodes in the suprasternal region.
- Tracheostomy is an operation in which the trachea is opened and a tube inserted into it to facilitate breathing. It is most commonly done in the retrothyroid region after retracting the isthmus of the thyroid gland (Fig. 12.8). A suprathyroid tracheostomy is liable to stricture, and an infrathyroid one is difficult due to the depth of the trachea and is also dangerous because numerous vessels lie anterior to the trachea here.
- Cut throat wounds are most commonly situated just above or just below the hyoid bone. The main vessels of the neck usually escape injury because they are pushed backwards to a deeper plane during voluntary extension of the neck.
- Skin incisions to be made parallel to natural creases or Langer's lines (Fig. 12.9).

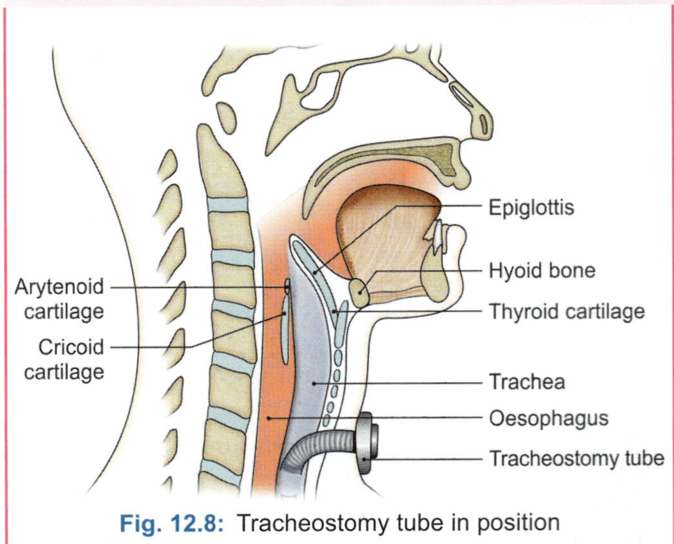

Fig. 12.8: Tracheostomy tube in position

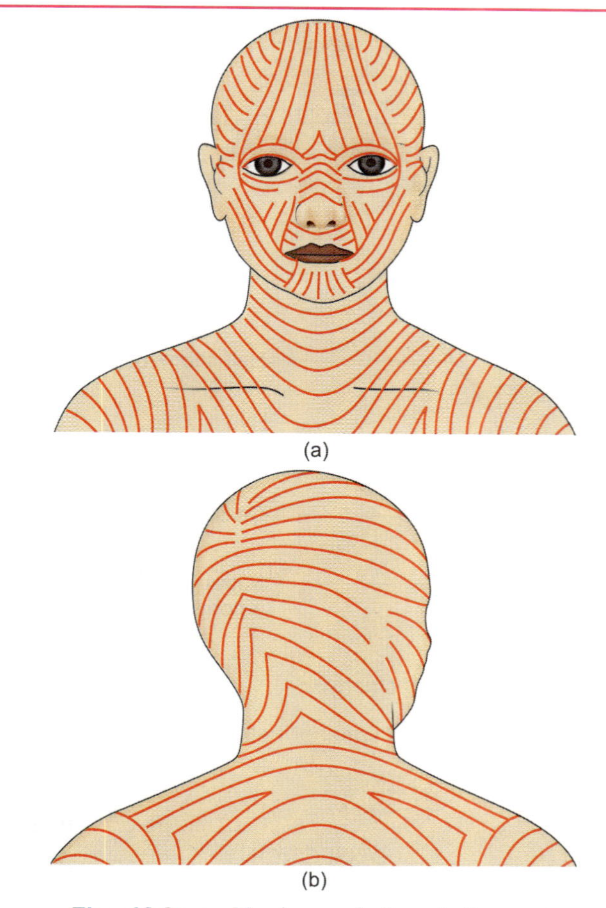

Figs 12.9a and b: Langer's lines in the neck

- Ludwig's angina is the cellulitis of the floor of the mouth. The infection spreads above the mylohyoid forcing the tongue upwards. Mylohyoid is pushed downwards. There is swelling within the mouth as well as below the chin.

ANTERIOR TRIANGLE

BOUNDARIES

The boundaries of the anterior triangle of neck are: The anterior median plane of the neck medially; sternocleidomastoid laterally; base of the mandible and a line joining the angle of the mandible to the mastoid process, superiorly (Fig. 12.10).

SUBDIVISIONS

The anterior triangle is subdivided (by the digastric muscle and the superior belly of the omohyoid) into:

a. Submental,
b. Digastric,
c. Carotid, and
d. Muscular triangles (Fig. 12.10).

SUBMENTAL TRIANGLE

This is a median triangle. It is bounded as follows.

On each side, there is the anterior belly of the corresponding digastric muscles. Its base is formed by the body of the hyoid bone. Its apex lies at the chin. The floor of the triangle is formed by the right and left mylohyoid muscles and the median raphe uniting them (Fig. 12.3).

Contents

1 Two to four small *submental lymph nodes* are situated in the superficial fascia between the anterior bellies of the digastric muscles (Fig. 12.3). They drain:
   a. Superficial tissues below the chin
   b. Central part of the lower lip
   c. The adjoining gums
   d. Anterior part of the floor of the mouth
   e. The tip of the tongue.

   Their efferents pass to the submandibular nodes.

2 Small submental veins join to form the anterior jugular veins.

DIGASTRIC TRIANGLE

The area between the body of the mandible and the hyoid bone is known as the submandibular region. The superficial structures of this region lie in the submental and digastric triangles. The deep structures of the floor of the mouth and root of the tongue will be studied separately at a later stage under the heading 'submandibular region' in Chapter 15.

Boundaries

The boundaries of the digastric triangle are as follows.

Anteroinferiorly: Anterior belly of digastric.

Posteroinferiorly: Posterior belly of digastric and the stylohyoid.

Superiorly or base: Base of the mandible and a line joining the angle of the mandible to the mastoid process (Fig. 12.10).

Roof

The roof of the triangle is formed by:

1 Skin

2 Superficial fascia, containing:
   a. The platysma
   b. The cervical branch of the facial nerve
   c. The ascending branch of the transverse or anterior cutaneous nerve of the neck.

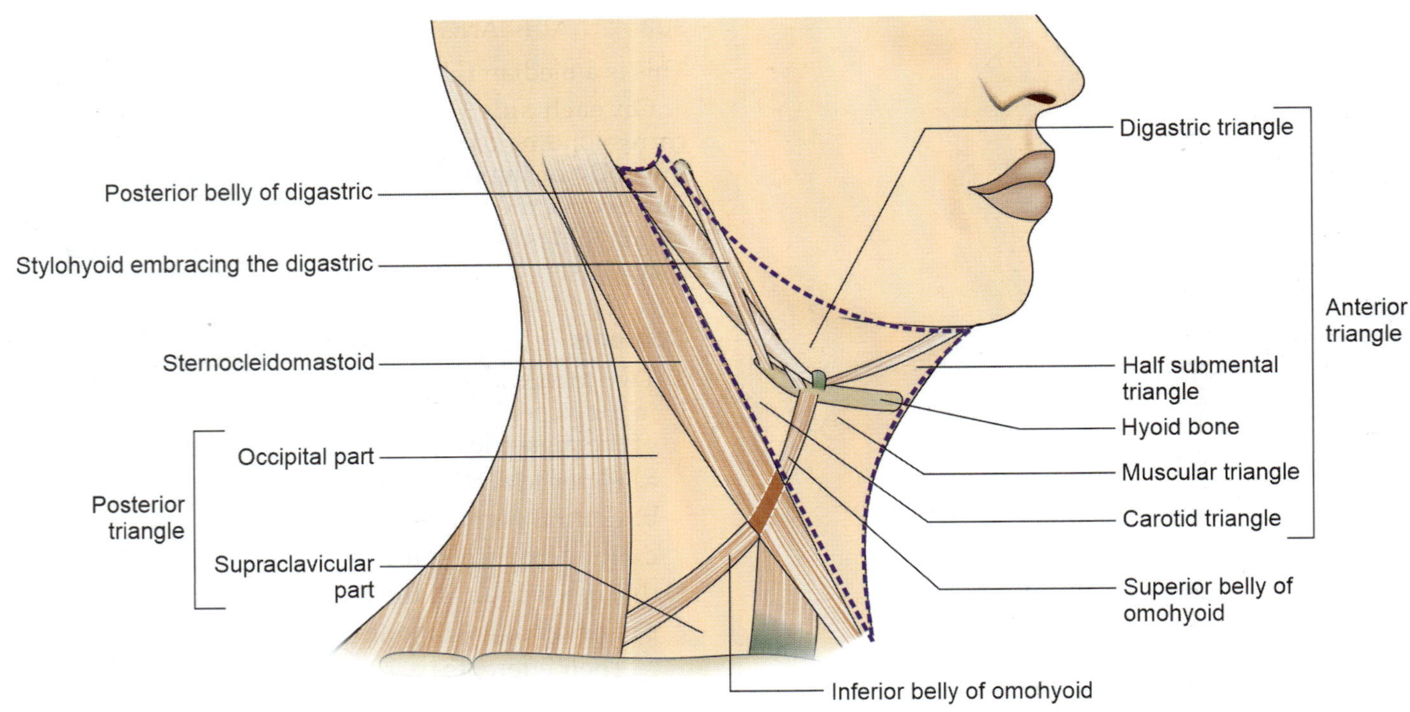

Fig. 12.10: The triangles of the neck. The anterior triangle is subdivided by digastrics and superior belly of omohyoid. Posterior triangle is subdivided by inferior belly of omohyoid

3 Deep fascia, which splits to enclose the submandibular salivary gland (*see* Fig. 15.6).

Floor

The *floor* is formed by the mylohyoid muscle anteriorly, and by the hyoglossus posteriorly. A small part of the middle constrictor muscle of the pharynx appears in the floor (Fig. 12.11).

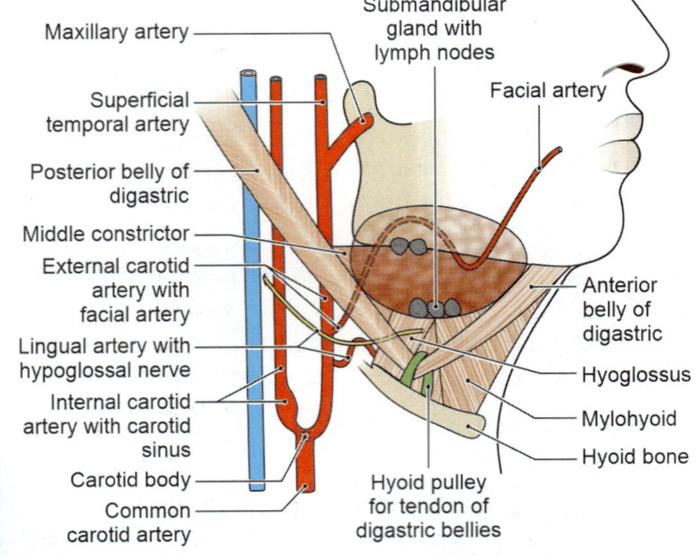

Fig. 12.11: Floor and contents of the digastric triangle

DISSECTION

Remove the deep fascia from anterior bellies of digastric muscles to expose parts of two mylohyoid muscles. Clean the boundaries and contents of the submental triangle.

Cut the deep fascia from the mandible and reflect it downwards to expose the submandibular gland. Identify and clean anterior and posterior bellies of digastric muscles, which form the boundaries of digastric triangle. Identify the intermediate tendon of digastric after pulling the submandibular gland laterally. Clean the stylohyoid muscle which envelops the tendon of digastric and is lying along with the posterior belly of digastric muscle (Fig. 12.10). Identify the contents of digastric triangle (*refer to BDC App*).

Contents

Anterior Part of the Triangle

Structures superficial to mylohyoid are:

1 Superficial part of the submandibular salivary gland (Fig. 12.3).
2 The facial vein and the submandibular lymph nodes are superficial to it and the facial artery is deep to it.
3 Submental artery.
4 Mylohyoid nerve and vessels (Fig. 12.4).
5 The hypoglossal nerve.

Other relations will be studied in the submandibular region.

Posterior Part of the Triangle

1 *Superficial structures* are:
   a. Lower part of the parotid gland.
   b. The external carotid artery before it enters the parotid gland.

2 *Deep structures,* passing between the external and internal carotid arteries, are:
   a. The styloglossus
   b. The stylopharyngeus
   c. The glossopharyngeal nerve (Fig. 12.13)
   d. The pharyngeal branch of the vagus nerve
   e. The styloid process
   f. A part of the parotid gland.

3 *Deepest structures* include:
   a. The internal carotid artery (Fig. 12.13)
   b. The internal jugular vein
   c. The vagus nerve (*see* Fig. 11.8b).

   Most of these structures will be studied later.

CAROTID TRIANGLE

Boundaries

Anterosuperiorly: Posterior belly of the digastric muscle; and the stylohyoid (Fig. 12.12).

DISSECTION

Clean the area situated between posterior belly of digastric and superior belly of omohyoid muscle, to expose the three carotid arteries with internal jugular vein. Trace IX, X, XI and XII nerves in relation to these vessels (Fig. 12.10).

Identify middle and inferior constrictors of pharynx and thyrohyoid membrane forming its floor (Fig. 12.12).

Carefully clean and preserve superior root, the loop and inferior root of ansa cervicalis in relation to anterior aspect of carotid sheath. Locate the sympathetic trunk situated posteromedial to the carotid sheath (*see* Fig. 3.8b). Dissect the branches of external carotid artery (Figs 12.13 and 12.16).

Identify and preserve internal laryngeal nerve in the thyrohyoid interval. Trace it posterosuperiorly till vagus. Also look for external laryngeal nerve supplying the cricothyroid muscle (Fig. 12.13).

The carotid triangle provides a good view of all the large vessels and nerves of the neck, particularly when its posterior boundary is retracted slightly backwards.

Anteroinferiorly: Superior belly of the omohyoid.

Posteriorly: Anterior border of the sternocleidomastoid muscle.

Roof

1 Skin
2 Superficial fascia containing:
   a. The plastysma

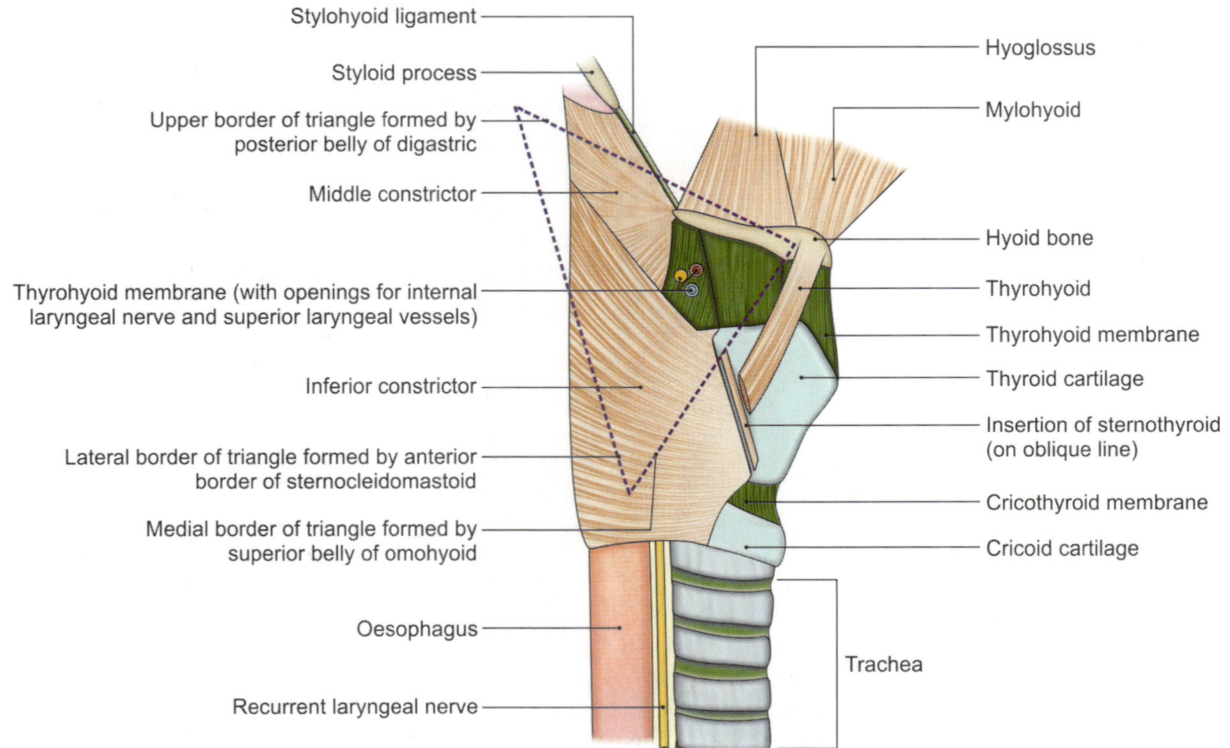

Fig. 12.12: Floor of the carotid triangle

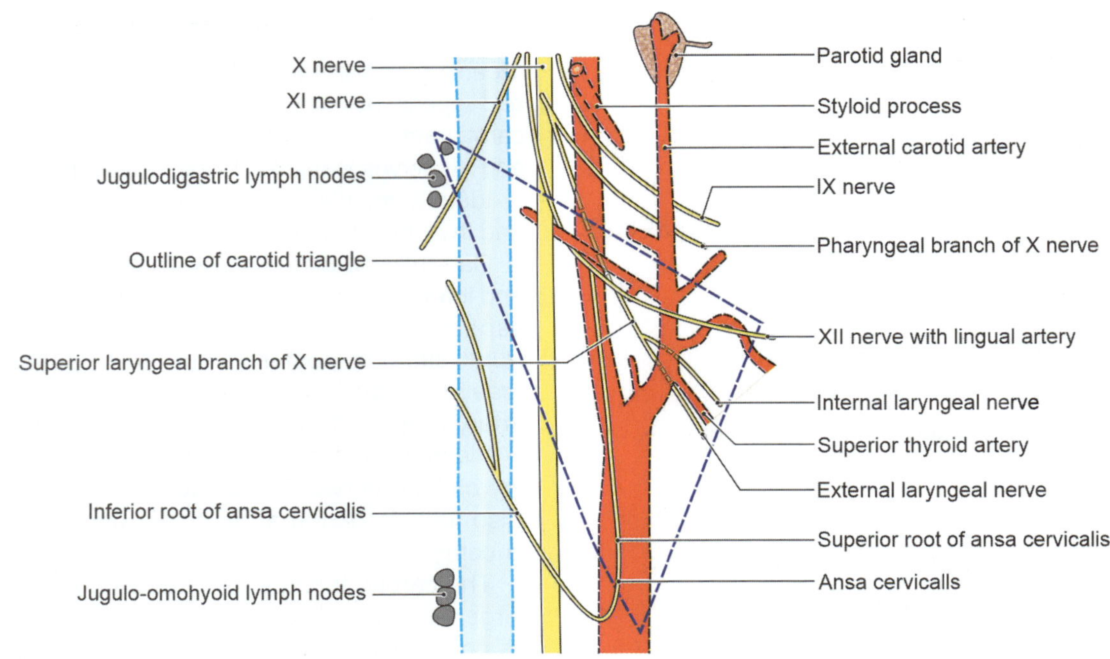

Fig. 12.13: The ninth, tenth, eleventh and twelfth cranial nerves and their branches related to the carotid arteries and to the internal jugular vein, in and around the left carotid triangle

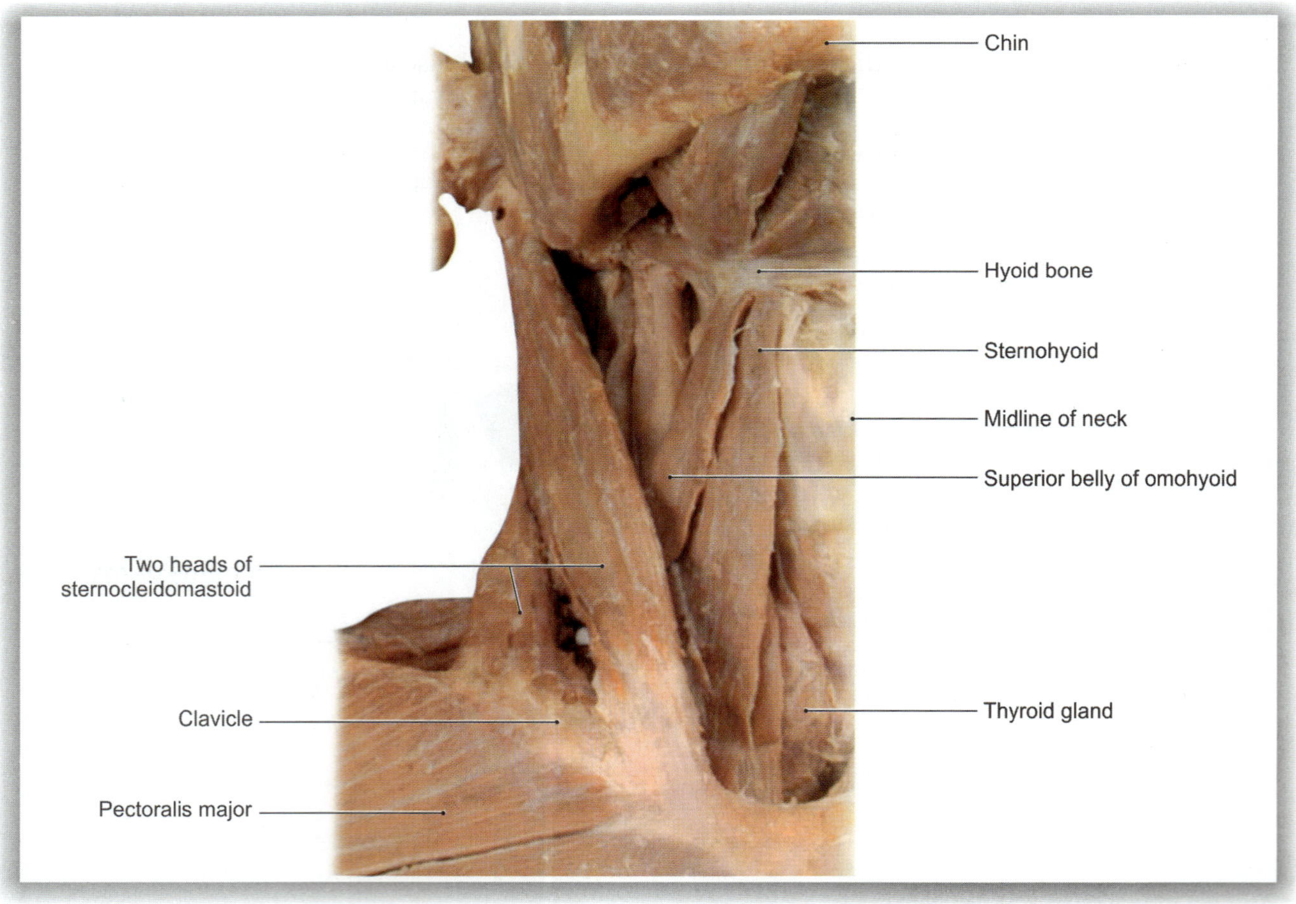

Fig. 12.14: Dissection of muscular triangle

b. The cervical branch of the facial nerve
c. The transverse cutaneous nerve of the neck.

3 Investing layer of deep cervical fascia.

Floor

It is formed by parts of:
a. The middle constrictor of pharynx
b. The inferior constrictor of the pharynx (Fig. 12.12)
c. Thyrohyoid membrane.

Contents

Arteries

1 The common carotid artery with the carotid sinus and the carotid body at its termination
2 Internal carotid artery
3 The external carotid artery with its superior thyroid, lingual, facial, ascending pharyngeal and occipital branches (Fig. 12.12).

Veins

1 The internal jugular vein
2 The common facial vein draining into the internal jugular vein.
3 A pharyngeal vein which usually ends in the internal jugular vein.
4 The lingual vein which usually terminates in the internal jugular vein.

Nerves

1 The vagus running vertically downwards.
2 The superior laryngeal branch of the vagus, dividing into the external and internal laryngeal nerves.
3 The spinal accessory nerve running backwards over the internal jugular vein.
4 The hypoglossal nerve running forwards over the external and internal carotid arteries. The hypoglossal nerve gives off the upper root of the ansa cervicalis or descendens hypoglossi, and another branch to the thyrohyoid (Fig. 12.15).
5 Sympathetic chain runs (*see* Fig. 11.8b) vertically downwards posterior to the carotid sheath.
6 *Carotid sheath* with its contents (*see* Fig. 11.8).

Lymph Nodes

The deep cervical lymph nodes are situated along the internal jugular vein, and include the jugulodigastric node below the posterior belly of the digastric and the jugulo-omohyoid node above the inferior belly of the omohyoid (*see* Fig. 16.31).

MUSCULAR TRIANGLE

Boundaries

Anteriorly: Anterior median line of the neck from the hyoid bone to the sternum.

Posterosuperiorly: Superior belly of the omohyoid muscle (Fig. 12.10).

Posteroinferiorly: Lower part of anterior border of the sternocleidomastoid muscle (Fig. 12.14).

DISSECTION

Identify the infrahyoid muscles on each side of the median plane. Cut through the origin of sternocleidomastoid muscle and reflect it upwards. Trace the nerve supply of infrahyoid muscles.

The superficial structures in the infrahyoid region are included in this triangle. The deeper structures (thyroid gland, trachea, oesophagus, etc.) will be studied separately at a later stage.

Contents

The infrahyoid muscles are the chief contents of the triangle. These muscles may also be regarded arbitrarily as forming the floor of the triangle (Fig. 12.6).

The *infrahyoid muscles* are:
a. Sternohyoid
b. Sternothyroid
c. Thyrohyoid
d. Omohyoid.

These ribbon muscles have the following general features.

a. They are arranged in two layers—superficial (sternohyoid and omohyoid) and deep (sternothyroid and thyrohyoid) (Fig. 12.6).
b. All of them are supplied by the ventral rami of first, second and third cervical spinal nerves.
c. Because of their attachment to the hyoid bone and to the thyroid cartilage, they move these structures.
d. Sternohyoid, superior belly of omohyoid, and sternothyroid lie superficial to the lateral or superficial convex surface of the thyroid gland (*see* Fig. 16.4).
e. The anterior surface of isthmus of thyroid gland is covered by right and left sternothyroid and sternohyoid muscles (*see* Fig. 11.3).

The specific details of infrahyoid muscles are shown in Table 12.1.

ANSA CERVICALIS OR ANSA HYPOGLOSSI

This is a thin nerve loop that lies embedded in the anterior wall of the carotid sheath over the lower part of the larynx. It supplies the infrahyoid muscles (Fig. 12.15).

Table 12.1: Infrahyoid muscles

Muscle	*Proximal attachment*	*Distal attachment*	*Nerve supply*	*Actions*
1. **Sternohyoid** (Fig. 12.6)	a. Posterior surface of manubrium sterni b. Adjoining parts of the clavicle and the posterior sternoclavicular ligament	Medial part of lower border of hyoid bone	Ansa cervicalis C1–C3	Depresses the hyoid bone following its elevation during swallowing and during vocal movements
2. **Sternothyroid:** It lies deep to the sternohyoid	a. Posterior surface of manubrium sterni b. Adjoining part of first costal cartilage	Oblique line on the lamina of the thyroid cartilage	Ansa cervicalis C1–C3	Depresses the larynx after it has been elevated in swallowing and in vocal movements
3. **Thyrohyoid:** It lies deep to the sternohyoid	Oblique line of thyroid cartilage	Lower border of the body and the greater cornua of the hyoid bone	C1 through hypoglossal nerve	a. Depresses the hyoid bone b. Elevates the larynx when the hyoid is fixed by the suprahyoid muscles
4. **Omohyoid:** It has an inferior belly, a common tendon and a superior belly. It arises by the inferior belly, and is inserted through the superior belly	a. Upper border of scapula near the suprascapular notch b. Adjoining part of suprascapular ligament	Lower border of body of hyoid bone lateral to the sternohyoid. The central tendon lies on the internal jugular vein at the level of the cricoid cartilage and is bound to the clavicle by a fascial pulley	Superior belly by the superior root of the ansa cervicalis, and inferior belly by inferior root of ansa cervicalis	Depresses the hyoid bone following its elevation during swallowing or in vocal movements

Formation

It is formed by a superior and an inferior root. The *superior root* is the continuation of the descending branch of the hypoglossal nerve. Its fibres are derived from the first cervical nerve. This root descends over the internal carotid artery and the common carotid artery.

The *inferior root* or descending cervical nerve is derived from second and third cervical spinal nerves. As this root descends, it winds around the internal jugular vein, and then continues anteroinferiorly to join the superior root in front of the common carotid artery (Fig. 12.15).

Distribution

Superior root: To the superior belly of the omohyoid.

Ansa cervicalis: To the sternohyoid, the sternothyroid.

Inferior root: To the inferior belly of the omohyoid.

Note that the thyrohyoid and geniohyoid are supplied by separate branches from the first cervical nerve through the hypoglossal nerve (Fig. 12.15).

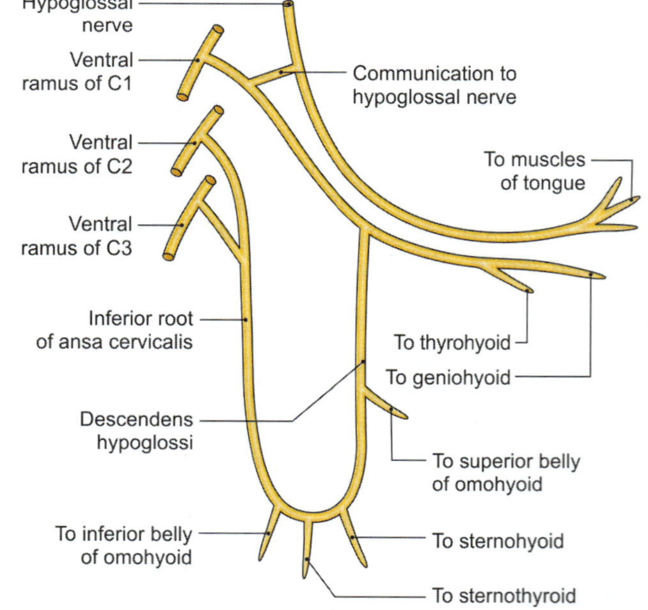

Fig. 12.15: Ansa cervicalis, and branches of the first cervical nerve distributed through the hypoglossal nerve

COMMON CAROTID ARTERY

The right common carotid artery is a branch of the brachiocephalic artery. It begins in the neck behind the right sternoclavicular joint (Fig. 12.16, also *see* Fig. 16.17). The left common carotid artery is branch of the arch of the aorta.

Carotid Sinus

The termination of the common carotid artery, or the beginning of the internal carotid artery shows a slight dilatation, known as the carotid sinus. In this region, the tunica media is thin, but the adventitia is relatively thick and receives a rich innervation from the glossopharyngeal and sympathetic nerves. The carotid sinus acts as a *baroreceptor* or *pressure receptor* and regulates blood pressure.

Carotid Body

Carotid body is a small, oval reddish brown structure situated behind the bifurcation of the common carotid artery. It receives a rich nerve supply mainly from the glossopharyngeal nerve, but also from the vagus and sympathetic nerves. It acts as a *chemoreceptor* and responds to changes in the oxygen, carbon dioxide and pH content of the blood.

Other *allied chemoreceptors* are found near the arch of the aorta, the ductus arteriosus, and the right subclavian artery. These are supplied by the vagus nerve.

CLINICAL ANATOMY

- The carotid sinus is richly supplied by nerves. In some persons, the sinus may be hypersensitive. In such persons, sudden rotation of the head may cause slowing of heart. This condition is called 'carotid sinus syndrome'.
- The supraventricular tachycardia may be controlled by carotid sinus massage, due to inhibitory effects of vagus nerve on the heart.
- The necktie should not be tied tightly, as it may compress both the internal carotid arteries, supplying the brain.

EXTERNAL CAROTID ARTERY

External carotid artery is one of the terminal branches of the common carotid artery. In general, it lies anterior to the internal carotid artery, and is the chief artery of supply to structures in the front of the neck and in the face (Fig. 12.16, also *see* Fig. 16.17).

Course and Relations

1 The external carotid artery begins in the carotid triangle at the level of the upper border of the thyroid cartilage opposite the disc between the third and fourth cervical vertebrae. It runs upwards and slightly backwards and laterally, and terminates behind the neck of the mandible by dividing into the maxillary and superficial temporal arteries.

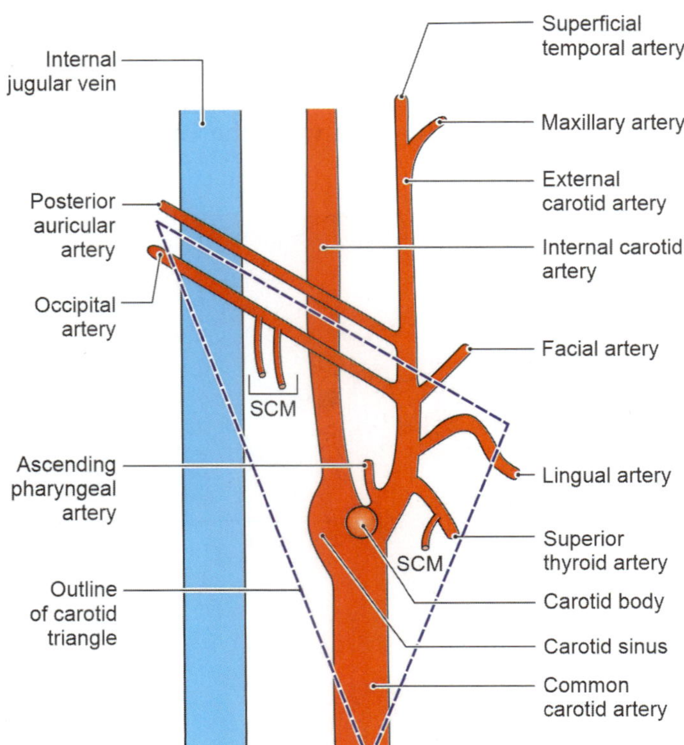

Fig. 12.16: Right carotid arteries including branches of the external carotid artery. (SCM: Sternocleidomastoid)

2 The external carotid artery has a *slightly curved course,* so that it is anteromedial to the internal carotid artery in its lower part, and anterolateral to the internal carotid artery in its upper part (*see* Fig. 16.16).
3 *In the carotid triangle,* the external carotid artery is comparatively superficial, and lies under cover of the anterior border of the sternocleidomastoid. The artery is crossed superficially by the cervical branch of the facial nerve, the hypoglossal nerve (Fig. 12.13) and the facial, lingual and superior thyroid veins. Deep to the artery, there are:
   a. The wall of the pharynx
   b. The superior laryngeal nerve which divides into the external and internal laryngeal nerves (Fig. 12.13).
   c. The ascending pharyngeal artery.
4 *Above the carotid triangle*, the external carotid artery lies deep in the substance of the parotid gland. Within the gland, it is related superficially to the retromandibular vein and the facial nerve (*see* Fig. 13.4). Deep to the external carotid artery, there are:
   a. The internal carotid artery.
   b. Structures passing between the external and internal carotid arteries; these being styloglossus, stylopharyngeus both arising from the styloid process, IX nerve, pharyngeal branch of X nerve (Fig. 12.13).
   c. Two structures deep to the internal carotid artery, namely the superior laryngeal nerve (Fig. 12.13) and the superior cervical sympathetic ganglion.

Branches

The external carotid artery gives off eight branches which may be grouped as follows. Though small parts of 1–4 and 6th branches lie in carotid triangle, these have been described completely.

Anterior
1 Superior thyroid (Fig. 12.16)
2 Lingual (Fig. 12.17)
3 Facial

Posterior
4 Occipital
5 Posterior auricular

Medial
6 Ascending pharyngeal

Terminal
7 Maxillary
8 Superficial temporal (Fig. 12.16).

Superior Thyroid Artery

The superior thyroid artery arises from the external carotid artery just below the level of the greater cornua of the hyoid bone.

It runs downwards and forwards parallel and just superficial to the external laryngeal nerve. It passes deep to the three long infrahyoid muscles to reach the upper pole of the lateral lobe of the thyroid gland.

Its relationship to the external laryngeal nerve, which supplies the cricothyroid muscle is important to the surgeon during thyroid surgery. The artery and nerve are close to each other higher up, but diverge slightly near the gland. To avoid injury to the nerve, the superior thyroid artery is ligated as near the gland as possible (*see* Fig. 16.7).

Apart from its terminal branches to the thyroid gland, it gives one important branch, the *superior laryngeal artery,* which pierces the thyrohyoid membrane in company with the internal laryngeal nerve (Fig. 12.7). The

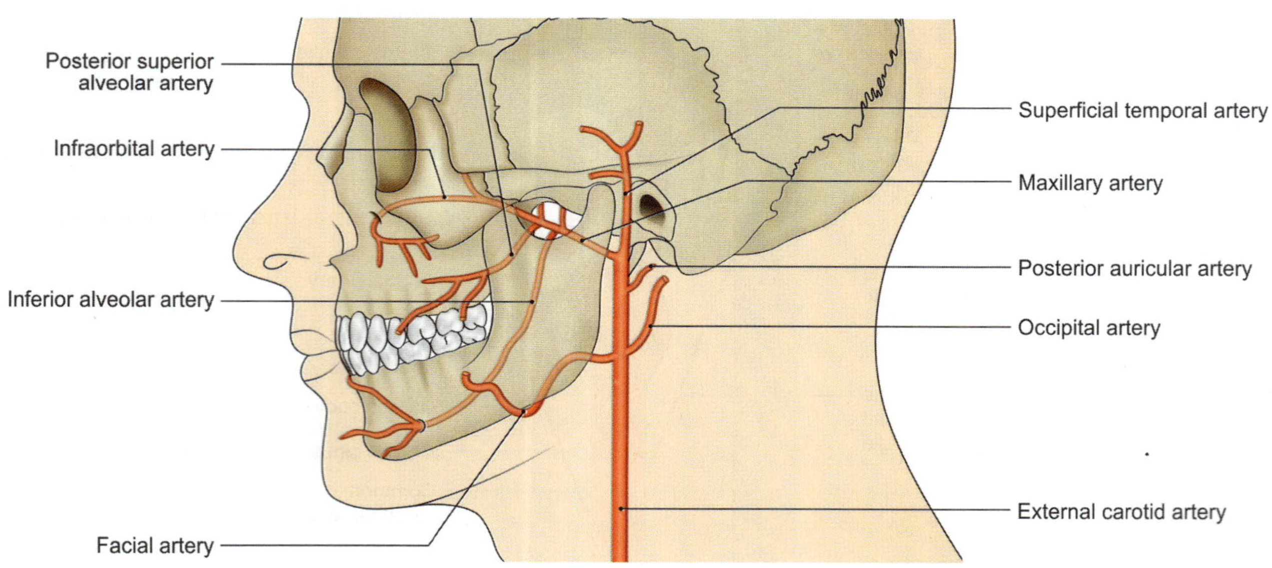

Fig. 12.17: Branches of external carotid and maxillary arteries

superior thyroid artery also gives a sternocleidomastoid branch to that muscle and a cricothyroid branch that anastomoses with the artery of the opposite side in front of the cricovocal membrane.

Lingual Artery

The lingual artery arises from the external carotid artery opposite the tip of the greater cornua of the hyoid bone. It is tortuous in its course (*see* Fig. 25.6).

Its course is divided into three parts by the hyoglossus muscle.

- The *first part* lies in the carotid triangle. It forms a characteristic upward loop which is crossed by the hypoglossal nerve. The lingual loop permits free movements of the hyoid bone.
- The *second part* lies deep to the hyoglossus along the upper border of hyoid bone. It is superficial to the middle constrictor of the pharynx.
- The *third part* is called the arteria profunda linguae, or the *deep lingual artery*. It runs upwards along the anterior border of the hyoglossus, and then horizontally forwards on the undersurface of the tongue as the *fourth part*. In its vertical course, it lies between the genioglossus medially and the inferior longitudinal muscle of the tongue laterally. The horizontal part of the artery is accompanied by the lingual nerve.

It gives branches: Suprahyoid, dorsal lingual, sublingual.

During surgical removal of the tongue, the first part of the artery is ligated before it gives any branch to the tongue or to the tonsil.

Facial Artery

The facial artery arises from the external carotid just above the tip of the greater cornua of the hyoid bone.

It runs upwards first in the neck as cervical part and then on the face as facial part. The course of the artery in both places is tortuous. The tortuosity in the neck allows free movements of the pharynx during deglutition. On the face, it allows free movements of the mandible, the lips and the cheek during mastication and during various facial expressions. The artery escapes traction and pressure during these movements.

The *cervical part* of the facial artery runs upwards on the superior constrictor of pharynx deep to the posterior belly of the digastric, stylohyoid and to the ramus of the mandible.

It grooves the posterior end of the submandibular salivary gland. Next the artery makes an S-bend (two loops) first winding down over the submandibular gland, and then up over the base of the mandible (*see* Fig. 15.7).

The *facial part* of the facial artery enters the face at anteroinferior angle of masseter muscle, runs upwards close to angle of mouth, side of nose till medial angle of eye. It is described in Chapter 10.

The cervical part of the facial artery gives off the ascending palatine, tonsillar, submental, and glandular branches for the submandibular salivary gland and lymph nodes.

The *ascending palatine artery* arises near the origin of the facial artery. It passes upwards between the styloglossus and the stylopharyngeus, crosses over the upper border of the superior constrictor and supplies the tonsil and the root of the tongue.

The *submental branch* is a large artery which accompanies the mylohyoid nerve, and supplies the submental triangle and the sublingual salivary gland (Fig. 12.3).

Occipital Artery

The occipital artery arises from the posterior aspect of the external carotid artery, opposite the origin of the facial artery.

It is crossed at its origin by the hypoglossal nerve.

In the carotid triangle, the artery gives two sternocleidomastoid branches. The upper branch accompanies the accessory nerve, and the lower branch arises near the origin of the occipital artery.

The further course of the artery in scalp has been described in Chapter 18.

Posterior Auricular Artery

The posterior auricular artery arises from the posterior aspect of the external carotid just above the posterior belly of the digastric (Fig. 12.16).

It runs upwards and backwards deep to the parotid gland, but superficial to the styloid process. It crosses the base of the mastoid process, and ascends behind the auricle.

It supplies the back of the auricle, the skin over the mastoid process, and over the back of the scalp. It is cut in incisions for mastoid operations. Its *stylomastoid branch* enters the stylomastoid foramen, and supplies the middle ear, the mastoid antrum and air cells, the semicircular canals, and the facial nerve.

Ascending Pharyngeal Artery

This is a small branch that arises from the medial side of the external carotid artery. It arises very close to the lower end of external carotid artery (Fig. 12.16).

It runs vertically upwards between the side wall of the pharynx, and the tonsil, medial wall of the middle ear and the auditory tube. It sends meningeal branches into the cranial cavity through the foramen lacerum, the jugular foramen and the hypoglossal canal.

Maxillary Artery

This is the larger terminal branch of the external carotid artery. It begins behind the neck of the mandible under cover of the parotid gland. It runs forwards deep to the neck of the mandible below the auriculotemporal nerve, and enters the infratemporal fossa where it will be studied at a later stage (*see* Chapter 14).

Superficial Temporal Artery

1 It is the smaller terminal branch of the external carotid artery. It begins, behind the neck of the mandible under cover of the parotid gland (*see* Fig. 13.5a).
2 It runs vertically upwards, crossing the root of the zygoma or preauricular point, where its *pulsations* can be easily felt. About 5 cm above the zygoma, it divides into anterior and posterior branches which supply the temple and scalp. The anterior branch anastomoses with the supraorbital and supratrochlear branches of the ophthalmic artery.
3 In addition to the branches which supply the temple, the scalp, the parotid gland, the auricle and the facial muscles, the superficial temporal artery gives off a *transverse facial artery,* already studied with the face, and a *middle temporal artery* which runs on the temporal fossa deep to the temporalis muscle.

POTENTIAL TISSUE SPACES IN HEAD AND NECK

Submental space: Lies below inferior border of mandible. Corresponds to submental triangle. It communicates with submandibular spaces of both sides.

Submandibular space: Lies between anterior and posterior bellies of digastric muscle and inferior border of mandible. It communicates with sublingual and submental spaces.

Parotid space: Localized around parotid gland behind ramus of mandible, communicates with retropharyngeal space and even mediastinum.

Parapharyngeal space: Lies in suprahyoid region of neck, lateral to pharynx. It is continuous with retropharyngeal space.

Retropharyngeal space: Lies between anteriorly placed buccopharyngeal fascia and posteriorly placed prevertebral fascia. It communicates with peritonsillar space, submental spaces and may reach mediastinum.

Peritonsillar space: Lies between anterior and posterior fauces of the palatine tonsil. It communicates with sublingual space.

Mnemonics

External carotid artery branches

Some **A**natomists **L**ike **F**reaking **O**ut **P**oor **M**edical **S**tudents

Superior thyroid (anterior)
Ascending pharyngeal (medial)
Lingual (anterior)
Facial (anterior)
Occipital (posterior)
Posterior auricular (posterior)
Maxillary (terminal)
Superficial temporal (terminal)

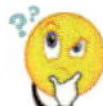

FACTS TO REMEMBER

- Apex of anterior triangle of neck is close to the sternum, while that of posterior triangle is close to the superior nuchal line.
- Submental triangle is half on each side of the midline.
- Maximum blood vessels are present in the carotid triangle.
- Superficial temporal artery can be palpated at the preauricular point.
- The necktie should not be tied tightly, as it may compress both the internal carotid arteries, supplying the brain.

CLINICOANATOMICAL PROBLEM

A patient is undergoing abdominal surgery. Anaesthetist is sitting at the head end of the table and monitoring patient's pulse by palpating arteries in the head and neck region

- What is the artery anaesthetist palpating?
- Name the other palpable arteries in the body.

Ans: The anaesthetist has been monitoring the pulse by palpating the common carotid artery at the anterior border of sternocleidomastoid muscle. He need not get up to feel the radial pulse repeatedly.

Other palpable arteries in head and neck are superficial temporal and facial. In upper limb, palpable arteries are third part of axillary artery, brachial artery and radial pulse.

In abdomen, one can feel abdominal aorta pulsation when one lies supine.

Palpable arteries in lower limb are femoral at head of femur, popliteal, dorsalis pedis and posterior tibial.

FURTHER READING

- Borges AE, Alexander JE. Relaxed skin tension lines, Z-plastics on scars, and fusiform excision of lesions. Br J Plast Surg 1962;15:242–54.
  A paper that provides the anatomical basis for every incision made on the face.
- Barker BCW, Davies PL. The applied anatomy of the pterygomandibular space. Br J Surg 1972;10:43–55.
  A description of the relationships of the structures within the pterygomandibular space, with particular reference to anaesthesia associated with an inferior alveolar nerve block.

Frequently Asked Questions

1. Describe carotid triangle under following headings:
   a. Boundaries b. Contents
   c. Nerves
   d. Arteries
2. Describe the boundaries and contents of digastric triangle.
3. Write short notes/enumerate:
   a. Branches of external carotid artery
   b. Infrahyoid muscles
   c. Ansa cervicalis
   d. Facial artery—cervical part
   e. Lingual artery

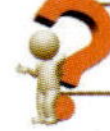

Multiple Choice Questions

1. Only medial branch of external carotid artery is:
   a. Superior thyroid
   b. Lingual
   c. Ascending pharyngeal
   d. Maxillary
2. All the following are branches of external carotid artery, *except*:
   a. Posterior ethmoidal b. Occipital
   c. Lingual d. Facial
3. All are the muscles forming boundaries of carotid triangle, *except*:
   a. Posterior belly of digastric
   b. Superior belly of omohyoid
   c. Inferior belly of omohyoid
   d. Sternocleidomastoid
4. Hyoid bone develops from:
   a. 1st and 2nd arches b. 2nd and 3rd arches
   c. 3rd and 4th arches d. 1st, 2nd and 3rd arches
5. Which of the following is not a palpable artery in head and neck?
   a. Facial artery b. Superficial temporal artery
   c. Lingual artery d. Common carotid artery
6. Which of the following is not a infrahyoid muscle?
   a. Sternohyoid b. Sternothyroid
   c. Thyrohyoid d. Omohyoid—inferior belly
7. Which of the following nerves runs with vagus between internal carotid artery and internal jugular vein till the angle of the mandible?
   a. Hypoglossal b. Accessory
   c. Glossopharyngeal d. Maxillary

Answers

1. c **2.** a **3.** c **4.** b **5.** c **6.** d **7.** a

VIVA VOCE

- Name the contents of submental triangle.
- Enumerate the boundaries of carotid triangle. Name the structures piercing the thyrohyoid membrane.
- Name the branches of external carotid artery given off in the carotid triangle.
- How is ansa cervicalis formed? What are its branches?
- Name the main contents of digastric triangle. How does hyoid bone develop?
- What are the arteries related to posterior belly of digastric muscle?

Anterior triangle of the neck

Chapter 13

Parotid Region

> "Eat, drink and feel no sorrow; For there may not be a tomorrow."
> —Anonymous

INTRODUCTION

Parotid region contains the largest serous salivary gland and the 'queen of the face', the facial nerve. Parotid gland contains vertically disposed blood vessels and horizontally situated facial nerve and its various branches. Parotid gland gets affected by virus of mumps, which can extend the territory of its attack up to gonads as well. One must be careful of the branches of facial nerve while incising the parotid abscess by giving horizontal incision. Facial nerve is described in detail in Chapter 4, *BD Chaurasia's Human Anatomy, Volume 4*. Its extracranial course is given in this chapter.

SALIVARY GLANDS

There are three pairs of large salivary glands—the parotid, submandibular and sublingual. In addition, there are numerous small glands in the tongue, the palate, the cheeks and the lips. These glands produce saliva which keeps the oral cavity moist, and helps in chewing and swallowing. The saliva also contains enzymes that aid digestion.

PAROTID GLAND

Features

(*Para* = around; *otic* = ear)

The parotid gland is the largest of the salivary glands. It weighs about 25 g. It is situated below the external acoustic meatus, between the ramus of the mandible and the sternocleidomastoid. The gland overlaps these structures. Anteriorly, the gland also overlaps the masseter muscle (Fig. 13.1). Skin over the gland is supplied by great auricular nerve (C2, C3).

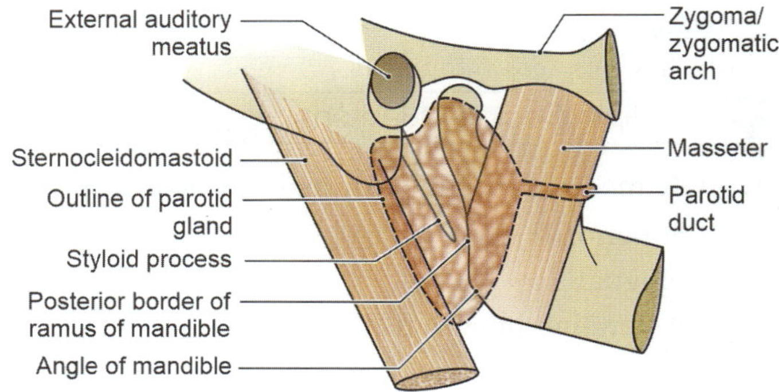

Fig. 13.1: Position of parotid gland

DISSECTION

Carefully cut through the fascial covering of the parotid gland from the zygomatic arch above to the angle of mandible below. While removing tough fascia, dissect the structures emerging at the periphery of the gland *(refer to BDC App)*.

Trace the duct of the parotid gland anteriorly till the buccinator muscle (*see* Fig. 10.20). Trace one or more of the branches of facial nerve till its trunk in the posterior part of the gland. The trunk can be followed till the stylomastoid foramen. Trace its posterior auricular branch. Trace the course of retromandibular vein and external carotid artery in the gland, removing the glands in pieces. Clean the facial nerve already dissected. Study the extracranial course of facial nerve.

Facial nerve is the main nerve of the face, supplying all the muscles of facial expression, carrying secretomotor fibres to submandibular, sublingual salivary glands, including those in tongue and floor of mouth. It is also secretomotor to glands in the nasal cavity, palate and the lacrimal gland. It is responsible enough for carrying the taste fibres from anterior two-thirds of tongue also except from the vallate papillae.

Capsule of Parotid Gland

The investing layer of the deep cervical fascia forms a capsule for the gland (Fig. 13.2). It is supplied by great auricular nerve. The fascia splits (between the angle of the mandible and the mastoid process) to enclose the gland. The superficial lamina/parotidomasseteric fascia, thick and adherent to the gland, is attached above to the zygomatic arch. The deep lamina is thin and is attached to the styloid process, tympanic plate, the angle and posterior border of the ramus of the mandible. A portion of the deep lamina, extending between the styloid process and the mandible, is thickened to form the *stylomandibular ligament* which separates the parotid gland from the submandibular salivary gland. The ligament is pierced by the external carotid artery (*see* Fig. 11.4a).

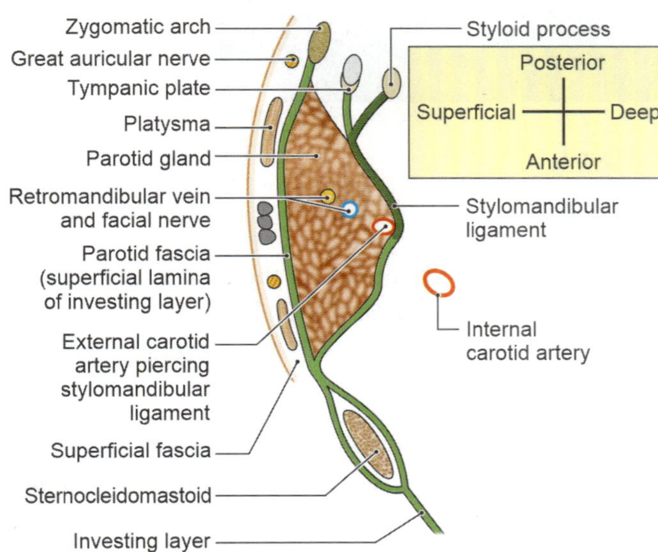

Fig. 13.2: Capsule of the parotid gland

CLINICAL ANATOMY

- *Parotid swellings* are very painful due to the unyielding nature of the parotid fascia.
- *Mumps* is an infectious disease of the salivary glands (usually the parotid) caused by a specific virus. Viral parotitis or mumps characteristically does not suppurate. Its complications are orchitis and pancreatitis.

External Features

The gland resembles a three-sided pyramid.

The apex of the pyramid is directed downwards (Figs 13.3a and b).

The gland has four surfaces:

a. Superior (base of the pyramid)
b. Superficial (Fig. 13.3a)
c. Anteromedial
d. Posteromedial (Fig. 13.4a).

The surfaces are separated by three borders:

a. Anterior (Fig. 13.4b)
b. Posterior
c. Medial/pharyngeal edge

Relations

The *apex* (Fig. 13.3a) overlaps the posterior belly of the digastric and the adjoining part of the carotid triangle.

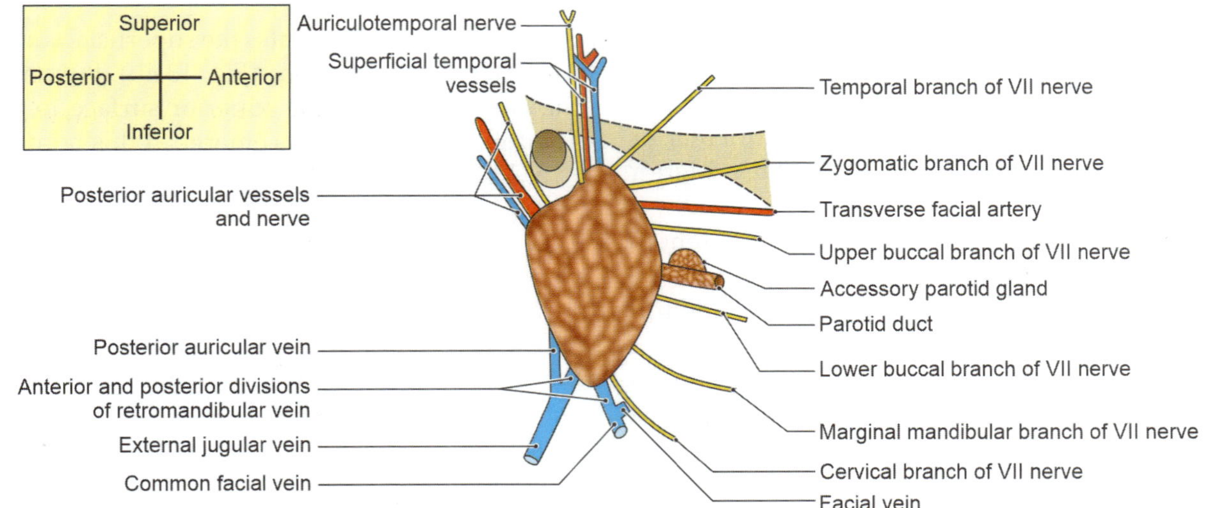

Fig. 13.3a: Structures emerging at the periphery of the parotid gland

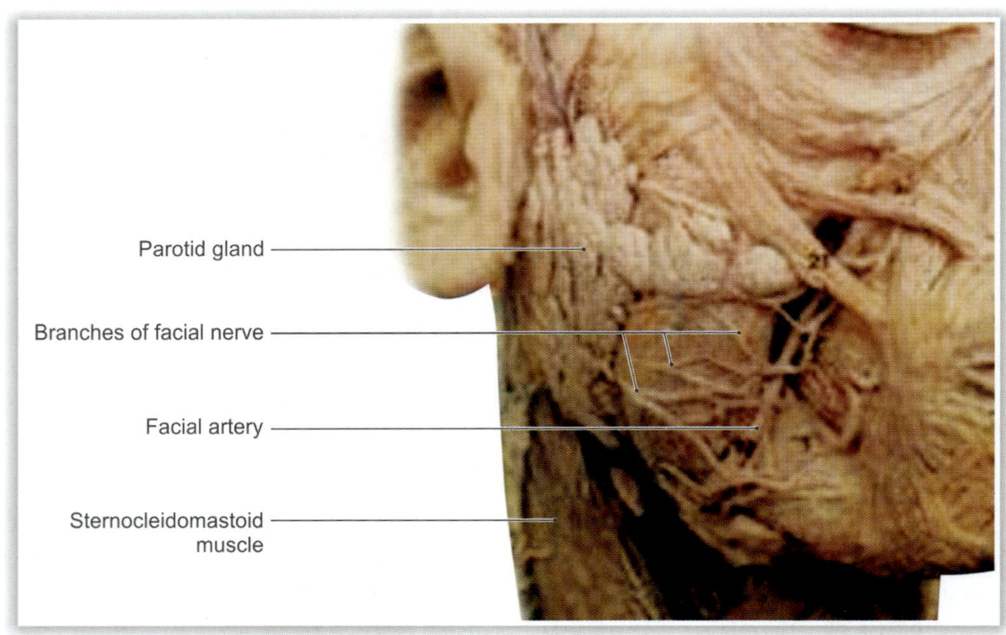

Fig. 13.3b: Parotid gland

The cervical branch of the facial nerve and the two divisions of the retromandibular vein emerge near the apex.

Surfaces

The *superior surface* or base forms the upper end of the gland which is small and concave. It is related to:

a. The cartilaginous part of the external acoustic meatus.
b. The posterior surface of the temporomandibular joint (Fig. 13.3b).
c. The superficial temporal vessels.
d. The auriculotemporal nerve (Fig. 13.3a).

The *superficial surface* is the largest of the four surfaces. It is covered with:

a. Skin
b. Superficial fascia containing the anterior branches of the great auricular nerve, the preauricular or superficial parotid lymph nodes and the posterior fibres of the platysma and risorius.
c. The parotid fascia which is thick and adherent to the gland (Fig. 13.2).
d. A few deep parotid lymph nodes embedded in the gland.

The *anteromedial surface* (Fig. 13.4a) is grooved by the posterior border of the ramus of the mandible. It is related to:

a. The masseter
b. The lateral surface of the temporomandibular joint
c. The posterior border of the ramus of the mandible
d. The medial pterygoid
e. The emerging branches of the facial nerve.

The *posteromedial surface* (Fig. 13.4a) is moulded to the mastoid and the styloid processes and the structures attached to them. Thus, it is related to:

a. The mastoid process, with the sternocleidomastoid and the posterior belly of the digastric.
b. The styloid process, with structures attached to it.
c. The external carotid artery and facial nerve enter the gland through this surface. The internal carotid artery lies deep to the styloid process (Fig. 13.4a).

Borders

The *anterior border* separates the superficial surface from the anteromedial surface (Fig. 13.4b). It extends from the anterior part of the superior surface to the apex. The following structures emerge at this border.

a. The parotid duct
b. Most of the terminal branches of the facial nerve
c. The transverse facial vessels.

In addition, the accessory parotid gland lies on the parotid duct close to this border (Fig. 13.3a).

The *posterior border* separates the superficial surface from the posteromedial surface. It overlaps the sternocleidomastoid (Fig. 13.4b).

The *medial edge* or *pharyngeal border* separates the anteromedial surface from the posteromedial surface. It is related to the lateral wall of the pharynx (Fig. 13.4a).

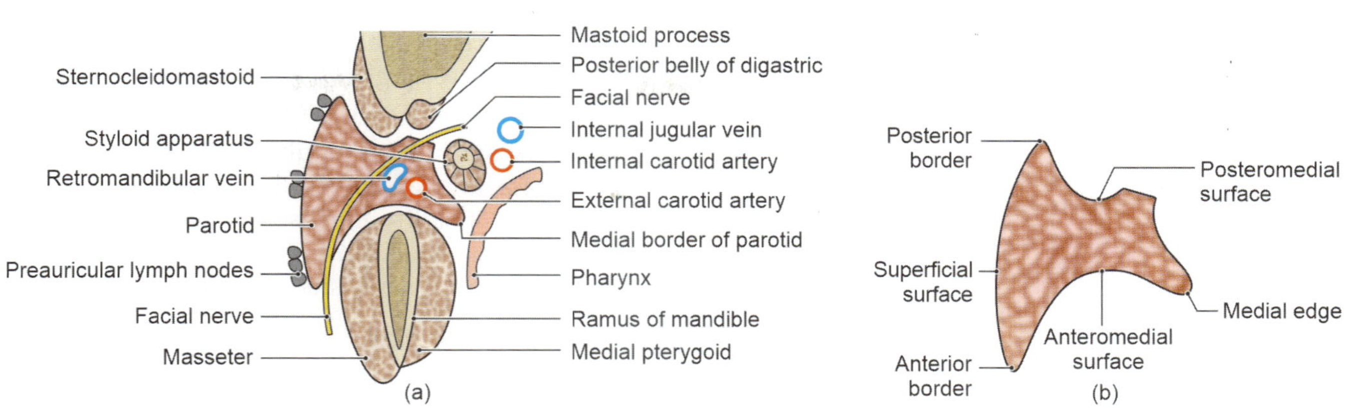

Figs 13.4a and b: (a) Horizontal section through the parotid gland showing its relations and the structures passing through it; (b) Gross features of parotid gland

Structures within the Parotid Gland

From medial to lateral side, these are as follows.

1 *Arteries:* The external carotid artery enters the gland through its posteromedial surface (Fig. 13.5a). The maxillary artery leaves the gland through its anteromedial surface. The superficial temporal artery gives transverse facial artery and emerges at the anterior part of the superior surface.

2 *Veins:* The retromandibular vein is formed within the gland by the union of the superficial temporal and maxillary veins. In the lower part of the gland, the vein divides into anterior and posterior divisions which emerge close to the apex (lower pole) of the gland (Fig. 13.5b).

3 Facial nerve is the nerve of the second branchial arch.

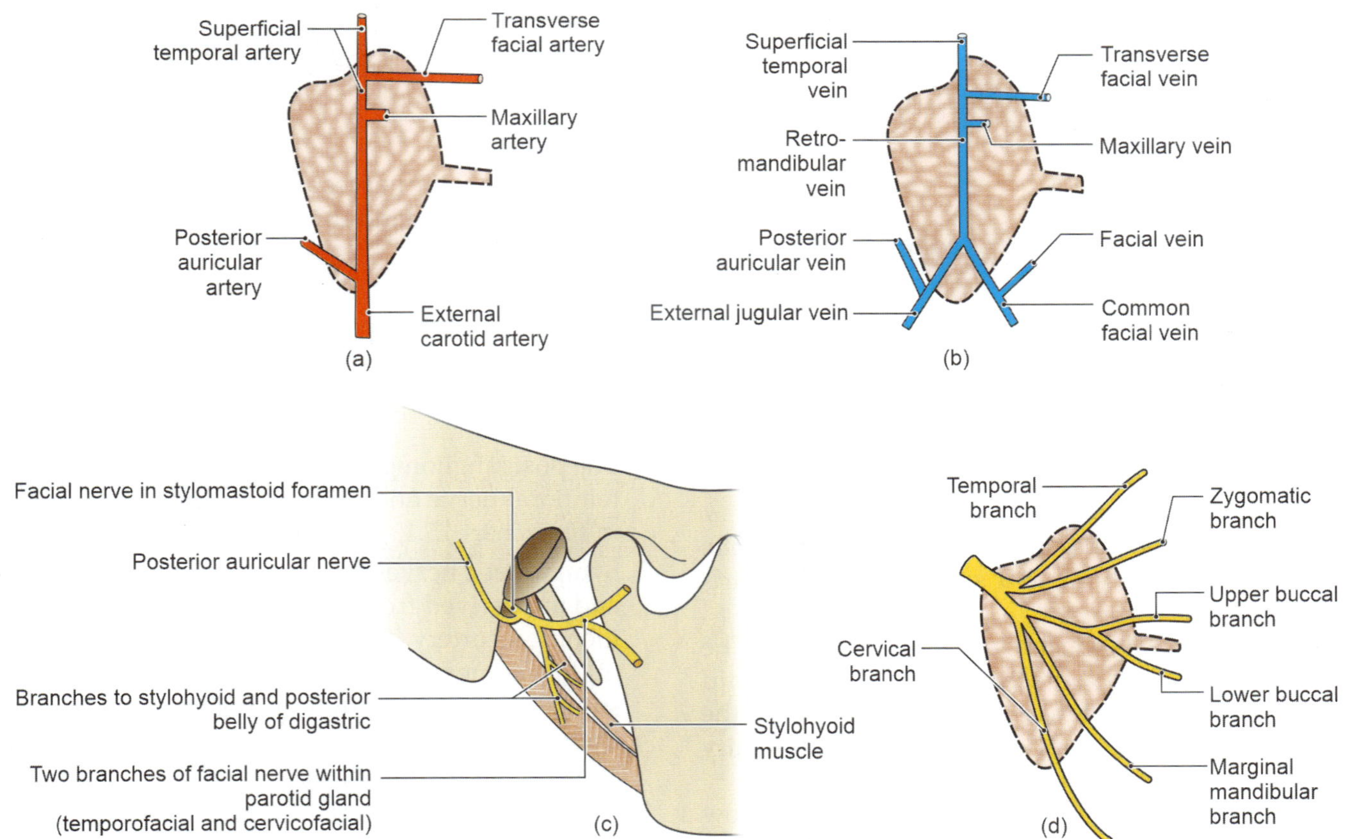

Figs 13.5a to d: Structures within the parotid gland: (a) Arteries; (b) Veins; (c) Branches of facial nerve at its exit; (d) Five terminal branches of facial nerve

The facial nerve leaves the skull by passing through the stylomastoid foramen.

In its extracranial course, the facial nerve crosses the lateral side of the base of the styloid process. Then the nerve enters the posteromedial surface of the parotid gland, runs forwards through the gland crossing the retromandibular vein and the external carotid artery. Behind the neck of the mandible, it divides into two branches—temporofacial and cervicofacial. Temporofacial gives temporal and zygomatic branches. Cervicofacial gives buccal, marginal mandibular and cervical branches. These five terminal branches emerge along the anterior border and apex of the parotid gland (Fig. 13.5d).

Branches at its exit from the stylomastoid foramen

i. Communicating branches with adjacent cranial and spinal nerves.
ii. The posterior auricular nerve arises just below the stylomastoid foramen. It ascends between the mastoid process and the external acoustic meatus, and supplies:
   a. Auricularis posterior
   b. Occipitalis
   c. Intrinsic muscles on the back of auricle.
iii. The digastric branch, arises close to the previous nerve. It is short and supplies the posterior belly of the digastric (Fig. 13.5c).
iv. The stylohyoid branch, arises with the digastric branch, is long and supplies the stylohyoid muscle.

Terminal branches

i. Temporal branches cross the zygomatic arch and supply:
   a. Auricularis anterior
   b. Auricularis superior
   c. Intrinsic muscles on the lateral side of the ear
   d. Frontalis
   e. Orbicularis oculi
   f. Corrugator supercilii.
ii. The zygomatic branches run across the zygomatic bone and supply the orbicularis oculi.
iii. The buccal branches are two in number. The upper buccal branch runs above the parotid duct and the lower buccal branch below the duct. They supply muscles in that vicinity especially the buccinator.
iv. The marginal mandibular branch runs below the angle of the mandible deep to the platysma. It crosses the body of the mandible and supplies muscles of the lower lip and chin.
v. The cervical branch emerges from the apex of the parotid gland, and runs downwards and forwards in the neck to supply the platysma.

Bell's palsy: Sudden paralysis of facial nerve at the stylomastoid foramen, results in asymmetry of corner of mouth, inability to close the eye, disappearance of nasolabial fold and loss of wrinkling of skin of forehead on the same side (*see* Fig. 10.14).

Patey's faciovenous plane

The gland is composed of a large superficial and a small deep part, the two being connected by an 'isthmus' around which facial nerve divides.

Accessory processes of parotid gland

- Facial process—along parotid duct. It lies between zygomatic arch and the parotid duct (Fig. 13.3a).
- Pterygoid process—between mandibular ramus and medial pterygoid.
- Glenoid process—between external acoustic meatus and temporomandibular joint
- Poststyloid process

Blood Supply

The parotid gland is supplied by the external carotid artery and its branches that arise within the gland. The veins drain into the external jugular vein and internal jugular vein.

Nerve Supply

1 Parasympathetic nerves are secretomotor (Fig. 13.6). They reach the gland through the auriculotemporal nerve.

   The preganglionic fibres begin in the inferior salivatory nucleus; pass through the glossopharyngeal nerve, its tympanic branch, the tympanic plexus and the lesser petrosal nerve; and relay in the otic ganglion.

   The postganglionic fibres pass through the auriculotemporal nerve and reach the gland. This is shown in Flowchart 13.1.

2 Sympathetic nerves are postganglionic, vasomotor, and are derived from the plexus around the middle meningeal artery. These fibres start from lateral horn of T1 segment of spinal cord. These synapse in superior cervical ganglion. Postganglionic fibres travel along branches of external carotid, maxillary arteries and their branches.

3 Sensory nerves to the gland come from the auriculotemporal nerve, but the parotid fascia is innervated by the sensory fibres of the great auricular nerve (C2, C3).

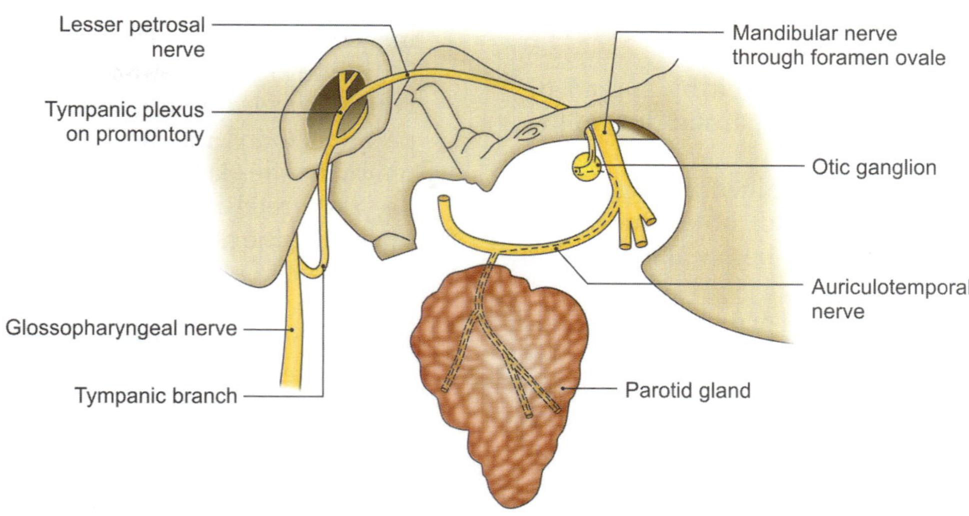

Fig. 13.6: Parasympathetic nerve supply to the parotid gland

Flowchart 13.1: Tracing nerve supply of parotid gland

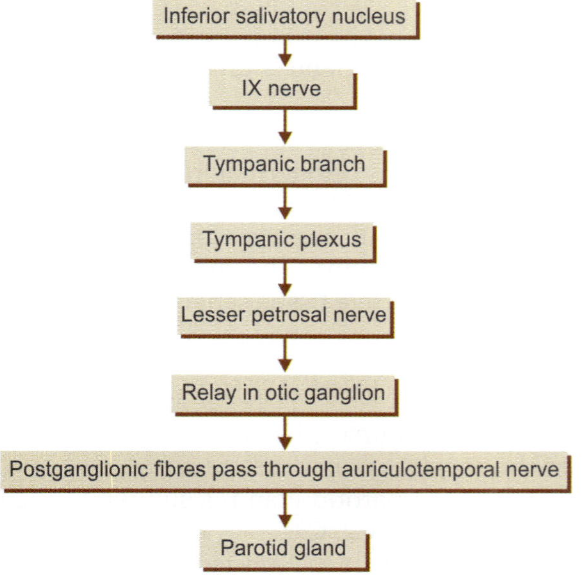

Lymphatic Drainage

Lymph drains first to the parotid nodes and from there to the upper deep cervical nodes.

Parotid Lymph Nodes

The parotid lymph nodes lie partly in the superficial fascia and partly deep to the deep fascia over the parotid gland (Fig. 13.4). They drain:

a. Temple
b. Side of the scalp
c. Lateral surface of the auricle
d. External acoustic meatus
e. Middle ear
f. Parotid gland
g. Upper part of the cheek
h. Parts of the eyelids and orbit.

Efferents from these nodes pass to the upper group of deep cervical nodes.

Parotid Duct/Stenson's Duct
(Dutch Anatomist, 1638–86)

Parotid duct is thick-walled and is about 5 cm long. It emerges from the middle of the anterior border of the gland (Fig. 13.1). It runs forwards and slightly downwards on the masseter. Here its relations are.

Superiorly

1 Accessory parotid gland
2 The transverse facial vessels (Fig. 13.3a)
3 Upper buccal branch of the facial nerve

Inferiorly

The lower buccal branch of the facial nerve.

At the anterior border of the masseter, the parotid duct turns medially and pierces:

a. The buccal pad of fat
b. The buccopharyngeal fascia
c. The buccinator (obliquely)

Because of the oblique course of the duct through the buccinator, inflation of the duct is prevented during blowing.

The duct runs forwards for a short distance between the buccinator and the oral mucosa. Finally, the duct turns medially and opens into the vestibule of the mouth (gingivobuccal vestibule) opposite the crown of the upper second molar tooth (Fig. 13.7).

CLINICAL ANATOMY

- A *parotid abscess* may be caused by spread of infection from the opening of parotid duct in the mouth cavity (Fig. 13.8).
- A parotid abscess is best drained by horizontal incision/making many small holes known as Hilton's method (Fig. 13.8) below the angle of mandible.
- Parotidectomy is the removal of the parotid gland. After this operation, at times, there may be aberrant regeneration of the secretomotor fibres in the auriculotemporal nerve which join the great auricular nerve. This causes stimulation of the sweat glands and hyperaemia in the area of its distribution, thus producing redness and sweating in the area of skin supplied by the nerve. This clinical entity is called *Frey's syndrome*. Whenever, such a person chews there is increased sweating in the region supplied by auriculotemporal nerve. So, it is also called 'auriculotemporal syndrome'.
- During surgical removal of the parotid gland or parotidectomy, the facial nerve is preserved by removing the gland in two parts—superficial and deep separately. The plane of cleavage is defined by tracing the nerve from behind forwards.
- *Mixed parotid tumour* is a slow growing lobulated painless tumour without any involvement of the facial nerve. Malignant change of such a tumour is indicated by pain, rapid growth, fixity with hardness, involvement of the facial nerve, and enlargement of cervical lymph nodes.
- The parotid calculi may get formed within the parotid gland or in its Stenson's duct. These can be located by injecting a radio-opaque dye through its opening in the vestibule of the mouth. The procedure is called 'Sialogram'. The duct can be examined by a spatula or bidigital examination.

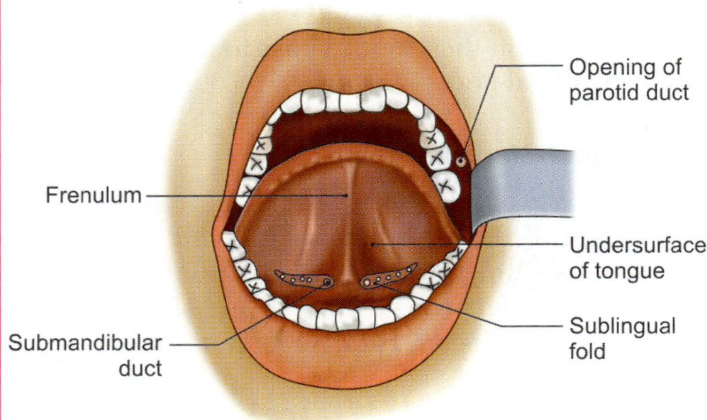

Fig. 13.7: Openings of salivary glands

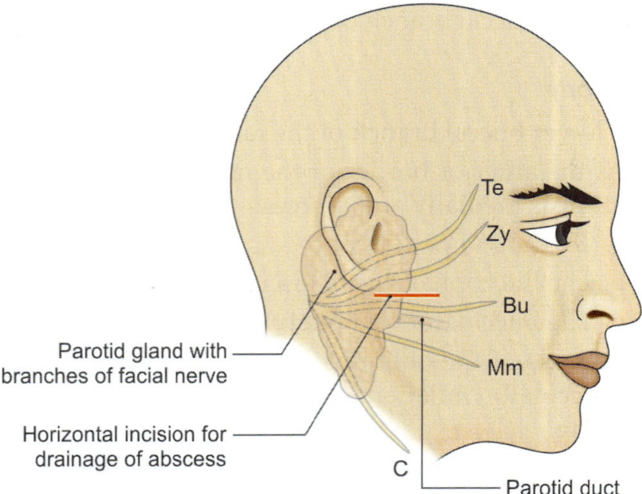

Fig. 13.8: Horizontal incision for draining parotid abscess. Branches of facial nerve also seen. Te—temporal; Zy—zygomatic, Bu—buccal; Mm—marginal mandibular; C—cervical

HISTOLOGY

Histology of parotid gland is given in Chapter 15.

DEVELOPMENT

The parotid gland is ectodermal in origin. It develops from the buccal epithelium just lateral to the angle of mouth. The outgrowth branches repeatedly to form the duct system and acini. The mesoderm forms the intervening connective tissue septa.

FACTS TO REMEMBER

- Facial nerve courses through the parotid gland, *without supplying any structure in it*.
- Skin over the parotid gland is supplied by great auricular nerve, C2, C3.
- Deepest structure in the substance of parotid gland is the external carotid artery.
- Otic ganglion is the only parasympathetic ganglion with four roots, including a motor root.
- Facial nerve divides into temporofacial and cervicofacial branches. The former gives temporal and zygomatic branches. The latter gives buccal, marginal mandibular and cervical branches.
- Facial nerve passes through two foramina of skull, i.e. internal acoustic meatus and stylomastoid foramen.

CLINICOANATOMICAL PROBLEM

A young man complained of fever and sore throat, noted a swelling and felt pain on both sides of his face in front of the ear. Within a few days, he noted swellings below his jaw and below his chin. He suddenly started looking very healthy by facial appearance. The pain increased while chewing or drinking lemon juice. The physician noted enlargement of all three salivary glands on both sides of the face.

- Where do the ducts of salivary glands open?
- Why did the pain increase while chewing?
- Why did the pain increase while drinking lemon juice?

Ans: The duct of the parotid gland opens at a papilla in the vestibule of mouth opposite the 2nd upper molar tooth. The duct of submandibular gland opens at the papilla on the sublingual fold. The sublingual gland opens by 10–12 ducts on the sublingual fold.

The investing layer of cervical fascia encloses both the parotid and the submandibular glands and is attached to the lower border of the mandible. As mandible moves during chewing, the fascia gets stretched which results in pain. The fascia and skin are supplied by the great auricular nerve.

While drinking lemon juice, there is a lot of pain, as the salivary secretion is stimulated by the acid present in the lemon juice.

The investing layer of cervical fascia encloses: Two muscles—the trapezius and the sternocleidomastoid; two spaces—the suprasternal space and the supraclavicular space; two glands—the parotid and the submandibular; and forms two pulleys—one for the intermediate tendon of digastric muscle and other for the intermediate tendon of omohyoid muscle.

FURTHER READING

- Mitz V, Peyronie M. The superficial musculo-aponeurotic system (SMAS) in the parotid and cheek area. Plast Reconstruct Surg 1976;58:80–88.
  A paper that provides the anatomical basis for all invasive aesthetic and reconstructive facelift surgery.
- Ziarah HA, Atkinson ME. The surgical anatomy of the mandibular distribution of the facial nerve. Br J Oral Surg 1981;19:159–70.
  An outline of how the mandibular branch of the facial nerve is at risk in all incisions at the lower border of the mandible, in submandibular gland excision, incision of space-occupying dental infections, and neck dissection. A detailed knowledge of this structure is essential.

Frequently Asked Questions

1. Describe parotid gland under the following headings:
   a. Gross anatomy
   b. Structures emerging at various borders, apex and base
   c. Nerve supply
   d. Clinical anatomy
2. Describe briefly the structures present within the parotid gland.
3. Write short notes on/enumerate:
   a. Parotid duct
   b. Histology of parotid gland

Multiple Choice Questions

1. Nerve carrying postganglionic parasympathetic fibres of the parotid gland is:
   a. Facial b. Auriculotemporal
   c. Inferior alveolar d. Buccal
2. Somata of postganglionic secretomotor fibres to parotid gland lie in:
   a. Ciliary ganglion
   b. Pterygopalatine ganglion
   c. Otic ganglion
   d. Submandibular ganglion
3. Which of the following arteries passes between the roots of the auriculotemporal nerve?
   a. Maxillary
   b. Middle meningeal
   c. Superficial temporal
   d. Accessory meningeal
4. Vein formed by union of posterior division of retromandibular and posterior auricular vein is:
   a. Internal jugular b. External jugular
   c. Common facial d. Anterior jugular
5. All of the following are peripheral parasympathetic ganglia, *except*:
   a. Otic b. Ciliary
   c. Pterygopalatine d. Geniculate
6. Which artery is not inside the parotid gland?
   a. External carotid
   b. Internal carotid
   c. Superficial temporal
   d. Maxillary
7. Which one of the following nerves is not related to parotid gland?
   a. Temporal branch of facial
   b. Zygomatic branch of facial
   c. Buccal branch of facial
   d. Posterior superior alveolar branch of maxillary
8. Pes anserinus is the arrangement in which of the following nerves?
   a. Vagus b. Trigeminal
   c. Facial d. Glossopharyngeal

Answers

1. b **2.** c **3.** b **4.** b **5.** d **6.** b **7.** d **8.** c

VIVA VOCE

- Enumerate the structures emerging from the anterior border of parotid gland.
- What structures lie within the parotid gland?
- Trace the secretomotor nerve supply of the parotid gland.
- What is the histological structure of parotid gland?
- What are the structures pierced by parotid duct and where do they open?
- Name the areas drained by parotid lymph nodes.
- What is Hilton's method of drainage of parotid abscess?

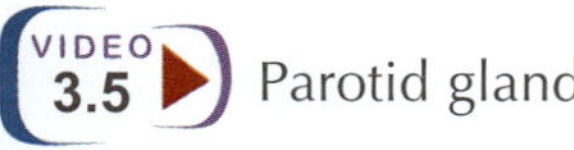

Parotid gland

Chapter

14

Temporal and Infratemporal Regions

"Best physicians are: Doctor Quiet, Doctor Rest, Doctor Diet and Doctor Merryman."
—Regimen of Salerno

INTRODUCTION

Temporal and infratemporal regions include muscles of mastication, which develop from mesoderm of first branchial arch. The muscles of mastication are innervated by mandibular branch of trigeminal nerve. Only one joint, the temporomandibular joint, is present on each side between the base of skull and mandible to allow movements during speech and mastication.

The parasympathetic ganglion is the otic ganglion, the only ganglion with four roots, i.e. sensory, sympathetic, motor and secretomotor or parasympathetic.

The blood supply of this region is through the maxillary artery. Middle meningeal artery is its most important branch, as its injury results in extradural haemorrhage (*see* Fig. 9.10).

TEMPORAL FOSSA

In order to understand these regions, the osteology of the temporal fossa, and the infratemporal fossa should be studied. The *temporal fossa* lies on the side of the skull, and is bounded by the superior temporal line and the zygomatic arch.

Boundaries

Anterior: Zygomatic and frontal bones (Fig. 14.1)

Posterior: Inferior temporal line and supramastoid crest

Superior: Superior temporal line

Inferior: Zygomatic arch

Floor: Parts of frontal, parietal, temporal and greater wing of sphenoid. Temporalis muscle is attached to the floor and inferior temporal line.

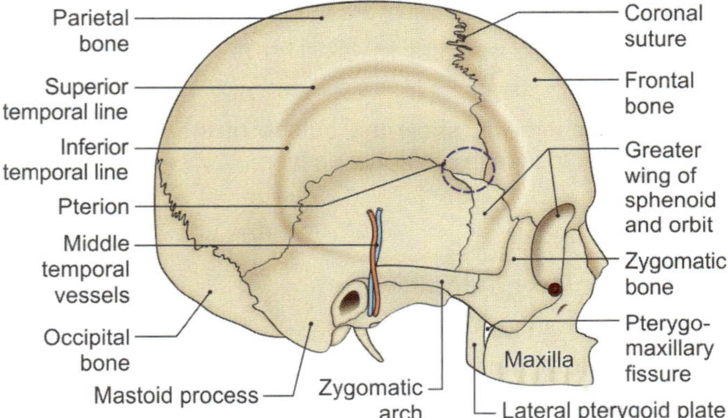

Fig. 14.1: Some features seen on the lateral side of the skull

Contents

1 Temporalis muscle
2 Middle temporal artery (branch of superficial temporal artery) (Fig. 14.1)
3 Zygomaticotemporal nerve and artery
4 Deep temporal nerves for supplying temporalis muscle
5 Deep temporal artery, branch of maxillary artery

INFRATEMPORAL FOSSA

It is an irregular space below zygomatic arch.

Boundaries

Anterior: Posterior surface of body of maxilla

Roof: Infratemporal surface of greater wing of sphenoid

Medial: Lateral pterygoid plate and pyramidal process of palatine bone

Lateral: Ramus of mandible (Fig. 14.2)

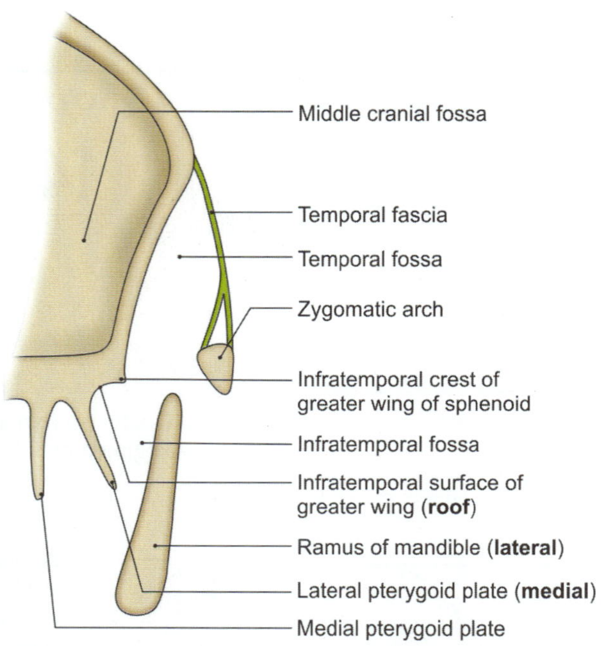

Fig. 14.2: Scheme to show the outline of the temporal and infratemporal fossae in a coronal section

Contents

1 Lateral pterygoid muscle
2 Medial pterygoid muscle
3 Mandibular nerve with its branches, otic ganglion
4 Posterior superior alveolar nerve branch of maxillary nerve (*see* Chapter 23)
5 Chorda tympani, branch of VII nerve
6 1st and 2nd parts of maxillary artery with their branches
7 Posterior superior alveolar artery, branch of 3rd part of maxillary artery
8 Accompanying veins

Landmarks on the lateral side of the head

The external ear or pinna is a prominent feature on the lateral aspect of the head.

1 The *zygomatic bone* forms the prominence of the cheek at the inferolateral corner of the orbit. The *zygomatic arch* bridges the gap between the eye and the ear.
2 The head of the mandible lies in front of the tragus. It is felt best during movements of the lower jaw.
3 The *mastoid process* is a large bony prominence situated behind the lower part of the auricle.
4 The superior *temporal line* forms the upper boundary of the temporal fossa which is filled up by the temporalis muscle.
5 The *pterion* is the area in the temporal fossa where four bones (frontal, parietal, temporal and greater wing of sphenoid) adjoin each other across an H-shaped suture (Fig. 14.1).
6 The junction of the back of the head with the neck is indicated by the external occipital protuberance and the superior nuchal lines.

MUSCLES OF MASTICATION

FEATURES

The muscles of mastication move the mandible during mastication and speech. They are the masseter, the temporalis, the lateral pterygoid and the medial pterygoid. They develop from the mesoderm of the first branchial arch, and are supplied by the mandibular nerve which is the nerve of that arch. The muscles are enumerated in Table 14.1 and shown in Figs 14.3 to 14.5. Temporal fascia and relations of lateral and medial pterygoid muscles are described.

TEMPORAL FASCIA

The temporal fascia is a thick aponeurotic sheet that roofs over the temporal fossa and covers the temporalis muscle. Superiorly, the fascia is single layered and is attached to the superior temporal line. Inferiorly, it splits into two layers which are attached to the inner and outer lips of the upper border of the zygomatic arch. The small gap between the two layers contains fat, a branch from the superficial temporal artery and the zygomaticotemporal nerve.

DISSECTION

Identify the masseter muscle extending from the zygomatic arch to the ramus of the mandible (Fig. 14.3). Cut the zygomatic arch in front of and behind the attachment of masseter muscle and reflect it downwards. Divide the nerve and blood vessels to the muscle. Clean the ramus of mandible by stripping off the masseter muscle from it *(refer to BDC App)*.

Give an oblique cut from the centre of mandibular notch to the lower end of anterior border of ramus of mandible. Turn this part of the bone including the insertion of temporalis muscle upwards. Strip the muscle from the skull and identify deep temporal nerves and vessels.

Make one cut through the neck of the mandible. Give another cut through the ramus at a distance of 4 cm from the neck. Remove the bone carefully in between these two cuts, avoiding injury to the underlying structures. The lateral pterygoid is exposed in the upper part and medial pterygoid in the lower part of the dissection (Fig. 14.5).

Table 14.1: Muscles of mastication

Muscle	*Origin*	*Fibres*	*Insertion*	*Nerve supply*	*Actions*
1. **Masseter** Quadrilateral, covers lateral surface of ramus of mandible, has three layers (Fig. 14.3)	a. *Superficial layer* (largest): From anterior two-thirds of lower border of zygomatic arch and adjoining zygomatic process of maxilla b. *Middle layer:* From lower border of posterior one-third of zyomatic arch c. *Deep layer:* From deep surface of zygomatic arch	a. Superficial fibres pass downwards and backwards at 45° b. Middle fibres pass vertically downwards c. Deep fibres pass vertically downwards	a. *Superficial layer* into the lower part of the lateral surface of ramus of mandible b. *Middle layer* into the central part of ramus of the mandible c. *Deep layer* into rest of the ramus of the mandible	Masseteric nerve, a branch of anterior division of mandibular nerve	a. Elevates mandible to close the mouth to bite b. Superficial fibres cause protrusion
2. **Temporalis** Fan-shaped, fills the temporal fossa (Fig. 14.4)	a. Temporal fossa, excluding zygomatic bone b. Temporal fascia	Anterior fibres run vertically, middle obliquely and posterior horizontally. All converge and pass through gap deep to zygomatic arch	a. Margins and deep surface of coronoid process. b. Anterior border of ramus of the mandible	Two deep temporal branches from anterior division of mandibular nerve	a. Elevates mandible b. Helps in side-to-side grinding movement c. Posterior fibres retract the protruded mandible
3. **Lateral pterygoid** Short, conical, has upper and lower heads (Fig. 14.5)	a. *Upper head* (small): From infratemporal surface and crest of greater wing of sphenoid bone b. *Lower head* (larger): From lateral surface of lateral pterygoid plate. Origin is medial to insertion	Fibres run backwards and laterally and converge for insertion	a. Pterygoid fovea on the anterior surface of neck of mandible b. Anterior margin of articular disc, and c. Capsule of temporo-mandibular joint. Insertion is postero-lateral and at a slightly higher level than origin	A branch from anterior division of mandibular nerve	a. Depress mandible to open mouth, with suprahyoid muscles. It is indispensible for actively opening the mouth b. Protrudes mandible c. Right lateral pterygoid turns the chin to left side
4. **Medial pterygoid** Quadrilateral, has a small superficial and a large deep head (Fig. 14.5)	a. *Superficial head* (small slip): From tuberosity of maxilla and adjoining bone b. *Deep head* (quite large): From medial surface of lateral pterygoid plate and adjoining process of palatine bone	Fibres run downwards, backwards and laterally. The two heads embrace part of the lower head of lateral pterygoid (Fig. 14.5)	Roughened area on the medial surface of angle and adjoining ramus of mandible, below and behind the mandibular foramen and mylohyoid groove	Nerve to medial pterygoid, branch of the main trunk of mandibular nerve	a. Elevates mandible b. Helps protrude mandible c. Right medial pterygoid with right lateral pterygoid turn the chin to left side as part of grinding movements

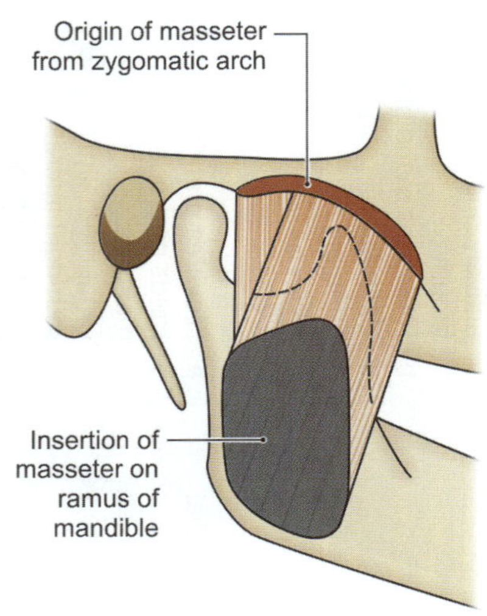

Fig. 14.3: Origin and insertion of the masseter muscle

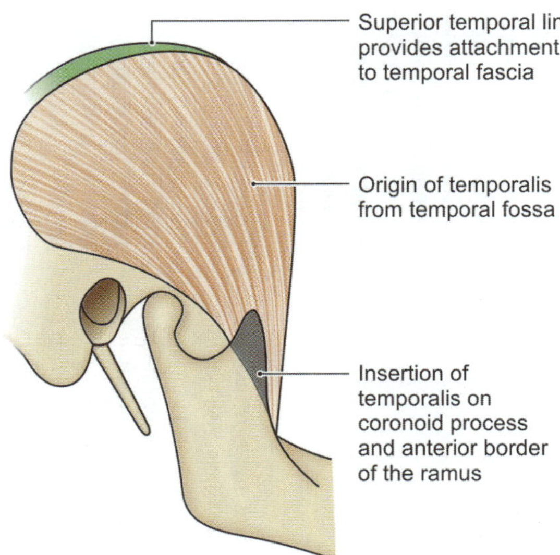

Fig. 14.4: Origin and insertion of the temporalis muscle

The superficial surface of the temporal fascia receives an expansion from the epicranial aponeurosis (*see* Fig. 10.3). This surface gives origin to the auricularis anterior and superior, and is related to the superficial temporal vessels, the auriculotemporal nerve, and the temporal branch of the facial nerve (*see* Fig. 13.3a). The deep surface of the temporal fascia gives origin to some fibres of the temporalis muscle.

The fascia is extremely dense. In some species (e.g. tortoise), the temporal fascia is replaced by bone.

RELATIONS OF LATERAL PTERYGOID

The lateral pterygoid may be regarded as the key muscle of this region because its relations provide a fair idea about the layout of structures in the infratemporal fossa. The relations are as follows:

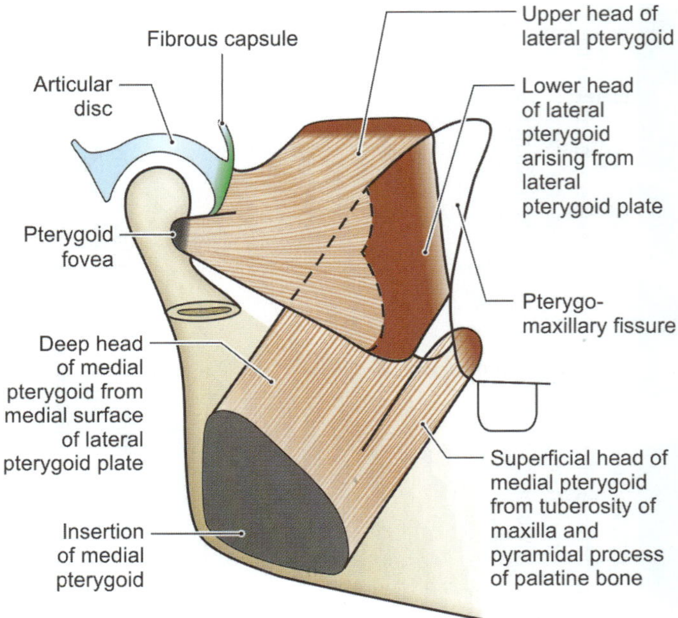

Fig. 14.5: The lateral and medial pterygoid muscles

Superficial Relations

1 Masseter
2 Ramus of the mandible
3 Tendon of the temporalis
4 The maxillary artery (Fig. 14.6)

Deep Relations

1 Mandibular nerve
2 Middle meningeal artery (Fig. 14.11)
3 Sphenomandibular ligament
4 Deep head of the medial pterygoid

Structures Emerging at the Upper Border

1 Deep temporal nerves (Fig. 14.6)
2 Masseteric nerve

Structures Emerging at the Lower Border

1 Lingual nerve and artery
2 Inferior alveolar nerve
3 The middle meningeal and accessory meningeal arteries pass upwards deep to it (Fig. 14.6).

Structures Passing through the Gap between the Two Heads

1 The maxillary artery enters the gap
2 The buccal branch of the mandibular nerve comes out through the gap (Fig. 14.6).

The pterygoid plexus of veins surrounds the lateral pterygoid.

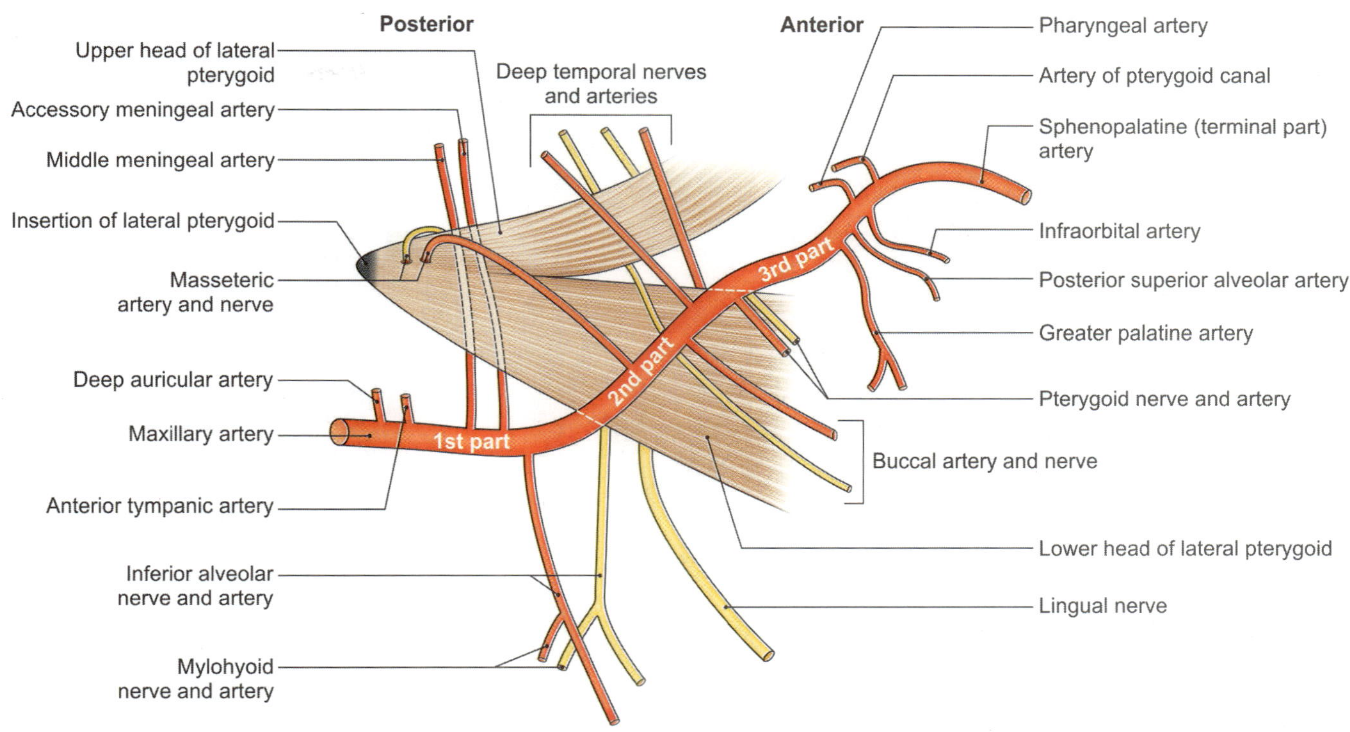

Fig. 14.6: Some relations of the lateral pterygoid muscle and branches of maxillary artery

RELATIONS OF MEDIAL PTERYGOID

The superficial and deep heads of medial pterygoid enclose the lower head of lateral pterygoid muscle (Fig. 14.5).

Superficial Relations

The upper part of the muscle is separated from the lateral pterygoid muscle by:

1. The lateral pterygoid plate
2. The lingual nerve (Fig. 14.5)
3. The inferior alveolar nerve.

Lower down the muscle is separated from the ramus of the mandible by the lingual and inferior alveolar nerves, the maxillary artery, and the sphenomandibular ligament.

Deep Relations

The relations are:

1. Tensor veli palatini
2. Superior constrictor of pharynx
3. Styloglossus
4. Stylopharyngeus attached to the styloid process.

CLINICAL ANATOMY

Temporalis and masseter muscles are palpated by requesting the person to clench the teeth. Medial and lateral pterygoid muscles can be tested by requesting the person to move the lower jaw from one side to other side.

MAXILLARY ARTERY

Features

This is the larger terminal branch of the external carotid artery, given off behind the neck of the mandible. It has a wide territory of distribution, and supplies:

1. The external and middle ears, and the auditory tube (Fig. 14.7)
2. The dura mater
3. The upper and lower jaws with their teeth (Fig. 14.6)
4. The muscles of the temporal and infratemporal regions
5. The nose and paranasal air sinuses
6. The palate
7. The root of the pharynx.

DISSECTION

External carotid artery divides into its two terminal branches, maxillary and superficial temporal on the anteromedial surface of the parotid gland (*see* Fig. 13.5a). The maxillary artery, appears in this region. Identify some of its branches. Most important to be identified is the middle meningeal artery. Learn its course and branches given in Chapter 20. Accompanying these branches are the veins and pterygoid venous plexus and the superficial content of infratemporal fossa. Remove these veins. Try to see its communication with the cavernous sinus and facial vein.

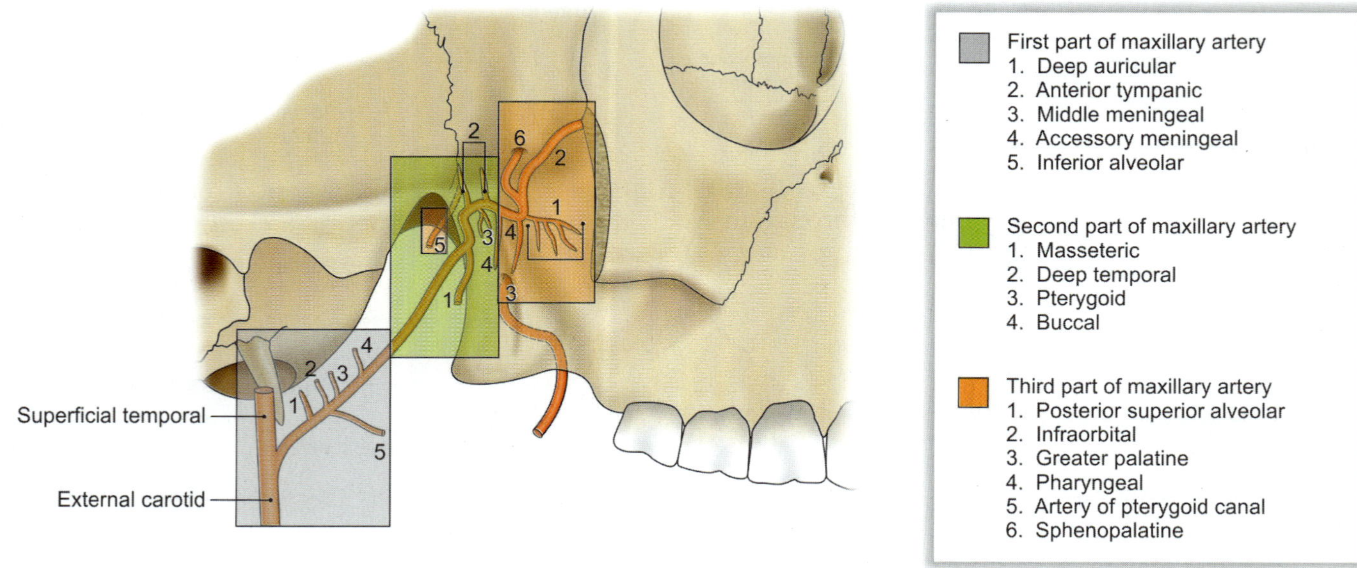

Fig. 14.7: Branches of three parts of the maxillary artery

Course and Relations

For descriptive purposes, the maxillary artery is divided into three parts (Fig. 14.7 and Table 14.2).

1 The *first (mandibular) part* runs horizontally forwards, first between the neck of the mandible and the sphenomandibular ligament, below the auriculo-

Table 14.2: Branches of maxillary artery (Figs 14.6 and 14.7)

Branches	*Foramina transmitting*	*Distribution*
A. Of first part		
1. Deep auricular	Foramen in the floor (cartilage or bone) of external acoustic meatus	Skin of external acoustic meatus, and outer surface of tympanic membrane
2. Anterior tympanic	Petrotympanic fissure	Inner surface of tympanic membrane
3. Middle meningeal	Foramen spinosum	Supplies more of bone and less of meninges; also 5th and 7th nerves, middle ear and tensor tympani
4. Accessory meningeal	Foramen ovale	Main distribution is extracranial to pterygoids
5. Inferior alveolar	Mandibular foramen	Lower 8 teeth and mylohyoid muscle
B. Of second part		
1. Masseteric	—	Masseter
2. Deep temporal	—	Temporalis (two branches)
3. Pterygoid	—	Lateral and medial pterygoids
4. Buccal	—	Skin of the cheek
C. Of third part		
1. Posterior superior alveolar	Alveolar canals in body of maxilla	Upper molar and premolar teeth and gums; maxillary sinus
2. Infraorbital	Inferior orbital fissure	Lower orbital muscles; lacrimal sac; maxillary sinus; upper incisor and canine teeth
3. Greater palatine	Greater palatine canal	Soft palate; tonsil; palatine glands and mucosa of upper gums
4. Pharyngeal	Pharyngeal (palatovaginal) canal	Roof of nose and pharynx; auditory tube; sphenoidal sinus
5. Artery of pterygoid canal	Pterygoid canal	Auditory tube; upper pharynx and middle ear
6. Sphenopalatine (terminal part)	Sphenopalatine foramen	Lateral and medial walls of nose and various air sinuses (artery of epistaxis)

temporal nerve, and then along the lower border of the lateral pterygoid.

2 The *second (pterygoid) part* runs upwards and forwards superficial to the lower head of the lateral pterygoid.
3 The *third (pterygopalatine) part* passes between the two heads of the lateral pterygoid and through the pterygomaxillary fissure, to enter the pterygopalatine fossa.

Branches of First Part of the Maxillary Artery

1 The *deep auricular artery* supplies the external acoustic meatus, the tympanic membrane and the temporomandibular joint (Fig. 14.7).
2 The *anterior tympanic* branch supplies the middle ear including the medial surface of the tympanic membrane.
3 The *middle meningeal artery* is described in Chapter 20. It lies between lateral pterygoid and sphenomandibular ligaments, then between two roots of auriculotemporal nerve, enters the skull through foramen spinosum to reach middle cranial fossa. It divides into a large frontal branch which courses towards the *pterion* and a smaller parietal branch (Fig. 14.11, also *see* Fig. 20.14).
4 The *accessory meningeal artery* enters the cranial cavity through the foramen ovale. Apart from the meninges, it supplies structures in the infratemporal fossa.
5 The *inferior alveolar artery* runs downwards and forwards medial to the ramus of the mandible to reach the mandibular foramen. Passing through this foramen, the artery enters the mandibular canal (within the body of the mandible) in which it runs downwards and then forwards.

   Before entering the mandibular canal, the artery gives off a lingual branch to the tongue; and a mylohyoid branch that descends in the mylohyoid groove (on the medial aspect of the mandible) and runs forwards above the mylohyoid muscle (*see* Fig. 9.25).

   Within the mandibular canal, the artery gives branches to the mandible and to the roots of the each tooth attached to the bone.

   It also gives off a mental branch that passes through the mental foramen to supply the chin (*see* Fig. 9.24).

Branches of Second Part of the Maxillary Artery

These are mainly muscular. These are:

1 Masseteric
2 Deep temporal (anterior and posterior)
3 Laterior pterygoid
4 Buccal for skin of cheek.

Branches of Third Part of the Maxillary Artery

1 The *posterior superior alveolar artery* arises just before the maxillary artery enters the pterygomaxillary fissure. It descends on the posterior surface of the maxilla and gives branches that enter canals in the bone to supply the molar and premolar teeth, and the maxillary air sinus.
2 The *infraorbital artery* also arises just before the maxillary artery enters the pterygomaxillary fissure. It enters the orbit through the inferior orbital fissure. It then runs forwards in relation to the floor of the orbit, first in the infraorbital groove and then in the infraorbital canal to emerge on the face through the infraorbital foramen. It gives off some *orbital branches*, for structures in the orbit; *middle superior alveolar branch* for premolar teeth and the *anterior superior alveolar* branches that enter apertures in the maxilla to reach the incisor and canine teeth attached to the bone.

   After emerging on the face, the infraorbital artery gives branches to the lacrimal sac, the nose and the upper lip.

   The remaining branches of the third part arise within the pterygopalatine fossa (Fig. 14.7).

3 The *greater palatine artery* runs downwards in the greater palatine canal to emerge on the posterolateral part of the hard palate through the greater palatine foramen. It then runs forwards near the lateral margin of the palate to reach the incisive canal (near the midline) through which some terminal branches enter the nasal cavity (*see* Fig. 9.12).

   Branches of the artery supply the palate and gums. While still within the greater palatine canal, it gives off the *lesser palatine arteries* that emerge on the palate through the lesser palatine foramina, and run backwards into the soft palate and tonsil.

4 The *pharyngeal branch* runs backwards through a canal related to the inferior aspect of the body of the sphenoid bone (pharyngeal or palatinovaginal canal). It supplies part of the nasopharynx, the auditory tube and the sphenoidal air sinus.
5 The *artery of the pterygoid canal* runs backwards in the canal of the same name and helps to supply the pharynx, the auditory tube and the tympanic cavity.
6 The *sphenopalatine artery* passes medially through the sphenopalatine foramen to enter the cavity of the nose. It gives off *posterolateral nasal* branches to the lateral wall of the nose and to the paranasal sinuses; and *posteromedial branches* to the nasal septum. Sphenopalatine artery is the artery of 'epistaxis' (*see* Fig. 23.5).

CLINICAL ANATOMY

- The anterior branch of middle meningeal artery is likely to be injured at the pterion in roadside accidents. It leads to extradural haemorrhage (*see* Fig. 9.10). The clot must be sucked out at the earliest, otherwise it may compress the motor area of brain.
- Bleeding from lower teeth is from branches of inferior alveolar artery (1st part of maxillary artery) and from upper teeth is from branches of 3rd part of maxillary artery. These are posterior superior alveolar and infraorbital arteries.
- Sphenopalatine is the terminal branch of 3rd part of maxillary artery. It anastomoses with neighbouring vessels to form large capillary plexus called Kiesselbach's plexus at the anteroinferior angle of the nasal septum. It is a common site of bleeding from nose or epistaxis and is known as Little's area. So sphenopalatine artery is called 'the artery of epistaxis'.

PTERYGOID PLEXUS OF VEINS

It lies around and within the lateral pterygoid muscle. The tributaries of the plexus correspond to the branches of the maxillary artery. The plexus is drained by the maxillary vein which begins at the posterior end of the plexus and unites with the superficial temporal vein to form the retromandibular vein. Thus, the maxillary vein accompanies only the first part of the maxillary artery.

The plexus communicates:

a. With the inferior ophthalmic vein through the inferior orbital fissure.
b. With the cavernous sinus through the emissary veins.
c. With the facial vein (FV) through the deep facial vein.

FV communicates with inferior ophthalmic vein. Thus infection from FV/inferior ophthalmic vein can reach cavernons sinus causing its thrombosis and palsy of cranial nerves in the sinus.

TEMPOROMANDIBULAR JOINT

Type of Joint

This is a synovial joint of the condylar variety.

Articular Surfaces

The upper articular surface is formed by the following parts of the temporal bone.

DISSECTION

Cut the lateral pterygoid muscle close to its insertion. Dislodge the head of mandible from the articular disc. Locate the articular cartilages covering the head of the mandible and the mandibular fossa. Take out the articular disc as well and study its shape and its role in increasing the varieties of movements.

1 Articular tubercle (anterior root of zygomatic arch).
2 Anterior part of mandibular fossa (Fig. 14.8).
3 Posterior non-articular part formed by the tympanic plate.

The inferior articular surface is formed by the head of the mandible.

The articular surfaces are covered with *fibrocartilage*. The joint cavity is divided into upper and lower parts by an intra-articular disc.

Ligaments

The ligaments are the fibrous capsule, the lateral temporomandibular ligament, the sphenomandibular ligament, the stylomandibular ligament and pterygomandibular ligament.

1 The *fibrous capsule* is attached *above* to the articular tubercle, the circumference of the mandibular fossa in front and the squamotympanic fissure behind, and *below* to the neck of the mandible. The capsule is loose above the intra-articular disc, and tight below it. The synovial membrane lines the fibrous capsule and the neck of the mandible (Fig. 14.9).
2 The *lateral temporomandibular ligament* reinforces and strengthens the lateral part of the capsular ligament. Its fibres are directed downwards and backwards. It is attached above to the articular tubercle, and

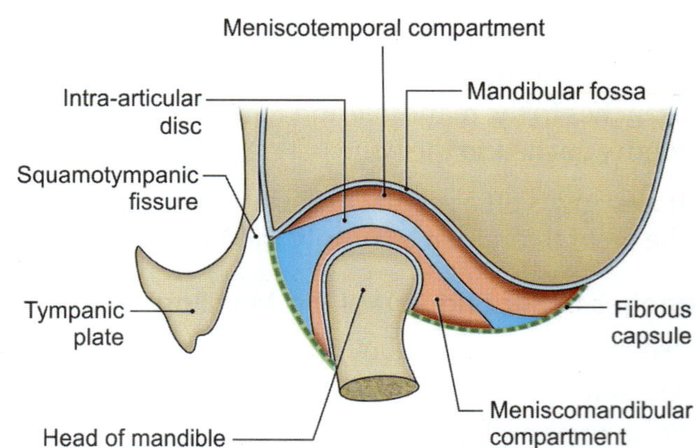

Fig. 14.8: Subdivisions and attachments of the articular disc of temporomandibular joint (TMJ)

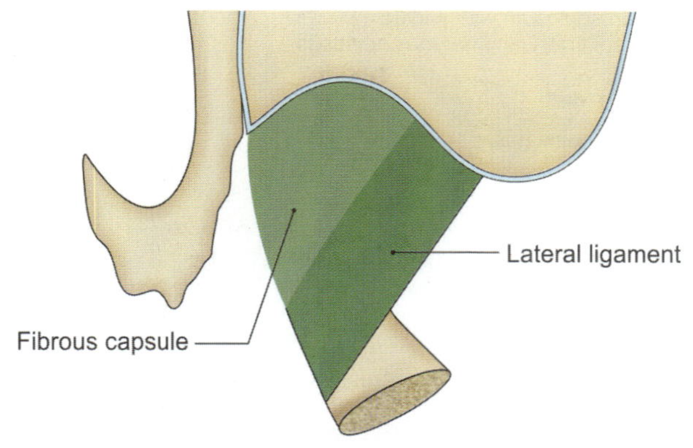

Fig. 14.9: Fibrous capsule and lateral ligament of the temporomandibular joint

below to the posterolateral aspect of the neck of the mandible.

3 The *sphenomandibular ligament* is an accessory ligament, that lies on a deep plane away from the fibrous capsule. It is attached superiorly to the spine of the sphenoid, and inferiorly to the lingula of the mandibular foramen. It is a remnant of the dorsal part of Meckel's cartilage.

The ligament is related *laterally* to:

a. Lateral pterygoid muscle (Fig. 14.10)
b. Auriculotemporal nerve
c. Maxillary artery (Fig. 14.11).

The ligament is related medially to:

a. Chorda tympani nerve
b. Wall of the pharynx.

Near its lower end, it is pierced by the mylohyoid nerve and vessels.

4 The *stylomandibular ligament* is another accessory ligament of the joint. It represents a thickened part of the *deep cervical fascia* which separates the parotid and submandibular salivary glands. It is attached above to the lateral surface of the styloid process, and below to the angle and adjacent part of posterior border of the ramus of the mandible (Fig. 14.11).

5 *Pterygomandibular ligament* is attached above to pterygoid hamulus at lower end of medial pterygoid plate and below to inner aspect of mandible just behind 3rd molar tooth.

Articular Disc

The *articular disc* is an oval predominantly fibrous plate that divides the joint into an upper and a lower compartments. The upper compartment permits *gliding* movements, and the lower, *rotatory* as well as *gliding* movements.

The disc has a concavoconvex superior surface, and a concave inferior surface. The periphery of the disc is attached to the fibrous capsule. The disc is composed of an anterior region, anterior thick band, intermediate region, posterior thick band and bilaminar region (Fig. 14.10) containing venous plexus. The disc represents the degenerated primitive insertion of lateral pterygoid. The disc prevents friction between the articulating surfaces.

It acts as a cushion and helps in shock absorption. It stabilises the condyle by filling up the space between articulating surfaces.

The proprioceptive fibres present in the disc help to regulate movements of the joint.

The disc helps in distribution of weight across the TMJ by increasing the area of contact.

Synovium: The capsule of TMJ is lined by synovium and the synovial fluid fills the joint cavity.

Synovial tissue is a vascular connective tissue lining the fibrous capsule. It extends till the boundaries of the articulating surfaces.

Synovial fluid is filtrate of plasma with additional proteins and mucins. Its main content is hyaluronic

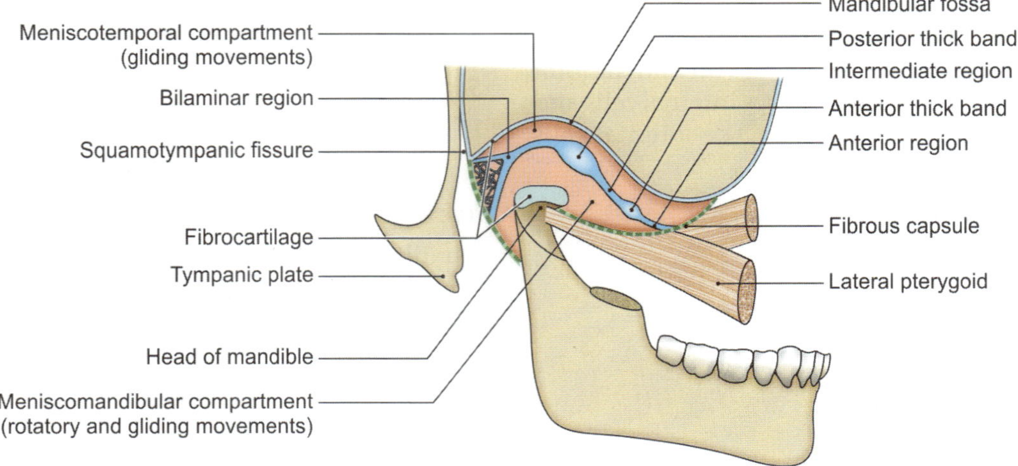

Fig. 14.10: Articular surfaces of the temporomandibular joint

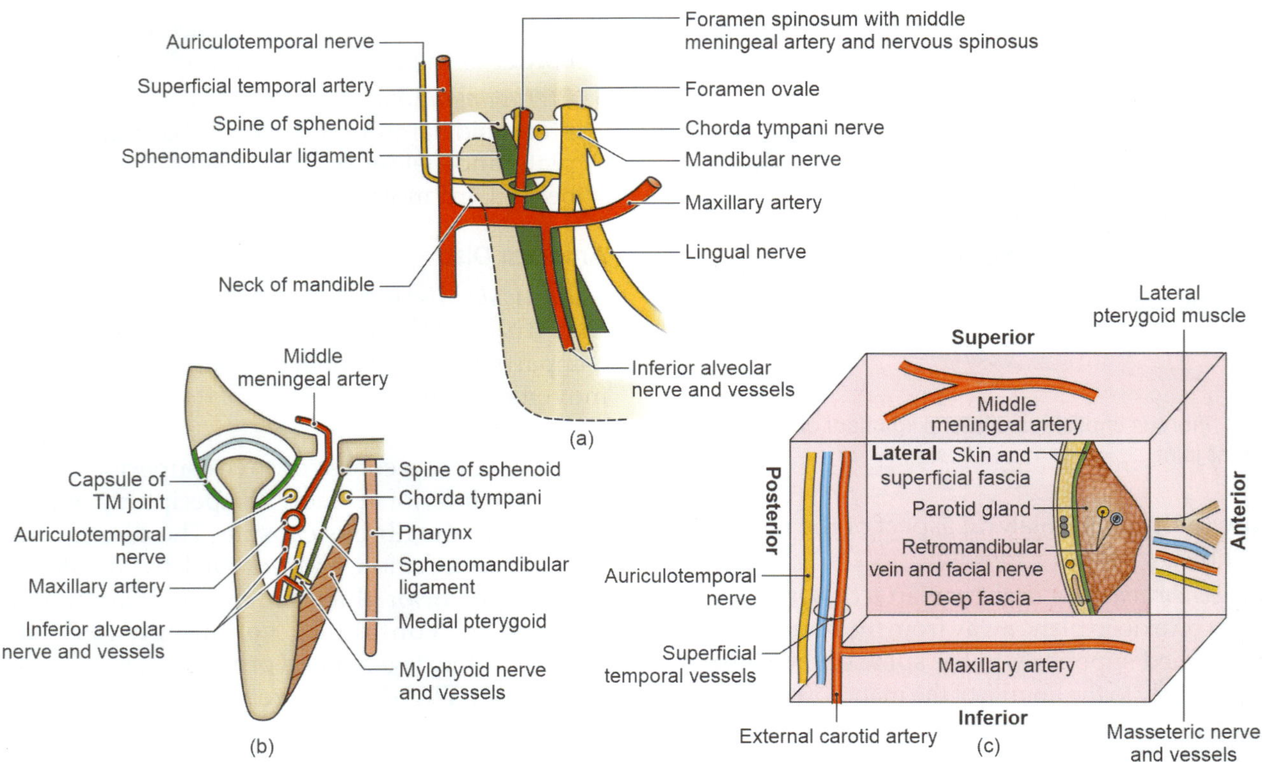

Figs 14.11a to c: (a and b) Superficial relations of the sphenomandibular ligament seen after removal of the lateral pterygoid; Medial relations of temporomandibular joint also seen; (c) Shows other relations of the joint

acid. The lining of fluid on the articulating surfaces decreases friction during joint motion and joint compression.

Histology: The condyle of mandible is composed of cancellous bone. It is covered by a thin layer of compact bone. The red bone marrow inside the condyle is cellular or myeloid in type.

The roof of the mandibular fossa consists of a thin layer of compact bone.

The articular eminence is also composed of cancellous bone covered by a layer of compact bone.

Articular disc: It is comprised of dense fibrous tissue with a few elastic fibres.

Synovial membrane: The synovial membrane lining the fibrous capsule folds to form synovial villi into the joint spaces. Synovial membrane comprises internal cells and sub-intimal connective tissue layer. The internal cells are like fibroblast, macrophage cells.

Relations of Temporomandibular Joint

Lateral

1 Skin and fasciae
2 Parotid gland (Fig. 14.11c)
3 Temporal branches of the facial nerve

Medial

1 The tympanic plate separates the joint from the internal carotid artery.
2 Spine of the sphenoid, with upper end of the sphenomandibular ligament attached to it (Fig. 14.11b).
3 Auriculotemporal and chorda tympani nerves.
4 Middle meningeal artery (Fig. 14.11a).

Anterior

1 Lateral pterygoid
2 Masseteric nerve and artery (Fig. 14.11c).

Posterior

1 The parotid gland separates the joint from the external auditory meatus.
2 Superficial temporal vessels
3 Auriculotemporal nerve (*see* Fig. 13.3a)

Superior

1 Middle cranial fossa
2 Middle meningeal vessels

Inferior

Maxillary artery and vein

Blood Supply

Branches from superficial temporal and maxillary arteries. Veins follow the arteries.

Nerve Supply

Auriculotemporal nerve and masseteric nerve.

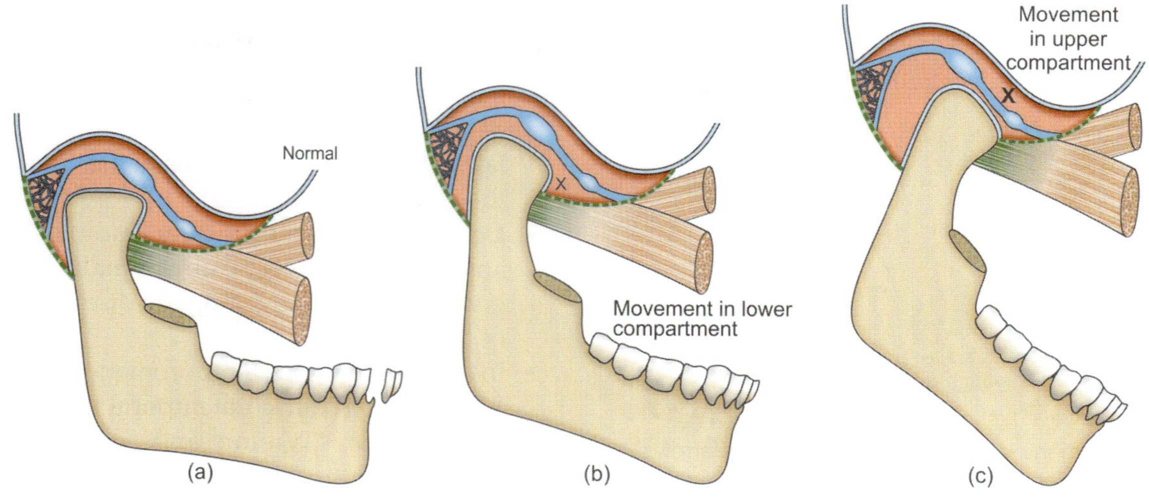

Figs 14.12a to c: Movements in lower and upper compartments during opening of the mouth

Movements

1 Depression (open mouth) (Figs 14.12a–c)
2 Elevation (closed mouth)
3 Protrusion (protraction of chin)
4 Retrusion (retraction of chin)
5 Lateral or side-to-side movements during chewing or grinding.

Movements of this joint can be palpated by putting finger at preauricular point or into external auditory meatus. The movements at the joint can be divided into those between the upper articular surface and the articular disc, i.e. meniscotemporal (upper) compartment and those between the disc and the head of the mandible, i.e. meniscomandibular (lower) compartment. Most movements occur simultaneously at the right and left temporomandibular joints.

In forward movement or protraction of the mandible, the articular disc with the head of the mandible glides forwards over the upper articular surface. Movement occurs in meniscotemporal compartment. In retraction, the articular disc glides backwards over the upper articular surface taking the head of mandible with it. Mandible rotates around a horizontal axis extending from left to right condyle.

In slight opening of the mouth or depression of the mandible, the head of the mandible moves on the undersurface of the disc like a hinge in lower compartment (Fig. 14.12b). The movement occurs around a vertical axis passing through the condyle and posterior border of the ramus of mandible. In wide opening of the mouth, this hinge-like movement is followed by gliding of the disc and the head of the mandible in upper compartment, as in protraction. At the end of this movement, the head comes to lie under the articular tubercle (Fig. 14.12c). These movements are reversed in closing the mouth or elevation of the mandible.

Chewing movements involve side-to-side movements of the mandible. In these movements, the head of (say) right side glides forwards along with the disc as in protraction, but the head of the left side merely rotates on a vertical axis. As a result of this, the chin moves forwards and to left side (the side on which no gliding has occurred). Alternate movements of this kind on the two sides result in side-to-side movements of the jaw. Here the mandible rotates around an imaginary axis running along the mid-sagittal plane.

Muscles Producing Movements

↓ *depression* is brought about mainly by the lateral pterygoid. The digastric, geniohyoid and mylohyoid muscles help when the mouth is opened wide or against resistance.

The origin of only lateral pterygoid is anterior, slightly lower and medial to its insertion. During contraction, it rotates the head of mandible and opens the mouth. During wide opening, it pulls the articular disc forwards. So, movement occurs in both the compartments. It is also done passively by gravity (Figs 14.10 and 14.13).

↑ *elevation* is brought about by the masseter, the anterior vertical, middle oblique fibres of temporalis, and the medial pterygoid muscles of both sides. These are antigravity muscles.

← *protrusion* is done by the lateral and medial pterygoids and superficial oblique fibres of masseter.

→ *retraction* is produced by the posterior horizontal fibres of the temporalis and deep vertical fibres of masseter.

Lateral or side-to-side movements, e.g. chewing from left side produced by right lateral pterygoid, right medial pterygoid which push the chin to left side. Then left temporalis (anterior fibres), left masseter (deep fibres) (↔) chew the food. Chewing from right side involves left lateral pterygoid, left medial

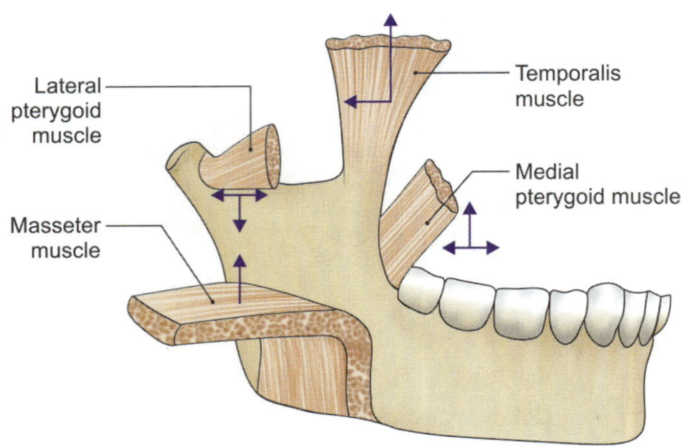

Fig. 14.13: Movements of temporomandibular joint (arrows) by muscles of mastication

pterygoid, right temporalis and right masseter. Since, so many muscles are involved, chewing becomes tiring.

Age Changes in TMJ

- The large marrow spaces in the condyle decrease in size as one advances in age.
- Red marrow gets replaced by fatty marrow.
- The trabeculae become thick
- The fibrocartilage covering the articular surface shows calcification.

TMJ Disorders

1. Inflammatory—arthritis
2. Congenital and developmental—hypoplasia, aplasia and hyperplasia
3. Related to intra articular disc—disc displacement, dislocation or deviation
4. Ankylosis—true/false/fibrous/bony
5. Neoplasia
6. Muscle related—spasm, myofascial pain

Myofascial Pain Dysfunction Syndrome (MPDS)

Features are:

1. Tenderness of muscles of mastication
2. Opening of mouth is limited
3. Joint sounds are produced
4. Seen more in females
5. May be related to stress
6. Occurs due to spasm of muscles of mastication
7. It is treated conservatively.

CLINICAL ANATOMY

- *Dislocation of mandible:* During excessive opening of the mouth, the head of the mandible of one or both sides may slip anteriorly into the infratemporal fossa, as a result of which there is inability to close the mouth. Reduction is done by depressing the jaw with the thumbs placed on the last molar teeth, and at the same time elevating the chin (Fig. 14.14).
- Derangement of the articular disc may result from any injury, like overclosure or malocclusion. This gives rise to clicking and pain during movements of the jaw.
- In operations on the temporomandibular joint, the VII nerve and auriculotemporal nerve, branch of mandibular division of V nerve should be preserved with care (Fig. 14.15).

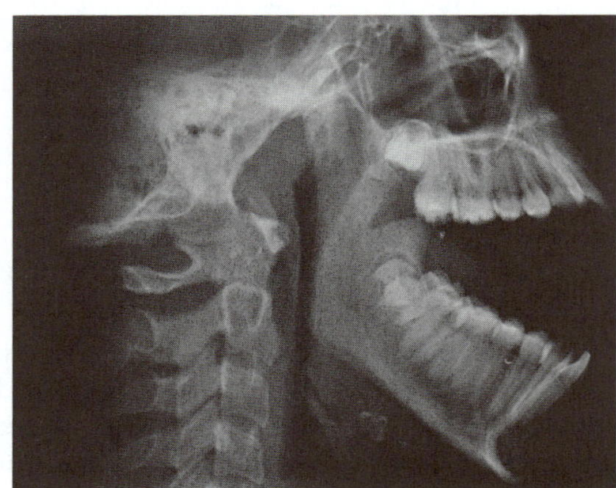

Fig. 14.14: Dislocation of the head of mandible

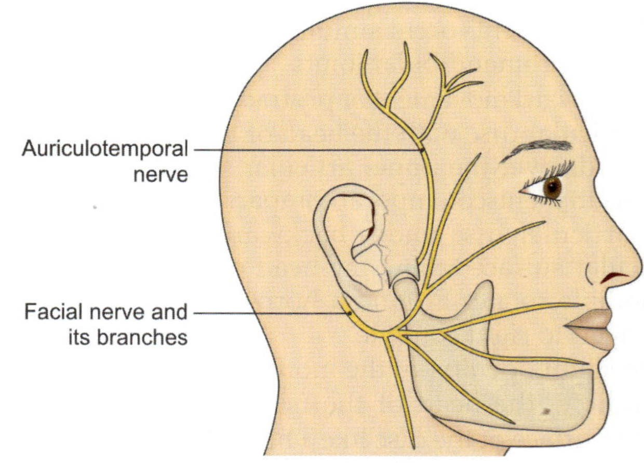

Fig. 14.15: Close relation of the two nerves to the temporomandibular joint

MANDIBULAR NERVE

This is the largest mixed branch of the trigeminal nerve. It is the nerve of the first branchial arch and supplies all structures derived from that arch. Otic and

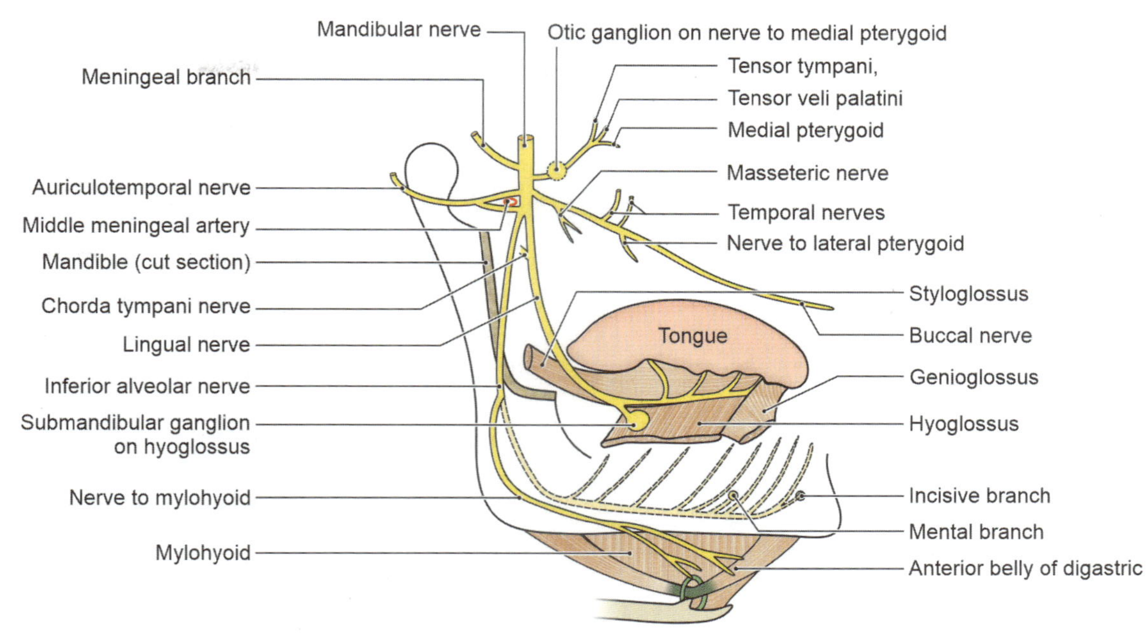

Fig. 14.16: Distribution of mandibular nerve (V3)

submandibular ganglia are associated with this nerve (Fig. 14.16).

Course and Relations

Mandibular nerve begins in the middle cranial fossa through a large sensory root and a small motor root. The sensory root arises from the lateral part of the trigeminal ganglion, and leaves the cranial cavity through the foramen ovale (Fig. 14.17).

The motor root lies deep to the trigeminal ganglion and to the sensory root. It also passes through the

DISSECTION

Identify middle meningeal artery arising from the maxillary artery and trace it till the foramen spinosum. Note the two roots of auriculotemporal nerve surrounding the artery. Trace the origin of the auriculotemporal nerve from mandibular nerve (Fig. 14.11). Dissect all the other branches of the nerve. Identify the chorda tympani nerve joining the lingual branch of mandibular nerve. Lift the trunk of mandibular nerve laterally and locate the otic ganglion *(refer to BDC App)*.

Trace all connections of the otic ganglion.

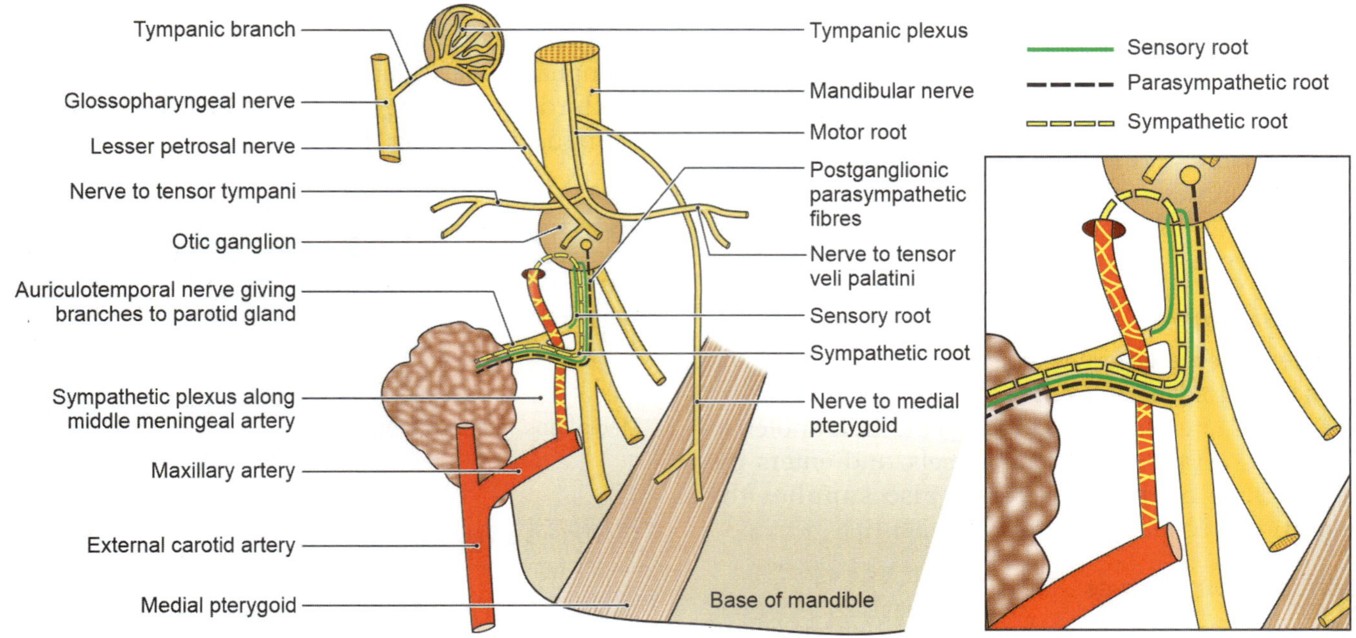

Fig. 14.17: Right otic ganglion seen from medial side

foramen ovale to join the sensory root just below the foramen thus forming the main trunk. The main trunk lies in the infratemporal fossa, on the tensor veli palatini, deep to the lateral pterygoid. After a short course, the main trunk divides into a small anterior trunk and a large posterior trunk (Fig. 14.16).

Branches

From the main trunk:

a. Meningeal branch
b. Nerve to the medial pterygoid.

From the anterior trunk:

a. A sensory branch—the buccal nerve
b. Motor branches—the masseteric and deep temporal nerves and the nerve to the lateral pterygoid.

From the posterior trunk:

a. Auriculotemporal,
b. Lingual, and
c. Inferior alveolar nerves.

Meningeal Branch or Nervus Spinosus

Meningeal branch enters the skull through the *foramen spinosum* with the middle meningeal artery and supplies the dura mater of the middle cranial fossa.

Nerve to Medial Pterygoid

Nerve to medial pterygoid arises close to the otic ganglion and supplies the medial pterygoid from its deep surface. This nerve gives a motor root to the otic ganglion which does not relay and supplies the tensor veli palatini, and the tensor tympani muscles (Fig. 14.17).

Buccal Nerve

Buccal nerve is the only sensory branch of the anterior division of the mandibular nerve. It passes between the two heads of the lateral pterygoid, runs downwards and forwards, and supplies the skin of cheek and mucous membrane related to the buccinator (Fig. 14.6). It also supplies the labial aspect of gums of molar and premolar teeth.

Masseteric Nerve

Masseteric nerve emerges at the upper border of the lateral pterygoid just in front of the temporomandibular joint, passes laterally through the mandibular notch in company with the masseteric vessels, and enters the deep surface of the masseter. It also supplies the temporomandibular joint (*see* Fig. 9.24).

Deep Temporal Nerves

Deep temporal nerves are two nerves—anterior and posterior. They pass between the skull and the lateral pterygoid, and enter the deep surface of the temporalis.

Nerve to Lateral Pterygoid

Nerve to lateral pterygoid enters the deep surface of the muscle.

Auriculotemporal Nerve

Auriculotemporal nerve arises by two roots which run backwards, encircle the middle meningeal artery, and unite to form a single trunk (Figs 14.11, 14.16 and 14.17). The nerve continues backwards between the neck of the mandible and the sphenomandibular ligament, above the maxillary artery. Behind the neck of the mandible, it turns upwards and ascends on the temple behind the superficial temporal vessels.

The *auricular part* of the nerve supplies the skin of the tragus; and the upper parts of the pinna, the external acoustic meatus and the tympanic membrane. (Note that the lower parts of these regions are supplied by the great auricular nerve and the auricular branch of the vagus nerve.) The *temporal part* supplies the skin of the temple (*see* Fig. 10.5). *In addition,* the auriculotemporal nerve also supplies the parotid gland (secretomotorand also sensory, Fig. 14.17) and the temporomandibular joint (*see* Table A.2).

Lingual Nerve

Lingual nerve (Table 14.3) is one of the two terminal branches of the posterior division of the mandibular nerve (Fig. 14.16). It is sensory to the anterior two-thirds of the tongue and to the floor of the mouth. However, the fibres of the chorda tympani (branch of facial nerve) which is secretomotor to the submandibular and sublingual salivary glands and gustatory to the anterior two-thirds of the tongue, are also distributed through the lingual nerve (Fig. 14.18).

Table 14.3: Branches of the mandibular nerve (CN V3)

Muscular	*Sensory*	*Others*
Temporalis and masseter	Meningeal Auriculotemporal	Carries taste fibres
Medial and lateral pterygoids	Inferior alveolar mental and incisive	Carries secreto-motor fibres
Tensor veli palatini and tensor tympani	Lingual	Articular
Mylohyoid and digastric (anterior belly)	Buccal	—

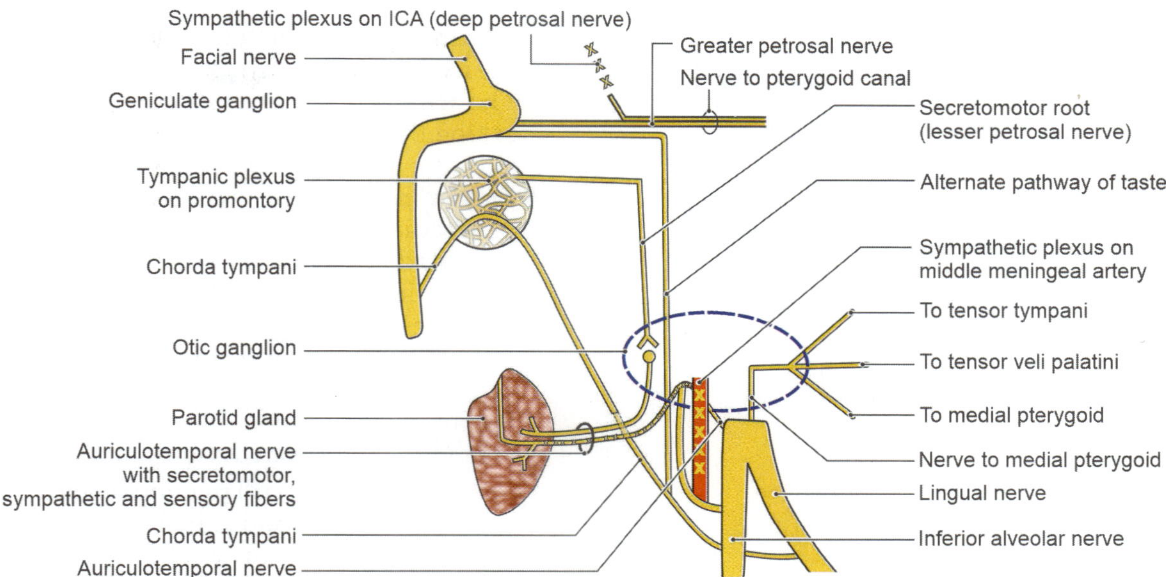

Fig. 14.18: Connections of otic ganglion (schematic)

Course

Lingual nerve begins 1 cm below the skull. About 2 cm below skull, it is joined by chorda tympani nerve at an acute angle. Then it lies in contact with mandible medial to 3rd *molar tooth*. Finally, it lies on surface of hyoglossus and genioglossus to reach the tongue.

Relations

It begins 1 cm below the skull. It runs first between the tensor veli palatini and the lateral pterygoid, and then between the lateral and medial pterygoids.

About 2 cm below the skull, it is joined by the chorda tympani nerve (Fig. 14.18).

Emerging at the lower border of the lateral pterygoid, the nerve runs downwards and forwards between the ramus of the mandible and the medial pterygoid. Next it lies in direct contact with the mandible, medial to the third molar tooth between the origins of the superior constrictor and the mylohyoid muscles (*see* Fig. 9.25).

It soon leaves the gum and runs over the hyoglossus deep to the mylohyoid. Finally, it lies on the surface of the genioglossus deep to the mylohyoid. Here it winds around the submandibular duct and divides into its terminal branches (*see* Fig. 15.4).

Inferior Alveolar Nerve

Inferior alveolar nerve is the larger terminal branch of the posterior division of the mandibular nerve (Fig. 14.16). It runs vertically downwards lateral to the medial pterygoid and to the sphenomandibular ligament. It enters the mandibular foramen and runs in the mandibular canal. It is accompanied by the inferior alveolar artery (*see* Fig. 9.25).

Branches

1. The *mylohyoid branch* contains all the motor fibres of the posterior division. It arises just before the inferior alveolar nerve and enters the mandibular foramen. It pierces the sphenomandibular ligament with the mylohyoid artery, runs in the mylohyoid groove, and supplies the mylohyoid muscle and the anterior belly of the digastric (Fig. 14.11b).
2. While running in the mandibular canal the inferior alveolar nerve gives branches that supply the lower teeth and gums.
3. The *mental nerve* emerges at the mental foramen and supplies the skin of the chin, and the skin and mucous membrane of the lower lip (Fig. 14.16).
4. Its incisive branch supplies the labial aspect of gums of canine and incisor teeth.

OTIC GANGLION

It is a peripheral parasympathetic ganglion which relays secretomotor fibres to the parotid gland. Topographically, it is intimately related to the mandibular nerve, but functionally, it is a part of the glossopharyngeal nerve (Figs 14.17 and 14.18).

Size and Situation

It is 2 to 3 mm in size, and is situated in the infratemporal fossa, just below the foramen ovale. It lies medial to the mandibular nerve, and lateral to the tensor veli palatini. It surrounds the origin of the nerve to the medial pterygoid (Fig. 14.16).

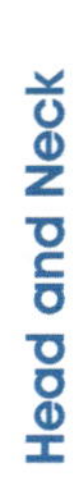

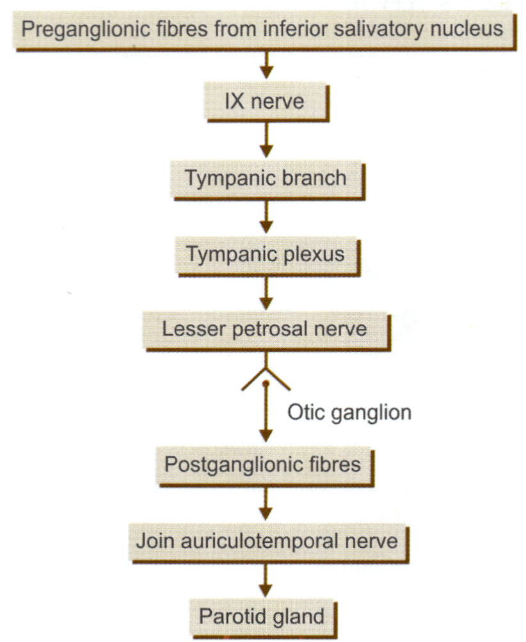

Flowchart 14.1: Secretomotor fibres for parotid gland

Connections and Branches

The secretomotor *motor or parasympathetic root* is formed by the lesser petrosal nerve. Its origin and course is shown in Flowchart 14.1.

The *sympathetic root* is derived from the plexus on the middle meningeal artery. It contains postganglionic fibres arising in the superior cervical ganglion. The fibres pass through the otic ganglion without relay and reach the parotid gland via the auriculotemporal nerve. They are vasomotor in function.

The *sensory root* comes from the auriculotemporal nerve and is sensory to the parotid gland.

Other fibres passing through the ganglion are as follows:

a. The nerve to medial pterygoid gives a motor root to the ganglion which passes through it without relay and supplies medially placed tensor veli palatini and laterally placed tensor tympani muscles.
b. The chorda tympani nerve is connected to the otic ganglion and also to the nerve of the pterygoid canal (Fig. 14.18). These connections provide an alternative pathway of taste from the anterior two-thirds of the tongue.

CLINICAL ANATOMY

- The motor part of the mandibular nerve is tested clinically by asking the patient to clench her/his teeth and then feeling for the contracting masseter and temporalis muscles on the two sides. If one masseter is paralysed, the jaw deviates to the paralysed side, on opening the mouth by the action of the normal lateral pterygoid of the opposite side. The activity of the pterygoid muscles is tested by asking the patient to move the chin from side-to-side.
- *Referred pain:* In cases with cancer of the tongue, pain radiates to the ear and to the temporal fossa, over the distribution of the auriculotemporal nerve as both lingual and auriculotemporal nerves are branches of mandibular nerve. Sometimes the lingual nerve is divided to relieve intractable pain of this kind. This may be done where the nerve lies in contact with the mandible below and behind the last molar tooth, covered only by mucous membrane.
- *Mandibular neuralgia:* Trigeminal neuralgia of the mandibular division is often difficult to treat. In such cases, the sensory root of the nerve may be divided behind the ganglion, and this is now the operation of choice when pain is confined to the distribution of the maxillary and mandibular nerves. During division, the ophthalmic fibres that lie in the superomedial part of the root are spared, to preserve the corneal reflex thus avoiding damage to the cornea (Fig. 14.19).
- Lingual nerve lies in contact with mandible, medial to the third molar tooth. In extraction of malplaced 'wisdom' tooth, care must be taken not to injure the lingual nerve (*see* Fig. 9.25). Its injury results in loss of all sensations from anterior two-thirds of the tongue.

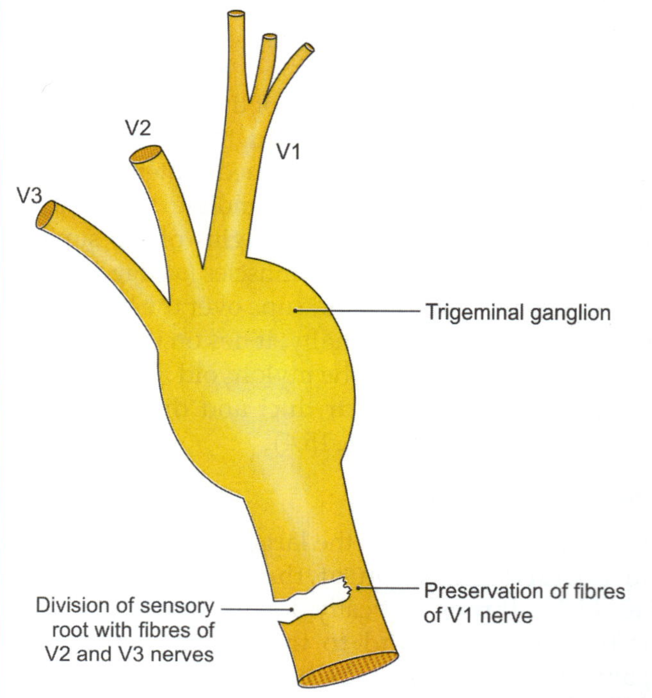

Fig. 14.19: Partial cutting of the sensory root of trigeminal nerve

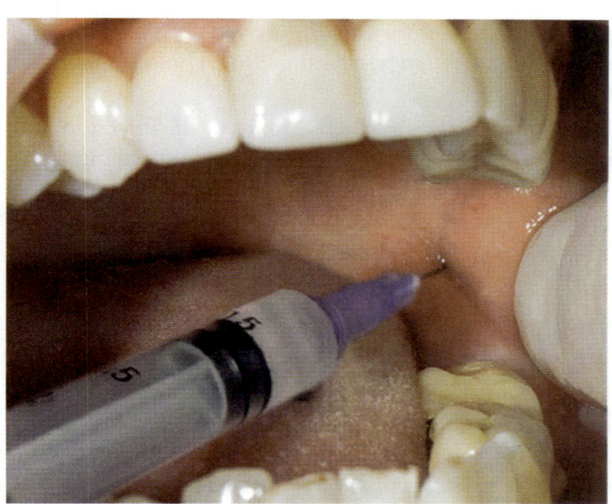

Fig. 14.20: Injection given in mandibular foramen for anaesthetising the inferior alveolar nerve before extraction of last molar tooth

- A lesion at the foramen ovale leads to paraesthesia along the mandible, tongue, temporal region and paralysis of the muscles of mastication. This also leads to loss of jaw-jerk reflex.
- The mandibular nerve supplies both the efferent and afferent loops of the jaw-jerk reflex, as it is a mixed nerve. Tapping the chin causes contraction of the pterygoid muscles.
- In extraction of mandibular teeth, inferior alveolar nerve needs to be anaesthetised. The drug is given into the nerve before it enters the mandibular canal (Fig. 14.20).
- *Inferior alveolar nerve:* Inferior alveolar nerve as it travels the mandibular canal can be damaged by the fracture of the mandible. This injury can be assessed by testing sensation over the chin.
- During extraction of the 3rd molar, the buccal nerve may get involved by the local anaesthesia causing temporary numbness of the cheek.

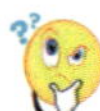

Mnemonics

Function of Lateral (La) vs. Medial (Me) pterygoid muscles

"La": Jaw is open, so lateral pterygoid opens mouth.
"Me": Jaw is closed, so medial pterygoid closes the mouth.

V3: Sensory branches

"**B**uccaneers **A**re **I**nferior **L**inguists"

Buccal
Auriculotemporal
Inferior alveolar
Lingual

Maxillary Artery Branches

"DAM I AM Piss Drunk But Stupid Drunk"

Deep auricular
Anterior tympanic
Middle meningeal
Inferior alveolar
Accessory meningeal
Masseteric
Pterygoid
Deep temporal
Buccal
Sphenopalatine
Descending palatine

V3 Innervated muscles (branchial arch 1 derivatives)

M.D. My TV

Mastication (masseter, temporalis, lateral and medial, pterygoids)
Digastric (anterior belly)
Mylohyoid
tensor **T**ympani
tensor **V**eli palatini

FACTS TO REMEMBER

- Mandibular nerve is the only mixed branch of trigeminal nerve.
- The nerve is associated with two parasympathetic ganglia, i.e. otic and submandibular ganglia.
- Maxillary artery gives many branches; some accompany branches of maxillary nerve and others branches of mandibular nerve as there is no mandibular artery.
- Only muscle of mastication which depresses the TMJ is the lateral pterygoid muscle.
- Spine of sphenoid is related to chorda tympani and auriculotemporal nerves. Injury to the spine will hamper the secretion of three salivary glands.
- Auriculotemporal nerve and branches of facial nerve are related to temporomandibular joint.

CLINICOANATOMICAL PROBLEM

A patient of carcinoma in anterior two-thirds of tongue complains of pain in his lower teeth, temporal region and the temporomandibular joint.

- Why is pain of tongue referred to lower teeth?
- Which are the other areas of referred pain?

Ans: Sensations from anterior two-thirds of the tongue are carried by lingual, branch of mandibular nerve. Since there are too many pain impulses due to disease, these impulses course through other branches of the nerve, where it gets referred. So pain is felt in lower teeth, from where sensations are carried by inferior alveolar nerve. The mandibular nerve also carries sensation from temporomandibular joint and temporal region so the pain also gets referred to these regions.

Examples of referred pain are:
- Pain of gallbladder is referred to right shoulder.
- Pain of myocardial ischaemia is felt in the chest and medial side of left arm.
- Pain of foregut-derived organs is felt in epigastrium.
- Pain of midgut-derived organs is felt in periumbilical region.
- Pain of hindgut-derived organs is felt in suprapubic region.

FURTHER READING

- Cheung LK. The vascular anatomy of the human temporalis muscle: Implications for surgical splitting techniques. Int J Oral Maxillofac Surg 1996;25:414–21.

  A cadaveric study of 15 cadavers/30 temporalis muscle specimens to assess the territory supplied by each of the three principal nutrient arteries (angiosomes) and the clinical implications of the results.
- Langdon J, Berkovitz BKB, Moxham BJ. Infection and the infratemporal fossa and associated tissue spaces. In: Langdon J, Berkovitz BKB, Moxham BJ (eds). Surgical Anatomy of the Infratemporal Fossa. London: M. Duniatz, 2002; pp 77–99.

  A chapter that describes the tissue spaces in the floor of the mouth and how they become involved in the spread of infection.
- Lang J. Mandible. In: Clinical Anatomy of the Masticatory Apparatus and Peripharyngeal Spaces. New York: Thieme; 1995; pp. 19–41.

  Detailed anatomical descriptions including measurements of the maxilla and mandible, the infratemporal fossa and its contents, and the temporomandibular joint, relating these to clinical practice.
- Nitzan DW. The process of lubrication impairment and its involvement in temporomandibular joint disc displacement. J Oral Maxillofac Surg 2001;59:36–45.

  An overview of the lubrication impairment and its possible role in disc displacement.

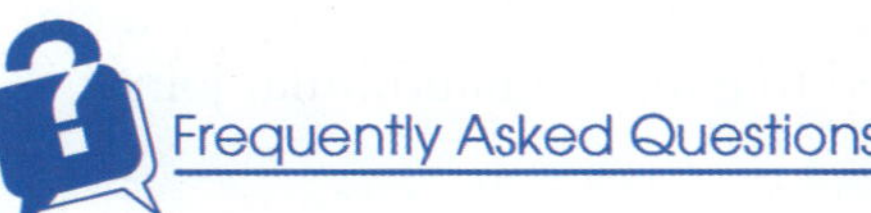

Frequently Asked Questions

1. Describe temporomandibular joint under the following headings:
   a. Bones taking part
   b. Capsule and ligaments
   c. Relations
   d. Movements and their muscles
   e. Clinical anatomy
2. Describe muscles of mastication under the following headings:
   a. Origin
   b. Insertion
   c. Actions
   d. Clinical anatomy
3. Write short notes on/enumerate:
   a. Otic ganglion and its connections
   b. Branches of 1st part of maxillary artery
   c. Branches of mandibular nerve
   d. Branches of 3rd part of maxillary artery
   e. Sphenomandibular ligament and the structures piercing it

Multiple Choice Questions

1. Action of lateral pterygoid muscle is:
   a. Elevation and retraction of mandible
   b. Depression and retraction of mandible
   c. Elevation and protrusion of mandible
   d. Depression and protrusion of mandible
2. Which of the following muscles is used for opening the mouth?
   a. Medial pterygoid b. Temporalis
   c. Lateral pterygoid d. Masseter
3. Which of the following ligaments is not a ligament of temporomandibular joint?
   a. Pterygomandibular
   b. Sphenomandibular
   c. Lateral ligament
   d. Stylomandibular
4. Which one is not a branch of maxillary artery?
   a. Anterior tympanic b. Anterior ethmoidal
   c. Middle meningeal d. Inferior alveolar
5. Which of the following is not a muscle of mastication?
   a. Medial pterygoid
   b. Masseter
   c. Temporalis
   d. Orbicularis oris
6. Dislocated mandible can be reversed by:
   a. Depressing the jaw posteriorly and elevating the chin
   b. Depressing the jaw and depressing the chin
   c. Elevating the jaw and elevating the chin
   d. Depressing the chin and elevating the jaw posteriorly
7. Nervus spinosus is a branch of:
   a. Maxillary nerve b. Mandibular nerve
   c. Ophthalmic nerve d. 2nd cervical nerve
8. Lingual nerve is the branch of:
   a. Facial nerve
   b. Glossopharyngeal nerve
   c. Mandibular nerve
   d. Hypoglossal nerve
9. Lingual nerve can be pressed against a bone inside the mouth near the roots of the:
   a. Third upper molar tooth
   b. Second upper molar tooth
   c. Third lower molar tooth
   d. First lower molar tooth
10. Nerve piercing sphenomandibular ligament is:
   a. Nerve to mylohyoid
   b. Inferior alveolar
   c. Buccal
   d. Lingual

Answers

1. d **2.** c **3.** a **4.** b **5.** d **6.** a **7.** b **8.** c **9.** c **10.** a

VIVA VOCE

- Which parasympathetic ganglion has four roots? Name four roots and branches of the ganglion.
- Which muscle of mastication acts to open the mouth?
- Name the branches of all the parts of the maxillary artery.
- Which is the artery of epistaxis?
- Name the two compartments of temporomandibular joint. What movements occur in these compartments?
- Name the muscles supplied by mandibular division of trigeminal nerve.
- What are the nerves related to the spine of sphenoid and what are their clinical importance?
- How does TMJ get dislocated? How can the dislocation be corrected?
- Which are the nerves related to TMJ?

VIDEO 3.6 Infratemporal fossa, muscles of mastication, mandibular nerve

Chapter 15

Submandibular Region

"Life is too short for men to take it too seriously."
—George Bernard Shaw

INTRODUCTION

Submandibular region includes deeper structures in the area between the mandible and hyoid bone including the floor of the mouth and the root of the tongue.

The submandibular region contains the suprahyoid muscles, submandibular and sublingual salivary glands and submandibular ganglion. Chorda tympani nerve from facial nerve provides preganglionic secretomotor fibres to the glands. Chorda tympani also carries fibres of sensation of taste from anterior two-thirds of tongue except from the circumvallate papillae. Taste from the circumvallate papillae is carried by the glosso-pharyngeal nerve.

SUPRAHYOID MUSCLES

Features

The suprahyoid muscles are the digastric, the stylohyoid, the mylohyoid and the geniohyoid. The muscles are in following layers.

1 First layer formed by *digastric* (Greek two bellies) and stylohyoid (Fig. 15.1).
2 Second layer formed by *mylohyoid* (Greek pertaining to hyoid bone) (Fig. 15.2).
3 Third layer formed by geniohyoid and hyoglossus (Fig. 15.4).
4 Fourth layer formed by genioglossus (Fig. 15.4). The muscles are described in Table 15.1.

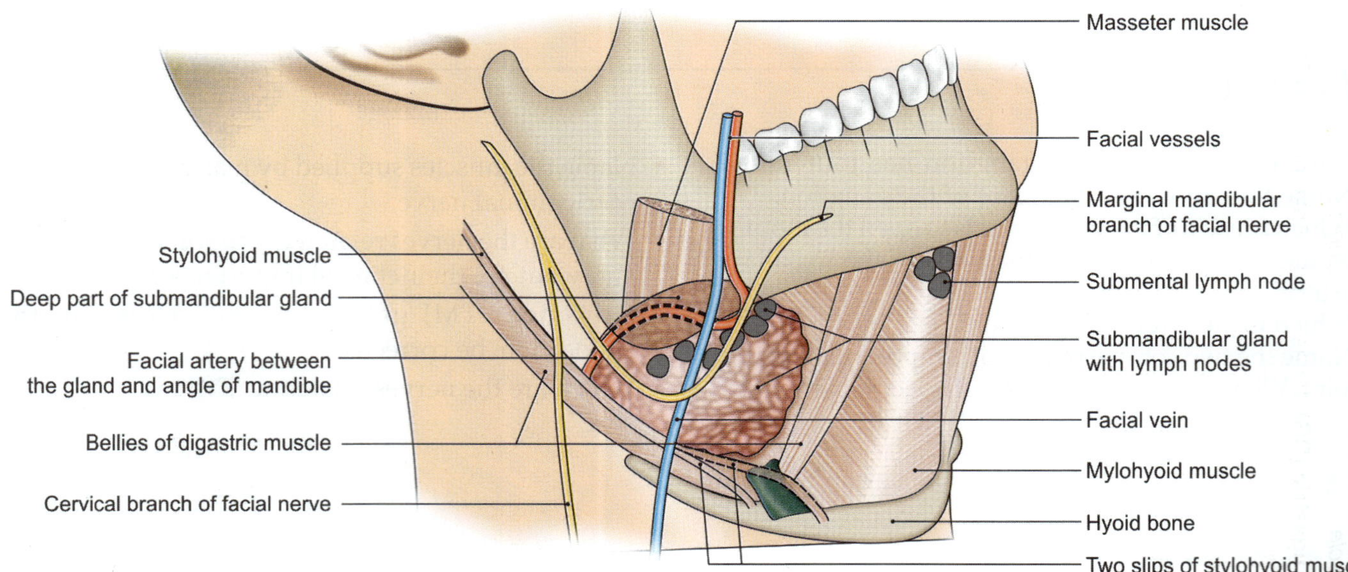

Fig. 15.1: Relation of marginal mandibular branch of facial nerve to the submandibular gland and its lymph nodes

Table 15.1: Suprahyoid muscles

Muscle	*Origin*	*Fibres*	*Insertion*	*Nerve supply*	*Actions*
1. **Digastric** (DG): It has two bellies united by an intermediate tendon (Figs 15.1 and 15.2)	a. Anterior belly (DGA): From digastric fossa of mandible b. Posterior belly (DGP): From mastoid notch of temporal bone	a. Anterior belly runs downwards and backwards b. Posterior belly runs downwards and forwards	Both heads meet at the intermediate tendon which perforates SH and is held by a fibrous pulley to the hyoid bone	a. Anterior belly by nerve to mylohyoid b. Posterior belly by facial nerve	a. Depresses mandible when mouth is opened widely or against resistance; it is secondary to lateral pterygoid b. Elevates hyoid bone
2. **Stylohyoid** (SH): Small muscle, lies on upper border of DGP (Fig. 15.2)	Posterior surface of styloid process	Tendon is perforated by DGP tendon	Junction of body and greater cornua of hyoid bone (*see* Fig. 9.47)	Facial nerve	a. Pulls hyoid bone upwards and backwards b. With other hyoid muscles, it fixes the hyoid bone
1 and 2 are muscles of 1st muscular plane					
3. **Mylohyoid** (MH): Flat, triangular muscle; two mylohyoids form floor of mouth cavity, deep to DGA (Figs 15.1 and 15.2)	Mylohyoid line of mandible (*see* Fig. 9.23b)	Fibres run medially and slightly downwards	a. Posterior fibres: Body of hyoid bone (*see* Fig. 9.47) b. Middle and anterior fibres; median raphe, between mandible and hyoid bone	Nerve to mylohyoid	a. Elevates floor of mouth in first stage of deglutition b. Helps in depression of mandible, and elevation of hyoid bone
3 is muscle of 2nd muscular plane					
4. **Geniohyoid** (GH): Short and narrow muscle; lies above medial part of MH (Fig. 15.4)	Inferior mental spine (genial tubercle)	Runs backwards and downwards	Anterior surface of body of hyoid bone	C1 through hypoglossal nerve	a. Elevates hyoid bone b. May depress mandible when hyoid is fixed
5. **Hyoglossus**: It is a muscle of tongue. It forms important landmark in this region (Fig. 15.4)	Whole length of greater cornua and lateral part of body of hyoid bone (*see* Fig. 9.47)	Fibres run upwards and forwards	Side of tongue between styloglossus and inferior longitudinal muscle of tongue	Hypoglossal (XII) nerve	Depresses tongue makes dorsum convex, retracts the protruded tongue
4 and 5 are muscles of 3rd muscular plane					
6. **Genioglossus:** It is the bulkiest muscle of tongue. It is fan-shaped	Upper genial tubercle of mandible	Fibres radiate	Upper fibres pass upwards and forwards to tip of tongue. Middle fibres along whole length of dorsum. Lower fibres into body of hyoid.	Hypoglossal (XII)	Pulls posterior part of tongue forwards, i.e. protrudes tongue. It is a life-saving muscle
6 is a muscle of 4th muscular plane.					

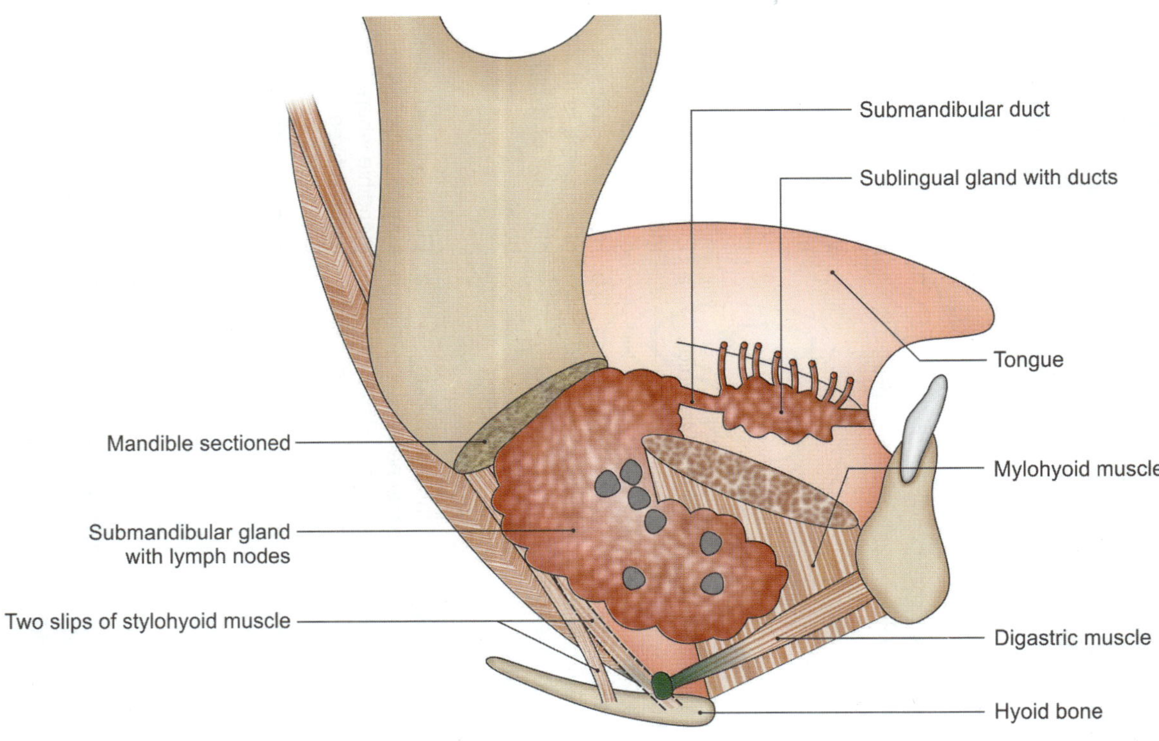

Fig. 15.2: Mylohyoid muscle dividing the gland into two parts

DISSECTION

Cut the facial artery and vein present at the anteroinferior angle of masseter muscle. Separate the origin of anterior belly of digastric muscle from the digastric fossa near the symphysis menti. Push the mandible upwards. Clean and expose the posterior belly of digastric muscle and its accompanying stylohyoid muscle. Identify the digastrics, stylohyoid, mylohyoid, geniohyoid, and hyoglossus *(refer to BDC App)*.

Relations of Posterior Belly of Digastric

Superficial

1 Mastoid process with the sternocleidomastoid, splenius capitis and the longissimus capitis (Fig. 15.3, also *see* Fig. 13.4a)
2 The stylohyoid
3 The parotid gland with retromandibular vein
4 Submandibular salivary gland (Fig. 15.3) and lymph nodes
5 Angle of the mandible with medial pterygoid

Deep

1 Transverse process of the atlas with superior oblique and the rectus capitis lateralis
2 Internal carotid, external carotid, lingual, facial and occipital arteries
3 Internal jugular vein
4 Vagus, accessory and hypoglossal cranial nerves (Fig. 15.3)
5 The hyoglossus muscle

Upper Border

1 The posterior auricular artery (*see* Fig. 12.14)
2 The stylohyoid muscle

Lower Border

Lower border is related to occipital artery (*see* Fig. 12.14).

Relations of Mylohyoid

Superficial

1 Anterior belly of digastric (Fig. 15.1)
2 Superficial part of the submandibular salivary gland
3 Mylohyoid nerve and vessels
4 Submental branch of the facial artery

Deep

1 Hyoglossus with its superficial relations, namely the styloglossus, the lingual nerve, the submandibular ganglion, the deep part of the submandibular salivary gland, the submandibular duct, the hypoglossal nerve, and the venae comitantes hypoglossi (Figs 15.2 and 15.4).
2 The genioglossus with its superficial relations, namely the sublingual salivary gland, the lingual nerve, submandibular duct, the lingual artery, and the hypoglossal nerve (Fig. 15.4).

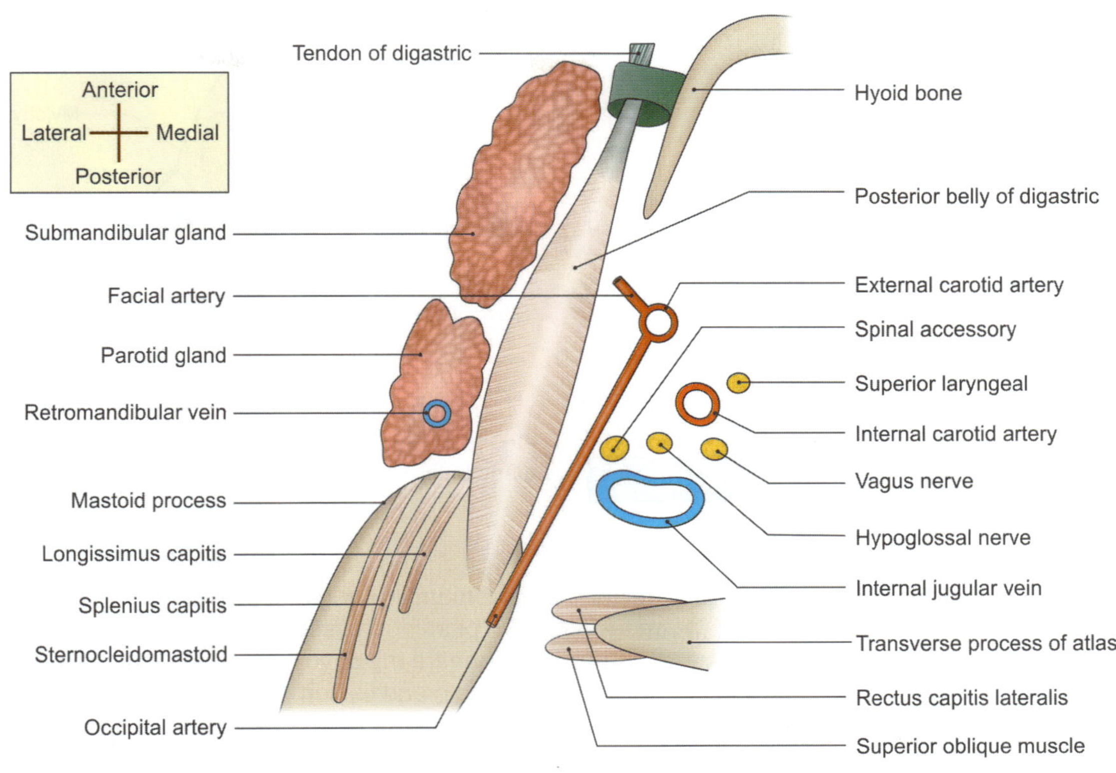

Fig. 15.3: Posterior belly of the digastric muscle, and structures related to it, seen from below

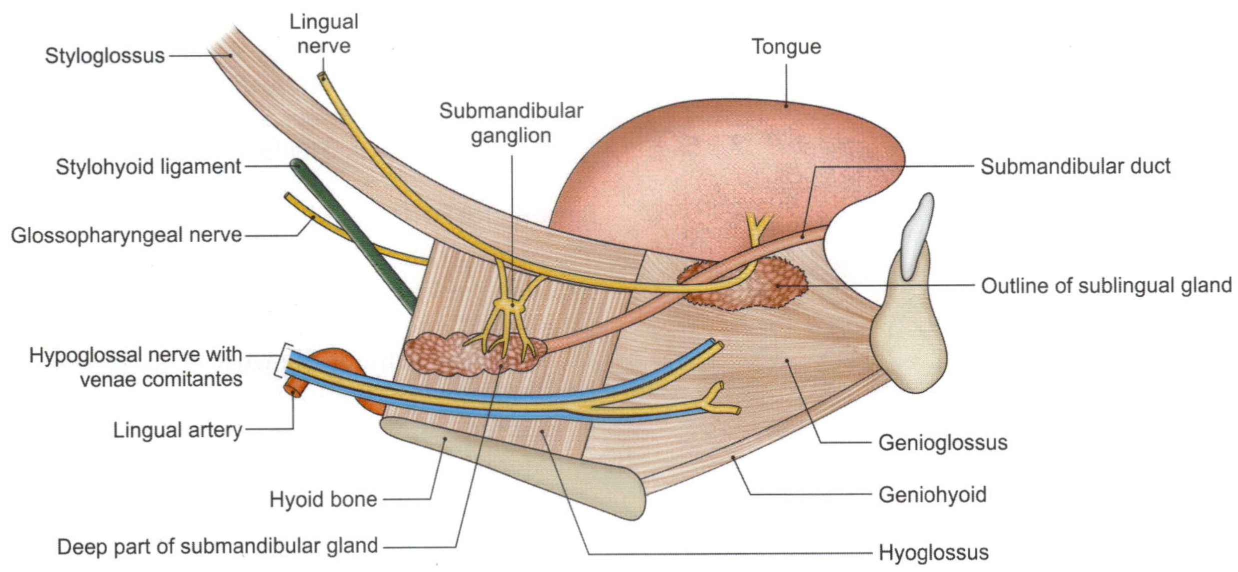

Fig. 15.4: Submandibular region showing the superficial relations of the hyoglossus and genioglossus muscles, the deep part of submandibular gland is also shown

Relations of Hyoglossus

Superficial

Styloglossus, lingual nerve, submandibular ganglion, deep part of submandibular gland, submandibular duct, hypoglossal nerve and veins accompanying it (Fig. 15.4).

Deep

1 Inferior longitudinal muscle of the tongue

2 Genioglossus
3 Middle constrictor of the pharynx
4 Glossopharyngeal nerve
5 Stylohyoid ligament
6 Lingual artery

Structures passing deep to posterior border of hyoglossus, from above downwards:

1 Glossopharyngeal nerve
2 Stylohyoid ligament
3 Lingual artery (Fig. 15.4).

SUBMANDIBULAR SALIVARY GLAND

Features

This is a large salivary gland, situated in the anterior part of the digastric triangle. The gland is about the size of a walnut weighing about 15 to 20 g. It is roughly J-shaped, being indented by the posterior border of the mylohyoid which divides it into a larger part superficial to the muscle, and a small part lying deep to the muscle (Fig. 15.5).

***Coverings*:** The gland is partially enclosed between two layers of deep cervical fascia. The superficial (Fig. 15.6) layer of fascia covers the inferior surface of the gland and is attached to the base of the mandible. The deep layer covers the medial surface of the gland and is superiorly to the mylohyoid line of the mandible (Fig. 15.6).

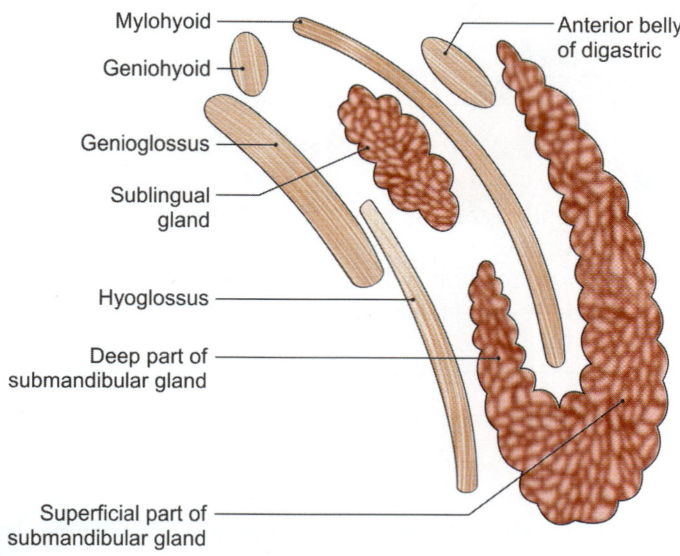

Fig. 15.5: Horizontal section through the submandibular region showing the location of the submandibular and sublingual glands

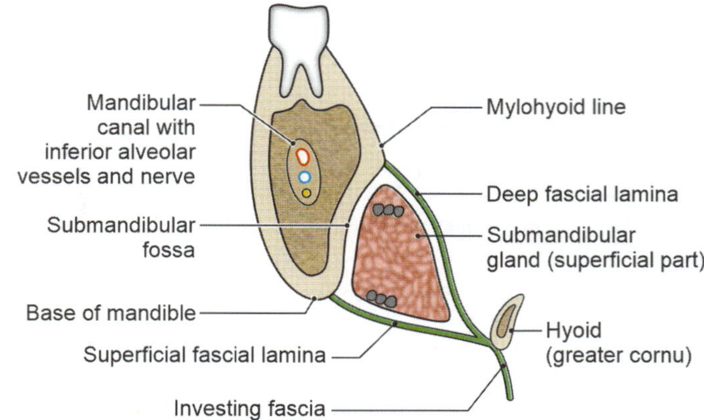

Fig. 15.6: Fascial coverings of the superficial part of the submandibular salivary gland

DISSECTION

Submandibular gland is seen in the digastric triangle. On pushing the superficial part of the gland posteriorly, the entire mylohyoid muscle is exposed. The deep part of the gland lies on the superior surface of the muscle. Separate the facial artery from the deep surface of gland and identify its branches in neck. The hyoglossus muscle is recognised as a quadrilateral muscle lying on deeper plane than mylohyoid muscle. Identify lingual nerve with submandibular ganglion, and hypoglossal nerve running on the hyoglossus muscle from lateral to the medial side. Deep part of gland and its duct are also visible on this surface of hyoglossus muscle (Fig. 15.4).

Carefully release the hyoglossus muscle from the hyoid bone and reflect it towards the tongue. Note the structures deep to the muscle, e.g. genioglossus muscle, lingual artery, vein and middle constrictor of the pharynx.

Superficial Part

This part of the gland fills the digastric triangle. It extends superiorly deep to the mandible up to the mylohyoid line. Inferiorly: It overlaps stylohyoid and the posterior belly of digastric (Figs 15.1 and 15.2). It has three surfaces:

a. Inferior (Fig. 15.1)
b. Lateral
c. Medial.

Relations

The **inferior surface** is covered by:

a. Skin
b. Platysma
c. Cervical branch of the facial nerve
d. Deep fascia
e. Facial vein (Fig. 15.7)
f. Submandibular lymph nodes (Fig. 15.1)

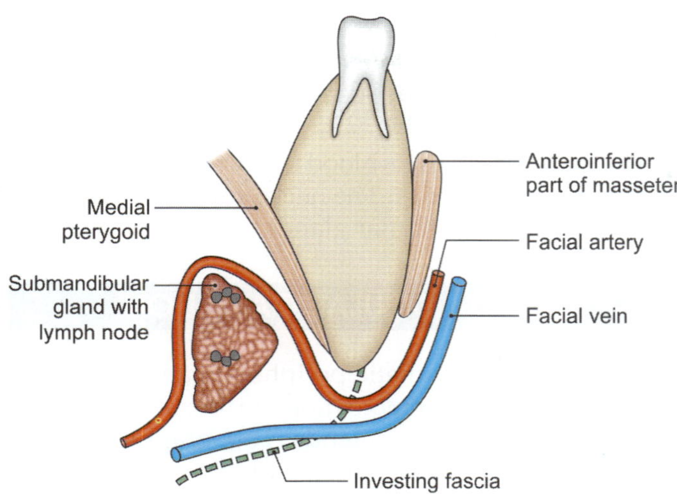

Fig. 15.7: Relationship of the facial vessels to the submandibular gland and to the mandible

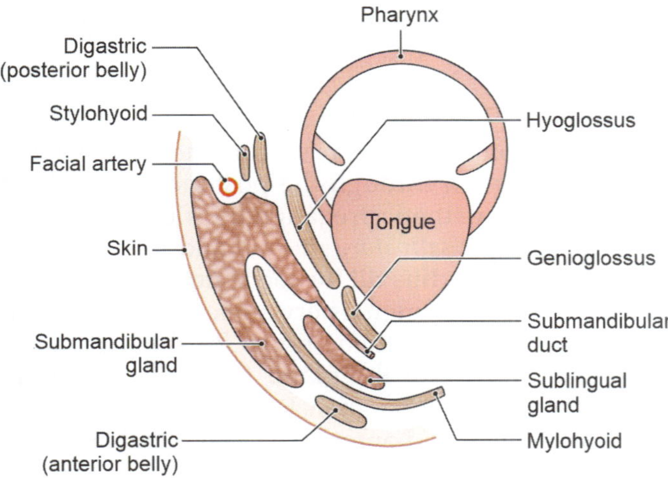

Fig. 15.8: Schematic horizontal section through the submandibular region

The **lateral surface** is related to:

a. The submandibular fossa on the mandible
b. Insertion of the medial pterygoid (Fig. 15.7)
c. The facial artery (Figs 15.7 and 15.8).

The **medial surface** is related to:

- *Anterior part:* Mylohyoid, submental branch of facial artery, mylohyoid nerve and vessels
- *Middle part:* Hyoglossus, styloglossus, lingual artery, XII nerve
- *Posterior part:* Stylohyoid, styloglossus, IX nerve.

Deep Part

This part is small in size. It lies deep to the mylohyoid, and superficial to the hyoglossus and the styloglossus (Fig. 15.4). Posteriorly, it is continuous with the superficial part around the posterior border of the mylohyoid (Fig. 15.5). Anteriorly, it extends up to the posterior end of the sublingual gland.

Relations

Present in between mylohyoid and hyoglossus.

Laterally – Mylohyoid
Medially – Hyoglossus
Above – Lingual nerve with submandibular ganglion
Below – Hypoglossal nerve

Blood Supply and Lymphatic Drainage

The submandibular gland is supplied by the facial artery.

The facial artery arises from the external carotid just above the tip of the greater cornua of the hyoid bone.

The *cervical part* of the facial artery runs upwards on the superior constrictor of pharynx deep to the posterior belly of the digastric, and stylohyoid to the ramus of the mandible. It grooves the posterior end of the submandibular salivary gland. Next the artery makes an S-bend (two loops) first winding down over the submandibular gland, and then up over the base of the mandible (Figs 15.7 and 15.8). Facial artery is palpable on the base of mandible at the anteroinferior angle of masseter muscle.

The veins drain into the common facial or lingual vein.

Lymph passes to submandibular lymph nodes.

Nerve Supply

It is supplied by branches from the submandibular ganglion. These branches convey:

1. Secretomotor fibres (Fig. 15.9)
2. Sensory fibres from the lingual nerve
3. Vasomotor sympathetic fibres from the plexus on the facial artery.

The secretomotor pathway is shown in Flowchart 15.1.

SUBMANDIBULAR DUCT/WHARTON'S DUCT (ENGLISH SCIENTIST: 1614–73)

It is thin walled, and is about 5 cm long. It emerges at the anterior end of the deep part of the gland and runs upwards and forwards on the hyoglossus, between the lingual and hypoglossal nerves. At the anterior border of the hyoglossus, the duct is crossed by the lingual nerve (Fig. 15.4). It opens on the floor of the mouth, on the summit of the sublingual papilla, at the side of the frenulum of the tongue (*see* Fig. 25.2).

SUBLINGUAL SALIVARY GLAND

This is smallest of the three salivary glands. It is almond-shaped and weighs about 3 to 4 g. It lies above the mylohyoid, below the mucosa of the floor of the

Flowchart 15.1: Secretomotor fibres to the glands

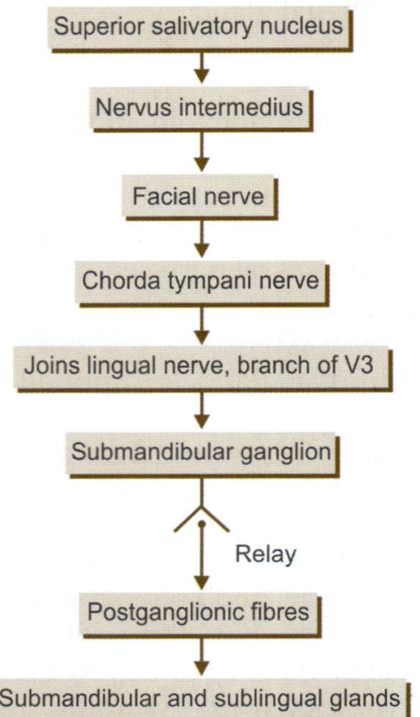

mouth, medial to the sublingual fossa of the mandible and lateral to the genioglossus (Figs 15.2, 15.4 and 15.8).

Relations

Front – Meets opposite side gland
Behind – Comes in contact with deeper part of submandibular gland
Above – Mucous membrane of mouth
Below – Mylohyoid muscle
Lateral – Sublingual fossa
Medial – Genioglossus muscles (Fig. 15.8)

About 15 ducts emerge from the gland. Most of them open directly into the floor of the mouth on the summit of the sublingual fold. A few of them join the submandibular duct (*see* Fig. 25.2).

The gland receives its blood supply from the lingual and submental arteries. The nerve supply is similar to that of the submandibular gland.

SUBMANDIBULAR GANGLION

This is a parasympathetic peripheral ganglion. It is a relay station for secretomotor fibres to the submandibular and sublingual salivary glands. Topographically, it is related to the lingual nerve, but functionally, it is connected to the chorda tympani branch of the facial nerve (Flowchart 15.1).

The fusiform ganglion lies on the hyoglossus muscle just above the deep part of the submandibular salivary gland, suspended from the lingual nerve by two roots (Fig. 15.9).

Connections and Branches

1 The secretomotor fibres pass from the lingual nerve to the ganglion through the posterior root. These are parasympathetic preganglionic fibres that arise in the *superior salivatory nucleus* and pass through nervus intermedius till the facial nerve, the chorda tympani and the lingual nerve to reach the ganglion for relay. Postganglionic fibres for the submandibular gland reach the gland through five or six branches from the ganglion. Postganglionic fibres for the sublingual and anterior lingual glands re-enter

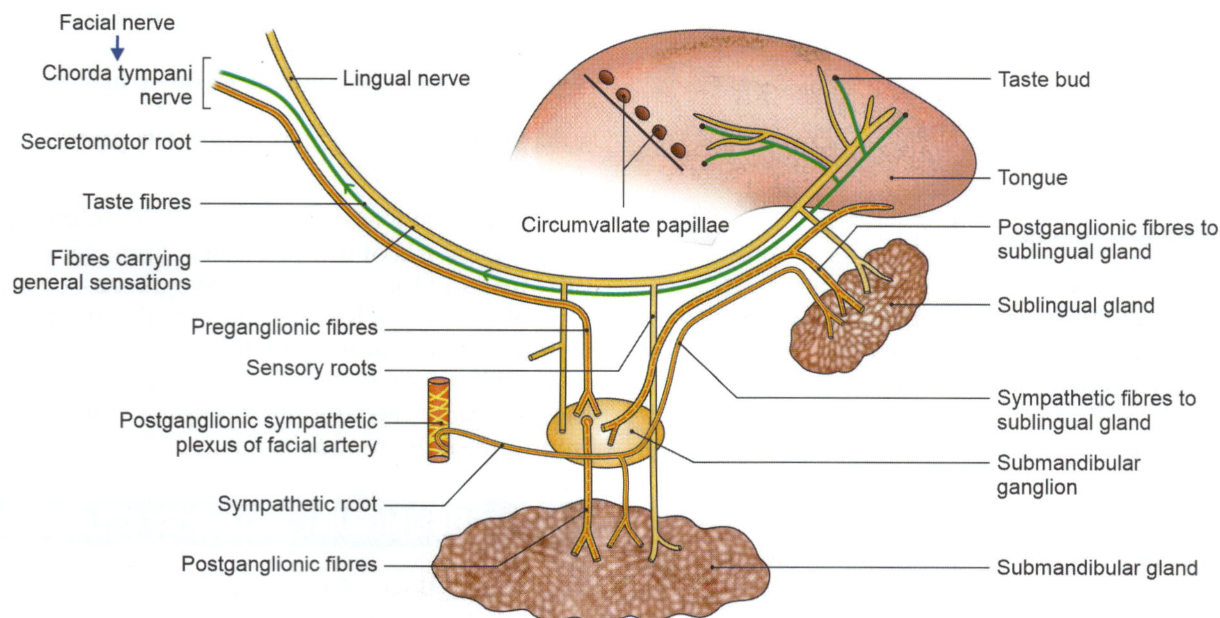

Fig. 15.9: Connection of the submandibular ganglion

the lingual nerve through the anterior root and travel to the gland through the distal part of the lingual nerve (Flowchart 15.1).

2 The sympathetic fibres are derived from the plexus around the facial artery. It contains postganglionic fibres arising in the superior cervical ganglion which arise from T1 segment of spinal cord and synapse in superior cervical sympathetic ganglion. They pass through submandibular ganglion without relay, and supply vasomotor fibres to the submandibular and sublingual glands (Fig. 15.9).

3 Sensory fibres reach the ganglion through the lingual nerve (Table 15.2). Comparison of three salivary glands is depicted in Table 15.2.

HISTOLOGY

The histological structure of parotid, submandibular and sublingual salivary glands is shown in Figs 15.10–15.12.

Table 15.2: Comparison of the three salivary glands

	Parotid	*Submandibular*	*Sublingual*
Location	In relation to external ear, angle of mandible, mastoid process (*see* Fig. 13.1)	Lies in submandibular fossa close to angle of mandible (Fig. 15.6)	Lies in sublingual fossa on the base of the mandible (Fig. 15.2)
Size	Largest	Medium sized	Smallest
Relation to fascia	Enclosed by investing layer of cervical fascia	Enclosed by investing layer of cervical fascia	Not enclosed
Type of gland	Purely serous secreting (Fig. 15.10)	Mixed, both serous and mucus secreting (Fig. 15.11)	Purely mucus secreting (Fig. 15.12)
Gross features	Comprises 3 surfaces, 3 borders, apex and base, one artery, one vein, one nerve and lymph nodes lie within the gland (*see* Chapter 13)	Comprises 3 surfaces, inferior, lateral and medial. One artery which indents the posterior end of the gland. Only lymph nodes lie within it	Related closely to lingual nerve and submandibular duct
Secretomotor root	From IX cranial nerve (Flowchart 13.1)	From VII cranial nerve (Flowchart 15.1)	From VII cranial nerve (Flowchart 15.1)
Sympathetic root	Plexus around middle meningeal artery	Plexus around facial artery	Same as submandibular gland
Sensory	Auriculotemporal nerve	Lingual nerve	Lingual nerve
Development	Ectoderm	Endoderm	Endoderm
Opening of the duct	Vestibule of mouth opposite 2nd upper molar tooth (*see* Fig. 13.7)	Papilla on sublingual fold in the floor of the mouth (*see* Fig. 25.2)	10–12 ducts open on sublingual fold in the floor of the mouth (*see* Fig. 25.2)

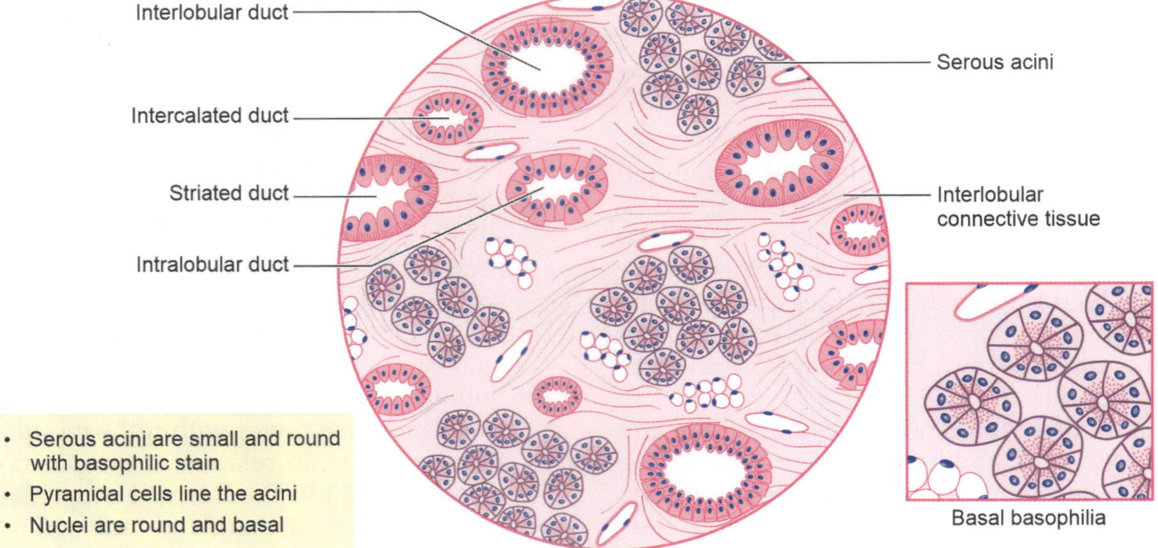

Fig. 15.10: Histology of parotid gland

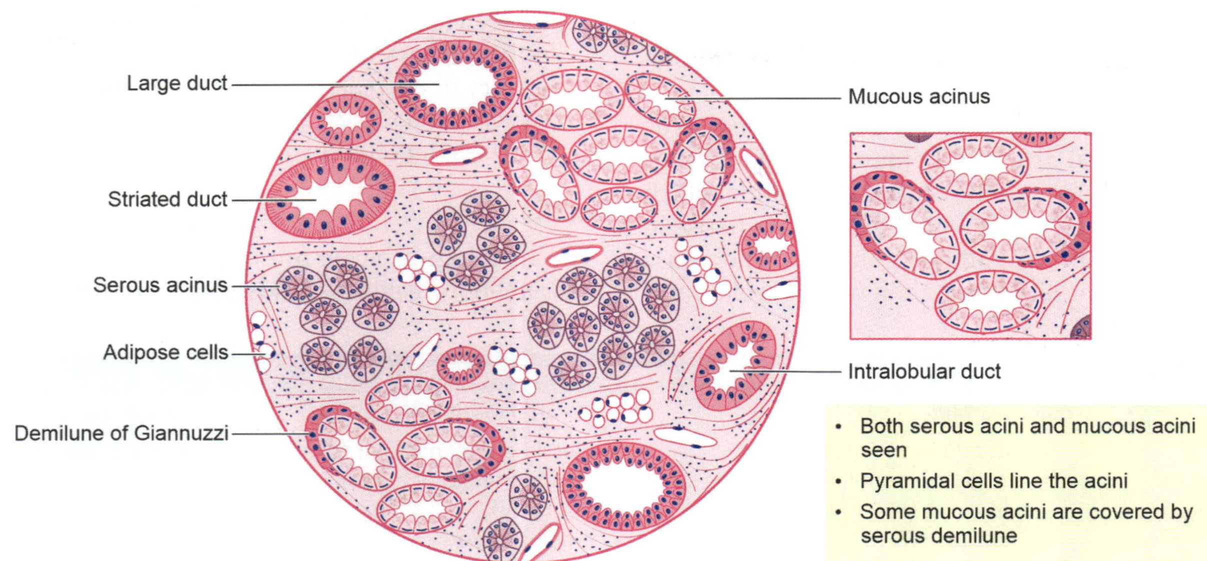

Fig. 15.11: Histology of submandibular gland

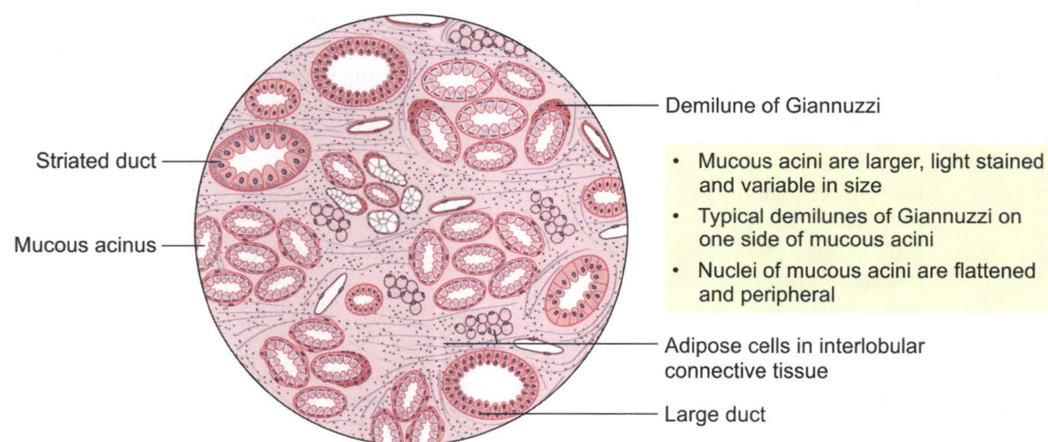

Fig. 15.12: Histology of sublingual gland

CLINICAL ANATOMY

- The chorda tympani nerve supplying secretomotor fibres to submandibular and sublingual salivary glands lies medial to the spine of sphenoid (*see* Fig. 9.11c). The auriculotemporal nerve supplying secretomotor fibres to the parotid gland is related to lateral aspect of spine of sphenoid. Injury to spine may involve both these nerves with loss of secretion from all three salivary glands.
- Submandibular lymph nodes lie both within and outside the submandibular salivary gland. The gland is to be removed, if lymph nodes are affected in any disease especially carcinoma of tongue (Fig. 15.1).
- Mylohyoid muscle divides the gland into superficial and deep parts (Fig. 15.5). Lymph nodes lie around and within the gland. Cancer of the tongue or of the gland may metastasise into the mandible also (Fig. 15.2).
- Secretion of submandibular gland is more viscous, so there are more chances of the gland getting calculi or small stones. The duct passes upwards against gravity, so flow is relatively slow.
- Submandibular gland can be manually palpated by putting one finger within the mouth and one finger outside, in relation to the position of the gland (Fig. 15.13). The enlarged lymph nodes lying on the surface of the gland and within its substance can also be palpated.

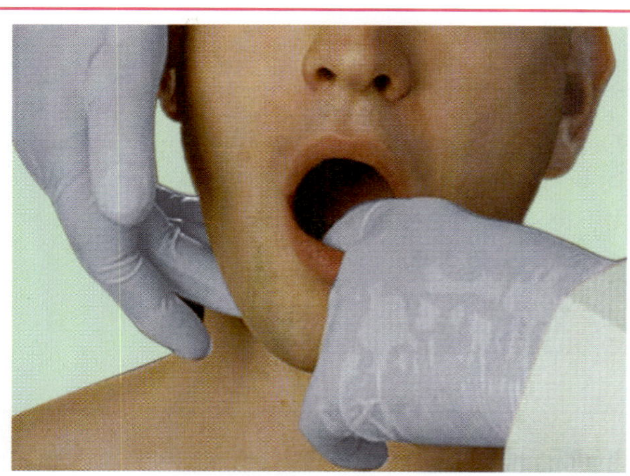

Fig. 15.13: Bimanual palpation of submandibular gland and lymph nodes

- The duct of submandibular gland may get impacted by a small stone, which can be demonstrated on radiographs.
- Excision of the submandibular gland for calculus or tumour is done by an incision below the angle of the jaw. Since the marginal mandibular branch of the facial nerve passes posteroinferior to the angle of the jaw before crossing it, the incision must be placed more than 4 cm below the angle to preserve the nerve (Fig. 15.1).

  The nerve also passes across the lymph nodes of submandibular region. One should be careful of the nerve while doing biopsy of lymph node.

FACTS TO REMEMBER

- Chorda tympani nerve carries secretomotor fibres to the submandibular ganglion. It also carries taste from most of the anterior two-thirds of the tongue.
- The submandibular lymph nodes are also present in the submandibular gland. In cancer of the tongue, this gland is also excised to get rid off the lymph nodes with secondaries from the tongue.
- Facial artery is tortuous to accommodate to the movements of pharynx. It is the chief artery of the palatine tonsil.
- Suprahyoid muscles are disposed in four layers:
  1st layer: Digastrics and stylohyoid
  2nd layer: Mylohyoid
  3rd layer: Geniohyoid and hyoglossus
  4th layer: Genioglossus (Fig. 15.8)

CLINICOANATOMICAL PROBLEM

A patient is diagnosed with cancer of the tongue. The lesion was on the dorsum of tongue close to its lateral border.

- Where does all the lymph from cancerous lesion drain?
- Which other parts have be removed during the surgery to remove the lesion?

Ans: The lymph from dorsum of tongue close to lateral border chiefly drains into the submandibular group of lymph nodes. A few lymph vessels may even cross the midline to drain into the opposite submandibular lymph nodes.

These lymph nodes are present within and outside the submandibular salivary gland. So during removal of lymph nodes this salivary gland is also to be removed.

The incision in the neck is to be placed about 4 cm below the angle of mandible, to preserve the marginal mandibular branch of facial nerve as it passes posteroinferior to the angle of the jaw before crossing it. If this branch is injured, muscles of lower lip would get paralysed (Fig. 15.1).

FURTHER READING

- Garrett JR, Ekstrom J, Anderson LC (eds). Neural Mechanisms of Salivary Secretion. Frontiers in Oral Bilogy, vol 11.Basel: Karger 1999.

  A book that contains much basic information concerning the role of nerves in the secretory process of salivary glands.
- Scott J. Structure and function in aging human salivary glands. Gerontology 1986;5:149–58.

  A paper that gives quantitative information on changes that occur in the parenchyma of the major salivary glands with age and discusses the results in terms of xerostomia.

Frequently Asked Questions

1. Describe the submandibular salivary gland under the following headings:
   a. Parts
   b. Relations
   c. Nerve supply
   d. Clinical anatomy
2. Describe the attachments, nerve supply and actions of both bellies of digastric muscle.
3. Write short notes on:
   a. Hyoglossus muscle
   b. Mylohyoid muscle
   c. Submandibular ganglion

Multiple Choice Questions

1. One of the following statements about chorda tympani nerve is not true:
   a. Branch of facial nerve
   b. Joins lingual nerve in infratemporal fossa
   c. Carries postganglionic parasympathetic fibres
   d. Carries taste fibres from most of the anterior two-thirds of tongue
2. Nerve carrying preganglionic parasympathetic fibres to submandibular ganglion:
   a. Greater petrosal b. Lesser petrosal
   c. Deep petrosal d. Chorda tympani
3. Which of the following nerves lies posteroinferior to angle of mandible?
   a. Zygomatic branch of facial
   b. Buccal branch of facial
   c. Marginal mandibular branch of facial
   d. Cervical branch of facial
4. Submandibular lymph nodes drain all of the following areas, *except:*
   a. Lateral side of tongue
   b. External nose, upper lip
   c. Lateral halves of eyelids
   d. Medial halves of eyelids
5. Which muscle divides the submandibular gland into a superficial and deep parts?
   a. Hyoglossus
   b. Mylohyoid
   c. Geniohyoid
   d. Anterior belly of digastric

Answers

1. c **2.** d **3.** c **4.** c **5.** b

VIVA VOCE

- Name the layers of suprahyoid muscles. Which nerves supply these muscles?
- Which muscle divides the submandibular gland into a superficial and deep part?
- Where does the duct of submandibular gland open?
- Name the roots of the submandibular ganglion. What are its branches?
- Trace the secretomotor fibres of the submandibular gland.
- Which areas are drained by the submandibular lymph nodes?
- Why are facial and lingual arteries tortuous?
- What are the main features of histological structure of submandibular gland?

Submandibular salivary gland

Chapter

16

Structures in the Neck

"The extirpation of the thyroid gland for goitre typifies perhaps better than any operation, the supreme triumphs of the surgeon's art."
—William S Halsted

INTRODUCTION

The thyroid gland lies in front of the neck. Skin incision for its surgery should be horizontal, for better healing and for cosmetic reasons. Branches of subclavian artery anastomose with those of axillary artery around the scapula.

Scalenus anterior is important. It may compress the subclavian artery to cause 'scalenus anterior syndrome'.

Lymph nodes are clinically important in deciding the prognosis and treatment of malignancies.

Contents: There are numerous structures in the neck. For convenience, they may be grouped as follows:

a. *Glands:* Thyroid and parathyroid.
b. *Thymus:* Involutes at puberty.
c. *Arteries:* Subclavian and carotid.
d. *Veins:* Subclavian, internal jugular and brachiocephalic.
e. *Nerves:* Glossopharyngeal, vagus, accessory (in this Chapter), and hypoglossal (described in Chapter 25).
f. *Sympathetic trunk:* It has three cervical ganglia.
g. Lymph nodes and thoracic duct.
h. Styloid apparatus.

GLANDS

THYROID GLAND

The thyroid (shield-like) is an endocrine gland with rich blood supply situated in the lower part of the front and sides of the neck. It regulates the basal metabolic rate, stimulates somatic and psychic growth, and plays an important role in calcium metabolism. Since it is placed superficially, it can easily be examined. This is the only gland using natural iodine for the synthesis of its hormones which are stored within the follicles to be used according to the needs of the body.

The gland consists of right and left *lobes* that are joined to each other by the *isthmus* (Fig. 16.1). A third, pyramidal lobe, may project upwards from the isthmus (or from one of the lobes). Sometimes a fibrous or fibromuscular band (levator glandulae thyroideae) descends from the body of the hyoid bone to the isthmus or to the pyramidal lobe (Fig. 16.2).

DISSECTION

Sternocleidomastoid muscle has already been reflected laterally from its origin. Cut the sternothyroid muscle near its origin and reflect it upwards. Clean the surface of trachea and identify inferior thyroid vein and remains of the thymus gland (darker in colour than fat).

Isthmus of the thyroid gland lies on the 2nd–4th tracheal rings. Pyramidal lobe, if present, projects from the upper border of the isthmus. On each side of isthmus is the lateral lobe of the gland. Clean the lobes and identify the vessels of thyroid gland. Identify the recurrent laryngeal nerves tucked between the lateral surfaces of trachea and oesophagus. Look for beaded thoracic duct present on the left of oesophagus. Trace the superior and inferior thyroid arteries. Identify cricothyroid and inferior constrictor muscles lying medial to the lobes of thyroid gland (Figs 16.1 to 16.6) *(refer to BDC App)*.

Thyroid gland (butterfly shaped)

Cut the isthmus of the thyroid gland and turn one of the lobes laterally. Locate an anastomosis between the posterior branch of superior thyroid and ascending branch of inferior thyroid arteries supplying the gland. Identify the two parathyroid glands on the sides of this anastomotic vessel (Figs 16.7 and 16.12).

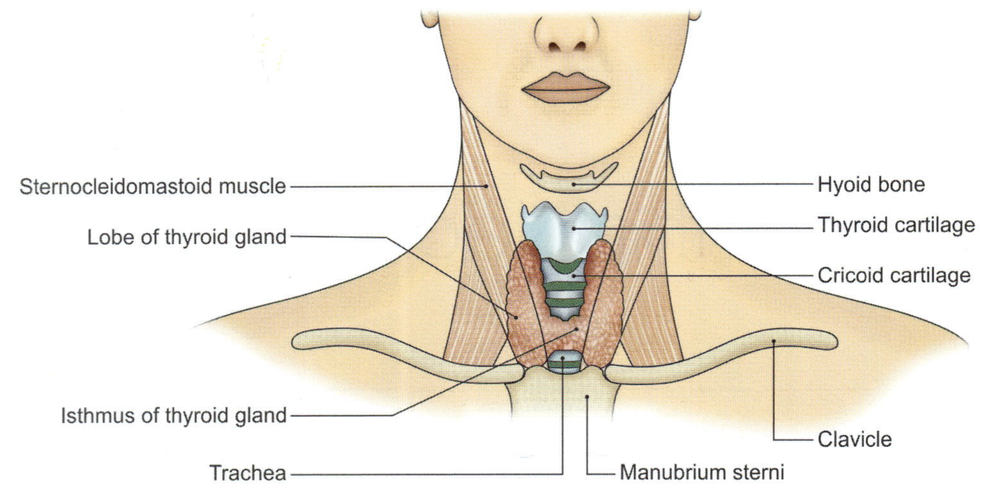

Fig. 16.1: Position of thyroid gland

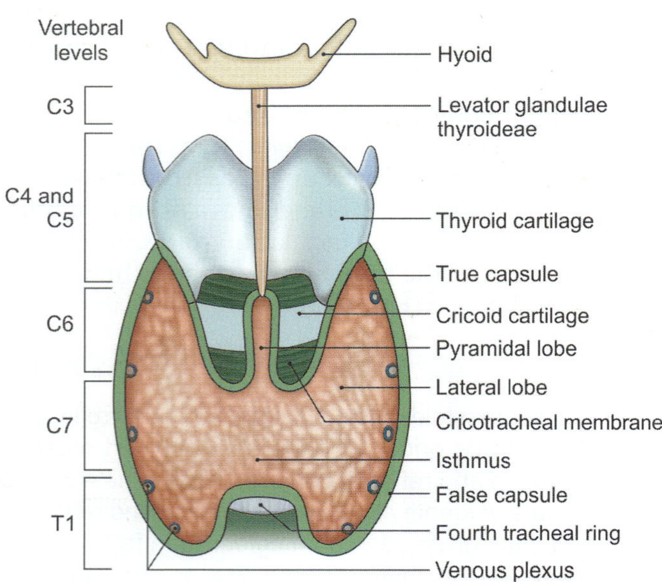

Fig. 16.2: Scheme to show the location and subdivisions of the thyroid gland including the false capsule

Situation and Extent

1 The gland lies against vertebrae C5–C7 and T1, embracing the upper part of the trachea (Fig. 16.2).
2 Each lobe extends from the middle of thyroid cartilage to the fourth or fifth tracheal ring.
3 The isthmus extends from the second to the fourth tracheal ring.

Dimensions and Weight

Each lobe measures about 5 × 2.5 × 2.5 cm, and the isthmus 1.2 × 1.2 cm. On an average, the gland weighs about 25 g. However, it is larger in females than in males, and further increases in size during menstruation and pregnancy.

Capsules of Thyroid

1 The *true capsule* is the peripheral condensation of the connective tissue of the gland.

A dense capillary plexus is present deep to the true capsule. To avoid haemorrhage during operations, the thyroid is removed along with the true capsule. It can be compared with the prostate in which the venous plexus lies between the two capsules of the gland, and therefore, during prostatectomy, both capsules are left behind (Figs 16.3a and b).

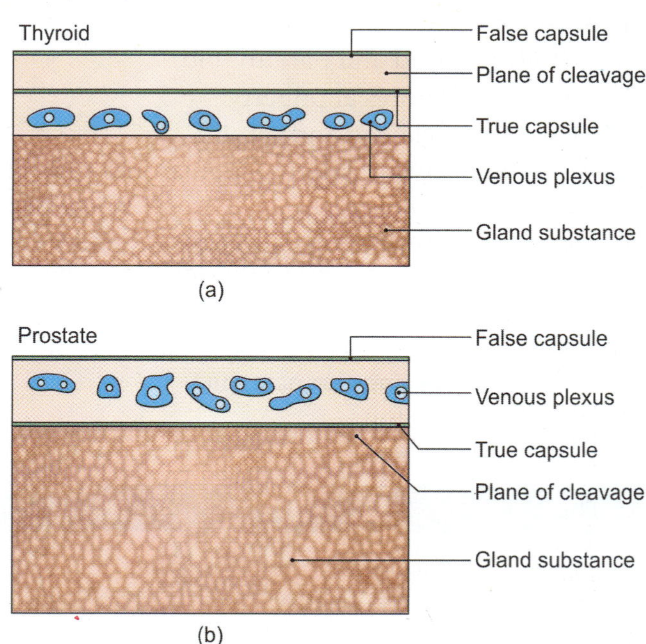

Figs 16.3a and b: Schemes of comparing the relationship of the venous plexuses related to: (a) The thyroid gland; (b) The prostate, with the true and false capsules around these organs. Note the plane of cleavage along which the organ is separated from neighbouring structures during surgical removal

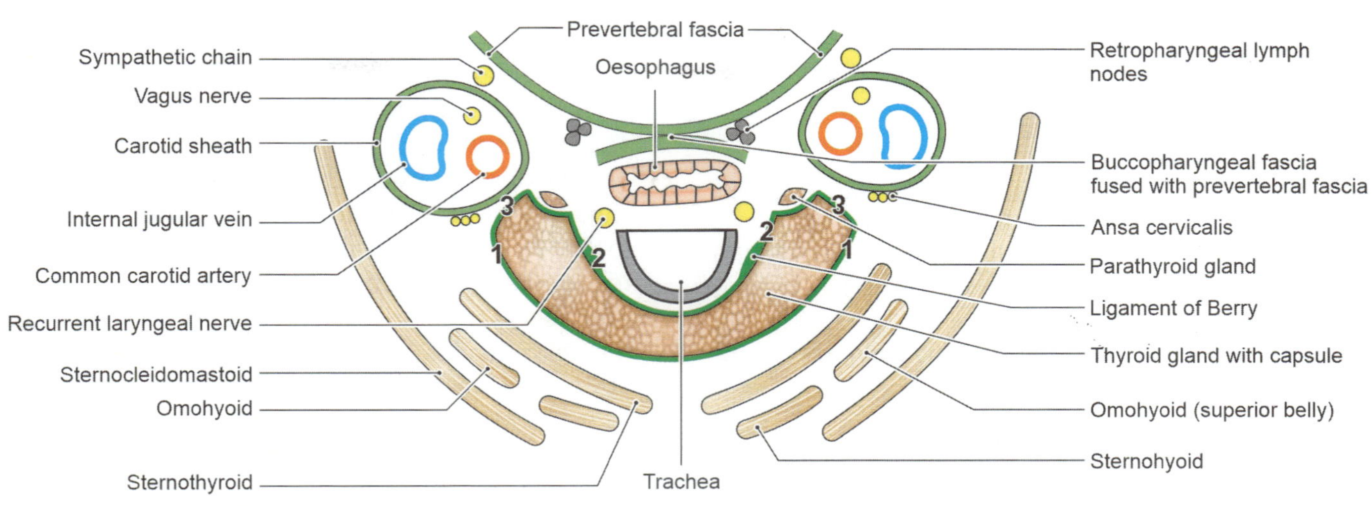

Fig. 16.4: Transverse section through the anterior part of the neck at the level of the isthmus of the thyroid gland; 1. Lateral surface; 2. Medial surface, 3. Posterior surface

2 The *false capsule* is derived from the pretracheal layer of the deep cervical fascia (Fig. 16.2). It is thin along the posterior border of the lobes, but thick on the inner surface of the gland where it forms a suspensory ligament (of Berry), which connects the lobe to the cricoid cartilage (Fig. 16.4).

Parts and Relations

The lobes are conical in shape having:

a. An apex
b. A base
c. Three surfaces: Lateral, medial and posterolateral.
d. Two borders: Anterior and posterior.

The *apex* is directed upwards and slightly laterally. It is limited superiorly by the attachment of the sternothyroid muscle to the oblique line of thyroid cartilage which is medial to the apex. The apex is related to superior thyroid artery and the external laryngeal nerve (Fig. 16.5).

The *base* is at level with the 4th or 5th tracheal ring. It is related to inferior thyroid artery and recurrent laryngeal nerve (Fig. 16.7).

The *lateral* or *superficial surface* is convex, and is covered by:

a. The sternohyoid
b. The superior belly of omohyoid
c. The sternothyroid
d. The anterior border of the sternocleidomastoid (Fig. 16.4).

The *medial surface* is related to:

a. Two tubes—trachea and oesophagus
b. Two muscles—inferior constrictor and cricothyroid
c. Two nerves—external laryngeal and recurrent laryngeal (Fig. 16.5).

The *posterolateral* or *posterior surface* is related to the carotid sheath and overlaps the common carotid artery (Fig. 16.4).

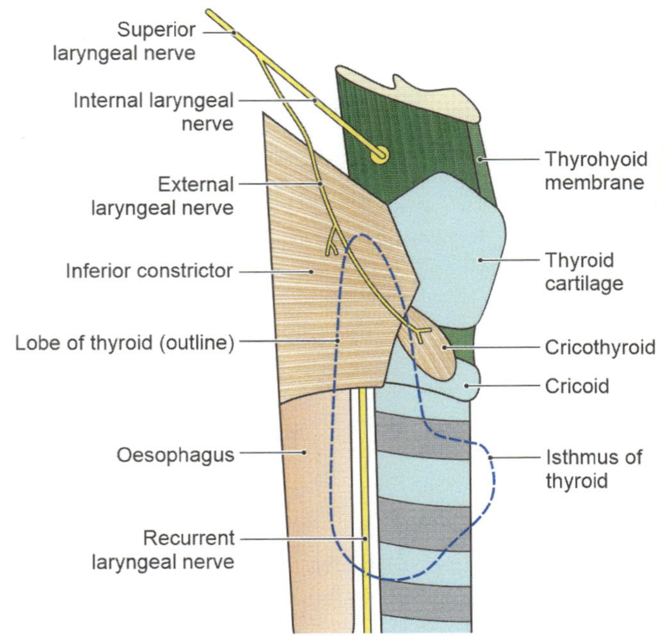

Fig. 16.5: Deep relations of the thyroid gland

The *anterior border* is thin and is related to the anterior branch of superior thyroid artery (Fig. 16.7).

The *posterior border* is thick and rounded and separates the medial and posterior surfaces. It is related to:

a. Inferior thyroid artery.
b. Anastomosis between the posterior branch of superior and ascending branch of inferior thyroid arteries.
c. Parathyroid glands.
d. Thoracic duct only on the left side (Fig. 16.7).

The *isthmus* connects the lower parts of the two lobes. It has:

a. Two surfaces: Anterior and posterior.
b. Two borders: Superior and inferior.

The *anterior surface* is covered by:

a. The right and left sternothyroid and sternohyoid muscles.
b. The anterior jugular veins.
c. Fascia and skin (Fig. 16.4).

The *posterior surface* is related to the second to fourth tracheal rings.

The *upper border* is related to anterior branches of the right and left superior thyroid arteries (Fig. 16.6) which anastomose here.

Lower border: Inferior thyroid veins leave the gland at this border (Fig. 16.8).

Arterial Supply

The thyroid gland is supplied by the superior and inferior thyroid arteries.

1 The *superior thyroid artery* is the first anterior branch of the external carotid artery (Figs 16.6 and 16.7). It runs downwards and forwards in intimate relation to the external laryngeal nerve. After giving branches to adjacent structures, the artery pierces the pretracheal fascia to reach the apex of the lobe where the nerve deviates medially. At the upper pole, the artery divides into anterior and posterior branches.

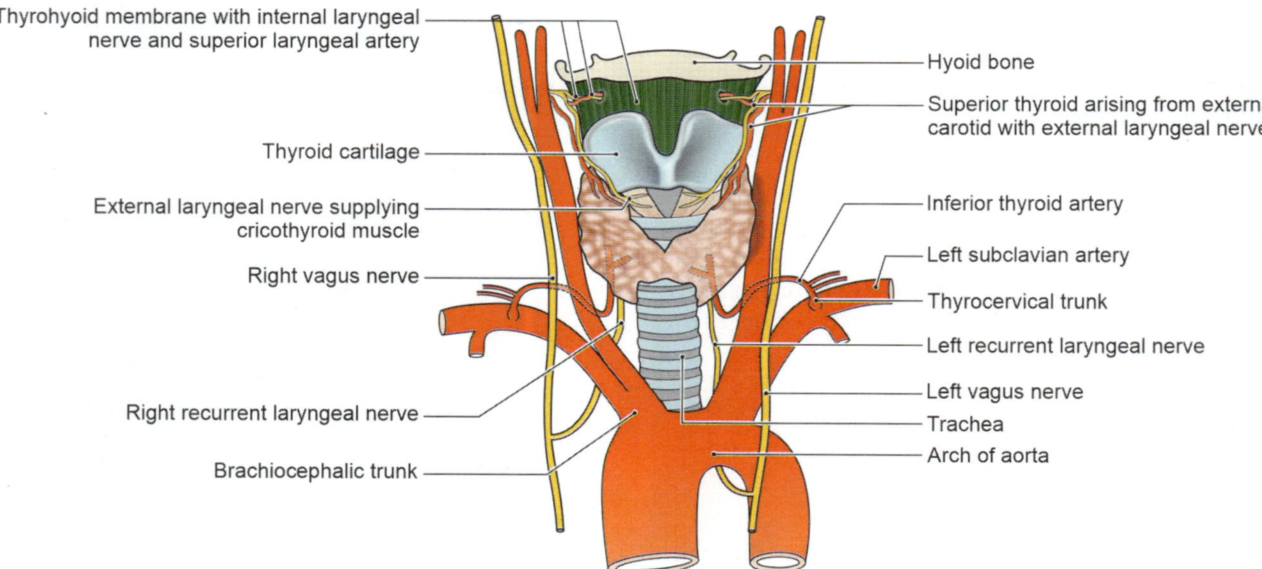

Fig. 16.6: Arterial supply of anterior aspect of thyroid gland

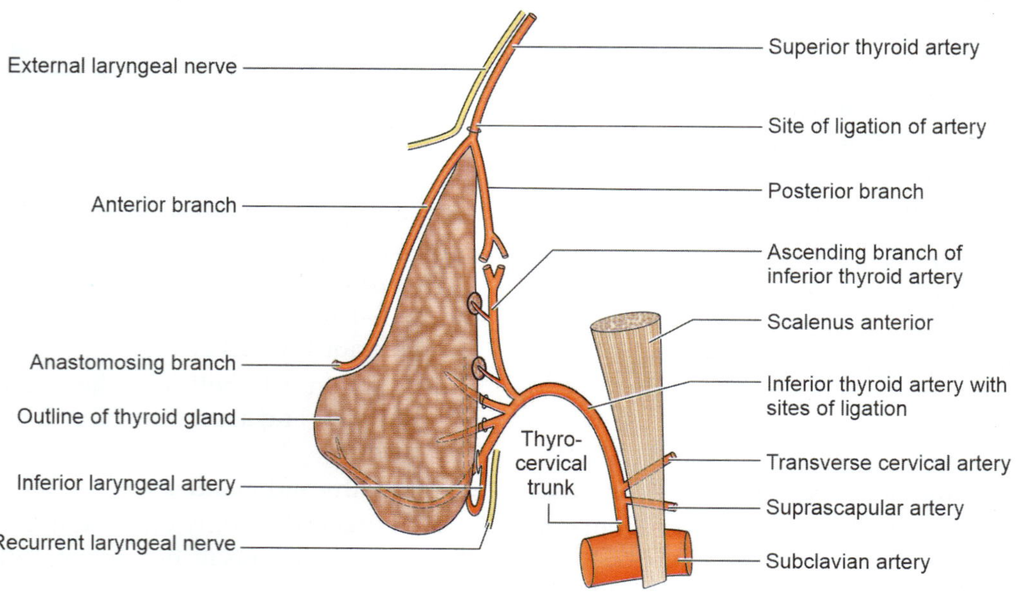

Fig. 16.7: Arterial supply of the surfaces of thyroid gland. Sites of ligatures of the superior and branches of inferior thyroid arteries are shown

The *anterior branch* descends on the anterior border of the lobe and continues along the upper border of the isthmus to anastomose with its fellow of the opposite side.

The *posterior branch* descends on the posterior border of the lobe and anastomoses with the ascending branch of inferior thyroid artery (Fig. 16.7).

2 The *inferior thyroid artery* is a branch of thyrocervical trunk (which arises from the subclavian artery).

It runs first upwards, then medially, and finally downwards to reach the base of the gland. During its course, it passes behind the carotid sheath and the middle cervical sympathetic ganglion; and in front of the vertebral vessels; and gives off branches to adjacent structures.

Its terminal part is intimately related to the recurrent laryngeal nerve, while proximal part is away from the nerve.

The artery divides into 4 to 5 glandular branches which pierce the fascia separately to reach the lower part of the gland. One *ascending branch* anastomoses with the posterior branch of the superior thyroid artery and supplies the parathyroid glands.

3 Sometimes (in 3% of individuals), the thyroid is also supplied by the *lowest thyroid artery (thyroidea ima artery)* which arises from the brachiocephalic trunk or directly from the arch of the aorta. It enters the lower part of the isthmus.

4 *Accessory thyroid arteries* arising from tracheal and oesophageal arteries also supply the thyroid.

Venous Drainage

The thyroid is drained by the superior, middle and inferior thyroid veins.

The *superior thyroid vein* emerges at the upper pole and accompanies the superior thyroid artery. It ends in the internal jugular vein (Fig. 16.8).

The *middle thyroid vein* is a short, wide channel which emerges at the middle of the lobe and soon enters the internal jugular vein.

The *inferior thyroid veins* emerge at the lower border of isthmus. They form a plexus in front of the trachea, and drain into the left brachiocephalic vein.

A *fourth thyroid vein* (Kocher) may emerge between the middle and inferior veins, and drain into the internal jugular vein.

Lymphatic Drainage

Lymph from the upper part of the gland reaches the upper deep cervical lymph nodes either directly or through the prelaryngeal nodes. Lymph from the lower part of the gland drains to the lower deep cervical nodes directly, and also through the pretracheal and paratracheal nodes.

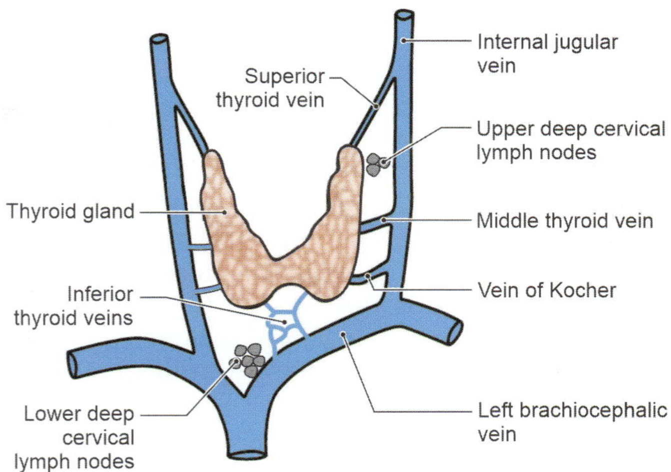

Fig. 16.8: Venous drainage and lymphatic drainage of the thyroid gland (lateral view). Deep cervical lymph nodes are also shown

Nerve Supply

Nerves are derived mainly from the middle cervical ganglion and partly from the superior and inferior cervical ganglia. These are vasoconstrictor.

CLINICAL ANATOMY

- Any swelling of the thyroid gland (goitre) should be palpated from behind (Fig. 16.9).
- Removal of the thyroid (thyroidectomy) with true capsule may be necessary in hyperthyroidism.

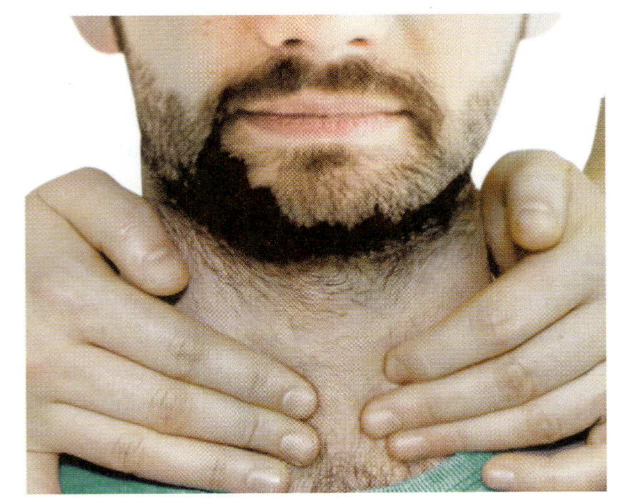

Fig. 16.9: Palpation of thyroid gland from behind

- In subtotal thyroidectomy, the posterior parts of both lobes are left behind. This avoids the risk of simultaneous removal of the parathyroids and also of postoperative myxoedema (caused by deficiency of thyroid hormones).
- During thyroidectomy, the superior thyroid artery is ligated near the gland to save the external laryngeal nerve. The stem of inferior thyroid artery is not ligated (Fig. 16.7). Its glandular branches are ligated separately. In this way, blood supply to parathyroid glands is maintained.
- Hypothyroidism causes cretinism in infants and myxoedema in adults.
- Benign tumours of the gland may displace and even compress neighbouring structures, like the carotid sheath, the trachea, etc. Malignant growths tend to invade and erode neighbouring structures. Pressure symptoms and nerve involvements are common in carcinoma of the gland giving rise to dyspnoea, dysphagia and dysphonia.

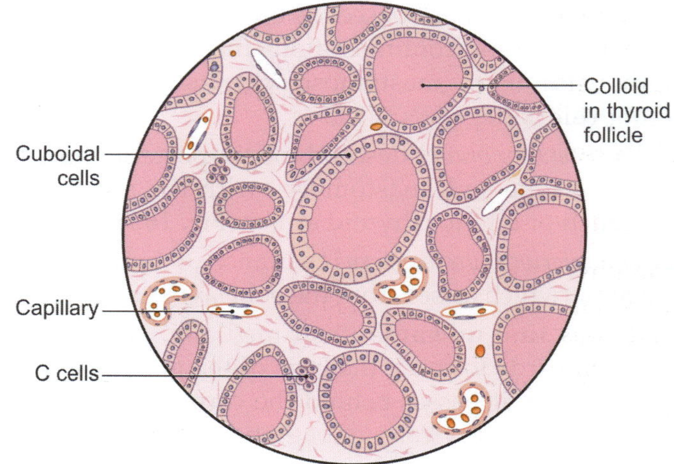

Fig. 16.10: Histology of thyroid gland

HISTOLOGY

The thyroid gland is made up of the following two types of secretory cells.

1 *Follicular cells* lining the follicles of the gland secrete tri-iodothyronin and tetraiodothyronin (thyroxin) which stimulate basal metabolic rate and somatic and psychic growth of the individual. During active phase, the lining of the follicles is columnar, while in resting phase, it is cuboidal. Follicles contain the colloid (the hormone) in their lumina (Fig. 16.10).

2 *Parafollicular cells (C cells)* are fewer and light cells. These lie in between the follicles. They secrete thyrocalcitonin which promotes deposition of calcium salts in skeletal and other tissues, and tends to produce hypocalcaemia. These effects are opposite to those of parathormone.

DEVELOPMENT

The thyroid gland develops from a *median endodermal thyroid diverticulum* which grows down in front of the neck from the floor of the primitive pharynx (foramen caecum), just caudal to the tuberculum impar (Figs 16.11a–d).

The lower end of the diverticulum enlarges to form the gland. The rest of the diverticulum remains narrow and is known as the *thyroglossal duct*. Most of the duct soon disappears. The position of the upper end is marked by the *foramen caecum* of the tongue, and the lower end often persists as the *pyramidal lobe*. The gland becomes functional during third month of development.

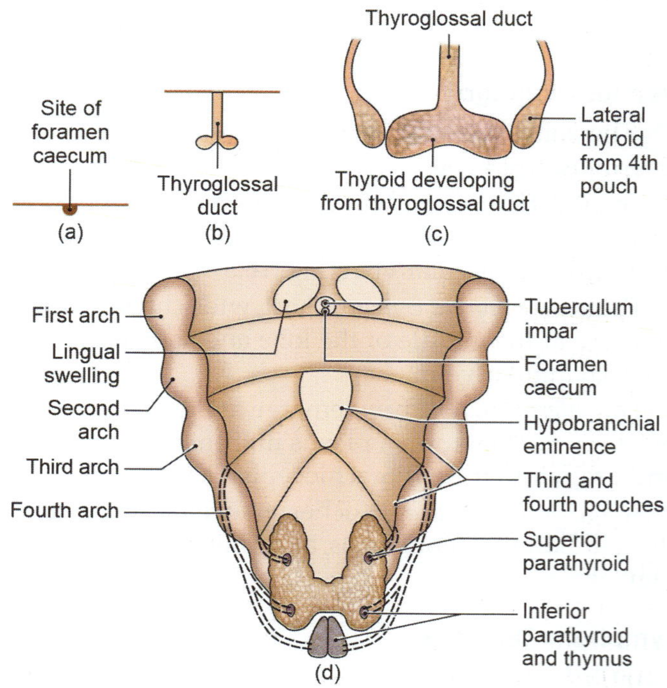

Figs 16.11a to d: Development of thyroid, parathyroid and thymus glands. Parathyroids are placed posteriorly

Remnants of the thyroglossal duct may form thyroglossal cysts, or a thyroglossal fistula. Thyroid tissue may develop at abnormal sites along the course of the duct resulting in lingual or retrosternal thyroids. Accessory thyroids may be present.

PARATHYROID GLANDS

Parathyroid glands are two pairs (superior and inferior) of small endocrine glands, that usually lie on the posterior border of the thyroid gland, within the false capsule (Figs 16.12a and b). The *superior parathyroids* are also referred to as *parathyroid IV* because they develop from the endoderm of the *fourth pharyngeal pouch*. The *inferior parathyroids*, similarly, are also called *parathyroid III* because they develop from the *third pouch* (Fig. 16.11d).

The parathyroids secrete the hormone *parathormone* which controls the metabolism of calcium and phosphorus along with thyrocalcitonin.

Each parathyroid gland is oval or lentiform in shape, measuring 6 × 4 × 2 mm (the size of a split pea). Each gland weighs about 50 mg.

Position

The anastomosis between the superior and inferior thyroid arteries is usually a good guide to the glands because they usually lie close to it (Fig. 16.12b).

The *superior parathyroid* is more constant in position and usually lies at the middle of the posterior border of the lobe of the thyroid gland. It is usually dorsal to the recurrent laryngeal nerve.

The *inferior parathyroid* is more variable in position. It may lie:

a. Within the thyroid capsule, below the inferior thyroid artery and near the lower pole of the thyroid lobe (Fig. 16.12a).
b. Behind and outside the thyroid capsule, immediately above the inferior thyroid artery.
c. Within the substance of the lobe near its posterior border. It is usually ventral to the recurrent laryngeal nerve.

Vascular Supply

The parathyroid glands receive a rich blood supply from the inferior thyroid artery and from the anastomosis between the superior and inferior thyroid arteries. The veins and lymphatics of the gland are associated with those of the thyroid and the thymus.

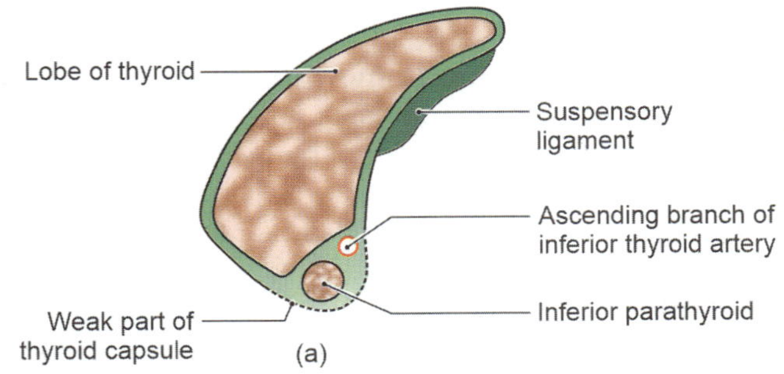

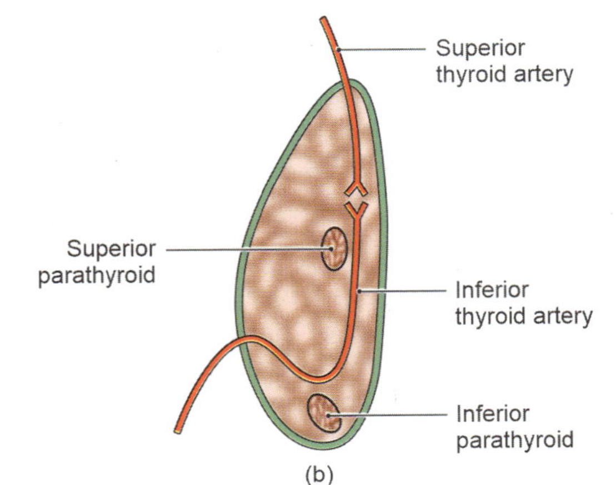

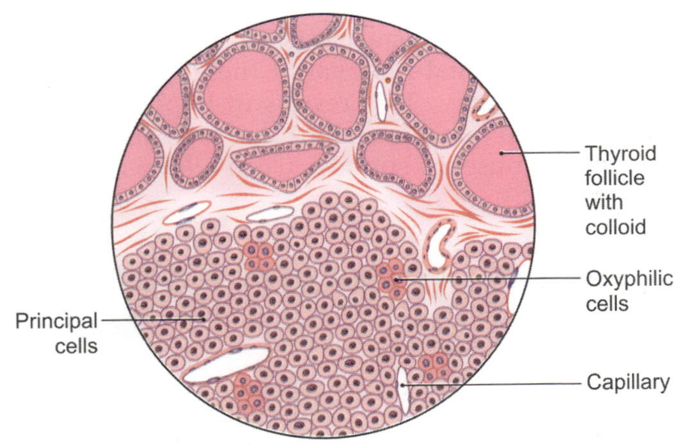

- Principal cells
- Oxyphilic cells
- Capsule separating the parathyroid from thyroid tissue

(c)

Figs 16.12a to c: Schemes to show the location of the parathyroid glands: (a) Transverse section through the left lobe of the thyroid gland; (b) Posterior view of the left lobe of the thyroid gland; (c) Histology of the parathyroid gland

Nerve Supply

Vasomotor nerves are derived from the middle and superior cervical ganglia. Parathyroid activity is controlled by blood calcium levels; low levels stimulate and high levels inhibit the activity of the glands.

HISTOLOGY

The reticular tissue forms framework of the parathyroid gland. The parenchyma consists of *principal cells* and *oxyphilic cells*. Principal cells or chief cells are arranged in sheets with numerous sinusoids and capillaries traversing them. The principal cells are polygonal or round with a centrally placed vesicular nuclei and a pale staining acidophilic cytoplasm (Fig. 16.12c).

Oxyphilic cells are a few in number, occur singly or in small groups. These are larger than principal cells. They have darkly staining nuclei and strongly acidophilic cytoplasm. Oxyphilic cells are seen to increase with age.

The principal or chief cells secrete *parathormone* responsible for maintaining the blood calcium level.

CLINICAL ANATOMY

- Tumours of the parathyroid glands lead to excessive secretion of parathormone (hyperparathyroidism). This leads to increased removal of calcium from bone, making them weak and liable to fracture. Calcium levels in blood increase (hypercalcaemia) and increased urinary excretion of calcium can lead to the formation of stones in the urinary tract.
- Hypoparathyroidism may occur spontaneously or from accidental removal of the glands during thyroidectomy. This results in hypocalcaemia leading to increased neuromuscular irritability causing muscular spasm and convulsions (tetany) (Fig. 16.13).

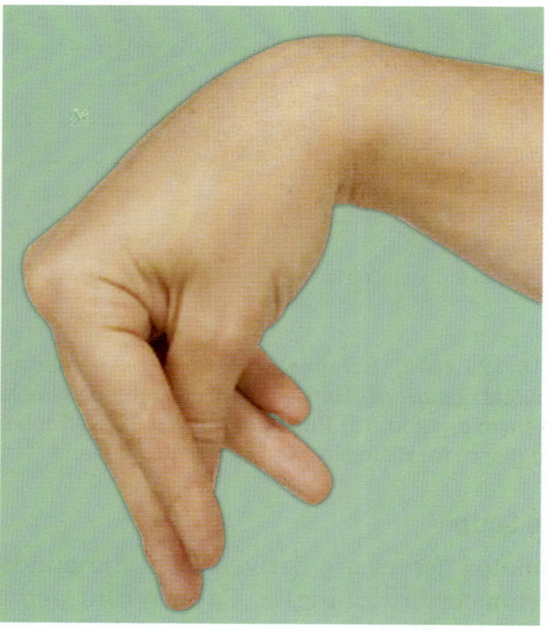

Fig. 16.13: Spasm in the hand due to tetany

- Parathyroid glands are tough glands and will continue to function, if these are transplanted from an excised thyroid gland into the sternocleidomastoid muscle.

THYMUS

The *thymus* (Greek thyme leaf) is an important lymphoid organ, situated in the anterior and superior mediastina of the thorax, extending above into the lower part of the neck. It is well developed at birth, continues to grow up to puberty, and thereafter, undergoes gradual atrophy and replacement by fat.

The thymus is a bilobed structure, made up of two pyramidal lobes of unequal size which are connected together by areolar tissue.

Each lobe develops from the endoderm of the third pharyngeal pouch. It lies on the pericardium, the great vessels of the superior mediastinum, and the trachea.

The thymus weighs 10–15 g at birth, 30–40 g at puberty, and only 10 g after mid-adult life. Thus, after puberty, it becomes inconspicuous due to replacement by fat.

Blood Supply

The thymus is supplied by branches from the internal thoracic and inferior thyroid arteries. Its veins drain into the left brachiocephalic, internal thoracic and inferior thyroid veins.

Nerve Supply

Vasomotor nerves are derived from the stellate ganglion. The capsule is supplied by the phrenic nerve and by the descendens cervicalis.

Functions

1. The thymus controls lymphopoiesis, and maintains an effective pool of circulating lymphocytes, competent to react to innumerable antigenic stimuli.
2. It controls development of the peripheral lymphoid tissues of the body during the neonatal period. By puberty, the main lymphoid tissues are fully developed.
3. The cortical lymphocytes of the thymus arise from stem cells of bone marrow origin. Most (95%) of the lymphocytes (T lymphocytes) produced are autoallergic (act against the host or 'self' antigens), short-lived (3–5 days) and never move out of the organ. They are destroyed within the thymus by phagocytes. Their remnants are seen as Hassall's corpuscles.

   The remaining 5% of the T lymphocytes are long-lived (3 months or more), and move out of the thymus to join the circulating pool of lymphocytes where they act as immunologically competent but uncommitted cells, i.e. they can react to any unfamiliar, new antigen. On the other hand, the other circulating lymphocytes (from lymph nodes, spleen, etc.) are committed cells, i.e. they can mount an immune response only when exposed to a particular antigen. Thymic lymphopoiesis, lympholysis and involution are all intrinsically controlled.

4 The medullary epithelial cells of the thymus are thought to secrete:
   a. *Lymphopoietin*, which stimulates lymphocyte production both in the cortex of the thymus and in peripheral lymphoid organs.
   b. The *competence-inducing factor*, which may be responsible for making new lymphocytes competent to react to antigenic stimuli.

5 Normally, there are no germinal centres in the thymic cortex. Such centres appear in autoimmune diseases. This may indicate a defect in the normal function of the thymus.

CLINICAL ANATOMY

- Involution of the thymus is enhanced by hypertrophy of the adrenal cortex, injection of cortisone or of androgenic hormone. The involution is delayed by castration and adrenalectomy.
- Thymic hyperplasia or tumours are often associated with myasthenia gravis, characterised by excessive fatigability of voluntary muscles.

  The precise role of the thymus in this disease is uncertain; it may influence, directly or indirectly, the transmission at the neuromuscular junction. Figure 16.14 shows drooping of eyelids.
- Thymic tumours may press on the trachea, oesophagus and the large veins of the neck, causing hoarseness, cough, dysphagia and cyanosis.

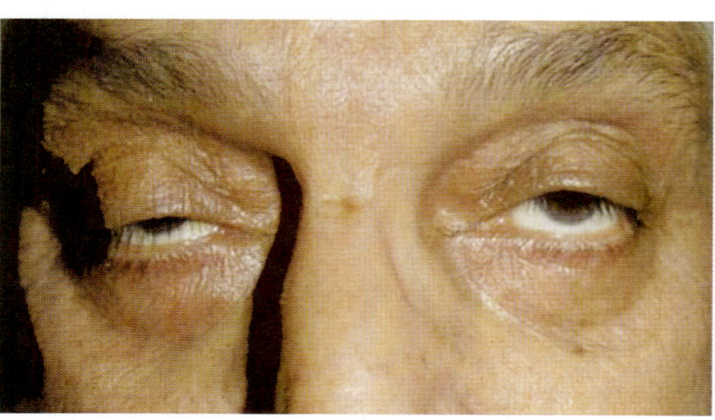

Fig. 16.14: Myasthenia gravis

HISTOLOGY OF THYMUS

Thymus consists of a thin outer fibrous covering known as the capsule. From the capsule extend many thin connective tissue septa dividing it incompletely into various lobules. Each lobule has a peripheral darker cortex and a central lighter medulla. The interlobular septa are partial and do not extend into the medulla, so that there is continuity of the medullary tissue of the various lobules (Fig. 16.15).

Chief cells present in thymus are:

a. *Thymic lymphocytes*: These are situated in the interstices of the thymic reticulum and are immunologically competent but uncommitted cells.

b. *Epithelial reticular cells*: These are flattened cells with pale nuclei. Their processes branch and lie in apposition with the processes of the adjoining cells forming thin membrane. These reticular cells develop from the endoderm of third pharyngeal pouch. These cells secrete hormones, thymosin, thymopoietin, thymulin and thymic humoral factor. These hormones are required for proliferation, differentiation, maturation of T lymphocytes. Hassall's corpuscles made up of concentric epithelial cells forming a hyaline mass is an important feature of the medulla.

DEVELOPMENT OF THYMUS AND PARATHYROID GLANDS

Development of Thymus

- Thymus develops from the endoderm of the ventral wing of the third pharyngeal pouch and from the mesenchyme into which the epithelial tubes grow.
- The bilateral primordia of the thymus lose their connections with the pharyngeal wall, come together in the median plane to form bilobed structure which

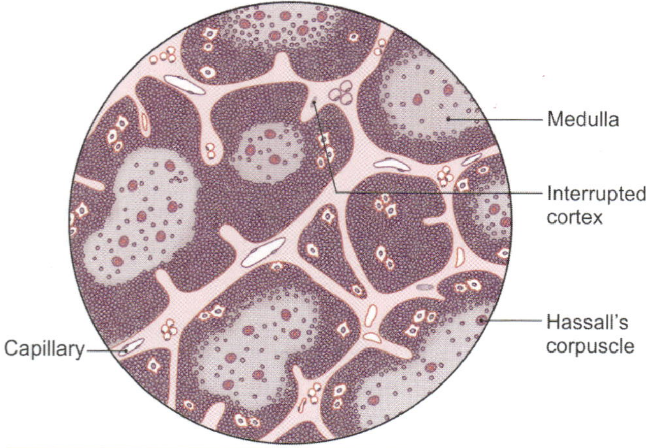

Fig. 16.15: Histology of thymus

migrates into the superior mediastinum part of the thoracic cavity.
- Thymus continues to grow after birth till puberty, after which it begins to undergo involution. Consequently, it is difficult to recognize in old age, as it is atrophied and replaced by fatty tissue.

Development of Parathyroid Glands

Inferior parathyroid glands are derived from the dorsal wing of the third pharyngeal pouch.
- Primordia of the inferior parathyroids along with primordia of thymus lose their connection with the pharyngeal wall.
- The downwards migrating thymus also pulls the inferior parathyroids with it, which finally come to rest on the inferior part of dorsal surface of the thyroid gland.

Superior parathyroid glands are derived from the endoderm of 4th pharyngeal pouch.
- The primordia of superior parathyroid glands, after losing connection with the pharyngeal wall, come to rest on the superior part of dorsal surface of the thyroid gland.
- As mentioned above, because of downwards migration with the thymus, the parathyroid glands derived from 3rd pouch become inferiorly located as compared to those derived from the 4th pouch.

BLOOD VESSELS OF THE NECK

SUBCLAVIAN ARTERY

This is the principal artery which continues as axillary artery for the upper limb. It also supplies a considerable part of the neck and brain through its branches (Fig. 16.16).

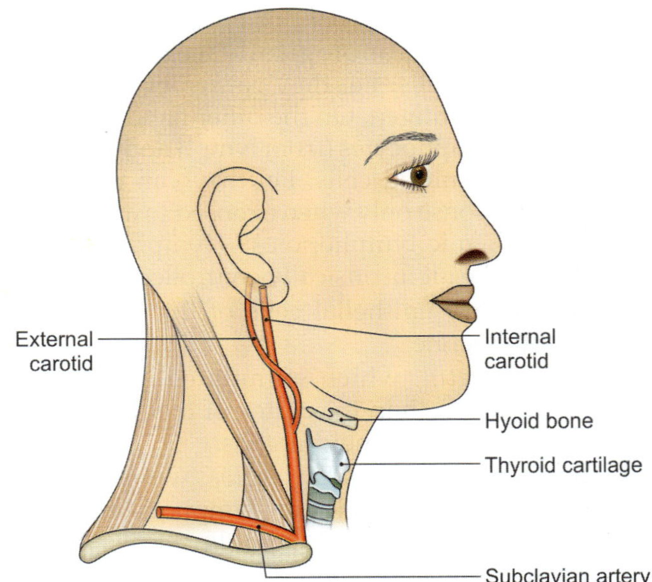

Fig. 16.16: Origin and course of the subclavian arteries

Origin

On the *right side*, it is branch of the brachiocephalic artery. It arises posterior to the sternoclavicular joint.

On the *left side*, it is a branch of the arch of the aorta. It ascends and enters the neck posterior to the left sternoclavicular joint. Both arteries pursue a similar course in the neck (Fig. 16.17).

DISSECTION

Identify scalenus anterior muscle in the anteroinferior part of the neck. Subclavian artery gets divided into three parts by this muscle. Identify vertebral, internal thoracic artery and the thyrocervical trunk with its branches arising from the first part of the artery, costocervical arising from second part and either dorsal scapular or none from the third part.

Course

1. Each artery arches laterally from the sternoclavicular joint to the outer border of the first rib where it ends by becoming continuous with the axillary artery (Fig. 16.17).
2. The scalenus anterior muscle crosses the artery anteriorly and divides it into three parts. The first part is medial, the second part posterior, and the third part lateral to scalenus anterior.

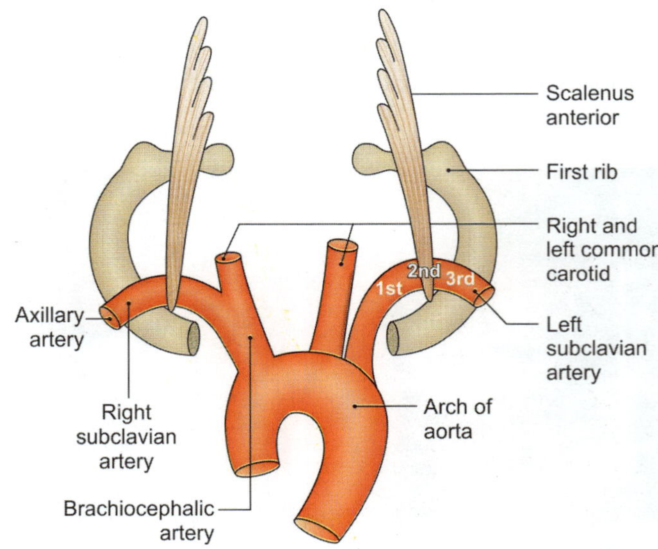

Fig. 16.17: Course of subclavian and carotid arteries

Relations of the First Part

Anterior

Immediate relations from medial to lateral side are:
1 Common carotid artery
2 Vagus
3 Internal jugular vein
4 The sternothyroid and the sternohyoid muscles
5 Sternocleidomastoid

Posterior (Posteroinferior)

1 Suprapleural membrane
2 Cervical pleura
3 Apex of lung (Fig. 16.18)

Relations of the Second Part

Anterior

1 Scalenus anterior
2 Right phrenic nerve deep to the prevertebral fascia
3 Sternocleidomastoid

Posterior (Posteroinferior)

1 Suprapleural membrane
2 Cervical pleura
3 Apex of lung

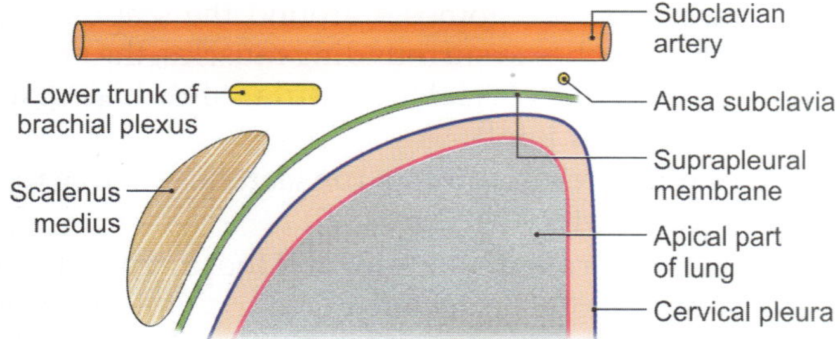

Fig. 16.18: Schematic transverse section through the lower part of neck to show the relations of the left subclavian artery

Superior

Upper and middle trunks of the brachial plexus.

Relations of the Third Part

Anterior

1 Middle one-third of the clavicle
2 The posterior border of the sternocleidomastoid

Posterior (Posteroinferior)

1 Scalenus medius
2 Lower trunk of brachial plexus
3 Suprapleural membrane
4 Cervical pleura
5 Apex of lung

Superior

Upper and middle trunks of brachial plexus

Inferior

First rib (Fig. 16.19)

Branches

From the first part

1 Vertebral artery (Fig. 16.19)
2 Internal thoracic artery
3 Thyrocervical trunk, which divides into three branches:
   a. Inferior thyroid (Fig. 16.20)
   b. Suprascapular
   c. Transverse cervical arteries.
4 Costocervical trunk, which divides into two branches:
   a. Superior intercostal
   b. Deep cervical arteries.
   This artery comes *from second part* on the right side.

From the third part: Dorsal scapular artery—occasionally.

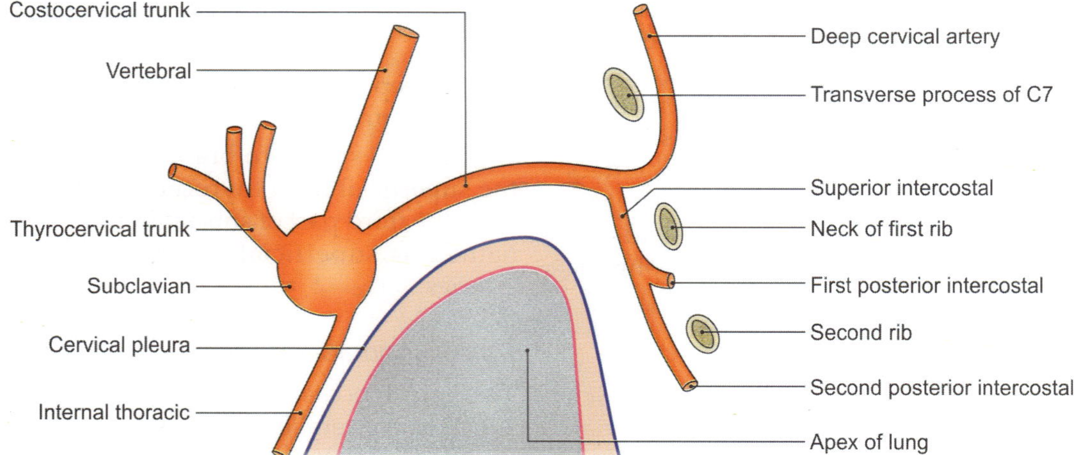

Fig. 16.19: Branches of the subclavian artery. Note that the branches actually arise at different levels, but are shown at same level schematically

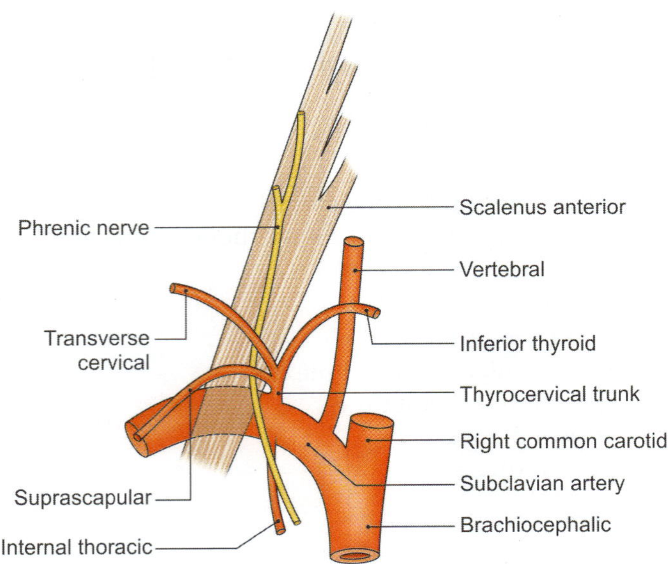

Fig. 16.20: Branches of the right subclavian artery

Vertebral Artery

Vertebral artery is the first and largest branch of the first part of the subclavian artery. It runs a long course and ends in the cranial cavity by supplying the brain.

It is divided into four parts. The *first part* extends from its origin to the foramen transversarium of the sixth cervical vertebra. This part runs upwards and backwards into the angle between the scalenus anterior and the longus colli muscles, behind the common carotid artery, the vertebral vein and the inferior thyroid artery (*see* Fig. 17.5). Details of all the four parts are described in the section on the prevertebral region (*see* Chapter 17).

Internal Thoracic Artery

Internal thoracic artery arises from the inferior aspect of the first part of the subclavian artery opposite the origin of the thyrocervical trunk. The origin lies near the medial border of the scalenus anterior (Fig. 16.20). The artery runs downwards and medially in front of the cervical pleura. Anteriorly, the artery is related to the sternal end of the clavicle. The artery enters the thorax by passing behind the first costal cartilage. It runs till 6th intercostal space where it ends by dividing into superior epigastric and musculophrenic arteries.

Thyrocervical Trunk

Thyrocervical trunk is a short, wide vessel which arises from the front of the first part of the subclavian artery, close to the medial border of the scalenus anterior, and between the phrenic and vagus nerves. It almost immediately divides into the inferior thyroid, suprascapular and transverse cervical arteries (Figs 16.19 and 16.20).

The *inferior thyroid artery* is described with the thyroid gland. In addition to glandular branches to the thyroid, it gives:

a. The ascending cervical artery which runs upwards in front of the transverse processes of cervical vertebrae.
b. The inferior laryngeal artery which accompanies the recurrent laryngeal nerve, and enters the larynx deep to the lower border of the inferior constrictor (Fig. 16.7).
c. Other branches which supply the pharynx, the trachea, the oesophagus and surrounding muscles.

The *suprascapular artery* runs laterally and downwards, and crosses the scalenus anterior and the phrenic nerve.

It lies behind the internal jugular vein and the sternocleidomastoid. It then crosses the trunks of the brachial plexus and runs in the posterior triangle, behind and parallel with the clavicle, to reach the superior border of the scapula (*see* Fig. 11.9).

It crosses above the suprascapular ligament and takes part in the anastomoses around the scapula. In addition to branches to surrounding muscles, the artery also supplies the clavicle, scapula, shoulder and acromioclavicular joints.

The *transverse cervical artery* runs laterally above the suprascapular artery (*see* Fig. 11.9).

It crosses the scalenus anterior and the phrenic nerve passing behind the internal jugular vein and the sternocleidomastoid.

It then crosses the brachial plexus and the floor of the posterior triangle to reach the anterior border of trapezius, where it divides into superficial and deep branches. The superficial branch accompanies the spinal root of accessory nerve till the lower end of the muscle.

The deep branch passes deep to levator scapulae and takes part in the anastomoses around the scapula.

Sometimes the two branches may arise separately; the superficial from thyrocervical trunk and the deep from the third part of subclavian artery. Then these are named as superficial cervical and dorsal scapular arteries.

Dorsal Scapular Artery

This artery occasionally arises from the third part of subclavian artery. If transverse cervical does not divide into superficial and deep branches but continues as superficial branch, the distribution of deep branch is taken over by dorsal scapular artery.

Costocervical Trunk

Costocervical trunk arises from the posterior surface of the second part of the subclavian artery on the right side; but from the first part of the artery on the left side. It arches backwards over the cervical pleura, and divides into the descending superior intercostal and ascending deep cervical arteries at the neck of the first rib (Fig. 16.19).

The *superior intercostal artery* descends in front of the neck of the first rib, and divides into the first and second posterior intercostal arteries.

The *deep cervical artery* is analogous to the posterior branch of a posterior intercostal artery. It passes backwards between the transverse process of the 7th cervical vertebra and the neck of the first rib. It then ascends between the semispinalis capitis and cervicis up to the axis vertebra. It anastomoses with the occipital and vertebral arteries.

CLINICAL ANATOMY

- The third part of the subclavian artery can be effectively compressed against the first rib after depressing the shoulder. The pressure is applied downwards, backwards, and medially in the angle between the sternocleidomastoid and the clavicle.
- A cervical rib may compress the subclavian artery, diminishing the radial pulse (Fig. 16.21).
- The right subclavian artery may arise from the descending thoracic aorta. In that case, it passes posterior to the oesophagus which may be compressed and the condition is known as dysphagia lusoria.
- An aneurysm may form in the third part of the subclavian artery. Its pressure on the brachial plexus causes pain, weakness, and numbness in the upper limb.
- Obstruction to the subclavian artery proximal to the origin of vertebral artery may lead to 'stealing of blood from the brain through the opposite vertebral artery'. This may provide necessary blood to the affected side. The nervous symptoms incurred are called 'subclavian steal syndrome' (Fig. 16.22).

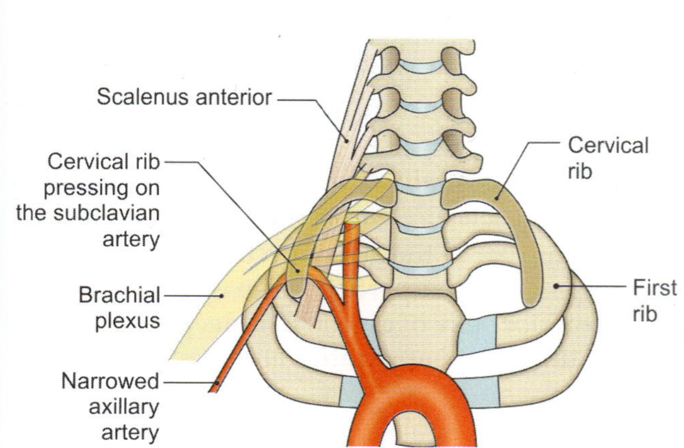

Fig. 16.21: The cervical rib pressing on the subclavian artery narrowing the axillary artery and diminishing the radial pulse

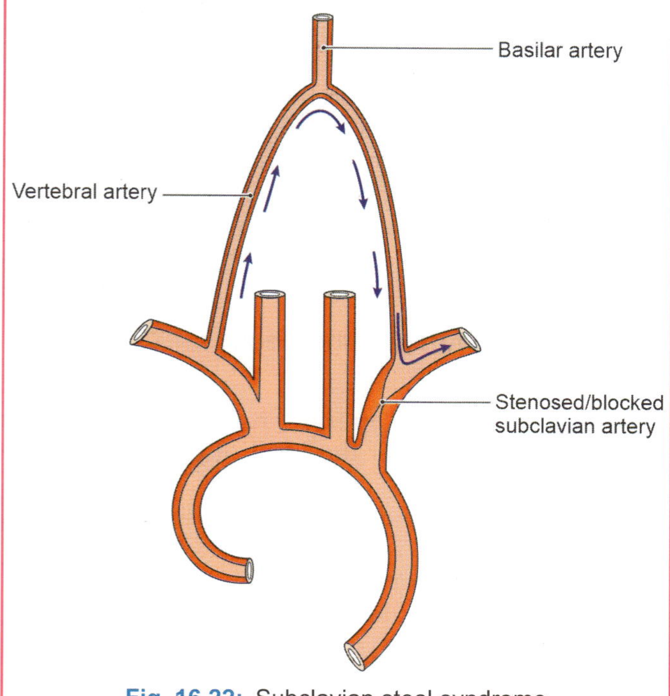

Fig. 16.22: Subclavian steal syndrome

COMMON CAROTID ARTERY

Features

The *origin* and *course* of the common carotid arteries has been described in Chapter 12. The common carotid artery is enclosed in the *carotid sheath.*

Course

Common carotid artery begins in the thorax in front of the trachea opposite a point a little to the left of the

DISSECTION

The common carotid artery has been exposed in the carotid triangle. Clean it in its entire course. Identify the internal carotid artery and trace it till it leaves the neck.

Veins

Identify the tributaries of subclavian, internal jugular and brachiocephalic veins.

centre of the manubrium. It ascends to the back of left sternoclavicular joint and enters the neck.

In the neck, both arteries have a similar course. Each artery runs upwards within the carotid sheath, under cover of the anterior border of the sternocleidomastoid. It lies in front of the lower four cervical transverse processes. At the level of the upper border of the thyroid cartilage, the artery ends by dividing into the external and internal carotid arteries. External carotid artery has been described in Chapter 11.

Relations of the Artery in the Neck

Anterior Relations

1 The common carotid artery is crossed by the superior belly of omohyoid at the level of cricoid cartilage (*see* Fig. 12.14).
2 Below the omohyoid, the artery is deeply situated, and is covered by:
   a. The sternocleidomastoid
   b. The anterior jugular vein
   c. The sternohyoid
   d. The sternothyroid and the middle thyroid vein.

Posterior Relations

1 Transverse process of vertebrae C4–C8, and the muscles attached to their anterior tubercles (longus colli, longus capitis, scalenus anterior).
2 The inferior thyroid artery crosses medially at the level of the cricoid cartilage.
3 Vertebral artery (Fig. 16.23)
4 On the left side, the thoracic duct crosses laterally behind the artery at the level of vertebra C7, in front of the vertebral vessels.

Medial Relations

1 Thyroid gland

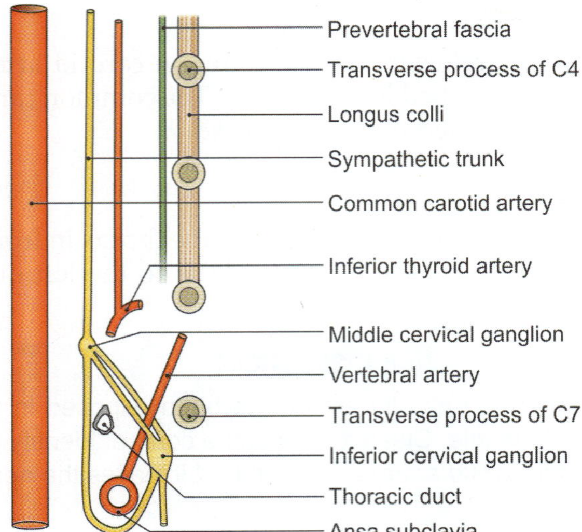

Fig. 16.23: Schematic sagittal section showing posterior relations of the common carotid artery

2 Larynx and pharynx; trachea, oesophagus and recurrent laryngeal nerve (Fig. 16.5).

Lateral Relation

Internal jugular vein.

Posterolateral Relation

Vagus nerve (Fig. 16.4).

CLINICAL ANATOMY

The pulsation of common carotid artery can be felt by compressing against the carotid tubercle, i.e. the anterior tubercle of the transverse process of vertebra C6 which lies at the level of the cricoid cartilage.

INTERNAL CAROTID ARTERY

The internal carotid artery is one of the two terminal branches of the common carotid artery. It begins at the level of the upper border of the thyroid cartilage opposite the disc between the third and fourth cervical vertebrae, and ends inside the cranial cavity by supplying the brain. This is the principal artery of the brain and the eye. It also supplies the related bones and meninges.

For convenience of description, the course of the artery is divided into four parts:

a. Cervical part, in the neck
b. Petrous part, within the petrous temporal bone (*see* Fig. 20.16)
c. Cavernous part, within the cavernous sinus
d. Cerebral part in relation to base of the brain.

Cervical Part

1 It ascends vertically in the neck from its origin to the base of the skull to reach the lower end of the carotid canal. This part is enclosed in the carotid sheath (with the internal jugular vein and the vagus nerve).
2 No branches arise from the internal carotid artery in the neck.
3 Its initial part usually shows a dilatation, the *carotid sinus* which acts as a baroreceptor (*see* Fig. 12.14).
4 The lower part of the artery (in the carotid triangle) is comparatively superficial. The upper part, above the posterior belly of digastric, is deep to the parotid gland, the styloid apparatus, and many other structures.

Relations

Anterior or superficial

1 In the carotid triangle:
   a. Anterior border of sternocleidomastoid

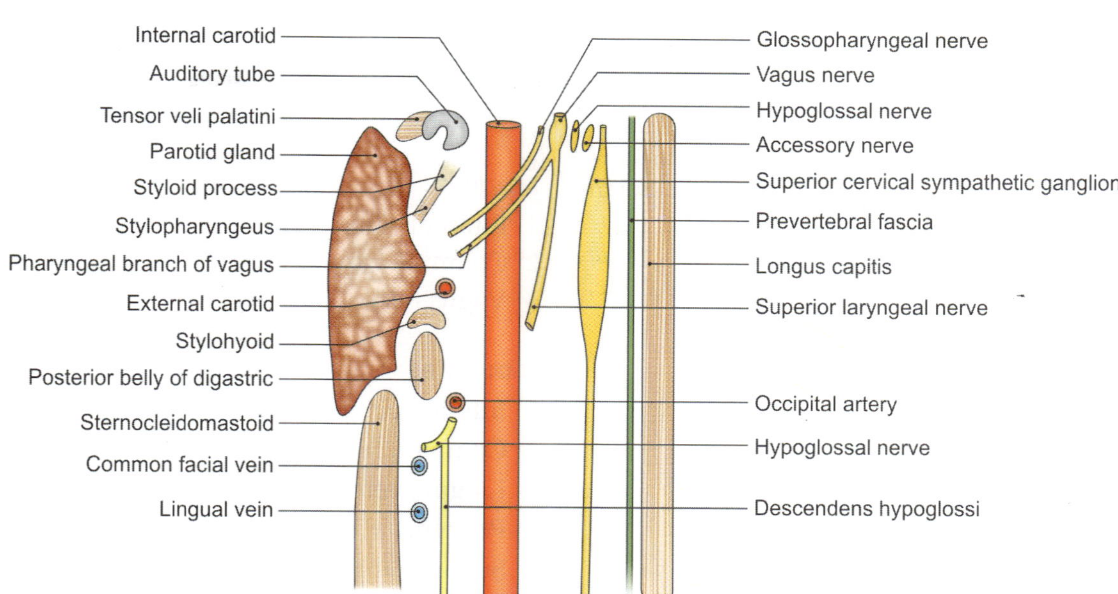

Fig. 16.24: Schematic sagittal section showing the anterior and posterior relations of the internal carotid artery

   b. The external carotid artery is anteromedial to it (Fig. 16.16).
2 Above the carotid triangle (*see* Fig. 12.13):
   a. Posterior belly of digastric
   b. Stylohyoid
   c. Stylopharyngeus
   d. Styloid process
   e. Parotid gland with structures within it.

Posterior

1 Superior cervical ganglion
2 Carotid sheath
3 The glossopharyngeal, vagus, accessory and hypoglossal nerves at the base of the skull.

Medial

1 Pharynx
2 The external carotid is anteromedial to it below the parotid.

Lateral

1 Internal jugular vein
2 Temporomandibular joint (at the base of the skull)

Petrous Part

1 In the carotid canal, the artery first runs upwards, and then turns forwards and medially at right angles. It emerges at the apex of the petrous temporal bone, in the posterior wall of the foramen lacerum where it turns upwards and medially.
2 *Relations:* The artery is surrounded by venous and sympathetic plexuses. It is related to the middle ear and the cochlea (posterosuperiorly); the auditory tube and tensor tympani (anterolaterally); and the trigeminal ganglion (superiorly) (*see* Fig. 20.14).
3 *Branches:*
   a. *Caroticotympanic* branches enter the middle ear, and anastomose with the anterior and posterior tympanic arteries (*see* Fig. 20.16).
   b. The *pterygoid branch* (small and inconstant) enters the pterygoid canal with the nerve of that canal and anastomoses with the greater palatine artery.

Cavernous and Cerebral Parts

Cavernous part runs in the cavernous sinus (*see* Fig. 20.6). Cerebral part lies at base of skull and gives ophthalmic, anterior cerebral, middle cerebral, posterior communicating and anterior choroidal arteries.

SUBCLAVIAN VEIN

Course

It is a continuation of the axillary vein. It begins at the outer border of the first rib, and ends at the medial border of the scalenus anterior by joining the internal jugular vein to form the brachiocephalic vein.

It lies:
   a. In front of the subclavian artery, the scalenus anterior and the right phrenic nerve
   b. Behind the clavicle and the subclavius
   c. Above the first rib and pleura.

Its tributaries are:
   a. The external jugular vein (Fig. 16.25)
   b. The dorsal scapular vein
   c. The thoracic duct on the left side
   d. The right lymphatic duct on the right side.

INTERNAL JUGULAR VEIN

Course

1 It is a direct continuation of the sigmoid sinus. It begins at the jugular foramen, and ends behind the sternal end of the clavicle by joining the subclavian vein to form the brachiocephalic vein.
2 The origin is marked by a dilation, the *superior bulb* which lies in the jugular fossa of the temporal bone, beneath the floor of the middle ear cavity. The termination of the vein is marked by the *inferior bulb* which lies beneath the lesser supraclavicular fossa.

Relations

Superficial

1 Sternocleidomastoid
2 Posterior belly of digastric
3 Superior belly of omohyoid
4 Parotid gland
5 Styloid process
6 The internal carotid artery, and the glossopharyngeal, vagus, accessory and hypoglossal cranial nerves (at the base of skull)

Posterior

1 Transverse process of atlas
2 Cervical plexus
3 Scalenus anterior
4 First part of subclavian artery

Medial

1 Internal carotid artery
2 Common carotid artery
3 Vagus nerve

Tributaries

1 Inferior petrosal sinus
2 Common facial vein
3 Lingual vein
4 Pharyngeal veins
5 Superior thyroid vein
6 Middle thyroid vein (Fig. 16.25)

The thoracic duct opens into the angle of union between the left internal jugular vein and the left subclavian vein. The right lymphatic duct opens similarly on the right side.

In the middle of the neck, the internal jugular vein may communicate with the external jugular vein through the oblique jugular vein which runs across the anterior border of the sternocleidomastoid.

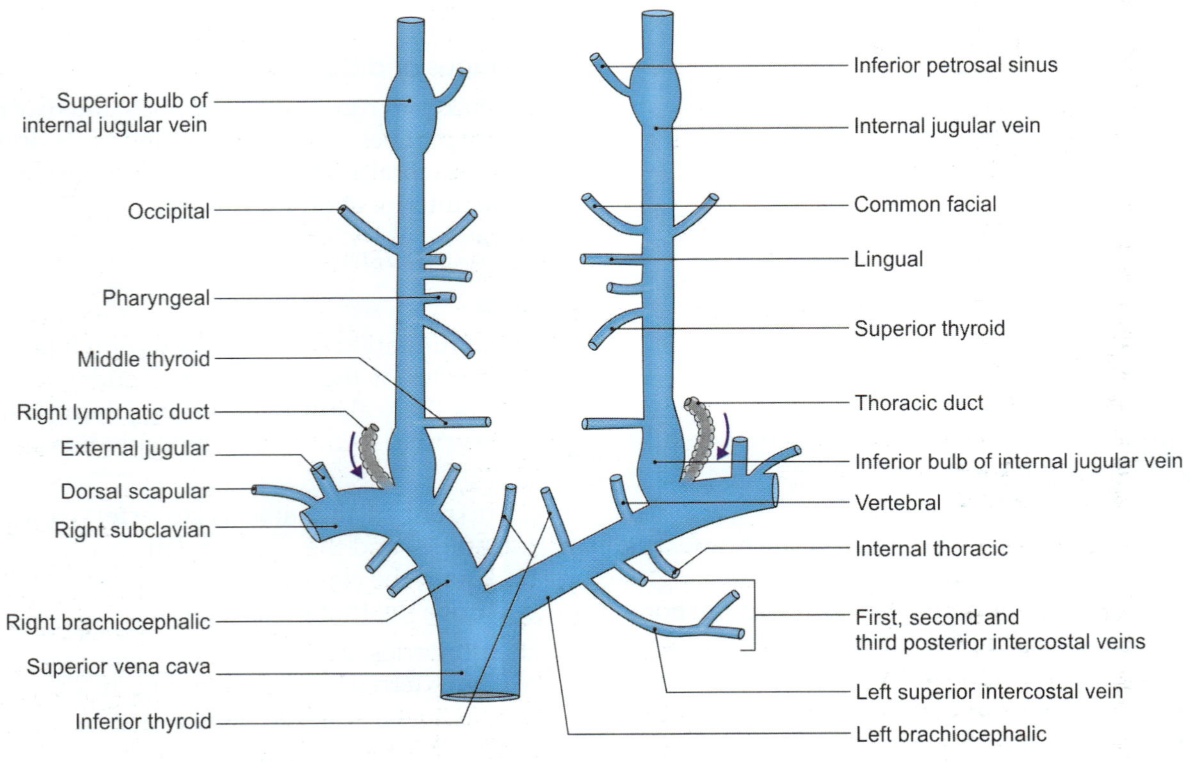

Fig. 16.25: The veins of the neck

CLINICAL ANATOMY

- Deep to the lesser supraclavicular fossa, the internal jugular vein is easily accessible for recording of venous pulse tracings. The vein can be cannulated by direct puncture in the interval between sternal and clavicular heads of sterno-cleidomastoid muscle.
- In congestive cardiac failure or any other disease where venous pressure is raised, the internal jugular vein is markedly dilated and engorged.

BRACHIOCEPHALIC VEIN

1 The right brachiocephalic vein (2.5 cm long) is shorter than the left (6 cm long) (Fig. 16.25).
2 Each vein is formed behind the sternoclavicular joint, by the union of the internal jugular vein and the subclavian vein.
3 The right vein runs vertically downwards. The left vein runs obliquely downwards and to the right behind the upper half of the manubrium sterni. The two brachiocephalic veins unite at the lower border of the right first costal cartilage to form the superior vena cava.
4 The *tributaries* correspond to the branches of the first part of the subclavian artery. These are as follows.

Right Brachiocephalic

a. Vertebral
b. Internal thoracic
c. Inferior thyroid
d. First posterior intercostal

Left Brachiocephalic

a. Vertebral (Fig. 16.25)
b. Internal thoracic
c. Inferior thyroid
d. First posterior intercostal
e. Left superior intercostal
f. Thymic and pericardial veins

NERVES OF THE NECK

GLOSSOPHARYNGEAL NERVE—IX NERVE

Glossopharyngeal nerve exits the cranial cavity via anterior part of jugular foramen.

Course

1 It runs between internal carotid artery and internal jugular vein, lying deep to the styloid process and muscles attached to the process.
2 Then it courses between internal carotid and external carotid arteries, where it curves round the lateral border of stylopharyngeus muscle.
3 As it reaches submandibular region, it passes deep to hyoglossus muscle to reach the area of palatine tonsil and base of the tongue (Fig. 16.26).

Branches

1 Tympanic branch courses through middle ear and gives secretomotor root to otic ganglion.
2 Carotid branch for carotid body and carotid sinus.
3 Muscular for stylopharyngeus muscle.
4 Carries taste from vallate papillae of tongue.
5 Carries general sensations from posterior one-third of tongue and palatine tonsil.
6 Branch to pharyngeal plexus.

VAGUS NERVE—X NERVE

Vagus leaves the cranial cavity through jugular foramen lying posterior to IX nerve. Soon it is joined course by cranial root of XI nerve. In the neck, the nerve lies in the carotid sheath, medial to internal jugular vein and posterior to internal carotid and common carotid arteries (Fig. 16.27).

Then it passes through thorax and abdomen.

Branches in Neck

- Meningeal
- Auricular
- Pharyngeal for most muscles of soft palate 4 out of 5 and pharynx 5 out of 6, carotid for carotid body and carotid sinus, superior laryngeal gives internal laryngeal for mucous membrane of larynx and external laryngeal for cricothyroid muscle.
- Right recurrent laryngeal is given off in neck while left one is given off in thorax. The nerves supply all intrinsic muscles of larynx, and sensory branches to mucous membrane of larynx below vocal cords.
- Cardiac branches for deep cardiac plexus.

ACCESSORY NERVE—XI NERVE

This nerve also leaves the cranial cavity through the jugular foramen. It is made up of a cranial root and a spinal root. The two roots join in jugular foramen, but again separate as it passes out of the foramen. Cranial root joins X nerve and gets distributed with it for 4 out of 5 palatal muscles, 5 out of 6 pharyngeal muscles and all laryngeal muscles (Fig. 16.27).

The spinal root descends between internal jugular vein and internal carotid artery for some distance.

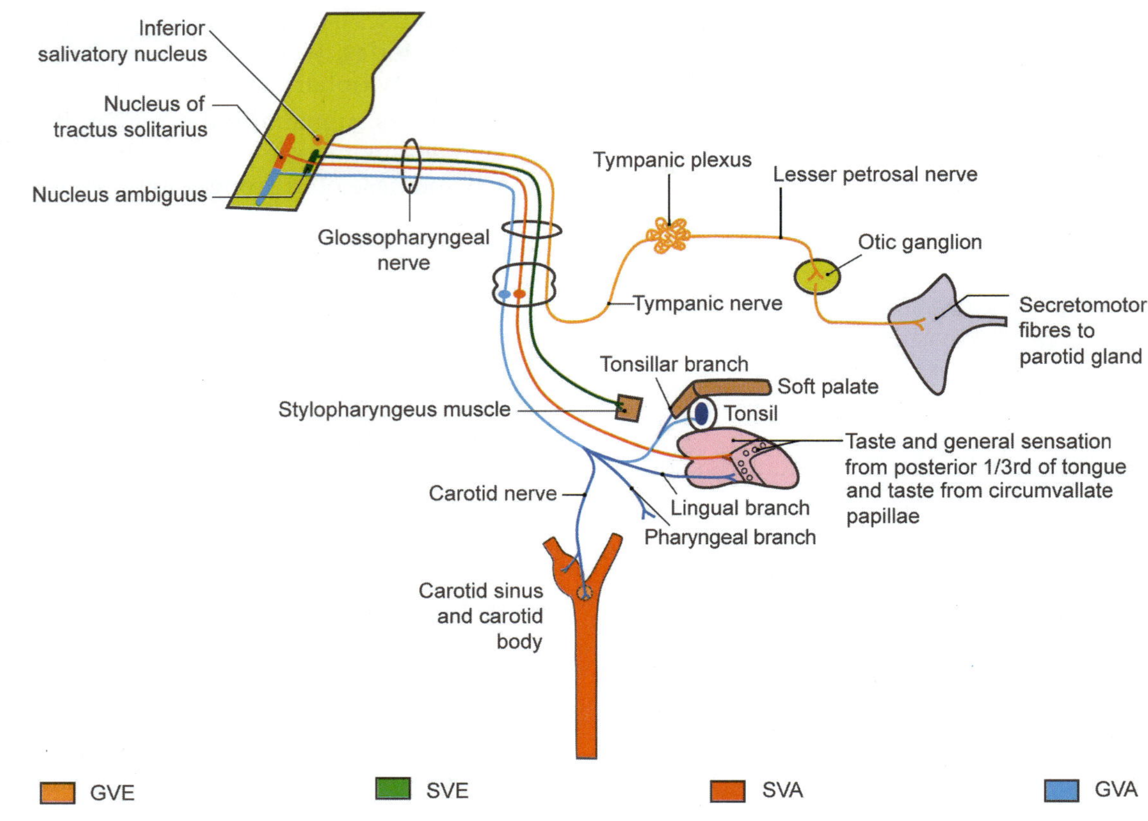

Fig. 16.26: Distribution of glossopharyngeal nerve

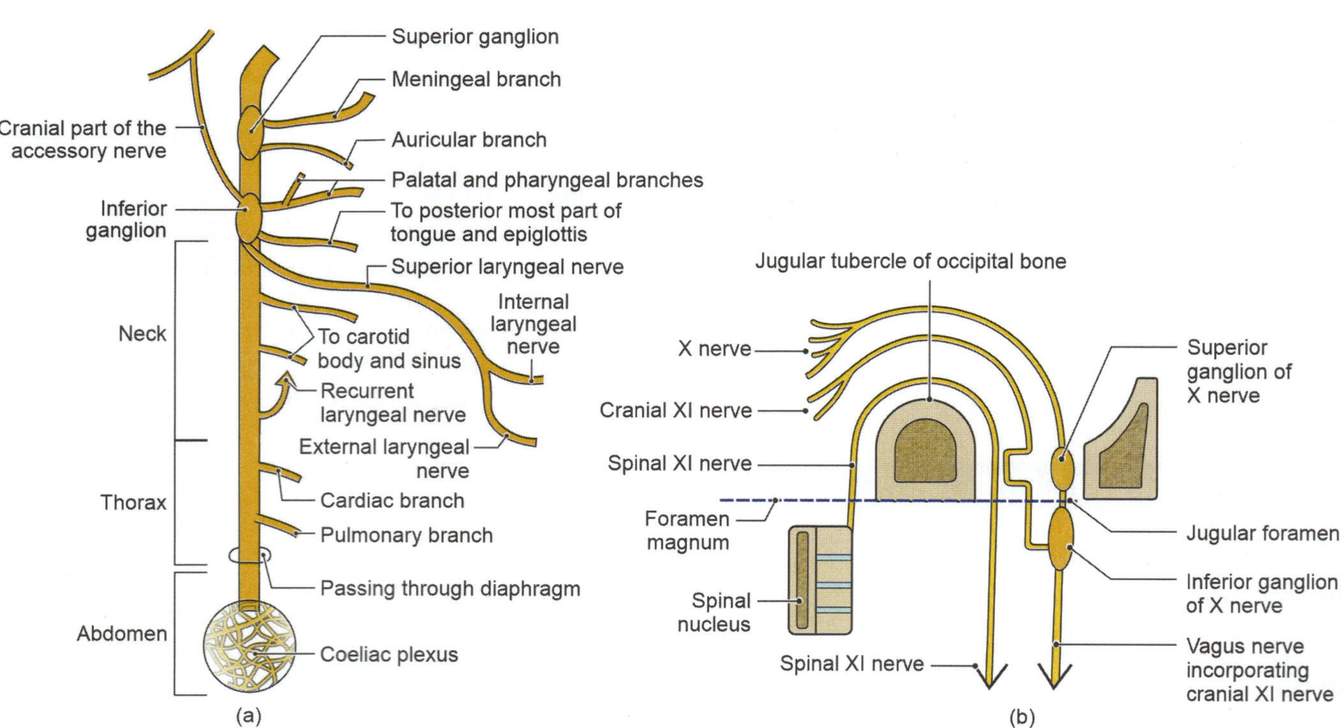

Figs 16.27a and b: (a) Distribution of vagus and cranial part of accessory nerves; (b) Cranial and spinal roots of accessory (XI) nerve

It then lies superficial to internal jugular vein to reach anterior border of sternocleidomastoid muscle. It enters the muscle, supplies it and leaves the muscle at its posterior border a little above its middle.

Then it passes downwards and backwards in the posterior triangle of neck. Finally, it leaves posterior triangle by passing deep to trapezius (*see* Fig. 11.10).

Thus the spinal root of XI nerve supplies: Sternocleidomastoid and trapezius muscles.

DISSECTION

The course of IX–XI cranial nerves has been seen in different chapters. Now trace these nerves and their branches.

The sympathetic trunk has been identified as lying posteromedial to the carotid sheath. Trace it upwards and downwards and locate the three cervical ganglia.

Dissect the formation and branches of the cervical plexus. Identify the phrenic nerve on the surface of scalenus anterior muscle behind the prevertebral fascia.

CERVICAL PART OF SYMPATHETIC TRUNK

Features

The cervical parts of the right and left sympathetic trunks are situated one on each side of the cervical part of the vertebral column, behind the carotid sheath (common carotid and internal carotid arteries) and in front of the prevertebral fascia.

FORMATION

There are *no white rami communicantes* (i.e. incoming root) in the neck and this part of the trunk is formed by fibres which emerge from segments T1 to T4 of the spinal cord, and then ascend into the neck (Fig. 16.28).

Grey rami communicantes (i.e. outgoing roots) are present.

Relations

Anterior

a. Internal carotid artery
b. Common carotid artery
c. Carotid sheath (Fig. 16.4)
d. Inferior thyroid artery

Posterior

a. Prevertebral fascia
b. Longus capitis and cervicis muscles
c. Transverse processes of the lower six cervical vertebrae.

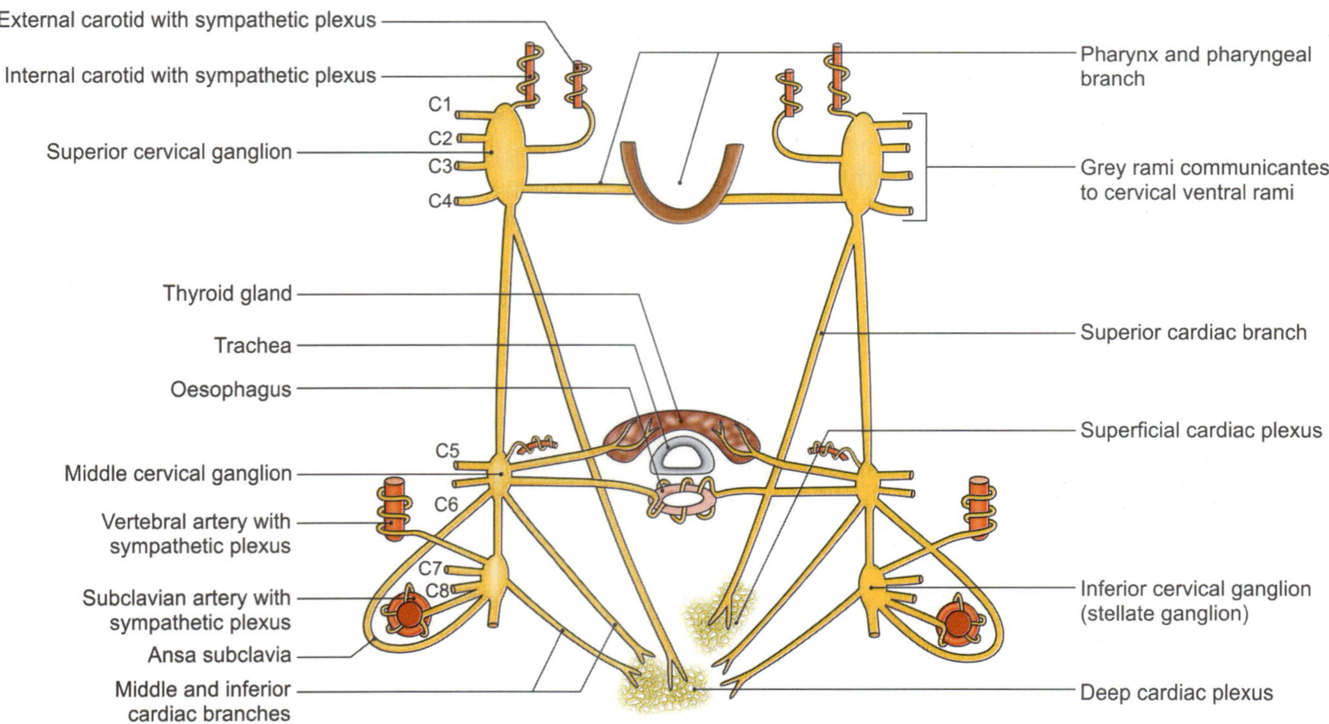

Fig. 16.28: The cervical sympathetic trunks and their branches

GANGLIA

Theoretically, there should be eight sympathetic ganglia corresponding to the eight cervical nerves, but due to fusion, there are only three ganglia—superior, middle and inferior.

Superior Cervical Ganglion

Size and Shape

This is the largest of the three ganglia. It is spindle-shaped, and about 2.5 cm long (Fig. 16.28).

Situation and Formation

It lies just below the skull, opposite the second and third cervical vertebrae, behind the carotid sheath and in front of the prevertebral fascia (longus capitis). It is formed by fusion of the upper 4 cervical ganglia.

Communications. With cranial nerves IX, X and XII, and with the external and recurrent laryngeal nerves.

Branches

1 Grey rami communicantes pass to the ventral rami of upper four cervical nerves (Fig. 16.28).
2 The internal carotid nerve arises from the upper end of the ganglion and forms a plexus around the internal carotid artery. A part of this plexus supplies the dilator pupillae (*see* Chapter 27). Some of these fibres form the deep petrosal nerve for pterygopalatine ganglion; others give fibres along long ciliary nerve for the ciliary ganglion.
3 The external carotid branches form a plexus around the external carotid artery. Some of these fibres form the sympathetic roots of the otic and submandibular ganglia (*see* Table A.2, Appendix).
4 Pharyngeal branches take part in the formation of the pharyngeal plexus.
5 The left superior cervical cardiac branch goes to the superficial cardiac plexus while the right branch goes to the deep cardiac plexus.

Middle Cervical Ganglion

Size and Shape

This ganglion is very small. It may be divided into 2 to 3 smaller parts, or may be absent.

Situation

It lies in the lower part of the neck, in front of vertebra C6 just above the inferior thyroid artery, behind the carotid sheath (Fig. 16.28).

Formation

It is formed by fusion of the fifth and sixth cervical ganglia connections. It is connected with the inferior cervical ganglion directly, and also through a loop that winds round the subclavian artery. This loop is called the ansa subclavia.

Branches

1 Grey rami communicantes are given to the ventral rami of the 5th and 6th cervical nerves.
2 Thyroid branches accompany the inferior thyroid artery to the thyroid gland. They also supply the parathyroid glands (Fig. 16.28).
3 Tracheal and oesophageal branches.
4 The middle cervical cardiac branch is the largest of the sympathetic cardiac branches. It goes to the deep cardiac plexus.

Inferior Cervical Ganglion

Size, Shape and Formation

It is formed by fusion of 7th and 8th cervical ganglia. This is often fused with the first thoracic ganglion and is then known as the *cervicothoracic ganglion* or *stellate ganglion* because it is star-shaped.

It is situated between the transverse process of vertebra C7 and the neck of the first rib. It lies behind the vertebral artery, and in front of ramus of spinal nerve C8. *A cervicothoracic ganglion extends in front of the neck of the first rib.*

Branches

1 Grey rami communicantes are given to the ventral rami of nerves C7 and C8.
2 Vertebral branches form a plexus around the vertebral artery.
3 Subclavian branches form a plexus around the subclavian artery. This plexus is joined by branches from the ansa subclavia (Fig. 16.28).
4 An inferior cervical cardiac branch goes to the deep cardiac plexus.

Branches of the cervical sympathetic ganglia are listed in Table 16.1.

CLINICAL ANATOMY

- The head and neck are supplied by sympathetic nerves arising from the upper four thoracic segments of the spinal cord. Most of these preganglionic fibres pass through the stellate ganglion to relay in the superior cervical ganglion.
- Injury to cervical sympathetic trunk produces Horner's syndrome. It is characterized by:
  a. Ptosis—drooping of the upper eyelid.
  b. Miosis—constriction of the pupil (Fig. 16.29).
  c. Anhydrosis—loss of sweating on that side of the face.

Table 16.1: Branches of cervical sympathetic ganglia			
	Superior cervical ganglion	*Middle cervical ganglion*	*Inferior cervical ganglion*
Arterial branches	i. Along internal carotid artery as internal carotid nerve ii. Along common carotid and external carotid arteries	Along inferior thyroid artery	Along subclavian and vertebral arteries
Grey rami communicantes	Along 1–4 cervical nerves	Along 5 and 6 cervical nerves	Along 7 and 8 cervical nerves
Along cranial nerves	Along cranial nerves IX, X, XI and XII	–	–
Visceral branches	Pharynx, cardiac	Thyroid, cardiac	Cardiac

d. Enophthalmos—retraction of the eyeball.
e. Loss of the ciliospinal reflex—pinching the skin on the nape of the neck does not produce dilatation of the pupil (which normally takes place).

- Horner's syndrome can also be caused by a lesion within the central nervous system anywhere at or above the first thoracic segment of the spinal cord involving sympathetic fibres.

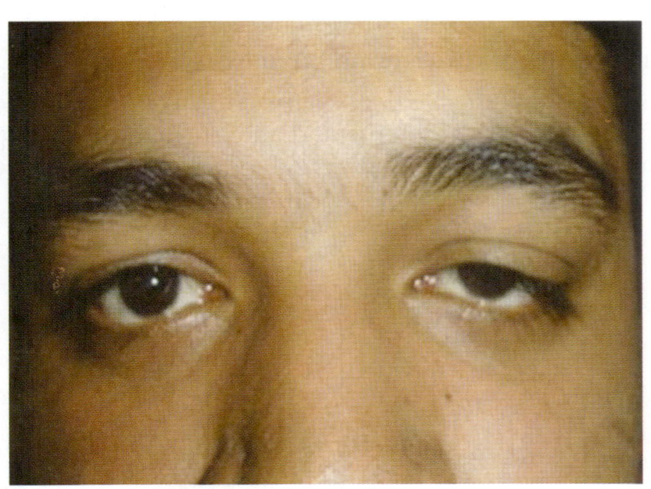

Fig. 16.29: Horner's syndrome on left side

LYMPHATIC DRAINAGE OF HEAD AND NECK

DISSECTION

Identify the lymph nodes in the submental, the submandibular, the parotid, the mastoid and the occipital regions including the deep cervical nodes. Dissect the main lymph trunk present at the root of the neck.

Features

Lymph nodes in head and neck are as follows:

a. Superficial group
b. Deep group
c. Deepest group

SUPERFICIAL GROUP

Buccal and Mandibular Nodes

The buccal node lies on the buccinator, and the mandibular node at the lower border of the mandible near the anteroinferior angle of the masseter, in close relation to the marginal mandibular branch of the facial nerve. They drain part of the cheek and the lower eyelid. Their efferents pass to the anterosuperior group of deep cervical nodes (Fig. 16.30).

Preauricular Nodes

Drain parotid gland, temporal region, middle ear, etc.

Postauricular (Mastoid) Nodes

The postauricular nodes lie on the mastoid process, superficial to the sternocleidomastoid and deep to the auricularis posterior. They drain a strip of scalp just above and behind the auricle, the upper half of the medial surface and margin of the auricle, and the posterior wall of the external acoustic meatus. Their efferents pass to the posterosuperior group of deep cervical nodes (Fig. 16.30).

Occipital Nodes

The occipital nodes lie at the apex of the posterior triangle superficial to the attachment of the trapezius. They drain the occipital region of the scalp. Their efferents pass to the supraclavicular members of the posteroinferior group of deep cervical nodes.

Anterior Superficial Cervical Nodes

The anterior cervical nodes lie along the *anterior jugular vein* and are unimportant. The suprasternal lymph node is a member of this group. They drain the skin of the

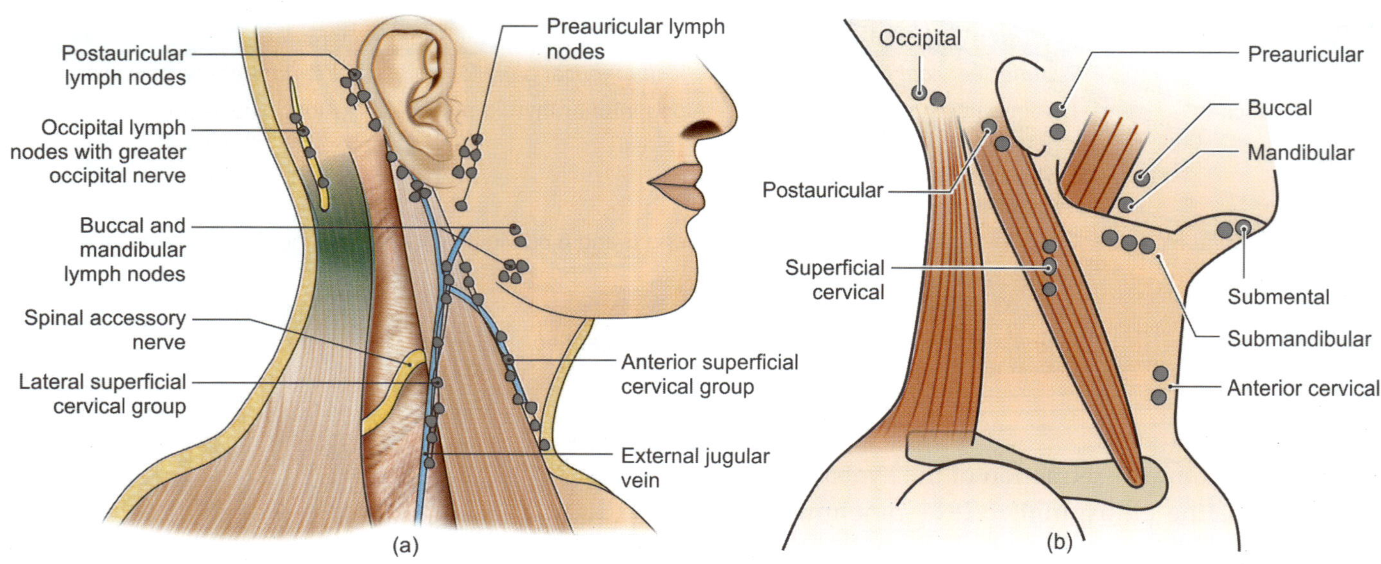

Figs 16.30a and b: Superficial lymph nodes of the neck

anterior part of the neck below the hyoid bone. Their efferents pass to the deep cervical nodes of both sides (Fig. 16.30).

Lateral Superficial Cervical Nodes

The superficial cervical nodes lie along the *external jugular vein* superficial to the sternocleidomastoid. They drain the lobule of the auricle, the floor of the external acoustic meatus, and the skin over the lower parotid region and the angle of the jaw. Their efferents pass round both borders of the muscle to reach the upper and lower deep cervical nodes.

DEEP GROUP

It comprises five levels of lymph nodes (Fig. 16.31).

Submental and Submandibular Nodes

Submental nodes lie deep to the chin. These drain the lymph from tip of tongue and anterior part of floor of mouth. The submandibular nodes drain lateral surface

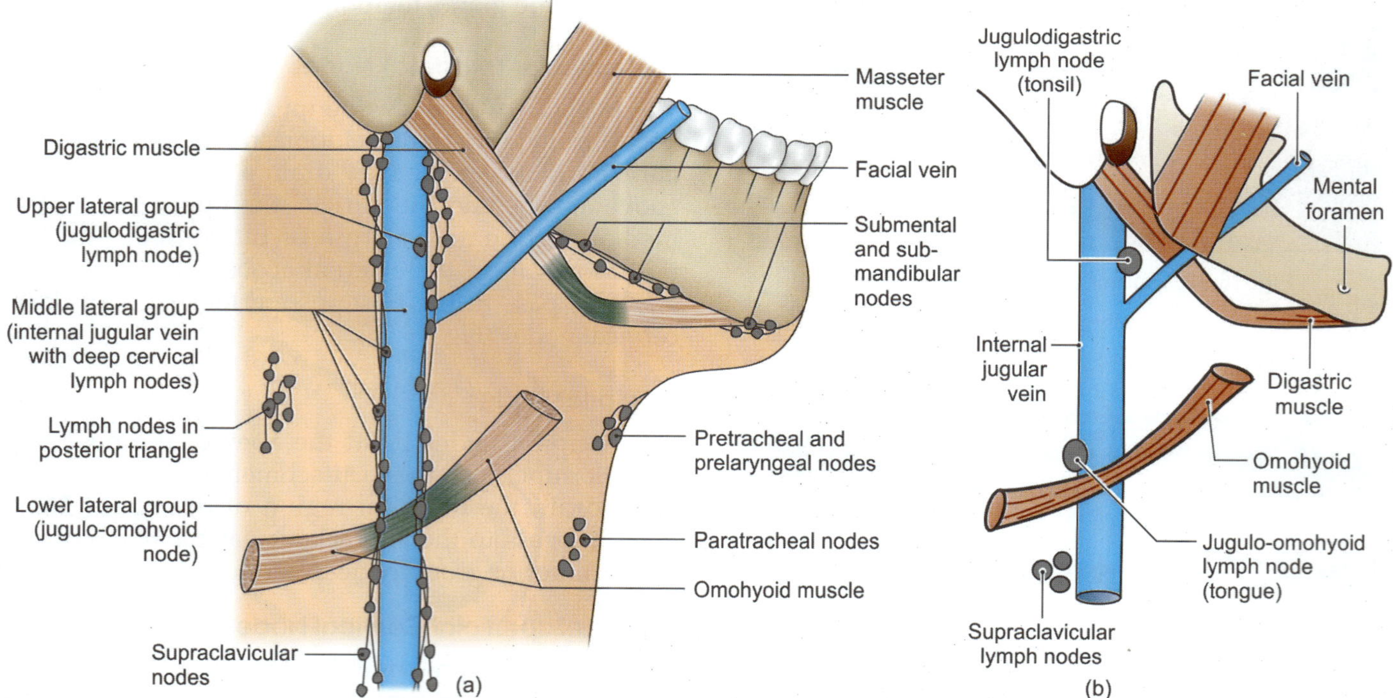

Figs 16.31a and b: Deep and deepest groups of lymph nodes in the neck

of tongue, lower gums and teeth and central area of forehead.

The *submandibular lymph nodes* are clinically very important because of their wide area of drainage. They are very commonly enlarged. The nodes lie beneath the deep cervical fascia on the surface of the submandibular salivary gland. They drain:

a. Centre of the forehead.
b. Nose with the frontal, maxillary and ethmoidal air sinuses.
c. The inner canthus of the eye.
d. The upper lip and the anterior part of the cheek with the underlying gum and teeth.
e. The outer part of the lower lip with the lower gums and teeth excluding the incisors.
f. The anterior two-thirds of the tongue excluding the tip, and the floor of the mouth. They also receive efferents from the submental lymph nodes.

The *efferents* from the submandibular nodes pass mostly to the jugulo-omohyoid node and partly to the jugulodigastric node. These nodes are situated along the internal jugular vein and are members of the deep cervical chain (Fig. 16.31).

Upper Lateral Nodes around Internal Jugular Vein

The *jugulodigastric node* (Fig. 16.29) is a member of this group. It lies below the posterior belly of digastric, between the angle of the mandible and anterior border of the sternocleidomastoid, in the triangle bounded by the posterior belly of digastric, the facial vein and the internal jugular vein. It is the main node draining the *tonsil*.

Middle Lateral Nodes around Internal Jugular Vein

These drain thyroid and parathyroid glands. They receive efferents from prelaryngeal, pretracheal and paratracheal lymph nodes.

Lower Lateral Nodes around Internal Jugular Vein

The *jugulo-omohyoid node* is a group of nodes. It lies just above the intermediate tendon of the omohyoid, under cover of the posterior border of the sternocleido-mastoid. It is the main lymph node of the *tongue*.

Lymph Nodes in Posterior Triangle

The lymph nodes are present around the spinal root of accessory nerve.

Efferents of the deep cervical lymph nodes join together to form the *jugular lymph trunks*, one on each side. The left jugular trunk opens into the thoracic duct. The right trunk may open either into the right lymphatic duct, or directly into the angle of junction between the internal jugular and subclavian veins.

DEEPEST GROUP

Prelaryngeal and Pretracheal Nodes

The prelaryngeal and pretracheal nodes lie deep to the investing fascia, the prelaryngeal nodes on the cricothyroid membrane, and the pretracheal in front of the trachea below the isthmus of the thyroid gland. They drain the larynx, the trachea and the isthmus of the thyroid. They also receive afferents from the anterior cervical nodes. Their efferents pass to the nearby deep cervical nodes.

Paratracheal Nodes

The paratracheal nodes lie on the sides of the trachea and oesophagus along the recurrent laryngeal nerves. They receive lymph from the oesophagus, the trachea and the larynx, and pass it onto the deep cervical nodes.

Retropharyngeal Nodes

The retropharyngeal nodes (Fig. 16.4) lie in front of the prevertebral fascia and behind the buccopharyngeal fascia covering the posterior wall of the pharynx. They extend laterally in front of the lateral mass of the atlas and along the lateral border of the longus capitis. They drain the pharynx, the auditory tube, the soft palate, the posterior part of the hard palate, and the nose. Their efferents pass to the upper lateral group of deep cervical nodes (Fig. 16.4).

Waldeyer's Ring

The ring comprises lingual, palatine, tubal and nasopharyngeal tonsils (*see* Fig. 22.13).

MAIN LYMPH TRUNKS AT THE ROOT OF THE NECK

1 The *thoracic duct* is the largest lymph trunk of the body. It begins in the abdomen from the upper end of the cisterna chyli enters the thorax through aortic opening, traverses the thorax, and ends on the left side of the root of the neck by opening into the angle of junction between the left internal jugular vein and the left subclavian vein (Fig. 16.25). Before its termination, it forms an arch at the level of the transverse process of vertebra C7 rising 3 to 4 cm above the clavicle. The relations of the arch are:

Anterior:
a. Left common carotid artery
b. Vagus
c. Internal jugular vein.

Posterior:
a. Vertebral artery and vein
b. Sympathetic trunk
c. Thyrocervical trunk and its branches

d. Prevertebral fascia
e. Phrenic nerve
f. Scalenus anterior.

Apart from its tributaries in the abdomen and thorax, the thoracic duct receives (in the neck):
a. The left jugular trunk
b. The left subclavian trunk
c. The left bronchomediastinal trunk.

It drains most of the body, except for the right upper limb, the right halves of the head, the neck and the thorax and the superior surface of the liver.

2 The right *jugular trunk* drains half of the head and neck.
3 The right *subclavian trunk* drains the upper limb.
4 The *bronchomediastinal trunk* drains the lung, half of the mediastinum and parts of the anterior walls of the thorax and abdomen.
5 On the right side, the subclavian, jugular and bronchomediastinal trunks unite to form the *right lymph trunk* which ends in a manner similar to the thoracic duct (Fig. 16.25).

Classification of Lymph Nodes

There are about 800 lymph nodes in the body and about 300 nodes are present in the region of neck.

American Joint Committee on Cancer has divided palpable lymph nodes into 7 levels. This is based on the extent and level of involvement in metastatic tumours.

Level I—it contains submental, submandibular present in digastric triangle bounded by anterior and posterior belly of digastrics, hyoid bone and body of mandible.

Level II—contains upper jugular lymph nodes. Extends from level of base of skull above to the level of hyoid bone below.

Level III—contains middle jugular lymph nodes from hyoid bone above to cricothyroid membrane below.

Level IV—contains lower jugular lymph nodes. Extends from cricothyroid membrane above to the clavicle below.

Level V—contains lymph nodes in the posterior triangle of neck, bounded by sternocleidomastoid muscle, trapezius muscle and middle third of clavicle.

Level VI—contains lymph nodes in the anterior compartment. Extends from hyoid bone above to suprasternal notch below. These lie between the medial borders of right and left carotid sheaths.

Level VII—contains lymph nodes below suprasternal notch in the superior mediastinum.

CLINICAL ANATOMY

- The deep cervical lymph nodes lie on the internal jugular vein. These nodes often become adherent to the vein in malignancy or in tuberculosis. Therefore, during operation on such patients, the vein is also resected. These are examined from behind with the neck slightly flexed.
- Superficial cervical, supraclavicular and lymph nodes of anterior triangle can easily be palpated (Fig. 16.32).
- Chronic infection of the palatine tonsil causes enlargement of jugulodigastric lymph nodes which adhere to the internal jugular vein.
- Painful enlargement of the submandibular lymph nodes is common because infections in tongue, mouth and cheek are quite common. These nodes may be affected by tubercular bacteria.
- Spinal root of accessory nerve may get entangled in the enlarged lymph nodes situated in the posterior triangle of neck. While taking biopsy of the lymph node, one must be careful not to injure the accessory nerve lest trapezius gets damaged (*see* Fig. 11.9).

The left supraclavicular nodes are called Virchow's lymph nodes. Cancer from stomach and testis may metastasize into these lymph nodes, which may become palpable.

Common causes of lymph node enlargement

a. *Local causes:* Acute infection, chronic infection, malignancy of any part of the body.
b. *General causes:* Tuberculosis, secondary syphilis, Hodgkin's disease, lymphatic leukaemia.

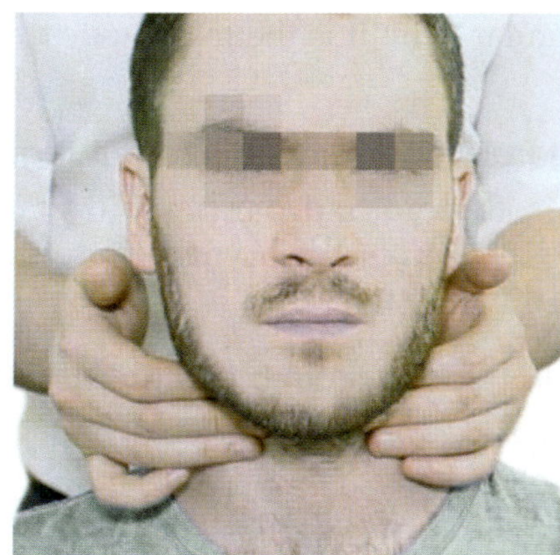

Fig. 16.32: Palpation of the lymph nodes

STYLOID APPARATUS

The styloid process with its attached structures is called the styloid apparatus. The structures attached to the process are three muscles and two ligaments. The muscles are the stylohyoid, styloglossus and stylopharyngeus and ligaments are the stylohyoid and stylomandibular (Figs 16.33a and b).

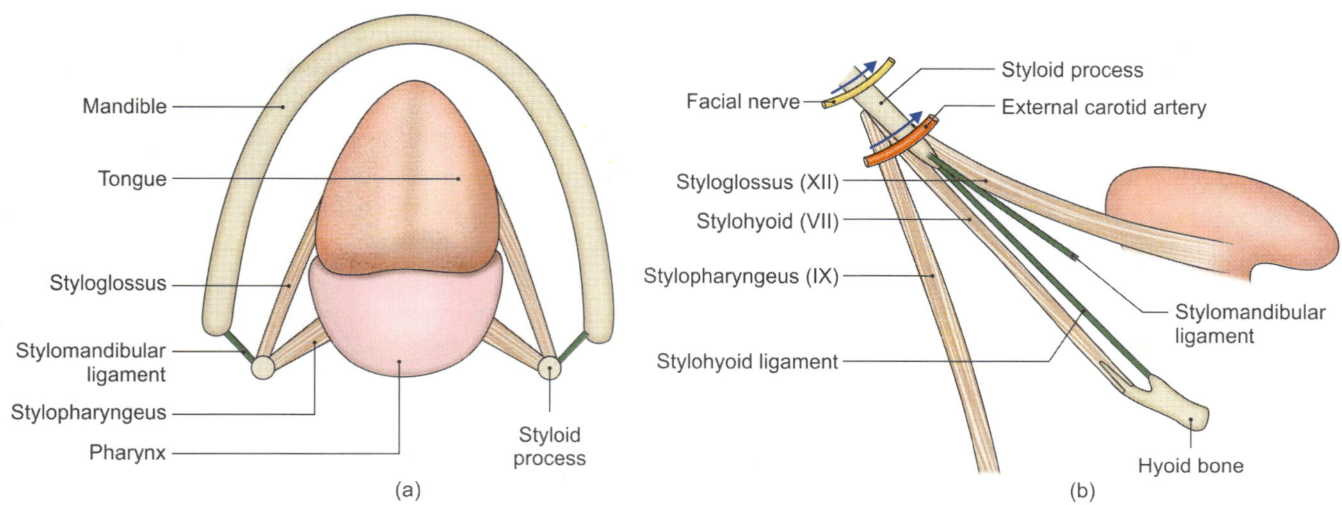

Figs 16.33a and b: The styloid apparatus: (a) Superior view; (b) Lateral view

The apparatus is of diverse origin. The styloid process, the stylohyoid ligament and stylohyoid muscle are derived from the second branchial arch; the stylopharyngeus from the third arch; the styloglossus from occipital myotomes; and the stylomandibular ligament from a part of the deep fascia of neck.

The *five attachments resemble the reins of a chariot*. Two of these reins (ligaments) are nonadjustable, whereas the other three (muscles) are adjustable and are controlled each by a separate cranial nerve—seventh, ninth and twelfth nerves.

The *styloid process* is a long, slender and pointed bony process projecting downwards, forwards and slightly medially from the temporal bone. It descends between the external and internal carotid arteries to reach the side of the pharynx. It is interposed between the parotid gland laterally and the internal jugular vein medially.

The *styloglossus muscle* arises from the anterior surface of the styloid process and is inserted into the side of the tongue.

The *stylopharyngeus muscle* arises from the medial surface of the base of the styloid process and is inserted on the posterior border of the lamina of the thyroid cartilage (*see* Fig. 22.23).

Stylohyoid extends between posterior surface of styloid process and hyoid bone. It splits at its lower end to enclose the intermediate tendon of digastric muscle.

The *stylomandibular ligament* is attached laterally to styloid process above and angle of mandible below.

The *stylohyoid ligament* extends from the tip of the styloid process to the lesser cornua of the hyoid bone.

Features

1 External carotid artery crosses tip of styloid process superficially and pierces stylomandibular ligament.
2 Facial nerve crosses the base of styloid process laterally after it emerges from stylomastoid foramen.

DEVELOPMENT OF THE ARTERIES

Brachoicephalic artery	:	Right aortic sac
Right subclavian artery	:	Proximal part from the right 4th aortic arch artery and remaining part from right 7th cervical intersegmental artery.
Left subclavian artery	:	Only left 7th cervical intersegmental artery.
Common carotid	:	Third aortic arch proximal to external carotid bud.
Internal carotid artery	:	Third aortic arch, distal to the external carotid bud and original dorsal aorta cranial to the attachment of third aortic arch.
External carotid artery	:	Develop as sprout from the third aortic arch.
Pulmonary trunk	:	Part of truncus arteriosus.
Arch of aorta	:	Left aortic sac
	:	Left 4th aortic arch
	:	Left dorsal aorta.

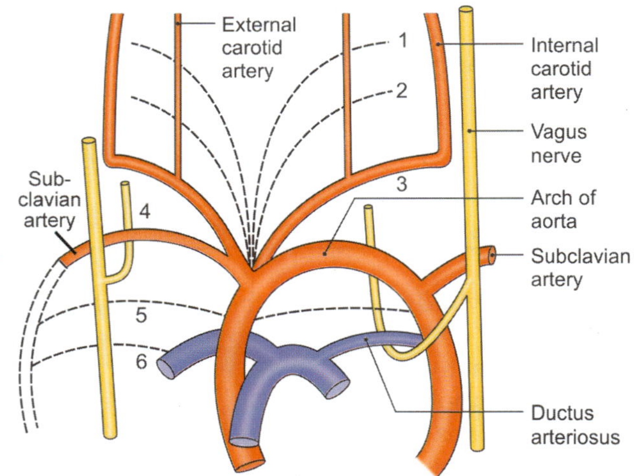

Fig. 16.34: Relation to recurrent laryngeal nerve

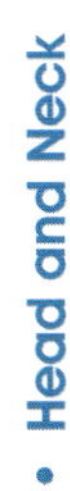

Relation to recurrent laryngeal nerve (Fig. 16.34). Recurrent laryngeal is given off from vagi in relation to distal part of 6th arch artery. Since this distal part forms ligamentum arteriosum on left side only, the recurrent laryngeal nerve hooks around this ligamentum in thorax to reach tracheo-oesophageal groove.

On the right side, there is no ligamentum arteriosum, the recurrent laryngeal nerve slips upwards in the neck and hooks around the right subclavian artery to reach the tracheo-oesophageal groove.

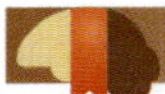

Mnemonics

Tributaries of Internal Jugular Vein

"**M**edical **S**chools **L**et **C**onfident **P**eople **I**n"

From inferior to superior:
Middle thyorid
Superior thyroid
Lingual
Common facial
Pharyngeal
Inferior petrosal sinus

FACTS TO REMEMBER

- Isthmus of thyroid gland acts as a shield for trachea.
- Parathyroid glands lie along the anastomotic channel between posterior branch of superior thyroid artery and ascending branch of inferior thyroid artery.
- Internal carotid artery comprises 4 parts: Cervical, petrous, cavernous and cerebral.
- Superior cervical ganglion gives grey rami communicantes (grc) to C1–C4 nerves.
- Middle cervical ganglion gives grc to C5, C6 nerves.
- Inferior cervical ganglion gives grc to C7, C8 nerves.
- Scalenus anterior can press upon the subclavian artery and brachial plexus, causing nervous and vascular changes in upper limb.
- Phrenic nerve (C4) supplies motor fibres to musculature of diaphragm. It carries sensory fibres from peritoneum underlying diaphragm, mediastinal pleura and pericardium.
- Styloid apparatus comprises styloglossus (XII), stylohyoid (VII), stylopharyngeus muscles (IX); and stylohyoid and stylomandibular ligaments.

CLINICOANATOMICAL PROBLEM

A 40-year-old woman complained of a swelling in front of her neck, nervousness and loss of weight. Her diagnosis was hyperthyroidism. Partial thyroidectomy was performed, and she complained of hoarseness after the operation.

- Why does thyroid swelling move up and down during deglutition?
- Why does she complain of hoarseness after the operation?
- Which other gland can be removed with thyroid?

Ans: The thyroid gland is suspended from cricoid cartilage by the pretracheal fascia and ligament of Berry. So all the swellings associated with thyroid gland move with deglutition.

She complains of hoarseness. It may be due to injury to the recurrent laryngeal nerve as it lies close to the inferior thyroid artery near the lower pole of the gland.

The parathyroid gland lying on the back of thyroid gland may be removed. Parathyroid controls calcium level in the blood.

FURTHER READING

- Mohebati A, Shaha AR. Anatomy of thyroid and parathyroid glands and neurovascular relations. Clin Anat 2012;25: 19–31.

A review of the pertinent anatomy and embryology of the thyroid and parathyroid glands and the critical structures that lie in their proximity.

Frequently Asked Questions

1. Describe thyroid gland under the following headings:
   a. Position
   b. Gross anatomy
   c. Blood supply
   d. Clinical anatomy
2. Enumerate the various group of lymph nodes in the neck. Mention the areas drained by these nodes.
3. Write short notes on/enumerate:
   a. Styloid apparatus
   b. Branches of subclavian artery
   c. Branches of superior cervical ganglion
   d. Horner's syndrome
   e. Tributaries of internal jugular vein

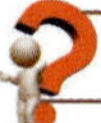

Multiple Choice Questions

1. Where should the superior thyroid artery be ligated during thyroidectomy?
   a. Close to its origin from external carotid artery
   b. Close to the upper pole of the lateral lobe
   c. Anterior and posterior branches separately
   d. Anywhere in its course
2. Where should inferior thyroid artery be ligated during thyroidectomy?
   a. Away from the gland
   b. At its distal or terminal part
   c. Anywhere in its course
   d. The branches ligated separately
3. Horner's syndrome produces all symptoms, *except:*
   a. Partial ptosis b. Miosis
   c. Anhydrosis d. Exophthalmos
4. Which of the following muscles is not supplied by ansa cervicalis?
   a. Sternohyoid
   b. Sternothyroid
   c. Inferior belly of omohyoid
   d. Geniohyoid
5. One of the following is not a branch of subclavian artery:
   a. Internal thoracic b. Vertebral
   c. Costocervical trunk d. Subscapular
6. One of the following symptoms is not seen in Horner's syndrome:
   a. Complete ptosis b. Miosis
   c. Anhydrosis d. Enophthalmos
7. One of the following statements about parathyroid gland is not true:
   a. Inferior parathyroid arises from 3rd pharyngeal pouch
   b. Parathyroid glands are supplied by superior thyroid artery
   c. Superior parathyroid arises from 4th pharyngeal pouch
   d. Thymus develops along with inferior parathyroid gland
8. Which one is not a branch of thyrocervical trunk?
   a. Inferior thyroid b. Suprascapular
   c. Transverse cervical d. Deep cervical
9. Which one is not a component of carotid sheath?
   a. Internal carotid artery
   b. Vagus nerve
   c. Sympathetic trunk
   d. Internal jugular vein

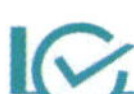

Answers

1. b **2.** a **3.** d **4.** d **5.** d **6.** a **7.** b **8.** d **9.** c

VIVA VOCE

- What does the word 'thyroid' mean?
- Where does the thyroid venous plexus lie in relation to its capsules?
- Where is superior thyroid artery ligated during thyroidectomy and why?
- Why is inferior thyroid artery not ligated during thyroidectomy and which of its branches are ligated?
- How many veins drain the thyroid gland?
- How does thyroid gland develop?
- Which artery is the guide to location of the parathyroid glands?
- What are the types of cells present in histological slide of parathyroid gland?
- Name the functions of thymus gland.
- Why is "parathyroid III" called the inferior parathyroid gland?
- Name the branches of arch of aorta.
- Name the branches of 1st part of subclavian artery.
- Name the branches of thyrocervical trunk.
- How many cervical sympathetic ganglia are there? Name the branches of superior cervical ganglion.
- Name the branches of inferior cervical ganglion.
- What are the features of Horner's syndrome?
- Which are the superficial group of cervical lymph nodes?
- Name the lymph nodes forming Waldeyer's ring.
- What are the structures attached to the styloid process? Give the nerve supply of these muscles.
- What are the areas innervated by phrenic nerve branches?
- Name the developmental components of arch of an aorta.
- Enumerate the muscles supplied by ansa cervicalis and its roots.

VIDEO 3.8 Thyroid gland

Chapter 17

Prevertebral and Paravertebral Regions

"I profess to learn and to teach anatomy not from books but from dissections, not from the tenets of philosophers but from the fabric of nature."
—William Harvey

INTRODUCTION

The prevertebral region contains four muscles, vertebral artery and joints of the neck. Vertebral artery, a branch of subclavian artery, comprises four parts—1st, 2nd and 3rd are in the neck and the fourth part passes through the foramen magnum to reach the subarachnoid space and the vertebral arteries of two sides unite to form a single median basilar artery which gives branches to supply a part of cerebral cortex, cerebellum, internal ear and pons. Congenital or acquired diseases of cervical vertebrae or their joints give rise to lots of symptoms related to branches of vertebral artery.

The apical ligament of dens is a continuation of notochord. Transverse ligament, which is a part of cruciate ligament, keeps the dens of axis in position. If this ligament is injured by disease or in 'capital punishment', there is immediate death due to injury to vasomotor centres in medulla oblongata. Trachea and oesophagus are contents of prevertebral region.

The paravertebral region contains three scalene muscles, cervical plexus, its branches including the phrenic nerve. This region also includes the cervical pleura.

PREVERTEBRAL MUSCLES (Anterior Vertebral Muscles)

The four prevertebral or anterior vertebral muscles are the longus colli (cervicis), the longus capitis, the rectus capitis anterior and the rectus capitis lateralis (Figs 17.1a and b). These are weak flexors of the head and neck. They extend from the base of the skull to the superior mediastinum. They partially cover the anterior aspect of the vertebral column. They are covered anteriorly by the thick prevertebral fascia. The muscles are described in Table 17.1.

VERTEBRAL ARTERY

Features

The vertebral artery is one of the two principal arteries which supply the brain. In addition, it also supplies the spinal cord, the meninges, and the surrounding muscles and bones. It arises from the posterosuperior aspect of the first part of the subclavian artery near its commencement. It runs a long course, and ends in the cranial cavity by supplying the brain (Fig. 17.2). The artery is divided into four parts.

First Part

The first part extends from the origin of the artery (from the subclavian artery) to the transverse process of the sixth cervical vertebra.

This part of the artery runs upwards and backwards in the triangular space between the scalenus anterior and the longus colli muscles called the scalenovertebral triangle (Fig. 17.3).

Relations

Anterior

1 Carotid sheath with common carotid artery
2 Vertebral vein

DISSECTION

Remove the scalenus anterior muscle. Identify deeply placed anterior and posterior intertransverse muscles. Cut through the anterior intertransverse muscles to expose the second part of vertebral artery. First part was seen as the branch arising from the first part of the subclavian artery. Its third part was seen in the suboccipital triangle. The fourth part lies in the cranial cavity.

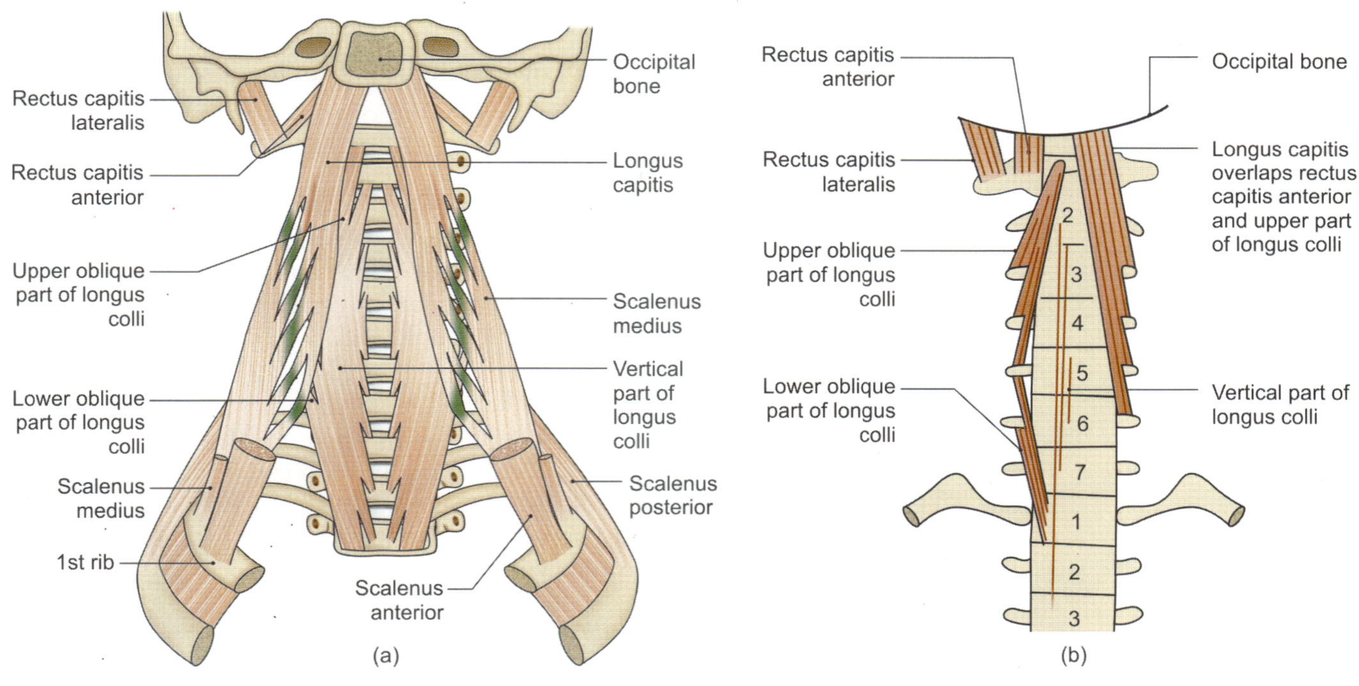

Figs 17.1a and b: The prevertebral muscles

Table 17.1: The prevertebral muscles

Muscle	*Origin*	*Insertion*	*Nerve supply*	*Actions*
1. **Longus colli (cervicis)** This muscle extends from the atlas to the third thoracic vertebra. It has upper and lower oblique parts and a middle vertical part (Fig. 17.1)	a. The upper oblique part is from the anterior tubercles of the transverse processes of cervical vertebrae 3, 4, 5 b. Lower oblique part is from bodies of upper 2–3 thoracic vertebrae c. Middle vertical part is from bodies of upper 3 thoracic and lower 3 cervical vertebrae	a. Upper oblique part is into the anterior tubercle of the atlas b. Lower oblique part is into the anterior tubercles of the transverse processes of 5th and 6th cervical vertebrae c. Middle vertical part is into bodies of 2, 3, 4 cervical vertebrae	Ventral rami of nerves C3–C8	a. Flexes the neck b. Oblique parts flex the neck laterally c. Lower oblique part rotates the neck to the opposite side
2. **Longus capitis** It overlaps the longus colli. It is thick above and narrow below	Anterior tubercles of transverse processes of cervical 3–6 vertebrae	Inferior surface of basilar part of occipital bone	Ventral rami of nerves C1–C3	Flexes the head
3. **Rectus capitis anterior** This is a very short and flat muscle. It lies deep to the longus capitis	Anterior surface of lateral mass of atlas in front of the occipital condyle	Basilar part of the occipital bone	Ventral ramus of nerve C1	Flexes the head
4. **Rectus capitis lateralis** This is a short, flat muscle	Upper surface of transverse process of atlas	Inferior surface of jugular process of the occipital bone	Ventral rami of nerves C1, C2	Flexes the head laterally

3 Inferior thyroid artery
4 Thoracic duct on left side (Fig. 17.5).

Posterior

1 Transverse process of 7th cervical vertebra (Fig. 17.2)
2 Stellate ganglion
3 Ventral rami of nerves C7, C8.

Scalenovertebral Triangle

The triangle is present at the root of the neck.

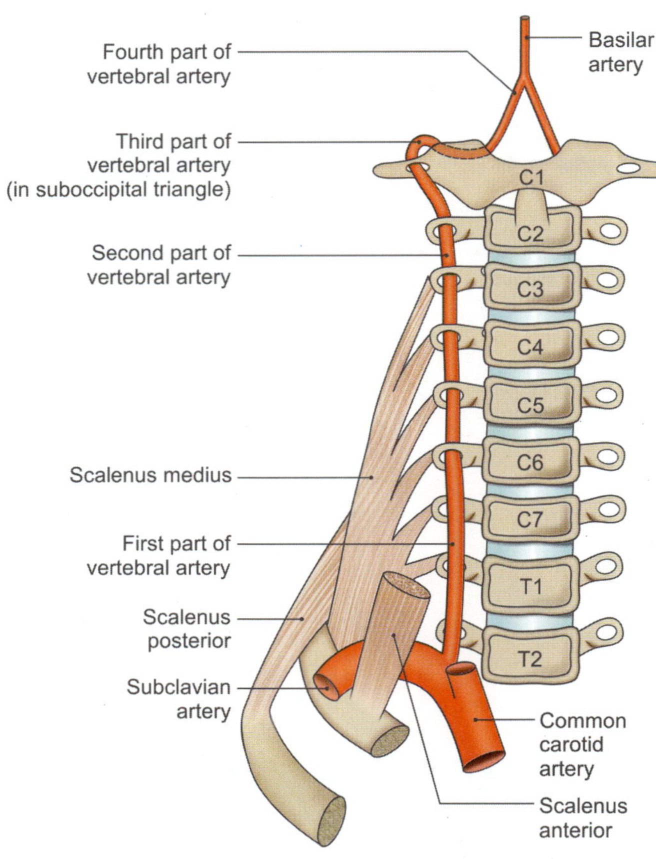

Fig. 17.2: Scheme showing parts of the vertebral artery, as seen from the front

Boundaries

Medial: Lower oblique part of longus colli

Lateral: Scalenus anterior

Apex: Transverse process of C6 vertebra

Base: 1st part of subclavian artery

Posterior wall: Transverse process of C7, ventral ramus of C8 nerve, neck of 1st rib and cupola of pleurae

Contents: First part of vertebral artery, cervical part of sympathetic trunk (Fig. 17.12).

Second Part

The second part runs through the foramina transversaria of the upper six cervical vertebrae. Its course is vertically up to the axis vertebra. It then runs upwards and laterally to reach the foramen transversarium of the atlas vertebra.

Relations

1. The ventral rami of second to sixth cervical nerves lie posterior to the vertebral artery.
2. The artery is accompanied by a venous plexus and a large branch from the stellate ganglion (*see* Fig. 16.28).

Third Part

Third part lies in the suboccipital triangle. Emerging from the foramen transversarium of the atlas, the artery

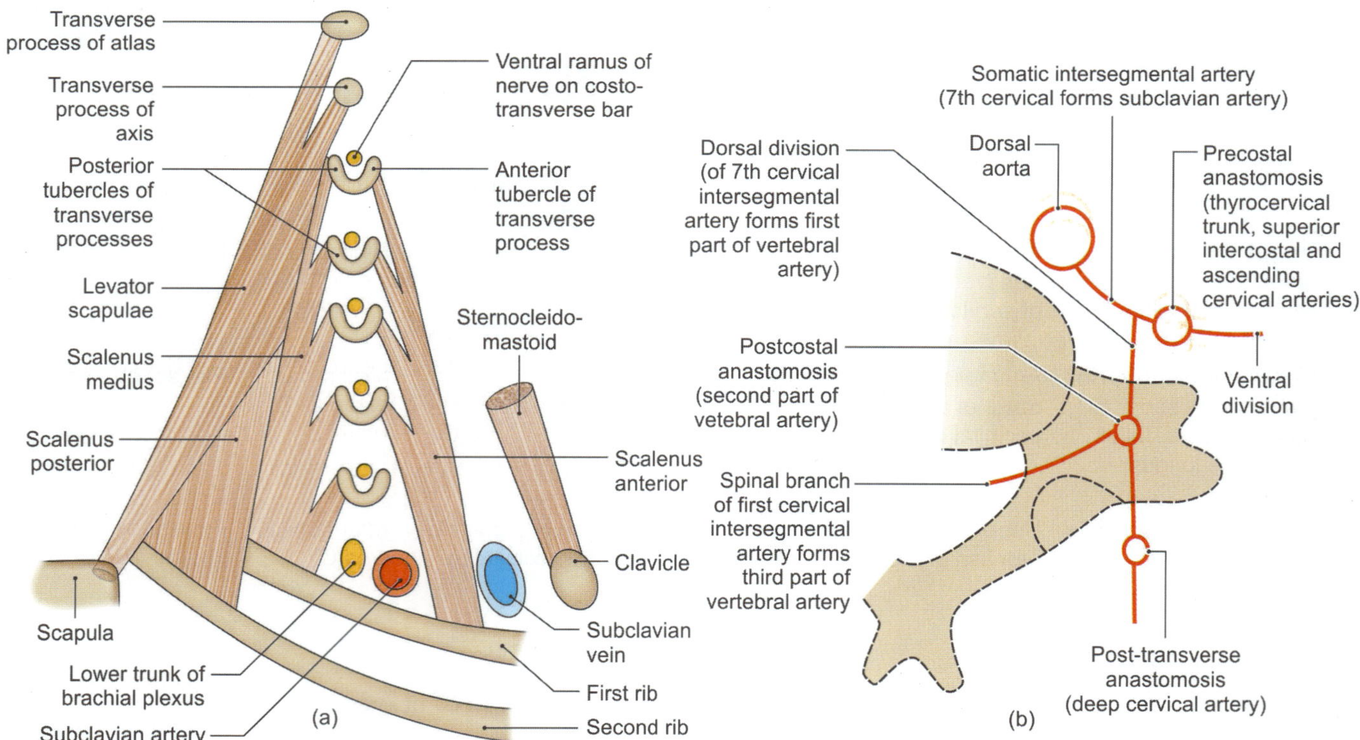

Figs 17.3a and b: (a) Schematic sagittal section through the left scalenus anterior to show its relations; (b) Development of vertebral artery

winds medially around the posterior aspect of the lateral mass of the atlas. It runs medially lying on the posterior arch of this bone, and enters the vertebral canal by passing deep to the lower arched margin of the posterior atlanto-occipital membrane.

Relations

Anterior: Lateral mass of atlas.

Posterior: Semispinalis capitis.

Lateral: Rectus capitis lateralis.

Medial: Ventral ramus of the first cervical nerve.

Inferior:
1 Dorsal ramus of the first cervical nerve (*see* Fig. 18.6)
2 The posterior arch of the atlas (*see* Fig. 18.6).

Fourth Part

1 The fourth part extends from the posterior atlanto-occipital membrane to the lower border of the pons.
2 In the vertebral canal, it pierces the dura and the arachnoid, and ascends in front of the roots of the hypoglossal nerve. As it ascends, it gradually inclines medially to reach the front of the medulla. At the lower border of the pons, it unites with its fellow of the opposite side to form the basilar artery (Fig. 17.2).

Branches of Vertebral Artery

First part has no branches.

Cervical Branches

1 Spinal branches from the *second part* enter the vertebral canal through the intervertebral foramina and supply the spinal cord, the meninges and the vertebrae.
2 Muscular branches arise from the *third part* and supply the suboccipital muscles.

Cranial Branches

These arise from the *fourth part*. They are:
1 *Meningeal* branches
2 The *posterior spinal* artery
3 The *anterior spinal* artery
4 The *posterior inferior cerebellar* artery
5 *Medullary* arteries
These are described in Chapter 36.

DEVELOPMENT OF VERTEBRAL ARTERY

Different parts of vertebral artery develop in the following ways.

First part: From a branch of dorsal division of 7th cervical intersegmental artery.

Second part: From postcostal anastomosis.

Third part: From spinal branch of the first cervical intersegmental artery.

Fourth part: From preneural branch of first cervical intersegmental artery.

TRACHEA

The trachea is a non-collapsible, wide tube, forming the beginning of the lower respiratory passages. It is kept patent because of the presence of C-shaped cartilaginous 'rings' in its wall. The cartilages are deficient posteriorly, this part of the wall-being made up of muscle (trachealis) and fibrous tissue. The soft posterior wall allows expansion of the oesophagus during passage of food.

Dimensions

The *trachea* (Latin rough air vessel) is about 10 to 15 cm long. Its upper half lies in the neck and its lower half in the superior mediastinum. The external diameter measures 2 cm in the male and 1.5 cm in the female. The lumen is smaller in the living than in cadavers. It is about 3 mm at 1 year of age, and corresponds to the age in years during childhood, with a maximum of 12 mm at puberty.

Cervical Part of Trachea

1 The trachea begins at the lower border of the cricoid cartilage opposite the lower border of vertebra C6. It runs downwards and slightly backwards in front of the oesophagus, follows the curvature of the spine, and enters the thorax in the median plane.
2 In the neck, the trachea is comparatively superficial and has the following relations.

Anterior

1 Isthmus of the thyroid gland covering the second and third tracheal rings (*see* Fig. 16.1).
2 Inferior thyroid veins below the isthmus (*see* Fig. 16.8).
3 Pretracheal fascia enclosing the thyroid and the inferior thyroid veins.
4 Sternohyoid and sternothyroid muscles (*see* Fig. 16.4).
5 Investing layer of the deep cervical fascia and the suprasternal space.
6 The skin and superficial fascia.
7 In children, the left brachiocephalic vein extends into the neck and then lies in front of the trachea.

Posterior

1 Oesophagus
2 Longus colli
3 Recurrent laryngeal nerve in the tracheo-oesophageal groove (*see* Fig. 16.5).

On Each Side

1 The corresponding lobe of the thyroid glands.
2 The common carotid artery within the carotid sheath (*see* Fig. 16.4).

Vessels and Nerves

The trachea is supplied by branches from the inferior thyroid arteries. Its veins drain into the left brachiocephalic vein. Lymphatics drain into the pretracheal and paratracheal nodes.

Parasympathetic nerves (from the vagus through the recurrent laryngeal nerve) are sensory and secretomotor to the mucous membrane, and motor to the trachealis muscle. Sympathetic nerves (from the cervical ganglion) are vasomotor.

CLINICAL ANATOMY

- The trachea may be compressed by pathological enlargements of the thyroid, the thymus, lymph nodes and the aortic arch. This causes dyspnoea, irritative cough, and often a husky voice.
- Tracheostomy is an emergency operation done in cases of laryngeal obstruction (foreign body, diphtheria, carcinoma, etc.). It is commonly done in the retrothyroid region after retracting the isthmus of the thyroid gland.

OESOPHAGUS

The oesophagus is a muscular food passage lying between the trachea and the vertebral column. Normally, its anterior and posterior walls are in contact. The oesophagus expands during the passage of food by pressing into the posterior muscular part of the trachea (*see* Fig. 16.4).

The oesophagus is a downward continuation of the pharynx and begins at the lower border of the cricoid cartilage, opposite the lower border of the body of vertebra C6. It passes downwards behind the trachea, traverses the superior and posterior mediastina of the thorax, and ends by opening into the cardiac end of the stomach in the abdomen. It is about 25 cm long.

The cervical part of the oesophagus is related:

a. *Anteriorly,* to the trachea and to the right and left recurrent laryngeal nerves.
b. *Posteriorly,* to the longus colli muscle and the vertebral column.
c. *On each side,* to the corresponding (*see* Fig. 16.5) lobe of the thyroid gland; and on the left side, to the thoracic duct.

The cervical part of the oesophagus is supplied by the inferior thyroid arteries. Its veins drain into the left brachiocephalic vein. Its lymphatics pass to the deep cervical lymph nodes. The oesophagus is narrowest at its junction with the pharynx, the junction being the narrowest part of the gastrointestinal tract, except for the vermiform appendix.

For thoracic part of oesophagus study, *see* Chapter 20, *BD Chaurasia's Human Anatomy, Volume 1.*

CLINICAL ANATOMY

Oesophagus has four natural constrictions. While passing any instrument, one must be careful at these sites (Fig. 17.4).

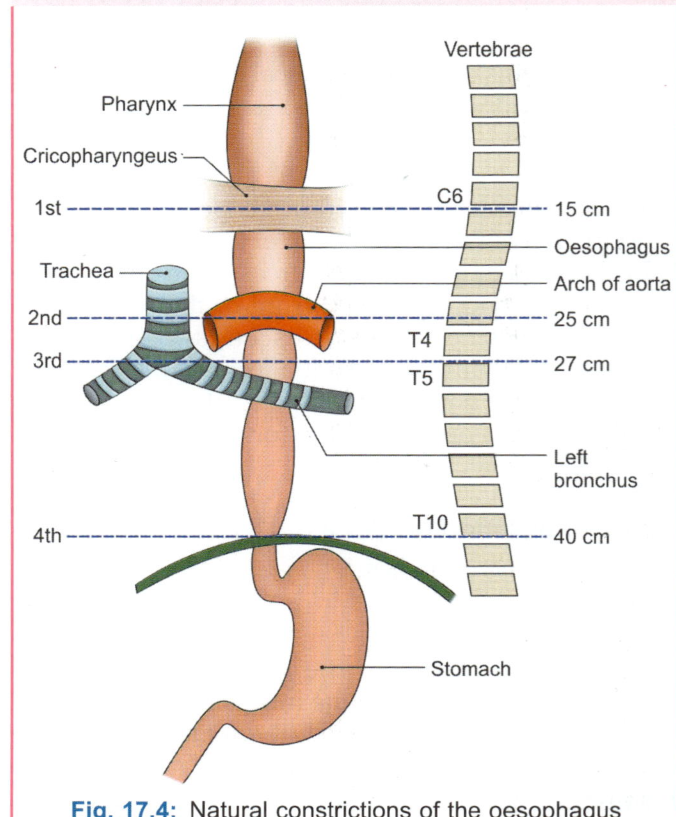

Fig. 17.4: Natural constrictions of the oesophagus

JOINTS OF THE NECK

Typical Cervical Joints between the Lower Six Cervical Vertebrae

The bodies of cervical vertebra are united by intervertebral disc. On each side of the disc are small synovial joints (Fig. 17.5a) called joints of Luschka or uncovertebral joints. The adjacent vertebrae are connected by several ligaments which are as follows.

1. The *anterior longitudinal ligament* passes from the anterior surface of the body of one vertebra to another. Its upper end reaches the basilar part of the occipital bone (Fig. 17.5b).
2. The *posterior longitudinal ligament* is present on the posterior surface of the vertebral bodies within the

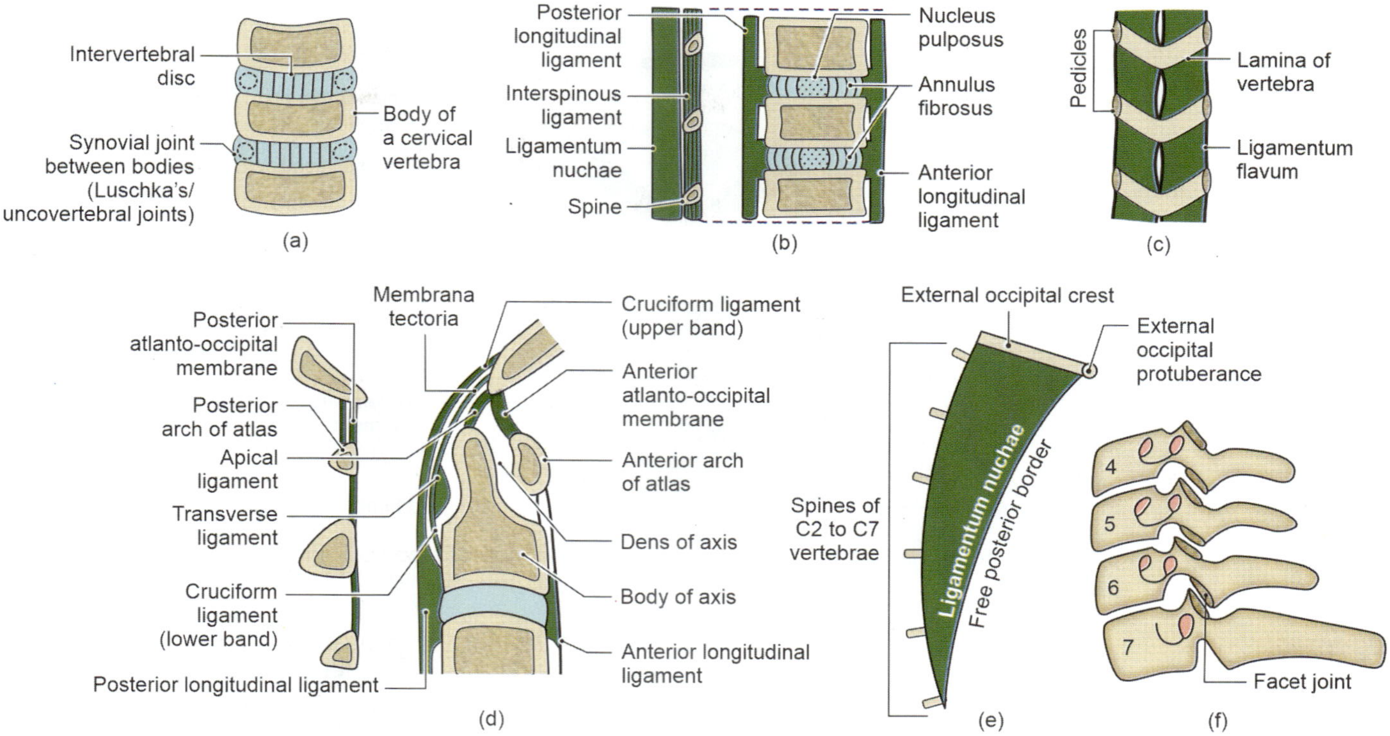

Figs 17.5a to f: (a) Joints between vertebral bodies as seen from front; (b) Side view showing the ligaments; (c) Anterior view of the ligamentum flava; (d) Median section through the foramen magnum and upper two cervical vertebrae showing the ligaments in this region; (e) Ligamentum nuchae; (f) Facet joint

vertebral canal. Its upper end reaches the body of the axis vertebra beyond which it continues as the *membrana tectoria* (Fig. 17.5b).

3. The *intertransverse ligaments* connect adjacent transverse processes.
4. The *interspinous ligaments* connect adjacent spines.
5. The *supraspinous ligaments* connect the tips of the spines of vertebrae from the seventh cervical to the sacrum. In the cervical region, they are replaced by the ligamentum nuchae.
6. *Joint between vertebral arches*: Joint between superior and inferior articular processes of adjacent vertebrae is plane joint of synovial variety. The articular processes slope inferiorly to allow rotation of neck. These are also called zygapophyseal/facet joints (Fig. 17.5f).
7. The laminae of adjacent vertebrae are united by ligamentum flava, made up of elastic fibres. It ends at C2 level (Fig. 17.5c).

   The *ligamentum nuchae* is triangular in shape. Its apex lies at the seventh cervical spine and its base at the external occipital crest. Its anterior border is attached to cervical spines, while the posterior border is free and provides attachment to the investing layer of deep cervical fascia. The ligament gives origin to the splenius, rhomboids and trapezius muscles (Fig. 17.5e).

Joints between Atlas, Axis and Occipital Bone

1 The atlanto-occipital and the atlantoaxial joints are designed to permit free movements of the head on the neck (vertebral column).

2 The axis vertebra and the occipital bone are connected together by very strong ligaments. Between these two bones, the atlas is held like a washer. The axis of movement between the atlas and skull is transverse, permitting flexion and extension (nodding), whereas the axis of movement between the axis and the atlas is vertical, permitting rotation of the head (Fig. 17.5d).

Atlanto-occipital Joints

Types and Articular Surfaces

These are synovial joints of the ellipsoid variety.

Above: The convex occipital condyles (Fig. 17.6).

Below: The superior articular facets of the atlas vertebra. These are concave. The articular surfaces are elongated, and are directed forwards and medially.

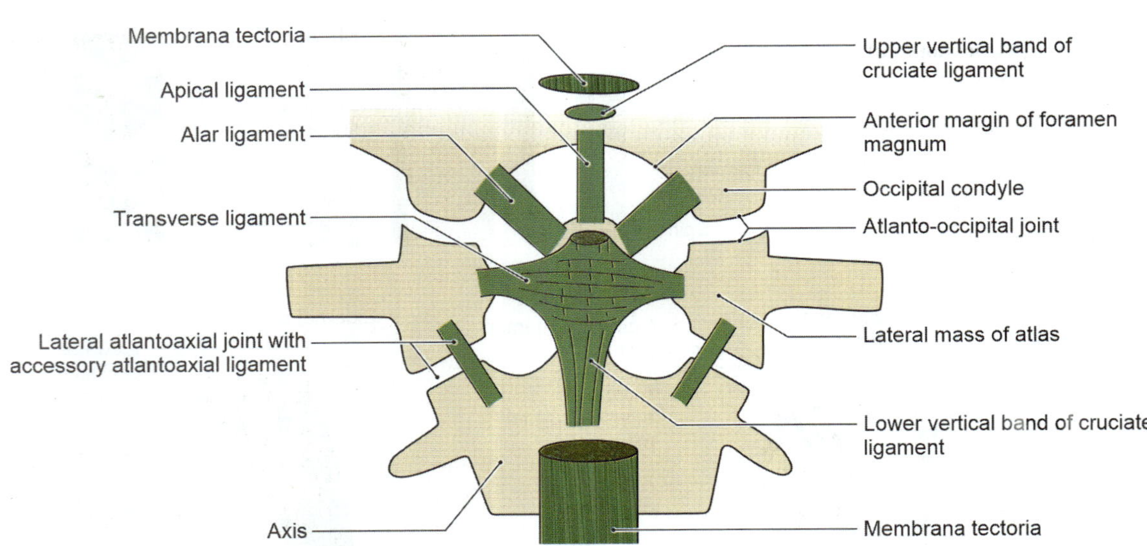

Fig. 17.6: Posterior view of the ligaments connecting the axis with the occipital bone

Ligaments

1 The *fibrous capsule (capsular ligament)* surrounds the joint. It is thick posterolaterally and thin anteromedially (Fig. 17.5d).

2 The *anterior atlanto-occipital membrane* extends from the anterior margin of the foramen magnum above, to the upper border of the anterior arch of the atlas below (Fig. 17.5d). Laterally, it is continuous with the anterior part of the capsular ligament, and anteriorly, it is strengthened by (the cord-like anterior longitudinal ligament.

3 The *posterior atlanto-occipital membrane* extends from the posterior margin of the foramen magnum above, to the upper border of the posterior arch of the atlas below (Fig. 17.5d). Inferolaterally, it has a free margin which arches over the vertebral artery and the first cervical nerve (*see* Fig. 18.5). Laterally, it is continuous with the posterior part of the capsular ligament.

Arterial and Nerve Supply

The joint is supplied by the vertebral artery and by the first cervical nerve.

Movements

Since these are ellipsoid joints, they permit movements around two axes. Flexion and extension (nodding) occur around a transverse axis. Slight lateral flexion is permitted around an anteroposterior axis.

1 *Flexion* is brought about by the longus capitis and the rectus capitis anterior.

2 *Extension* is done by the rectus capitis posterior major and minor, the obliquus capitis superior, the semispinalis capitis, the splenius capitis, and the upper part of the trapezius.

3 *Lateral bending* is produced by the rectus capitis lateralis, the semispinalis capitis, the splenius capitis, the sternocleidomastoid, and the trapezius (Fig. 17.7).

Atlantoaxial Joints

Types and Articular Surfaces

These joints comprise:

1 A pair of lateral atlantoaxial joints between the inferior facets of the atlas and the superior facets of the axis. These are plane joints.

2 A median atlantoaxial joint between the dens (odontoid process) and the anterior arch and between dens and transverse ligament of the atlas. It is a pivot joint. The joint has two separate synovial cavities— anterior and posterior (Figs 17.5 and 17.6).

Ligaments

The lateral atlantoaxial joints are supported by:

a. A capsular ligament all around.
b. The lateral part of the anterior longitudinal ligament.
c. The ligamentum flavum.
   Accessory atlantoaxial ligament.

The median atlantoaxial joint is strengthened by the following.

a. The anterior smaller part of the joint between the anterior arch of the atlas and the dens is surrounded by a loose capsular ligament (Fig. 17.5).
b. The posterior larger part of the joint between the dens and transverse ligament (often called a bursa) is often continuous with one of the atlanto-occipital joints. Its main support is the transverse ligament which forms a part of the cruciform ligament of the atlas (Fig. 17.6).

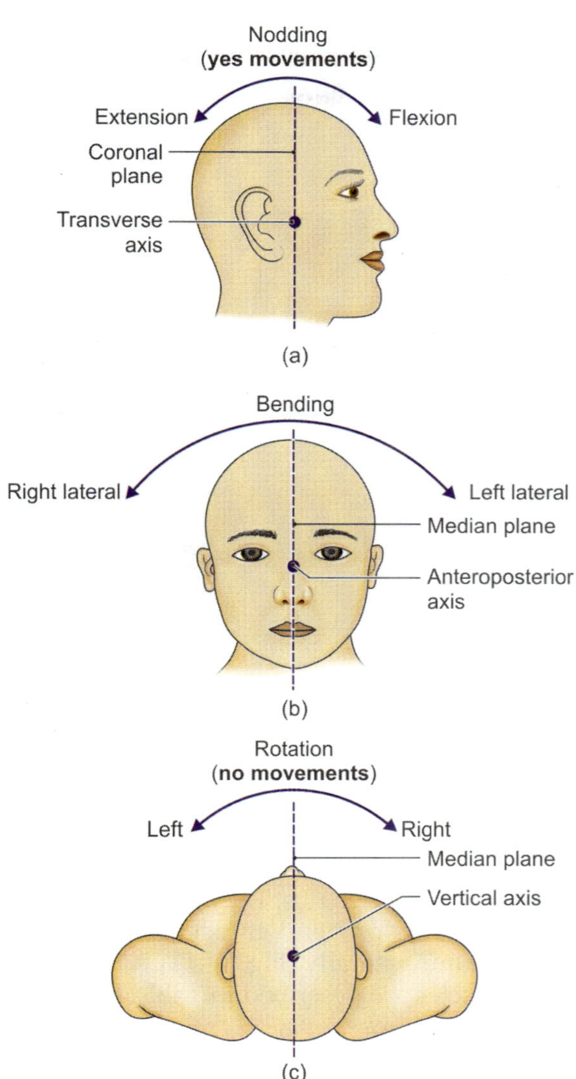

Figs 17.7a to c: Various movements of the neck

The *transverse ligament* (Fig. 17.6) is attached on each side to the medial surface of the lateral mass of the atlas. In the median plane, its fibres are prolonged upwards to the basiocciput and downwards to the body of the axis, thus forming the *cruciform ligament of the atlas vertebra*. The transverse ligament embraces the narrow neck of the dens, and prevents its dislocation.

Movements

Movements at all three joints are rotatory and take place around a vertical axis. The dens forms a pivot around which the atlas rotates (carrying the skull with it). The movement is limited by the alar ligaments (Figs 17.6 and 17.7a–c).

The rotatory movements are brought about by the obliquus capitis inferior, the rectus capitis posterior major and the splenius capitis of one side (*see* Fig. 18.5), acting with the sternocleidomastoid of the opposite side.

Ligaments Connecting Axis with Occipital Bone

These ligaments are the membrana tectoria, the cruciate ligament, the apical ligament of the dens and the alar ligaments. They support both the atlanto-occipital and atlantoaxial joints.

1 The *membrana tectoria* is an upward continuation of the posterior longitudinal ligament. It lies posterior to the transverse ligament. It is attached inferiorly to the posterior surface of the body of the axis and superiorly to the basiocciput (within the foramen magnum) (Fig. 17.5d).
2 *Cruciate ligament* (*see* transverse ligament).
3 The *apical ligament of the dens* extends from the apex of the dens to the basiocciput inferior to the attachment of the cruciate ligament. It is the continuation of the notochord (Fig. 17.5d).
4 The *alar ligament*, one on each side, extends from the upper part of the lateral surface of the dens to the medial surface of the occipital condyles. These are strong ligaments which limit the rotation and flexion of the head. They are relaxed during extension (Fig. 17.6).

CLINICAL ANATOMY

- Death in execution by hanging is due to dislocation of the dens following rupture of the transverse ligament of the dens, which then crushes the spinal cord and medulla. However, hanging can also cause fracture through the axis, or separation of the axis from the third cervical vertebra (Fig. 17.8).
- *Cervical spondylosis:* Injury or degenerative changes of old age may rupture the thin lateral parts of the annulus fibrosus (of the intervertebral disc) resulting in prolapse of the nucleus pulposus. This

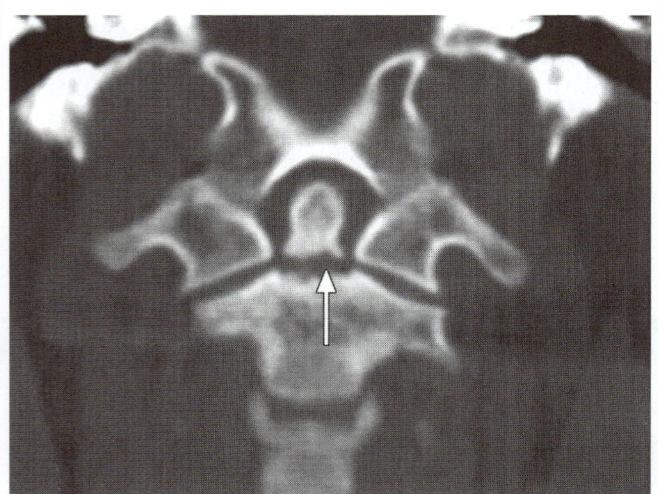

Fig. 17.8: Fracture of the dens during hanging

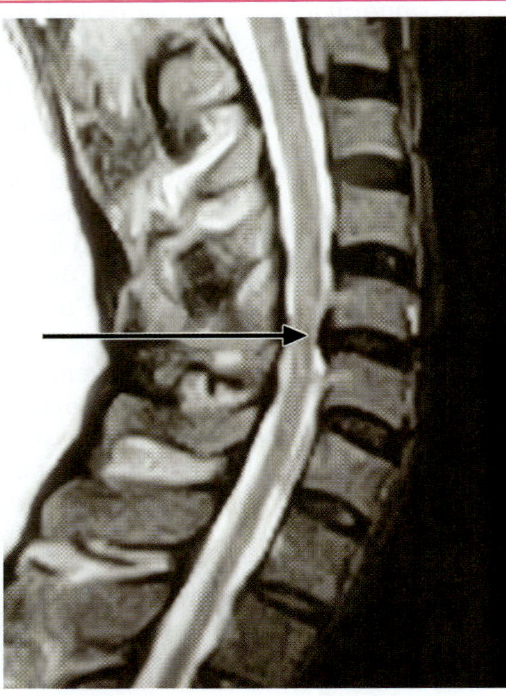

Fig. 17.9: Posterior intervertebral disc prolapse

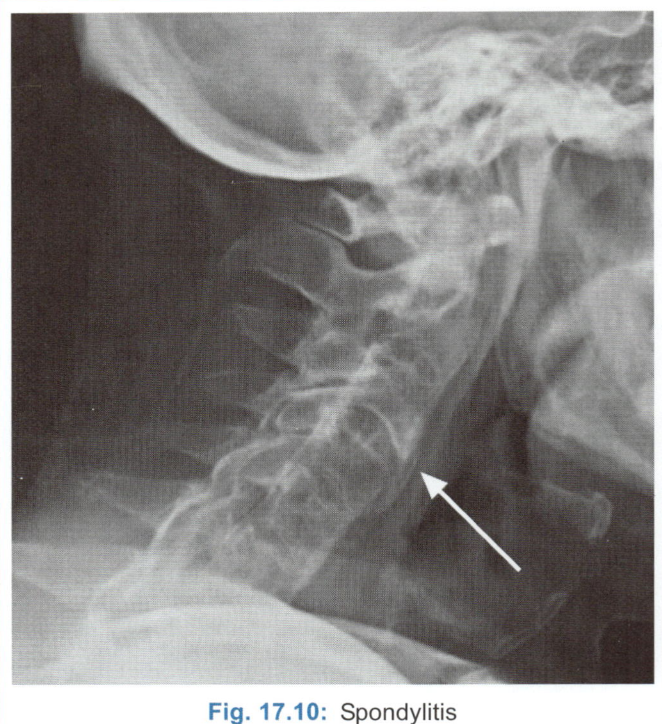

Fig. 17.10: Spondylitis

is known as disc prolapse or spondylosis and may be lateral or median (Fig. 17.9). Although, it is commonest in the lumbar region, it may occur in the lower cervical region. This causes shooting pain along the distribution of the cervical nerve pressed. A direct posterior prolapse may compress the spinal cord.

- Cervical vertebrae may be fractured, or dislocated by a fall on the head with acute flexion of the neck. In the cervical region, the vertebrae can dislocate without any fracture of the articular processes due to their horizontal position.
- Pithing of frog takes place when the cruciate ligament of median atlantoaxial joint ruptures, crushing the vital centres in medulla oblongata, resulting in immediate death. This occurs in judicial hanging as well.
- The degenerative changes or spondylitis may occur in the cervical spine, leading to narrowed intervertebral foramen, causing pressure on the spinal nerves (Fig. 17.10).

PARAVERTEBRAL REGION

SCALENE MUSCLES

Features

There are usually three scalene muscles, the scalenus anterior, the scalenus medius and the scalenus posterior. The scalenus medius is the largest, and the scalenus posterior the smallest, of three. These muscles extend from the transverse processes of cervical vertebrae to the first two ribs. They can, therefore, either elevate these ribs or bend the cervical part of the vertebral column laterally (Fig. 17.11).

These muscles are described in Table 17.2.

Additional Features of the Scalene Muscles

1. Sometimes a fourth, rudimentary scalene muscle, the *scalenus minimus* is present. It arises from the anterior border of the transverse process of vertebra C7 and is inserted into the inner border of the first rib behind the groove for the subclavian artery and into the dome of the cervical pleura. The *suprapleural membrane* is regarded as the expansion of this muscle. Contraction of the scalenus minimus pulls the dome of the cervical pleura.
2. *Relations of scalenus anterior.* The scalenus anterior is a *key* muscle of the lower part of the neck because of

DISSECTION

Clean and define the cervical parts of the trachea and oesophagus.

Scalenus anterior has been seen in relation to subclavian artery. Scalenus medius is one of the muscles forming floor of posterior triangle of neck. Scalenus posterior lies deep to the medius (Fig. 17.3).

The relations of the cervical pleura are shown in Fig. 17.11.

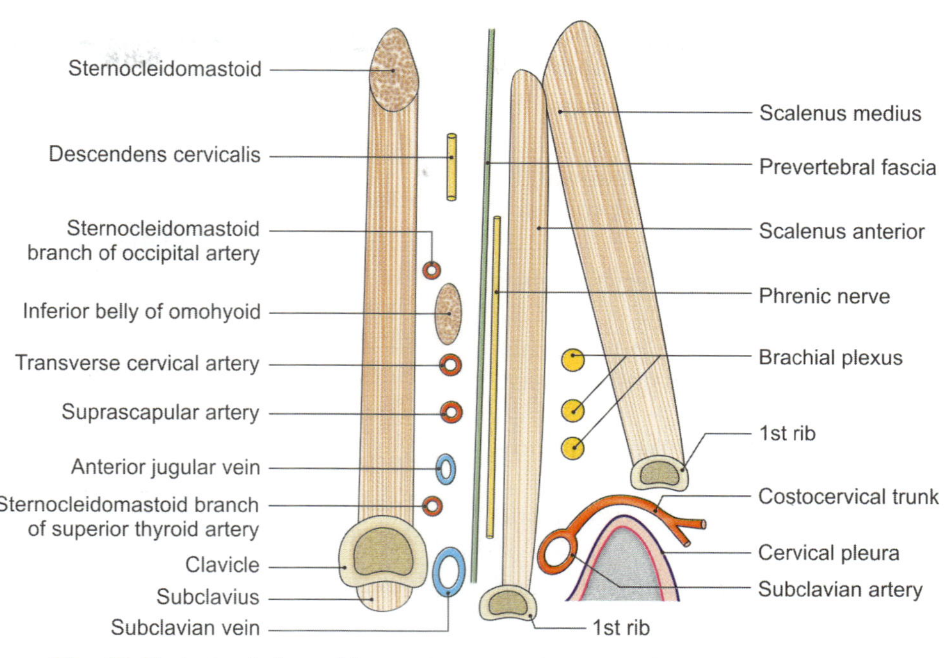

Fig. 17.11: Lateral view of the scalene muscles with a few related structures

Table 17.2: The scalene muscles

Muscle	*Origin*	*Insertion*	*Nerve supply*	*Actions*
1. **Scalenus anterior** (Fig. 17.11)	Anterior tubercles of transverse processes of cervical vertebrae 3 to 6	Scalene tubercle and adjoining ridge on the superior surface of the first rib (between subclavian artery and vein)	Ventral rami of nerves C4–C6	a. Anterolateral flexion of cervical spine b. Rotates cervical spine to opposite side c. Elevates the first rib during inspiration d. Stabilises the neck along with other muscles
2. **Scalenus medius** (Fig. 17.3)	a. Posterior tubercles of transverse processes of cervical vertebrae 3 to 7 b. Transverse process of axis and sometimes also of the atlas vertebra	Superior surface of the first rib behind the groove for the subclavian artery	Ventral rami of nerves C3–C8	a. Lateral flexion of the cervical spine. b. Elevation of first rib c. Stabilises neck along with other muscles
3. **Scalenus posterior** (Fig. 17.3)	Posterior tubercles of transverse processes of cervical vertebrae 4 to 6	Outer surface of the second rib behind the tubercle for the serratus anterior	Ventral rami of nerves C6–C8	a. Lateral flexion of cervical spine b. Elevation of the second rib c. Stabilises neck along with other muscles

its intimate relations to many important structures in this region. It is a useful surgical landmark.

Anterior

a. Phrenic nerve covered by prevertebral fascia
b. Lateral part of carotid sheath containing the internal jugular vein
c. Sternocleidomastoid (Fig. 17.11)
d. Clavicle

Posterior

a. Brachial plexus (Fig. 17.11)
b. Subclavian artery
c. Scalenus medius
d. Cervical pleura covered by the suprapleural membrane (Fig. 17.13)

The *medial border* of the muscle is related:

a. In its lower part to an inverted V-shaped interval, formed by the diverging borders of the scalenus anterior and the longus colli. This interval contains many important structures as follows:

i. Vertebral vessels running vertically from the base to the apex of this space.
ii. Inferior thyroid artery arching medially at the level of the 6th cervical transverse process.
iii. Sympathetic trunk.
iv. The first part of the subclavian artery traverses the lower part of the gap.
v. On the left side, the thoracic duct arches laterally at the level of the seventh cervical transverse process (Fig. 17.12).
vi. The carotid sheath covers all the structures mentioned above.
vii. The sternocleidomastoid covers the carotid sheath (*see* Fig. 16.4).

b. In its upper part, the scalenus anterior is separated from the longus capitis by the ascending cervical artery.

The *lateral border* of the muscle is related to the trunks of the brachial plexus and the subclavian artery which emerges at this border and enter the posterior triangle (Fig. 17.11).

CERVICAL PLEURA

The cervical pleura covers the apex of the lung. It rises into the root of the neck, about 5 cm above the first costal cartilage and 2.5 cm above the medial one-third of the clavicle. The pleural dome is strengthened on its outer surface by the suprapleural membrane, so that the root of the neck is not puffed up and down during respiration.

Relations

Anterior

1 Subclavian artery and its branches
2 Scalenus anterior (Fig. 17.13).

Posterior

Neck of the first rib and the following structures in front of it.

1 Sympathetic trunk
2 First posterior intercostal vein (Fig. 17.13)
3 Superior intercostal artery
4 The first thoracic nerve

Lateral

1 Scalenus medius
2 Lower trunk of the brachial plexus

Medial

1 Vertebral bodies
2 Oesophagus (Fig. 17.13)
3 Trachea
4 Left recurrent laryngeal nerve
5 Thoracic duct (on left side)
6 Large arteries and veins of the neck

CERVICAL PLEXUS

Formation

The cervical plexus is formed by the ventral rami of the upper four cervical nerves (Fig. 17.14). The rami emerge between the anterior and posterior tubercles of the cervical transverse processes, grooving the costotransverse bars. The four roots are connected with one another to form three loops (Fig. 17.15).

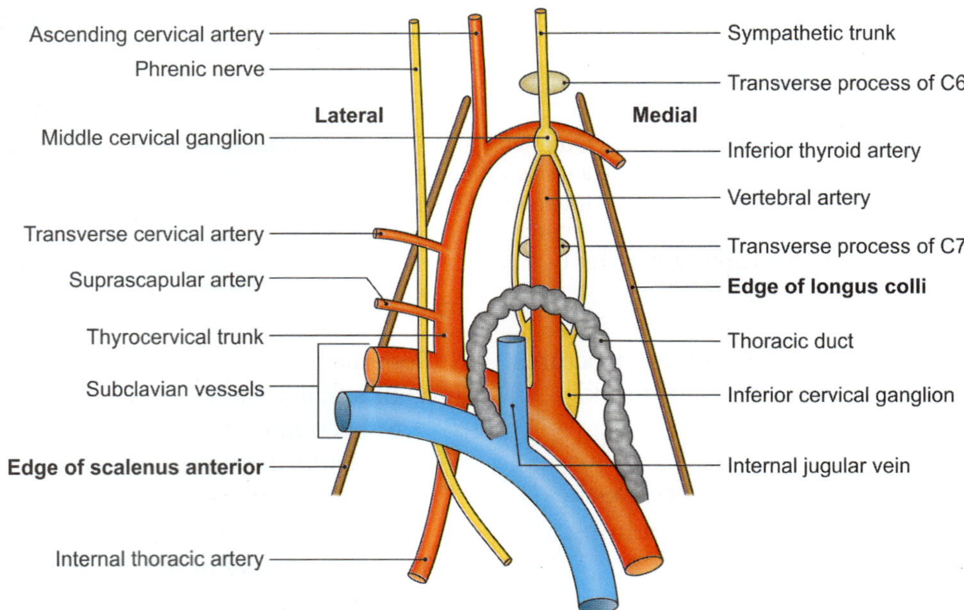

Fig. 17.12: Structures present in the triangular interval between scalenus anterior and the longus colli, i.e. scalenovertebral triangle

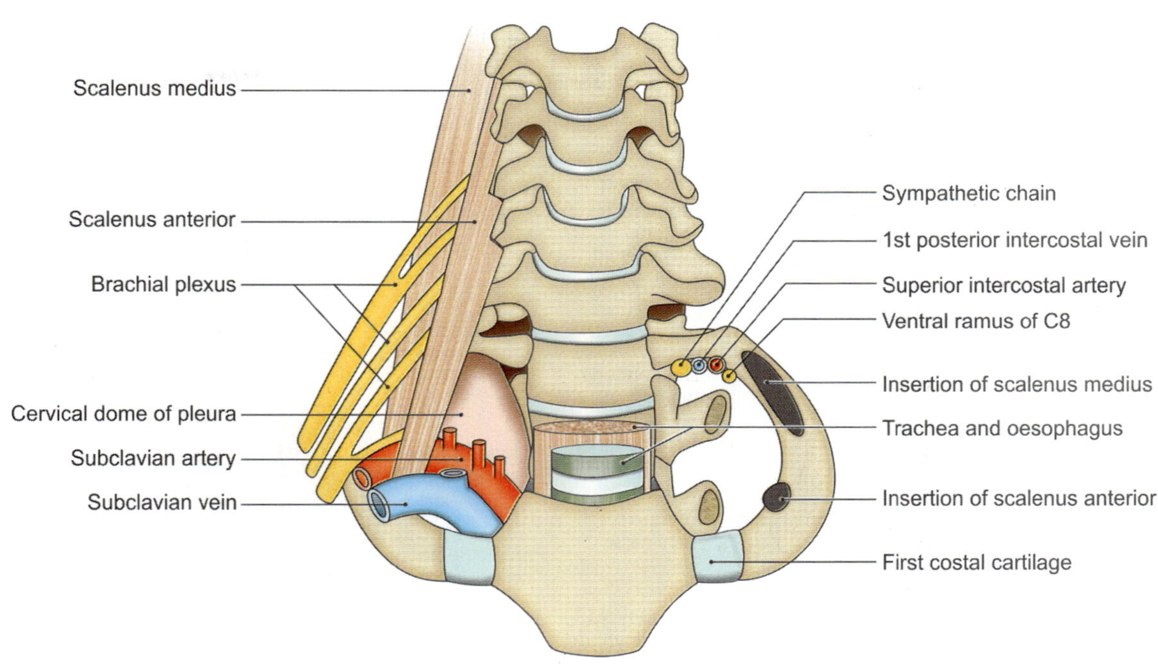

Fig. 17.13: Relations of the cervical pleura

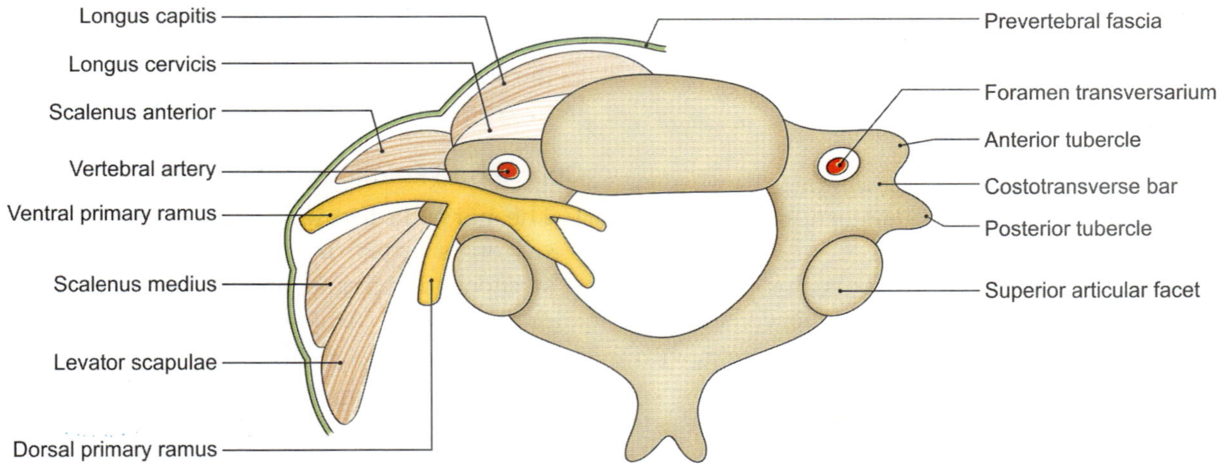

Fig. 17.14: Scheme to show the position of a cervical nerve relative to the muscles of the region

Position and Relations of the Plexus

The plexus is related:

1 *Posteriorly,* to the muscles which arise from the posterior tubercles of the transverse processes, i.e. the levator scapulae and the scalenus medius.
2 *Anteriorly,* to the prevertebral fascia, the internal jugular vein and the sternocleidomastoid.

Branches

Superficial (Cutaneous) Branches

1 Lesser occipital (C2)
2 Great auricular (C2, C3)
3 Transverse (anterior) cutaneous nerve of the neck (C2, C3)
4 Supraclavicular (C3, C4)

These are described in Chapter 11.

Deep Branches

Communicating branches

1 Grey rami pass from the superior cervical ganglion to the roots of C1–C4 nerves.
2 A branch from C1 joins the hypoglossal nerve and carries fibres for supply of the thyrohyoid and geniohyoid muscles (directly) and the superior belly of the omohyoid through the ansa cervicalis.
3 A branch each from C2, C3 to the sternocleidomastoid and branches from C3 and C4 to the trapezius communicate with the accessory nerve.

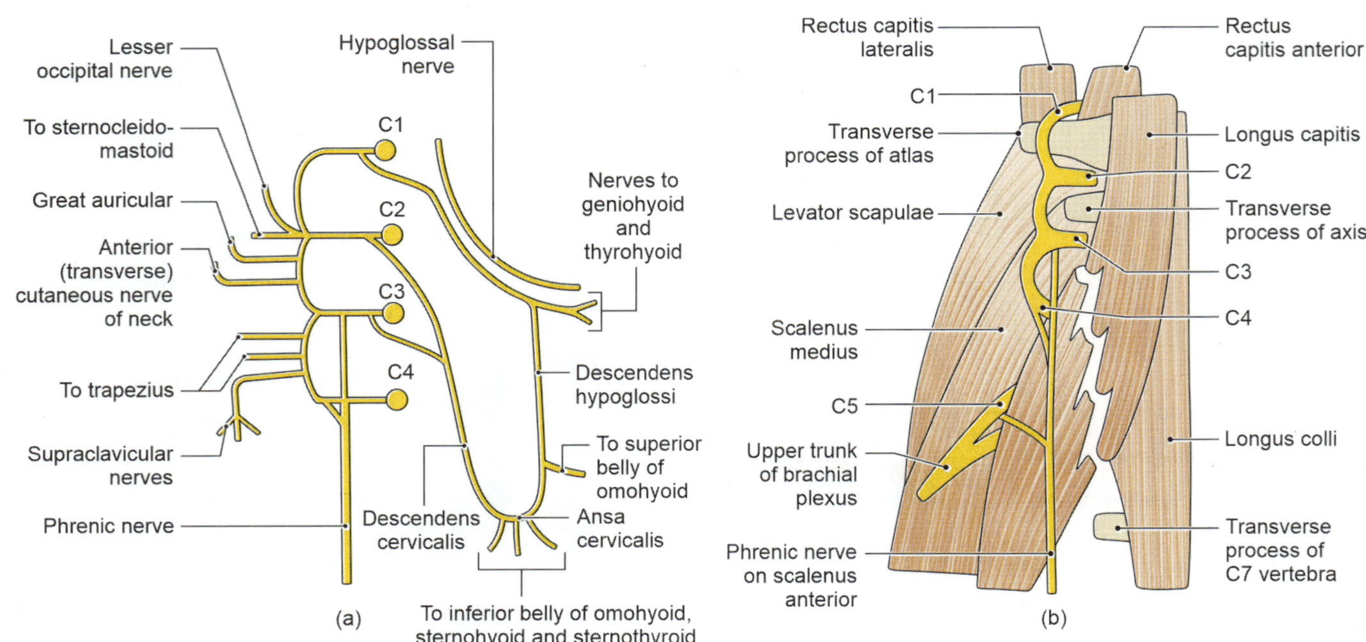

Fig. 17.15: Right cervical plexus and its branches

Muscular branches

Muscles supplied solely by cervical plexus:

1 Rectus capitis anterior from C1.
2 Rectus capitis lateralis from C1, C2.
3 Longus capitis from C1 to C3.
4 Lower root of ansa cervicalis (descendens cervicalis) from C2, C3 (to sternohyoid, sternothyroid and inferior belly of omohyoid).

Muscles supplied by cervical plexus along with the brachial plexus or the spinal accessory nerve:

a. Sternocleidomastoid from C2 to C3 along with accessory nerve (Fig. 17.15).
b. Trapezius from C3 to C4 along with accessory nerve.
c. Levator scapulae from C3 to C5 (dorsal scapular nerve).
d. The diaphragm from phrenic nerve from C3 to C5.
e. Longus colli from C3 to C8.
f. Scalenus medius from C3 to C8.
g. Scalenus anterior from C4 to C6.
h. Scalenus posterior from C6 to C8.

PHRENIC NERVE

This is a mixed nerve carrying motor fibres to the diaphragm and sensory fibres from the diaphragm, pleura, pericardium, and part of the peritoneum (Fig. 17.15).

Origin

Phrenic nerve arises chiefly from the fourth cervical nerve but receives contributions from third and fifth cervical nerves. The contribution from C5 may come directly from the root or indirectly through the nerve to the subclavius. In the latter case, the contribution is known as the *accessory phrenic nerve.*

Course and Relations in the Neck

1 The nerve is formed at the lateral border of the scalenus anterior, opposite the middle of the sternocleidomastoid, at the level of the upper border of the thyroid cartilage.
2 It runs vertically downwards on the anterior surface of the scalenus anterior (Fig. 17.16). Since the muscle is oblique, the nerve appears to cross it obliquely from lateral to medial border. In this part of its course, the nerve is related anteriorly to the prevertebral fascia, the inferior belly of the omohyoid, the transverse cervical artery, the suprascapular artery, the internal jugular vein, the sternocleidomastoid, and the thoracic duct on left side (Fig. 17.12).
3 After leaving the anterior surface of scalenus anterior, the nerve runs downwards on the cervical pleura behind the commencement of the brachiocephalic vein. Here it crosses the internal thoracic artery (either anteriorly or posteriorly) from lateral to medial side, and enters the thorax behind the first costal cartilage. On the left side, the nerve leaves (crosses) the medial margin of the scalenus anterior at a higher level and crosses in front of the first part of the subclavian artery.

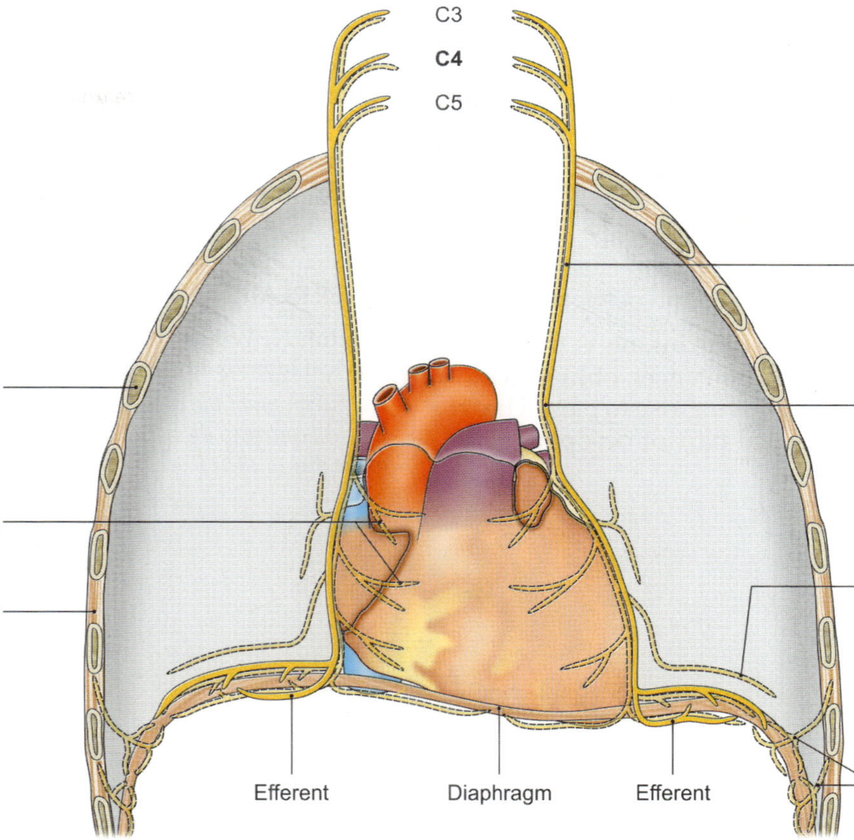

Fig. 17.16: Formation, course and distribution of phrenic nerve

CLINICAL ANATOMY

The accessory phrenic nerve is commonly a branch from the nerve to the subclavius. It lies lateral to the phrenic nerve and descends behind, or sometimes in front of the subclavian vein. It joins the main nerve usually near the first rib, but occasionally the union may even be below the root of the lung.

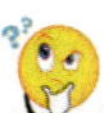

FACTS TO REMEMBER

- Vertebral artery comprises 4 parts:
  a. First part in neck
  b. Second part in forearm transversaria of C6 to C1 vertebrae
  c. Third part on the posterior arch of atlas.
  d. Fourth part through foramen magnum in the cranial cavity.
- Apical ligament is a remnant of notochord.
- Median atlantoaxial joint is a pivot type of joint, permitting movement of 'No'
- Atlanto-occipital joint is an ellipsoid joint permitting movement of 'Yes'.
- Transverse ligament of atlas is part of the cruciate ligament. It keeps the dens of axis in position.

CLINICOANATOMICAL PROBLEMS

Case 1

A person is to be hanged till death for his most unusual and rare crime.

- What anatomical changes occur during this procedure?
- Name the ligaments of median atlantoaxial joint.

Ans: Death in execution by hanging is due to dislocation of the dens of the axis vertebra following rupture of the transverse ligament of the dens. Dens all of a sudden is pushed backwards with great force, crushing the lowest part of medulla oblongata which houses the vasomotor centres

The ligaments of atlantoaxial joint are:

- Transverse ligament of dens
- Upper part of vertical band
- Lower part of vertical band

These three parts form cruciform ligament of the atlas vertebra.

There are two joint cavities. The anterior one between the posterior surface of anterior arch of atlas and dens. It is surrounded by loose capsular ligament.

The posterior, larger one is between the dens and the transverse ligament of the dens (Fig. 17.5).

Case 2

A man aged 55 years complained of dysphagia in eating solid and even soft food and liquids. There was a large lymph node felt at the anterior border of sternocleidomastoid muscle. The diagnosis on biopsy was cancer of cervical part of oesophagus.

- How was the large lymph node formed?
- Why did the patient have dysphagia?
- Where can the cancer spread around oesophagus?

Ans: The pain during eating or drinking is due to cancer of the oesophagus. The cancer obliterates increasing part of the lumen, giving rise to pain. The lymphatic drainage of cervical part of oesophagus goes to inferior group of deep cervical lymph nodes. These had metastasized to the lymph node at the anterior border of sternocleidomastoid muscle. Since trachea lies just anterior to oesophagus, the cancer can spread to trachea or any of the principal bronchi. It may even cause narrowing of trachea or bronchi.

FURTHER READING

- Bogduk N, Windsor M, Inglis A. The innervation of the cervical intervertebral discs. Spine 1988;13:2–8.

  A description of the cervical sinuvertebral nerves, which have an upward course in the vertebral canal, supplying the lateral aspects of the disc at their level of entry and the disc.

Frequently Asked Questions

1. Describe median atlantoaxial joint. Name the movements which occur here with their muscles.
2. Describe atlanto-occipital joint briefly.
3. Write short notes on/enumerate:
   a. Ligaments connecting axis to the skull
   b. Cruciate ligament
   c. Parts of vertebral artery

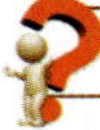

Multiple Choice Questions

1. How many synovial cavities are there in median atlantoaxial joint?
   a. One b. Three
   c. Two d. Four
2. Which of the following ligaments is the upward continuation of membrana tectoria?
   a. Posterior longitudinal
   b. Ligamentum nuchae
   c. Ligamentum flava
   d. Anterior longitudinal
3. Which ligament mentioned below is chiefly elastic?
   a. Anterior longitudinal
   b. Ligamenta flava
   c. Ligamentum nuchae
   d. Posterior longitudinal
4. Where is the intervertebral disc absent?
   a. Between first and second cervical vertebrae
   b. Between thoracic twelve and first lumbar vertebrae
   c. Between thoracic one and cervical seven vertebrae
   d. Between lumbar five and first sacral vertebrae
5. Which of the following joints do not have a fibrocartilaginous intra-articular disc?
   a. Temporomandibular
   b. Shoulder
   c. Sternoclavicular
   d. Inferior radioulnar

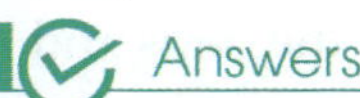

Answers

1. c **2.** a **3.** b **4.** a **5.** b

VIVA VOCE

- Name the boundaries and contents of scaleno-vertebral triangle.
- Where are the various parts of vertebral artery placed?
- What is the relation of scalenus anterior muscle to the subclavian artery?
- What structure forms the posterior relation of the cervical pleura?
- What is tracheostomy and where is it performed?
- Name the ligaments between occipital bone and axis vertebra.
- Give the attachment of posterior atlanto-occipital membrane. What structures lie under its free margin?
- Give the attachments of cruciate ligament of the atlas vertebra.
- What are the attachments of apical ligament of dens and alar ligament?
- What happens during judicial hanging?
- What type of joint is median atlantoaxial joint?
- What type of joint is atlanto-occipital joint?

Chapter

18

Back of the Neck

"I bend, but do not break."
—Anonymous

INTRODUCTION

The vertebral column at back provides a median axis for the body. The joints of neck are described in Chapter 17. There are big muscles from the sacrum to the skull in different strata which keep the spine straight. The uppermost part of back of neck is the suboccipital region. This region contains the suboccipital triangle containing the third part of the vertebral artery, which enters the skull to supply the brain. If it gets pressed, many symptoms appear.

DISSECTION

Extend the incision from external occipital protuberance (i), to the spine of the seventh cervical vertebra. Give a horizontal incision from spine of 7th cervical vertebra or vertebra prominens (iv), till the acromion process (v). This will expose the upper part and apex of posterior triangle of neck. Look for the occipital artery at its apex.

Extend the incision from vertebra prominens to spine of lumbar 5 vertebra. Reflect the skin laterally along an oblique line from spine of T12 (ii), till the deltoid tuberosity (iii) (Fig. 18.1).

Close to the median plane in the superficial fascia are seen the greater occipital nerve and occipital artery.

Cut through trapezius muscle vertically at a distance of 2 cm from the median plane. Reflect it laterally and identify the accessory nerve, superficial branch of transverse cervical artery and ventral rami of 3rd and 4th cervical nerves *(refer to BDC App)*.

Latissimus dorsi has already been exposed by the students dissecting the upper limb. Otherwise extend the incision from T12 spine till L5 spine. Reflect the skin till lateral side of the trunk and define the margins of broad thin latissimus dorsi. This muscle and trapezius form the first layer of muscles.

The second layer comprises splenius muscle, levator scapulae, rhomboid major, rhomboid minor, serratus posterior superior and serratus posterior inferior muscles. The splenius is the highest of these muscles.

Levator scapulae forms part of the muscular floor of the posterior triangle. It is positioned between scalenus medius below and splenius capitis above. Follow its nerve and blood supply from dorsal scapular nerve and deep branch of transverse cervical artery, respectively.

Spinal root of accessory nerve and fibres from C3 and C4 to trapezius muscle lie on the levator scapulae.

Rhomboid minor and major lie on same plane as levator scapulae. Both are supplied by dorsal scapular nerve (C5).

Deep to the two rhomboid muscles is thin aponeurotic serratus posterior superior muscle from spines of C7 and T1–T2 vertebrae to be inserted into 2nd–5th ribs. Serratus posterior inferior muscle arises from T11 to T12 spines and thoracolumbar fascia and is inserted into 9th–12th ribs.

The third layer is composed of erector spinae or sacrospinalis with its three subdivisions and semispinalis with its three divisions (Figs 18.2a to c).

Erector spinae arises from the dorsal surface of sacrum and ascends up the lumbar region. There it divides into three subdivisions, the medial one is spinalis—inserted into the spines, the intermediate one is longissimus—inserted into the transverse processes, and the lateral one is iliocostalis—inserted into the ribs. Each of these divisions is made of short parts, fresh slips arising from the area where the lower slips are inserted (Fig. 18.3).

Deep to erector spinae is the semispinalis again made up of three parts: Semispinalis thoracis, semispinalis cervicis, and semispinalis capitis.

Both these muscles are innervated by the dorsal rami of cervical, thoracic, lumbar and sacral nerves.

Muscles of fourth layer are the multifidus, rotatores, interspinales, intertransversarii and suboccipital muscles (Fig. 18.4).

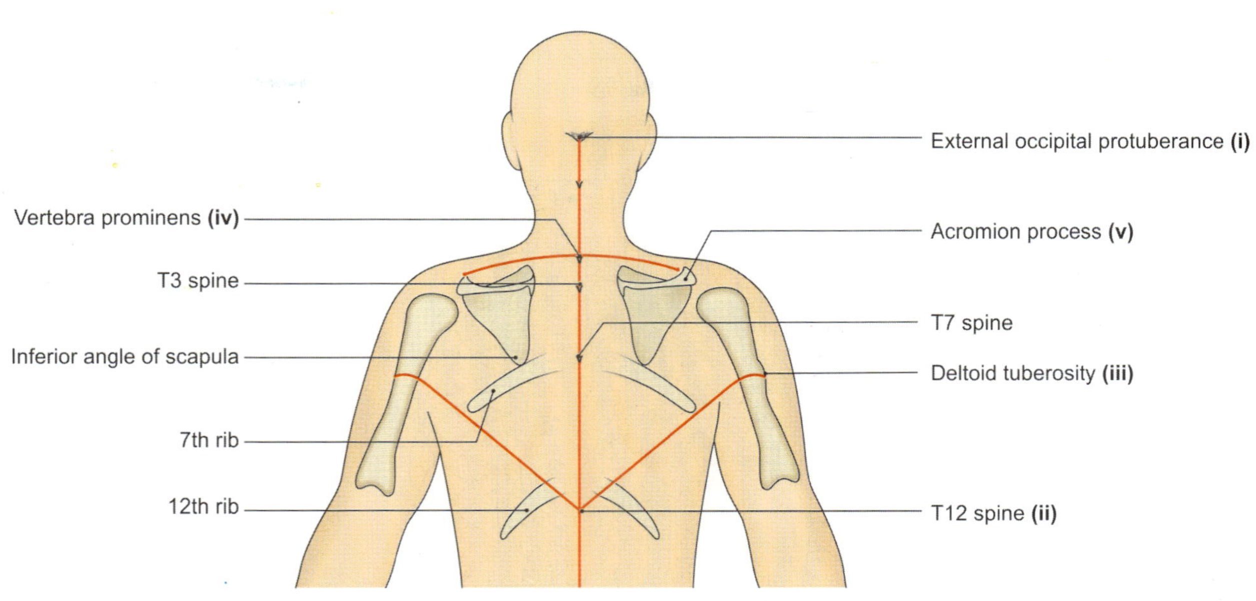

Fig. 18.1: Lines of dissection of back

NERVE SUPPLY OF SKIN

The skin of the nape or back of the neck, and of the back of the scalp (Fig. 18.2) is supplied by medial branches of the dorsal rami of C2 the *greater occipital nerve;* C3 the *third occipital nerve.* Each posterior primary ramus divides into a medial branch and a lateral branch, both of which supply the intrinsic muscles of the back. The medial branch in this region supplies the skin as well. The *dorsal ramus of C1* does not divide into medial and lateral branches, and is distributed only to the muscles bounding the suboccipital triangle.

The *ligamentum nuchae* is a triangular fibrous sheet that separates muscles of the two sides of the neck. It is better developed and is more elastic in quadrupeds in whom, it has to support a heavy head.

MUSCLES OF THE BACK

The *muscles* of the entire back can be grouped into the following four layers from superficial to the deeper plane.

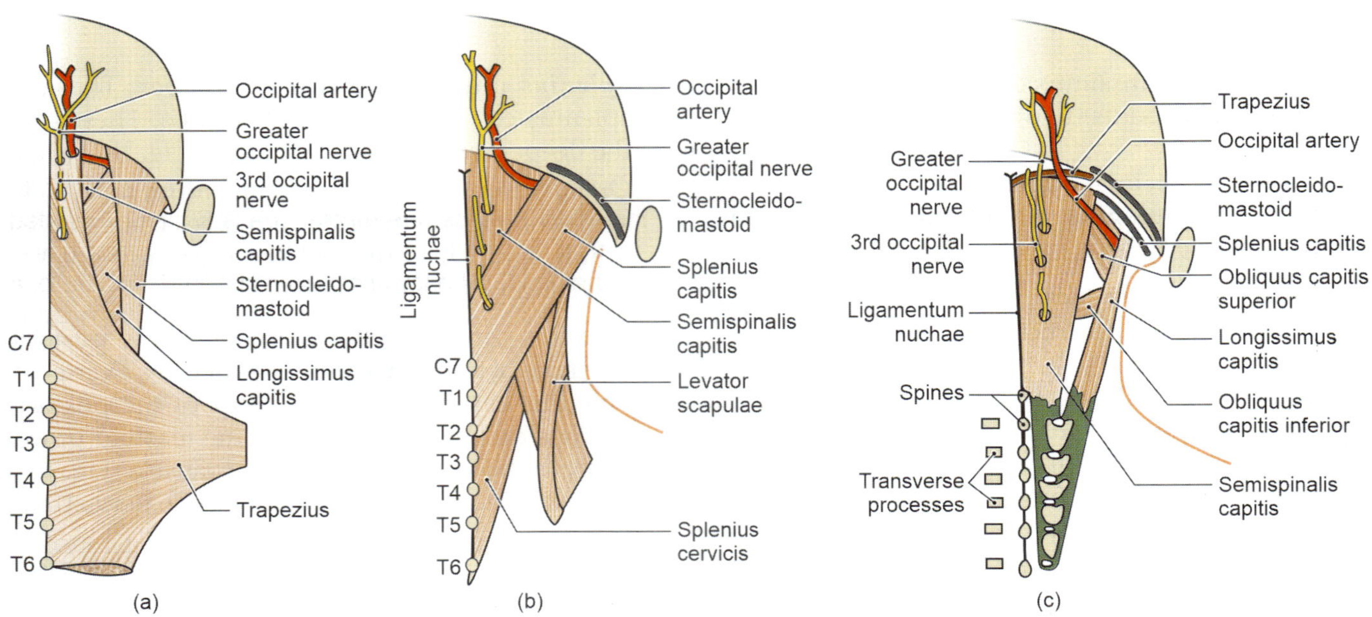

Figs 18.2a to c: Muscles of first, second and third layers: (a) First layer; (b) Second layer; (c) Third layer

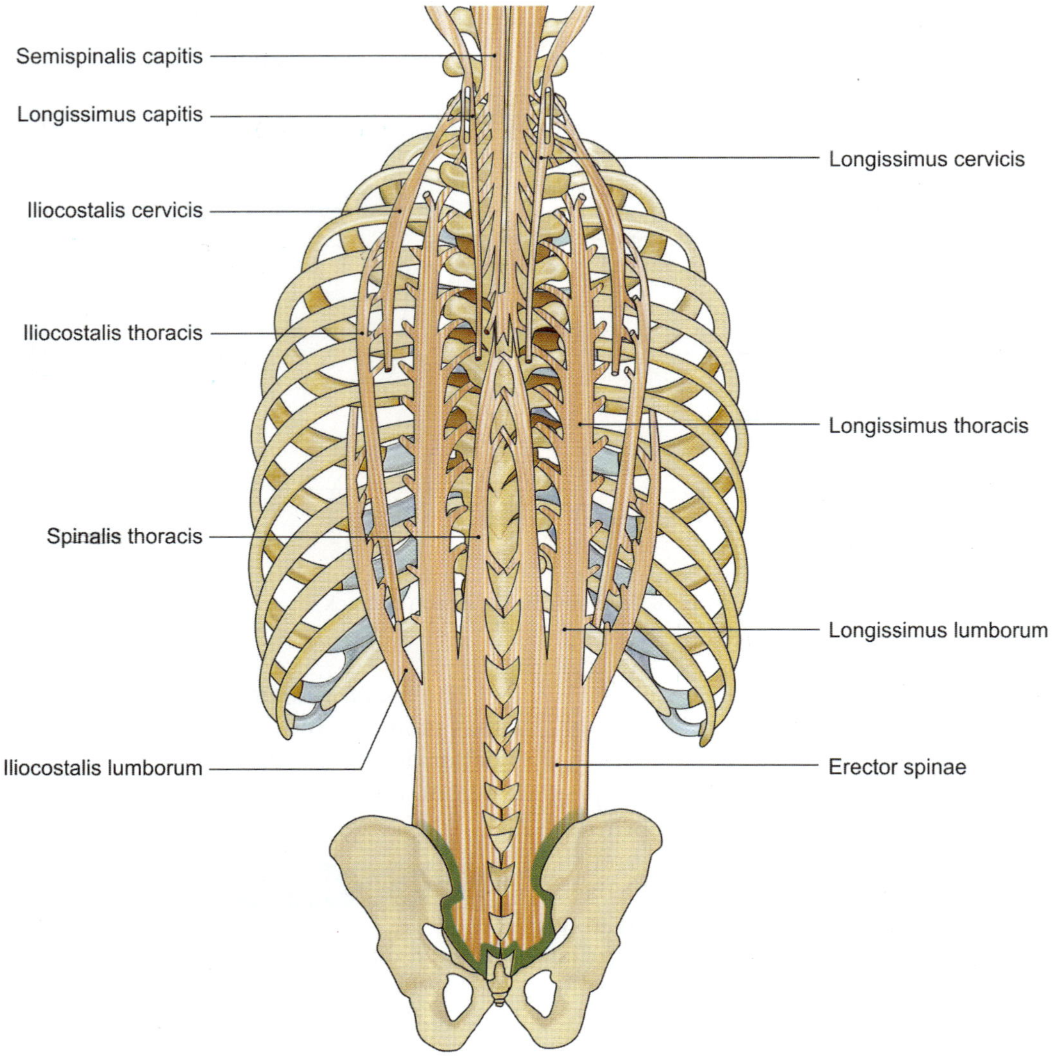

Fig. 18.3: Third layer—the erector spinae/sacrospinalis muscle with its three columns

1 Trapezius and latissimus dorsi (Fig. 18.2a), levator scapulae, rhomboids (two) (Fig. 18.2b) (Tables 18.1 and 18.2).

2 Serratus posterior superior, serratus posterior inferior and splenius. These small muscles are described briefly here.

Serratus posterior superior

Origin: Ligamentum nuchae, spines of T1–T3 vertebrae.
Insertion: Upper borders of 2nd–5th ribs.
Nerve supply: 2nd–5th intercostal nerves
Action: Elevates 2nd–5th ribs.

Serratus posterior inferior

Origin: Spines of T11–L2 vertebrae.
Insertion: Lower borders of 9th–12th ribs.
Nerve supply: 9th–12th intercostal nerves.
Action: Depress the lower ribs.

Splenius muscles are two in number. These are splenius cervicis and splenius capitis. These cover the deeper muscles like a bandage (Fig. 18.2c).

Origin: From lower half of ligamentum nuchae and spines of upper 6 thoracic vertebrae. These curve in a half spiral fashion and separate into splenius cervicis and splenius capitis.

Splenius cervicis gets inserted into the posterior tubercles of transverse processes of C1–C4 vertebrae. Splenius capitis forms the floor of the posterior triangle and gets inserted into the mastoid process beneath the sternocleidomastoid muscle (Fig. 18.5). It is supplied by dorsal rami of C1–C6 nerves.

3 a. *Erector spinae* or *sacrospinalis* is the true muscle of the back, supplied by posterior rami of the spinal nerves. It extends from the sacrum to the skull (Fig. 18.3).

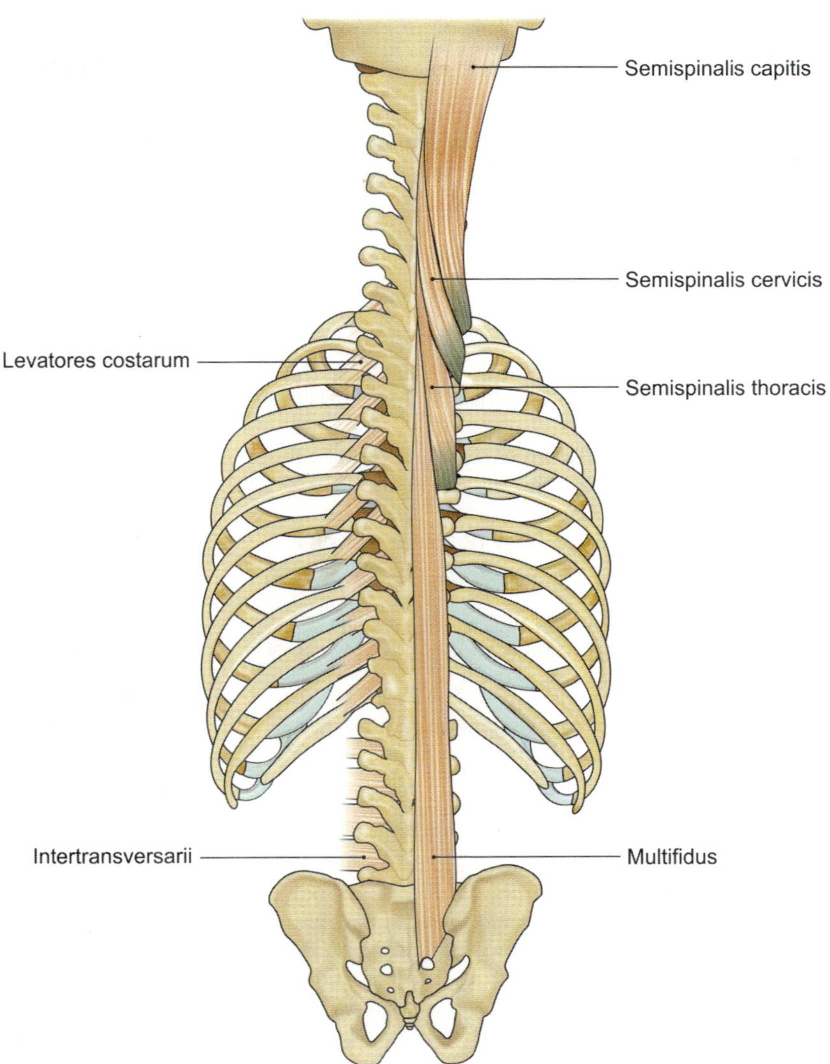

Fig. 18.4: Third layer—three parts of semispinalis. Fourth layer—the multifidus, levator costarum and intertransversarii muscles

Origin: Mainly from the back of sacrum between median and lateral sacral crests, from the dorsal segment of iliac crest and related ligaments. Soon it splits into three columns: Iliocostalis, longissimus, and spinalis.

i. *Iliocostalis* is the lateral column and comprises iliocostalis lumborum, iliocostalis thoracis and iliocostalis cervicis.

   These are short slips and are inserted into angles of the ribs and posterior tubercles of cervical transverse process. Origin of the higher slips is medial to the insertion of the lower slips.

ii. *Longissimus* is the middle column and is composed of:

   Longissimus lumborum

   Longissimus thoracis—inserted into transverse processes of thoracic vertebrae.

   Longissimus cervicis—inserted into transverse process of C2–C6 vertebrae.

   Longissimus capitis—inserted into mastoid process (Fig. 18.3).

iii. *Spinalis* is the medial column, extending between lumbar and cervical spines. Its parts are: Spinalis lumborum, spinalis thoracis, and spinalis cervicis.

b. The other muscle of this layer is semispinalis extending between transverse processes and spines of the vertebrae. It has three parts:

   i. Semispinalis thoracis (Fig. 18.4).
   ii. Semispinalis cervicis
   iii. Semispinalis capitis

It only lies in the upper half of vertebral column. Semispinalis capitis is its biggest component. It arises from transverse processes of C3–T4

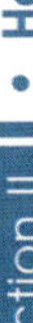

Table 18.1: Attachments of muscles connecting the upper limb to the vertebral column

Muscle	*Origin*	*Insertion*
Trapezius The right and left muscles together form a trapezium that covers the upper half of the back (Fig. 18.2a)	• Medial one-third of superior nuchal line • External occipital protuberance • Ligamentum nuchae • C7 spine • T1–T12 spines • Corresponding supraspinous ligaments	• Upper fibres into the posterior border and adjoining surfaces of lateral one-third of clavicle • Middle fibres into the medial margin of the acromion process and upper lip of the crest of spine of the scapula • Lower fibres on the apex of triangular area at the medial end of the spine, with a bursa intervening
Latissimus dorsi It covers a large area of the lower back, and is overlapped by the trapezius (Fig. 18.2a)	• Posterior one-third of the outer lip of iliac crest • Posterior layer of lumbar fascia; thus attaching the muscle to the lumbar and sacral spines • Spines of T7–T12, lower four ribs • Inferior angle of the scapula	The muscle winds round the lower border of the teres major, and forms the posterior fold of the axilla The tendon is twisted upside down and is inserted into floor of the intertubercular sulcus
Levator scapulae (Fig. 18.2b)	• Transverse processes of C1, C2 • Posterior tubercles of the transverse processes of C3, C4	Superior angle and upper part of medial border (up to triangular area) of the scapula
Rhomboid minor	• Lower part of ligamentum nuchae • Spines C7 and T1	Base of the triangular area at the root of the spine of the scapula
Rhomboid major	• Spines of T2–T5 • Supraspinous ligaments	Medial border of scapula below the root of the spine

Table 18.2: Nerve supply and actions of muscles connecting the upper limb to the vertebral column

Muscle	*Nerve supply*	*Actions*
Trapezius	• Spinal part of accessory nerve (XI) • Branches from C3, C4	• Upper fibres act with levator scapulae, and elevate the scapula, as in shrugging. Upper fibres of both sides extend the neck • Middle fibres act with rhomboids, and retract the scapula • Upper and lower fibres act with serratus anterior, and rotate the scapula forwards around the chest wall thus playing an important role in abduction of the arm beyond 90° • Steadies the scapula
Latissimus dorsi	Thoracodorsal nerve (C6–C8) (nerve to latissimus dorsi)	• Adduction, extension, and medial rotation of the shoulder as in swimming, rowing, climbing, pulling, folding the arm behind the back, and scratching the opposite scapula • Helps in violent expiratory effort like coughing, sneezing, etc. • Essentially a climbing muscle • Hold inferior angle of the scapula in place
Levator scapulae	• A branch from dorsal scapular nerve (C5) • Branches from C3, C4	• Helps in elevation of scapula • Steadies the scapula during movements of the arm
Rhomboid minor	Dorsal scapular nerve (C5)	• Retraction of scapula
Rhomboid major	Dorsal scapular nerve (C5)	• Retraction of scapula

vertebrae, passes up next to the median plane, and gets inserted into the medial area between superior and inferior nuchal lines of the occipital bone.

4 *Multifidus, rotatores, interspinales, intertransversarii* and *suboccipital* muscles. Multifidus is one of the oblique deep muscles. It arises from mammillary process of lumbar vertebrae to be inserted into 2–3 higher spinous processes. Rotatores are the deepest group. These pass from root of transverse process to the root of the spinous process. These are well developed in thoracic region. Interspinales lie between the adjacent spines of the vertebrae. These are better developed in cervical and lumbar regions. Intertransversarii connect the transverse processes of the adjacent vertebrae.

SUBOCCIPITAL REGION

Muscle Layers in Neck (Fig. 18.4)

In the *suboccipital region* between the occiput and the spine of the axis vertebra, the four muscular layers are represented by:

- Trapezius
- Splenius capitis
- Semispinalis capitis and longissimus capitis
- The four suboccipital muscles.

The *arteries* found in the back of the neck are:

a. Occipital
b. Deep cervical
c. Third part of the vertebral artery
d. Minute twigs from the second part of the vertebral artery.

The *suboccipital venous plexus* is known for its extensive layout and complex connections.

DISSECTION

It is deep triangle in the area between the occiput and the spine of second cervical (the axis) vertebra. The deepest muscles are the muscles of suboccipital triangle.

Cut the attachments of trapezius from superior nuchal line and reflect it towards the spine of scapula. Cut the splenius capitis from its attachment on the mastoid process and reflect it downwards. Clean the superficial fascia over the semispinalis capitis medially and longissimus capitis laterally. Reflect longissimus capitis downwards from the mastoid process.

Cut through semispinalis capitis and turn it towards lateral side. Define the boundaries and contents of the suboccipital triangle.

Suboccipital Muscles

The suboccipital muscles are described in Table 18.3.

The suboccipital triangle is a muscular space situated deep in the suboccipital region.

Exposure of Suboccipital Triangle

In order to expose the triangle, the following layers are reflected (Fig. 18.5).

1 The *skin* is very thick.

2 The *superficial fascia* is fibrous and dense. It contains:

   a. The greater and third occipital nerves.
   b. The terminal part of the occipital artery, with accompanying veins.

3 The fibres of the *trapezius* run downwards and laterally over the triangle. The sternocleidomastoid overlaps the region laterally.

Table 18.3: The suboccipital muscles

Muscle	*Origin*	*Insertion*	*Nerve supply*	*Actions*
1. **Rectus capitis posterior major** (Fig. 18.5)	Spine of axis	Lateral part of the area below the inferior nuchal line	Suboccipital nerve or dorsal ramus C1	1. Mainly postural 2. Acting alone, it turns the chin to the same side 3. Acting together, the two muscles extend the head
2. **Rectus capitis posterior minor** (Fig. 18.5)	Posterior tubercle of atlas	Medial part of the area below the inferior nuchal line	"	1. Mainly postural 2. Extends the head
3. **Obliquus capitis superior** (superior oblique)	Transverse process of atlas	Lateral area between the nuchal lines	"	1. Mainly postural 2. Extends the head 3. Flexes the head laterally
4. **Obliquus capitis inferior** (inferior oblique; Fig. 18.5)	Spine of axis	Transverse process of atlas	"	1. Mainly postural 2. Turns chin to the same side

4 The *splenius capitis* runs upwards and laterally for insertion into the mastoid process deep to the sternocleidomastoid.

5 The *semispinalis capitis* runs vertically upwards for insertion into the medial part of the area between the superior and inferior nuchal lines. In the same plane laterally, there lies the *longissimus capitis* which is inserted into the mastoid process deep to the splenius.

Reflection of the semispinalis capitis exposes the *suboccipital triangle.*

Boundaries

Superomedially

Rectus capitis posterior major muscle supplemented by the *rectus capitis posterior minor* (Fig. 18.5).

Superolaterally

Obliquus capitis superior muscle.

Inferiorly

Obliquus capitis inferior muscle.

Roof

Medially
Dense fibrous tissue covered by the *semispinalis capitis.*

Laterally
Longissimus capitis and occasionally the *splenius capitis.*

Floor

1 Posterior arch of atlas.
2 Posterior atlanto-occipital membrane.

Contents

1 Third part of vertebral artery (Fig. 18.6).
2 Dorsal ramus of nerve C1—suboccipital nerve.
3 Suboccipital plexus of veins.

Vertebral Artery

It is the first and largest branch of the first part of the subclavian artery, destined chiefly to supply the brain. Out of its four parts, only the third part appears in the suboccipital triangle (Figs 18.5 and 18.6). This part appears at the foramen transversarium of the atlas, grooves the atlas, and leaves the triangle by passing deep to the lateral edge of the posterior atlanto-occipital membrane. The artery is separated from the posterior arch of the atlas by the first cervical nerve and its dorsal and ventral rami. For complete description of the vertebral artery, *see* Chapter 17.

Dorsal Ramus of First Cervical Nerve

It emerges between the posterior arch of the atlas and the vertebral artery, and soon breaks up into branches which supply the four suboccipital muscles and the semispinalis capitis. The nerve to the inferior oblique gives off a communicating branch to the greater occipital nerve capitis (Figs 18.5 and 18.6).

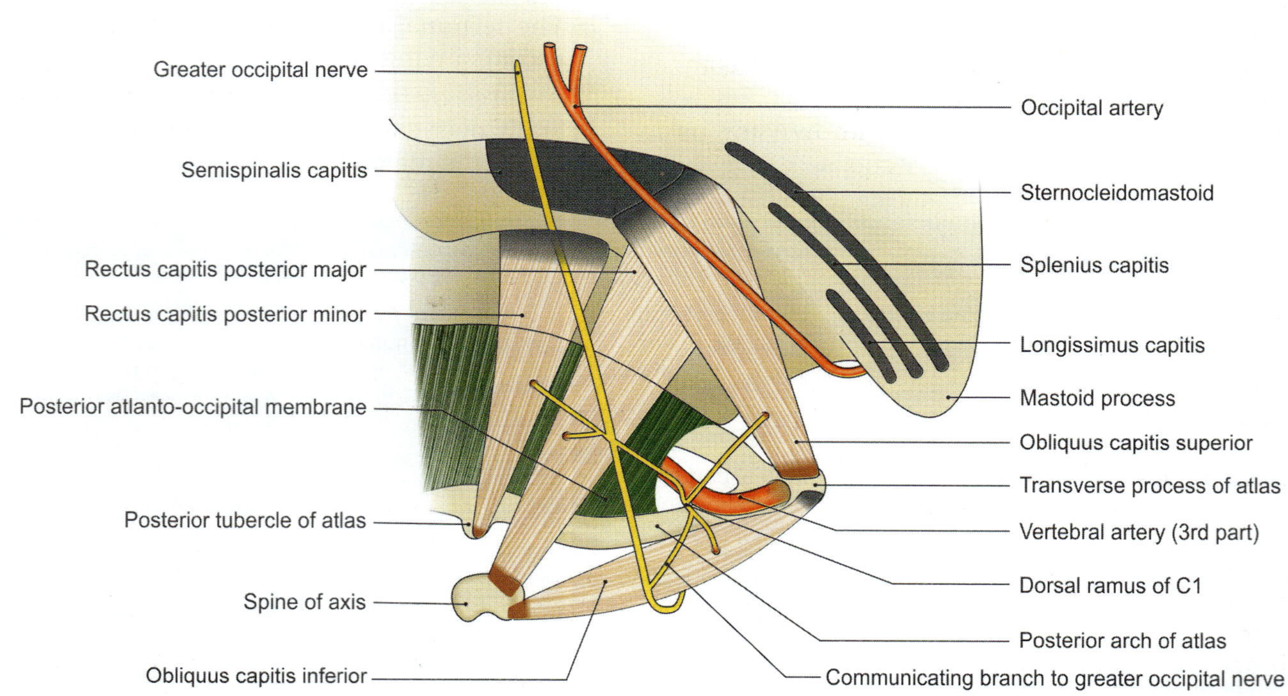

Fig. 18.5: Right suboccipital triangle: Boundaries, floor and contents

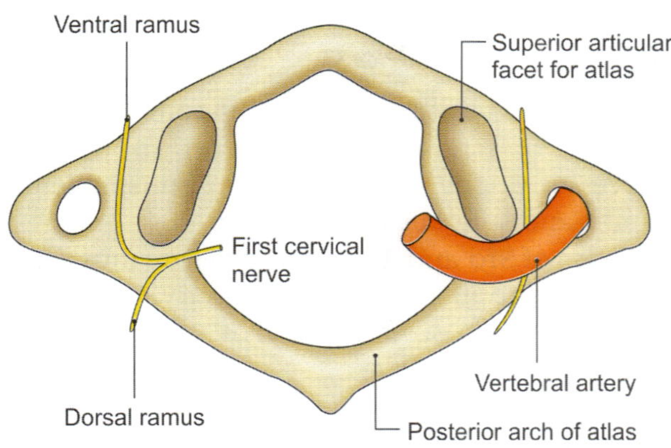

Fig. 18.6: Relationship of the vertebral artery to the atlas vertebra and to the first cervical nerve, as seen from above

Suboccipital Plexus of Veins

It lies in and around the suboccipital triangle, and drains the:

1 Muscular veins
2 Occipital veins
3 Internal vertebral venous plexus
4 Condylar emissary vein.

It itself drains into the deep cervical and vertebral plexus of veins.

Other Related Structures

Greater Occipital Nerve

It is the large medial branch of the dorsal ramus of the second cervical nerve. It is the *thickest cutaneous nerve* in the body. It winds round the middle of the lower border of the inferior oblique muscle, and runs upwards and medially. It crosses the suboccipital triangle and pierces the semispinalis capitis and trapezius muscles to ramify on the back of the head reaching up to the vertex. It supplies the semispinalis capitis in addition to the scalp (Fig. 18.2c).

Third Occipital Nerve

It is the slender medial branch of the dorsal ramus of the third cervical nerve. After piercing the semispinalis capitis and the trapezius, it ascends medial to the greater occipital nerve. It supplies the skin to the back of the neck up to the external occipital protuberance.

Occipital Artery

It arises from the external carotid artery, opposite the origin of the facial artery (Figs 18.2 and 18.5). It runs backwards and upwards deep to the lower border of the posterior belly of the digastric, crossing the carotid sheath, and the accessory and hypoglossal nerves. Next it runs deep to the mastoid process and to the muscles attached to it—the sternocleidomastoid, digastric, splenius capitis and longissimus capitis. The artery then crosses the rectus capitis lateralis, the superior oblique and the semispinalis capitis muscles at the apex of the posterior triangle. Finally, it pierces the trapezius 2.5 cm from the midline and comes to lie along the greater occipital nerve. In the superficial fascia of the scalp, it has a tortuous course.

Its branches in this region are:

a. Mastoid
b. Meningeal
c. Muscular.

One of the muscular branches is large, it is called the *descending branch* and has superficial and deep branches. The superficial branch anastomoses with the superficial branch of the transverse cervical artery; while the deep branch descends between the semispinalis capitis and cervicis, and anastomoses with the vertebral and deep cervical arteries. It also gives two branches to sternocleidomastoid muscle.

Deep Cervical Artery

It is a branch of the costocervical trunk of the subclavian artery. It passes into the back of the neck just above the neck of the first rib. It ascends deep to the *semispinalis capitis* and anastomoses with the descending branch of the occipital artery (*see* Fig. 16.19).

CLINICAL ANATOMY

- Neck rigidity, seen in cases with meningitis, is due to spasm of the extensor muscles. This is caused by irritation of the nerve roots during their passage through the subarachnoid space which is infected. Passive flexion of neck and straight leg raising test cause pain as the nerves are stretched (Figs 18.7a and b).
- Cisternal puncture is done when lumbar puncture fails. The patient either sits up or lies

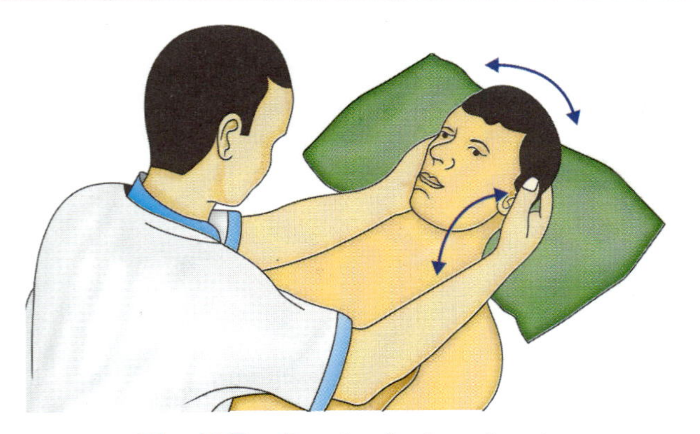

Fig. 18.7a: Passive flexion of neck

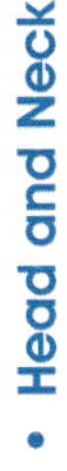

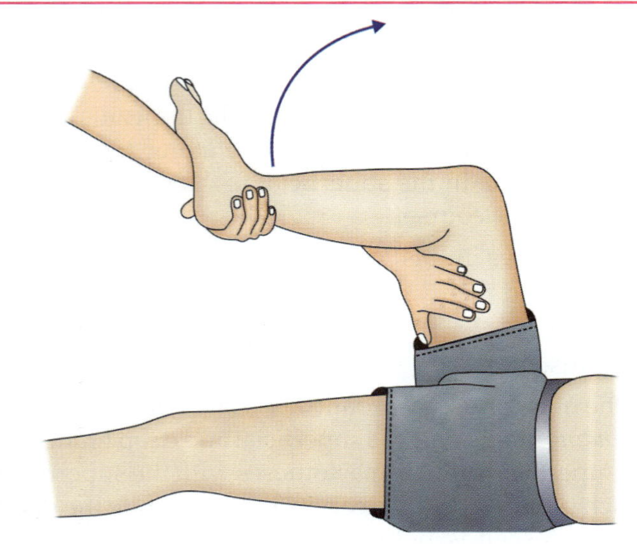

Fig. 18.7b: Straight leg raising test causes pain in meningitis

down in the left lateral position. A needle is introduced in the midline above the spine of axis in forward and upward direction parallel to an imaginary line extending from external acoustic meatus to nasion. It passes through the posterior atlanto-occipital membrane between the posterior arch of atlas and the posterior margin of foramen magnum. The needle enters the cerebellomedullary cistern and small amount of CSF is withdrawn.

- Neurosurgeons approach the posterior cranial fossa through this region.

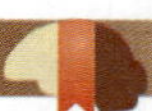

Mnemonics

"I Love Sunshine"

From inferior to superior:

Iliocostalis

Longissimus

Spinalis

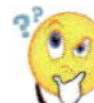

FACTS TO REMEMBER

Muscles of the back are disposed in four layers:

- Muscles of 1st and 2nd layers are supplied by nerves of upper limb except trapezius, splenius capitis and splenius cervicis.
- Muscles of 3rd and 4th layers are true muscles of the back, supplied by dorsal primary rami.
- Artery lying on posterior arch of atlas is the third part of vertebral artery.
- Greater occipital nerve is the thickest cutaneous nerve of the body.

CLINICOANATOMICAL PROBLEM

A child aged 8 years has been having high grade fever with bad throat. On 4th day, he could not move his neck during drinking water or milk as there was severe pain in the neck.

- Why is there pain even in drinking water?
- How has it become such a serious condition?

Ans: Due to bad throat, the infection from pharynx reached middle ear via pharyngotympanic tube, from where it infected the meninges of the brain. This is a serious condition and is called meningitis. The child shows neck rigidity. It is due to spasm of the extensor muscles and is caused by irritation of nerve roots during their passage through subarachnoid space, which is infected.

Passive flexion of neck and straight leg raising test result in pain as the nerves are stretched.

FURTHER READING

- Adams MA, Bogduk, Burton K, et al. The Biomechanics of Back Pain. 2nd ed. Edinburgh: Elsevier, Churchill Livingstone 2006.

  A comprehensive and detailed source of information on the functional anatomy, tissue biology and biomechanics of the lumbar spine.
- Groen GJ, Baljet, Drukker J. Nerves and nerve plexuses of the human vertebral column. Am J Anat 1990;188:282–96.

  An acetylcholinesterase whole-mount study of human fetal material giving detail of the perivertebral nerve plexuses and of the sinuvertebral nerves.

Frequently Asked Questions

1. Enumerate the boundaries and contents of the suboccipital triangle. Name the muscles supplied by dorsal ramus of 1st cervical nerve.
2. Name the various parts of sacrospinalis/erector spinae muscle.
3. Write short notes on:
   a. Occipital artery
   b. Meningitis

Multiple Choice Questions

1. Which action is not done by trapezius muscles?
   a. Protraction of scapula
   b. Shrugging of shoulder
   c. Retraction of scapula
   d. Overhead abduction of scapula
2. Sacrospinalis does not form:
   a. Spinalis
   b. Longissimus
   c. Iliocostalis
   d. Splenius
3. Which part of vertebral artery lies in the suboccipital triangle?
   a. 1st
   b. 3rd
   c. 2nd
   d. 4th
4. Dorsal ramus of which of the cervical nerves has no cutaneous branch?
   a. 1st
   b. 2nd
   c. 3rd
   d. 4th
5. Which is the thickest cutaneous nerve of the body?
   a. Greater occipital
   b. Lesser occipital
   c. Great auricular
   d. Third occipital
6. Which of the following cervical nerves is known as suboccipital nerve?
   a. 1st
   b. 2nd
   c. 3rd
   d. 4th

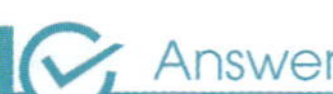

Answers

1. a **2.** d **3.** b **4.** a **5.** a **6.** a

VIVA VOCE

- Name the muscles in all 4 layers of the back.
- What are the parts of erector spinae muscle?
- What are the boundaries of suboccipital triangle and name its contents?
- Name the thickest cutaneous nerve of the body.
- What are the parts of semispinalis muscle? Which nerves supply this muscle?

VIDEO 3.10 Muscles of the back

Chapter 19

Contents of Vertebral Canal

"Remember that your patient is a human being like yourself. Your knowledge of anatomy may save his or her life."
—Richard Snell

INTRODUCTION

When the vertebrae are put in a sequence, their vertebral foramina lie one below the other forming a continuous canal which is called the *vertebral canal*. This canal contains the three meninges with their spaces and the spinal cord including the cauda equina. The intervertebral foramina are a pair of foramina between the pedicles of the adjacent vertebrae. Each foramen contains dorsal and ventral roots, trunk and dorsal and ventral primary rami of the spinal nerve, and spinal vessels.

CONTENTS

The vertebral canal contains the following structures from without inwards (Fig. 19.1).

1 Epidural or extradural space
2 Thick dura mater or pachymeninx
3 Subdural capillary space
4 Delicate arachnoid mater
5 Wide subarachnoid space containing cerebrospinal fluid (CSF)
6 Firm pia mater. The arachnoid and pia together form the leptomeninges.
7 Spinal cord or spinal medulla and the cauda equina.

The spinal cord is considered in Chapter 31. The other contents are described below.

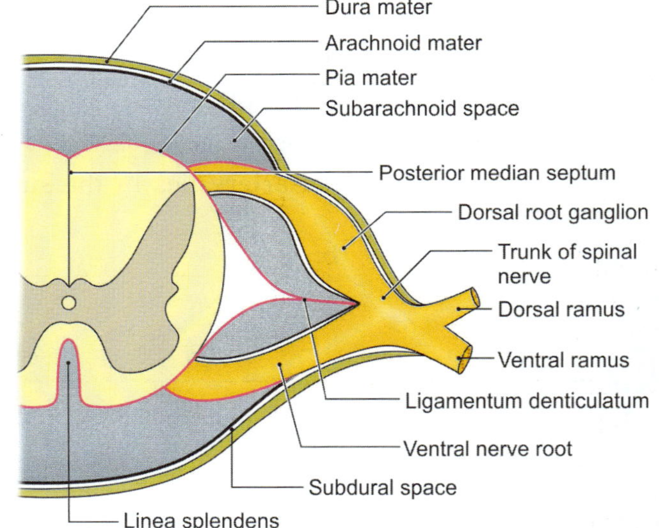

Fig. 19.1: Schematic transverse section showing the spinal meninges

DISSECTION

Clean the spines and laminae of the entire vertebral column by removing all the muscles attached to them. Trace the dorsal rami of spinal nerves towards the intervertebral foramina. Saw through the spines and laminae of the vertebrae carefully and detach them so that the spinal medulla/spinal cord encased in the meninges becomes visible.

Clean the external surface of dura mater enveloping the spinal cord by removing fat and epidural plexus of veins. Carefully cut through a small part of the dura mater by a fine median incision. Extend this incision above and below. See the delicate arachnoid mater. Incise it. Push the spinal cord to one side and try to identify the ligamentum denticulatum. Define the attachments of the dorsal and ventral nerve roots on the surface of spinal cord and their union to form the trunk of the spinal nerve. Cut the trunk of all spinal nerves on both the sides. Gently pull the spinal cord with cauda equina out from the vertebral canal.

Epidural Space

Epidural space lies between the spinal dura mater, and the periosteum with ligaments lining the vertebral canal.

It contains:

a. Loose areolar tissue
b. Semiliquid fat
c. Spinal arteries on their way to supply the deeper contents
d. The internal vertebral venous plexus.

The *spinal arteries* arise from different sources at different levels; they enter the vertebral canal through the intervertebral foramina, and supply the spinal cord, the spinal nerve roots, the meninges, the periosteum and ligaments.

Venous blood from the spinal cord drains into the epidural or internal vertebral plexus.

Spinal Dura Mater

Spinal dura mater is a thick, tough fibrous membrane which forms a loose sheath around the spinal cord (Fig. 19.2). It is continuous with the meningeal layer of the cerebral dura mater. The spinal dura extends from the foramen magnum to the lower border of the second sacral vertebra; whereas the spinal cord ends at the lower border of first lumbar vertebra. The dura gives tubular prolongations to the dorsal and ventral nerve roots and to the spinal nerves as they pass through the intervertebral foramina.

Subdural Space

Subdural space is a capillary or potential space between the dura and the arachnoid, containing a thin film of serous fluid. This space permits movements of the dura over the arachnoid. The space is continued for a short distance onto the spinal nerves, and is in free communication with the lymph spaces of the nerves.

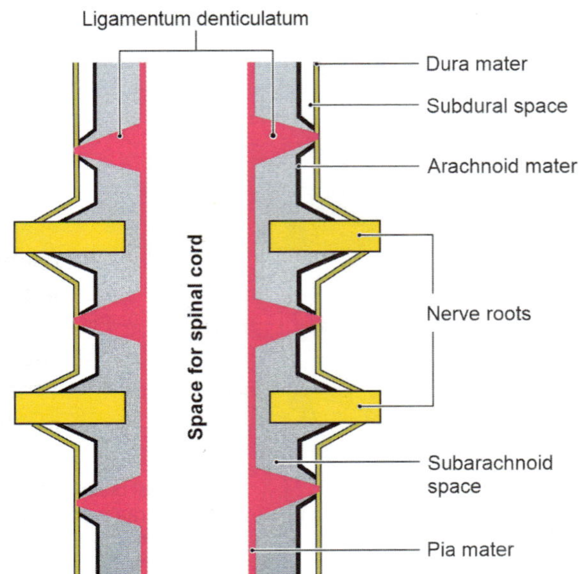

Fig. 19.2: Ligamentum denticulatum and its relationship to the dura mater and to the arachnoid mater

Arachnoid Mater

Arachnoid mater is a thin, delicate and transparent membrane that loosely invests the entire central nervous system (Fig. 19.2). Inferiorly, it extends, like the dura, up to the lower border of the second sacral vertebra. It is adherent to the dura only where some structures pierce the membrane, and where the ligamentum denticulata are attached to the dura mater.

Subarachnoid Space

Subarachnoid space is a wide space between the pia and the arachnoid, filled with cerebrospinal fluid (CSF). It surrounds the brain and spinal cord like a water cushion. The spinal subarachnoid space is wider than the space around the brain. It is widest below the lower end of the spinal cord where it encloses the cauda equina. *Lumbar puncture* is usually done in the lower widest part of the space, between third and fourth lumbar vertebrae.

Spinal Pia Mater

Spinal pia mater is thicker, firmer, and less vascular than the cerebral pia, but both are made up of two layers:

a. An outer *epi-pia* containing larger vessels.
b. An inner *pia-glia or pia-intima* which is in contact with nervous tissue.

Between the two layers, there are many small blood vessels and also cleft-like spaces which communicate with the subarachnoid space. The pia mater closely invests the spinal cord, and is continued below the spinal cord as the *filum terminale.*

Posteriorly, the pia is adherent to the posterior median septum of the spinal cord, and is also connected to the arachnoid by a fenestrated *subarachnoid septum.*

Anteriorly, the pia is folded into the anterior median fissure of the spinal cord. It thickens at the mouth of the fissure to form a median, longitudinal glistening band, called the *linea splendens* (Fig. 19.1).

On each side between the ventral and dorsal nerve roots, the pia forms a narrow vertical ridge, called the *ligamentum denticulatum*. This is so-called because it gives off a series of triangular tooth-like processes which project from its lateral free border (Fig. 19.3). Each ligament has 21 processes; the first at the level of the foramen magnum, and the last between twelfth thoracic and first lumbar spinal nerves. Each process passes through the arachnoid to the dura between two *adjacent spinal nerves*. The processes suspend the spinal cord in the middle of the subarachnoid space.

The *filum terminale* is a delicate, thread-like structure about 20 cm long. It extends from the apex of the conus medullaris to the dorsum of the first piece of the

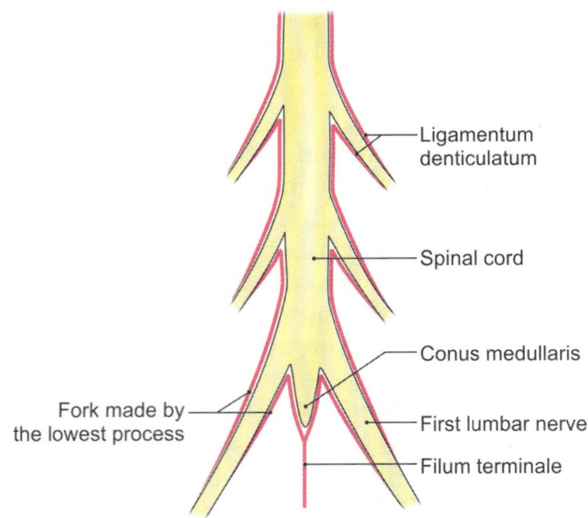

Fig. 19.3: Ligamentum denticulatum

coccyx. It is composed chiefly of pia mater, although a few nerve fibres rudiments of 2nd and 3rd coccygeal nerves are found adherent to the upper part of its outer surface. The central canal of the spinal cord extends into it for about 5 mm.

The filum terminale is subdivided into a part lying within the dural sheath called the *filum terminale internum*; and a part lying outside the dural sheath, below the level of the second sacral vertebra called the *filum terminale externum*. The filum terminale internum is 15 cm long, and the externum is 5 cm long.

Pial sheaths surround the nerve roots crossing the subarachnoid space, and the vessels entering the substance of the spinal cord.

CLINICAL ANATOMY

Leptomeningitis

- Inflammation due to infection of leptomeninges, i.e. pia mater and arachnoid mater is known as *meningitis*. This is commonly tubercular or pyogenic. It is characterized by fever, marked headache, neck rigidity, often accompanied by delirium and convulsions, and a changed biochemistry of CSF. CSF pressure is raised, its proteins and cell content are increased, and sugars and chloride are selectively diminished.
- *Lumbar puncture in adult:* Patient is lying on side with maximally flexed spine. A line is taken between highest points of iliac spine at L4 level. Skin locally anaesthetized, and lumbar puncture needle with trocar inserted carefully between L3 and L4 spines. Needle courses through skin fat, supraspinous and interspinous ligaments, ligamentum flava, epidural space, dura, arachnoid, subarachnoid space to release CSF (Fig. 19.4).
- *Lumbar puncture in infant/children:* During 2nd month of life, spinal cord usually reaches L3 level. Lumbar puncture needle is introduced in flexed spine between L4 and L5.
- *Cisternal puncture:* This procedure is rather difficult and dangerous. Cerebellomedullary cistern is approached through posterior atlanto-occipital membrane.
- *Lumbar epidural:* The epidural space is the space between vertebral canal and dura mater. The epidural space is deeper in the midline. The procedure is same as lumbar puncture, the needle should reach only in the epidural space and not deep to it in the dura mater. Epidural space is utilized for giving anaesthesia or analgesia (Fig. 19.5).

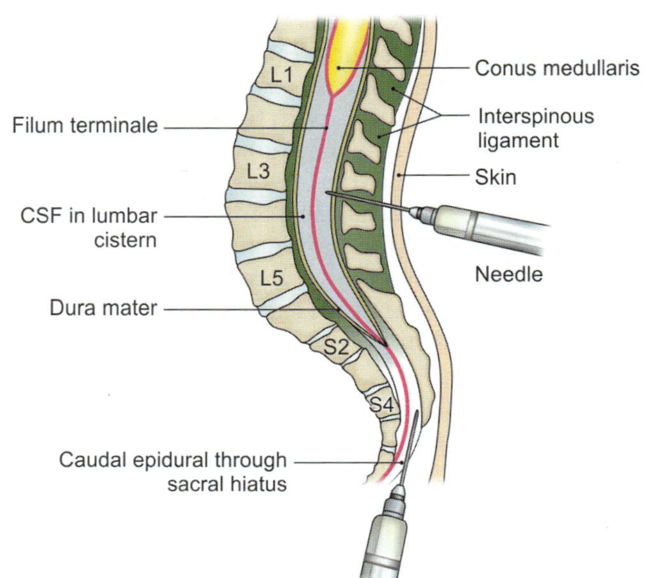

Fig. 19.4: Lumbar puncture in an adult

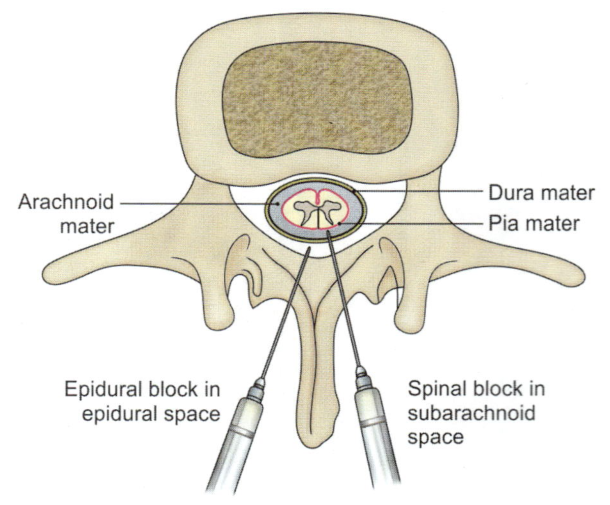

Fig. 19.5: Lumbar epidural anaesthesia and spinal block

- *Caudal epidural:* The needle is passed through sacral hiatus, which lies equidistant from the right and left posterior superior iliac spines. The needle passes through posterior sacrococcygeal ligament and enters the sacral canal. Then the hub of needle is lowered so that it passes along sacral canal. This space lies below S2 (Fig. 19.4).

SPINAL NERVES

The spinal cord gives rise to 31 pairs of *spinal nerves:* Eight cervical, twelve thoracic, five lumbar, five sacral, and one coccygeal. Each nerve is attached to the cord by two roots—ventral motor and dorsal sensory. Each dorsal nerve root bears a ganglion. The *ventral and dorsal nerve roots* unite in the intervertebral foramen to form the *nerve trunk* which soon divides into ventral and dorsal *rami* (Fig. 19.6).

The uppermost nerve roots pass horizontally from the spinal cord to reach the intervertebral foramina (Fig. 19.7). Lower down they have to pass with increasing obliquity, as the spinal cord is much shorter than the vertebral column. Below the termination of the spinal cord at the level of first lumbar vertebra, the obliquity becomes more marked.

Below the lower end of the spinal cord, the roots form a bundle known as the *cauda equina* because of its resemblance to the tail of a horse.

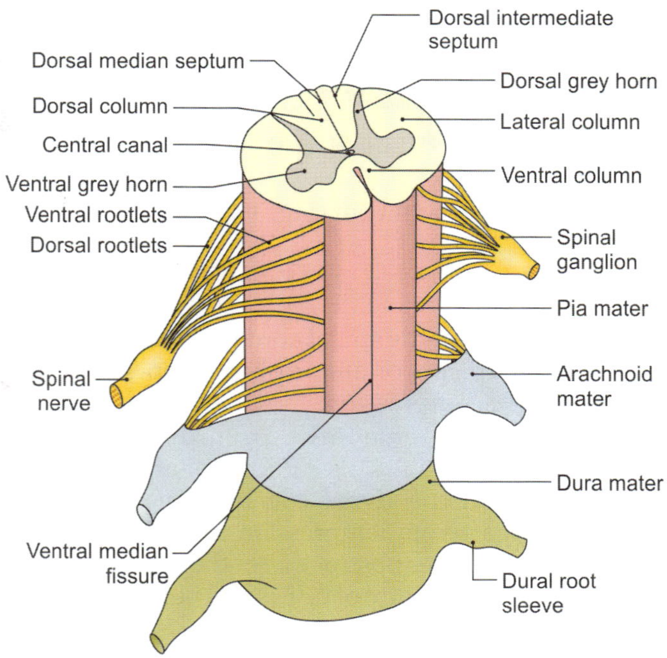

Fig. 19.6: Formation of spinal nerve

The roots of spinal nerves are surrounded by sheaths derived from the meninges. The *pial and arachnoid sheaths* extend up to the dura mater. The *dural sheath* encloses the terminal parts of the roots, continues over the nerve trunk, and is lost by merging with the epineurium of the nerve.

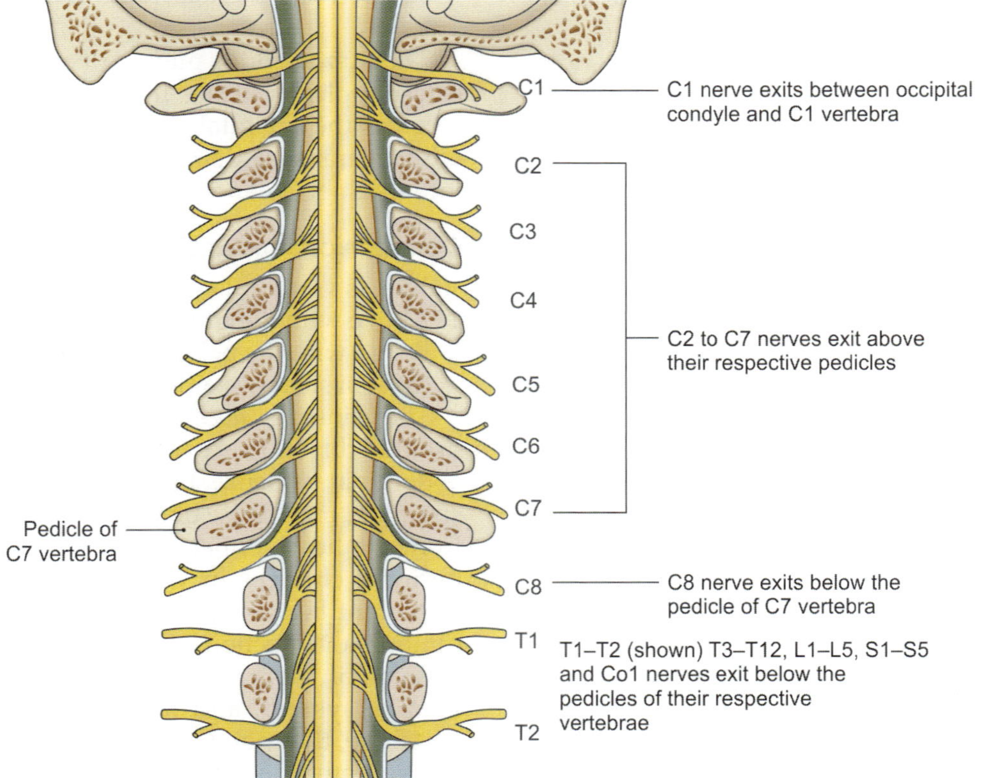

Fig. 19.7: Nomenclature of spinal nerves

An intervertebral foramen contains:
a. The ends of the nerve roots
b. The dorsal root ganglion
c. The nerve trunk
d. The beginning of the dorsal and ventral rami
e. A spinal artery
f. An intervertebral vein (Fig. 19.1).

CLINICAL ANATOMY

- Compression of the spinal cord by a tumour gives rise to paraplegia or quadriplegia, depending on the level of compression.
- Spinal tumours may arise from dura mater—meningioma, glial cells—glioma, nerve roots—neurofibroma, ependyma–ependymoma, and other tissues. Apart from compression of the spinal cord, the tumour causes obstruction of the subarachnoid space so that pressure of CSF is low below the level of lesion (*Froin's syndrome*). There is yellowish discolouration of CSF below the level of obstruction. CSF reveals high level of protein but the cell content is normal. *Queckenstedt's test* does not show a sudden rise and a sudden fall of CSF pressure by coughing or by brief pressure over the jugular veins. Spinal block can be confirmed either by myelography, CT scan or MRI scan.
- Compression of the cauda equina gives rise to flaccid paraplegia, saddle anaesthesia and sphincter disturbances. This is called the *cauda equina syndrome*.
- Compression of roots of spinal nerves may be caused by prolapse of an intervertebral disc, by osteophytes (formed in osteoarthritis), by a cervical rib, or by an extramedullary tumour. Such compression results in shooting pain along the distribution of the nerve.

VERTEBRAL SYSTEM OF VEINS

The vertebral venous plexus assumes importance in cases of:
1 Carcinoma of the prostate causing secondaries in the vertebral column and the skull.
2 Chronic empyema (collection of pus in the pleural cavity) causing brain abscess by septic emboli.

Anatomy of the Vertebral Venous Plexus

The vertebral venous system is made up of a valveless, complicated network of veins with a longitudinal pattern. It runs parallel to and anastomoses with the superior and inferior venae cavae. This network has three intercommunicating subdivisions (Fig. 19.8).

1 *The epidural plexus:* Lies in the vertebral canal outside the dura mater. The plexus consists of a postcentral and a prelaminar portion. Each portion is drained by two vessels. The plexus drains the structures in the vertebral canal, and is itself drained at regular intervals by segmental veins—vertebral, posterior intercostal, lumbar and lateral sacral.

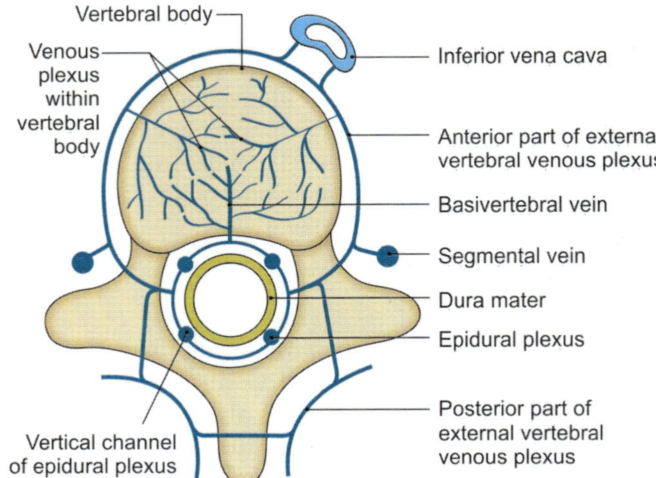

Fig. 19.8: The vertebral system of veins

2 *Plexus within the vertebral bodies:* It drains backwards into the epidural plexus, and anterolaterally into the external vertebral plexus.
3 *External vertebral venous plexus:* It consists of anterior vessels lying in front of the vertebral bodies, and the posterior vessels on the back of the vertebral arches and on adjacent muscles. It is drained by segmental veins.

The suboccipital plexus of veins is a part of the external plexus. It lies in the suboccipital triangle. It receives the occipital veins of the scalp, is connected with the transverse sinus by emissary veins, and drains into the subclavian veins.

Communications and Implications

Valveless vertebral system of veins communicates:
1 Above with the intracranial venous sinuses.
2 Below with the pelvic veins, the portal vein, and the caval system of veins.

The veins are *valveless* and the blood can flow in them in either direction. An increase in intrathoracic or intra-abdominal pressure, brought about by coughing and straining, may cause blood to flow in the plexus away from the heart, either upwards or downwards. Such periodic changes in venous pressure are clinically important because they make possible the spread of tumours or infections. For example, cells from pelvic, abdominal, thoracic and breast tumours may enter the venous system, and may ultimately lodge in the vertebrae, the spinal cord, the skull, or the brain.

The common primary sites of tumours causing secondaries in vertebrae are the breast and the prostate.

FACTS TO REMEMBER

- Spinal cord in adult ends at lower border of lumbar one vertebra.
- Spinal dura mater and arachnoid mater extend till second sacral vertebra.
- Spinal pia mater comprises an outer epi-pia and an inner pia-intima.
- Ligamenta denticulata of pia mater are two vertical ridges with 21 tooth-like processes which suspend the spinal cord in the subarachnoid space.

  The lowest or 21st process lies between T12 and L1 spinal nerves.
- Through the vertebral venous plexus, secondaries of prostate or breast can reach up to the cranial cavity.

CLINICOANATOMICAL PROBLEM

A patient suffering from cancer of prostate gland has developed secondaries in the brain.

- What is the route taken by cancer cells to reach the brain from the prostate gland, a pelvic organ?

Ans: The veins from prostate drain into prostatic venous plexus which communicates with the pelvic veins. These veins send small tributaries through pelvic sacral foramina into the vertebral canal. The vertebral canal lodges vertebral venous plexus which continues up the whole height of the vertebral canal and drains into segmental veins in abdominal cavity, thoracic cavity, in the neck and in basilar venous plexus. Thus, cancer cells 'climb' up to reach basilar venous plexus which has connections with cerebral veins. These cells travel through the cerebral veins to settle in brain resulting in secondaries. This plexus is valveless and dangerous.

Frequently Asked Questions

1. Write short notes on:
   a. Cauda equina
   b. Ligamentum denticulatum
   c. Filum terminale
   d. Typical spinal nerve
   e. Caudal anaesthesia

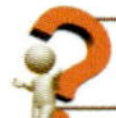

Multiple Choice Questions

1. Where does main part of vertebral venous plexus lie?
   a. Subdural space
   b. Epidural space
   c. Subarachnoid space
   d. Outside the vertebrae

2. Following are the contents of thoracic part of vertebral canal, *except*:
   a. Dura mater
   b. Arachnoid mater
   c. Pia mater
   d. Cauda equina

3. Intervertebral foramen contains all, *except*:
   a. Ends of nerve roots
   b. Nerve trunk
   c. Sympathetic ganglion
   d. Spinal artery

4. Subarachnoid space extends till:
   a. S1 vertebra b. S2 vertebra
   c. L1 vertebra d. L3 vertebra

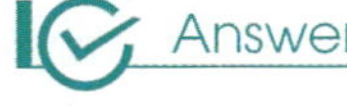

Answers

1. b **2.** d **3.** c **4.** b

VIVA VOCE

- Name the supports of the spinal cord.
- Where is lumbar puncture done in a child and an adult and why?
- What is ligamentum denticulatum?
- Name the types of spinal nerves.
- Name the contents of an intervertebral foramen.
- What are the symptoms of 'cauda equina syndrome'?
- Where does spinal cord end in an adult?
- Where do arachnoid and dura maters end?
- Name the parts of vertebral venous plexus.

Chapter 20

Cranial Cavity

"Happiness is when head, heart and hand work in harmony."
—Krishna Garg

INTRODUCTION

Cranial cavity, the highest placed cavity, contains the brain, meninges, venous sinuses, all cranial nerves, four petrosal nerves, parts of internal carotid artery and a part of the vertebral artery besides the special senses. The anterior branch of middle meningeal artery lies at the pterion and is prone to rupture resulting in extradural haemorrhage.

CONTENTS OF CRANIAL CAVITY

The convex upper wall of the cranial cavity is called the *vault*. It is uniform and smooth. The base of the cranial cavity is uneven and presents three cranial fossae (anterior, middle and posterior) lodging the uneven base of the brain.

The cranial cavity contains the brain and meninges—the outer dura mater, the middle arachnoid mater, and the inner pia mater. The dura mater is the thickest of the three meninges. It encloses the cranial venous sinuses, and has a distinct blood supply and nerve supply. The dura is separated from the arachnoid by a potential subdural space. The arachnoid is separated from the pia by a wider subarachnoid space filled with cerebrospinal fluid (CSF). The arachnoid, pia, subarachnoid space and CSF are dealt with the brain; the dura is described here. This chapter also includes hypophysis cerebri, trigeminal ganglion, middle meningeal artery and other structures seen after removal of the brain, e.g. various cranial nerves and internal carotid artery.

DISSECTION

Detach the epicranial aponeurosis, if not already done, laterally till the inferior temporal line. In the region of the temple, detach the temporalis muscle with its overlying fascia and reflect these downwards over the pinna.

Removal of skull cap or calvaria

Draw a horizontal line across the skull 1 cm above the orbital margins and 1 cm above the inion. Saw through the skull. Be careful in the temporal region as skull is rather thin there. Separate the inner table of skull from the fused endosteum and dura mater.

Removal of the brain

To remove the brain and its enveloping meninges, the structures leaving or entering the brain through various foramina of the skull have to be carefully detached/incised. Start from the anterior aspect by detaching falx cerebri from the crista galli.

Put 2–3 blocks under the shoulders so that head falls backwards. This will expose the olfactory bulb, which may be lifted from the underlying anterior cranial fossa. Identify optic nerve, internal carotid artery, infundibulum passing towards hypophysis cerebri. Divide all three structures. Cut through the oculomotor and trochlear nerves in relation to free margin of tentorium cerebelli. Divide the attachment of tentorium from the petrous temporal bone.

Identify and divide trigeminal, abducent, facial, and vestibulocochlear nerves. Then cut glossopharyngeal, vagus, accessory and hypoglossal nerves. All these nerves have to be cut first on one side and then on the other side. Lastly identify the two vertebral arteries entering the skull through foramen magnum on each side of the spinal medulla. With a sharp knife, cut through these structures. Thus the whole brain with the meninges can be gently removed from the skull. Preserve it in 5% formaldehyde.

Cut through the dura mater on the ventral aspect of brain till the inferolateral borders along the superciliary margin. Pull upwards the fold of dura mater present between the adjacent medial surfaces of cerebral hemispheres. This will be possible till the occipital lobe of brain. Pull backwards a similar but much smaller fold between two lobes of cerebellum, i.e. falx cerebelli.

Separating the cerebrum from the cerebellum is a double fold of dura mater called tentorium cerebelli. Pull it out in a horizontal plane by giving incision along the petrous temporal bone.

Learn about the folds of dura mater, i.e. falx cerebri, tentorium cerebelli, falx cerebelli, diaphragma sellae including trigeminal cave from the specimen with the help of base of skull. Make a paper model of these dural folds for recapitulation *(refer to BDC App)*.

CEREBRAL DURA MATER

The dura mater is the outermost, thickest and toughest membrane covering the brain (*dura* = hard) (*mater* = mother).

There are two layers of dura:

a. An outer or *endosteal layer* which serves as an internal periosteum or endosteum or endocranium for the skull bones.
b. An inner or *meningeal layer* which surrounds the brain. The meningeal layer is continuous with the spinal dura mater.

The two layers are fused to each other at all places, except where the cranial venous sinuses are enclosed between them.

Endosteal Layer or Endocranium

1 The endocranium is continuous:
   a. With the periosteum lining the outside of the skull or pericranium through the sutures and foramina.
   b. With the periosteal lining of the orbit through the superior orbital fissure.
2 It provides sheaths for the cranial nerves, the sheaths fuse with the epineurium outside the skull. Over the optic nerve, the dura forms a sheath which becomes continuous with the sclera.
3 Its outer surface is adherent to the inner surface of the cranial bones by a number of fine fibrous and vascular processes. The adhesion is most marked at the sutures, on the base of the skull and around the foramen magnum.

Meningeal Layer

At places, the meningeal layer of dura mater is folded on itself to form partitions which divide the cranial cavity into compartments which lodge different parts of the brain (Fig. 20.1). The folds are:

- Falx cerebri
- Tentorium cerebelli (Fig. 20.2)
- Falx cerebelli
- Diaphragma sellae.

Falx Cerebri

The falx cerebri is a large sickle-shaped fold of dura mater occupying the median longitudinal fissure between the two cerebral hemispheres (Fig. 20.1). It has two ends:

1 The *anterior end* is narrow, and is attached to the crista galli.

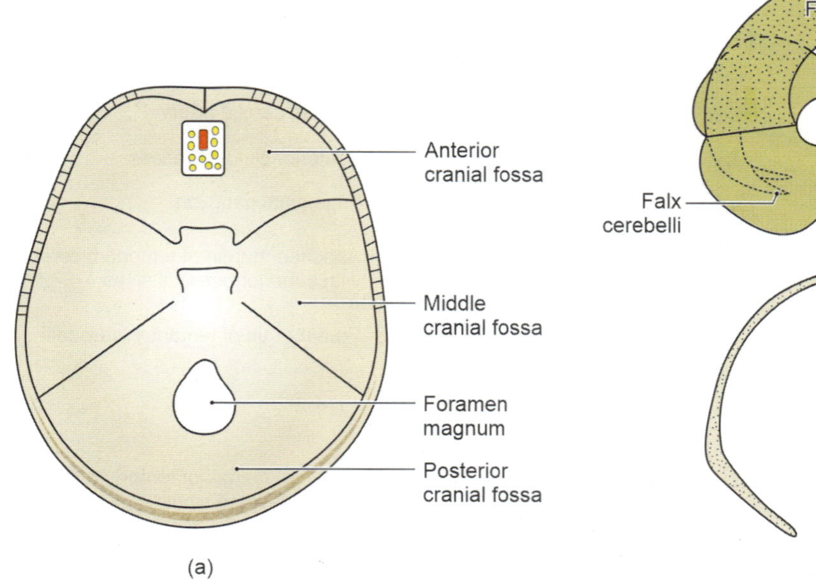

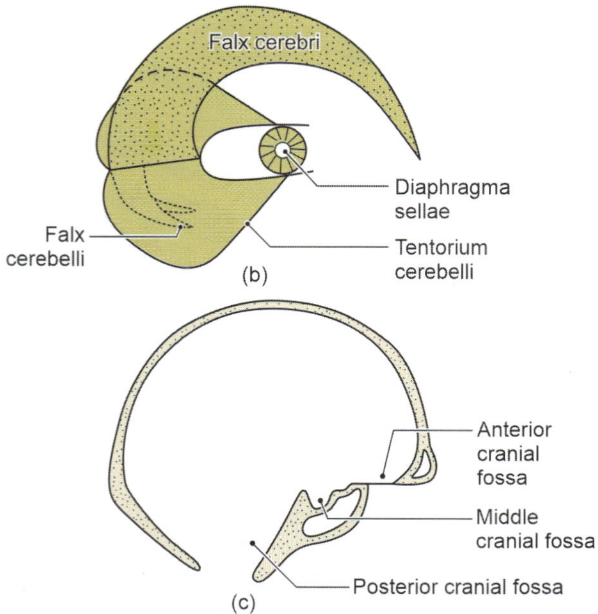

Fig. 20.1: Folds of meningeal layer of dura mater

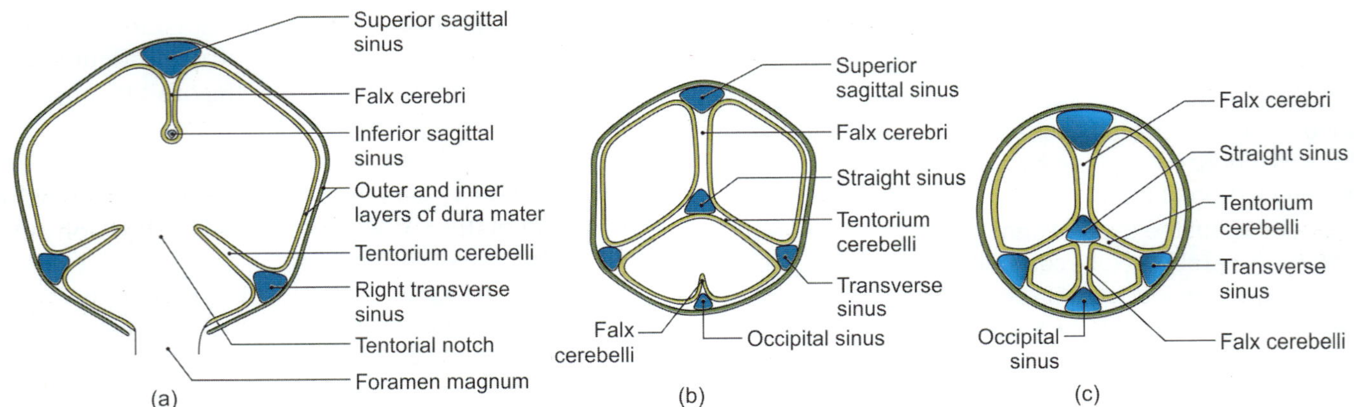

Figs 20.2a to c: Coronal sections through the posterior cranial fossa showing folds of dura mater and the venous sinuses enclosed in them: (a) Section through the tentorial notch (anterior part of the fossa); (b) Section through the middle part of the fossa; (c) Section through the posteriormost part

2 The *posterior end* is broad, and is attached along the median plane to the upper surface of the tentorium cerebelli.

The falx cerebri has two margins:

1 The *upper margin* is convex and is attached to the lips of the sagittal sulcus.
2 The *lower margin* is concave and free.

The falx cerebri has right and left surfaces each of which is related to the medial surface of the corresponding cerebral hemisphere.

Three important venous sinuses are present in relation to this fold. The *superior sagittal sinus* lies along the upper margin; the *inferior sagittal* sinus along the lower margin; and the *straight sinus* along the line of attachment of the falx to the tentorium cerebelli (Figs 20.2a–c).

Tentorium Cerebelli

The tentorium cerebelli is a tent-shaped fold of dura mater, forming the roof of the posterior cranial fossa. It separates the cerebellum from the occipital lobes of the cerebrum, and broadly divides the cranial cavity into supratentorial and infratentorial compartments. The infratentorial compartment is the posterior cranial fossa containing the hindbrain and the lower part of the midbrain.

The tentorium cerebelli has a free margin and an attached margin (Fig. 20.3). The *anterior free margin* is U-shaped and free. The ends of the 'U' are attached anteriorly to the anterior clinoid processes. This margin bounds the *tentorial notch* which is occupied by the midbrain and the anterior part of the superior vermis. The *outer or attached margin* is convex. Posterolaterally,

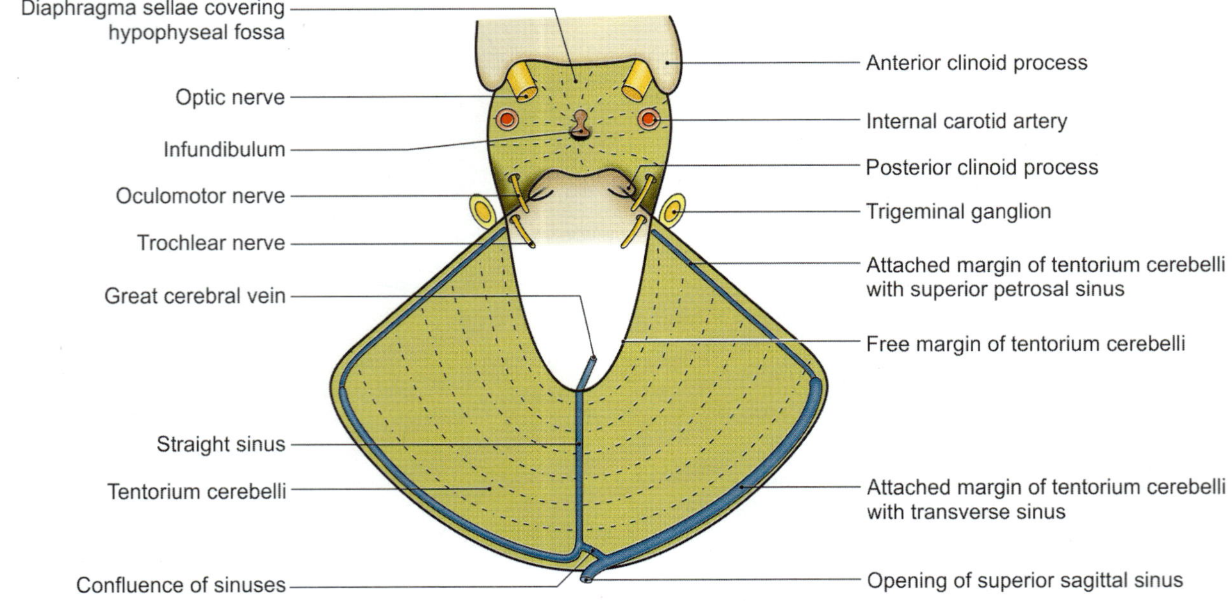

Fig. 20.3: Tentorium cerebelli and diaphragma sellae seen from above

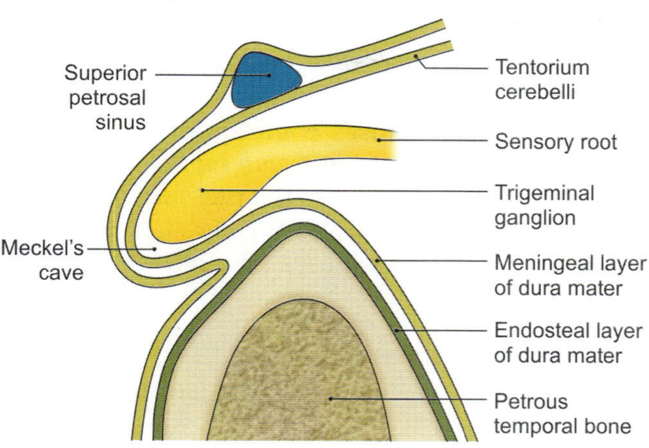

Fig. 20.4: Parasagittal section through the petrous temporal bone and meninges to show the formation of the trigeminal cave

it is attached to the lips of the transverse sulci on the occipital bone, and on the posteroinferior angle of the parietal bone. Anterolaterally, it is attached to the superior border of the petrous temporal bone and to the posterior clinoid processes. Along the attached margin, there are the transverse and superior petrosal venous sinuses.

The *trigeminal* or *Meckel's cave* is a recess of dura mater present in relation to the attached margin of the tentorium. It is formed by evagination of the inferior layer of the tentorium over the trigeminal impression on the petrous temporal bone. It contains the trigeminal ganglion (Fig. 20.4).

The free and attached margins of the tentorium cerebelli cross each other near the apex of the petrous temporal bone. Anterior to the point of crossing, there is a triangular area which forms the posterior part of the roof of the cavernous sinus, and is pierced by the third and fourth cranial nerves.

The tentorium cerebelli has two surfaces—superior and inferior. The *superior surface* is convex and slopes to either side from the median plane. The falx cerebri is attached to this surface, in the midline; the straight sinus lies along the line of this attachment. The superior surface is related to the occipital lobes of the cerebrum. The *inferior surface* is concave and fits the convex superior surface of the cerebellum. The falx cerebelli is attached to its posterior part (Fig. 20.2c).

Falx Cerebelli

The falx cerebelli is a small sickle-shaped fold of dura mater projecting forwards into the posterior cerebellar notch (Fig. 20.2c).

The *base* of the sickle is attached to the posterior part of the inferior surface of the tentorium cerebelli in the median plane. The *apex* of the sickle is frequently divided into two parts which are lost on the sides of the foramen magnum.

The *posterior margin* is convex and is attached to the internal occipital crest. It encloses the occipital sinus. The *anterior margin* is concave and free.

Diaphragma Sellae

The diaphragma sellae is a small circular, horizontal fold of dura mater forming the roof of the hypophyseal fossa.

Anteriorly, it is attached to the tuberculum sellae. Posteriorly, it is attached to the dorsum sellae. On each side, it is continuous with the dura mater of the middle cranial fossa (Fig. 20.5).

The diaphragma has a central aperture through which the stalk of the hypophysis cerebri passes.

Blood Supply

The outer layer is richly vascular. The inner meningeal layer is more fibrous and requires a little blood supply.

1 The vault or supratentorial space is supplied by the middle meningeal artery.
2 The anterior cranial fossa and the dural lining is supplied by meningeal branches of the anterior ethmoidal, posterior ethmoidal and ophthalmic arteries.
3 The middle cranial fossa is supplied by the middle meningeal, accessory meningeal, and internal carotid arteries; and by meningeal branches of the ascending pharyngeal artery.
4 The posterior cranial fossa is supplied by meningeal branches of the vertebral, occipital and ascending pharyngeal arteries.

Nerve Supply

1 The dura of the *vault* has only a few sensory nerves which are derived mostly from the ophthalmic division of the trigeminal nerve.

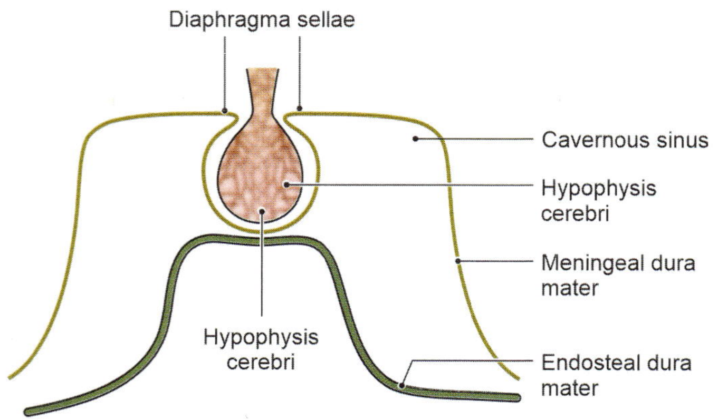

Fig. 20.5: Diaphragma sellae as seen in a sagittal section through the hypophyseal fossa

2 The dura of the floor has a rich nerve supply and is quite sensitive to pain.
   a. The *anterior cranial fossa* is supplied mostly by the anterior ethmoidal nerve and partly by the maxillary nerve.
   b. The *middle cranial fossa* is supplied by the maxillary nerve in its anterior half, and by branches of the mandibular nerve and from the trigeminal ganglion in its posterior half.
   c. The *posterior cranial fossa* is supplied chiefly by recurrent branches from first, second and third cervical spinal nerves and partly by meningeal branches of the ninth and tenth cranial nerves.

CLINICAL ANATOMY

- *Pain-sensitive intracranial structures* are:
  a. The large cranial venous sinuses and their tributaries from the surface of the brain
  b. Dural arteries
  c. The dural floor of the anterior and posterior cranial fossae
  d. Arteries at the base of the brain.
- *Headache* may be caused by:
  a. Dilatation of intracranial arteries
  b. Dilatation of extracranial arteries
  c. Traction or distension of intracranial pain-sensitive structures
  d. Infection and inflammation of intracranial and extracranial structures supplied by the sensory, cranial and cervical nerves.
- *Extradural and subdural haemorrhages* both are common. An extradural haemorrhage can be distinguished from a subdural haemorrhage because of the following differences.
  a. The extradural haemorrhage is arterial due to injury to middle meningeal artery, whereas subdural haemorrhage is venous in nature.
  b. Symptoms of cerebral compression are late in extradural haemorrhage.
  c. In an extradural haemorrhage, paralysis first appears in the face and then spreads to the lower parts of the body. In a subdural haemorrhage, the progress of paralysis is haphazard.
  d. In an extradural haemorrhage, there is no blood in the CSF, while it is a common feature of subdural haemorrhage.

VENOUS SINUSES OF DURA MATER

These are venous spaces, the walls of which are formed by dura mater. They have an inner lining of endothelium. There is no muscle in their walls. They have no valves.

Venous sinuses receive venous blood from the brain, the meninges, and bones of the skull. Cerebrospinal fluid is poured into some of them.

Cranial venous sinuses communicate with veins outside the skull through *emissary veins*. These communications help to keep the pressure of blood in the sinuses constant (*see* Table 9.1).

There are 23 venous sinuses, of which 8 are paired and 7 are unpaired.

Paired Venous Sinuses

There is one sinus each on right and left side.

1 Cavernous sinus
2 Superior petrosal sinus (Fig. 20.4)
3 Inferior petrosal sinus
4 Transverse sinus (Fig. 20.2)
5 Sigmoid sinus
6 Sphenoparietal sinus
7 Petrosquamous sinus
8 Middle meningeal sinus/veins

Unpaired Venous Sinuses

These are median in position

1 Superior sagittal sinus (Fig. 20.2)
2 Inferior sagittal sinus
3 Straight sinus (Fig. 20.3)
4 Occipital sinus
5 Anterior intercavernous sinus
6 Posterior intercavernous sinus
7 Basilar plexus of veins

Cavernous Sinus

Each cavernous sinus is a large venous space situated in the middle cranial fossa, on either side of the body of the sphenoid bone. Its interior is divided into a number of spaces or caverns by trabeculae. The trabeculae are much less conspicuous in the living than in the dead (Fig. 20.6).

The floor and medial wall of the sinus is formed by the endosteal dura mater. The lateral wall, and roof are formed by the meningeal dura mater.

Anteriorly, the sinus extends up to the medial end of the superior orbital fissure and *posteriorly*, up to the apex of the petrous temporal bone. It is about 2 cm long, and 1 cm wide.

DISSECTION

Define the cavernous sinuses situated on each side of the body of the sphenoid bone. Cut through it between the anterior and posterior ends and locate its contents. Define its connections with the other venous sinuses and veins *(refer to BDC App)*.

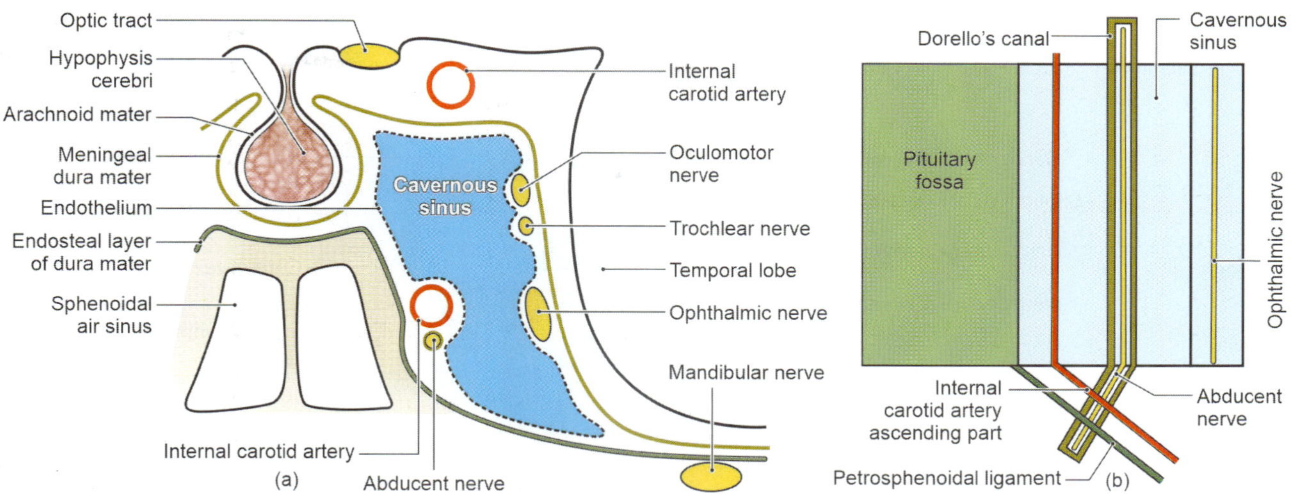

Fig. 20.6a and b: a. Coronal section through the middle cranial fossa showing the relations of the cavernous sinus; b. Dorello's canal (*Courtesy:* Dr SN Kazi)

Relations

Structures outside the sinus

1. *Superiorly:* Optic tract, optic chiasma, olfactory tract, internal carotid artery and anterior perforated substance.
2. *Inferiorly:* Foramen lacerum and the junction of the body and greater wing of the sphenoid bone (*see* Fig. 9.18).
3. *Medially:* Hypophysis cerebri and sphenoidal air sinus (Fig. 20.6).
4. *Laterally:* Temporal lobe with uncus.
5. *Below laterally:* Mandibular nerve
6. *Anteriorly:* Superior orbital fissure and the apex of the orbit.
7. *Posteriorly:* Apex of the petrous temporal and the crus cerebri of the midbrain.

Structures within the lateral wall of the sinus, from above downwards

1. *Oculomotor nerve*: In the anterior part of the sinus, it divides into superior and inferior divisions which leave the sinus by passing through the superior orbital fissure.
2. *Trochlear nerve:* In the anterior part of the sinus, it crosses superficial to the oculomotor nerve, and enters the orbit through the superior orbital fissure.
3. *Ophthalmic nerve:* In the anterior part of the sinus, it divides into the lacrimal, frontal and nasociliary nerves (*see* Figs 21.4 and 21.6).

Structures passing through the medial aspect of the sinus

Internal carotid artery with the venous and sympathetic plexus around it.

Abducent nerve, inferolateral to the internal carotid artery.

Abducent nerve enters the cavernous sinus by passing inferior to the petrosphenoidal ligament within a dural tunnel (Dorello's canal) just posterior to the short ascending portion of the cavernous carotid artery, and then runs on the inferolateral side of the horizontal portion of the cavernous carotid artery, just medial to the ophthalmic nerve at the lateral wall of the sinus, known as the infratrochlear or Parkinson's triangle. It gives access to the horizontal portion of the cavernous carotid artery and the abducent nerve (Fig. 20.6b).

The structures in the lateral wall and on the medial aspect of the sinus are separated from blood by the endothelial lining.

Maxillary nerve does not pass through cavernous sinus. It courses beneath the dura mater of middle cranial fossa, i.e. passes below the level of cavernous sinus.

Tributaries or Incoming Channels

From the orbit

1. The superior ophthalmic vein.
2. A branch of the inferior ophthalmic vein or sometimes the vein itself.
3. The central vein of the retina may drain either into the superior ophthalmic vein or into the cavernous sinus (Fig. 20.7).

From the brain

1. Superficial middle cerebral vein.
2. Inferior cerebral veins from the temporal lobe (Fig. 20.8).

From the meninges

1. Sphenoparietal sinus.
2. The frontal trunk of the middle meningeal vein may drain either into the pterygoid plexus through the foramen ovale or into the sphenoparietal or cavernous sinus.

Draining Channels or Communications

The cavernous sinus drains:

1. Into the transverse sinus through the superior petrosal sinus.

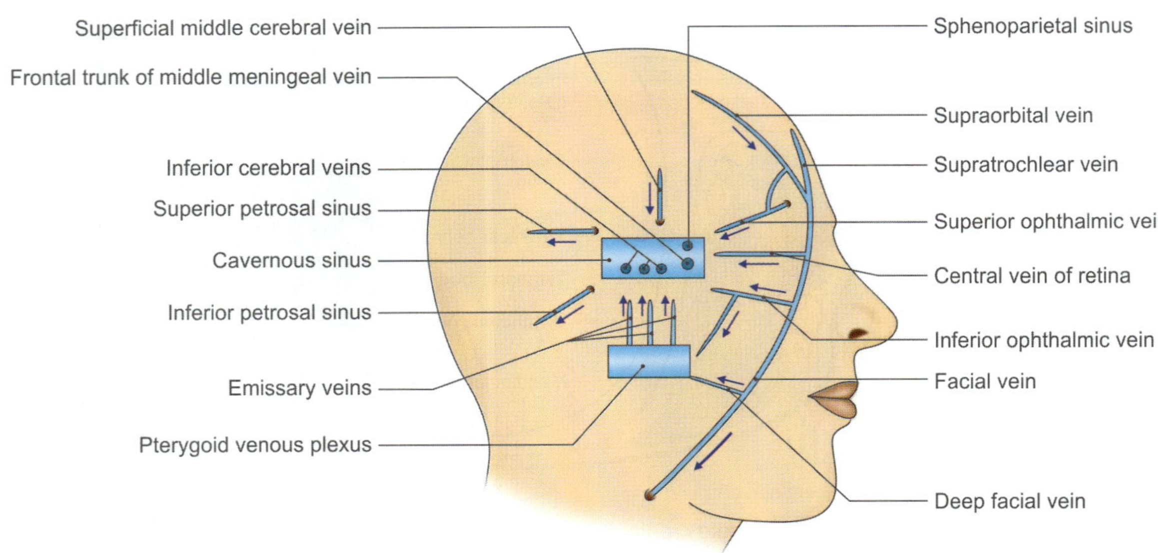

Fig. 20.7: Side view of the tributaries and communications of the cavernous sinus. Arrows show the direction of blood flow

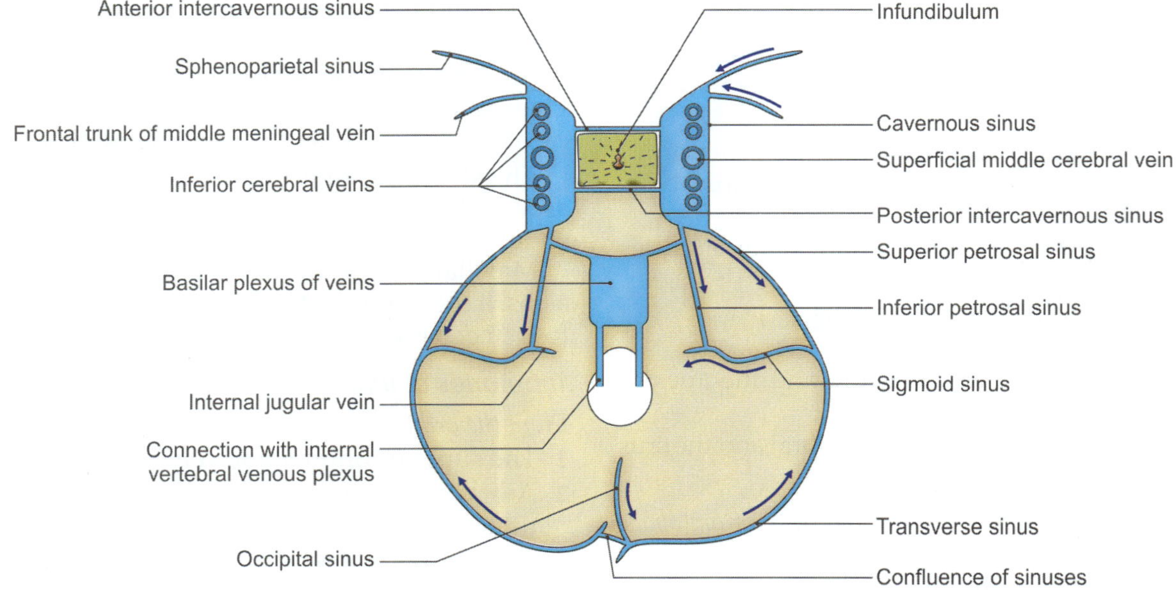

Fig. 20.8: Superior view of the tributaries and communications of the cavernous sinus. Arrows show the direction of blood flow

2 Into the internal jugular vein through the inferior petrosal sinus and through a plexus around the internal carotid artery.
3 Into the pterygoid plexus of veins through the emissary veins passing through the foramen ovale, the foramen lacerum and the emissary sphenoidal foramen (Table 20.1).
4 Into the facial vein through the superior ophthalmic vein.
5 The right and left cavernous sinuses communicate with each other through the anterior and posterior intercavernous sinuses and through the basilar plexus of veins (Fig. 20.8).

All these communications are valveless, and blood can flow through them in either direction.

Factors Helping Expulsion of Blood from the Sinus

1 Expansile pulsations of the internal carotid artery within the sinus
2 Gravity
3 Position of the head

CLINICAL ANATOMY

- *Thrombosis of the cavernous sinus* may be caused by sepsis in the dangerous area of the face, in nasal cavities, and in paranasal air sinuses. This gives rise to the following symptoms.

a. *Nervous symptoms:*
   – Severe pain in the eye and forehead in the area of distribution of ophthalmic nerve.
   – Involvement of the third, fourth and sixth cranial nerves resulting in paralysis of the muscles supplied.
b. *Venous symptoms:* Marked oedema of eyelids, cornea and root of the nose, with exophthalmos due to congestion of the orbital veins.

- A communication between the cavernous sinus and the internal carotid artery may be produced by head injury. When this happens the eyeball protrudes and pulsates with each heart beat. It is called the *pulsating exophthalmos*.

Superior Sagittal Sinus

The superior sagittal sinus occupies the upper convex, attached margin of the falx cerebri (Figs 20.9 and 20.10).

It begins anteriorly at the crista galli by the union of tiny meningeal veins. Here it communicates with the veins of the frontal sinus, and occasionally with the veins of the nose, through the foramen caecum. As the sinus runs upwards and backwards, it becomes progressively larger in size. It is triangular on cross-section. It ends near the internal occipital protuberance by turning to one side, usually the right, and becomes continuous with the right transverse sinus (Fig. 20.9). It generally communicates with the opposite sinus. The junction of all these sinuses is called the *confluence of sinuses*.

The *interior* of the sinus shows:

a. Openings of the superior cerebral veins.
b. Openings of venous lacunae, usually three on each side.
c. Arachnoid villi and granulations projecting into the lacunae as well as into the sinus (Fig. 20.10).
d. Numerous fibrous bands crossing the inferior angle of the sinus.

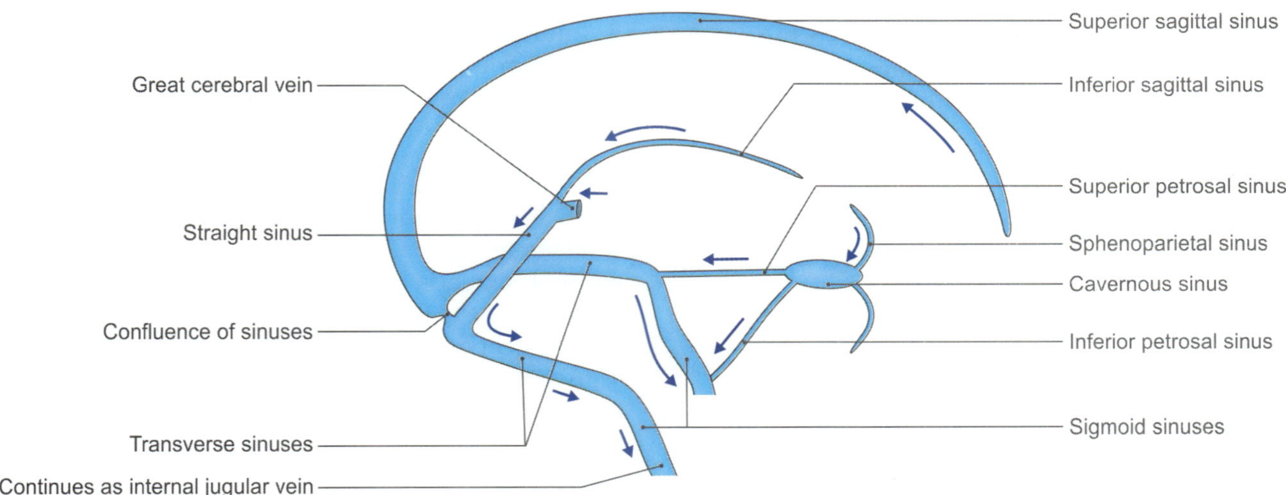

Fig. 20.9: Scheme to show the lateral view of the intracranial venous sinuses. Arrows show the direction of blood flow

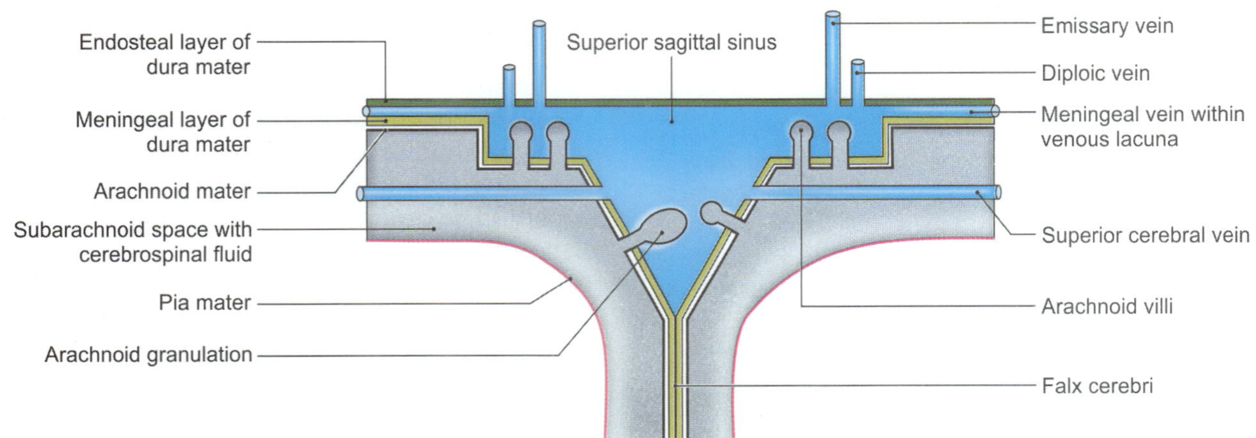

Fig. 20.10: Coronal section through superior sagittal sinus showing arrangement of the meninges, the arachnoid villi and granulations, and the various (emissary, diploic, meningeal and cerebral) veins in its relation

Tributaries

The superior sagittal sinus receives following tributaries.

a. Superior cerebral veins which never open into the venous lacunae (Fig. 20.10).
b. Parietal emissary veins (Table 20.1).
c. Venous lacunae, usually three on each side which first, receive the diploic and meningeal veins, and then open into the sinus.
d. Occasionally, a vein from the nose opens into the sinus when the foramen caecum is patent.

CLINICAL ANATOMY

Thrombosis of the superior sagittal sinus may be caused by spread of infection from the nose, scalp and diploe. This gives rise to:

a. A considerable rise in intracranial tension due to defective absorption of CSF.
b. Delirium and sometimes convulsions due to congestion of the superior cerebral veins.
c. Paraplegia of the upper motor neuron type due to bilateral involvement of the paracentral lobules of cerebrum where the lower limbs and perineum are represented.

Inferior Sagittal Sinus

The inferior sagittal sinus, a small channel, lies in the posterior two-thirds of the lower, concave free margin of the falx cerebri. It ends by joining the great cerebral vein to form the straight sinus (Fig. 20.9).

Straight Sinus

The straight sinus lies in the median plane within the junction of falx cerebri and the tentorium cerebelli. It is formed anteriorly by the union of the inferior sagittal sinus with the great cerebral vein, and ends at the internal occipital protuberance by continuing as the transverse sinus usually left (Fig. 20.9). In addition to the veins forming it, also receives a few of the superior cerebellar veins.

At the termination of the great cerebral vein into the sinus, there exists a ball valve mechanism, formed by a sinusoidal plexus of blood vessels, which regulates the secretion of CSF.

Table 20.1: Emissary veins: Valveless and communicate intracranial with extracranial veins

Sinus	*Connection*	*Veins*
Superior sagittal sinus	Parietal emissary vein	Veins of scalp,
	Foramen caecum	nasal veins
	Middle meningeal vein	Pterygoid veins
Transverse sinus	Petrosquamous	External jugular
Sigmoid sinus	Mastoid vein	Posterior auricular
	Hypoglossal vein	IJV
	Posterior condylar vein	Suboccipital vein
Cavernous sinus	Emissary veins	Pterygoid veins
	Veins around ICA	IJV
	Ophthalmic vein	Facial vein
	Inferior petrosal	IJV

ICA: Internal carotid artery; IJV: Internal jugular vein

Transverse Sinuses

The transverse sinuses are large sinuses (Fig. 20.8). The right sinus usually larger than the left, is situated in the posterior part of the attached margin of the tentorium cerebelli. The right transverse sinus is usually a continuation of the superior sagittal sinus, and the left sinus a continuation of the straight sinus. Each sinus extends from the internal occipital protuberance to the posteroinferior angle of the parietal bone at the base of mastoid process where it bends downwards and becomes the sigmoid sinus. Its *tributaries* are:

1. Superior petrosal sinus
2. Inferior cerebral veins
3. Inferior cerebellar veins
4. Diploic (posterior temporal) vein
5. Inferior anastomotic vein.

Sigmoid Sinuses

Each sinus, right or left, is the direct continuation of the transverse sinus (Fig. 20.9). It is S-shaped, hence the name. It extends from the posteroinferior angle of the parietal bone to the posterior part of the jugular foramen where it becomes the superior bulb of the internal jugular vein. It grooves the mastoid part of the temporal bone, where *it is separated anteriorly from the mastoid antrum and mastoid air cells by only a thin plate of bone.* Its tributaries are:

1. The mastoid and condylar emissary veins
2. Cerebellar veins
3. The internal auditory vein.

CLINICAL ANATOMY

- *Thrombosis of the sigmoid sinus* is always secondary to infection in the middle ear or otitis media, or in the mastoid process called mastoiditis.
- During operations on the mastoid process, one should be careful about the sigmoid sinus, so that it is not exposed.
- Spread of infection or thrombosis from the sigmoid and transverse sinuses to the superior sagittal sinus may cause impaired CSF drainage into the latter and may, therefore, lead to the development of hydrocephalus. Such a hydrocephalus associated with sinus thrombosis following ear infection is known as *otitic hydrocephalus.*

Other Sinuses

The *occipital sinus* is small, and lies in the attached margin of the falx cerebelli. It begins near the foramen magnum and ends in the confluence of sinuses (Figs 20.2 and 20.8).

The *sphenoparietal sinuses,* right and left, lie along the posterior free margin of the lesser wing of the sphenoid bone, and drain into the anterior part of the cavernous sinus. Each sinus may receive the frontal trunk of the middle meningeal vein (Fig. 20.9).

The *superior petrosal sinuses* lie in the anterior part of the attached margin of the tentorium cerebelli along the upper border of the petrous temporal bone. It drains the cavernous sinus into the transverse sinus (Fig. 20.8).

The *inferior petrosal sinuses,* right and left, lie in the corresponding petro-occipital fissure, and drain the cavernous sinus into the superior bulb of the internal jugular vein.

The *basilar plexus of veins* lies over the clivus of the skull. It connects the two inferior petrosal sinuses and communicates with the internal vertebral venous plexus.

The *middle meningeal veins* form two main trunks, one frontal or anterior and one parietal or posterior, which accompany the two branches of the middle meningeal artery. The *frontal trunk* may end either in the pterygoid plexus through the foramen ovale, or in the spheno-parietal or cavernous sinus. The *parietal trunk* usually ends in the pterygoid plexus through the foramen spinosum. The meningeal veins are nearer to the bone than the arteries, and are, therefore, more liable to injury in fractures of the skull.

The anterior and posterior *intercavernous sinuses* connect the cavernous sinuses. They pass through the diaphragma sellae, one in front and the other behind the infundibulum (Fig. 20.8).

HYPOPHYSIS CEREBRI (PITUITARY GLAND)

The hypophysis cerebri is a small endocrine gland situated in relation to the base of the brain. It is often called the master of the endocrine orchestra because it produces a number of hormones which control the secretions of many other endocrine glands of the body (Fig. 20.11).

The gland lies in the hypophyseal fossa or sella turcica or pituitary fossa. The fossa is roofed by the diaphragma sellae. The stalk of the hypophysis cerebri pierces the diaphragma sellae and is attached above to the floor of the third ventricle.

The gland is oval in shape, and measures 8 mm anteroposteriorly and 12 mm transversely. It weighs about 500 mg.

DISSECTION

Identify diaphragma sellae over the hypophyseal fossa. Incise it radially and locate the hypophysis cerebri lodged in its fossa. Take it out and examine it in detail with the hand lens (Figs 20.11 and 20.12a).

Relations

Superiorly

1 Diaphragma sellae (Fig. 20.5)
2 Optic chiasma
3 Tubercinerium
4 Infundibular recess of the third ventricle

Inferiorly

1 Irregular venous channels between the two layers of dura mater lining the floor of the hypophyseal fossa.

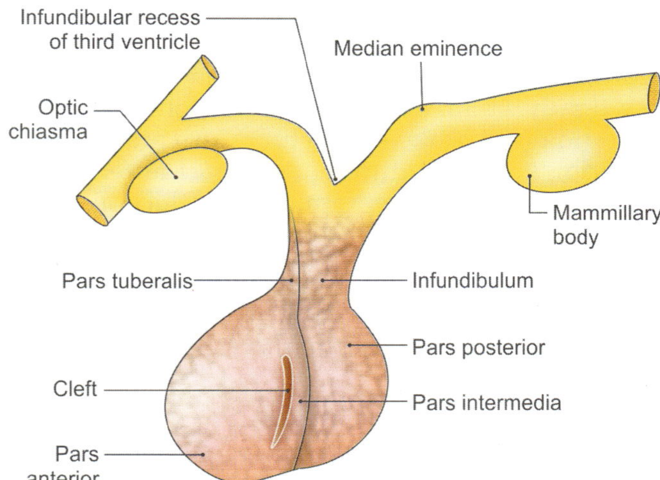

Fig. 20.11: Parts of the hypophysis cerebri as seen in a sagittal section

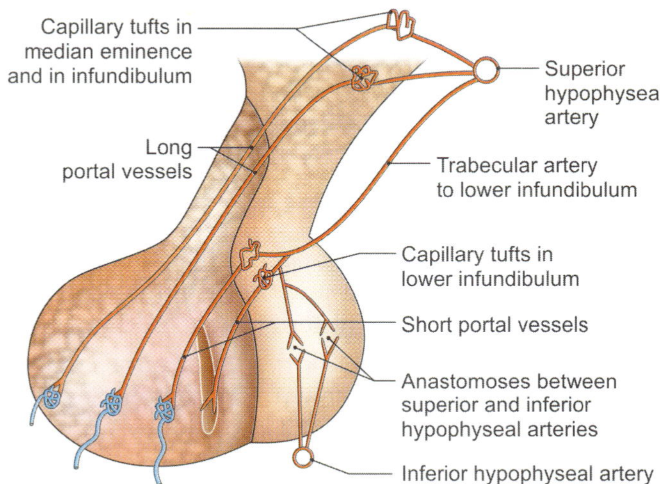

Fig. 20.12a: Arterial supply of the hypophysis cerebri. Note that the neurohypophysis is supplied by the superior and inferior hypophyseal arteries, and the adenohypophysis, exclusively by the portal vessels

2 Hypophyseal fossa.
3 Sphenoidal air sinuses (Fig. 20.6).

On each side

The cavernous sinus with its contents (Fig. 20.6).

Subdivisions/Parts and Development

The gland has two main parts: *Adenohypophysis* and *neurohypophysis* which differ from each other embryologically, morphologically and functionally.

The adenohypophysis develops as an upward growth called the Rathke's pouch from the ectodermal roof of the stomodeum. The neurohypophysis develops as a downward growth from the floor of the diencephalon, and is connected to the hypothalamus by neural pathways.

Molecular Regulation

Expression of transcription factors and growth factors in a tightly regulated pattern is responsible for the formation of Rathke's pouch, its orientation with posterior lobe, cell differentiation of anterior and posterior lobes and the hormonal production by the gland. Dysregulation of expression of these factors leads to congenital anomalies of pituitary and hormonal imbalance.

The subdivisions of each part are given below.

Adenohypophysis

1 *Anterior lobe* or *pars anterior, pars distalis, or pars glandularis:* This is the largest part of the gland (Fig. 20.11).
2 *Intermediate lobe* or *pars intermedia:* This is in the form of a thin strip which is separated from the anterior lobe by an intraglandular cleft, a remnant of the lumen of Rathke's pouch.
3 *Tuberal lobe* or *pars tuberalis:* It is an upward extension of the anterior lobe that surrounds and forms part of the infundibulum.

Neurohypophysis

1 *Posterior lobe* or *neural lobe, pars posterior:* It is smaller than the anterior lobe and lies in the posterior concavity of the larger anterior lobe.
2 *Infundibular stem,* which contains the neural connections of the posterior lobe with the hypothalamus.
3 *Median eminence* of the tubercinerium which is continuous with the infundibular stem.

Arterial Supply

The hypophysis cerebri is supplied by the following branches of the internal carotid artery.

1 One superior hypophyseal artery on each side (Fig. 20.12a).
2 One inferior hypophyseal artery on each side.

Each superior hypophyseal artery supplies:

a. Ventral part of the hypothalamus
b. Upper part of the infundibulum
c. Lower part of the infundibulum through a separate long descending branch, called the trabecular artery.

Each inferior hypophyseal artery divides into medial and lateral branches which join one another to form an arterial ring around the posterior lobe. Branches from this ring supply the posterior lobe and also anastomose with branches from the superior hypophyseal artery.

The anterior lobe or pars distalis is supplied exclusively by *portal vessels* arising from capillary tufts formed by the superior hypophyseal arteries (Fig. 20.12). The long portal vessels drain the median eminence and the upper infundibulum, and the short portal vessels drain the lower infundibulum. The portal vessels are of great functional importance because they carry the *hormone releasing factors* from the hypothalamus to the anterior lobe where they control the secretory cycles of different glandular cells.

Venous Drainage

Short veins emerge on the surface of the gland and drain into neighbouring dural venous sinuses. The hormones pass out of the gland through the venous blood, and are carried to their target cells.

HISTOLOGY

Anterior Lobe (Fig. 20.12b)

Chromophilic cells 50%

1 *Acidophils/alpha cells;* about 43%
   a. Somatotrophs: Secrete growth hormone (STH, GH).
   b. Mammotrophs (prolactin cells): Secrete lactogenic hormone.
2 *Basophils/beta cells,* about 7% of cells
   a. Thyrotrophs: Secrete thyroid-stimulating hormone (TSH).
   b. Corticotrophs: Secrete adrenocorticotrophic hormone (ACTH).
   c. Gonadotrophs: Secrete follicle-stimulating hormone (FSH).
   d. Luteotrophs: Secrete luteinising hormone (LH).

Chromophobic cells 50% represent the non-secretory phase of the other cell types, or their precursors.

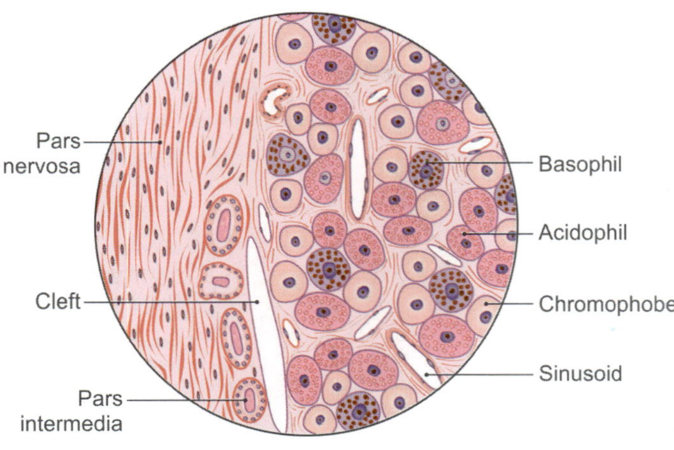

- Pars anterior contains acidophil, basophil and chromophobe cells
- Pars intermedia contains vesicles
- Pars posterior contains nerve fibres and pituicytes

Fig. 20.12b: Histology of hypophysis cerebri, 400X

Intermediate Lobe

It is made up of numerous basophil cells, and chromophobe cells surrounding masses of colloid material. It secretes the melanocyte-stimulating hormone (MSH).

Posterior Lobe

It is composed of:

1 A large number of nonmyelinated fibres forming hypothalamohypophyseal tract.

2 Modified neurological cells, called *pituicytes*. They have many dendrites which terminate on or near the sinusoids (Fig. 20.12b).

Hypothalamohypophyseal Portal System

The hypothalamohypophyseal tract begins in the preoptic and paraventricular nuclei of the hypothalamus. Its short fibres terminate in relation to capillary tufts of portal vessels, providing the possibility for a neural control of the secretory activity of the anterior lobe. The long fibres of the neurosecretory tract pass to the posterior lobe and terminate near vascular sinusoids.

The hormones related to the posterior lobe are:

a. *Vasopressin*, antidiuretic hormone (ADH) which acts on kidney tubules.

b. *Oxytocin*, which promotes contraction of the uterine and mammary smooth muscle.

These hormones are actually secreted by the hypothalamus, from where these are transported through the hypothalamohypophyseal tract to the posterior lobe of the gland.

CLINICAL ANATOMY

Pituitary tumours give rise to two main categories of symptoms:

A. *General symptoms* due to pressure over surrounding structures:
   a. The sella turcica is enlarged in size.
   b. Pressure over the central part of optic chiasma causes bitemporal hemianopia (Fig. 20.13).
   c. Pressure over the hypothalamus may cause one of the hypothalamic syndromes like obesity of Frolich's syndrome in cases with Rathke's pouch tumours.
   d. A large tumour may press upon the third ventricle, causing a rise in intracranial pressure.

B. *Specific symptoms* depending on the cell type of the tumour.
   a. Acidophil or eosinophil adenoma causes acromegaly in adults and gigantism in younger patients.
   b. Basophil adenoma causes Cushing's syndrome.
   c. Chromophobe adenoma causes effects of hypopituitarism.
   d. Posterior lobe damage causes diabetes insipidus, although the lesion in these cases usually lies in the hypothalamus.

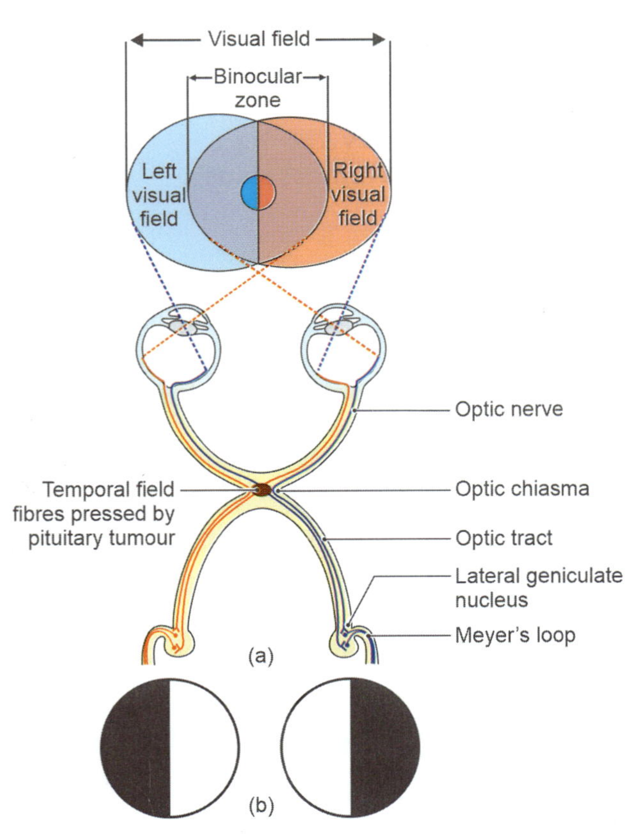

Fig. 20.13: Bitemporal hemianopia due to pressure of pituitary tumour on the central part of optic chiasma

TRIGEMINAL GANGLION

This is the *sensory ganglion* (*gasserian ganglion*) of the fifth cranial nerve. It is homologous with the dorsal nerve root ganglia of spinal nerves. All such ganglia are made up of pseudounipolar nerve cells, with a 'T'-shaped arrangement of their process; one process arises from the cell body which then divides into a central and a peripheral process.

The ganglion is crescentic or semilunar in shape, with its convexity directed anterolaterally. The three divisions of the trigeminal nerve—ophthalmic V1 (*see* Chapter 21), maxillary V2 (*see* Chapter 23) and mandibular V3 (*see* Chapter 14) emerge from this convexity. The posterior concavity of the ganglion receives the sensory root of the nerve (Fig. 20.13).

Situation and Meningeal Relations

The ganglion lies on the *trigeminal impression,* on the anterior surface of the petrous temporal bone near its apex. It occupies a special space of dura mater, called the *trigeminal or Meckel's cave.* There are two layers of dura below the ganglion (Fig. 20.4). The cave is lined by pia-arachnoid, so that the ganglion along with the motor root of the trigeminal nerve is surrounded by CSF. The ganglion lies at a depth of about 5 cm from the preauricular point.

Relations

Medially

1 Internal carotid artery
2 Posterior part of cavernous sinus

Laterally

Middle meningeal artery

Superiorly

Parahippocampal gyrus

Inferiorly

1 Motor root of trigeminal nerve
2 Greater petrosal nerve (Fig. 20.14)
3 Apex of the petrous temporal bone
4 The foramen lacerum.

Associated Root and Branches

The central processes of the ganglion cells form the large *sensory root* of the trigeminal nerve which is

DISSECTION

Identify trigeminal ganglion situated on the anterior surface of petrous temporal bone near its apex. Define the three branches emerging from its convex anterior surface.

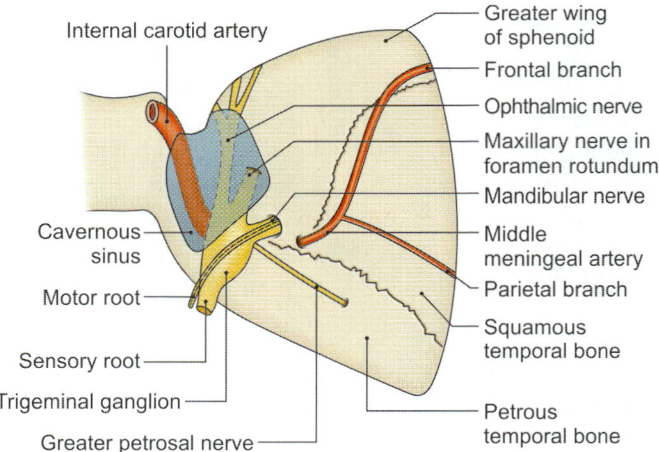

Fig. 20.14: Superior view of the middle cranial fossa showing some of its contents

attached to pons at its junction with the middle cerebellar peduncle.

The peripheral processes of the ganglion cells form three divisions of the trigeminal nerve, namely the *ophthalmic, maxillary and mandibular.*

The small *motor root* of the trigeminal nerve is attached to the pons superomedial to the sensory root. It passes under the ganglion from its medial to the lateral side, and joins the mandibular nerve at the foramen ovale.

Blood Supply

The ganglion is supplied by twigs from:

1 Internal carotid
2 Middle meningeal
3 Accessory meningeal arteries
4 By the meningeal branch of the ascending pharyngeal artery.

Trigeminal Nerve

Fifth cranial nerve is the largest cranial nerve. It comprises three branches, two of which are purely sensory and third, the largest branch is mixed nerve. Trigeminal nerve is the nerve of first brachial arch.

Branches of this nerve provide sensory fibres to the four parasympathetic ganglia associated with cranial outflow of parasympathetic nervous system. These are ciliary, pterygopalatine, otic and submandibular.

Ophthalmic, the first division, carries sensory fibres from the structures derived from frontonasal process. Maxillary, the second division, conveys afferent fibres from structures derived from maxillary process. Mandibular, the third mixed division, carries sensory fibres derives from mandibular process.

Sensory Components of V Nerve

Sensations of pain, temperature, touch and pressure from skin of face, mucous membrane of nose, most of the tongue, paranasal air sinuses travel along axons. Their cell bodies lie in the V ganglion or semilunar ganglion or Gasserian ganglion. This ganglion is equivalent to the spinal ganglia of other nerves. It lies at the apex of petrous temporal bone in a dural cave—the Meckel's cave. Peripheral processes form the three nerves.

Motor Component for the Muscles

The motor nucleus receives impulses from the right and left cerebral hemispheres, red nucleus and fibres of motor root supply four muscles of mastication—temporalis, masseter, lateral pterygoid and medial pterygoid and four other muscles which are tensor veli palatini, tensor tympani, mylohyoid and anterior belly of digastric.

In injury to:

- *Ophthalmic nerve:* There is loss of corneal blink reflex. This reflex is mediated by V_1 which is afferent pathway and VII nerve which subserves as efferent pathway.
- *Maxillary nerve:* There is loss of sneeze reflex. This branch is the afferent path of sneeze reflex. Efferent pathway of sneeze reflex is nucleus ambiguus, respiratory centre in medulla oblongata, phrenic nerve nucleus, motor cells of spinal cord for intercostal muscles.
- *Mandibular nerve:* There is loss of jaw jerk reflex.

  Flaccid paralysis of muscles of mastication in injury of mandibular nerve leads to decrease strength for biting.

CLINICAL ANATOMY

- Intractable facial pain due to trigeminal neuralgia or carcinomatosis may be abolished by injecting alcohol into the ganglion. Sometimes cutting of the sensory root is necessary (Fig. 20.15).
- Congenital cutaneous naevi on the face (port wine stains) map out accurately the areas supplied by one or more divisions of the V cranial nerve.

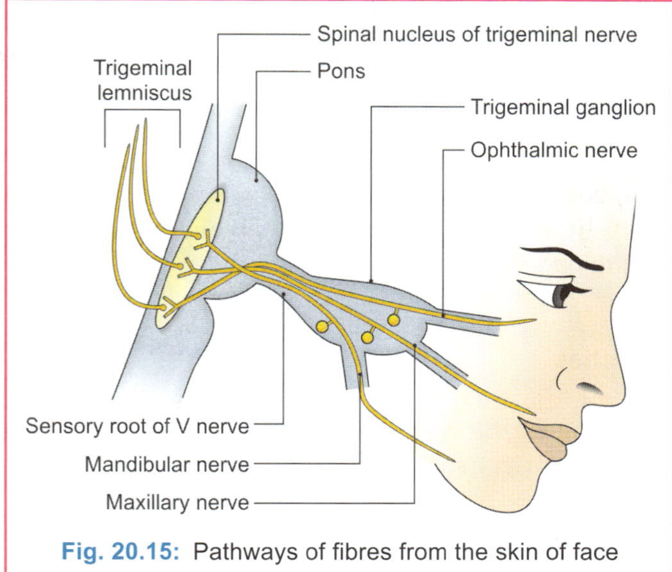

Fig. 20.15: Pathways of fibres from the skin of face

MIDDLE MENINGEAL ARTERY

The middle meningeal artery is important to the surgeon because this artery is the commonest source of extradural haemorrhage, which is an acute surgical emergency (Fig. 20.14).

Origin

The artery is a branch of the first part of the maxillary artery, given off in the infratemporal fossa (*see* Figs 14.6 and 14.7).

Course and Relations

1 In the infratemporal fossa, the artery runs upwards and medially deep to the lateral pterygoid muscle and superficial to the sphenomandibular ligament. Here it passes through a loop formed by the two roots of the auriculotemporal nerve (*see* Fig. 14.11).

2 It enters the middle cranial fossa through the foramen spinosum (Fig. 20.14).

3 In the middle cranial fossa, the artery has an extradural course, but the middle meningeal veins are closer to the bone than the artery. Here the artery runs forwards and laterally for a variable distance, grooving the squamous temporal bone, and divides into a frontal and parietal branch (Fig. 20.14).

4 The *frontal* or *anterior branch* is larger than the parietal branch. First it runs forwards and laterally towards the lateral end of the lesser wing of the sphenoid crossing the inner aspect of pterion (meeting point of frontal, parietal, squamous temporal and greater wing of sphenoid). Then it runs obliquely upwards and backwards, parallel to, and a little in front of the central sulcus of the cerebral hemisphere. Thus after crossing the pterion, the artery is closely related to the motor area of the cerebral cortex (*see* Fig. 9.8).

5 The *parietal* or *posterior branch* runs backwards over, or near the superior temporal sulcus of the cerebrum, about 4 cm above the level of the zygomatic arch. It ends in front of the posteroinferior angle of the parietal bone by dividing into branches.

DISSECTION

Dissect the middle meningeal artery which enters the skull through foramen spinosum. It is an important artery for the supply of endocranium, inner table of skull and diploe. Examine the other structures seen in cranial fossae after removal of brain. These are the cranial nerves, internal carotid artery, petrosal nerves and fourth part of vertebral artery.

Branches

The middle meningeal artery supplies only small branches to the dura mater. It is predominantly a periosteal artery supplying bone and red bone marrow in the diploe.

Within the cranial cavity, it gives off:

a. The *ganglionic branches* to the trigeminal ganglion.
b. A *petrosal branch* to the hiatus for the greater petrosal nerve.
c. A *superior tympanic branch* to the tensor tympani.
d. *Temporal branches* to the temporal fossa.
e. *Anastomotic branch* that enters the orbit and anastomoses with the lacrimal artery.

CLINICAL ANATOMY

- The middle meningeal artery is of great surgical importance because it can be torn in head injuries resulting in *extradural haemorrhage. The frontal* or *anterior branch* is commonly involved. The haematoma presses on the motor area, giving rise to hemiplegia of the opposite side. The anterior division can be approached surgically by making a hole in the skull over the pterion, 4 cm above the midpoint of the zygomatic arch (*see* Fig. 9.8).
- Rarely, the parietal or posterior branch is implicated, causing contralateral deafness. In this case, the hole is made at a point 4 cm above and 4 cm behind the external acoustic meatus.

OTHER STRUCTURES SEEN IN CRANIAL FOSSAE AFTER REMOVAL OF BRAIN

Various Structures

The structures seen after removal of the brain are: 12 cranial nerves, cavernous part of internal carotid artery, four petrosal nerves and fourth part of the vertebral artery.

DISSECTION

Following structures are seen in the anterior cranial fossa: Crista galli, cribriform plate of ethmoid, orbital part of frontal bone, and lesser wing of sphenoid.

Following structures are seen in the middle cranial fossa: Middle meningeal vessels, diaphragma sellae pierced by infundibulum, oculomotor nerves, internal carotid arteries, optic nerve, posterior cerebral artery, and great cerebral vein.

Following structures are seen in the posterior cranial fossa: Facial, vestibulocochlear, glossopharyngeal, vagus, accessory, hypoglossal nerves, vertebral arteries, and spinal root of accessory nerve.

Internal Carotid Artery

Internal carotid artery begins in the neck as one of the terminal branches of the common carotid artery at the level of the upper border of the thyroid cartilage. Its course is divided into the four parts (Fig. 20.16): Cervical, pertous, cavernous and cerebral.

Cervical part

In the neck, it lies within the carotid sheath. This part gives no branches (*see* Fig. 11.8).

Petrous part

Within the carotid canal situated in petrous part of the temporal bone. It gives caroticotympanic branches and artery of pterygoid canal (Fig. 20.16).

Cavernous part

Within the cavernous sinus (Fig. 20.6). This part of the artery gives off:

1 Cavernous branches to the trigeminal ganglion.
2 The superior and inferior hypophyseal branches to the hypophysis cerebri.

Cerebral part

This part lies at the base of the brain after emerging from the cavernous sinus. It gives off the following arteries:

1 Ophthalmic
2 Anterior cerebral
3 Middle cerebral
4 Posterior communicating
5 Anterior choroidal.

Of these, the ophthalmic artery supplies structures in the orbit; while the others supply the brain.

The curvatures of the petrous, cavernous and cerebral parts of the internal carotid artery together form an S-shaped figure, the carotid siphon of angiograms.

Cranial Nerves

The *first* or *olfactory nerve* is seen in the form of 15 to 20 filaments on each side that pierce the cribriform plate of the ethmoid bone.

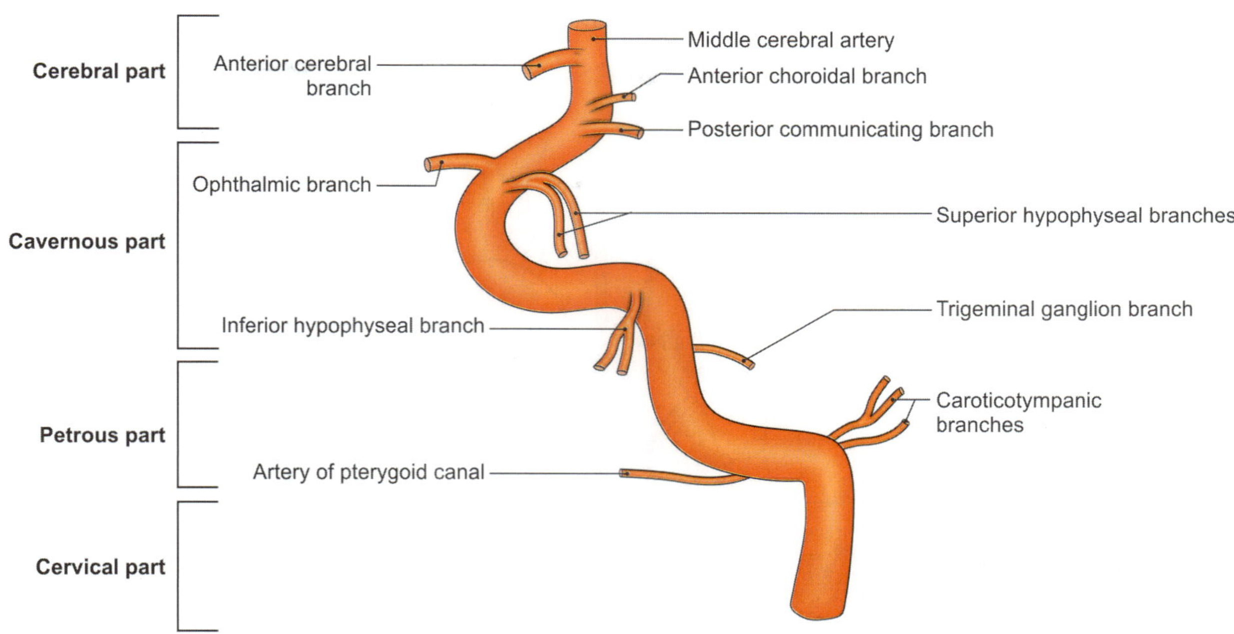

Fig. 20.16: Various parts of internal carotid artery

The *second* or *optic nerve* passes through the optic canal with the ophthalmic artery (Fig. 20.17).

The *third* or *oculomotor* and *fourth* or *trochlear nerves* pierce the posterior part of the roof of the cavernous sinus formed by crossing of the free and attached margins of the tentorium cerebelli; next they run in the lateral wall of the cavernous sinus. They enter the orbit through the superior orbital fissure (*see* Fig. 21.4).

The *fifth* or *trigeminal nerve* has a large sensory root and a small motor root. The roots cross the apex of the petrous temporal bone beneath the superior petrosal sinus, to enter the middle cranial fossa (Fig. 20.14).

The *sixth* or *abducent nerve* pierces the lower part of the posterior wall of the cavernous sinus near the apex of the petrous temporal bone. It runs forwards by the side of the dorsum sellae beneath the petrosphenoidal ligament to reach the centre of the cavernous sinus (Fig. 20.6).

The *seventh* or *facial* and *eighth* or *statoacoustic* or *vestibulocochlear nerves* pass through the internal acoustic meatus with the labyrinthine vessels.

The *ninth* or *glossopharyngeal, tenth* or *vagus* and *eleventh* or *accessory nerves* pierce the dura mater at the jugular foramen and pass out through it. The *glossopharyngeal* nerve is enclosed in a separate sheath of dura mater, while vagus and accessory nerves are enclosed in one sheath. The spinal part of the accessory nerve first enters the posterior cranial fossa through the foramen magnum, and then passes out through the jugular foramen along with cranial part.

The two parts of the *twelfth* or *hypoglossal nerve* pierce the dura mater separately opposite the hypoglossal canal and then pass out through it.

Petrosal Nerves

1. The *greater petrosal nerve* (Fig. 20.14) carries gustatory and parasympathetic fibres. It arises from the geniculate ganglion of the facial nerve, and enters the middle cranial fossa through the hiatus for the greater petrosal nerve on the anterior surface of the petrous temporal bone. It proceeds towards the foramen lacerum, where it joins the deep petrosal nerve which carries sympathetic fibres to form the nerve of the pterygoid canal (*see* Table A.2 in Appendix).

   The nerve of the pterygoid canal passes through the pterygoid canal to reach the pterygopalatine ganglion. The parasympathetic fibres relay in this ganglion. Postganglionic parasympathetic fibres arising in the ganglion ultimately supply the lacrimal gland and the mucosal glands of the nose, palate and pharynx (*see* Fig. 23.16b). The gustatory or taste fibres do not relay in the ganglion and are distributed to the palate.
2. The *deep petrosal nerve*, sympathetic in nature, is a branch of the sympathetic plexus around the internal carotid artery. It contains postganglionic fibres from the superior cervical sympathetic ganglion. The nerve joins the greater petrosal nerve to form the nerve of the pterygoid canal. The sympathetic fibres are distributed through the branches of the pterygopalatine ganglion (*see* Table A.2 in Appendix).
3. The *lesser petrosal nerve*, parasympathetic in nature, is a branch of the tympanic plexus, deriving its preganglionic parasympathetic fibres from the tympanic branch of the glossopharyngeal nerve. It emerges

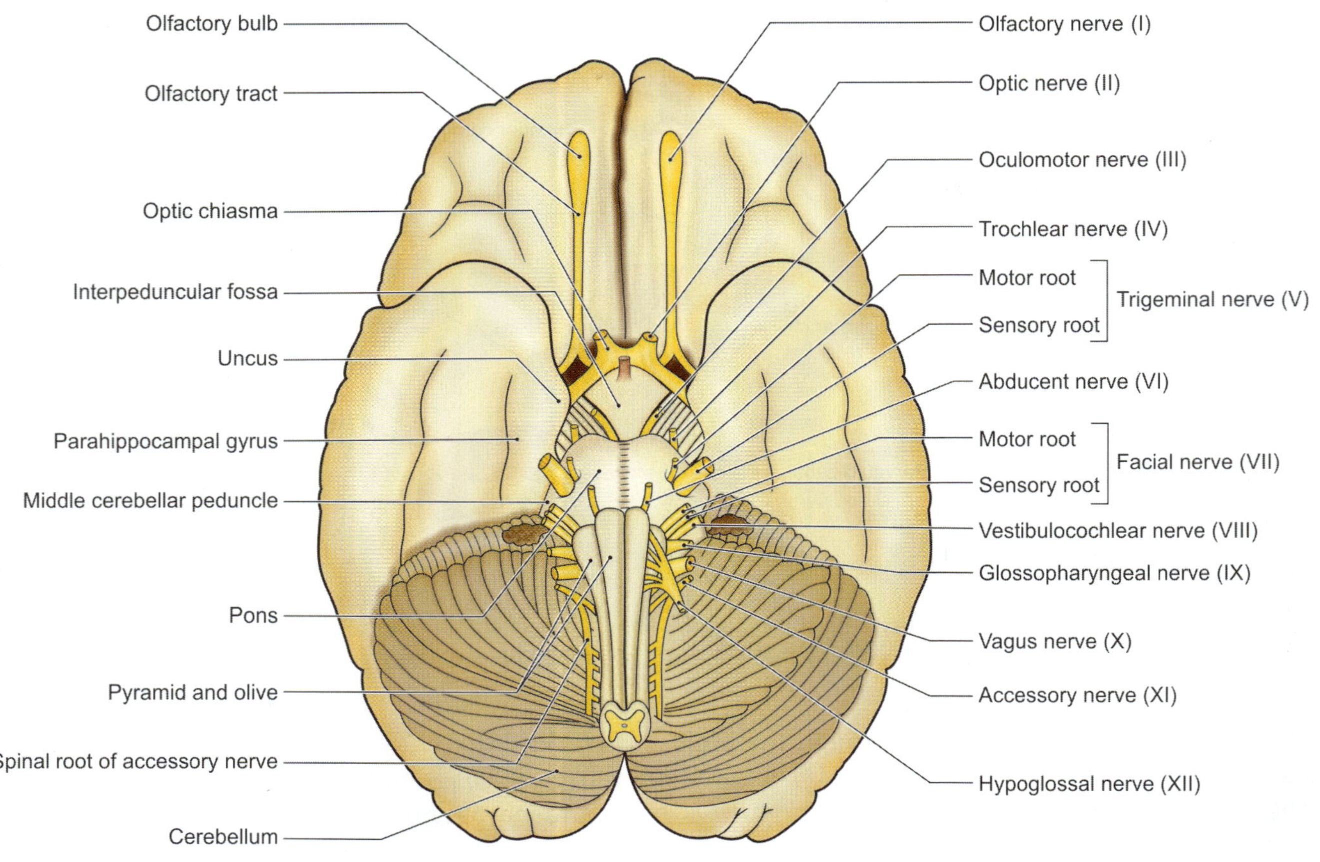

Fig. 20.17: Highlights of the cranial nerves

through the hiatus for the lesser petrosal nerve, situated just lateral to the hiatus for the greater petrosal nerve, passes out of the skull through the foramen ovale, and ends in the otic ganglion (*see* Fig. 14.17). Post-ganglionic fibres arising in the ganglion supply the parotid gland through the auriculotemporal nerve (*see* Table A.2 in Appendix).

4 The *external petrosal nerve,* sympathetic in nature, is an inconstant branch from the sympathetic plexus around the middle meningeal artery to the geniculate ganglion of the facial nerve.

Fourth Part of the Vertebral Artery

It enters the posterior cranial fossa through the foramen magnum after piercing the dura mater near the skull. It has been studied in Chapter 17.

Mnemonics

Cavernous sinus contents: O TOM CAT

Oculomotor nerve (III)
Trochlear nerve (IV)
Ophthalmic nerve (V1)
Maxillary nerve (V2)
Carotid artery (internal)
Abducent nerve (VI)
T: Nothing

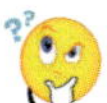

FACTS TO REMEMBER

- Meningeal layer of dura mater forms falx cerebri and falx cerebelli in sagittal plane and tentorium cerebelli and diaphragma sellae in horizontal plane.
- Only spinal ganglia present in the cranial cavity is the trigeminal ganglion.
- Only mixed branch of trigeminal is the mandibular branch. The other two are purely sensory.
- Anterior branch of middle meningeal artery lies on the inner aspect of *pterion* and is liable to injury, leading to extradural haemorrhage.

CLINICOANATOMICAL PROBLEM

A young person complains of a little painful papules on the right side of forehead along a nerve on the right side. There is redness of the eyes with severe pain.

- What is the diagnosis?
- Trace the pathway of pain impulses.

Ans: The diagnosis is 'herpes zoster'.

The pathway of pain impulses is shown in Flowchart 20.1.

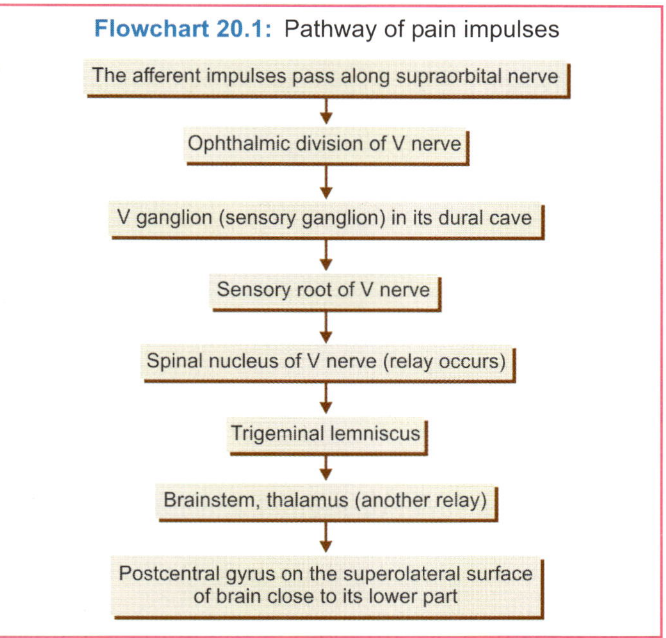

Flowchart 20.1: Pathway of pain impulses

FURTHER READING

- Rhoton AL. Cranial Anatomy and Surgical Approaches. Baltimore: Lippincortt Williams & Wilkins 2007.
  An essential masterpiece in microsurgical neuroanatomy and surgical approaches developed by Professor Rhoton after 40 years devoted to the field.

Frequently Asked Questions

1. Describe cavernous venous sinus under the following headings:
   a. Extent
   b. Relations
   c. Tributaries and communications
   d. Clinical anatomy
2. Write short notes on:
   a. Falx cerebri
   b. Superior sagittal sinus
   c. Hypophysis cerebri
   d. Middle meningeal artery
   e. Tentorium cerebelli
   f. Trigeminal ganglion

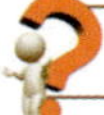

Multiple Choice Questions

1. One of the following structures is not related to cavernous sinus:
   a. Trochlear nerve
   b. Oculomotor nerve
   c. Optic nerve
   d. Ophthalmic nerve
2. Which is true about cavernous sinus?
   a. Oculomotor nerve in medial wall
   b. Trochlear nerve on medial wall
   c. Optic tract inferiorly
   d. Drains into transverse sinus
3. What is the correct position of VI nerve in relation to internal carotid artery in cavernous sinus?
   a. Medial b. Lateral
   c. Inferolateral d. Posterior
4. If III, IV, VI and ophthalmic nerves are paralysed, the infection is localised to:
   a. Brainstem
   b. Base of skull
   c. Cavernous sinus
   d. Apex of orbit
5. Which is not a part of internal carotid artery?
   a. Cervical b. Petrous
   c. Cerebral d. Ophthalmic
6. Rupture of which commonly injured artery causes extradural haemorrhage is:
   a. Trunk of middle meningeal artery
   b. Anterior branch of middle meningeal artery
   c. Posterior branch of middle meningeal artery
   d. None of the above

7. Which of the petrosal nerves carries preganglionic fibres to the otic ganglion?
   a. Greater
   b. Deep
   c. Lesser
   d. External

8. Arachnoid villi drain into which of the following sinuses?
   a. Transverse
   b. Straight
   c. Superior sagittal
   d. Sigmoid

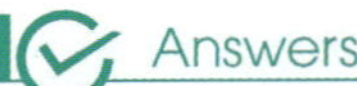

Answers

1. c **2.** d **3.** c **4.** c **5.** d **6.** b **7.** c **8.** c

VIVA VOCE

- Where does superior sagittal and inferior sagittal venous sinuses lie?
- What sinuses are present in relation to the tentorium cerebelli?
- How many roots are there in trigeminal ganglion? Name its branches.
- Name the structures present in the lateral wall of cavernous sinus.
- Name the tributaries of cavernous sinus.
- Name four emissary veins. What is their function and what is their clinical importance?
- Name the parts of adenohypophysis.
- Name the parts of neurohypophysis.
- Name the cranial nerves in order.
- Name the four parts of internal carotid artery.
- Which artery lies on the inner aspect of the pterion?
- Which is the mixed branch of trigeminal nerve?

VIDEO 3.12 **Cranial cavity:** Introduction, dura mater, venous sinuses, cavernous sinus

Chapter

21

Contents of the Orbit

"My heart leaps up when I behold a rainbow in the sky."
—William Wordsworth

INTRODUCTION

The orbits are bony cavities lodging the eyeballs, extraocular muscles, nerves, blood vessels and lacrimal gland. Out of 12 pairs of cranial nerves; II, III, IV, VI, a part of V, and some sympathetic fibres are dedicated to the contents of orbit only. Nature has provided orbit for the safety of the eyeball. We must also try and look after our orbits and their contents.

ORBITS

Features

The orbits are pyramidal cavities, situated one on each side of the root of the nose. They provide sockets for rotatory movements of the eyeball. The long axis of the each orbit passes backwards and medially. The medial walls are parallel to each other at a distance of 2.5 cm but the lateral walls are set at right angles to each other (*see* Fig. 9.21).

Contents

1 *Eyeball:* Eyeball occupies anterior one-third of orbit. It is described in Chapter 27.
2 *Fascia:* Orbital and bulbar.
3 *Muscles:* Extraocular and intraocular.
4 *Vessels:* Ophthalmic artery, superior and inferior ophthalmic veins, and lymphatics.
5 *Nerves:* Optic, oculomotor, trochlear and abducent; branches of ophthalmic and maxillary nerves, and sympathetic nerves.
6 *Lacrimal gland:* It has already been studied in Chapter 10.
7 *Orbital fat.*

Visual Axis and Orbital Axis

Axis passing through centres of anterior and posterior poles of the eyeball is known as visual axis. It makes an angle of 20–25° with the orbital axis (*see* Fig. 9.19), i.e. line passing through optic canal and centre of base of orbit, i.e. opening on the face.

DISSECTION

Strip the endosteum from the floor of the anterior cranial fossa. Gently break the orbital plate of frontal bone forming the roof of the orbit and remove it in pieces so that orbital periosteum is clearly visible. Medially, the ethmoidal vessels and nerves should be preserved. Posteriorly, identify the optic canal and superior orbital fissure and structures traversing these. Define the orbital fascia and fascial sheath of eyeball.

Divide the orbital periosteum along the middle of the orbit anteroposteriorly. Cut through it horizontally close to anterior margin of orbit *(refer to BDC App)*.

Orbital Fascia or Periorbita

It forms the *periosteum* of the bony orbit. Due to the loose connection to bone, it can be easily stripped. Posteriorly, it is continuous with the dura mater and with the sheath of the optic nerve. Anteriorly, it is continuous with the periosteum lining the bones around the orbital margin (Fig. 21.1).

There is a gap in the periorbita over the inferior orbital fissure. This gap is bridged by connective tissue with some smooth muscle fibres in it. These fibres constitute the orbitalis muscle.

a. At the upper and lower margins of the orbit, the orbital fascia sends off flap-like continuations into the eyelids. These extensions form the *orbital septum.*
b. A process of the fascia holds the fibrous pulley of the tendon of the superior oblique muscle in place.
c. Another process forms the *lacrimal fascia* which bridges the lacrimal groove.

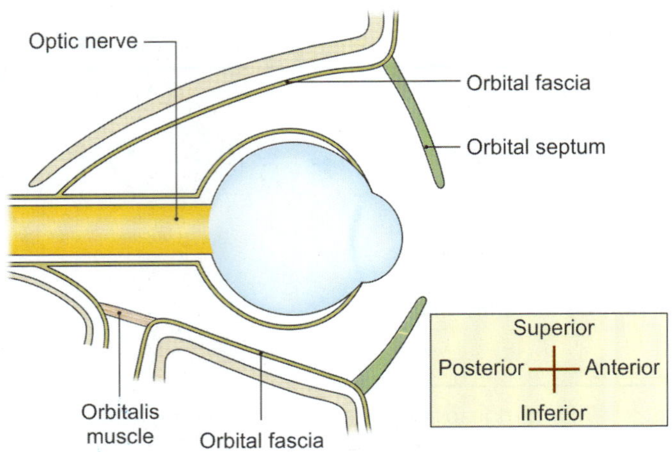

Fig. 21.1: Orbital fascia and fascial sheath of the eyeball as seen in a parasagittal section

Fascial Sheath of Eyeball or Bulbar Fascia

1 *Tenon's capsule* forms a thin, loose membranous sheath around the eyeball, extending from the optic nerve to the sclerocorneal junction or limbus. It is separated from the sclera by the episcleral space which is traversed by delicate fibrous bands. The eyeball can freely move within this sheath.
2 The *sheath* is pierced by:
   a. Tendons of the various extraocular muscles.
   b. Ciliary vessels and nerves around the entrance of the optic nerve.
3 The sheath gives off a number of expansions.
   a. A *tubular sheath* covers each orbital muscle.
   b. The *medial check ligament* is a strong triangular expansion from the sheath of the medial rectus muscle; it is attached to the lacrimal bone.
   c. The *lateral check ligament* is a strong triangular expansion from the sheath of the lateral rectus muscle; it is attached to the zygomatic bone (Fig. 21.2).
4 The lower part of Tenon's capsule is thickened, and is named the *suspensory ligament of the eye* or the *suspensory ligament of Lockwood* (Fig. 21.3). It is expanded in the centre and narrow at its extremities, and is slung like a hammock below the eyeball. It is formed by union of the margins of the sheaths of the inferior rectus and the inferior oblique muscles with the medial and lateral check ligaments.

EXTRAOCULAR MUSCLES

Involuntary Muscles

1 The superior tarsal muscle is the deeper portion of the levator palpebrae superioris. It is inserted on the upper margin of the superior tarsus. It elevates the upper eyelid.
2 The inferior tarsal muscle extends from the fascial sheath of the inferior rectus and inferior oblique to the lower margin of the inferior tarsus. It possibly depresses the lower eyelid.
3 The orbitalis bridges the inferior orbital fissure. Its action is uncertain (Fig. 21.1).

DISSECTION

Identify and preserve the trochlear nerve entering the superior oblique muscle in the superomedial angle of the orbit. Find the frontal nerve lying in the midline on the levator palpebrae superioris. It divides into two terminal divisions in the anterior part of orbit.

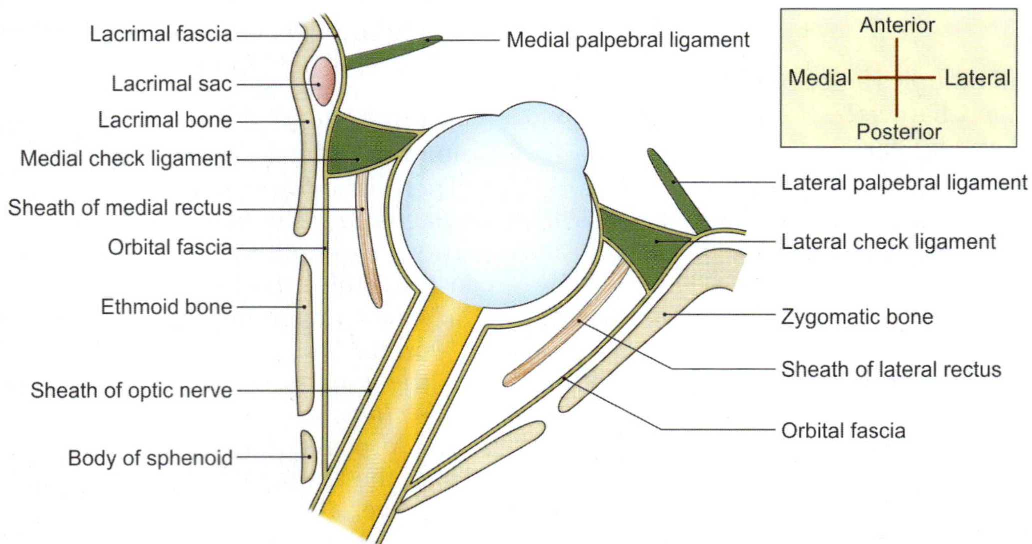

Fig. 21.2: Orbital fascia and fascial sheath of the eyeball as seen in transverse section

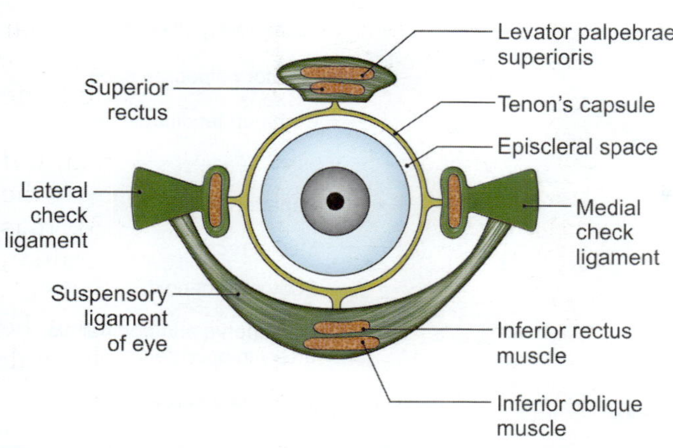

Fig. 21.3: Fascial sheath of the eyeball as seen in coronal section

Beneath the levator palpebrae superioris is the superior rectus muscle. The upper division of oculomotor nerve lies between these two muscles, supplying both of them. Along the lateral wall of the orbit, look for lacrimal nerve and artery to reach the superolateral corner of the orbit.

Follow the tendon of superior oblique muscle passing superolaterally beneath the superior rectus to be inserted into sclera behind the equator. After identification, divide frontal nerve, levator palpebrae superioris and superior rectus in the middle of the orbit and reflect them apart. Identify the optic nerve and other structures crossing it. These are nasociliary nerve, ophthalmic artery and superior ophthalmic vein. With the optic nerve find two long ciliary nerves and 12–20 short ciliary nerves. Remove the orbital fat and look carefully in the posterior part of the interval between the optic nerve and lateral rectus muscle along the lateral wall of the orbit and identify the pinhead-sized ciliary ganglion. Trace the roots connecting it to the nasociliary nerve and nerve to inferior oblique muscle.

Lastly, identify the abducent nerve closely adherent to the medial surface of lateral rectus muscle.

Incise the inferior fornix of conjunctiva and palpebral fascia. Elevate the eyeball and remove the fat and fascia to identify the origin of inferior oblique muscle from the floor of the orbit anteriorly.

Identify the levator palpebrae superioris and superior rectus above the eyeball, superior oblique superomedially, medial rectus medially, lateral rectus laterally, and inferior rectus inferiorly.

The voluntary muscles are miniature ribbon muscles, having short tendons of origin and long tendons of insertion.

Voluntary Extraocular Muscles

1 Four recti:
   a. Superior rectus
   b. Inferior rectus
   c. Medial rectus
   d. Lateral rectus
2 Two obliques:
   a. Superior oblique
   b. Inferior oblique
3 The levator palpebrae superioris elevates the upper eyelid.

Origin

1 The four recti arise from a *common annular tendon* or *tendinous ring* of Zinn. The ring is attached to the middle part of superior orbital fissure (Fig. 21.4). The lateral rectus has an additional small tendinous head which arises from the orbital surface of the greater wing of the sphenoid bone lateral to the tendinous ring. Through the gap between the two heads abducent nerve passes.
2 The superior oblique arises from the undersurface of lesser wing of the sphenoid, superomedial to the optic canal.
3 The inferior oblique arises from the orbital surface of the maxilla, lateral to the lacrimal groove. The muscle is situated near the anterior margin of the orbit.
4 The levator palpebrae superioris arises from the orbital surface of the lesser wing of the sphenoid bone, anterosuperior to the optic canal and to the origin of the superior rectus.

Insertion

1 The recti are inserted into the sclera, a little posterior to the limbus (corneoscleral junction). The average distances of the insertions from the cornea are: Superior 7.7 mm; inferior 6.5 mm, medial 5.5 mm; lateral 6.9 mm (Fig. 21.5).
2 The tendon of the superior oblique passes through a fibrocartilaginous pulley attached to the trochlear fossa of the frontal bone. The tendon then passes laterally, downwards and backward below the superior rectus. It is inserted into the sclera behind the equator of the eyeball, between the superior rectus and the lateral rectus.
3 The inferior oblique is fleshy throughout. It passes laterally, upwards and backwards below the inferior rectus and then deep to the lateral rectus. The inferior oblique is inserted close to the superior oblique a little below and posterior to the latter.
4 The flat tendon of the levator splits into a superior or voluntary and an inferior or involuntary lamellae. Superior lamella of the levator is inserted into the anterior surface of the superior tarsus, and into

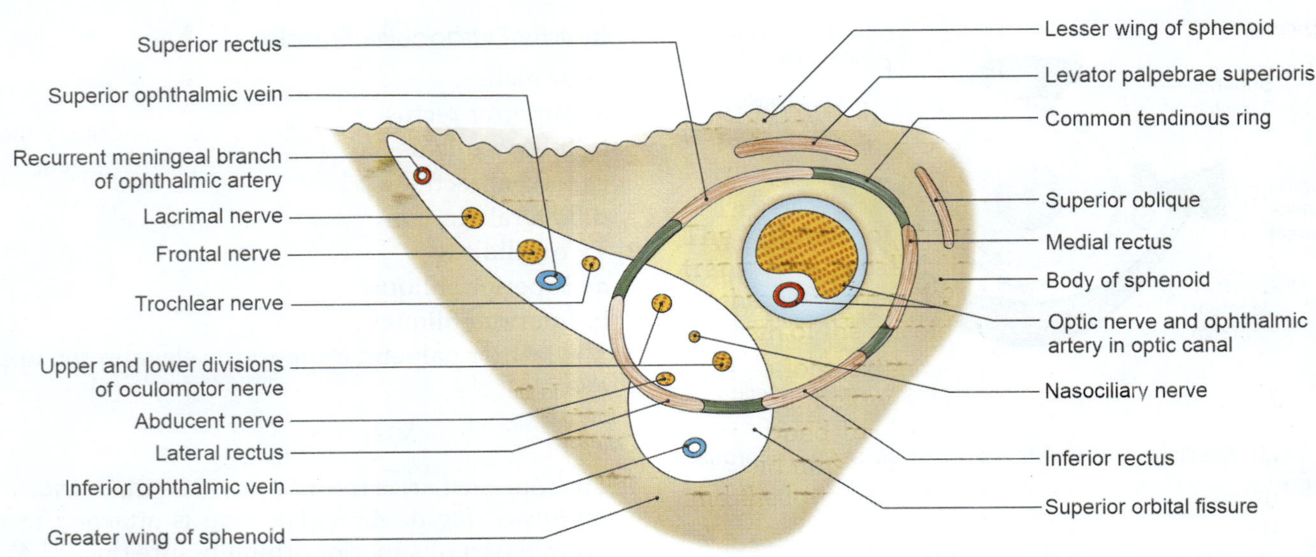

Fig. 21.4: Apical part of the orbit showing the origin of the extraocular muscles, the common tendinous ring and the structures passing through superior orbital fissure

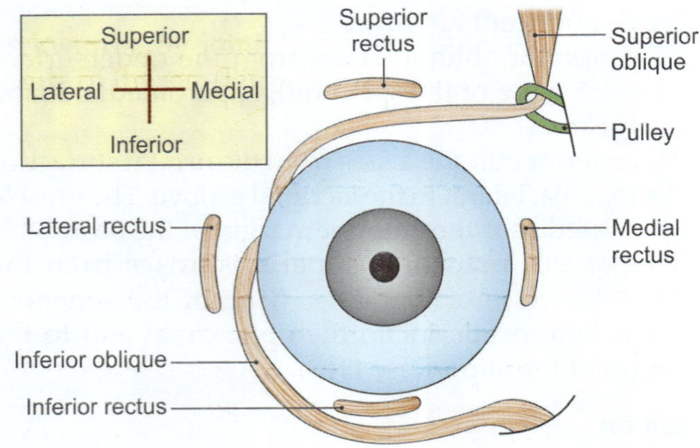

Fig. 21.5: Scheme to show the insertion of the oblique muscles of the eyeball

the skin of the upper eyelid. The inferior lamella (smooth part) is inserted into the upper margin of the superior tarsus (*see* Fig. 10.21b) and into superior conjunctival fornix.

Nerve Supply

1 The superior oblique is supplied by the IV cranial or trochlear nerve (SO4) (Fig. 21.6).
2 The lateral rectus is supplied by the VI cranial or abducent nerve (LR6).
3 The remaining four and a half extraocular muscles; superior, inferior and medial recti; inferior oblique and part of levator palpebrae superioris are all supplied by the III cranial or oculomotor nerve.

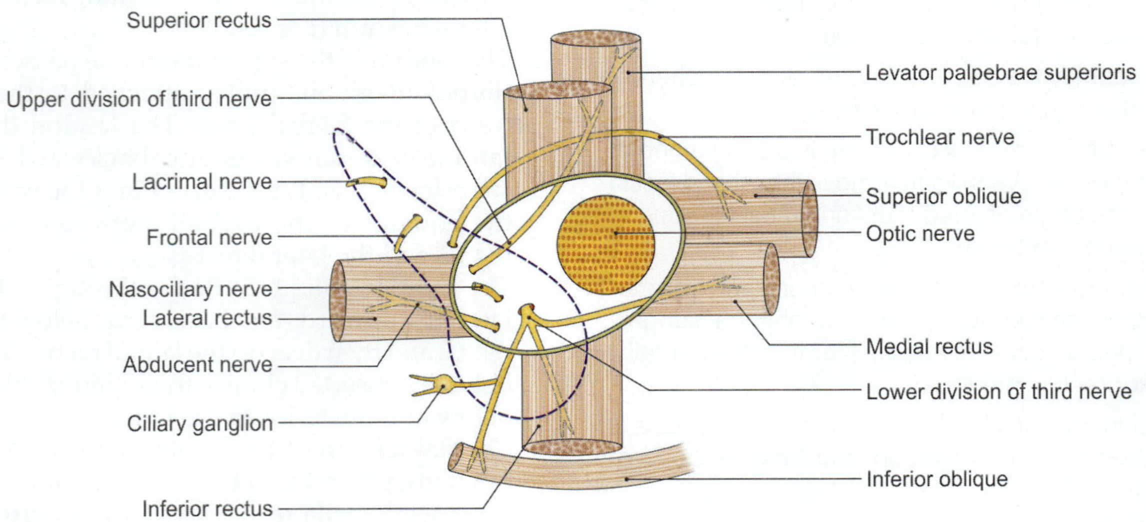

Fig. 21.6: Scheme showing the nerve supply of the extraocular muscles

Actions

1 The *movements of the eyeball* are as follows.
   a. *Around a transverse axis:*
      - Upward rotation or elevation (33°)
      - Downwards rotation or depression (33°)
   b. *Around a vertical axis:*
      - Medial rotation or adduction (50°)
      - Lateral rotation or abduction (50°)
   c. *Around an anteroposterior axis:*
      - Intorsion
      - Extorsion

      The rotatory movements of the eyeball upwards, downwards, medially or laterally, are defined in terms of the direction of movement of the centre of the pupil. The torsions are defined in terms of the direction of movement of the upper margin of the pupil at 12 o'clock position.
   d. The movements given above can take place in various combinations.

2 *Actions of individual muscles* are shown in Fig. 21.7a and Tables 21.1 and 21.2.

3 *Single* or *pure movements* are produced by combined actions of muscles. Similar actions get added

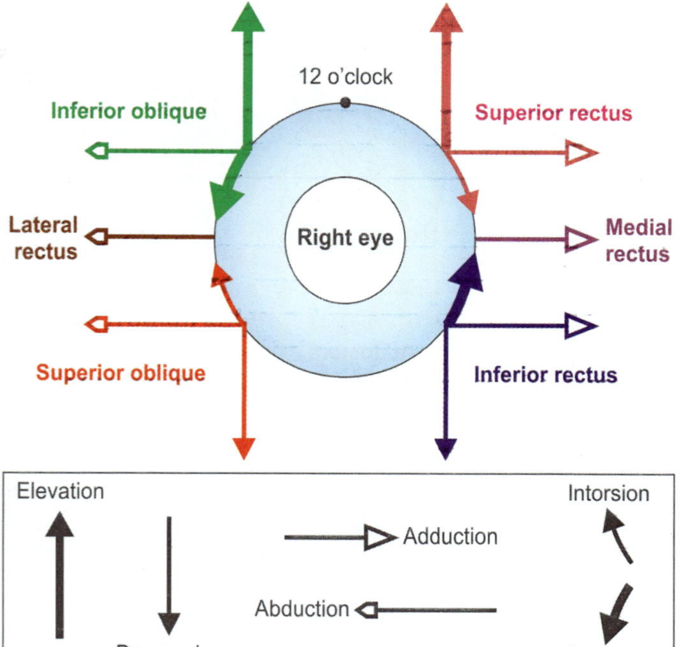

Fig. 21.7a: Scheme to show the actions of the extraocular muscles

Table 21.1: Actions of individual muscles according to their axes

Muscle	*Transverse axis*	*Vertical axis*	*Anteroposterior axis*
Superior rectus (SR)	Elevates	Adducts	Rotates medially (intorsion)
Inferior rectus (IR)	Depresses	Adducts	Rotates laterally (extorsion)
Superior oblique (SO)	Depresses	Abducts	Rotates medially (intorsion)
Inferior oblique (IO)	Elevates	Abducts	Rotates laterally (extorsion)
Medial rectus (MR)	—	Adducts	—
Lateral rectus (LR)	—	Abducts	—

Table 21.2: Action of individual muscles according to the position of eye

Muscle	*In primary position*	*Abducted eye*	*Adducted eye*
1. Superior oblique	Depression Abduction Intorsion	Only intorsion	Only depression
2. Inferior oblique	Elevation Abduction Extorsion	Only extorsion	Only elevation
3. Inferior rectus	Depression Adduction Extorsion	Only depression	Only extorsion
4. Superior rectus	Elevation Adduction Intorsion	Only elevation	Only intorsion
5. Medial rectus	Only adduction	—	—
6. Lateral rectus	Only abduction	—	—

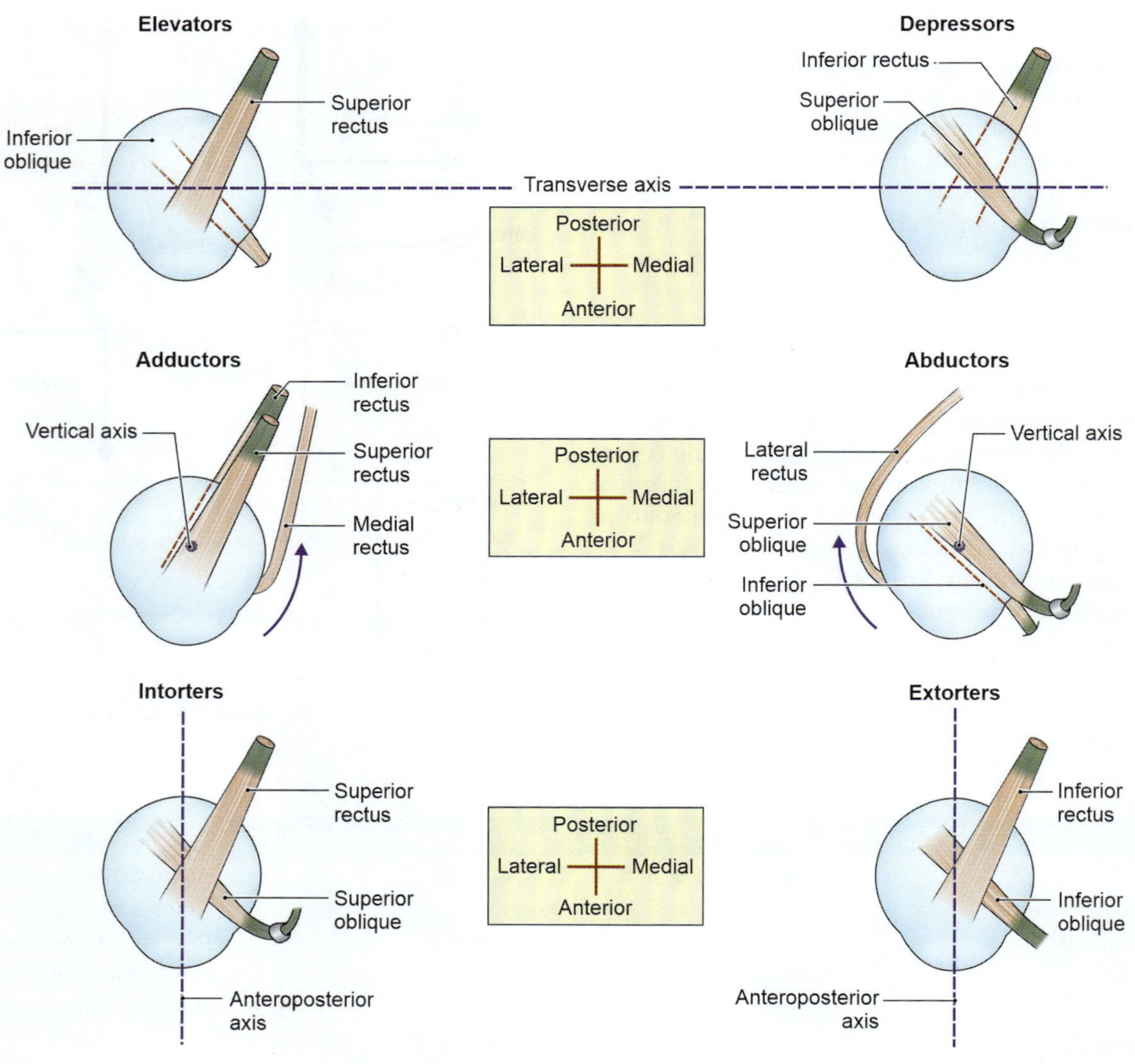

Fig. 21.7b: Single movement of the eye

together, while opposing actions cancel each other enabling pure movements (Fig. 21.7b).

a. *Upward rotation or elevation:* By the superior rectus and the inferior oblique.
b. *Downward rotation or depression:* By the inferior rectus and the superior oblique.
c. *Medial rotation or adduction:* By the medial rectus, the superior rectus and the inferior rectus.
d. *Lateral rotation or abduction:* By the lateral rectus, the superior oblique and the inferior oblique.
e. *Intorsion:* By the superior oblique and the superior rectus.
f. *Extorsion:* By the inferior oblique and the inferior rectus.

4 *Combined movements of the eyes*

Normally, movements of the two eyes are harmoniously coordinated. Such coordinated movements of both eyes are called *conjugate ocular movements* (Fig. 21.7c).

CLINICAL ANATOMY

- Weakness or paralysis of a muscle causes squint or strabismus, which may be concomitant or paralytic. Concomitant squint is congenital; there is no limitation of movement, and no diplopia (Fig. 21.8).

  In paralytic squint, movements are limited, diplopia and vertigo are present, head is turned in the direction of the function of paralysed muscle, and there is a false orientation of the field of vision.

- Nystagmus is characterized by involuntary, rhythmical oscillatory movements of the eyes. This is due to incoordination of the ocular muscles. It may be either vestibular or cerebellar, or even congenital.

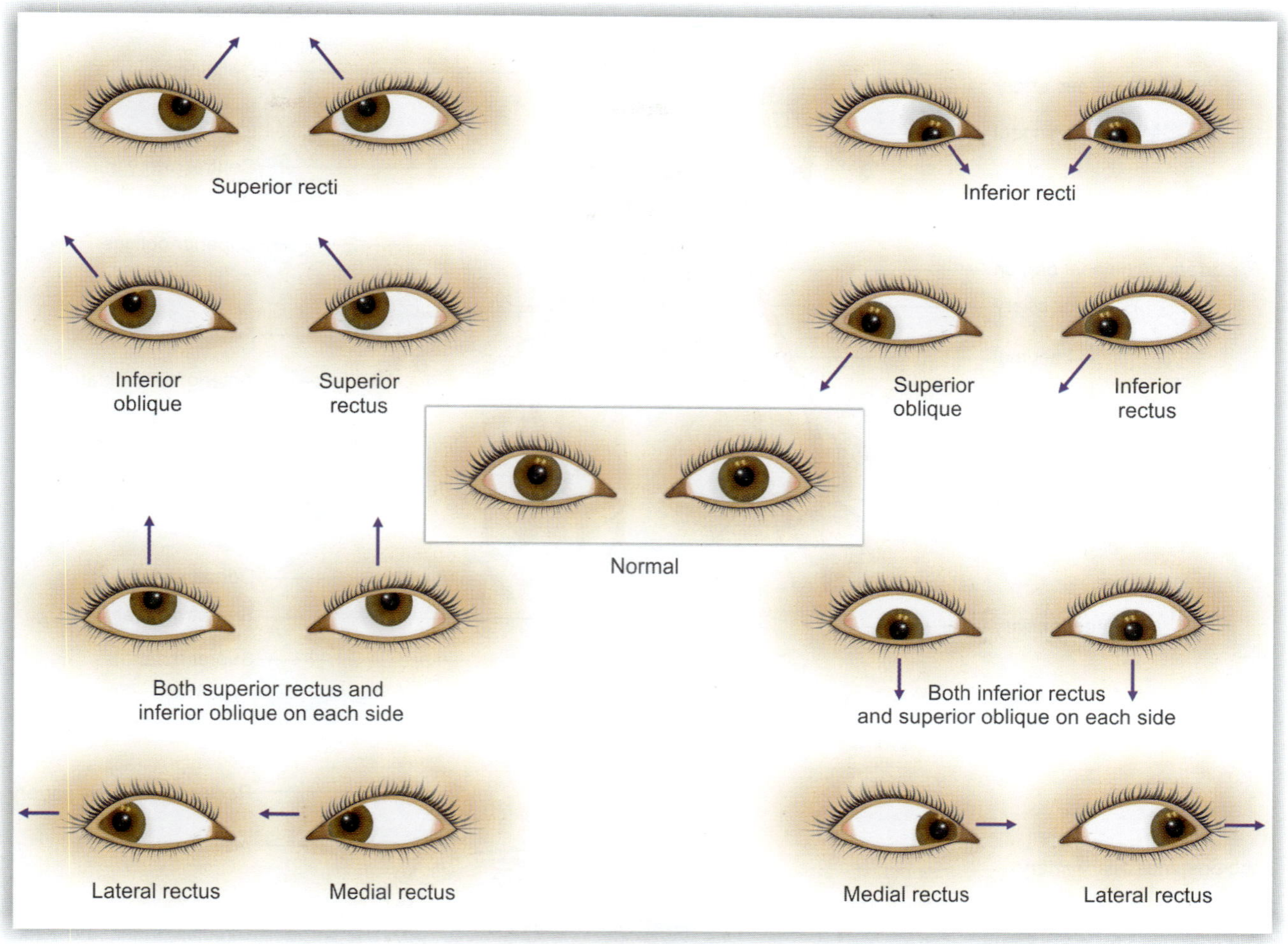

Fig. 21.7c: Muscles for conjugate movements of the eyes

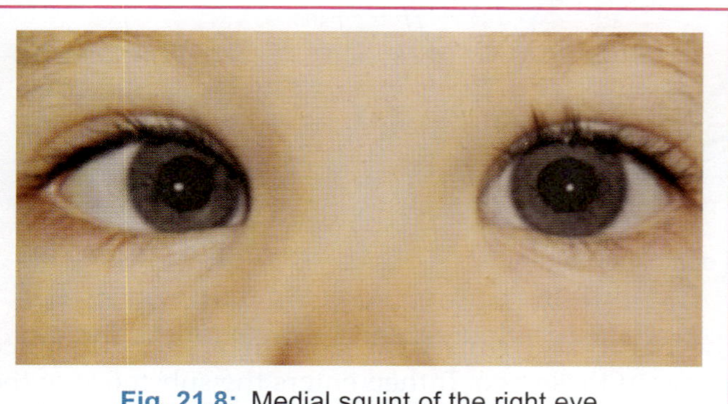

Fig. 21.8: Medial squint of the right eye

VESSELS OF THE ORBIT

OPHTHALMIC ARTERY

Origin

The ophthalmic artery is a branch of the cerebral part of the internal carotid artery, given off medial to the anterior clinoid process close to the optic canal (Figs 21.9 and 21.10).

Course and Relations

1 The artery enters the orbit through the optic canal, lying inferolateral to the optic nerve. Both the artery and nerve lie in a common dural sheath.

2 In the orbit, the artery pierces the dura mater, ascends over the lateral side of the optic nerve, and crosses above the nerve from lateral to medial side along with the nasociliary nerve. It then runs forwards along the medial wall of the orbit between the superior oblique and the medial rectus muscles and parallel to the nasociliary nerve.

3 It terminates near the medial angle of the eye by dividing into the supratrochlear and dorsal nasal branches (Fig. 21.9).

DISSECTION

Trace the ophthalmic artery after it was seen to cross over the optic nerve along with nasociliary nerve and superior ophthalmic vein. Identify its branches especially the central artery of the retina which is an 'end artery'.

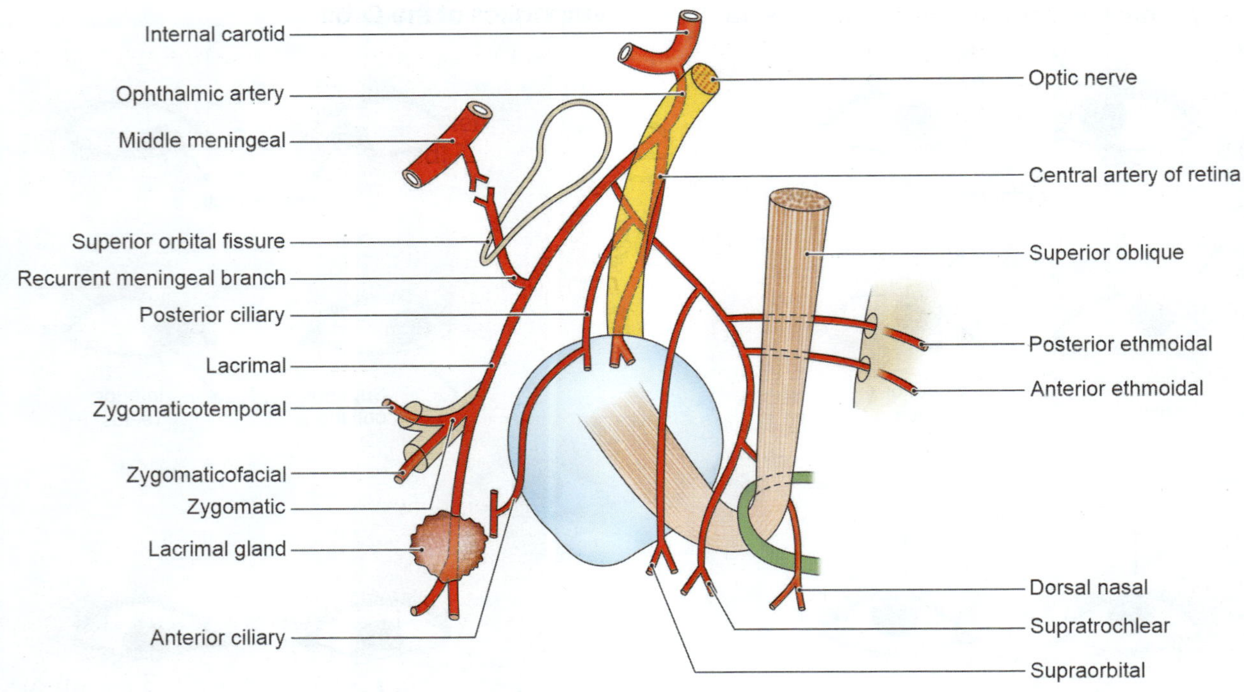

Fig. 21.9: The arteries of the eyeball

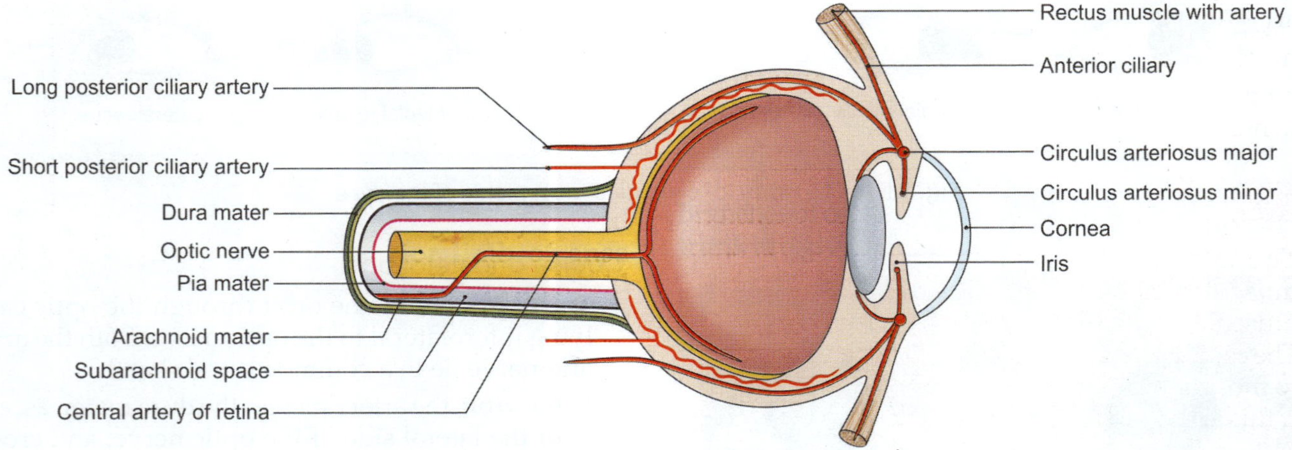

Fig. 21.10: Branches of ophthalmic artery

Branches

While still within the dural sheath, the ophthalmic artery gives off the *central artery of the retina*. After piercing the dura mater, it gives off a large lacrimal branch that runs along the lateral wall of the orbit. The main artery runs towards the medial wall of the orbit giving off a number of branches. The various branches are described below.

Central Artery of Retina

The central artery of retina (Fig. 21.10) is the first and most important branch of the ophthalmic artery. It first lies below the optic nerve. It pierces the dural sheath of the nerve and runs forwards for a short distance between these two. It then enters the substance of the nerve and runs forwards in its centre to reach the optic disc (Fig. 21.9). Here it divides into branches that supply the retina (*see* Fig. 27.11).

The central artery of the retina is an *end artery*. It does not have effective anastomoses with other arteries. Occlusion of the artery results in blindness. The intraocular part of the artery can be seen, in the living, through an ophthalmoscope (*see* Fig. 27.17).

Branches Arising from the Lacrimal Artery

1 Branches are given to the lacrimal gland.

2 Two zygomatic branches enter canals in the zygomatic bone. One branch appears on the face through the zygomaticofacial foramen. The other appears on the temporal surface of the bone through the zygomaticotemporal foramen.
3 Lateral palpebral branches supply the eyelids.
4 A recurrent meningeal branch runs backwards to enter the middle cranial fossa through the superior orbital fissure.
5 Muscular branches supply the muscles of the orbit.

Branches Arising from the Main Trunk

1 The posterior (long and short) ciliary arteries supply chiefly the choroid and iris. The eyeball is also supplied through anterior ciliary branches which are given off from arteries supplying muscles attached to the eyeball (Fig. 21.10).
2 The supraorbital and supratrochlear branches supply the skin of the forehead.
3 The anterior and posterior ethmoidal branches enter foramina in the medial wall of the orbit to supply the ethmoidal air sinuses. They then enter the anterior cranial fossa. The terminal branches of the anterior ethmoidal artery enter the nose and supply part of it.
4 The medial palpebral branches supply the eyelids.
5 The dorsal nasal branch supplies the upper part of the nose.

CLINICAL ANATOMY

- The anterior ciliary arteries arise from the muscular branches of ophthalmic artery. The muscular arteries are important in this respect.
- The central artery of retina is the only arterial supply to most of the nervous layer, the retina of the eye. If this artery is blocked, there is sudden blindness.

OPHTHALMIC VEINS

Superior ophthalmic vein: It accompanies the ophthalmic artery. It lies above the optic nerve. It receives tributaries corresponding to the branches of the artery, passes through the superior orbital fissure, and drains into the cavernous sinus. It communicates anteriorly with the supraorbital and angular veins (*see* Fig. 10.6).

Inferior ophthalmic vein: It runs below the optic nerve. It receives tributaries from the lacrimal sac, the lower orbital muscles, and the eyelids, and ends either by joining the superior ophthalmic vein or drains directly into the cavernous sinus. It communicates with the pterygoid plexus of veins by small veins passing through the inferior orbital fissure.

Lymphatics of the Orbit

The lymphatics drain into the preauricular parotid lymph nodes (*see* Fig. 10.25).

NERVES OF THE ORBIT

These are:
1 Optic II (Fig. 21.10)
2 Ciliary ganglion (Fig. 21.11)
3 Oculomotor (III) and trochlear (IV) (Figs 21.12 and 21.13)
4 Abducent (VI) (Fig. 21.14)
5 Branches of ophthalmic (V1) and maxillary divisions (V2) of the trigeminal nerve (Figs 21.15 and 21.16)
6 Sympathetic nerves.

OPTIC NERVE

The optic nerve is the nerve of sight. It is made up of the axons of cells in the ganglionic layer of the retina. It emerges from the eyeball 3 or 4 mm nasal to its posterior pole. It runs backwards and medially, and passes through the optic canal to enter the middle cranial fossa where it joins the optic chiasma (*see* Fig. 20.13).

The nerve is about 4 cm long, out of which 25 mm are intraorbital, 5 mm intracanalicular, and 10 mm intracranial. The entire nerve is enclosed in three meningeal sheaths. The subarachnoid space extends around the nerve up to the eyeball (Fig. 21.10).

Relations in the Orbit

1 At the apex of the orbit, the nerve is closely surrounded by the recti muscles. The ciliary ganglion lies between the optic nerve and the lateral rectus.
2 The central artery and vein of the retina pierce the optic nerve inferomedially about 1.25 cm behind the eyeball (Fig. 21.9).
3 The optic nerve is crossed superiorly by the ophthalmic artery, the nasociliary nerve and the superior ophthalmic vein.
4 The optic nerve is crossed inferiorly by the nerve to the medial rectus.
5 Near the eyeball, the nerve is surrounded by fat containing the ciliary vessels and nerves (*see* Fig. 27.2).

Structure

1 There are about 1.2 million myelinated fibres in each optic nerve, out of which about 53% cross in the optic chiasma.
2 The optic nerve is not a nerve in the strict sense as there is no neurolemmal sheath. It is actually a tract. It cannot regenerate, if it is cut. Developmentally,

the optic nerve and the retina are a direct prolongation of the brain.

CLINICAL ANATOMY

- The anastomoses between tributaries of facial vein and ophthalmic veins may result in spread of infection from the orbital and nasal regions to the cavernous sinus leading to its thrombosis.
- Optic neuritis is characterized by pain in and behind the eye on ocular movements and on pressure. The papilloedema is less but loss of vision is more. When the optic disc is normal as seen by an ophthalmoscope the same condition is called retrobulbar neuritis.
  The common causes are demyelinating diseases of the central nervous system, any septic focus in the teeth or paranasal sinuses, meningitis, encephalitis, syphilis, and even vitamin B deficiency.
- Optic nerve has no neurilemmal sheath, and has no power of regeneration. It is a tract and not a nerve.
- Optic atrophy may be caused by a variety of diseases. It may be primary or secondary.

CILIARY GANGLION

Ciliary ganglion is a peripheral parasympathetic ganglion placed in the course of the oculomotor nerve. It lies near the apex of the orbit between the optic nerve and the tendon of the lateral rectus muscle. It has parasympathetic, sensory and sympathetic roots.

The *parasympathetic root* arises from the nerve to the inferior oblique (Fig. 21.11). It contains preganglionic fibres that begin in the *Edinger-Westphal nucleus*. The fibres relay in the ciliary ganglion. Postganglionic fibres arising in the ganglion pass through the short ciliary nerves and supply the sphincter pupillae and the ciliaris muscle (*see* Appendix Flowchart A.4). These intraocular muscles are used in accommodation.

The *sensory root* comes from the nasociliary nerve. It contains sensory fibres for the eyeball. The fibres do not relay in the ganglion (Fig. 21.11).

The *sympathetic root* is a branch from the internal carotid plexus. It contains postganglionic fibres arising in the superior cervical ganglion (preganglionic fibres reach the ganglion from lateral horn of T1 spinal segment) which pass along internal carotid, ophthalmic and long ciliary arteries. They pass out of the ciliary ganglion without relay in the short ciliary nerves to supply the blood vessels of the eyeball. They also supply the dilator pupillae.

Branches

The ganglion gives off 8 to 10 short ciliary nerves which divide into 15 to 20 branches, and then pierce

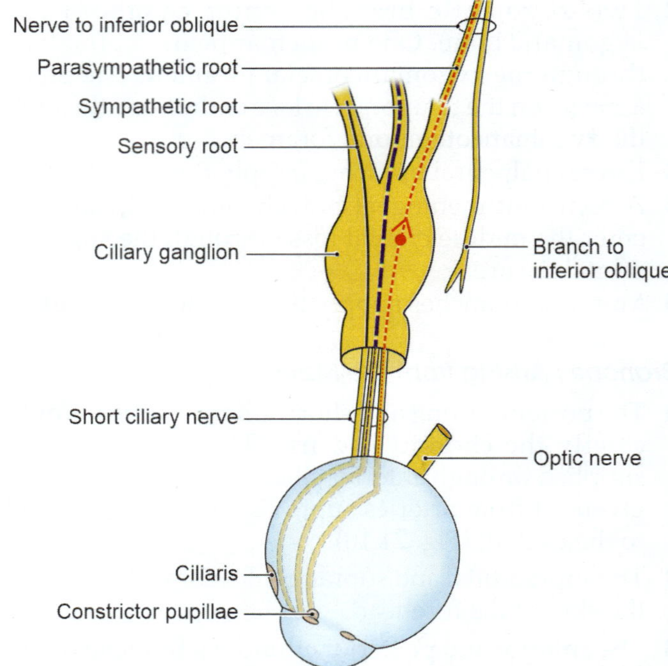

Fig. 21.11: Roots and branches of ciliary ganglion

the sclera around the entrance of the optic nerve. They contain fibres from all the three roots of the ganglion.

OCULOMOTOR NERVE

Course of oculomotor (III) nerve is shown by Flowchart 21.1 and Fig. 21.12.

Flowchart 21.1: Oculomotor nerve—III nerve

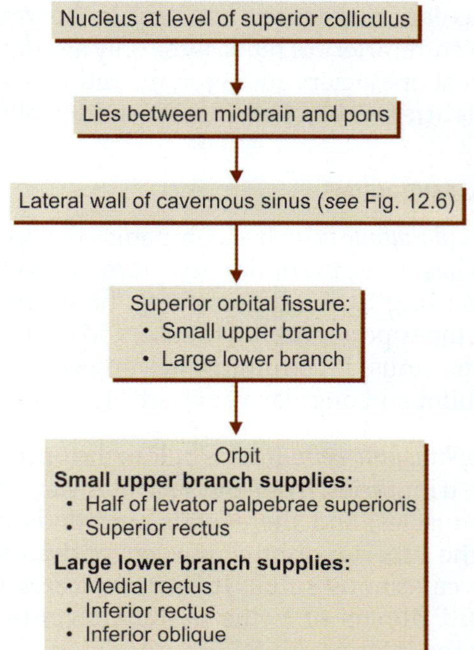

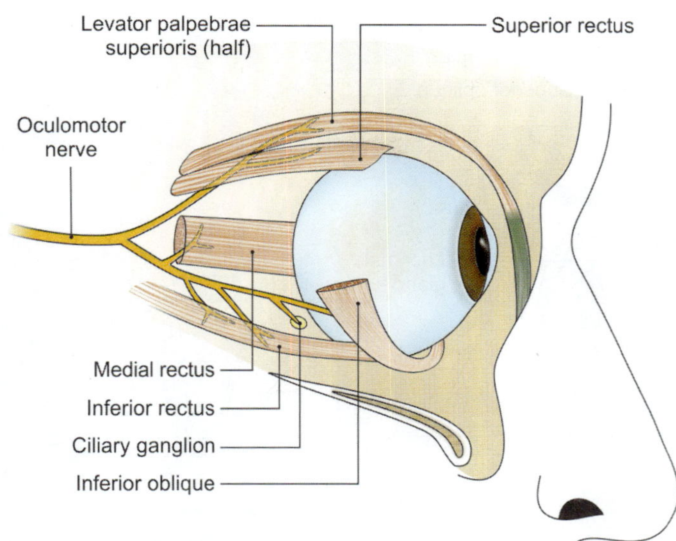

Fig. 21.12: Distribution of oculomotor nerve

TROCHLEAR NERVE

Course of trochlear (IV) nerve is shown by Flowchart 21.2 and Fig. 21.13.

Flowchart 21.2: Trochlear—IV nerve

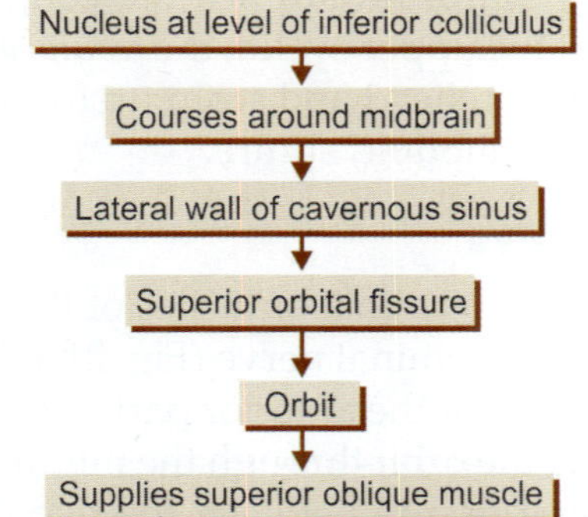

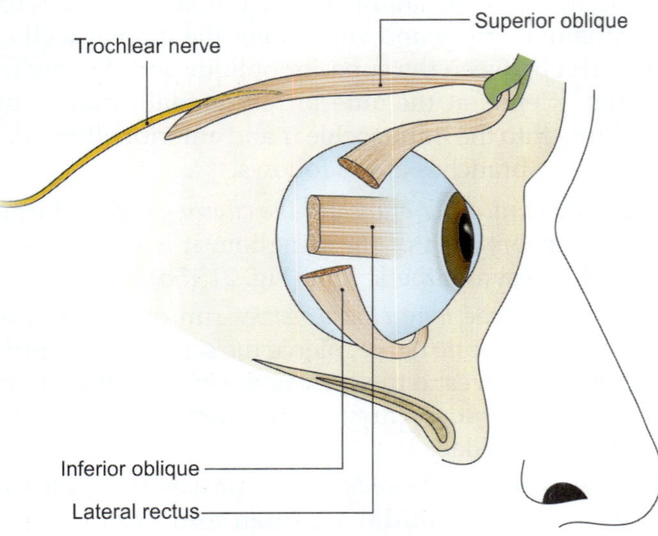

Fig. 21.13: Course of trochlear nerve

ABDUCENT NERVE

Course of abducent (VI) nerve is depicted by Flowchart 21.3 and Fig. 21.14.

Flowchart 21.3: Abducent nerve—VI nerve

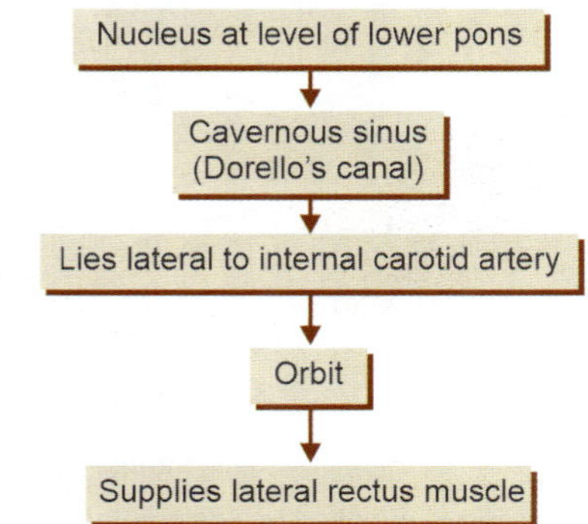

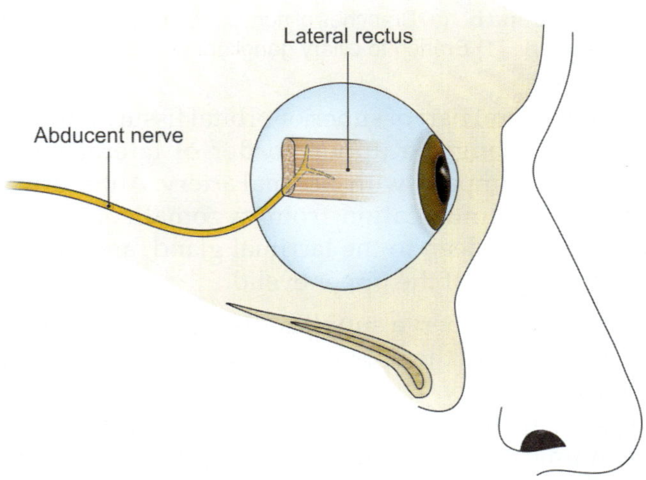

Fig. 21.14: Distribution of abducent nerve

BRANCHES OF OPHTHALMIC DIVISION OF TRIGEMINAL NERVE

Following are the branches of ophthalmic division of trigeminal nerve (Fig. 21.15).

1 Frontal	Supratrochlear Supraorbital
2 Nasociliary	Branch to ciliary ganglion 2–3 long ciliary nerves Posterior ethmoidal Infratrochlear Anterior ethmoidal
3 Lacrimal	Branch to the upper eyelid and secretomotor fibres to lacrimal gland.

Lacrimal Nerve

This is the smallest of the three terminal branches of ophthalmic nerve (Fig. 21.15a). It enters the orbit

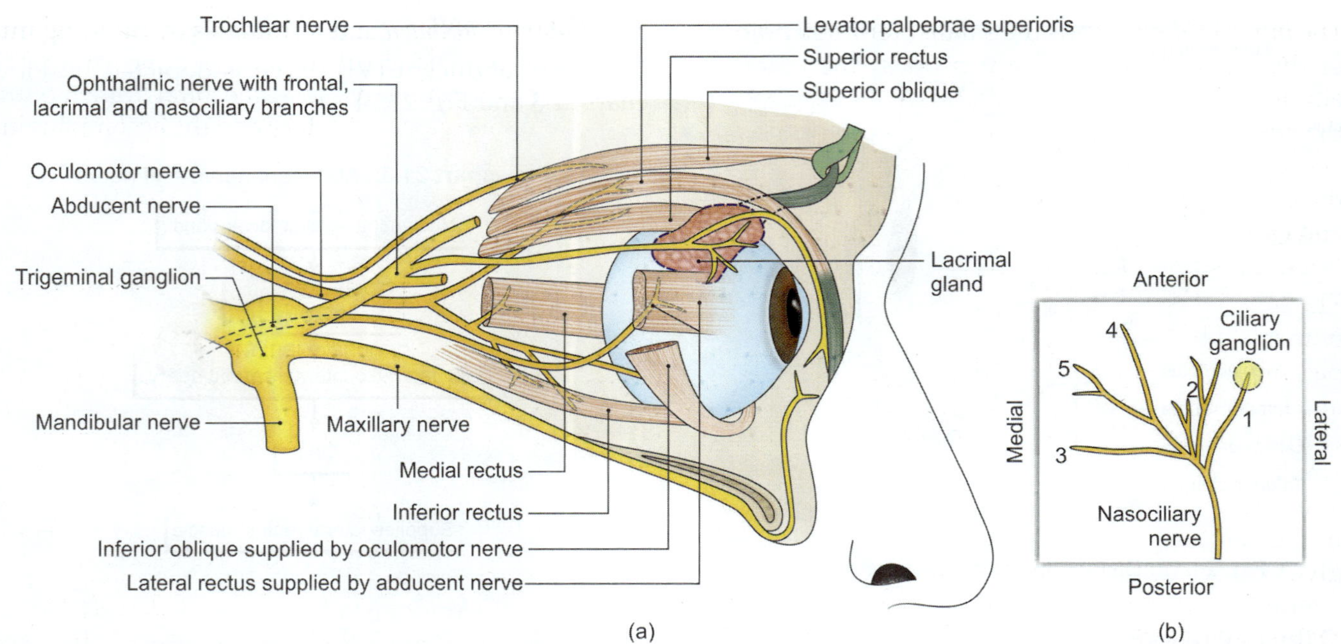

Figs 21.15a and b: (a) Branches of right ophthalmic nerve including III, IV, VI cranial nerves and the extraocular muscles, and (b) branches of nasociliary: (1) Branch to ciliary ganglion; (2) Long ciliary; (3) Posterior ethmoidal; (4) Infratrochlear; (5) Anterior ethmoidal

through lateral part of superior orbital fissure and runs forwards along the upper border of lateral rectus muscle, in company with lacrimal artery. Anteriorly, it receives communication from zygomaticotemporal nerve, passes deep to the lacrimal gland, and ends in the lateral part of the upper eyelid.

The lacrimal nerve supplies the lacrimal gland, the conjunctiva and the upper eyelid. Its own fibres to the gland are sensory. The secretomotor fibres to the gland come from the greater petrosal nerve through its communication with the zygomaticotemporal nerve (*see* Flowchart 10.2).

Frontal Nerve

This is the largest of the three terminal branches of the ophthalmic nerve (Figs 21.15a and b). It begins in the lateral wall of the anterior part of the cavernous sinus. It enters the orbit through the lateral part of the superior orbital fissure, and runs forwards on the superior surface of the levator palpebrae superioris. At the middle of the orbit, it divides into a small supratrochlear branch and a large supraorbital branch.

The *supratrochlear nerve* emerges from the orbit above the trochlea about one finger breadth from the median plane. It supplies the conjunctiva, the upper eyelid, and a small area of the skin of the forehead above the root of the nose (*see* Figs 10.5 and 10.16).

The *supraorbital nerve* emerges from the orbit through the supraorbital notch or foramen about two fingers breadth from the median plane. It divides into medial and lateral branches which runs upwards over the forehead and scalp. It supplies the conjunctiva, the central part of the upper eyelid, the *frontal air sinus* and the skin of the forehead and scalp up to the vertex, or even up to the lambdoid suture.

Nasociliary Nerve

This is one of the terminal branches of the ophthalmic division of the trigeminal nerve (Fig. 21.15b). It begins in the lateral wall of the anterior part of the cavernous sinus. It enters the orbit through the middle part of the superior orbital fissure between the two divisions of the oculomotor nerve (Fig. 21.4). It crosses above the optic nerve from lateral to medial side along with ophthalmic artery and runs along the medial wall of the orbit between the superior oblique and the medial rectus. It ends at the anterior ethmoidal foramen by dividing into the infratrochlear and anterior ethmoidal nerves. Its branches are as follows.

1. A *communicating branch to the ciliary ganglion* forms the sensory root of the ganglion. It is often mixed with the sympathetic root (Fig. 21.15b).
2. Two or three *long ciliary nerves* run on the medial side of the optic nerve, pierce the sclera, and supply sensory nerves to the cornea, the iris and the ciliary body. They also carry sympathetic nerves to the dilator pupillae.
3. The *posterior ethmoidal nerve* passes through the posterior ethmoidal foramen and supplies the ethmoidal and sphenoidal air sinuses.

4 The *infratrochlear nerve* is the smaller terminal branch of the nasociliary nerve given off at the anterior ethmoidal foramen. It emerges from the orbit below the trochlea for the tendon of the superior oblique and appears on the face above the medial angle of the eye. It supplies the conjunctiva, the lacrimal sac and caruncle, the medial ends of the eyelids and the upper half of the external nose (*see* Fig. 10.16).

5 The *anterior ethmoidal nerve* is the larger terminal branch of the nasociliary nerve. It leaves the orbit by passing through the anterior ethmoidal foramen. It appears, for a very short distance, in the anterior cranial fossa, above the cribriform plate of the ethmoid bone. It then descends into the nose through a slit at the side of the anterior part of the crista galli. In the nasal cavity, it lies deep to the nasal bone. It gives off two *internal nasal branches*—medial and lateral to the mucosa of the nose. Finally, it emerges at the lower border of the nasal bone as the *external nasal nerve* which supplies the skin of the lower half of the nose.

SOME BRANCHES OF MAXILLARY DIVISION OF THE TRIGEMINAL NERVE

Infraorbital Nerve

It is the continuation of the maxillary nerve. It enters the orbit through the *inferior orbital fissure*. It then runs forwards on the floor of the orbit or the roof of the maxillary sinus, at first in the *infraorbital groove* and then in the *infraorbital canal* remaining outside the periosteum of the orbit. It emerges on the face through the *infraorbital foramen* and terminates by dividing into palpebral, nasal and labial branches (*see* Fig. 10.16). The nerve is accompanied by the infraorbital branch of the third part of the maxillary artery and the accompanying vein (Fig. 21.16).

Branches

1 The *middle superior alveolar nerve* arises in the infraorbital groove, runs in the lateral wall of the maxillary sinus, and supplies the upper premolar teeth.

2 The *anterior superior alveolar nerve* arises in the infraorbital canal, and runs in a sinuous canal having a complicated course in the anterior wall of the maxillary sinus. It supplies the upper incisor and canine teeth, the maxillary sinus, and the antero-inferior part of the nasal cavity where it communicates with branches of anterior ethmoidal and anterior palatine nerves (*see* Fig. 23.16).

3 *Terminal branches—palpebral, nasal and labial* which supply a large area of skin on the face. They also supply the mucous membrane of the upper lip and cheek (*see* Fig. 10.16).

Zygomatic Nerve

It is a branch of the maxillary nerve, given off in the pterygopalatine fossa. It enters the orbit through the lateral end of the inferior orbital fissure, and runs along the lateral wall, outside the periosteum, to enter the zygomatic bone. Just before or after entering the bone, it divides into its two terminal branches, the *zygomaticofacial* and *zygomaticotemporal nerves* which supply the skin of the face and of the anterior part of the temple (*see* Fig. 10.16). The communicating branch to the

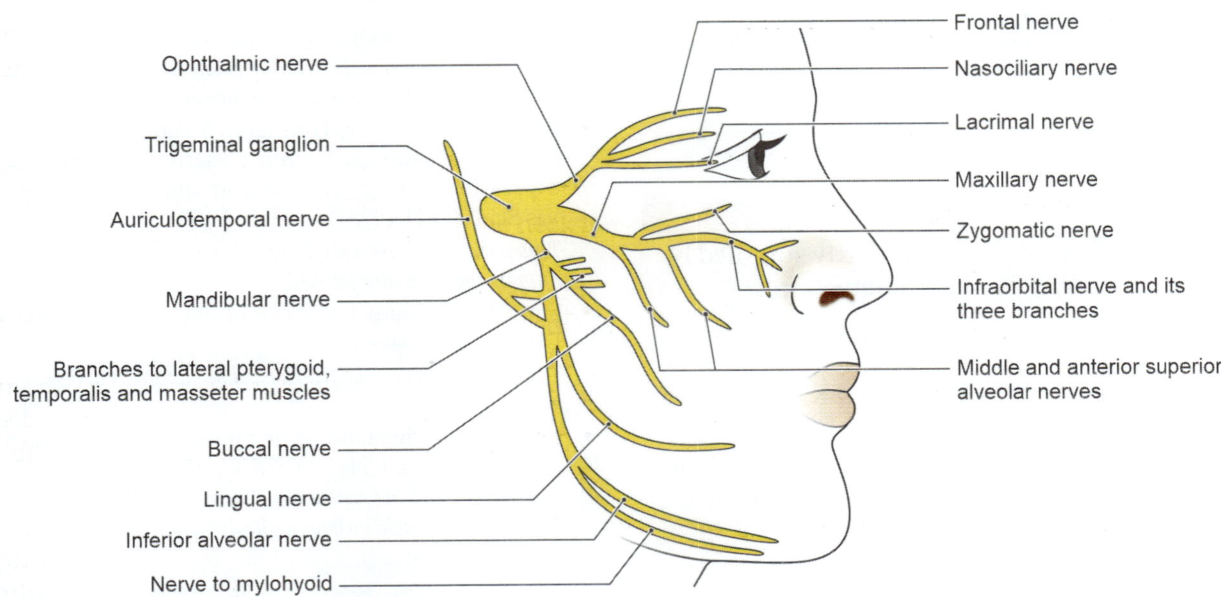

Fig. 21.16: Some branches of ophthalmic, maxillary and mandibular branches of trigeminal nerve

lacrimal nerve, which contains secretomotor fibres to the lacrimal gland, arises from the zygomaticotemporal nerve, and runs in the lateral wall of the orbit (*see* Chapter 10). Detailed description is given in Chapter 23.

Some Branches of Mandibular Division of Trigeminal Nerve

1. Anterior division gives muscular branches to masseter, temporalis and lateral pterygoid muscles.
2. Posterior division gives auriculotemporal nerve and then divides into lingual and inferior alveolar nerves. Details are given in Chapter 14.

SYMPATHETIC NERVES OF THE ORBIT

Sympathetic nerves arise from the internal carotid plexus and enter the orbit through the following sources.

1. The dilator pupillae of the iris is supplied by sympathetic nerves that pass through the ophthalmic nerve, the nasociliary nerve, and its long ciliary branches.
2. Other sympathetic nerves enter the orbit as follows:
   a. A plexus surrounds the ophthalmic artery.
   b. A direct branch from the internal carotid plexus passes through the superior orbital fissure and joins the ciliary ganglion.
   c. Other filaments pass along the oculomotor, trochlear, abducent, and ophthalmic nerves. All these sympathetic nerves are vasomotor in function.

Mnemonics

Extraocular muscles; cranial nerve innervation "LR6SO4 rest 3"

Lateral **r**ectus by **VI**

Superior **o**blique by **IV**

Rest are by **III** cranial nerve, i.e. half of levator palpebrae superioris, superior rectus (SR), medial rectus (MR), inferior rectus (IR) and inferior oblique (IO).

FACTS TO REMEMBER

- Levator palpebrae superioris is partly supplied by III nerve and partly by sympathetic fibres.
- Central artery of retina is an end artery.
- Nerve supply of extraocular muscles is LR6, SO4, rest (part of levator palpebrae sup., SR, MR, IR and IO) by III.
- Edinger-Westphal is the nucleus for the supply of ciliaris muscles and constrictor pupillae muscles.

The fibres supply these muscles after relaying in the ciliary ganglion.

- Elevation and depression of the cornea occur around a transverse axis.
- Adduction and abduction of the cornea take place around a vertical axis.
- Intorsion and extorsion occur around an antero-posterior axis.

CLINICOANATOMICAL PROBLEM

A hypertensive and diabetic lady with high cholesterol and lipids develops sudden blindness in her right eye.

- What has caused blindness in this particular case?
- Name the other end arteries in the body.

Ans: Hypertension causes atheromatous changes in the arteries. Most of the nervous layers of retina are supplied by a single 'end artery' with no anastomoses with any other artery. This artery is also vulnerable to blockage due to various changes in blood chemistry. If it gets blocked, the result is blindness of that eye.

Other end arteries are:

- Labyrinthine artery for the inner ear
- Coronary arteries are functional end arteries though these do anastomose
- Central branches of cerebral arteries
- Segmental branches of the kidney and spleen

FURTHER READING

- Graw J. Eye development. Curr Top Dev Biol 2010;90:343–86.
  This paper presents the transcription factors in eye development and discusses their relevance to human eye disorders.
- Pedrosa-Domellof F, Holmgren Y, Lucas CA, et al. Human extraocular muscles: Unique pattern of myosin heavy chain expression during myotube formation. Invest Ophthalmol Vis Sci 2000;41:1608–16.
  This paper presents a study of extraocular muscle development in human embryos and fetuses.
- Sinn R, Wittbrodt J. An eye of eye development. Mech of Dev 2013;130:347–58.
  This paper reviews the transcription factors in development of the eye.
- Miller JM. Understanding and misunderstanding extraocular muscle pulleys. J Vis 2007;7:10:1–15.
  A discussion of the issues and controversies regarding the role of extraocular muscle pulleys in health and disease.

Frequently Asked Questions

1. Describe extraocular muscles under the following headings:
   a. Origin
   b. Insertion
   c. Actions
   d. Nerve supply
   e. Clinical importance
2. Write short notes on:
   a. Ciliary ganglion
   b. Levator palpebrae superioris
   c. Ophthalmic artery
   d. Actions of oblique muscles

Multiple Choice Questions

1. Which nucleus is related to ciliary ganglion?
   a. Superior salivatory
   b. Lacrimatory
   c. Inferior salivatory
   d. Edinger-Westphal
2. Ophthalmic artery is a branch of which of the following arteries?
   a. Internal carotid
   b. External carotid
   c. Maxillary
   d. Vertebral
3. Supraorbital artery is a branch of:
   a. Maxillary
   b. External carotid
   c. Ophthalmic
   d. Internal carotid
4. Which of the following is true about ocular muscles?
   a. Medial rectus is supplied by III nerve
   b. Superior oblique turns the centre of cornea upwards and laterally
   c. Inferior oblique arises from medial wall of the orbit
   d. Lateral rectus is supplied by IV nerve
5. Which nerve does not transverse the middle part of superior orbital fissure?
   a. Two divisions of III nerve
   b. Frontal nerve
   c. VI nerve
   d. Nasociliary nerve
6. Which of the following arteries is an end-artery?
   a. Lacrimal artery
   b. Zygomaticotemporal artery
   c. Central artery of retina
   d. Anterior ethmoidal artery

Answers

1. d **2.** a **3.** c **4.** a **5.** b **6.** c

VIVA VOCE

- Name the extraocular muscles with their nerve supply.
- What nerves course through superior orbital fissure?
- Which muscles are attached behind the equator of the eyeball?
- What type of artery is 'central artery of retina' and why?
- Name the roots and branches of the ciliary ganglion.
- What is the course of nerve to inferior oblique?
- Name the branches of ophthalmic division of V nerve.
- What are the nerve supply and insertions of levator palpebrae superioris muscle?
- Which are the muscles innervated by fibres of Edinger-Westphal nucleus?

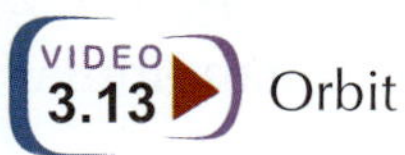

Orbit

Chapter 22

Mouth and Pharynx

"At times it is better to keep your mouth shut and let people wonder if you are a fool than to open it and remove all their doubts."
—James Sinclaire

ORAL CAVITY

Oral cavity is used for ingestion of food and fluids. It is continued posteriorly into the oropharynx, the middle part of the muscular pharynx. In its upper part, opens the posterior part of the nasal cavity and the inlet of larynx opens into its lower part. Roof of oral cavity is formed by the hard and the soft palates. Tongue is the biggest occupant of the oral cavity, described in Chapter 25. The cavity also contains 32 teeth in an adult.

Identification

Identify the structures in your own oral cavity. These are the vestibule, lips, cheeks, oral cavity proper and teeth.

Divisions

The oral or mouth cavity is divided into an outer, smaller portion, the vestibule, and an inner larger part, the oral cavity proper.

VESTIBULE

1 The vestibule of the mouth is a narrow space *bounded* externally by the lips and cheeks, and internally by the teeth and gums (Fig. 22.1).

2 It *communicates:*
   a. With the exterior through the oral fissure.
   b. With the mouth open, it communicates freely with the oral cavity proper. Even when the teeth are occluded a small communication remains behind the third molar tooth.

3 The *parotid duct* opens on the inner surface of the cheek opposite the crown of the upper second molar tooth (Fig. 22.1). Numerous *labial and buccal glands* (mucous) situated in the submucosa of the lips and cheeks open into the vestibule. Four or five *molar glands* (mucous), situated on the buccopharyngeal fascia, also open into the vestibule.

4 Except for the teeth, the entire vestibule is lined by mucous membrane. The mucous membrane forms median folds that pass from the lips to the gums, and are called the *frenula of the lips*.

CLINICAL ANATOMY

- The papilla of the parotid duct in the vestibule of the mouth provides access to the parotid duct for the injection of the radio-opaque dye to locate calculi in the duct system or the gland (Fig. 22.1).
- Koplik's spots are seen as white pinpoint spots around the opening of the parotid duct in measles. These are diagnostic of the disease.

Lips

1 The lips are fleshy folds lined externally by skin and internally by mucous membrane. The *mucocutaneous junction* lines the 'edge' of the lip, part of the mucosal surface is also normally seen.

2 Each lip is *composed* of:
   a. Skin
   b. Superficial fascia
   c. The orbicularis oris muscle
   d. The submucosa, containing mucous labial glands and blood vessels
   e. Mucous membrane.

3 The lips bound the *oral fissure*. They meet laterally at the angles of the mouth. The inner surface of each lip is supported by a *frenulum* which ties it to the gum. Philtrum is a median vertical groove on the outer surface of the upper lip.

4 *Lymphatics* of the central part of the lower lip drain to the submental nodes; the lymphatics from the rest of the lower lip pass to the submandibular nodes.

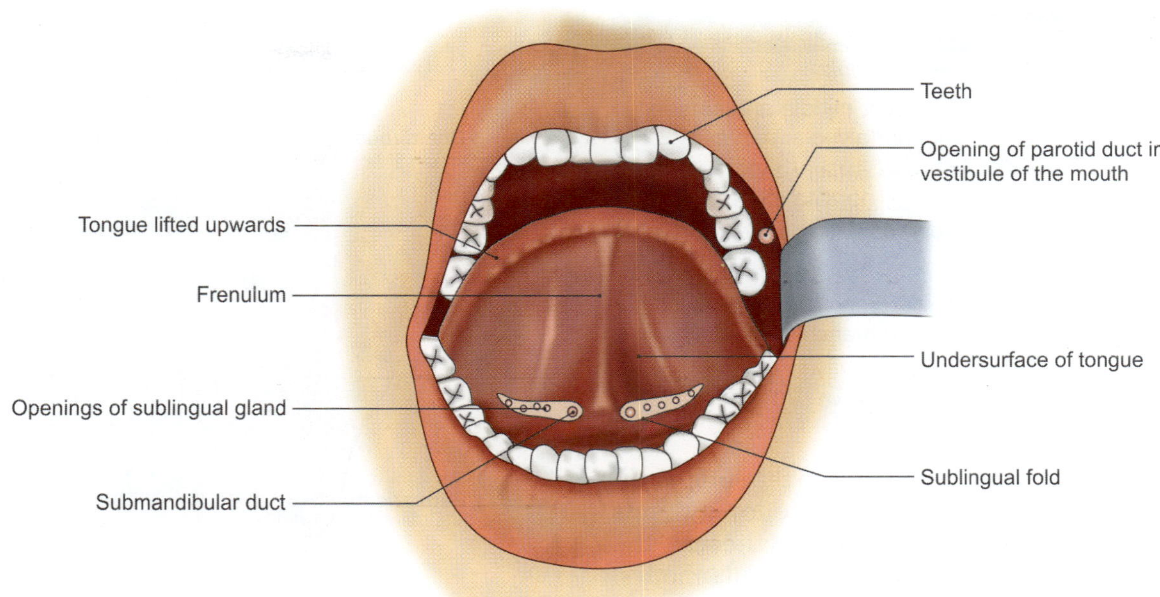

Fig. 22.1: Interior of the mouth cavity

Cheeks (Buccae)

1 The cheeks are fleshy flaps, forming a large part of each side of the face. They are continuous in front with the lips, and the junction is indicated by the *nasolabial sulcus (furrow)* which extends from the side of the nose to the angle of the mouth.

2 Each cheek is *composed of:*
   a. Skin
   b. Superficial fascia containing some facial muscles, the parotid duct, mucous molar glands, vessels and nerves.
   c. The buccinator covered by buccopharyngeal fascia and pierced by the parotid duct.
   d. Submucosa, with mucous buccal glands.
   e. Mucous membrane.

3 The *buccal pad of fat* is best developed in infants. It lies on the buccinator partly deep to the masseter and partly in front of it.

4 The *lymphatics* of the cheek drain chiefly into the submandibular and preauricular nodes, and partly also to the buccal and mandibular nodes.

ORAL CAVITY PROPER

1 It is *bounded* anterolaterally by the teeth, the gums and the alveolar arches of the jaws. The roof is formed by the hard palate and the soft palate. The *floor* is occupied by the tongue posteriorly, and presents the sublingual region anteriorly, below the tip of the tongue. Posteriorly, the cavity communicates with the pharynx through the *oropharyngeal isthmus (isthmus of fauces)* which is bounded superiorly by the soft palate, inferiorly by the tongue, and on each side by the palatoglossal arches.

2 The sublingual region presents the following features:
   a. In the median plane, there is a fold of mucosa passing from the inferior aspect of the tongue to the floor of the mouth. This is the *frenulum* of the tongue.
   b. On each side of the frenulum, there is a *sublingual papilla*. On the summit of this papilla, there is the opening of submandibular duct.
   c. Running laterally and backwards from the *sublingual papilla*, there is the sublingual fold which overlies the sublingual gland. A few sublingual ducts open on the edge of this fold.

3 *Lymphatics* from the anterior part of the floor of the mouth pass to the submental nodes. Those from the hard palate and soft palate pass to the retropharyngeal and upper deep cervical nodes. The gums and the rest of the floor drain into the submandibular nodes.

Gums (Gingivae)

1 The gums are the soft tissues which envelop the alveolar processes of the upper and lower jaws and surround the necks of the teeth. These are composed of dense fibrous tissue covered by stratified squamous epithelium.

2 Each gum has two parts:
   a. The free part surrounds the neck of the tooth like a collar.
   b. The *attached part* is firmly fixed to the alveolar arch of the jaw. The fibrous tissue of the gum is continuous with the periosteum lining the alveoli (periodontal membrane).

3 Nerve supply of gums is shown in Table 22.1.

Table 22.1: Nerve supply of gums

Upper gums	*Nerve supply*
Labial side (Fig. 22.4)	Posterior, middle and anterior superior alveolar nerves (V2)
Lingual side (*see* Fig. 23.16)	Anterior palatine and nasopalatine nerves (from pterygopalatine ganglion)
Lower gums	
Labial side	Buccal branch of mandibular and incisive branch of mental nerve (V3)
Lingual side	Lingual nerve (V3)

4 *Lymphatics* of the upper gums pass to the submandibular nodes. The anterior part of the lower gums drains into the submental nodes, whereas the posterior part drains into the submandibular nodes.

CLINICAL ANATOMY

Ludwig's angina is the cellulitis of the floor of the mouth. The tongue is forced upwards leading to swelling both below the chin and within the mouth. The disease is usually caused due to a carious molar tooth.

TEETH

The teeth form part of the masticatory apparatus and are fixed to the jaws. In man, the teeth are replaced only once *(diphyodont)* in contrast with non-mammallian vertebrates where teeth are constantly replaced throughout life (*polyphyodont*). The teeth of the first set (dentition) are known as *milk*, or *deciduous teeth*, and the second set, as *permanent teeth*.

The deciduous teeth are 20 in number. In each half of each jaw, there are two incisors, one canine, and two molars.

The permanent teeth are 32 in number, and consist of two incisors (Latin *to cut*), one canine (Latin *dog*), two premolars (Latin *millstone*), and three molars in each half of each jaw (Fig. 22.2).

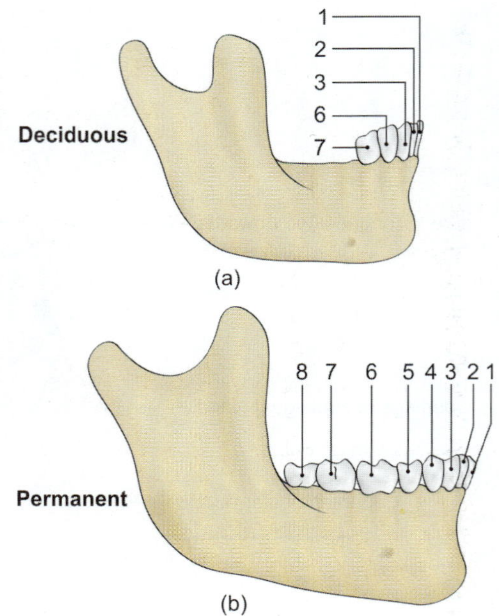

Figs 22.2a and b: Deciduous and permanent teeth. (1) Central incisor; (2) Lateral incisor; (3) Canine; (4) 1st premolar; (5) 2nd premolar; (6) 1st molar; (7) 2nd molar; (8) 3rd molar

Parts of a Tooth

Each tooth has three parts:

1 A *crown*, projecting above or below the gum.
2 A *root*, embedded in the jaw beneath the gum.
3 A *neck*, between the crown and root and surrounded by the gum (Fig. 22.3).

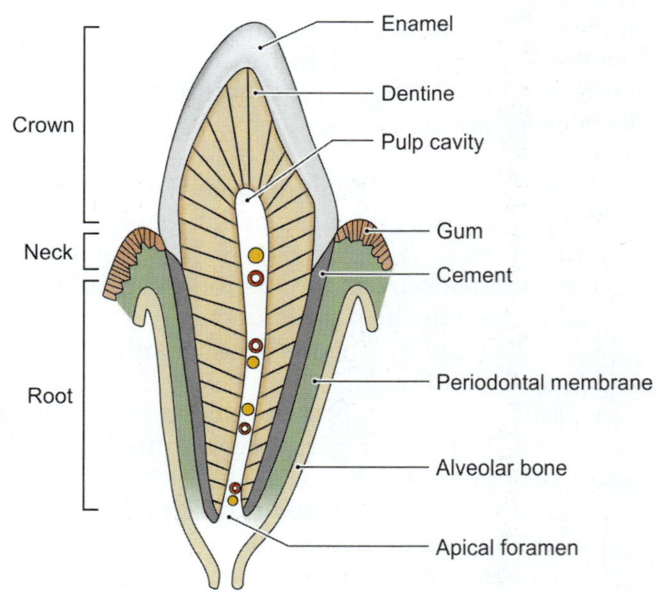

Fig. 22.3: Parts of a tooth

Structure

Structurally, each tooth is composed of:

1 The pulp in the centre
2 The dentine surrounding the pulp.
3 The enamel covering the projecting part of dentine, or crown.
4 The cementum surrounding the embedded part of the dentine.
5 The periodontal membrane.

The *pulp* is loose fibrous tissue containing vessels, nerves and lymphatics, all of which enter the pulp cavity through the apical foramen. The pulp is covered by a layer of tall columnar cells, known as *odontoblasts* which are capable of replacing dentine any time in life.

The *dentine* is a calcified material containing spiral tubules radiating from the pulp cavity. Each tubule is occupied by a protoplasmic process from one of the odontoblasts. The calcium and organic matter are in the same proportion as in bone.

The *enamel* is the hardest substance in the body. It is made up of crystalline prisms lying roughly at right angles to the surface of the tooth.

The *cementum* resembles bone in structure, but like enamel and dentine, there is neither any blood supply nor any nerve supply. Over the neck, the cementum commonly overlaps the cervical end of enamel; or, less commonly, it may just meet the enamel. Rarely, it stops short of the enamel (10%) leaving the cervical dentine covered only by gum.

The *periodontal membrane (ligament)* holds the root in its socket. This membrane acts as a periosteum to both the cementum as well as the bony socket.

Form and Function (Crowns and Roots)

1 The shape of a tooth is adapted to its function. The *incisors are cutting teeth,* with chisel-like crowns. The upper and lower incisors overlap each other like the blades of a pair of scissors. *The canines are holding and tearing teeth,* with conical and rugged crowns. These are better developed in carnivores. Each *premolar* has two cusps and is, therefore, also called a *bicuspid* tooth. The *molars are grinding teeth,* with square crowns, bearing four or five cusps on their crowns.

2 The incisors, canines and premolars have single roots, with the exception of the first upper premolar which has a bifid root. The upper molars have three roots, of which two are lateral and one is medial. The lower molars have only two roots—an anterior and a posterior.

Eruption of Teeth

The *deciduous teeth* begin to erupt at about the sixth month, and all get erupted by the end of the second year or soon after. The teeth of the lower jaw erupt slightly earlier than those of the upper jaw. The approximate ages of eruption of deciduous and permanent teeth are given in Table 22.2. Blood supply of teeth—both upper and lower are supplied by branches of maxillary artery.

Nerve Supply of Teeth

The pulp and periodontal membrane have the same nerve supply which is as follows:

The *upper teeth* are supplied by the posterior superior alveolar, middle superior alveolar, and the anterior superior alveolar nerves (maxillary nerve).

Table 22.2: Usual time of eruption of teeth and time of shedding of deciduous teeth

Tooth	*Eruption time*	*Shedding time*
Deciduous (Fig. 22.2a)		
Medial incisor	6–8 months	6–7 years
Lateral incisor	8–10 months	7–8 years
First molar	12–16 months	8–9 years
Canine	16–20 months	10–12 years
Second molar	20–24 months	10–12 years
Permanent (Fig. 22.2b)		
First molar	6–7 years	
Medial incisor	7–8 years	
Lateral incisor	8–9 years	
First premolar	10–11 years	
Second premolar	11–12 years	
Canine	12–13 years	
Second molar	13–14 years	
Third molar	17–25 years	

The *lower teeth* are supplied by the inferior alveolar nerve (mandibular nerve) (Fig. 22.4).

CLINICAL ANATOMY

- Being the hardest and chemically the most stable tissues in the body, the teeth are selectively preserved after death and may be fossilized. Because of this, the teeth are very helpful in medicolegal practice for identification of otherwise unrecognizable dead bodies. The teeth also provide by far the best data to study evolutionary changes and the relationship between ontogeny and phylogeny.
- In scurvy (caused by deficiency of vitamin C), the gums are swollen and spongy, and bleed on touch. In gingivitis, the edges of the gums are red and bleed easily.
- Improper oral hygiene may cause gingivitis and suppuration with pocket formation between the teeth and gums. This results in a chronic pus discharge at the margin of the gums. The condition is known as *pyorrhoea alveolaris* (chronic periodontitis). Pyorrhoea is common cause of foul breath for which the patient hardly ever consults a dentist because the condition is painless.
- Decalcification of enamel and dentine with consequent softening and gradual destruction of the tooth is known as *dental caries*. A caries tooth is tender on mastication.
- Infection of apex of root (apical abscess) occurs only when the pulp is dead. The condition can be recognized in a good radiograph.

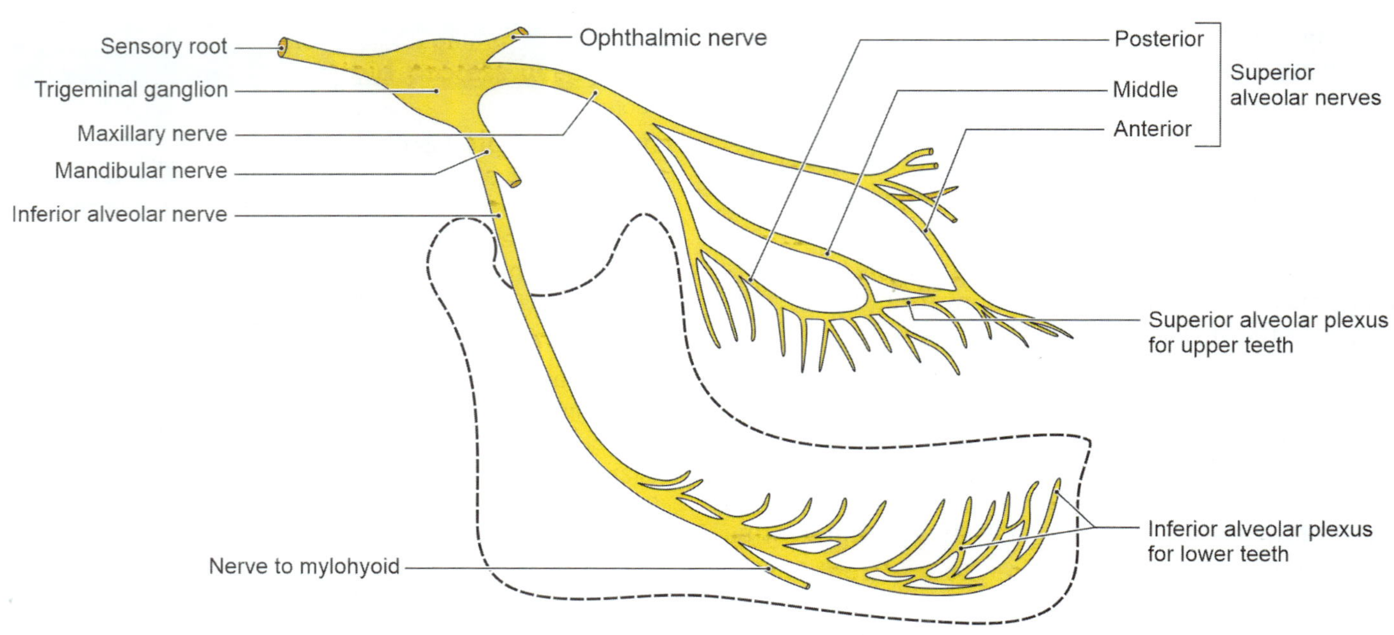

Fig. 22.4: Nerve supply of teeth

- Irregular dentition is common in rickets and the upper permanent incisors may be notched, the notching corresponds to a small segment of a large circle. Even in congenital syphilis, the same teeth are notched, but the notching corresponds to a large segment of a small circle (*Hutchinson's teeth*).
- The third molar teeth, also called *wisdom teeth,* usually erupt between 18 and 20 years. These may not erupt normally due to less space and may get impacted causing enormous pain.
- Time of eruption of the teeth helps in assessing the age of the person.
- The upper canine teeth are called as the 'eye teeth' as these have long roots which reach up to the medial angle of the eye. Infection of these roots may spread in the facial vein and even lead to thrombosis of the cavernous sinus.
- The upper teeth need separate injections of the anaesthetic on both the buccal and palatal surfaces of the maxillary process just distal to the tooth. The thin layer of bone permits rapid diffusion of the drug up to the tooth.

STAGES OF DEVELOPMENT OF DECIDUOUS TEETH

1. By 6th week of development, the epithelium covering the convex border of alveolar process of upper and lower jaws becomes thickened to form C-shaped dental lamina, which projects into the underlying mesoderm.
2. Dental laminae of upper and lower jaws develop 10 centres of proliferation from which dental buds grow into underlying mesenchyme. This is the *bud stage* (Figs 22.5a and b).
3. The deeper enlarged parts of the tooth bud is called *enamel organ*.
4. The enamel organ of dental bud is invaginated by mesenchyme of dental papilla making it cap-shaped. This is the *cap stage* (Fig. 22.5c).

   The dental papilla together with enamel organ is known as the tooth germ. The cell of enamel organ adjacent to dental papilla cells get columnar and are known as *ameloblasts*.

The mesenchymal cells now arrange themselves along the ameloblasts and are called odontoblasts. The two cell layers are separated by a basement membrane. The rest of the mesenchymal cells form the 'pulp of the tooth'. This is the *bell stage* (Fig. 22.5d).

Now ameloblasts lay enamel on the outer aspect, while odontoblasts lay dentine on the inner aspect. Later ameloblasts disappear while odontoblasts remain.

The root of the tooth is formed by laying down of layers of dentine, narrowing the pulp space to a canal for the passage of nerve and blood vessels only (Fig. 22.5e). The dentine in the root is covered by mesenchymal cells which differentiate into cementoblasts for laying down the cementum. Outside, this is the periodontal ligament connecting root to the socket in the bone.

Ectoderm forms enamel of tooth. Neural crest cells form dentine, dental pulp, cementum and periodontal ligament.

Formation of permanent teeth: These develop from the dental buds arising from the dental lamina and lie on the medial side of each developing milk tooth.

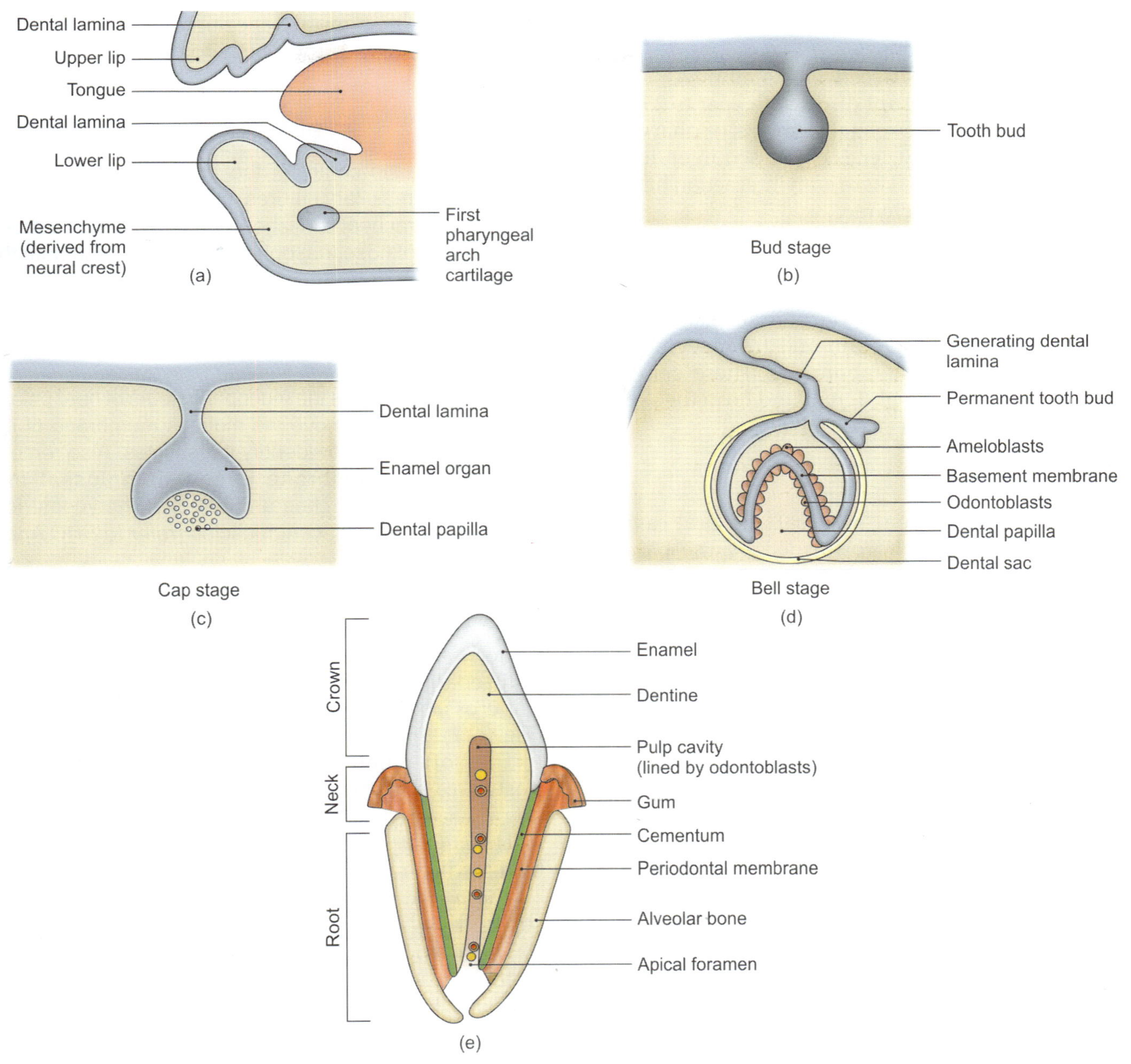

Figs 22.5a to e: Development of tooth

Molecular Regulation of Tooth Development

Tooth development is an example of epithelial–mesenchymal interaction. The mesenchyme is of neural-crest origin.

Tooth pattering from incisors to molars is an expression of HOX genes from mesenchyme. The epithelium causes differentiation to the bud stage. Then the mesenchyme causes the crest of the development. Various factors needed are WNTs, bone morphogenetic proteins, BMP and fibroblast growth factors (FGFs). The transcription factors are MSX1 and 2 which interact to produce cell differentiation of each tooth.

Teeth may also be having a 'signaling centre' like an organizer. This organizer region is called 'enamel knot' and appears in the dental epithelium at the tips of the tooth buds. This enamel knot enlarges at the 'cap stage' but disappears at the end of this stage. During the time of presence of the enamel knot, it expresses SHH, FGF4 and BMP2 and 4. FGF4 could be regulating outgrowth of cusps; while BMP4 may regulate timing of apoptosis in the knot cells. Many factors affect tooth development, including genetic and environmental factors.

Enamel—ameloblasts lies on a thick layer of dentine.

Dentine—odontoblasts—neural crest derivative

Cementum—cementoblast; mesenchymal derivative found in the root of teeth.

Milk teeth—erupt between 6 to 24 months

Permanent teeth—erupt during 6th year to 25 years

Pharyngeal arches: Skeletal elements of pharyngeal arches are regulated by genes expressed in endoderm of pharyngeal pouches. There is an interaction between epithelium and mesenchyme.

Mesenchyme expression of genes is determined by homeodomain containing transcription factors OTX2 and HOX genes carried to pharyngeal arches by migrating neural crest cells. The neural crest cells arise from caudal part of midbrain and from segments in hindbrain known as rhombomeres. These genes are controlled by endodermal signals and form the skeletal elements from the respective arches.

HARD PALATE

It is a partition between the nasal and oral cavities. Its anterior two-thirds are formed by the palatine processes of the maxillae; and its posterior one-third by the horizontal plates of the palatine bones (Fig. 22.6).

The *anterolateral margins* of the palate are continuous with the alveolar arches and gums.

The *posterior margin* gives attachment to the soft palate.

The *superior surface* forms the floor of the nose.

The *inferior surface* forms the roof of the oral cavity.

Vessels and Nerves

Arteries: Greater palatine branch of maxillary artery (*see* Figs 14.6 and 14.7).

Veins: Drain into the pterygoid plexus of veins.

Nerves: Greater palatine and nasopalatine branches of the pterygopalatine ganglion suspended by the maxillary nerve.

Lymphatics: The lymphatics drain mostly to the upper deep cervical nodes and partly to the retropharyngeal nodes.

DISSECTION

Cut through the centre of the frontal bone, internasal suture, intermaxillary sutures, chin, hyoid bone, thyroid, cricoid and tracheal cartilages; carry the incision through the septum of nose, nasopharynx, tongue, and both the palates.

Cut through the centre of the remaining occipital bone and cervical vertebrae. This will complete the *sagittal section of head and neck*.

Hard palate: Strip the mucoperiosteum of hard palate.

Soft palate: Remove the mucous membrane of the soft palate in order to identify its muscles. Also remove the mucous membrane over palatoglossal and palatopharyngeal arches and salpingopharyngeal fold to visualise the subjacent muscles *(refer to BDC App)*.

SOFT PALATE

It is a movable, muscular fold, suspended from the posterior border of the hard palate.

It separates the nasopharynx from the oropharynx, the crossroads between the food and air passages (Fig. 22.7).

The soft palate has two surfaces—anterior and posterior; and two borders—superior and inferior (Fig. 22.8a).

The *anterior (oral) surface* is concave and is marked by a median raphe.

The *posterior surface* is convex, and is continuous superiorly with the floor of the nasal cavity.

The *superior border* is attached to the posterior border of the hard palate, blending on each side with the pharynx (Figs 22.9a and b).

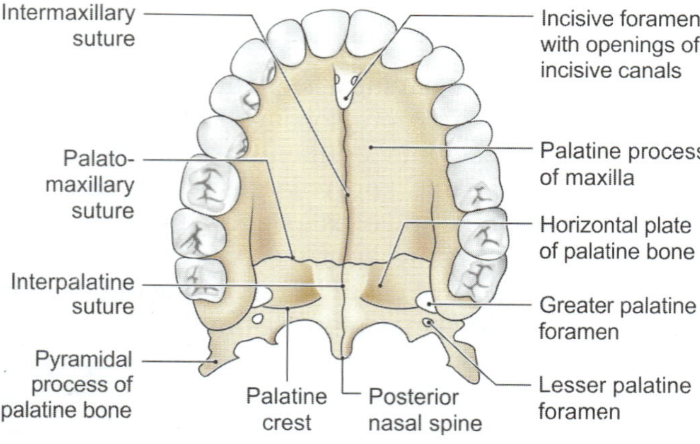

Fig. 22.6: Hard palate

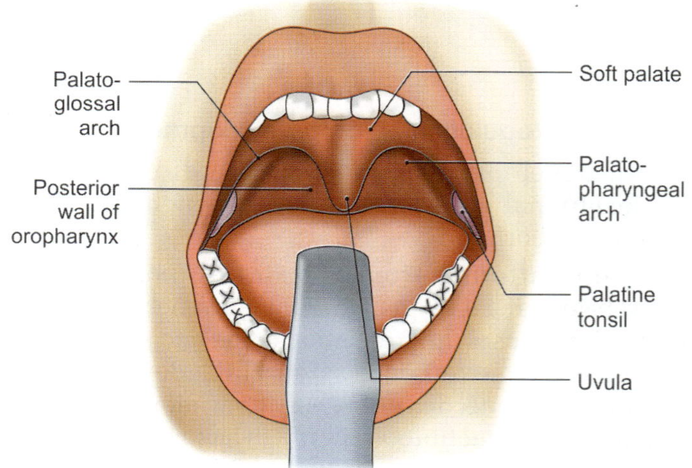

Fig. 22.7: Soft palate with palatine tonsils

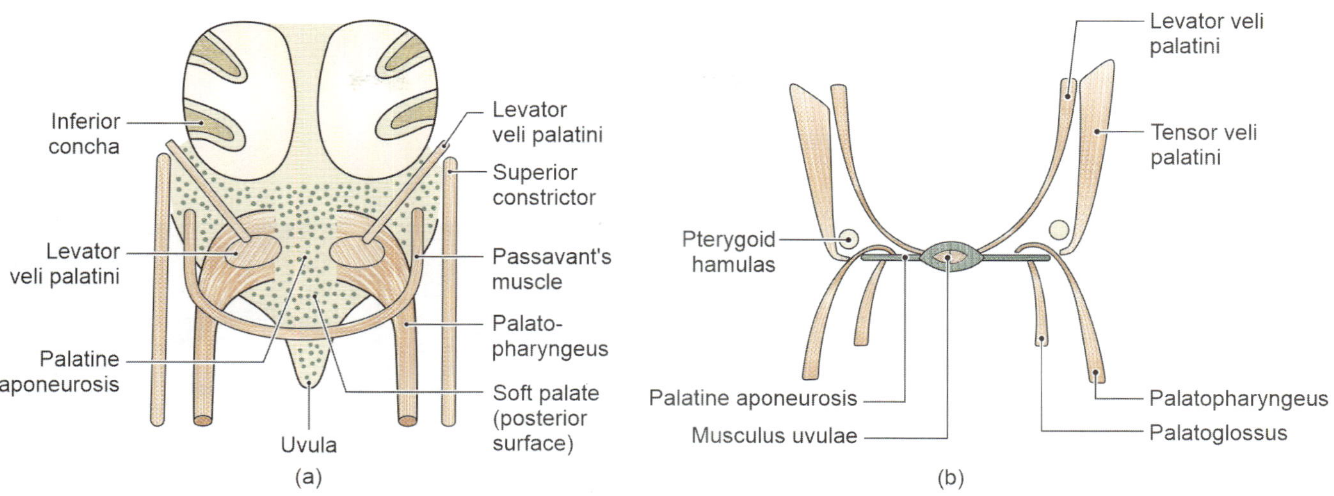

Figs 22.8a and b: (a) Attachment of the muscles of the soft palate; (b) Muscles of soft palate

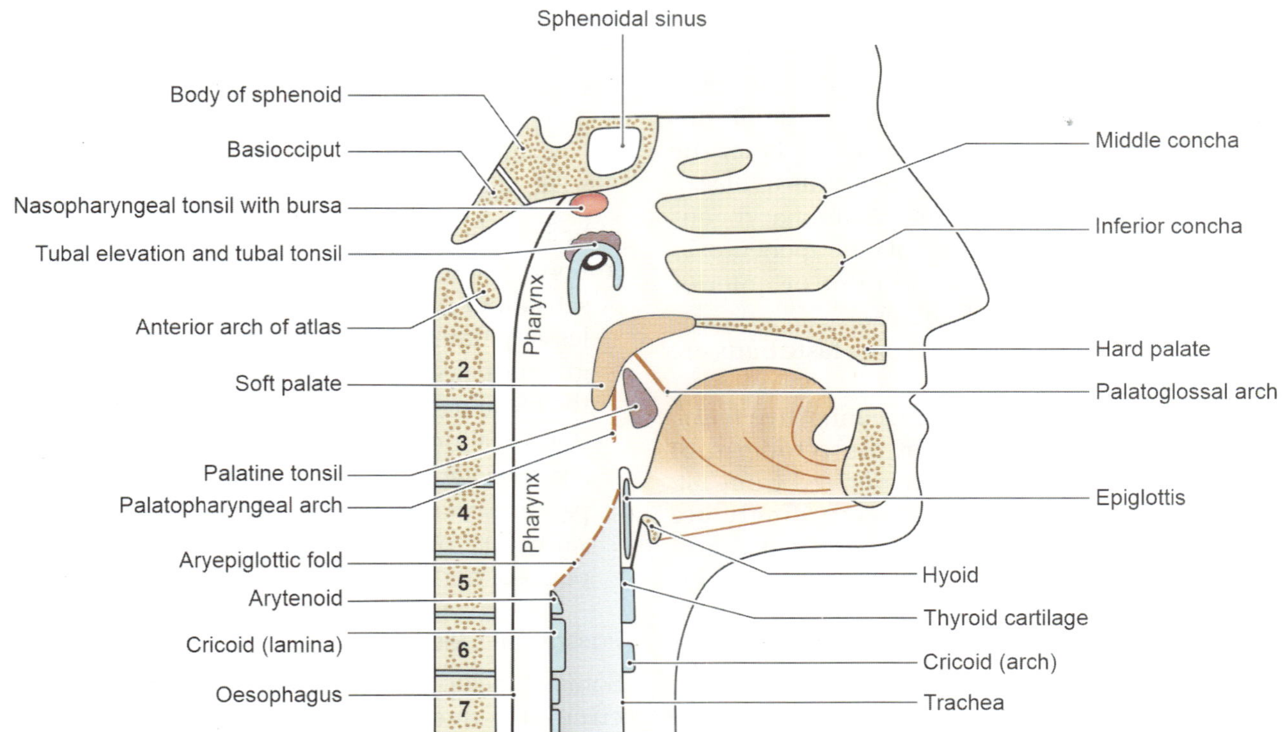

Fig. 22.9a: Sagittal section through the pharynx, the nose, the mouth and the larynx

The *inferior border* is free and bounds the pharyngeal isthmus. From its middle, there hangs a conical projection, called the uvula (Fig. 22.7). From each side of the base of the uvula (Latin *small grape*), two curved folds of mucous membrane extend laterally and downwards. The anterior fold is called the *palatoglossal arch* or anterior pillar of fauces. It contains the palatoglossus muscle and reaches the side of the tongue at the junction of its oral and pharyngeal parts. This fold forms the lateral boundary of the oropharyngeal isthmus or isthmus of fauces. The posterior fold is called the *palatopharyngeal* arch or posterior pillar of fauces. It contains the palatopharyngeus muscle. It forms the posterior boundary of the tonsillar fossa, and merges inferiorly with the lateral wall of the pharynx (Figs 22.8a and b).

Structure

The soft palate is a fold of mucous membrane containing the following parts.

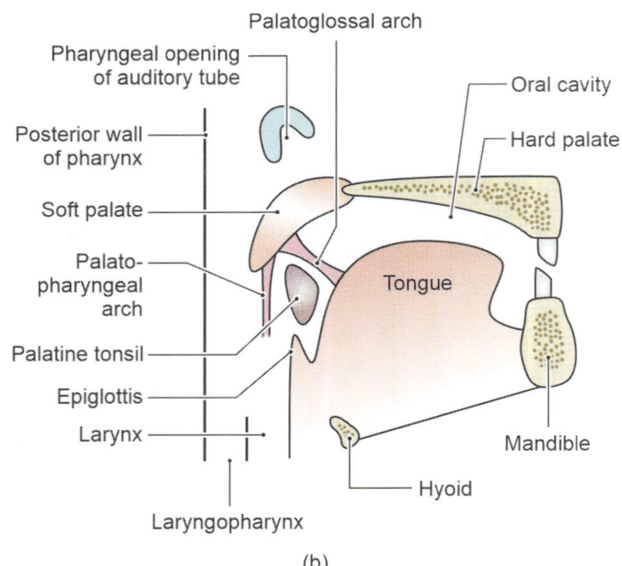

(b)

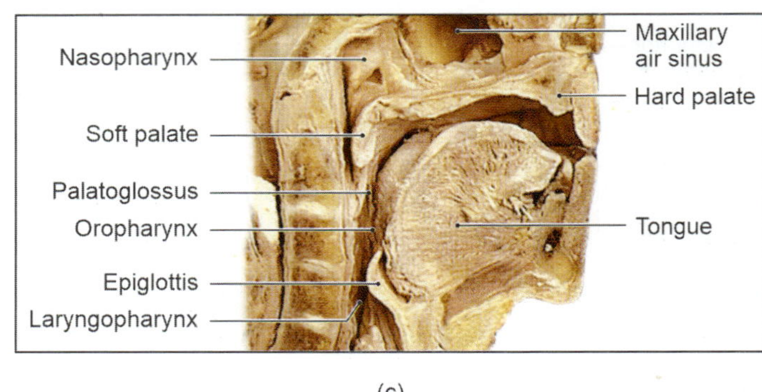

(c)

Fig. 22.9b and c: Sagittal section of pharynx

- The palatine aponeurosis which is the flattened tendon of the tensor veli palatini forms the fibrous basis of the palate. Near the median plane, the aponeurosis splits to enclose the musculus uvulae.
- The levator veli palatini and the palatopharyngeus lie on the superior surface of the palatine aponeurosis.
- The palatoglossus lies on the inferior or anterior surface of the palatine aponeurosis.
- Numerous mucous glands, and some taste buds are present.

Soft palate comprises epithelium, connective tissue and muscles. Epithelium is from the ectoderm of maxillary process. The muscles are derived from 1st, 4th and 6th branchial arches and accordingly are innervated by mandibular, superior laryngeal and recurrent laryngeal nerves.

Muscles of the Soft Palate

They are as follows:

1 Tensor palati (tensor veli palatini) (Figs 22.8a and b)
2 Levator palati (levator veli palatini)
3 Musculus uvulae
4 Palatoglossus
5 Palatopharyngeus.

Details of the muscles are given in Table 22.3.

Nerve Supply

1 *Motor nerves.* All muscles of the soft palate except the tensor veli palatini are supplied by the pharyngeal plexus. The fibres of this plexus are derived from the cranial part of the accessory nerve through the vagus. The tensor veli palatini is supplied by the mandibular nerve.
2 General *sensory nerves* are derived from:
   a. The middle and posterior lesser palatine nerves, which are branches of the maxillary nerve through the pterygopalatine ganglion (*see* Fig. 23.16).
   b. The glossopharyngeal nerve.
3 Special sensory or *gustatory nerves* carrying taste sensations from the oral surface are contained in the lesser palatine nerves. The fibres travel through the greater petrosal nerve to the geniculate ganglion of the facial nerve and from there to the nucleus of the tractus solitarius (Flowchart 22.1).
4 *Secretomotor nerves* are also contained in the lesser palatine nerves. They are derived from the superior salivatory nucleus and travel through the greater petrosal nerve (Flowchart 22.2).

Passavant's Ridge

Some of the upper fibres of the palatopharyngeus pass circularly deep to the mucous membrane of the pharynx, to form a sphincter internal to the superior constrictor. These fibres constitute Passavant's muscle which on contraction raises a ridge called the Passavant's ridge on the posterior wall of the naso-pharynx. When the soft palate is elevated it comes in contact with this ridge, the two together closing the pharyngeal isthmus between the nasopharynx and the oropharynx.

Morphology of Palatopharyngeus

In mammals with an acute sense of smell, the epiglottis lies above the level of the soft palate, and is supported by two vertical muscles (stylopharyngeus and

Table 22.3: Muscles of the soft palate			
Muscle	*Origin*	*Insertion*	*Actions*
1. **Tensor veli palatini** This is a thin, triangular muscle (Figs 22.8a and b)	a. Lateral side of auditory tube b. Adjoining part of the base of the skull (greater wing and scaphoid fossa of sphenoid bone)	Muscle descends, converges to form a delicate tendon which winds round the pterygoid hamulus, passes through the origin of the buccinator, and flattens out to form the palatine aponeurosis. Aponeurosis is attached to: a. Posterior border of hard palate b. Inferior surface of palate behind the palatine crest	a. Tightens the soft palate, chiefly the anterior part b. Opens the auditory tube to equalize air pressure between the middle ear and the nasopharynx
2. **Levator veli palatini** This is a cylindrical muscle that lies deep to the tensor veli palatini	a. Inferior aspect of auditory tube b. Adjoining part of inferior surface of petrous temporal bone	Muscle enters the pharynx by passing over the upper concave margin of the superior constrictor, runs downwards and medially and spreads out in the soft palate. It is inserted into the upper surface of the palatine aponeurosis	a. Elevates soft palate and closes the pharyngeal isthmus b. Opens the auditory tube-like the tensor veli palatini
3. **Musculus uvulae** This is a longitudinal strip placed on each side of the median plane, within the palatine aponeurosis	a. Posterior nasal spine b. Palatine aponeurosis	Mucous membrane of uvula	Pulls up the uvula
4. **Palatoglossus** (Figs 22.9a and b)	Oral surface of palatine aponeurosis	Descends in the palatoglossal arch, to the side of the tongue at the junction of its oral and pharyngeal parts	Pulls up the root of the tongue, approximates the palatoglossal arches, and thus closes the oropharyngeal isthmus
5. **Palatopharyngeus** It consists of two fasciculi that are separated by the levator veli palatini (also *see* Passavant's ridge)	a. Anterior fasciculus from posterior border of hard palate b. Posterior fasciculus from the palatine aponeurosis	Descends in the palatopharyngeal arch and spreads out to form the greater part of longitudinal muscle coat of pharynx. It is inserted into: a. Posterior border of the lamina of the thyroid cartilage b. Wall of the pharynx and its median raphe	Pulls up the wall of the pharynx and shortens it during swallowing

Flowchart 22.1: Gustatory nerves

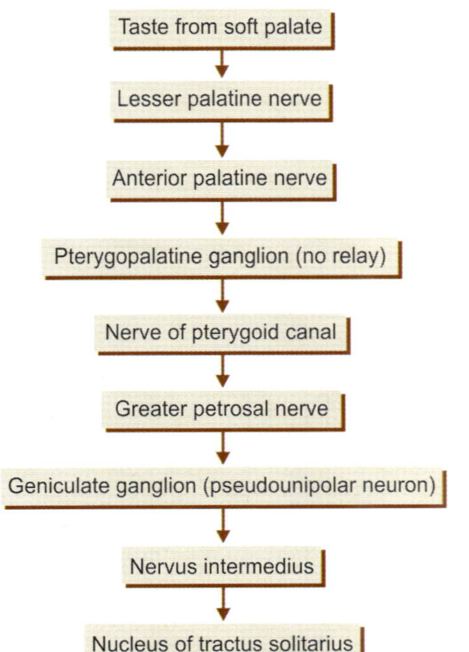

Flowchart 22.2: Secretomotor nerves

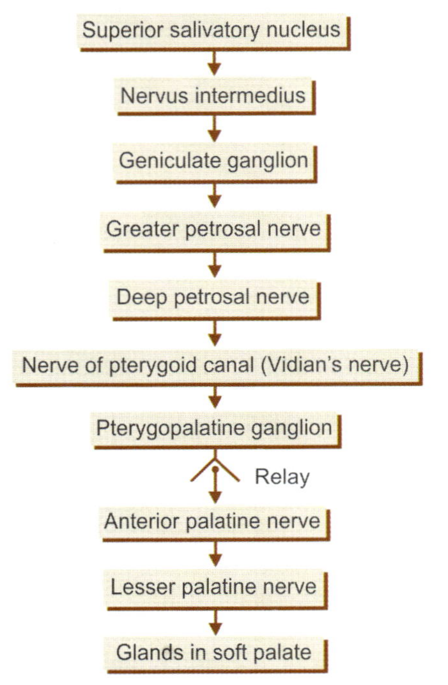

salpingopharyngeus) and by a sphincter formed by palatopharyngeus. The palatopharyngeal sphincter clasps the inlet of the larynx.

In man, the larynx descends and pulls the sphincter downwards leading to the formation of the human palatopharyngeus muscle. However, some fibres of the sphincter are left behind and form a sphincter inner to the superior constrictor at the level of the hard palate. These fibres constitute Passavant's muscle. Passavant's muscle is best developed in cases of cleft palate, as this compensates to some extent for the deficiency in the palate.

Movements and Functions of the Soft Palate

The palate controls two gates—upper airway or the pharyngeal isthmus and the upper food way or oropharyngeal isthmus. The upper airway crosses the upper food way (Figs 22.10a and b). The soft palate can completely close them, or can regulate their sizes according to requirements. Through these movements, the soft palate plays an important role in chewing, swallowing, speech, coughing, sneezing, etc. A few specific roles are given below.

1. It isolates the mouth from the oropharynx during chewing, so that breathing is unaffected.
2. It separates the oropharynx from the nasopharynx by locking Passavant's ridge during the second stage of swallowing, so that food does not enter the nose.
3. By varying the degree of closure of the pharyngeal isthmus, the quality of voice can be modified and various consonants are correctly pronounced.
4. During sneezing, the blast of air is appropriately divided and directed through the nasal and oral cavities without damaging the narrow nose. Similarly during coughing, it directs air and sputum into the mouth and not into the nose (Figs 22.10a and b).

Blood Supply

Arteries

1. Greater palatine branch of maxillary artery (*see* Fig. 14.6).
2. Ascending palatine branch of facial artery.
3. Palatine branch of ascending pharyngeal artery.

Veins

They pass to the pterygoid and tonsillar plexuses of veins.

Lymphatics

Drain into the upper deep cervical and retropharyngeal lymph nodes.

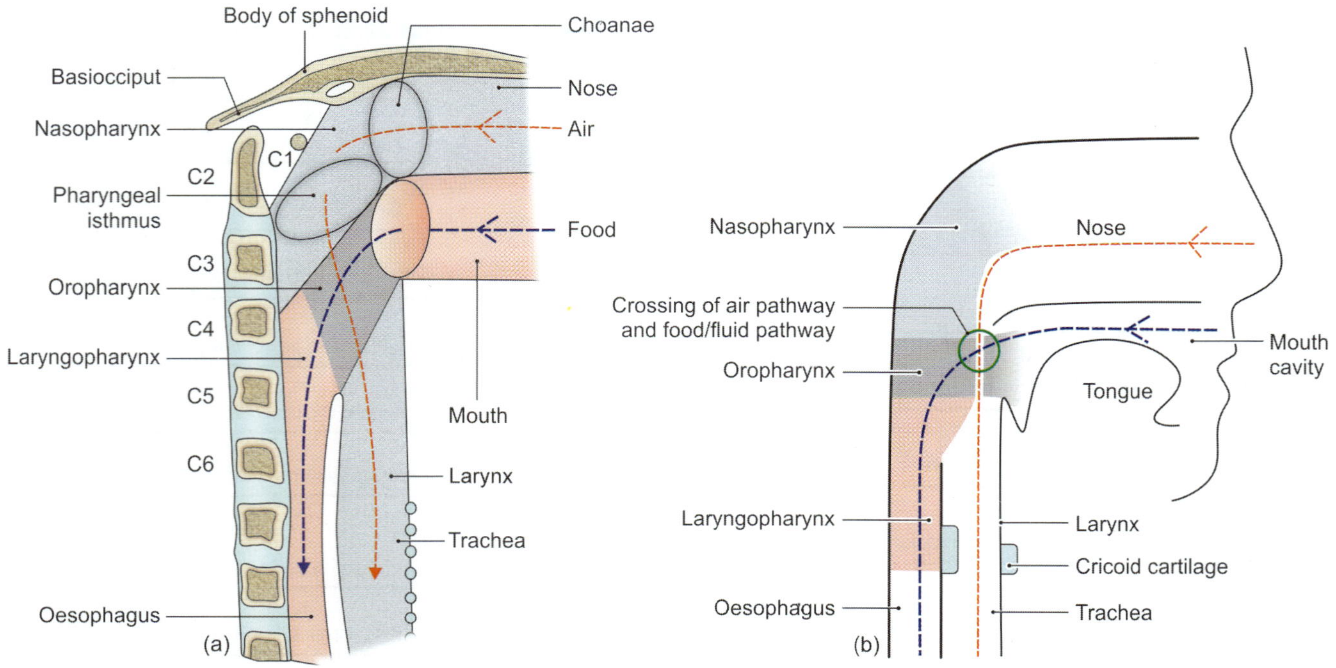

Figs 22.10a and b: Crossing of upper airway and upper food passages

CLINICAL ANATOMY

- Cleft palate is a congenital defect caused by non-fusion of the right and left palatal processes. It may be of different degrees. In the least severe type, the defect is confined to the soft palate. In the most severe cases, the cleft in the palate is continuous with harelip (Fig. 22.11).
- Paralysis of the soft palate in lesions of the vagus nerve produces:
  a. Nasal regurgitation of liquids
  b. Nasal twang in voice
  c. Flattening of the palatal arch
  d. Deviation of uvula to normal side (Fig. 22.12).
- Choking by food/fluid causes laryngeal obstruction and asphyxia. Heimlich maneuver can remove the obstruction.

Heimlich Manoeuvre

Stand behind the patient. Pass your arm under his arm. Put hand in his epigastrium; one hand made into a fist and other hand over fist. Give 3–4 abdominal thrusts directed upwards and backwards. This helps in squeezing residual air from lungs in trachea, and larynx, dislodges the foreign body and relieves laryngeal obstruction.

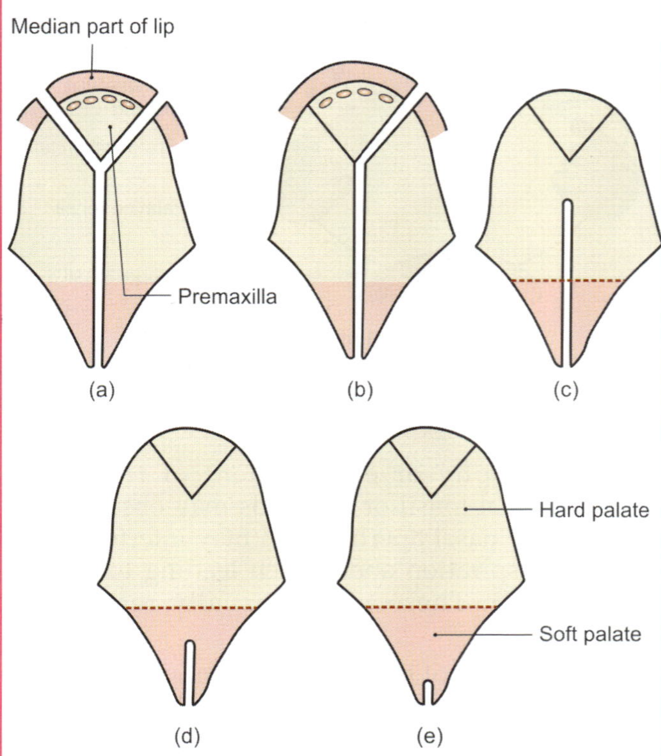

Figs 22.11a to e: Types of congenital cleft palate: (a) Bilateral complete; (b) Unilateral complete cleft palate; (c) Partial midline cleft; (d) Cleft of soft palate; (e) Bifid uvula

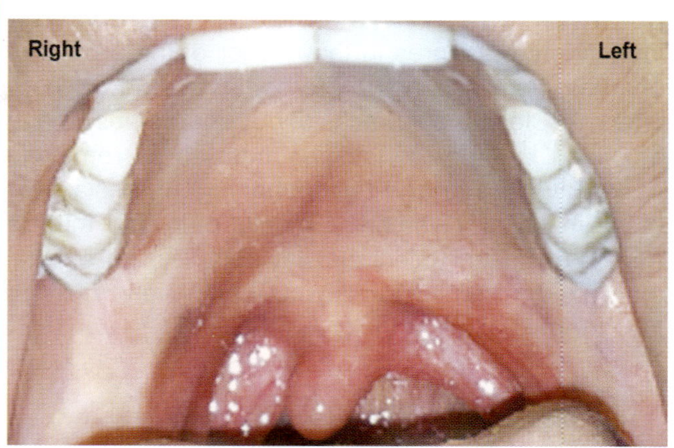

Fig. 22.12: Uvula deviated to right side in paralysis of left vagus nerve

DEVELOPMENT OF PALATE

The premaxilla or primitive palate carrying upper four incisor teeth is formed by the fusion of medial nasal folds, which are folds of frontonasal process.

The rest of the palate is formed by the shelf-like palatine processes of maxilla and horizontal plates of palatine bone. Most of the palate gets ossified to form the hard palate. The unossified posterior part of fused palatal processes forms the soft palate.

PHARYNX

The *pharynx* (Latin throat) is a wide muscular tube, situated behind the nose, the mouth and the larynx. Clinically, it is a part of the upper respiratory passages where infections are common. The upper part of the pharynx transmits only air, the lower part (below the inlet of the larynx), only food, but the middle part is a common passage for both air and food (Figs 22.9 and 22.10). The nasopharynx part of pharynx is connected to the middle ear via the pharyngotympanic tube.

Dimensions of Pharynx

Length: About 12 cm.

Width:

1. Upper part is widest (3.5 cm) and non-collapsible
2. Middle part is narrow
3. The lower end is the narrowest part of the gastro-intestinal tract (except for the vermiform).

DISSECTION

Identify the structures in the interior of three parts of pharynx, i.e. nasopharynx, oropharynx and laryngopharynx. Clean the surfaces of buccinator muscle and adjoining superior constrictor muscles by removing connective tissue and buccopharyngeal fascia over these muscles. Detach the medial pterygoid muscle from its origin and reflect it downwards. This will expose the superior constrictor muscle completely *(refer to BDC App)*.

Boundaries

Superiorly

Base of the skull, including the posterior part of the body of the sphenoid and the basilar part of the occipital bone, in front of the pharyngeal tubercle.

Inferiorly

The pharynx is continuous with the oesophagus at the level of the sixth cervical vertebra, corresponding to the lower border of the cricoid cartilage.

Posteriorly

The pharynx glides freely on the prevertebral fascia which separates it from the cervical vertebral bodies.

Anteriorly

It communicates with the nasal cavity, the oral cavity and the larynx. Thus, the anterior wall of the pharynx is incomplete.

On Each Side

1 The pharynx is attached to:
   a. Medial pterygoid plate
   b. Pterygomandibular raphe
   c. Mandible
   d. Tongue
   e. Hyoid bone
   f. Thyroid and cricoid cartilages.
2 It communicates on each side with the middle ear cavity through the auditory tube.
3 The pharynx is related on either side to:
   a. The styloid process and the muscles attached to it.
   b. The common carotid, internal carotid, and external carotid arteries, and the cranial nerves related to them.

Parts of the Pharynx

The cavity of the pharynx is divided into:

1 The nasal part—nasopharynx (Figs 22.9a and b)
2 The oral part—oropharynx (Table 22.3)
3 The laryngeal part—laryngopharynx (Fig. 22.18).

Comparison between nasopharynx, oropharynx and laryngopharynx shown in Table 22.4.

Waldeyer's Lymphatic Ring

In relation to the naso-oropharyngeal isthmus, there are several aggregations of lymphoid tissue that constitute Waldeyer's lymphatic ring (Fig. 22.13). The most important aggregations are the right and left palatine tonsils usually referred to simply as the tonsils. Posteriorly and above, there is the nasopharyngeal tonsil; laterally and above, there are the tubal tonsils, and inferiorly, there is the lingual tonsil over the posterior part of the dorsum of the tongue.

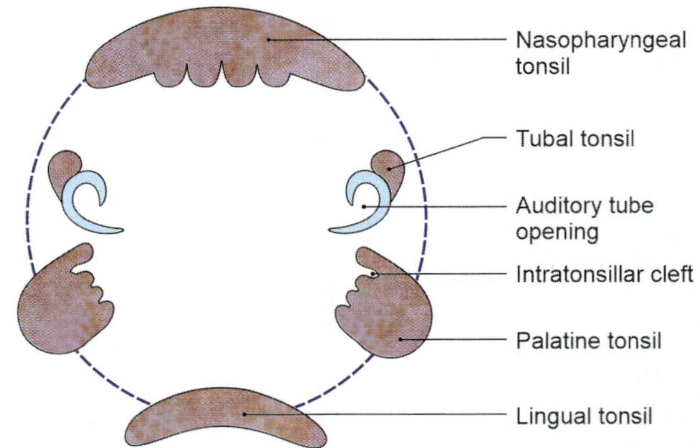

Fig. 22.13: Waldeyer's lymphatic ring

CLINICAL ANATOMY

- Hypertrophy or enlargement of the nasopharyngeal tonsil or adenoids may obstruct the posterior nasal aperture and may interfere with nasal respiration and speech leading to mouth breathing. These tonsils usually regress by puberty.
- Hypertrophy of the tubal tonsil may occlude the auditory or pharyngotympanic tube leading to middle ear problems.

Table 22.4: Comparison between nasopharynx, oropharynx and laryngopharynx

Particulars	*Nasopharynx*	*Oropharynx*	*Laryngopharynx*
a. Situation	Behind nose	Behind oral cavity	Behind larynx
b. Extent	Base of skull (body of sphenoid) to soft palate	Soft palate to upper border of epiglottis (Figs 22.9a and b)	Upper border of epiglottis to lower border of cricoid cartilage
c. Communications	Anteriorly with nose (Fig. 22.9a) Below with oropharynx	1. Anteriorly with oral cavity 2. Above with nasopharynx 3. Below with laryngopharynx	Inferiorly with oesophagus Anteriorly with larynx (Fig.22.9b) Above with oropharynx
d. Nerve supply	Pharyngeal branches of pterygopalatine ganglion	IX and X nerves	IX and X nerves
e. Relations:			
i. Anterior	Posterior nasal aperture	Oral cavity	1. Inlet of larynx 2. Posterior surface of cricoid cartilage 3. Arytenoid cartilage
ii. Posterior and roof	Body of sphenoid bone and basiocciput and anterior arch of atlas. Presence of: a. Nasopharyngeal tonsil prominent in children b. Nasopharyngeal bursa—mucus diverticulum	Body of second and third cervical vertebrae	Fourth and fifth cervical vertebrae
iii. Lateral wall	Opening of auditory tube above tube is tubal elevation with tubal tonsil	Tonsillar fossa containing palatine tonsils	Piriform fossa on each side of inlet of larynx, bounded by aryepiglottic fold medially and thyroid cartilage laterally.
f. Lining epithelium	Ciliated columnar epithelium	Stratified squamous nonkeratinised epithelium	Stratified squamous nonkeratinised epithelium
g. Function	Passage for air (respiratory function)	Passage for air and food	Passage for food

PALATINE TONSIL (THE TONSIL)

Features

The palatine tonsil (Latin *swelling*) occupies the tonsillar sinus or fossa between the palatoglossal and palatopharyngeal arches (Figs 22.7, 22.13 and 22.14). It can be seen through the mouth.

The tonsil is almond-shaped. It has two surfaces—medial and lateral; two borders—anterior and posterior; and two poles—upper and lower.

The *medial surface* is covered by stratified squamous epithelium continuous with that of the mouth. This surface has 12 to 15 crypts. The largest of these is called the *intratonsillar cleft* (Fig. 22.13).

The *lateral surface* is covered by a sheet of fascia which forms the hemicapsule of the tonsil. The capsule is an extension of the pharyngobasilar fascia. It is only loosely attached to the muscular wall of the pharynx, formed here by the superior constrictor and by the styloglossus, but anteroinferiorly the capsule is firmly adherent to the side of the tongue (suspensory ligament of tonsil) just in front of the insertion of the palatoglossus and the palatopharyngeus muscle. This firm attachment keeps the tonsil in place during swallowing (Fig. 22.15).

The tonsillar artery enters the tonsil by piercing the superior constrictor just behind the firm attachment (Fig. 22.15).

The palatine vein or external palatine or paratonsillar vein descends from the palate in the loose areolar tissue on the lateral surface of the capsule, and crosses the tonsil before piercing the wall of the pharynx. The vein may be injured during removal of the tonsil or tonsillectomy (Fig. 22.15).

The bed of the tonsil is formed from within outwards by:

a. The pharyngobasilar fascia (Fig. 22.14)
b. The superior constrictor and palatopharyngeus muscles
c. The buccopharyngeal fascia
d. In the lower part, the styloglossus
e. The glossopharyngeal nerve.

Still more laterally, there are the facial artery with its tonsillar and ascending palatine branches. The internal carotid artery is 2.5 cm posterolateral to the tonsil.

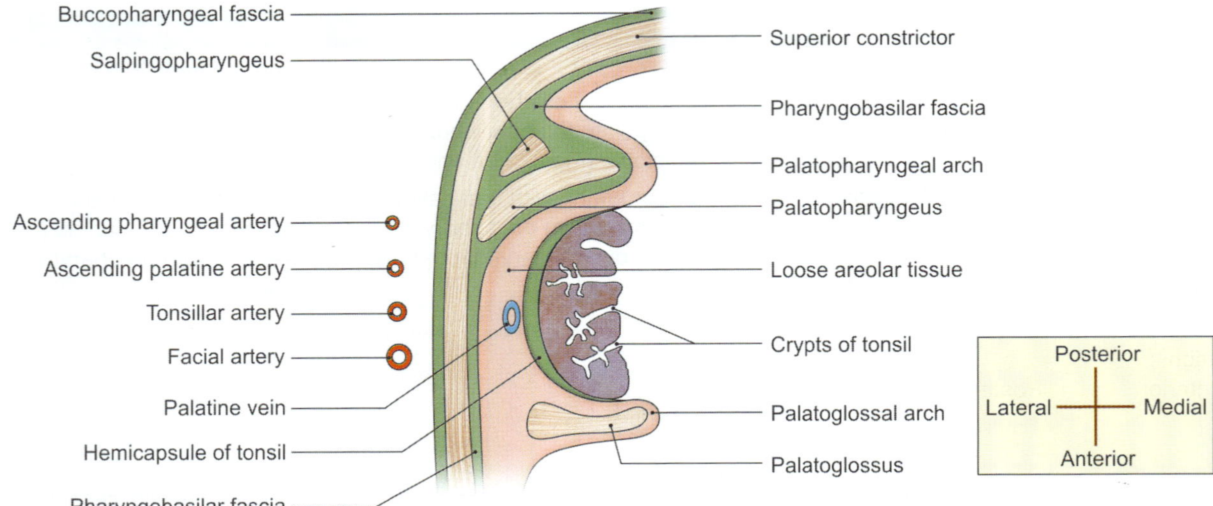

Fig. 22.14: Horizontal section through the tonsil showing its deep relations

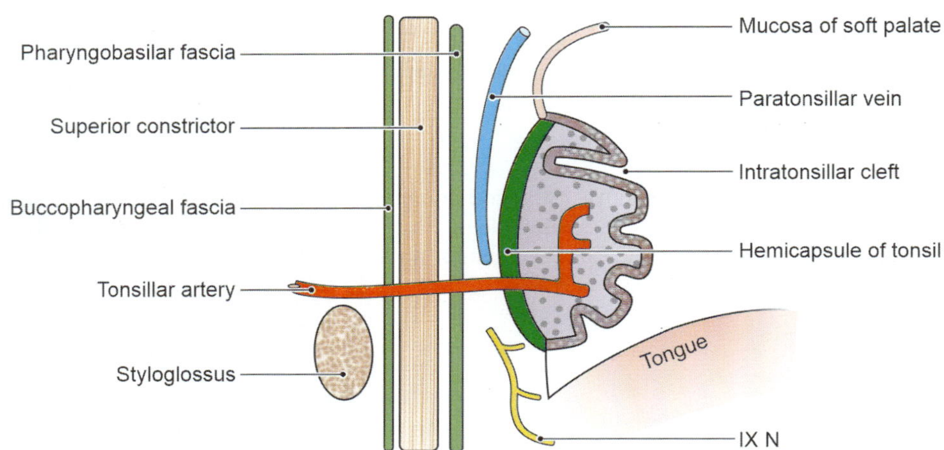

Fig. 22.15: Vertical section through the tonsil, showing its deep relations

The *anterior border* is related to the palatoglossal arch with its muscle (Fig. 22.7).

The *posterior border* is related to the palatopharyngeal arch with its muscle.

The *upper pole* is related to the soft palate, and the *lower pole*, to the tongue (Fig. 22.15).

The *plica triangularis* is a triangular vestigial fold of mucous membrane covering the anteroinferior part of the tonsil. The *plica semilunaris* is a similar semilunar fold that may cross the upper part of the tonsillar sinus.

The *intratonsillar cleft* is the largest crypt of the tonsil. It is present in its upper part (Fig. 22.13). It is sometimes wrongly named the supratonsillar fossa. The mouth of cleft is semilunar in shape and parallel to dorsum of tongue. It represents the internal opening of the second pharyngeal pouch. A peritonsillar abscess or quinsy often begins in this cleft.

Arterial Supply of Tonsil

1. Main source: Tonsillar branch of facial artery.
2. Additional sources:
   a. Ascending palatine branch of facial artery
   b. Dorsal lingual branches of the lingual artery
   c. Ascending pharyngeal branch of the external carotid artery
   d. The greater palatine branch of the maxillary artery (Fig. 22.16).

Venous Drainage

One or more veins leave the lower part of deep surface of the tonsil, pierce the superior constrictor, and join the palatine, pharyngeal, or facial veins.

Lymphatic Drainage

Lymphatics pass to jugulodigastric node (*see* Fig. 16.28).

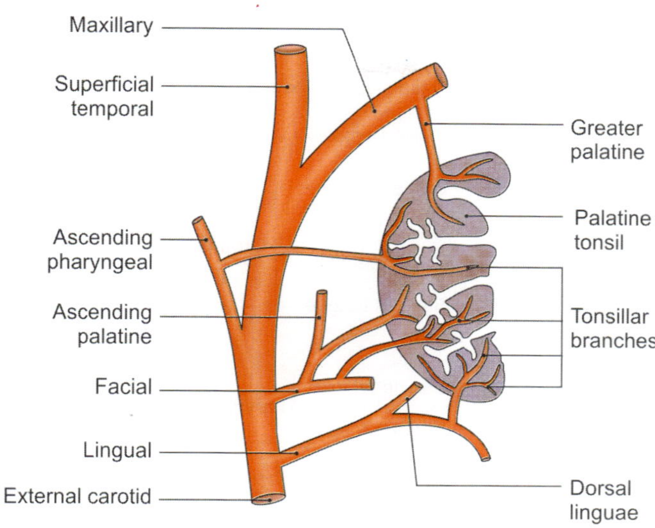

Fig. 22.16: Arterial supply of the palatine tonsil

There are no afferent lymphatics to the tonsil.

Nerve Supply

Glossopharyngeal and lesser palatine nerves.

CLINICAL ANATOMY

- The tonsils are large in children. They retrogress after puberty.
- The tonsils are frequently sites of infection, specially in children. Infection may spread to surrounding tissue forming a peritonsillar abscess.
- Enlarged and infected tonsils often require surgical removal. The operation is called *tonsillectomy*. A knowledge of the relationship of the tonsil is of importance to the surgeon.
- Tonsillectomy is usually done by the guillotine method. Haemorrhage after tonsillectomy is checked by removal of clot from the raw tonsillar bed. This is to be compared with the method for checking postpartum haemorrhage from the uterus. These are the only two organs in the body where bleeding is checked by removal of clots. In other parts of the body, clot formation is encouraged.
- Tonsillitis may cause referred pain in the ear as glossopharyngeal nerve supplies both these areas.
- Suppuration in the peritonsillar area is called *quinsy*. A peritonsillar abscess is drained by making an incision in the most prominent point of the abscess.
- Tonsils are often sites of a septic focus. Such a focus can lead to serious disease like pulmonary tuberculosis, meningitis, etc. and is often the cause of general ill health.

HISTOLOGY

The palatine tonsil is situated at the oropharyngeal isthmus. Its oral aspect is covered with stratified squamous nonkeratinised epithelium, which dips into the underlying tissue to form the crypts. The lymphocytes lie on the sides of the crypts in the form of nodules. The structure of tonsil is not differentiated into cortex and medulla (Fig. 22.17).

DEVELOPMENT

The tonsil develops from endoderm of ventral part of second pharyngeal pouch. Some part persists as the intratonsillar cleft. The lymphocytes are mesodermal in origin.

LARYNGEAL PART OF PHARYNX (LARYNGOPHARYNX)

This is the lower part of the pharynx situated behind the larynx. It extends from the upper border of the epiglottis to the lower border of the cricoid cartilage.

The *anterior wall* presents:

a. The inlet of the larynx (Fig. 22.18)
b. The posterior surfaces of the cricoid and arytenoid cartilages.

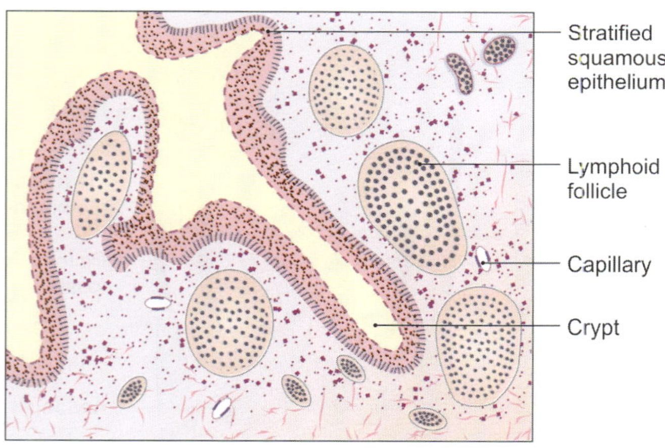

- Capsule shows stratified squamous non-keratinised epithelium on its oral aspect
- The epithelium forms crypts
- No differentiation into cortex and medulla

Fig. 22.17: Histology of palatine tonsil

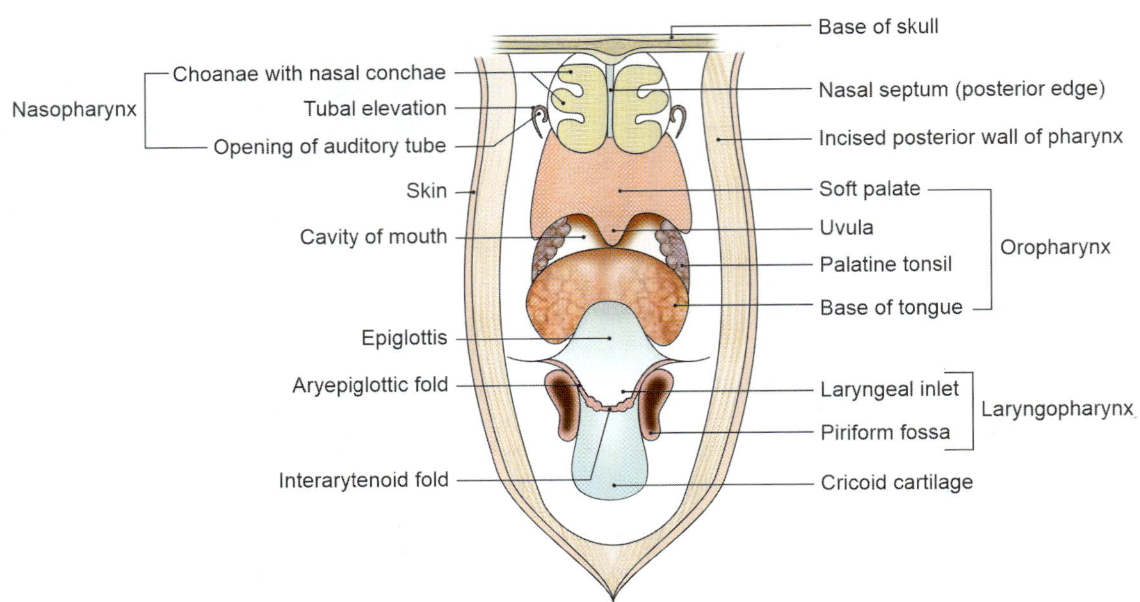

Fig. 22.18: The three regions of the pharynx

The *posterior wall* is supported mainly by the fourth and fifth cervical vertebrae, and partly by the third and sixth vertebrae. In this region, the posterior wall of the pharynx is formed by the superior, middle and inferior constrictors of the pharynx.

The *lateral wall* presents a depression called the *piriform fossa*, one on each side of the inlet of the larynx (Fig. 22.18). The fossa is bounded medially by the aryepiglottic fold, and laterally by the thyroid cartilage and the thyrohyoid membrane. Beneath the mucosa of fossa, there lies the internal laryngeal nerve. Removal of foreign bodies from the piriform fossa may damage the internal laryngeal nerve, leading to anaesthesia in the supraglottic part of the larynx (Fig. 22.19).

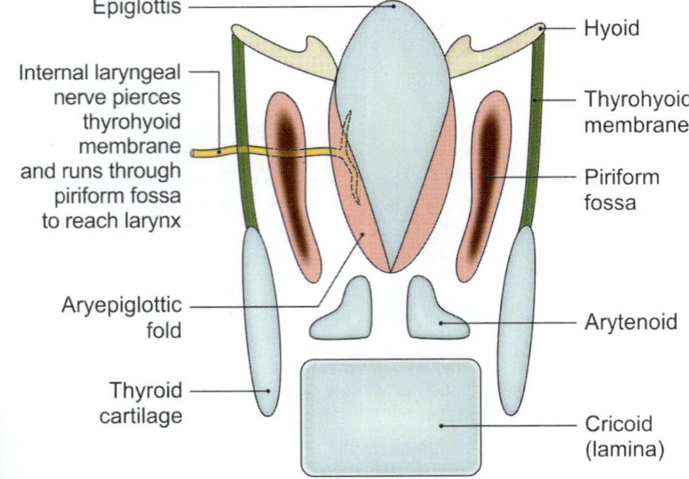

Fig. 22.19: Posterior view of the piriform fossa after removal of the tongue: Internal laryngeal nerve is shown only on left side

STRUCTURE OF PHARYNX

The wall of the pharynx is composed of the following five layers (Fig. 22.20) from within outwards.

1. *Mucosa*
2. *Submucosa*
3. *Pharyngobasilar fascia* or pharyngeal aponeurosis. This is a fibrous sheet internal to the pharyngeal muscles. It is thickest in the upper part where it fills the gap between the upper border of the superior constrictor and the base of the skull, and also posteriorly where it forms pharyngeal raphe. Superiorly, the fascia is attached to basiocciput, the petrous temporal bone, the auditory tube, posterior border of the medial pterygoid plate, and pterygomandibular raphe. Inferiorly, it is gradually lost deep to muscles, and hardly extend beyond the superior constrictor.
4. The *muscular coat* consists of an outer circular layer made up of the three constrictors (*superior, middle* and *inferior*) and an inner longitudinal layer made up of the stylopharyngeus, the salpingopharyngeus and the palatopharyngeus muscles. These muscles are described later.
5. The *buccopharyngeal fascia* covers the outer surface of the constrictors of the pharynx and extends forwards across the pterygomandibular raphe to cover the buccinator. Like the pharyngobasilar fascia, the buccopharyngeal fascia is best developed in the upper part of the pharynx.

Between the buccopharyngeal fascia and the muscular coat, there are the pharyngeal plexuses of veins and nerves (Fig. 22.20).

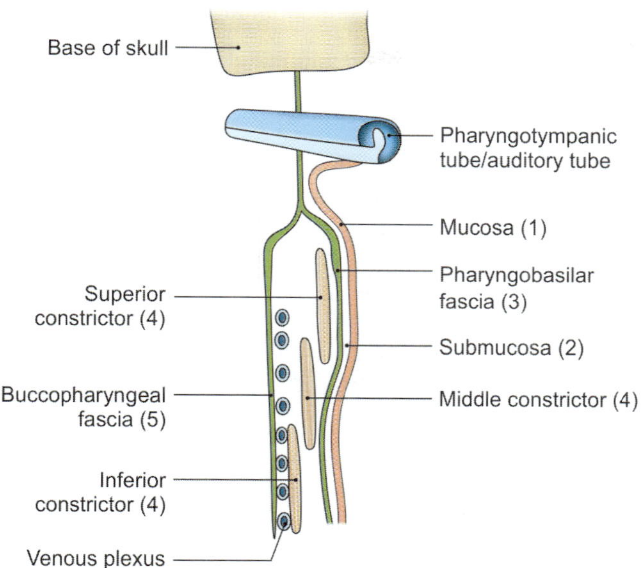

Fig. 22.20: Structure of the pharynx

MUSCLES OF THE PHARYNX (REFER TO BDC APP)

Preliminary Remarks about the Constrictors of the Pharynx

The muscular basis of the wall of the pharynx is formed mainly by the three pairs of constrictors—superior, middle and inferior. The origins of the constrictors are situated anteriorly in relation to the posterior openings of the nose—the mouth and the larynx. From here their fibres pass into the lateral and posterior walls of the pharynx, the fibres of the two sides meeting in the midline in a fibrous raphe.

The three constrictors are so arranged that the inferior overlaps middle which in turn overlaps the superior. The fibres of the superior constrictor reach the base of skull posteriorly, in the middle line. On the sides, however, there is a gap between the base of the skull and the upper edge of the superior constrictor. This gap is closed by the pharyngobasilar fascia which is thickened in this situation (Fig. 22.21). The lower edge of the inferior constrictor becomes continuous with the circular muscle of the oesophagus. These muscles develop from IV and VI pharyngeal arches (*see* Table A.5 in Appendix).

Origin of Constrictors

1 The *superior constrictor* takes origin (Fig. 22.21) from the following (from above downwards):
   a. Pterygoid hamulus (pterygopharyngeus)
   b. Pterygomandibular raphe (buccopharyngeus)
   c. Medial surface of the mandible at the posterior end of the mylohyoid line, i.e. near the lower attach-

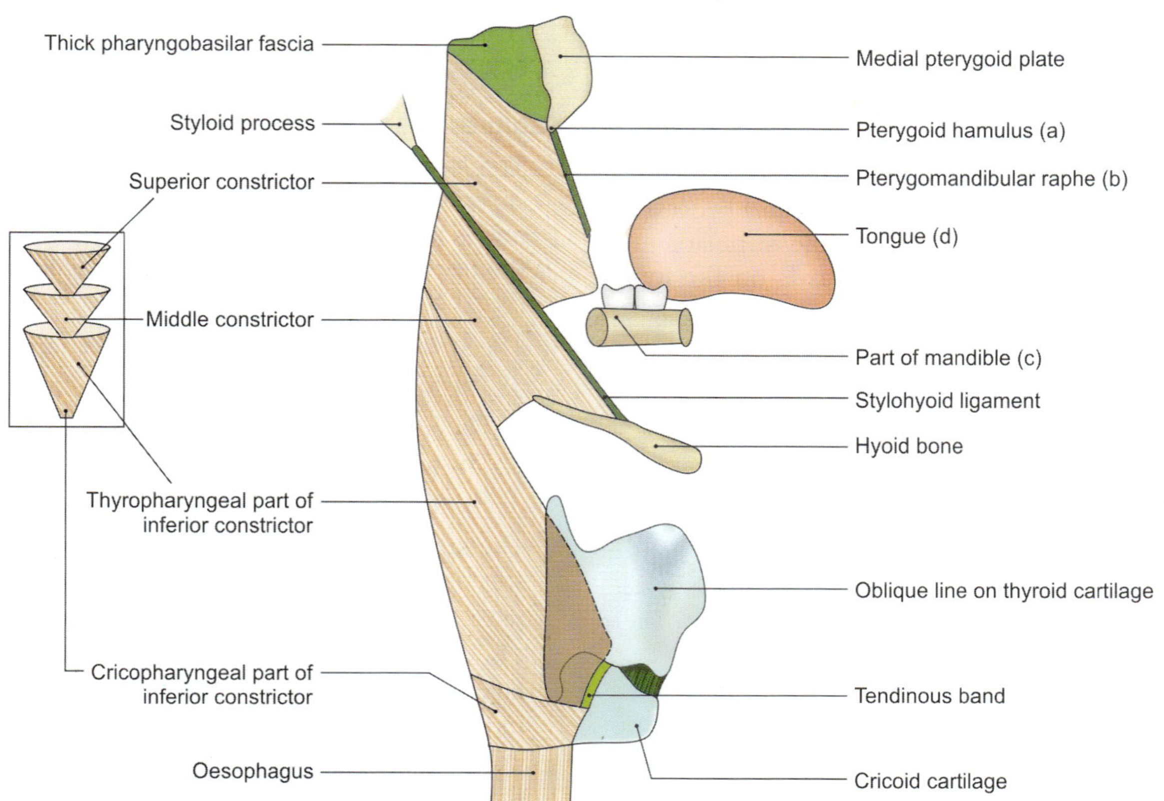

Fig. 22.21: Origin of the constrictors of the pharynx

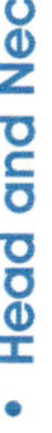

ment of the pterygomandibular raphe (*see* Fig. 9.25) (mylopharyngeus).

d. Side of posterior part of tongue (glossopharyngeus).

2 The *middle constrictor* takes origin from:

a. The lower part of the stylohyoid ligament

b. Lesser cornua of hyoid bone

c. Upper border of the greater cornua of the hyoid bone (*see* Fig. 9.47).

3 The *inferior constrictor* consists of two parts. One part, the *thyropharyngeus,* arises from the thyroid cartilage. The other part, the *cricopharyngeus,* arises from the cricoid cartilage.

The thyropharyngeus arises from:

a. The oblique line on the lamina of thyroid cartilage, including the inferior tubercle (Fig. 22.21).

b. A tendinous band that crosses the cricothyroid muscle and is attached above to the inferior tubercle of the thyroid cartilage.

c. The inferior cornua of the thyroid cartilage.

The cricopharyngeus arises from the cricoid cartilage behind the origin of the cricothyroid muscle.

Insertion of Constrictors

All the constrictors of the pharynx are inserted into a median raphe on the posterior wall of the pharynx. The upper end of the raphe reaches the base of the skull where it is attached to the pharyngeal tubercle on the basilar part of the occipital bone (Fig. 22.22).

Longitudinal Muscle Coat

The pharynx has three muscles that run longitudinally. The *stylopharyngeus* arises from the styloid process. It passes through the gap between the superior and middle constrictors to run downwards on the inner

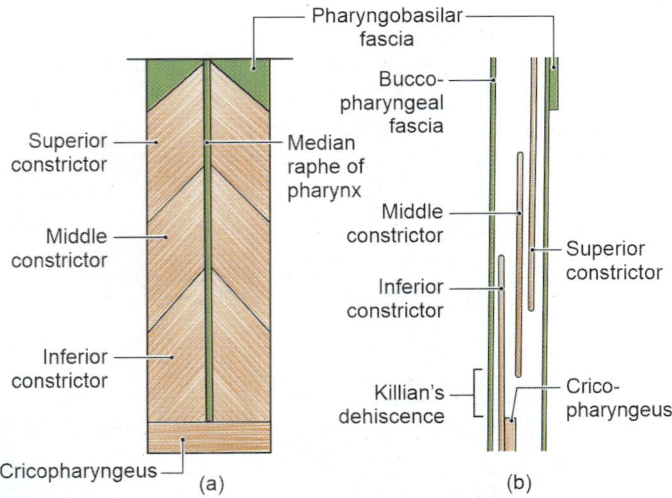

Fig. 22.22: Insertion of the constrictors of pharynx

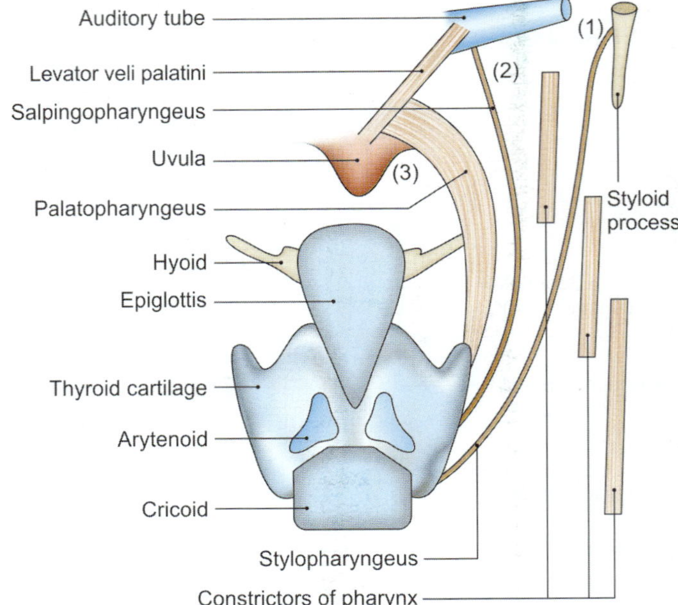

Fig. 22.23: Longitudinal muscles of pharynx: (1) Stylopharyngeus; (2) Salpingopharyngeus; (3) Palatopharyngeus

surface of the middle and inferior constrictors. The fibres of the *palatopharyngeus* descend from the sides of the palate and run longitudinally on the inner aspect of the constrictors (Fig. 22.23). The *salpingopharyngeus* descends from the auditory tube to merge with palatopharyngeus.

STRUCTURES IN BETWEEN PHARYNGEAL MUSCLES

Features

1 The *large gap between the upper concave border of the superior constrictor and the base of the skull* is semilunar and is known as the *sinus of Morgagni.* It is closed by the upper strong part of the pharyngobasilar fascia (Fig. 22.24).

The structures passing through this gap are:

a. The auditory tube

b. The levator veli palatini muscle

c. The ascending palatine artery (Fig. 22.24)

d. Palatine branch of ascending pharyngeal artery.

2 The structures passing through the *gap between the superior and middle constrictors* are: The stylopharyngeus muscle and the glossopharyngeal nerve.

3 The internal laryngeal nerve and the superior laryngeal vessels pierce the thyrohyoid membrane in the *gap between the middle and inferior constrictors.*

4 The recurrent laryngeal nerve and the inferior laryngeal vessels pass through the *gap between the lower border of the inferior constrictor and the oesophagus.*

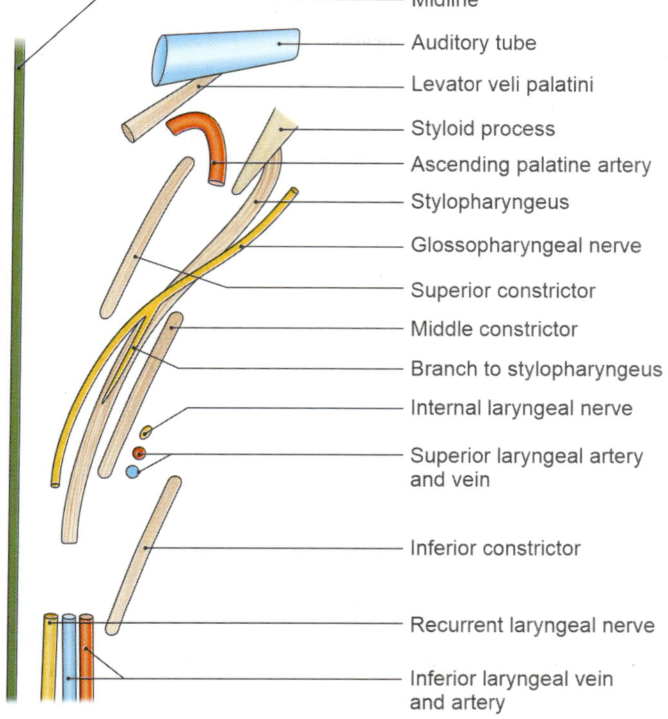

Fig. 22.24: Schematic coronal section through the pharynx, showing the gaps between pharyngeal muscles and the structures related to them

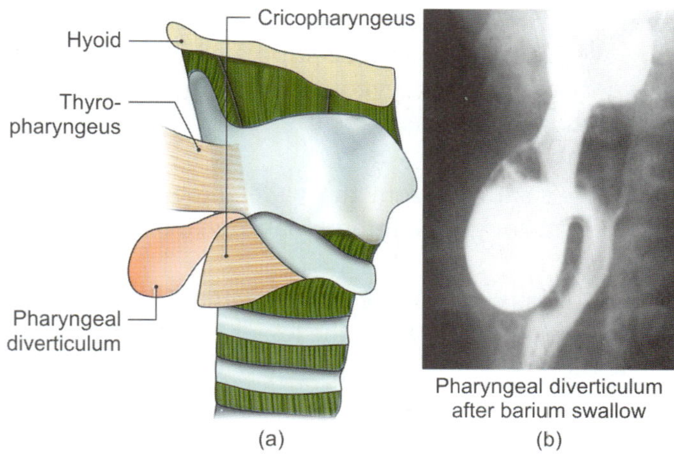

Figs 22.25a and b: (a) Pharyngeal diverticulum, and (b) pharyngeal diverticulum after barium swallow

DISSECTION

Define the attachments of middle and inferior constrictors of pharynx, and the structures situated traversing through the gaps between the three constrictor muscles. Identify structures above the superior constrictor muscle and below the inferior constrictor muscle.

Cut through the tensor veli palatini and reflect it downwards. Remove the fascia and identify the mandibular nerve again with otic ganglion medial to it. Identify the branches of the mandibular nerve. Locate the middle meningeal artery at the foramen spinosum, as it lies just posterior to mandibular nerve.

Killian's Dehiscence

In the posterior wall of the pharynx, the lower part of the thyropharyngeus is a single sheet of muscle, not overlapped internally by the superior and middle constrictors. This weak part lies below the level of the vocal folds or upper border of the cricoid lamina and is limited inferiorly by the thick cricopharyngeal sphincter. This area is known as *Killian's dehiscence*. Pharyngeal diverticula are formed by outpouching of the dehiscence (Figs 22.25a and b). Such diverticula are normal in the pig. Pharyngeal diverticula are often attributed to neuromuscular incoordination in this region which may be due to the fact that different nerves supply the two parts of the inferior constrictor (Fig. 22.22). The propulsive thyropharyngeus is supplied by the pharyngeal plexus, and sphincteric cricopharyngeus by the recurrent laryngeal nerve. If the cricopharyngeus fails to relax when the thyropharyngeus contracts, the bolus of food is pushed backwards, and tends to produce a diverticulum.

CLINICAL ANATOMY

- Difficulty in swallowing is known as dysphagia.
- *Pharyngeal diverticulum:* Read Killian's dehiscence (Fig. 22.25a).

NERVE SUPPLY OF PHARYNX

The pharynx is supplied by the pharyngeal plexus of nerves which lies chiefly on the middle constrictor. The plexus is formed by:

1. The pharyngeal branch of the vagus carrying fibres of the cranial accessory nerve.
2. The pharyngeal branches of the glossopharyngeal nerve.
3. The pharyngeal branches of the superior cervical sympathetic ganglion.

Motor fibres are derived from the cranial accessory nerve through the branches of the vagus. They supply all muscles of pharynx, except the stylopharyngeus which is supplied by the glossopharyngeal nerve.

The inferior constrictor receives an additional supply from the external and recurrent laryngeal nerves.

Sensory fibres or general visceral afferent from the pharynx travel mostly through the glossopharyngeal nerve, and partly through the vagus. However, the nasopharynx is supplied by the maxillary nerve through the pterygopalatine ganglion; and the soft palate and tonsil by the lesser palatine and glossopharyngeal nerves.

Taste sensations from the vallecula and epiglottic area pass through the internal laryngeal branch of the vagus.

The parasympathetic *secretomotor* fibres to the pharynx are derived from the lesser palatine branches of the pterygopalatine ganglion (*see* Fig. 23.15).

BLOOD SUPPLY OF PHARYNX

The arteries supplying the pharynx are almost the same as those supplying the tonsil. These are as follows:

1 Ascending pharyngeal branch of the external carotid artery.
2 Ascending palatine and tonsillar branches of the facial artery.
3 Dorsal lingual branches of the lingual artery.
4 The greater palatine, pharyngeal and pterygoid branches of the maxillary artery.

The veins form a plexus on the posterolateral aspect of the pharynx. The plexus receives blood from the pharynx, the soft palate and the prevertebral region. It drains into the internal jugular and facial veins.

LYMPHATIC DRAINAGE OF PHARYNX

Lymph from the pharynx drains into the retropharyngeal and deep cervical lymph nodes.

DEGLUTITION (SWALLOWING)

Swallowing of food occurs in three stages described below. Muscles of pharynx act during swallowing.

First Stage

1 This stage is voluntary in character.
2 The anterior part of the tongue is raised and pressed against the hard palate by the intrinsic muscles of the tongue, especially the superior longitudinal and transverse muscles. The movement takes place from anterior to the posterior side. This pushes the food bolus (Greek *lump*) into the posterior part of the oral cavity.
3 The soft palate closes down onto the back of the tongue, and helps to form the bolus.
4 Next, the hyoid bone is moved upwards and forwards by the suprahyoid muscles. The posterior part of the tongue is elevated upwards and backwards by the styloglossi; and the palatoglossal arches are approximated by the palatoglossi. This pushes the bolus through the oropharyngeal isthmus to the oropharynx, and the second stage begins.

Second Stage

1 It is involuntary in character. During this stage, the food is pushed from the oropharynx to the lower part of the laryngopharynx.
2 The nasopharyngeal isthmus is closed by elevation of the soft palate by levator veli palatini and tensor veli palatini and by approximation to it of the posterior pharyngeal wall (ridge of Passavant). This prevents the food bolus from entering the nose.
3 The inlet of larynx is closed by approximation of the aryepiglottic folds by aryepiglottic and oblique arytenoid. This prevents the food bolus from entering the larynx (*see* Fig. 24.10).
4 Next, the larynx and pharynx are elevated behind the hyoid bone by the longitudinal muscles of the pharynx. Then the bolus is pushed down over the posterior surface of the epiglottis, the closed inlet of the larynx and the posterior surface of the arytenoid cartilages, by gravity, and by contraction of the superior and middle constrictors and the palatopharyngeus.

Third Stage

1 This is also involuntary in character. In this stage, food passes from the lower part of the pharynx to the oesophagus.
2 This is brought about by the inferior constrictors of the pharynx.

DEVELOPMENT

The primitive gut extends from the buccopharyngeal membrane cranially, to the cloacal membrane caudally. It is divided into four parts—the pharynx, the foregut, the midgut and the hindgut. The pharynx extends from buccopharyngeal membrane to the tracheobronchial diverticulum. It is divided into upper part, the nasopharynx; middle part, the oropharynx; and the lower part, the laryngopharynx.

PHARYNGOTYMPANIC TUBE

Auditory tube is also known as the pharyngotympanic tube or the eustachian tube.

The auditory tube is a trumpet-shaped channel which connects the middle ear cavity with the nasopharynx. It is about 4 cm long, and is directed downwards, forwards and medially. It forms an angle of 45° with the sagittal plane and 30° with the horizontal plane. The tube is divided into bony and cartilaginous parts (Fig. 22.26).

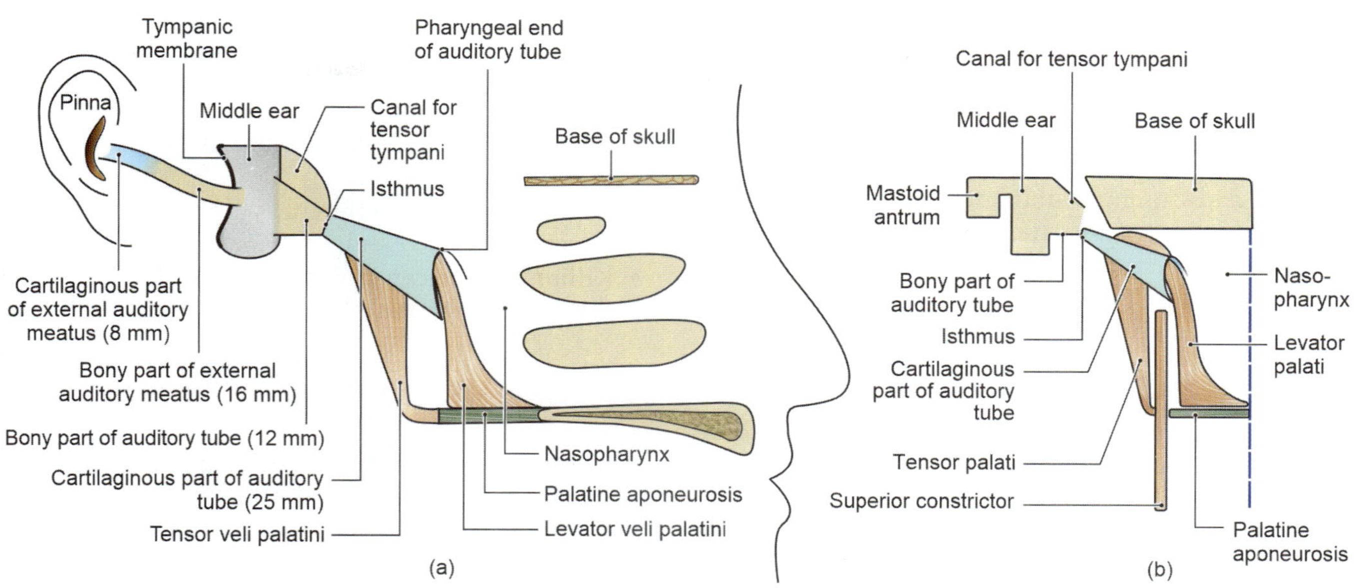

Fig. 22.26: Scheme showing anatomy of auditory tube and external auditory meatus

Bony Part

The bony part forms the posterior and lateral one-third of the tube. It is 12 mm long, and lies in the petrous temporal bone near the tympanic plate. Its lateral end is wide and opens on the anterior wall of the middle ear cavity. The medial end is narrow (isthmus) and is jagged for attachment of the cartilaginous part. The lumen of the tube is oblong being widest from side-to-side.

Relations

1 *Superior:* Canal for the tensor tympani (*see* Fig. 26.13).
2 *Medial:* Carotid canal.
3 *Lateral:* Chorda tympani, spine of sphenoid, auriculotemporal nerve (Fig. 22.8) and the temporomandibular joint.

Cartilaginous Part

The cartilaginous part forms the anterior and medial two-thirds of the tube. It is 25 mm long, and lies in the sulcus tubae, a groove between the greater wing of the sphenoid and the apex of the petrous temporal.

It is made up of a triangular plate of cartilage which is curled to form the superior and medial walls of the tube. The lateral wall and floor are completed by a fibrous membrane. The apex of the plate is attached to the medial end of the bony part. The base is free and forms the tubal elevation in the nasopharynx (Fig. 22.9).

Relations

1 *Anterolaterally:* Tensor veli palatini, mandibular nerve and its branches, otic ganglion, chorda tympani, middle meningeal artery and medial pterygoid plate (*see* Fig. 14.17).
2 *Posteromedially:* Petrous temporal and levator veli palatini.
3 The levator veli palatini is attached to its inferior surface, and the salpingopharyngeus to lower part near the pharyngeal opening.

Vascular Supply

The arterial supply of the tube is derived from the ascending pharyngeal and middle meningeal arteries and the artery of the pterygoid canal.

The veins drain into the pharyngeal and pterygoid plexuses of veins. Lymphatics pass to the retropharyngeal nodes.

Nerve Supply

1 At the ostium, by the pharyngeal branch of the pterygopalatine ganglion suspended by the maxillary nerve.
2 Cartilaginous part, by the nervus spinosus branch of mandibular nerve.
3 Bony part, by the tympanic plexus formed by glossopharyngeal nerve.

Function

The tube provides a communication of the middle ear cavity with the exterior, thus ensuring equal air pressure on both sides of the tympanic membrane.

The tube is usually closed. It opens during swallowing, yawning and sneezing, by the actions of the tensor and levator veli palatini muscles.

CLINICAL ANATOMY

- Infections may pass from the throat to the middle ear through the auditory tube. This is more common in children because the tube is shorter, wider and straighter in them (Fig. 22.27).
- Inflammation of the auditory tube (Eustachian catarrh) is often secondary to an attack of common cold, or of sore throat. This causes pain in the ear which is aggravated by swallowing, due to blockage of the tube. Pain is relieved by instillation of decongestant drops in the nose, which help to open the ostium. The ostium is commonly blocked in children by enlargement of the tubal tonsil.
- Pharyngeal spaces (*see* Chapter 11).

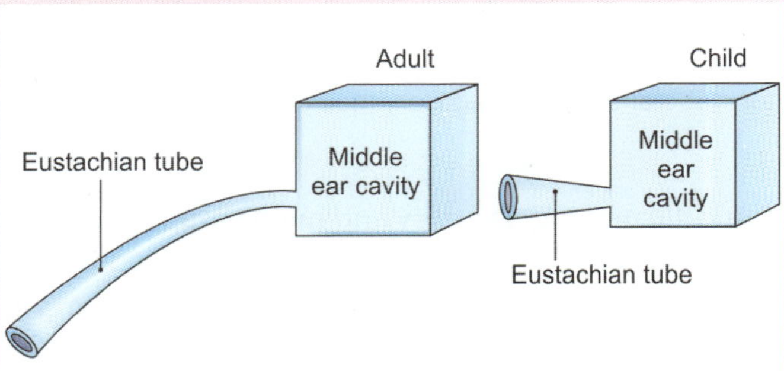

Fig. 22.27: Differences in Eustachian tube in adult and child

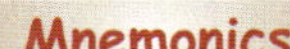

Mnemonics

Tonsils: The four types "PPLT (people) have tonsils"

Pharyngeal
Palatine
Lingual
Tubal

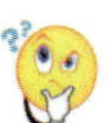

FACTS TO REMEMBER

- Both the maxillary and mandibular teeth are supplied by the branches of maxillary artery only.
- Upper teeth are supplied by branches of maxillary nerve.
- Lower teeth are supplied by branches of mandibular nerve.
- Waldeyer's ring consists of lingual tonsil, palatine tonsils, tubal tonsils and nasopharyngeal tonsils.
- All the 3 constrictors and 2 longitudinal muscles of pharynx are supplied by vagoaccessory complex, only stylopharyngeus is supplied by IX nerve.
- All the muscles of soft palate are supplied by vagoaccessory complex except tensor veli palatini, supplied by V3 nerve.
- Tonsillar branch of facial artery is the main artery of the palatine tonsil.
- Tonsils have only efferent lymph vessels but no afferent lymph vessel.
- Killian's dehiscence is a potential gap between thyropharyngeus and cricopharyngeus.

CLINICOANATOMICAL PROBLEM

A 12-year-old boy complained of sore throat and earache. He had 102°F temperature and difficulty in swallowing. He was also a mouth breather.

- What is Waldeyer's lymphatic ring?
- Explain the basis of boy's earache.
- What lymph node would likely to be swollen and tender?

Ans: Major collections of lymphoid tissue at the oropharyngeal junction are called the tonsils. These lie in a ring form called the Waldeyer's lymphatic ring. The components of this ring are lingual tonsil anteriorly, palatine tonsil laterally, tubal tonsil posterolaterally and pharyngeal tonsil posteriorly.

The earache may be due to infection of the throat reaching the middle ear. The pharyngotympanic tube from the region of nasopharynx communicates with the anterior wall of the middle ear cavity carrying the infection from pharynx to the ear causing the earache. IX nerve supplies both the pharynx and the middle ear. So the pain of pharynx is referred to the ear.

The jugulodigastric lymph node belonging to upper group of deep cervical group is most likely to be tender and swollen, as the lymphatics from the tonsil penetrate the wall of the pharynx to reach these lymph nodes.

FURTHER READING

- Berkovitz BKB, Holland GR, Moxham BJ. Oral Anatomy, Histology and Embryology, 4th ed. Edinburgh: Mosby, 2009.
  A textbook that describes in detail the gross morphology, histology and development of human teeth.
- Graney DO, Retruzzelli GJ, Myers EW. Anatomy. In: Cummings CW, Fredrickson JM, Harker LA, et al (eds). Otolaryngology: Head and Neck Surgery, vol 2, 3rd end. St Louis: Elsevier, Mosby; 1998; pp. 1327–48
  A concise account of the anatomy of the pharynx, highlighting features of clinical relevance.
- Hollinshead WH. Anatomy for Surgeons, Vol 1: The Head and Neck, 3rd ed. Philadelphia: Harper & Row, 1982.
  An older textbook that provides a valuable account of the anatomy of the pharynx and of tissue spaces in the neck. It is also a through guide to the earlier literature.

Frequently Asked Questions

1. Describe the nerve supply and actions of the muscles of soft palate. Add a note on its development including congenital anomalies.
2. Enumerate the components of Waldeyer's ring. Describe the palatine tonsil in detail. Add a note on its clinical importance.
3. Describe the attachments of the constrictor muscles of pharynx. Enumerate the structures lying in between these constrictor muscles.
4. Enumerate the length, parts, extent, relations and functions of auditory tube.

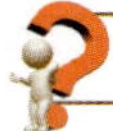

Multiple Choice Questions

1. The communication between vestibule and oral cavity proper lies:
   a. Behind 1st molar tooth
   b. Behind 2nd molar tooth
   c. Behind 3rd molar tooth
   d. No communication
2. The joint between tooth and gum is:
   a. Syndesmosis
   b. Gomphosis
   c. Sutures
   d. Primary cartilaginous joint
3. The first permanent tooth to erupt is:
   a. First molar
   b. First premolar
   c. Second molar
   d. Canine
4. Most of the muscles of soft palate are supplied by vagoaccessory complex, *except*:
   a. Levator veli palatini
   b. Tensor veli palatini
   c. Palatoglossus
   d. Musculus uvulae
5. Which one of the following is not a component of Waldeyer's ring?
   a. Tubal tonsil
   b. Pharyngeal tonsil
   c. Palatine tonsil
   d. Submental lymph nodes
6. Which of the following structures does not form bed of the tonsil?
   a. Superior constrictor
   b. Pharyngobasilar fascia
   c. Buccinator muscle
   d. Buccopharyngeal fascia
7. Which one of the following muscles of pharynx is not supplied by vagoaccessory complex?
   a. Superior constrictor
   b. Stylopharyngeus
   c. Palatopharyngeus
   d. Salpingopharyngeus
8. Which walls of cartilaginous part of auditory tube are formed by fibrous membrane?
   a. Lateral wall and floor
   b. Medial wall and floor
   c. Superior wall and medial wall
   d. Superior wall and floor
9. Paralysis of unilateral soft palate results in following effects, *except:*
   a. Depressed palatal arch
   b. Uvula deviated to paralysed side
   c. Nasal twang of voice
   d. Nasal regurgitation of liquids
10. Tonsillitis pain is referred to pain in ear as both are supplied by:
    a. Auricular branch of vagus
    b. Glossopharyngeal nerve
    c. Sympathetic fibres
    d. Cranial root of XI nerve

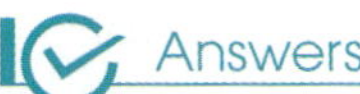

Answers

1. c **2.** b **3.** a **4.** b **5.** d **6.** c **7.** b **8.** a **9.** b **10.** b

VIVA VOCE

- Give the nerve supply of all the gums.
- What are the parts of a tooth?
- Which nerves supply the teeth?
- Name the muscles of the soft palate and give their nerve supply.
- Name the longitudinal and circular muscles of the pharynx with their nerve supply.
- Name the deep relations of the palatine tonsil.
- Which arteries supply the palatine tonsil?
- What is the function of auditory/pharyngotympanic tube? Name its parts and their length.
- What is Killian's dehiscence and what is its importance?

VIDEO 3.14 **Pharynx:** Introduction, muscles of pharynx, palate

Chapter 23

Nose, Paranasal Sinuses and Pterygopalatine Fossa

"Did God give us flowers and trees and also provide the allergies?"
—E Y Harburg

INTRODUCTION

Sense of smell perceived in the upper part of nasal cavity by olfactory nerve rootlets ends in olfactory bulb, which is connected to uncus and also to the dorsal nucleus of vagus in medulla oblongata. Good smell of food, thus stimulates secretion of gastric juice through vagus nerve.

Most of the mucous membrane of the nasal cavity is respiratory and is continuous with various paranasal sinuses. Since nose is the most projecting part of the face, its integrity must be maintained.

Environmental pollution causes inhalation of unwanted gases and particles, leading to frequent attacks of sinusitis, respiratory diseases including asthma.

Nasal mucous membrane is quite vascular. Sometimes picking of the nose may cause bleeding from 'Little's area'. Bleeding from nose is called *epistaxis*.

NOSE

The nose performs two functions. It is a respiratory passage. It is also the organ of smell. The receptors for smell are placed in the upper one-third of the nasal cavity. This part is lined by olfactory mucosa. The rest of the nasal cavity is lined by respiratory mucosa. The respiratory mucosa is highly vascular and warms the inspired air.

The secretions of numerous serous glands make the air moist; while the secretions of mucous glands trap dust and other particles. Thus the nose acts as an air conditioner where the inspired air is warmed, moistened and cleansed before it is passed onto the delicate lungs.

The *olfactory mucosa* lines the upper one-third of the nasal cavity including the roof formed by cribriform plate and the medial and lateral walls up to the level of the superior concha. It is thin and less vascular than the respiratory mucosa. It contains receptors called olfactory cells.

For descriptive purposes, the nose is divided into two main parts, the external nose and nasal cavity.

EXTERNAL NOSE

Some features of the external nose have been described in Chapter 10. These are root, dorsum, tip, anterior nares, nasal septum and columella.

The external nose has a skeletal framework that is partly bony and partly cartilaginous. The bones are the nasal bones, which form the bridge of the nose, and the frontal processes of the maxillae. The cartilages are the superior and inferior nasal cartilages, the septal cartilage, and small alar cartilages (Figs 23.1a and b). The skin over the external nose is supplied by the external nasal, infratrochlear and infraorbital nerves (*see* Fig. 10.16).

NASAL CAVITY

The nasal cavity extends from the external nares or nostrils to the posterior nasal apertures, and is subdivided into right and left halves by the nasal septum (Figs 23.2 and 23.4). Each half has a roof, a floor, and medial and lateral walls. Each half measures about 5 cm in height, 5–7 cm in length, and 1.5 cm in width near the floor. The width near the roof is only 1–2 mm.

The *roof* is about 7 cm long and 2 mm wide. It slopes downwards, both in front and behind. The middle horizontal part is formed by the cribriform plate of the ethmoid. The anterior slope is formed by the nasal part of the frontal bone, nasal bone, and the nasal cartilages. The posterior slope is formed by the inferior surface of the body of the sphenoid bone (Fig. 23.4).

The *floor* is about 5 cm long and 1.5 cm wide. It is formed by the palatine process of the maxilla and the

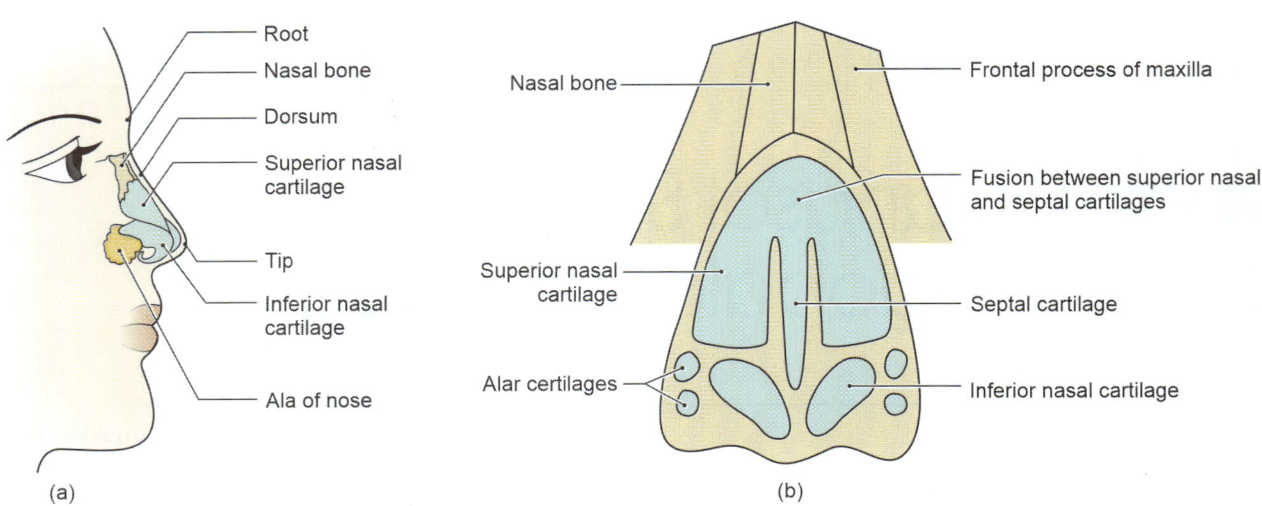

Figs 23.1a and b: (a) Skeleton of the external nose; (b) Anterior view

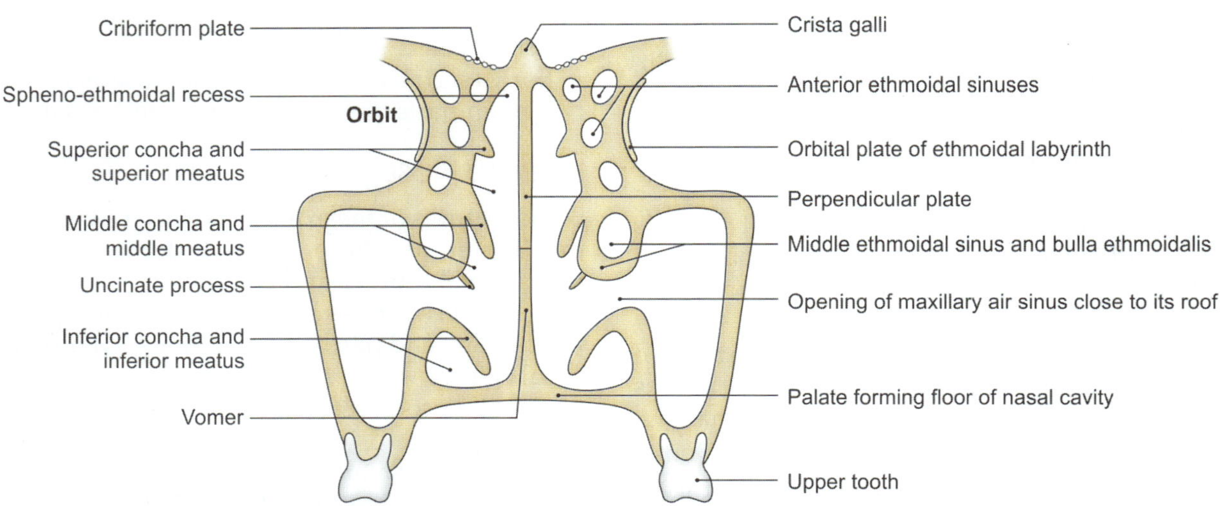

Fig. 23.2: Coronal section through the nasal cavity and the maxillary air sinuses

horizontal plate of the palatine bone. It is concave from side-to-side and is slightly higher anteriorly than posteriorly (Fig. 23.2).

CLINICAL ANATOMY

- Common cold or rhinitis is the commonest infection of the nose. It may be infective or allergic or both. It commonly occurs during change of the seasons.
- The paranasal air sinuses may get infected from the nose. Maxillary sinusitis is the commonest of such infections.
- The relations of the nose to the anterior cranial fossa through the cribriform plate (Fig. 23.12), and to the lacrimal apparatus through the nasolacrimal duct are important in the spread of infection (*see* Fig. 10.22a).
- Fracture of cribriform plate of ethmoid with tearing off of the meninges may tear the olfactory nerve rootlets (Fig. 23.3). In such cases, CSF may drip from the nasal cavity. It is called CSF rhinorrhoea.

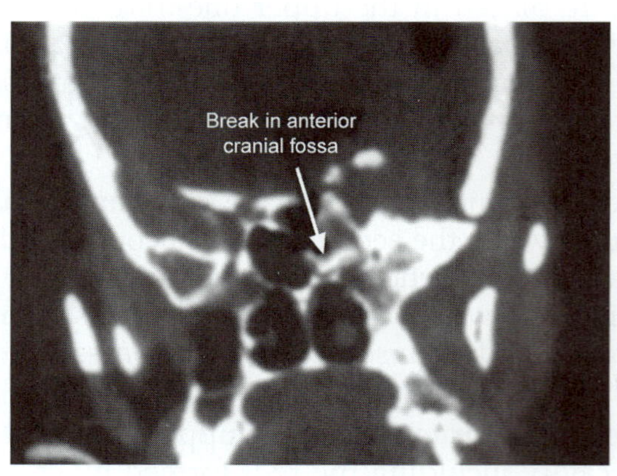

Fig. 23.3: CSF rhinorrhoea

NASAL SEPTUM

Features

The *nasal septum* is a median osseocartilaginous partition between the two halves of the nasal cavity. On each side, it is covered by mucous membrane and forms the medial wall of both nasal cavities.

The *bony part* is formed almost entirely by:

a. The vomer
b. The perpendicular plate of ethmoid. However, its margins receive contributions from the nasal spine of the frontal bone, the rostrum of the sphenoid, and the nasal crests of the nasal, palatine and maxillary bones (Fig. 23.4).

The *cartilaginous part* is formed by:

a. The septal cartilage
b. The septal processes of the inferior nasal cartilages (Fig. 23.1b).

The *cuticular part* or lower end is formed by fibrofatty tissue covered by skin. The lower margin of the septum is called the *columella*.

The nasal septum is rarely strictly median. Its central part is usually *deflected* to one or the other side. The deflection is produced by overgrowth of one or more of the constituent parts.

DISSECTION

Take the sagittal section of head and neck, prepared in Chapter 22.

Dissect and remove mucous membrane of the septum of nose in small pieces. The mucous membrane is covering both surfaces of the septum of the nose.

Dissect and preserve the nerves lying in the mucous membrane. Remove the entire mucous membrane to see the details in the interior of the nasal cavity *(refer to BDC App)*.

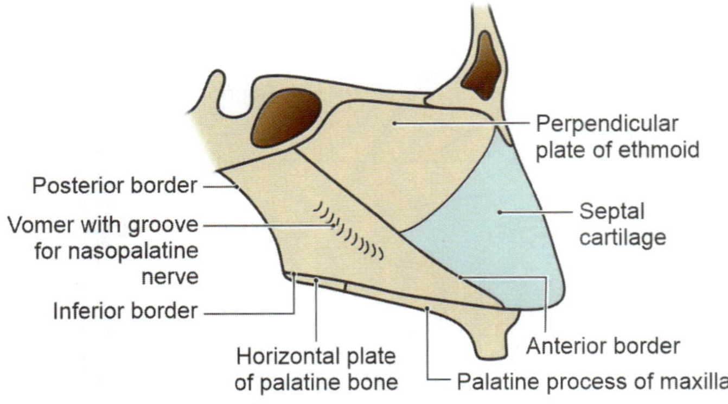

Fig. 23.4: Formation of the nasal septum

The septum has:

a. Four borders—superior, inferior, anterior and posterior.
b. Two surfaces—right and left.

Arterial Supply

Anterosuperior part is supplied by the anterior and posterior ethmoidal artery (Fig. 23.5).

Anteroinferior part is supplied by the septal branch of superior labial branch of facial artery.

Posterosuperior part is supplied by the sphenopalatine artery. *It is the main artery.*

The anteroinferior part or vestibule of the septum contains anastomoses between all branches, e.g. the septal branch of the superior labial branch of the facial artery, sphenopalatine artery, and anterior ethmoidal artery. These form a large capillary network called the *Kiesselbach's plexus*. This is a common site of bleeding from the nose or epistaxis, and is known as *Little's area.*

Venous Drainage

The veins form a plexus which is more marked in the lower part of septum or Little's area. The plexus drains anteriorly into the facial vein, and posteriorly through the sphenopalatine vein to pterygoid venous plexus.

Nerve Supply

1 *General sensory nerves,* arising from trigeminal nerve, are distributed to whole of the septum (Fig. 23.6).
   a. The anterosuperior part of the septum is supplied by the internal nasal branches of the anterior ethmoidal nerve.
   b. The posteroinferior part is supplied by the nasopalatine branch of the pterygopalatine ganglion. *It is the main nerve.*
2 *Special sensory nerves* or *olfactory* nerves are confined to the upper part or olfactory area.

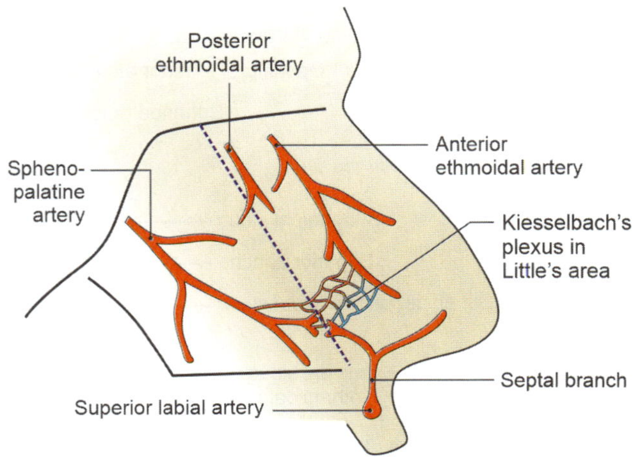

Fig. 23.5: Roof of the nasal cavity and arterial supply of nasal septum

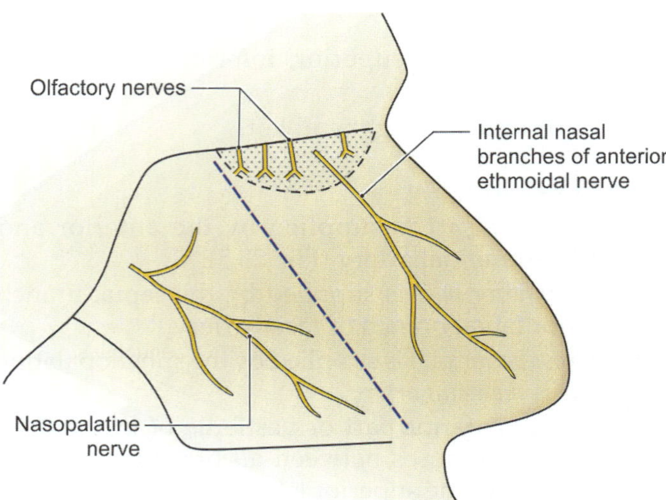

Fig. 23.6: Nerve supply of nasal septum

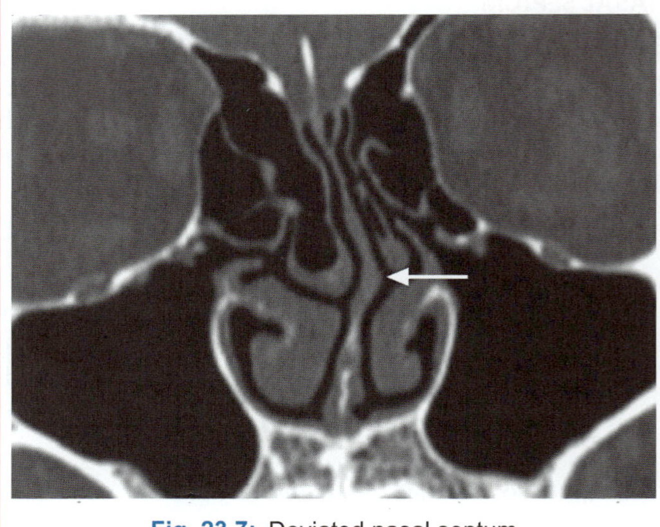

Fig. 23.7: Deviated nasal septum

Lymphatic Drainage

Anterior half to the submandibular nodes.

Posterior half to the retropharyngeal and deep cervical nodes.

CLINICAL ANATOMY

- Sphenopalatine artery is the artery of epistaxis.
- Little's area on the septum is a common site of bleeding from the nose or epistaxis (Fig. 23.5).
- Pathological deviation of the nasal septum is often responsible for repeated attacks of common cold, allergic rhinitis, sinusitis, etc. It requires surgical correction (Fig. 23.7).

LATERAL WALL OF NOSE

Features

The lateral wall of the nose is irregular owing to the presence of three shelf-like bony projections called *conchae*. The conchae increase the surface area of the nose for effective air-conditioning of the inspired air (Fig. 23.2).

The lateral wall separates the nose:

a. From the orbit above, with the ethmoidal air sinuses intervening.
b. From the maxillary sinus below.
c. From the lacrimal sac and nasolacrimal duct in front (*see* Fig. 10.22a).

The lateral wall can be subdivided into three parts:

a. A small depressed area in the anterior part is called the vestibule. It is lined by modified skin containing short, stiff, curved hairs called *vibrissae*.
b. The middle part is known as the *atrium* of the middle meatus.
c. The posterior part contains the conchae. Spaces separating the conchae are called meatuses (Fig. 23.8).

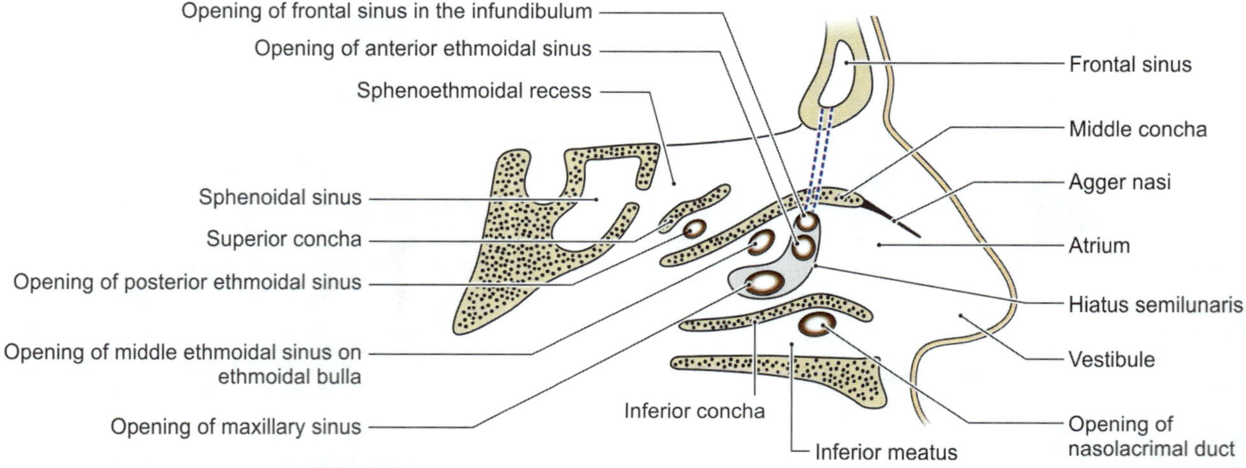

Fig. 23.8: Lateral wall of the nasal cavity seen after removing the conchae

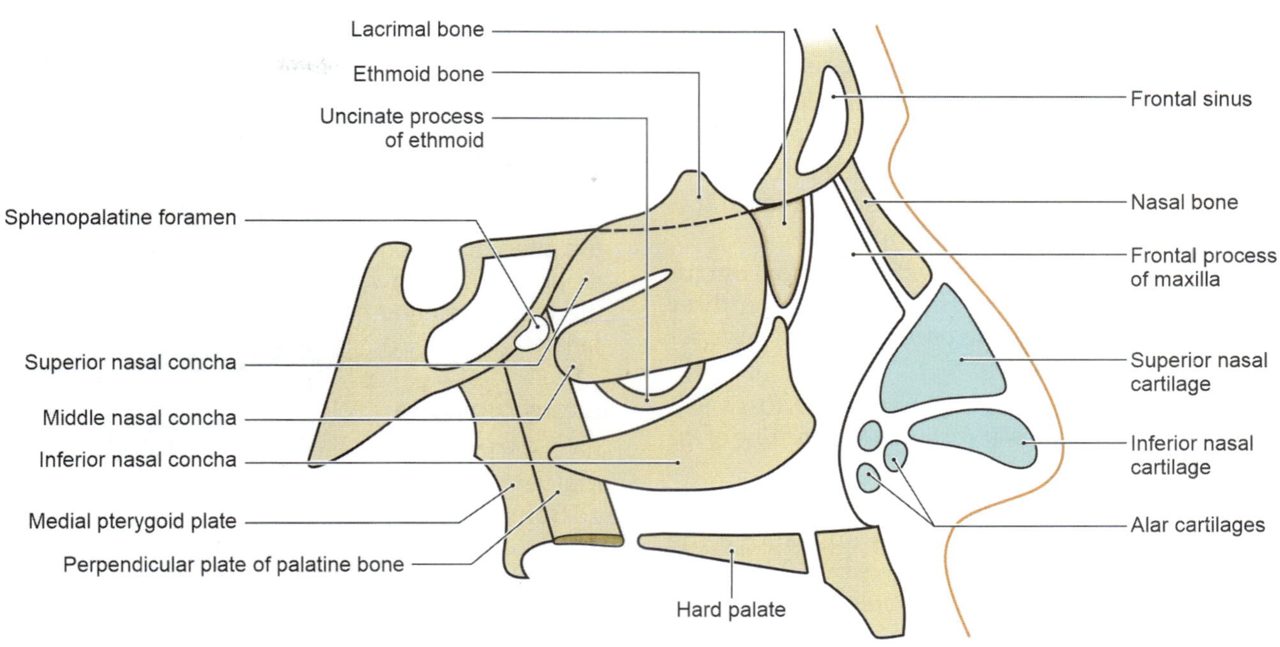

Fig. 23.9: Formation of the lateral wall of the nasal cavity

The *skeleton of the lateral wall* is partly bony, partly cartilaginous, and partly made up only of soft tissues.

The *bony part* is formed from before backwards by the following bones:

a. Nasal
b. Frontal process of maxilla (*see* Figs 9.22a and b)
c. Lacrimal
d. Labyrinth of ethmoid with superior and middle conchae
e. Inferior nasal concha, made up of spongy bone only (Fig. 23.9)
f. Perpendicular plate of palatine bone together with its orbital and sphenoidal processes
g. Medial pterygoid plate.

The *cartilaginous part* is formed by:

a. The superior nasal cartilage (Fig. 23.1).
b. The inferior nasal cartilage.
c. 3 or 4 small cartilages of the ala.

The *cuticular lower part* is formed by fibrofatty tissue covered with skin.

DISSECTION

Remove with scissors the anterior part of inferior nasal concha. This will reveal the opening of the nasolacrimal duct. Pass a thin probe upwards through the nasolacrimal duct into the lacrimal sac at the medial angle of the eye. Remove all the three nasal conchae to expose the meatuses lying below the respective concha. This will expose the openings of the sinuses present there *(refer to BDC App)*.

CONCHAE AND MEATUSES

Features

The *nasal conchae* are curved bony projections directed downwards and medially. The following three conchae are usually found:

1 The *inferior concha* (Latin *shell)* is an independent bone.
2 The *middle concha* is a projection from the medial surface of ethmoidal labyrinth (Fig. 23.8).
3 The *superior concha* is also a projection from the medial surface of the ethmoidal labyrinth. This is the smallest concha situated just above the posterior part of the middle concha (Fig. 23.8).

The *meatuses of the nose* are passages beneath the overhanging conchae. Each meatus communicates freely with the nasal cavity proper (Fig. 23.9).

1 The *inferior meatus* lies underneath the inferior concha, and is the largest of the three meatuses. The nasolacrimal duct opens into it at the junction of its anterior one-third and posterior two-thirds. The opening is guarded by the lacrimal fold, or *Hasner's valve.*
2 The *middle meatus* lies underneath the middle concha. It presents the following features:
   a. The *ethmoidal bulla* is a rounded elevation produced by the underlying middle ethmoidal sinuses which open at upper margin of bulla.
   b. The *hiatus semilunaris* is a deep semicircular sulcus below the bulla.
   c. The *infundibulum* is a short passage at the anterior end of the hiatus.

   d. The *opening of frontal air sinus* is seen in the anterior part of hiatus semilunaris (Fig. 23.8).
   e. The *opening of the anterior ethmoidal air sinus* is present behind the opening of frontal air sinus.
   f. The *opening of maxillary air sinus* is located in posterior part of the hiatus semilunaris. It is often represented by two openings.
3. The *superior meatus* lies below the superior concha. This is the shortest and shallowest of the three meatuses. It receives the *openings of the posterior ethmoidal air sinuses.*

The *sphenoethmoidal recess* is a triangular fossa just above the superior concha. It receives the *opening of the sphenoidal air sinus* (Fig. 23.8).

The *atrium of the middle meatus* is a shallow depression just in front of the middle meatus and above the vestibule of the nose. It is limited above by a faint ridge of mucous membrane, the *agger nasi*, which runs forwards and downwards from the upper end of the anterior border of the middle concha (Fig. 23.8).

Arterial Supply

1. The *anterosuperior quadrant* is supplied by the anterior ethmoidal artery assisted by the posterior ethmoidal artery.
2. The *anteroinferior quadrant* is supplied by branches from the facial artery (Fig. 23.10).
3. The *posterosuperior quadrant* is supplied by a few branches of the sphenopalatine artery.
4. The *posteroinferior quadrant* is supplied by branches from greater palatine artery which pierce the perpendicular plate of palatine bone and passes up through the incisive fossa.

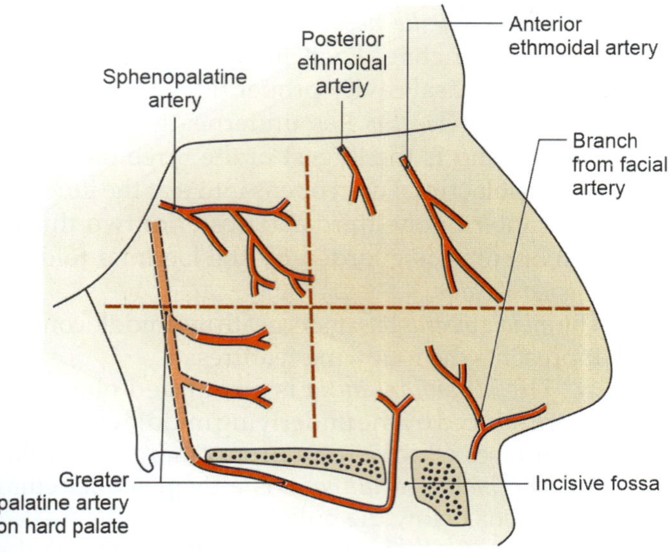

Fig. 23.10: Arteries supplying lateral wall of the nasal cavity

DISSECTION

Trace the nasopalatine nerve till the sphenopalatine foramen. Try to find a few nasal branches of the greater palatine nerve.

Gently break the perpendicular plate of palatine bone to expose the greater palatine nerve, branch of the pterygopalatine ganglion. Follow the nerve and its accompanying vessels to the hard palate. Identify the lesser palatine nerves and trace them till the soft palate.

Venous Drainage

The veins form a plexus which drains anteriorly into the facial vein; posteriorly, into the pharyngeal plexus of veins; and from the middle part, to the pterygoid plexus of veins.

Nerve Supply

1. *General sensory nerves* derived from the branches of trigeminal nerve are distributed to whole of the lateral wall:
   a. *Anterosuperior quadrant* is supplied by the anterior ethmoidal nerve branch of ophthalmic nerve (Fig. 23.11).
   b. *Anteroinferior quadrant* is supplied by the anterior superior alveolar nerve, branch of infraorbital, continuation of maxillary nerve.
   c. *Posterosuperior quadrant* is supplied by the lateral posterior superior nasal branches from the pterygopalatine ganglion.
   d. *Posteroinferior quadrant* is supplied by the anterior palatine branch from the pterygopalatine ganglion.
2. *Special sensory nerves* or *olfactory nerves* are distributed to the upper part of the lateral wall just below the cribriform plate of the ethmoid up to the superior concha.

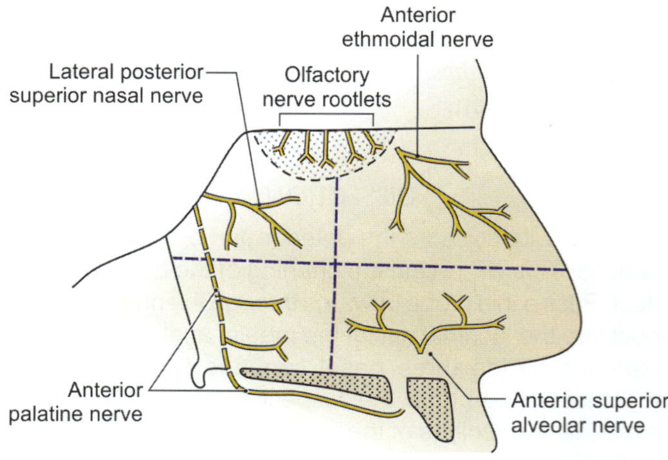

Fig. 23.11: Nerve supply of lateral wall of the nasal cavity

Note that the olfactory mucosa lies partly on the lateral walls and partly on the nasal septum.

Lymphatic Drainage

Lymphatics from the anterior half of the lateral wall pass to the submandibular nodes, and from the posterior half, to the retropharyngeal and upper deep cervical nodes.

CLINICAL ANATOMY

Hypertrophy of the mucosa over the inferior nasal concha is a common feature of allergic rhinitis, which is characterised by sneezing, nasal blockage and excessive watery discharge from the nose.

OLFACTORY NERVE—1ST NERVE

1 The *olfactory cells* (16–20 million in man) are bipolar neurons. They lie in the olfactory part of the nasal mucosa, and serve both as receptors as well as the first neurons in the olfactory pathway (Fig. 23.12).
2 The *olfactory* nerves, about 20 in number, represent central processes of the olfactory cells. They pass through the cribriform plate of ethmoid and make synaptic glomeruli with cells of olfactory bulb.

The mitral and tufted cells in the olfactory bulb give off fibres that form the *olfactory tract* and reach the anterior perforated substance and uncus.

CLINICAL ANATOMY

- Anosmia: Loss of olfactory fibres with ageing.
- Sense of smell is tested separately in each nostril.
- Allergic rhinitis causes temporary olfactory impairment.

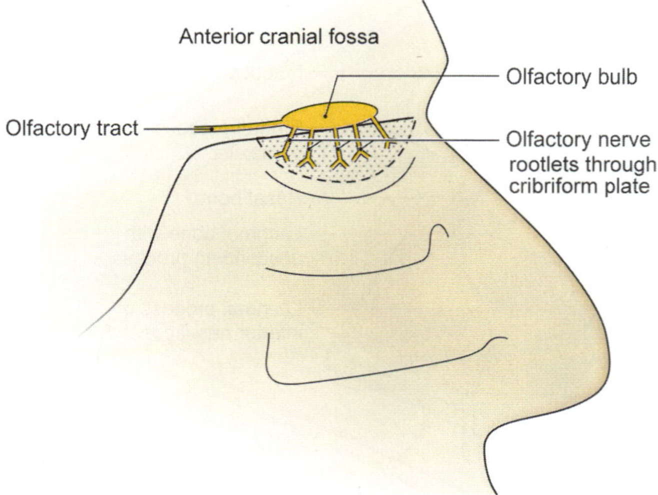

Fig. 23.12: Olfactory nerve rootlets in lateral wall of nose

PARANASAL SINUSES

Features

Paranasal sinuses are air-filled spaces present within some bones around the nasal cavities. The sinuses are *frontal, maxillary, sphenoidal and ethmoidal.* All of them open into the nasal cavity through its lateral wall (Fig. 23.13). The *function* of the sinuses is to make the skull lighter, warm up and humidify the inspired air. These also add resonance to the voice. In infections of the sinuses or *sinusitis,* the voice is altered.

The sinuses are rudimentary, or even absent at birth. They enlarge rapidly during the ages of 6 to 7 years, i.e. time of eruption of permanent teeth and then after puberty. From birth to adult life, the growth of the sinuses is due to enlargement of the bones; in old age, it is due to resorption of the surrounding cancellous bone.

The anatomy of individual sinuses is important as they are frequently infected.

Frontal Sinus

1 The frontal sinus lies in the frontal bone deep to the superciliary arch. It extends upwards above the medial end of the eyebrow, and backwards into the medial part of the roof of the orbit (Fig. 23.13).
2 It *opens* into the middle meatus of nose at the anterior end of the hiatus semilunaris either through the infundibulum or through the frontonasal duct (Fig. 23.8).
3 The right and left sinuses are usually unequal in size; and rarely one or both may be absent. Their *average* height, width and anteroposterior depth are each about 2.5 cm. The sinuses are better developed in males than in females.

DISSECTION

Remove the thin medial walls of the ethmoidal air cells, and look for the continuity with the mucous membrane of the nose. Remove the medial wall of maxillary air sinus extending anteriorly from opening of nasolacrimal duct till the greater palatine canal posteriorly. Now maxillary air sinus can be seen. Remove part of the roof of maxillary air sinus so that the maxillary nerve and pterygopalatine ganglion are identifiable in the pterygopalatine fossa.

Trace the infraorbital nerve in infraorbital canal in floor of orbit. Try to locate the sinuous course of anterior superior alveolar nerve into the upper incisor teeth.

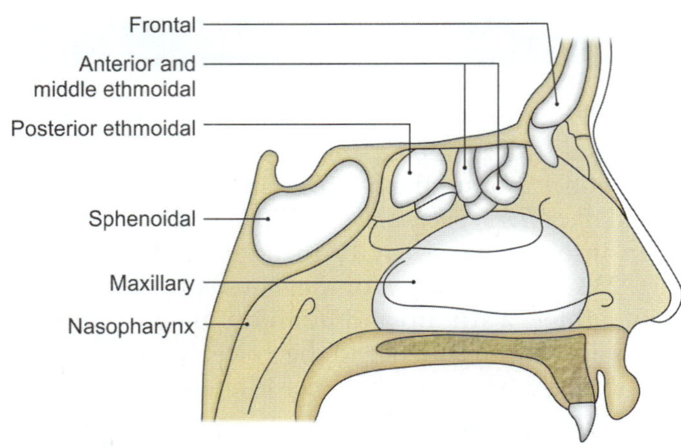

Fig. 23.13: Lateral wall of nasal cavity with location of paranasal sinuses

4 They are rudimentary or absent at birth. They are well developed between 7 and 8 years of age, but reach full size only after puberty.

5 *Arterial supply:* Supraorbital artery.

Venous drainage: Into the supraorbital and superior ophthalmic veins.

Lymphatic drainage: To submandibular nodes.

Nerve supply: Supraorbital nerve.

Maxillary Sinus

1 The maxillary sinus lies in the body of the maxilla (Fig. 23.2), and is the largest of all the paranasal sinuses. It is pyramidal in shape, with its base directed medially towards the lateral wall of the nose, and the apex directed laterally in the zygomatic process of the maxilla.

2 It *opens* into the middle meatus of the nose in the lower part of the hiatus semilunaris (Fig. 23.8). *The opening/hiatus is nearer the roof* (Fig. 23.2).

3 In an isolated maxilla, the opening or hiatus of the maxillary sinus is large. However, in the intact skull, the size of opening is reduced to 3 or 4 mm as it is overlapped by the following:

a. From above, by the uncinate process of the ethmoid, and the descending part of lacrimal bone.

b. From below, by lacrimal and ethmoidal processes of the inferior nasal concha.

c. From behind, by the perpendicular plate of the palatine bone (Fig. 23.14). It is further reduced in size by the thick mucosa of nose.

4 The size of sinus is variable. Average measurements are: Height—3.5 cm, width—2.5 cm and antero-posterior depth—3.5 cm (Fig. 23.13).

5 Its *roof* is formed by the floor of orbit, and is traversed by the infraorbital nerve. The *floor* is formed by the alveolar process of maxilla, and lies about 1 cm below the level of floor of the nose. The level corresponds to the level of lower border of the ala of nose.

The floor is marked by several conical elevations produced by the roots of upper molar and premolar teeth.

The roots may even penetrate the bony floor to lie beneath the mucous lining. The canine tooth may project into the anterolateral wall.

6 The maxillary sinus is the first paranasal sinus to *develop*.

7 *Arterial supply:* Facial, infraorbital and greater palatine arteries.

Venous drainage into the facial vein and the pterygoid plexus of veins.

Lymphatic drainage into the submandibular nodes.

Nerve supply: Posterior superior alveolar branches from maxillary nerve and anterior and middle superior alveolar branches from infraorbital nerve.

Sphenoidal Sinus

1 The right and left sphenoidal sinuses lie within the body of sphenoid bone (Fig. 23.13). They are

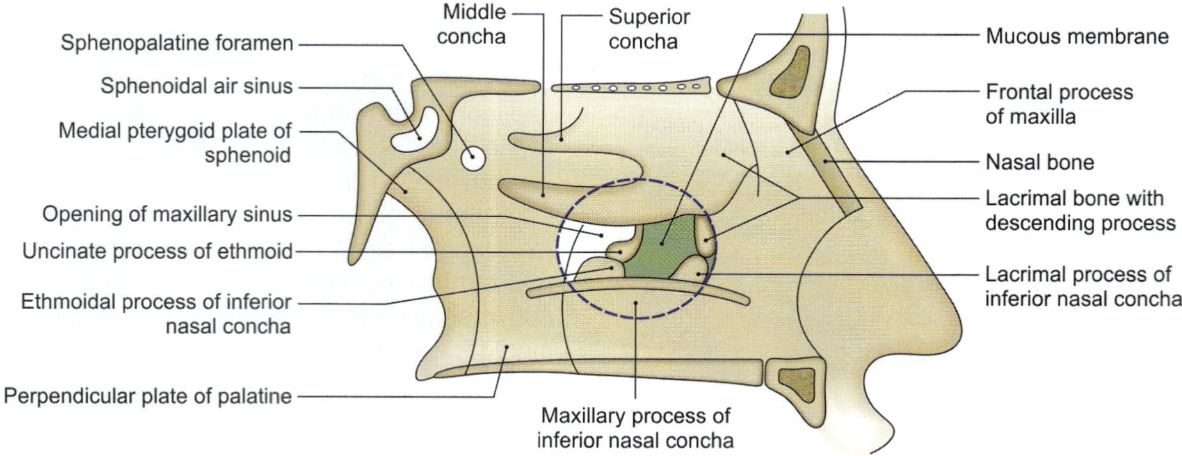

Fig. 23.14: Reduced size of maxillary air sinus

separated by a septum. The two sinuses are usually unequal in size. Each sinus opens into the spheno-ethmoidal recess of corresponding half of the nasal cavity (Fig. 23.8).

2 Each sinus is related superiorly to the optic chiasma and the hypophysis cerebri; and laterally to the internal carotid artery and the cavernous sinus (*see* Fig. 20.5).

3 *Arterial supply:* Posterior ethmoidal and internal carotid arteries.

Venous drainage: Into pterygoid venous plexus and cavernous sinus.

Lymphatic drainage: To the retropharyngeal nodes.

Nerve supply: Posterior ethmoidal nerve and orbital branches of pterygopalatine ganglion.

Ethmoidal Sinuses

1 Ethmoidal sinuses are numerous small intercommunicating spaces which lie within the labyrinth of the ethmoid bone (Fig. 23.2). They are completed from above by the orbital plate of the frontal bone, from behind by the sphenoidal conchae and the orbital process of the palatine bone, and anteriorly by the lacrimal bone. The sinuses are divided into anterior, middle and posterior groups (Fig. 23.13).

2 The *anterior ethmoidal sinus* is made up of 1 to 11 air cells, opens into the anterior part of the hiatus semilunaris of the nose. It is supplied by the anterior ethmoidal nerve and vessels. Its lymphatics drain into the submandibular nodes.

3 The *middle ethmoidal sinus* consisting of 1 to 7 air cells open into the middle meatus of the nose. It is supplied by the anterior ethmoidal nerve and vessels and the orbital branches of the pterygopalatine ganglion. Lymphatics drain into the submandibular nodes (Fig. 23.8).

4 The *posterior ethmoidal sinus* consisting of 1 to 7 air cells open into the superior meatus of the nose. It is supplied by the posterior ethmoidal nerve and vessels and the orbital branches of the pterygopalatine ganglion. Lymphatics drain into the retropharyngeal nodes.

CLINICAL ANATOMY

- Infection of a sinus is known as sinusitis. It causes headache and persistent, thick, purulent discharge from the nose. Diagnosis is assisted by transillumination and radiography. A diseased sinus is opaque.
- The maxillary sinus is most commonly involved. It may be infected from the nose or from a caries tooth. Drainage of the sinus is difficult because its ostium lies at a higher level than its floor. Hence, the sinus is drained surgically by making an artificial opening near the floor in one of the following two ways:
  a. Antrum puncture can be done by breaking the lateral wall of the inferior meatus and pushing in fluid and letting it drain through the natural orifice with head in dependent position (Fig. 23.15).
  b. An opening can be made at the canine fossa through the vestibule of the mouth, deep to the upper lip (Caldwell-Luc operation).
- Carcinoma of the maxillary sinus arises from the mucosal lining. Symptoms depend on the direction of growth.
  a. Invasion of the orbit causes proptosis and diplopia. If the infraorbital nerve is involved, there is facial pain and anaesthesia of the skin over the maxilla.
  b. Invasion of the floor may produce a bulging and even ulceration of the palate.
  c. Forward growth obliterates the canine fossa and produces a swelling of the face.
  d. Backward growth may involve the palatine nerves and produce severe pain referred to the upper teeth.
  e. Growth in a medial direction produces nasal obstruction, epistaxis and epiphora.
  f. Growth in a lateral direction produces a swelling on the face and a palpable mass in the labiogingival groove.

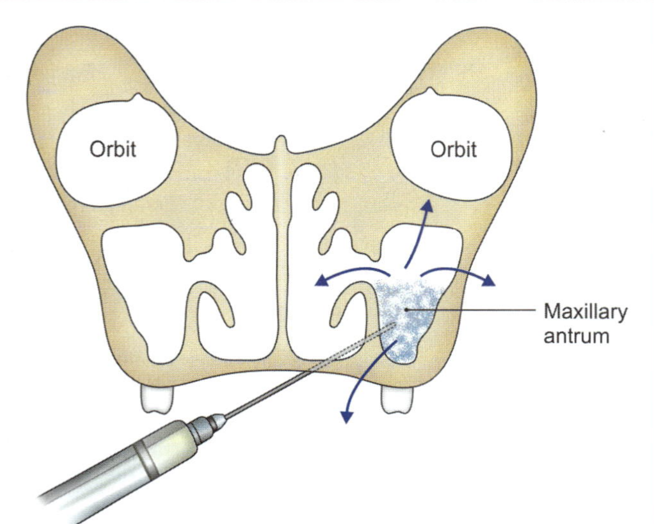

Fig. 23.15: Antrum puncture. Directions showing the invasion of the carcinoma of maxillary sinus

- Frontal sinusitis and ethmoiditis can cause oedema of the lids secondary to infection of the sinuses.
- Pain from ethmoid air sinus may be referred to forehead, as both are supplied by ophthalmic division of trigeminal nerve.
- Pain of maxillary sinusitis may be referred to upper teeth and infraorbital skin as all these are supplied by the maxillary nerve.

PTERYGOPALATINE FOSSA

This is small pyramidal space situated deeply, below the apex of the orbit (Fig. 23.16).

Boundaries

Study the boundaries on the skull.

Anterior: Superomedial part of the posterior surface of the maxilla.

Posterior: Root of the pterygoid process and adjoining part of the anterior surface of the greater wing of the sphenoid.

Medial: Upper part of the perpendicular plate of the palatine bone. The orbital and sphenoidal processes of the bone also take part.

Lateral: The fossa opens into the infratemporal fossa through the pterygomaxillary fissure.

Superior: Undersurface of the body of sphenoid.

Inferior: Closed by the pyramidal process of the palatine bone in the angle between the maxilla and the pterygoid process.

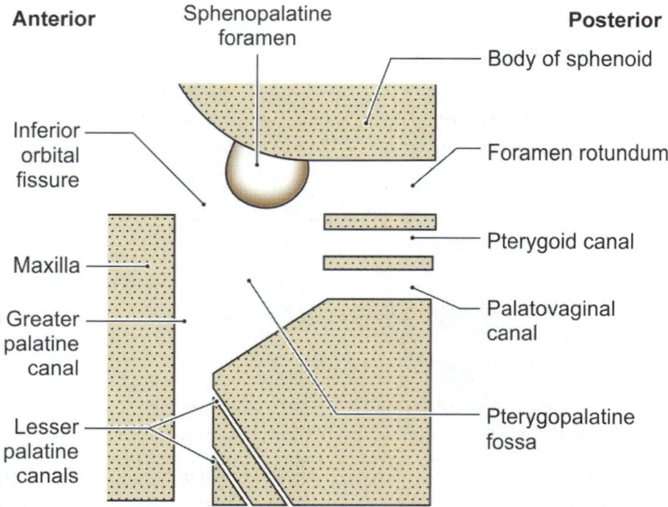

Fig. 23.16: Scheme to show the pterygopalatine fossa and its communications

Communications

Anteriorly: With the orbit through the medial end of the inferior orbital fissure (Fig. 23.16).

Posteriorly

1. Middle cranial fossa through the foramen rotundum.
2. Foramen lacerum through the pterygoid canal.
3. Pharynx through the palatinovaginal canal.

Medially: With the nose through sphenopalatine foramen.

Laterally: With the infratemporal fossa through the pterygomaxillary fissure.

Inferiorly: With the oral cavity through the greater and lesser palatine canals.

Contents

1. Third part of the maxillary artery and its branches which bear the same names as the branches of the pterygopalatine ganglia and accompany all of them (*see* Chapter 14; Figs 14.6 and 14.7).
2. Maxillary nerve and its branches—ganglionic, zygomatic and posterior superior alveolar.
3. Pterygopalatine ganglion and its numerous branches containing fibres of the maxillary nerve mixed with autonomic nerves (described below).

Maxillary Nerve

It arises from the trigeminal ganglion, runs forwards in the lateral wall of the cavernous sinus below the ophthalmic nerve, and leaves the middle cranial fossa by passing through the foramen rotundum (*see* Fig. 20.14). Next, the nerve crosses the upper part of pterygopalatine fossa, beyond which it is continued as the infraorbital nerve.

In the middle cranial fossa, maxillary nerve gives a meningeal branch.

In the pterygopalatine fossa, the nerve is related to the pterygopalatine ganglion, and gives off the ganglionic, posterior superior alveolar and zygomatic nerves.

Ganglionic Branches

The pterygopalatine ganglion is suspended by the ganglionic branches.

Posterior Superior Alveolar Nerve

It enters the posterior surface of the body of the maxilla, and supplies the three upper molar teeth and the adjoining part of the gum.

Zygomatic Nerve

It is a branch of the maxillary nerve, given off in the pterygopalatine fossa. It enters the orbit through the

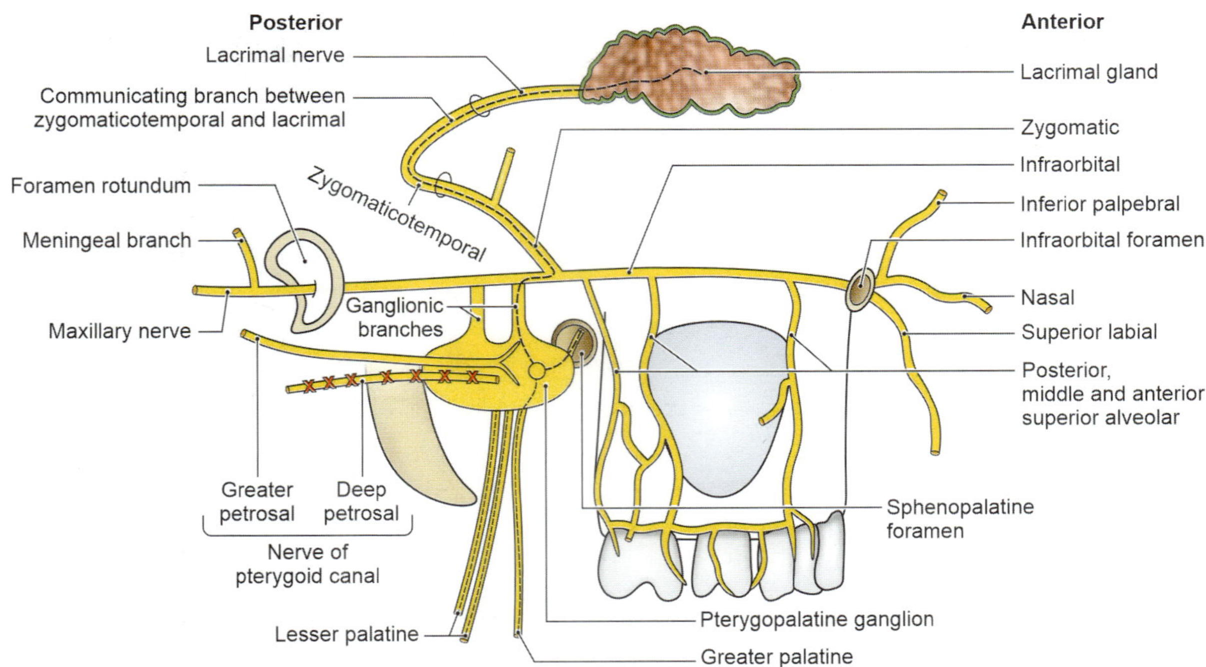

Fig. 23.17: Branches of maxillary nerve with pterygopalatine ganglion

lateral end of the inferior orbital fissure, and runs along the lateral wall, outside the periosteum, to enter the zygomatic bone. Just before or after entering the bone, it divides into two terminal branches, the *zygomaticofacial* and *zygomaticotemporal nerves* which supply the skin of the face and of the anterior part of the temple (*see* Fig. 10.16). The communicating branch to the lacrimal nerve, which contains secretomotor fibres to the lacrimal gland, arises from the zygomaticotemporal nerve, and runs in the lateral wall of the orbit (Fig. 23.17 and inset).

Infraorbital Nerve

It is the continuation of the maxillary nerve. It enters the orbit through the *inferior orbital fissure*. It then runs forwards on the floor of the orbit or the roof of the maxillary sinus, at first in the *infraorbital groove* and then in the *infraorbital canal* remaining outside the periosteum of the orbit. It emerges on the face through the *infraorbital foramen* and terminates by dividing into palpebral, nasal and labial branches. The nerve is accompanied by the infraorbital branch of the third part of the maxillary artery and the accompanying vein (*see* Fig. 10.16).

Branches

1 The *middle superior alveolar nerve* arises in the infraorbital groove, runs in the lateral wall of the maxillary sinus, and supplies the upper premolar teeth.
2 The *anterior superior alveolar nerve* arises in the infraorbital canal, and runs in a sinuous canal having a complicated course in the anterior wall of the maxillary sinus. It supplies the upper incisor and canine teeth, the maxillary sinus, and the antero-inferior part of the nasal cavity.
3 *Terminal branches—palpebral, nasal and labial* supply a large area of skin on the face. They also supply the mucous membrane of the upper lip and cheek (Fig. 23.17).

PTERYGOPALATINE GANGLION/SPHENOPALATINE GANGLION/GANGLION OF HAY FEVER/MECKEL'S GANGLION

Features

Pterygopalatine is the largest parasympathetic peripheral ganglion. It serves as a relay station for secretomotor fibres to the lacrimal gland and to the mucous glands of the nose, paranasal sinuses, palate and pharynx. Topographically, it is related to the maxillary nerve, but functionally it is connected to facial nerve through its greater petrosal branch.

The flattened ganglion lies in the pterygopalatine fossa just below the maxillary nerve, in front of the pterygoid canal and lateral to the sphenopalatine foramen (Figs 23.17 and 23.18).

Connections

1 The *parasympathetic root* of the ganglion is formed by the nerve of the pterygoid canal. It carries preganglionic fibres that arise from neurons present near the *superior salivatory* and *lacrimatory nuclei*, and

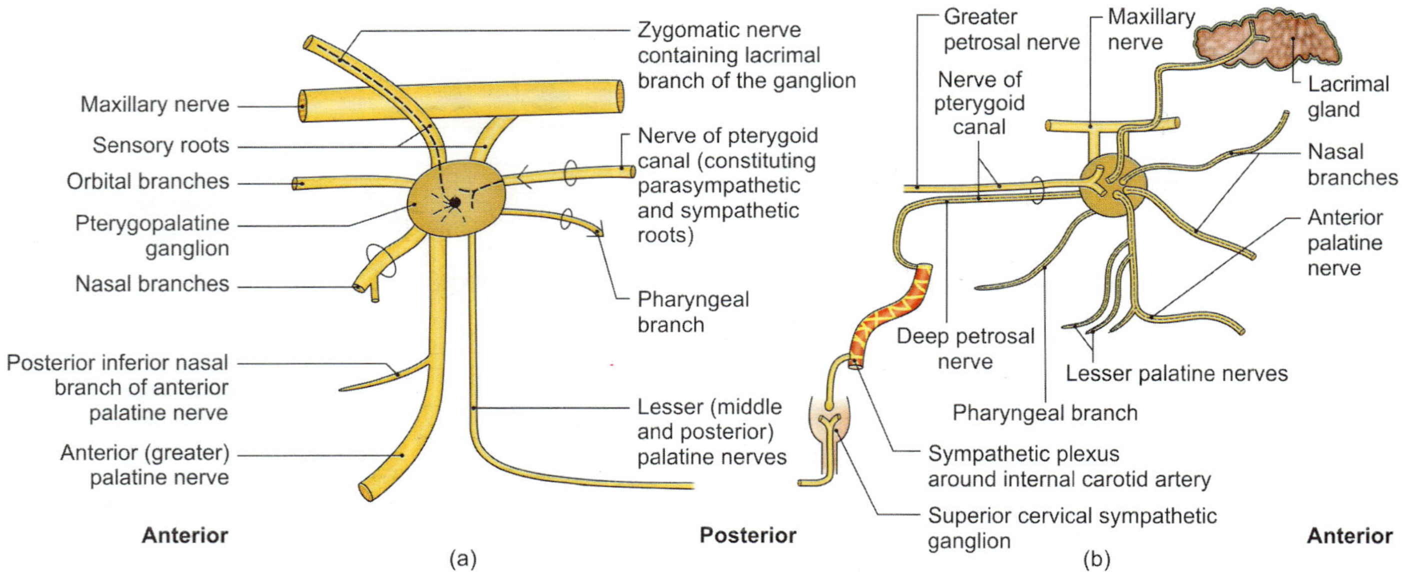

Figs 23.18a and b: (a) Connections and branches; (b) Roots and branches of pterygopalatine ganglion

pass through the *nervus intermedius*, the *facial nerve*, the *geniculate ganglion*, the *greater petrosal* nerve and the *nerve of the pterygoid canal* to reach the *ganglion*. The fibres relay in the ganglion. Postganglionic fibres arise in the ganglion to supply secretomotor nerves to the lacrimal gland and to the mucous glands of the nose, the paranasal sinuses, the palate and the nasopharynx (Fig. 23.2).

2 The *sympathetic root* is also derived from the nerve of the pterygoid canal. It contains postganglionic fibres arising in the *superior cervical sympathetic ganglion* which pass through the internal carotid plexus, the *deep petrosal nerve* and the *nerve of the pterygoid canal* to reach the ganglion. The fibres pass through the ganglion without relay, and supply vasomotor nerves to the mucous membrane of the nose, the paranasal sinuses, the palate and the nasopharynx (*see* Table A2 in Appendix).

3 The *sensory roots* come from the maxillary nerve. Its fibres pass through the ganglion without relay. They emerge in the branches (Fig. 23.17) described below.

Branches

The branches of the ganglion are actually branches of the maxillary nerve. They also carry parasympathetic and sympathetic fibres which pass through the ganglion. The branches are:

1 *Orbital branches* pass through the inferior orbital fissure, and supply the periosteum of the orbit, and the orbitalis muscle which is involuntary (Fig. 23.18).

2 *Palatine branches, the greater or anterior palatine nerve* descends through the greater palatine canal, and supplies the hard palate and the labial aspect of the upper gums. The *lesser or middle and posterior palatine nerves* supply the soft palate and the tonsil (Figs 23.18a and b).

3 *Nasal branches* enter the nasal cavity through the sphenopalatine foramen (Figs 23.17 and 23.18). The *lateral posterior superior nasal branches,* about six in number, supply the posterior parts of the superior and middle conchae (Fig. 23.11).

The *medial posterior superior nasal branches,* two or three in number, supply the posterior part of the roof of the nose and of the nasal septum (Fig. 23.6). The largest of these nerves is known as the *nasopalatine nerve* which descends up to the anterior part of the hard palate through the incisive foramen (Fig. 23.6).

4 The *pharyngeal branch* passes through the palatinovaginal canal and supplies the part of the nasopharynx behind the auditory tube (Figs 23.18a and b).

5 *Lacrimal branch*: The postganglionic fibres pass back into the maxillary nerve to leave it through its zygomatic nerve and its zygomaticotemporal branch, a communicating branch to lacrimal nerve to supply the secretomotor fibres to the lacrimal gland (Fig. 23.17).

Flowchart 23.1 shows the pathway for secretomotor fibres to lacrimal gland.

DISSECTION

Trace the connections, and branches of pterygopalatine ganglion. It is responsible for supplying secretomotor fibres to the glands of nasal cavity, palate, pharynx and the lacrimal gland. It is also called *hay fever ganglion* as inflammation of the ganglion causes allergic sinusitis.

Flowchart 23.1: The secretomotor fibres for lacrimal gland

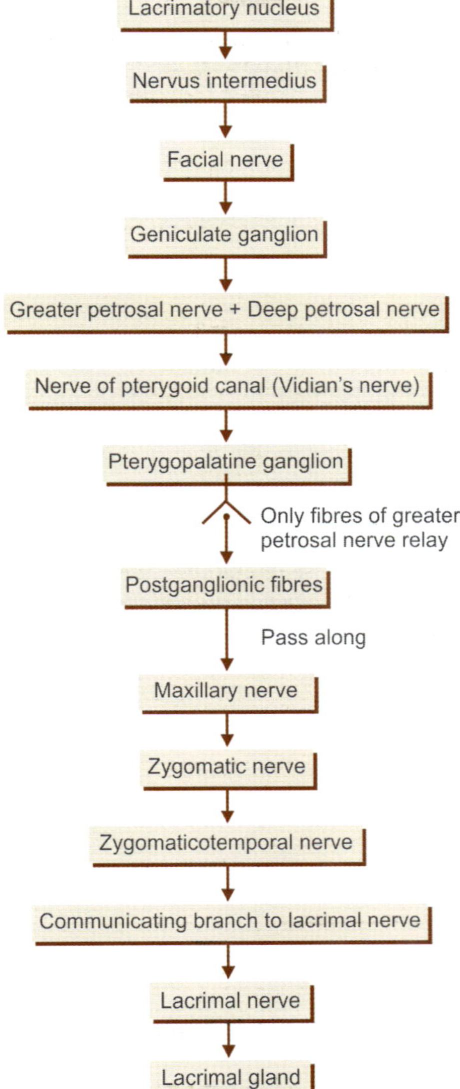

CLINICAL ANATOMY

- Trigeminal neuralgia affecting its maxillary branch produces symptoms in the area of its distribution. The nerve can be anaesthetised at the foramen rotundum.
- The pterygopalatine ganglion, if irritated or infected, causes congestion of the glands of palate and nose including the lacrimal gland producing running nose and lacrimation. The condition is called hay fever. The ganglion is called '*ganglion of hay fever*.
- Maxillary nerve carries the afferent limb fibres of the sneeze reflex as it carries general sensation from the nasal mucous membrane.

SUMMARY OF PTERYGOPALATINE FOSSA

It contains three or multiple of three structures:

Three contents:
- Maxillary nerve
- 3rd part of maxillary artery
- Pterygopalatine ganglion.

Three names of ganglion:
- Sphenopalatine
- Pterygopalatine
- Ganglion of hay fever/Meckel's ganglion.

Three structures traversing in openings in posterior wall:
- Maxillary nerve through foramen rotundum.
- Nerve of pterygoid canal through pterygoid canal.
- Pharyngeal branch through palatinovaginal canal.

Three structures through inferior orbital fissure:
- Infraorbital nerve.
- Zygomatic nerve.
- Orbital branches of the ganglion.

Three structures through inferior openings:
- One anterior palatine nerve with greater palatine vessels.
- Two posterior palatine nerves including lesser palatine vessels.

Three structures through medial opening:
- Nasopalatine nerve and sphenopalatine vessels.
- Medial posterior superior nasal branches.
- Lateral posterior superior nasal branches.

Three roots of the ganglion: Sensory, sympathetic and secretomotor.

3 × 2 branches of the ganglion: Orbital, pharyngeal, for lacrimal gland, anterior palatine, posterior palatine and nasopalatine branches.

3 × 2 branches of 3rd part of maxillary artery: Posterior superior alveolar, infraorbital, *sphenopalatine*, pharyngeal, artery of pterygoid canal and greater palatine.

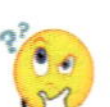

FACTS TO REMEMBER

- Artery of epistaxis is sphenopalatine.
- Upper few mm of lateral wall of nose and septum of nose are lined by olfactory epithelium with bipolar neurons in it.
- Most of the nerves and blood vessels to the lateral wall of nose and septum of nose are common. The difference is in their magnitude.
- Maxillary sinusitis is the commonest chronic sinusitis.
- Into the middle meatus of nose drain 4 sets of air sinuses.
- Sinusitis may occur due to air pollution.
- Pterygopalatine ganglion is the ganglion of 'hay fever'. It gives secretomotor fibres to lacrimal, nasal, palatal and pharyngeal glands.

- Pain of maxillary sinusitis is referred to upper teeth; of ethmoidal sinusitis to medial side of orbit and of frontal sinusitis to forehead.

CLINICOANATOMICAL PROBLEM

A child during hot summer months is playing in the park. He picks up his nose, and it starts bleeding

- What is the source of the bleeding?
- Name the arteries supplying septum of the nose.

Ans: The source of the nasal bleeding or epistaxis is injury to the large capillary plexus situated at the anteroinferior part of the septum of nose. It is called Kiesselbach's plexus and the area is also known as Little's area.

The arteries supplying the septum of nose are:

1. Anterior ethmoidal, branch of ophthalmic artery which is a branch of internal carotid.
2. Superior labial, a branch of facial artery, which in turn is a branch of external carotid artery.
3. Large sphenopalatine artery. This is the continuation of 3rd part of maxillary artery, one of the terminal branches of external carotid artery.
4. Some branches from greater palatine artery, a branch of maxillary artery.

FURTHER READING

- Becker S. Applied anatomy of the paranasal sinuses with emphasis on endoscopic sinus surgery. Ann ORL 1994;103:3–32.
  A review of serial cadaveric sections in three planes, analysed with specific attention to the anatomy of the paranasal sinuses as it pertains to endoscopic sinus surgery.
- Jafek BW. Ultrastructure of human nasal mucosa. Laryngoscope 1983;93:1579–99.
  A study that characterizes the normal ultrastructure of human nasal mucosa, emphasizing the differences between olfactory and respiratory epithelia.
- Lang J. Clinical Anatomy of the Nose, Nasal Cavity and Paranasal Sinuses, Stuttgart: Thieme. 1989.
  A study with the emphasis on exact measurements between surgical landmarks, with application to surgical procedures.
- Navarro JAC. The Nasal Cavity and Paranasal sinuses: Surgical Anatomy Berlin: Springer, 1997.
  A study that emphasizes anatomical variations and their surgical importance, with CT imaging accompanying three-place dissections.

Frequently Asked Questions

1. Classify paranasal air sinuses. Describe the maxillary air sinus with its clinical importance.
2. Describe the course and branches of maxillary nerve.
3. Write short notes on:
   a. Lateral wall of nose
   b. Pterygopalatine ganglion with its roots and branches
   c. Nerve supply of lacrimal gland
   d. Nerve supply of septum of nose
   e. Artery of epistaxis

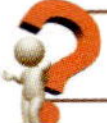

Multiple Choice Questions

1. Which of the following is the artery of epistaxis?
   a. Anterior ethmoidal
   b. Greater palatine
   c. Sphenopalatine
   d. Superior labial
2. Which one of the following air sinuses does not drain in the middle meatus of nose?
   a. Anterior ethmoidal
   b. Middle ethmoidal
   c. Posterior ethmoidal
   d. Maxillary
3. Which of the following air sinuses is first to develop?
   a. Maxillary
   b. Ethmoidal
   c. Frontal
   d. Sphenoidal
4. Nerve to pterygoid canal is formed by which nerves?
   a. Greater petrosal and deep petrosal
   b. Lesser petrosal and deep petrosal
   c. Greater petrosal and external petrosal
   d. Lesser petrosal and external petrosal
5. Which air sinus is most commonly infected?
   a. Ethmoidal
   b. Frontal
   c. Maxillary
   d. Sphenoidal
6. What is the length of auditory tube in adult person in mm?
   a. 36
   b. 3.6
   c. 46
   d. 48

Answers

1. c **2.** c **3.** a **4.** a **5.** c **6.** a

VIVA VOCE

- Name the boundaries of nasal cavity.
- Name the structures forming the nasal septum.
- Which nerves supply the nasal septum?
- What is Little's area? Which arteries anastomose in this area?
- Name the openings in the middle meatus of nose.
- How many air sinuses are there? What are their functions?
- Why does maxillary sinusitis become chronic?
- Which bones reduce the size of maxillary hiatus?
- Name the communications of pterygopalatine fossa.
- What are the roots of pterygopalatine ganglion? Name the branches of the pterygopalatine ganglion.
- Trace the pathway of secretomotor fibres to the lacrimal gland.
- How much of nasal cavity is lined by olfactory epithelium?

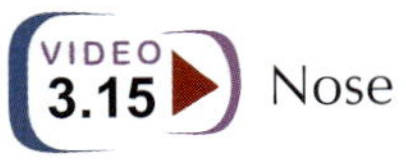

Nose

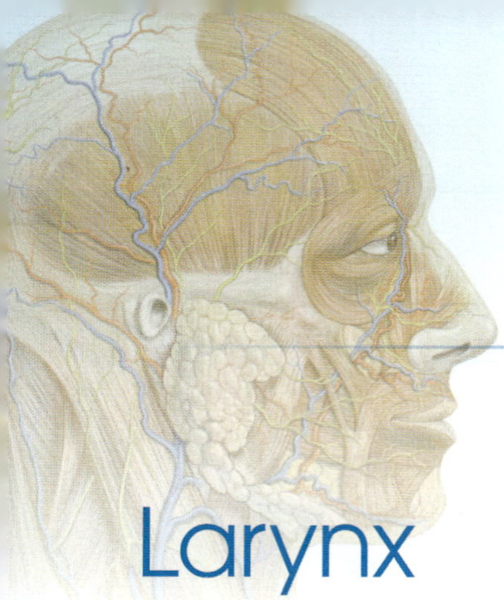

Larynx

Chapter

24

"Always laugh with others, never at them."
—Thackery

INTRODUCTION

The larynx (Latin *upper windpipe*) is the organ for production of voice or phonation. It is also an air passage, and acts as a sphincter at the inlet of the lower respiratory passages. The upper respiratory passages include the nose, the nasopharynx and the oropharynx.

Larynx or voice box is well developed in humans. Its capabilities are greatly enhanced by the large 'vocalisation area' in the lower part of motor cortex. Our speech is guided and controlled by the cerebral cortex. God has given us two ears and one mouth; to hear more, contemplate and speak less according to time and need.

A man's language is an 'index of intellect'. One speaks during the expiratory phase of respiration. Larynx is a part of the respiratory system allowing two-way flow of gases. It is kept patent because an adult is breathing about 15 times per minute, unlike the oesophagus which opens at the time of eating or drinking only.

Situation and Extent

The larynx lies in the anterior midline of the neck, extending from the root of the tongue to the trachea. In the adult male, it lies in front of the third to sixth cervical vertebrae, but in children and in the adult female, it lies at a little higher level (at C1 to C4 level) (Figs 24.1a to c).

Size

The length of the larynx is 44 mm in males and 36 mm in females. At puberty, the male larynx grows rapidly and becomes larger, seen as prominent angle of thyroid cartilage (Adam's apple); which makes his voice louder and low pitched. The pubertal growth of the female larynx is negligible, and her voice is high pitched. Internal diameter—up to 3 years, it is 3 mm; and in an adult, it is 12 mm.

CONSTITUTION OF LARYNX

The larynx is made up of a skeletal framework of cartilages. The cartilages are connected by joints, ligaments and membranes; and are moved by a number of muscles. The cavity of the larynx is lined by mucous membrane.

DISSECTION

Identify sternothyroid muscle in the sagittal section of head and neck and define its attachments on the thyroid cartilage. Define the attachments of inferior constrictor muscle from both cricoid and thyroid cartilages including the fascia overlying the cricothyroid muscle.

Cut through the inferior constrictor muscle to locate articulation of inferior horn of thyroid cartilage with cricoid cartilage, i.e. cricothyroid joint. Define the median cricothyroid ligament *(refer to BDC App)*.

Identify thyrohyoid muscle. Remove this muscle to identify thyrohyoid membrane. Identify superior laryngeal vessels and internal laryngeal nerve piercing this membrane. Identify epiglottis, thyroepiglottic and hyoepiglottic ligaments.

Strip the mucous membrane from the posterior surfaces of arytenoid and cricoid cartilages. Identify posterior cricoarytenoid, transverse arytenoid and oblique arytenoid muscles.

Recurrent laryngeal nerve was seen to enter larynx deep to the inferior constrictor muscle.

Identify cricothyroid muscle, which is the only intrinsic muscle of larynx placed on the external aspect of larynx. Remove the lower half of lamina of thyroid cartilage including the inferior horn of thyroid cartilage. Visualise the thyroarytenoid muscle in the vocal fold.

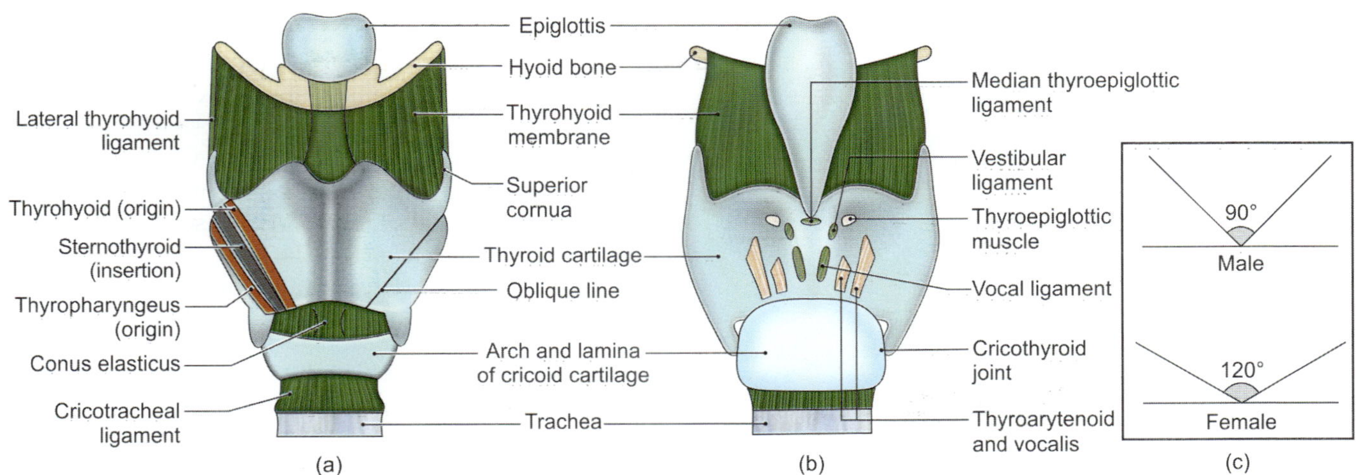

Figs 24.1a to c: Skeleton of the larynx: (a) Anterior view; (b) Posterior view; (c) Angle of thyroid laminae in male and female

CARTILAGES OF LARYNX

The larynx contains nine cartilages, of which three are unpaired and three are paired.

Unpaired cartilages

1. *Thyroid* (Greek shield-like)
2. *Cricoid* (Greek ring-like)
3. *Epiglottis* (Greek leaf-like) (Fig. 24.1a)

Paired cartilages

1. *Arytenoid* (Greek cup-shaped) (Fig. 24.1b)
2. *Corniculate* (Latin horn-shaped)
3. *Cuneiform* (Latin wedge-shaped)

Thyroid Cartilage

This cartilage is V-shaped in cross-section. It consists of right and left laminae (Fig. 24.1a). Each lamina is roughly quadrilateral. The laminae are placed obliquely relative to the midline, their posterior borders are far apart, but the anterior borders approach each other at an angle that is about 90° in the male and about 120° in the female (Fig. 24.1c).

The lower parts of the anterior borders of the right and left laminae fuse and form a median projection called the *laryngeal prominence.* The upper parts of the anterior borders do not meet. They are separated by the *thyroid notch.* The posterior borders are free. They are prolonged upwards and downwards as the superior and inferior cornua or horns. The superior cornua is connected with the greater cornua of the hyoid bone by the lateral *thyrohyoid ligament*.

The inferior cornua articulates with the cricoid cartilage to form the *cricothyroid joint* (Fig. 24.2).

The inferior border of the thyroid cartilage is convex in front and concave behind. In the median plane, it is connected to the cricoid cartilage by the *conus elasticus*.

The *outer surface* of each lamina is marked by an oblique line which extends from the superior thyroid tubercle in front of the root of superior cornua to the inferior thyroid tubercle behind the middle of inferior border. The (i) thyrohyoid, (ii) sternothyroid and (iii) thyropharyngeus part of inferior constrictor of pharynx are attached to the oblique line (Fig. 24.1a).

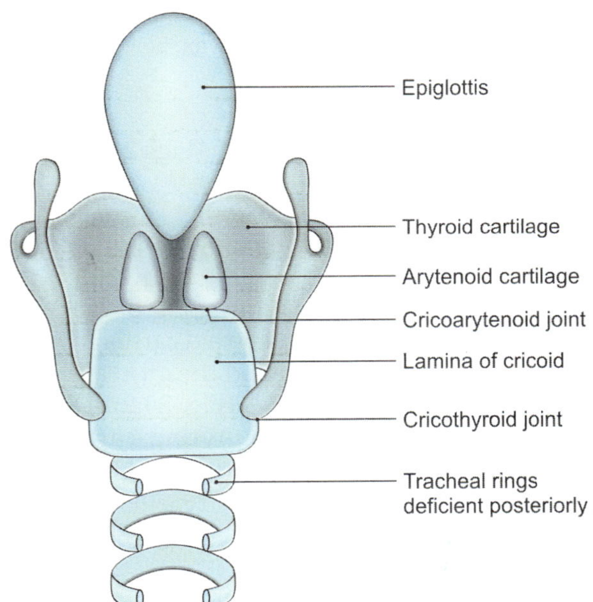

Fig. 24.2: Cartilages of the larynx: Posterior view

Attachments

Lower border and inferior cornua give insertion to triangular cricothyroid. Along the posterior border connecting superior and inferior cornua are the insertion of (i) palatopharyngeus, (ii) salpingopharyngeus, (iii) stylopharyngeus (Fig. 24.3).

On inner aspect are attached:

a. Median thyroepiglottic ligament
b. Thyroepiglottic muscle on each side
c. Vestibular fold on each side
d. Vocal fold on each side

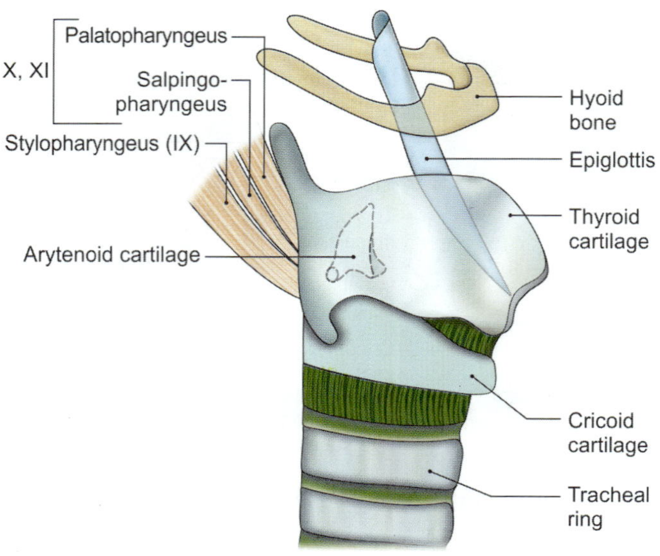

Fig. 24.3: Cartilages of the larynx: Lateral view

e. Thyroarytenoid
f. Vocalis muscle on each side (Figs 24.1 and 24.4).

Cricoid Cartilage

This cartilage is shaped like a ring and is a complete cartilage. It encircles the larynx below the thyroid cartilage and forms foundation stone of larynx. It is thicker and stronger than the thyroid cartilage. The ring has a narrow anterior part called the *arch,* and a broad posterior part, called the *lamina* (Fig. 24.2). The lamina projects upwards behind the thyroid cartilage, and articulates superiorly with the arytenoid cartilages.

The inferior cornua of the thyroid cartilage articulates with the side of the cricoid cartilage at the junction of the arch and lamina.

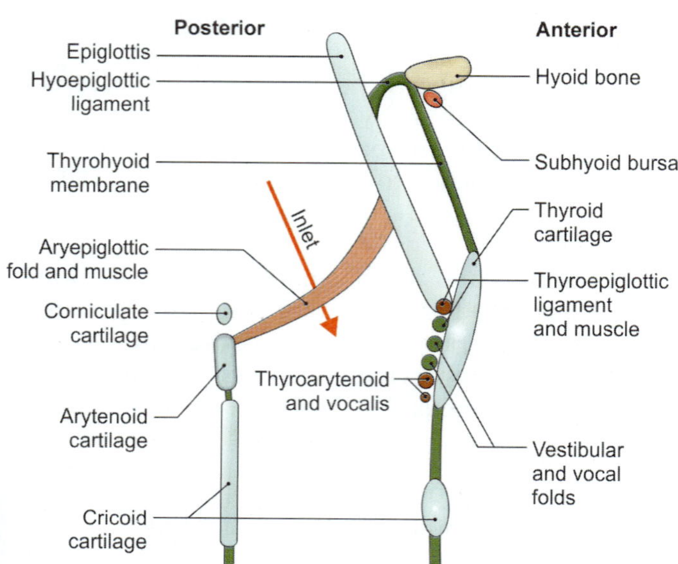

Fig. 24.4: Cartilages of the larynx as seen in sagittal section

Attachments

Anterior part of arch of cricoid gives origin to triangular *cricothyroid muscle,* a tensor of vocal cord (Fig. 24.9c).

Anterolateral aspect of arch gives origin to *lateral cricoarytenoid muscle,* an adductor of vocal cord.

Lamina of cricoid cartilage on its outer aspects gives origin to a very important 'safety muscle', the posterior cricoarytenoid muscle (Fig. 24.10).

Cricothyroid and quadrate membranes are also attached (Fig. 24.5a).

Epiglottic Cartilage/Epiglottis

This is a *leaf-shaped* cartilage placed in the anterior wall of the upper part of the larynx. Its *upper end* is broad and free, and projects upwards behind the hyoid bone and the tongue (Fig. 24.5b).

The *lower end* or thyroepiglottic ligament is pointed and is attached to the upper part of the angle between the two laminae of the thyroid cartilage (Figs 24.1b and 24.4).

Attachments

The right and left margins of the cartilage provide attachment to the aryepiglottic folds. Its *anterior surface* is connected:

a. To the tongue by a median *glossoepiglottic fold* (*see* Fig. 25.1)
b. To the hyoid bone by the hyoepiglottic ligament (Fig. 24.4). The *posterior surface* is covered with mucous membrane, and presents a tubercle in the lower part (Fig. 24.15).

Thyroepiglottic muscle is attached between thyroid cartilage and margins of epiglottis. It keeps the inlet of larynx patent for breathing.

Aryepiglottic muscle closes inlet during swallowing (Fig. 24.11a).

Arytenoid Cartilage

These are two small *pyramid-shaped* cartilages lying on the upper border of the lamina of the cricoid cartilage. The *apex* of the arytenoid cartilage is curved posteromedially and articulates with the corniculate cartilage. Its *base* is concave and articulates with the lateral part of the upper border of the cricoid lamina. Base is prolonged anteriorly to form the *vocal process,* and laterally to form the *muscular process* (Fig. 24.3). The *surfaces* of the cartilage are anterolateral, medial and posterior (Figs 24.2 to 24.4 and 24.5c).

Attachments

Vocal process: Vocal fold and vocalis muscle is attached.

Above vocal process: Vestibular fold attached.

Muscular process: Posterior aspect gives insertion to posterior cricoarytenoid.

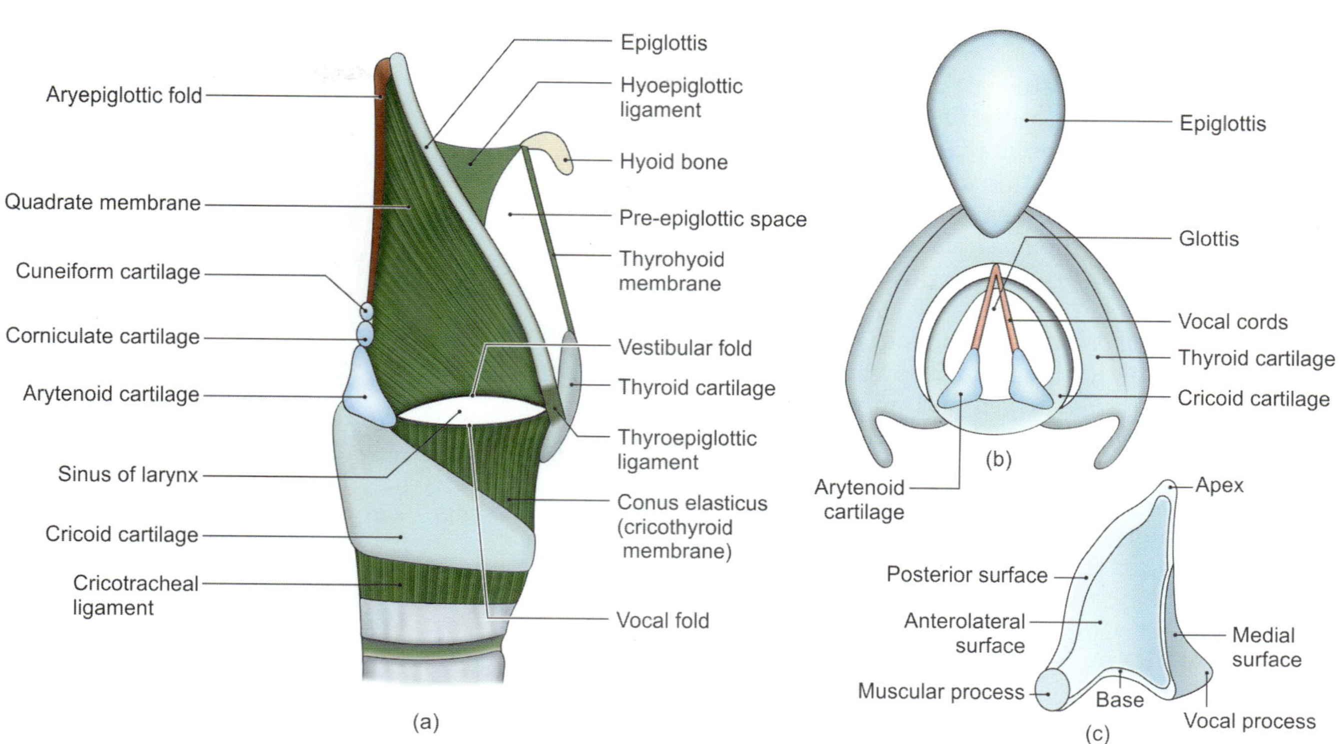

Figs 24.5a and b: (a) Ligaments and membranes of the larynx. Note the quadrate membrane and the conus elasticus, (b) vocal cords and inlet of larynx seen, and (c) arytenoid cartilage

Anterior aspect gives insertion to lateral crico-arytenoid.

Posterior surface: Transverse arytenoid across the two cartilages.

Between base and apex of arytenoid is *oblique arytenoid* which continues as *aryepiglottic muscle* into two sides of epiglottis.

Quadrangular or quadrate membrane is attached between arytenoid, epiglottis and thyroid cartilages.

Corniculate/Santorini Cartilages

These are two small conical nodules which articulate with the apex of the arytenoid cartilages, and are directed posteromedially. They lie in the posterior parts of the aryepiglottic folds (Fig. 24.5a).

Cuneiform/Wrisberg Cartilages

These are two small rod-shaped pieces of cartilage placed in the aryepiglottic folds just ventral to the corniculate cartilages (Fig. 24.5a).

Histology of Laryngeal Cartilages

The thyroid, cricoid cartilages, and the basal parts of the arytenoid cartilages are made up of the hyaline cartilage. They may ossify after the age of 25 years. The other cartilages of the larynx, e.g. epiglottis, corniculate, cuneiform and processes of the arytenoid are made of the elastic cartilage and do not ossify.

LARYNGEAL JOINTS

The *cricothyroid joint* is a *synovial* joint between the inferior cornua of the thyroid cartilage and the side of the cricoid cartilage. It permits rotatory movements around a transverse axis passing through both cricothyroid joints permitting tension and relaxation of vocal cords. There are some gliding movements also in different directions (Fig. 24.2).

The *cricoarytenoid joint* is also a *synovial* joint between the base of the arytenoid cartilage and the upper border of the lamina of the cricoid cartilage. It permits rotatory movements around a vertical axis permitting adduction and abduction of the vocal cords and also gliding movements in all directions (Fig. 24.2).

LARYNGEAL LIGAMENTS AND MEMBRANES

Extrinsic

1. The *thyrohyoid membrane* connects the thyroid cartilage to the hyoid bone. Its median and lateral parts are thickened to form the median and lateral thyrohyoid ligaments (Fig. 24.5a). The membrane is pierced by the internal laryngeal nerve, and by the superior laryngeal vessels.
2. The *hyoepiglottic ligament* connects the upper end of the epiglottic cartilage to the hyoid bone (Fig. 24.4).
3. The *cricotracheal ligament* connects the cricoid cartilage to the upper end of the trachea (Fig. 24.1).

Intrinsic

The intrinsic ligaments are part of a broad sheet of fibroelastic tissue, known as the *fibroelastic membrane of the larynx*. This membrane is placed just outside the mucous membrane. It is interrupted on each side by the sinus of the larynx. The part of the membrane above the sinus is known as the *quadrate membrane*, and the part below the sinus is called the *conus elasticus* (Fig. 24.5a).

The *quadrate membrane* extends from the arytenoid cartilage to the epiglottis. It has a lower free border which forms the *vestibular fold* and an upper border which forms the *aryepiglottic fold*.

The *conus elasticus* or *cricovocal membrane* extends upwards and medially from the arch of the cricoid cartilage. The anterior part is thick and is known as the *cricothyroid ligament*. The upper free border of the conus elasticus forms the *vocal fold* (Fig. 24.5b).

CAVITY OF LARYNX

1 The cavity of the larynx extends from the inlet of the larynx to the lower border of the cricoid cartilage. The *inlet of the larynx* is placed obliquely. It looks backwards and upwards, and opens into the laryngopharynx. The inlet is *bounded anteriorly*, by the epiglottis; *posteriorly*, by the interarytenoid fold of mucous membrane; and *on each side*, by the aryepiglottic fold (Figs 24.5a and b).

   Internal diameter: Up to 3 years, 3 mm; every year it increases by 1 mm up to 12 years.

2 Within the cavity of larynx, there are two folds of mucous membrane on each side. The upper fold is the *vestibular fold*, and the lower fold is the *vocal fold*. The space between the right and left vestibular folds is the *rima vestibuli*; and the space between the vocal folds is the *rima glottidis* (Fig. 24.6).

   The vocal fold is attached anteriorly to the middle of the angle of the thyroid cartilage on its posterior aspect; and posteriorly to the vocal process of the arytenoid cartilage (Fig. 24.11b).

   The rima is limited posteriorly by an interarytenoid fold of mucous membrane.

   The rima glottidis, therefore, has an anterior intermembranous part (three-fifths) and a posterior intercartilaginous part (Fig. 24.15a).

   The rima is the narrowest part of the larynx. It is longer (23 mm) in males than in females (17 mm).

3 The vestibular and vocal folds divide the cavity of the larynx into three parts:
   a. The part above the vestibular fold is called the *vestibule* of the larynx or supraglottis.
   b. The part between the vestibular and vocal folds is called the sinus or *ventricle* of the larynx (Fig. 24.6).

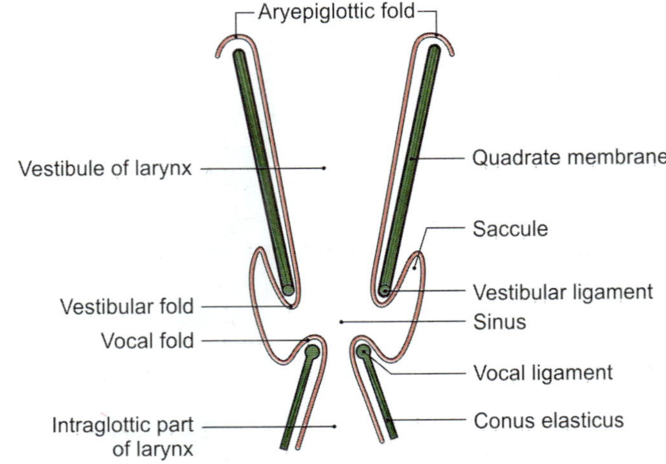

Fig. 24.6: Cavity of the larynx

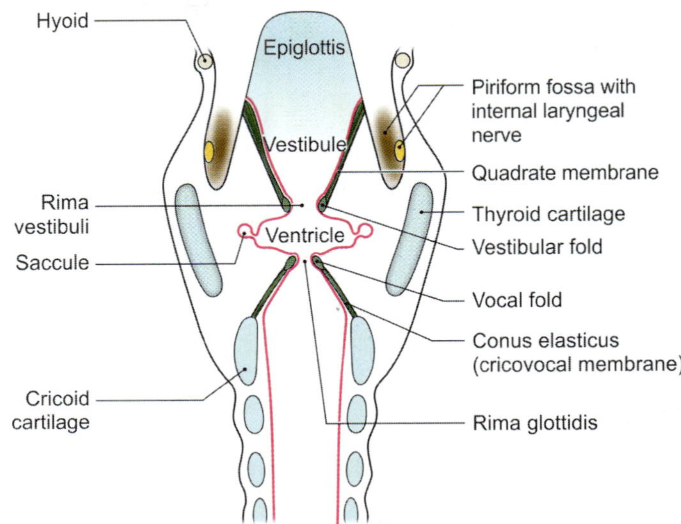

Fig. 24.7: Cavity of larynx and position of piriform fossa

   c. The part below the vocal folds is called the *infraglottis* (Fig. 24.7).

The *sinus of Morgagni or ventricle of the larynx* is a narrow fusiform cleft between the vestibular and vocal folds. The anterior part of the sinus is prolonged upwards as a diverticulum between the vestibular fold and the lamina of the thyroid cartilage. This extension is known as the *saccule of the larynx*. The saccule contains mucous glands which help to lubricate the vocal folds. It is often called *oil can of larynx*.

MUCOUS MEMBRANE OF LARYNX

1 The anterior surface and upper half of the posterior surface of the epiglottis, the upper parts of the aryepiglottic folds, and the vocal folds are lined by the *stratified squamous epithelium*. The rest of the laryngeal mucous membrane is covered with the *ciliated columnar epithelium*.

2 The mucous membrane is loosely attached to the cartilages of the larynx except over the vocal ligaments and over the posterior surface of the epiglottis where it is thin and firmly adherent.

3 The *mucous glands* are absent over the vocal cords, but are plentiful over the anterior surface of the epiglottis, around the cuneiform cartilages and in the vestibular folds. The glands are scattered over the rest of the larynx.

CLINICAL ANATOMY

- Since the larynx or glottis is the narrowest part of the respiratory passages, foreign bodies are usually lodged here.
- Infection of the larynx is called laryngitis. It is characterized by hoarseness of voice.
- Laryngeal oedema may occur due to a variety of causes. This can cause obstruction to breathing.
- Misuse of the vocal cords may produce nodules on the vocal cords mostly at the junction of anterior one-third and posterior two-thirds. These are called Singer's nodules or Teacher's nodules (Fig. 24.8).
- *Fibreoptic flexible laryngoscopy:* Under local anaesthesia, flexible laryngoscope is passed and larynx well visualised.
- *Microlaryngoscopy:* This procedure is performed under operating microscope. Vocal cord tumors and diseases are excised by this method.
- *External examination of larynx:* Head is flexed in sitting position. Examiner stands behind and palpates larynx and neck with finger tips for tumour, swelling, lymphadenitis, etc.
- Speech analysis is also necessary in laryngeal diseases.
- *Foreign body in larynx:* At times fish bones may get impacted in the vallecula or piriform fossa. Often these bones just scratch the mucosa on their way down, and the person gets a feeling of foreign body sensation, due to a dull visceral pain caused by the scratch.
- Piriform fossa lies between quadrate membrane and medial side of thyroid cartilage. It is traversed by internal laryngeal nerve. Piriform fossa is used to smuggle out precious stones, diamonds, etc. It is called *smuggler's fossa* (Fig. 24.7).
- The mucous membrane of the larynx is supplied by X nerve through superior laryngeal or recurrent laryngeal nerves. So laryngeal tumours may also cause referred pain in the ear partly supplied by auricular branch of X nerve.
- Large foreign bodies may block laryngeal inlet leading to suffocation.
- Small foreign bodies may lodge in laryngeal ventricle, cause reflex closure of the glottis and suffocation.
- Inflammation of upper larynx may cause oedema of supraglottis part. It does not extend below vocal cords because mucosa is adherent to vocal ligament.

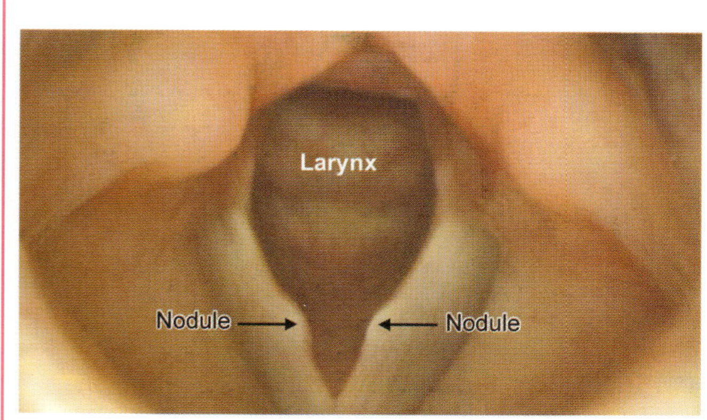

Fig. 24.8: Indirect laryngoscopic examination

INTRINSIC MUSCLES OF LARYNX

The attachments of intrinsic muscles of larynx are presented in Table 24.1 and their main action shown in Table 24.2.

Nerve Supply

All intrinsic muscles of the larynx are supplied by the recurrent laryngeal nerve except for the cricothyroid which is supplied by the external laryngeal nerve.

Actions

The vocal and muscular processes move in opposite directions. Any muscle which pulls the muscular process medially, pushes the vocal process laterally, resulting in abduction of vocal cords. This is done by only one pair of muscle, the posterior cricoarytenoid (Fig. 24.9a).

Muscles which pull the muscular process forward and laterally will push the vocal process medially (Fig. 24.9b) causing adduction of vocal cords. This is done by lateral cricoarytenoid and transverse arytenoid.

The cricothyroid causes rocking movement of thyroid forwards and downwards at cricothyroid joints, thus tensing and lengthening the vocal cords (Fig. 24.9c).

The thyroarytenoid pulls the arytenoid forward, relaxing the vocal cords (Table 24.2 and Fig. 24.11).

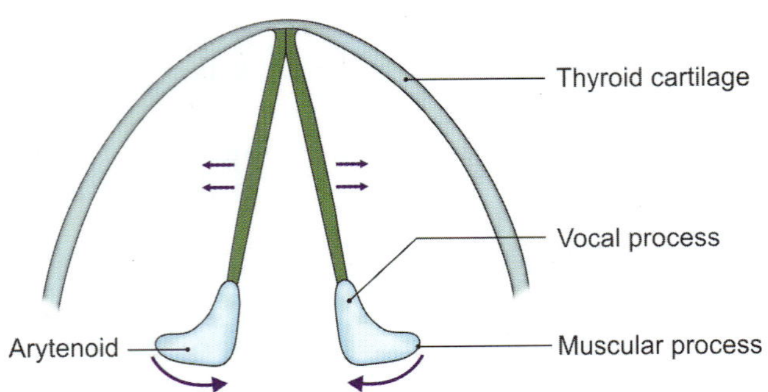

Fig. 24.9a: Abduction of vocal cords

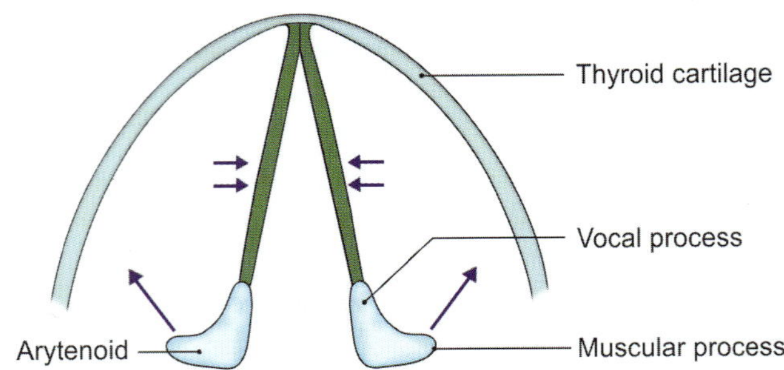

Fig. 24.9b: Adduction of vocal cords

Table 24.1: Intrinsic muscles of the larynx

Muscle	*Origin*	*Fibres*	*Insertion*
1. **Cricothyroid** The only muscle outside the larynx (Fig. 24.9c)	Lower border and lateral surface of cricoid	Fibres pass backwards and upwards	Inferior cornua and lower border of thyroid cartilage. It is called 'tuning fork of larynx'
2. **Posterior cricoarytenoid triangular** (Fig. 24.10)	Posterior surface of the lamina of cricoid	Upwards and laterally	Posterior aspect of muscular process of arytenoid
3. **Lateral cricoarytenoid** (Figs 24.11a and b)	Lateral part of upper border of arch of cricoid	Upwards and backwards	Anterior aspect of muscular process of arytenoid
4. **Transverse arytenoid** Unpaired muscle (Fig. 24.10)	Posterior surface of one arytenoid	Transverse	Posterior surface of another arytenoid
5,6. **Oblique arytenoid** and **aryepiglottic** (Fig. 24.10)	Muscular process of one arytenoid	Oblique	Apex of the other arytenoid. Some fibres are continued as *aryepiglottic* muscle to the edge of the epiglottis
7,8. **Thyroarytenoid** and **thyroepiglottic** (Figs 24.11a and b)	Thyroid angle and adjacent cricothyroid ligament	Backwards and upwards	Anterolateral surface of arytenoid cartilage. Some of the upper fibres of thyroarytenoid curve upwards into the aryepiglottic fold to reach the edge of epiglottis, known as *thyroepiglottic*
9. **Vocalis** (Fig. 24.12)	Vocal process of arytenoid cartilage	Pass forwards	Vocal ligament and thyroid angle

Table 24.2: Muscles acting on the larynx

Movement	*Muscle*
1. Elevation of larynx	Thyrohyoid, mylohyoid
2. Depression of larynx	Sternothyroid, sternohyoid
3. Opening inlet of larynx	Thyroepiglottic
4. Closing inlet of larynx	Aryepiglottic
5. Abductor of vocal cords	Posterior cricoarytenoid only
6. Adductor of vocal cords	Lateral cricoarytenoid, transverse and oblique arytenoids
7. Tensor of vocal cords and modulation of voice	Cricothyroid
8. Relaxor of vocal cords	Thyroarytenoid and vocalis

a. Muscles which abduct the vocal cords: Only posterior cricoarytenoids (safety muscle of larynx).

b. Muscles which adduct the vocal cords:

   i. Lateral cricoarytenoids

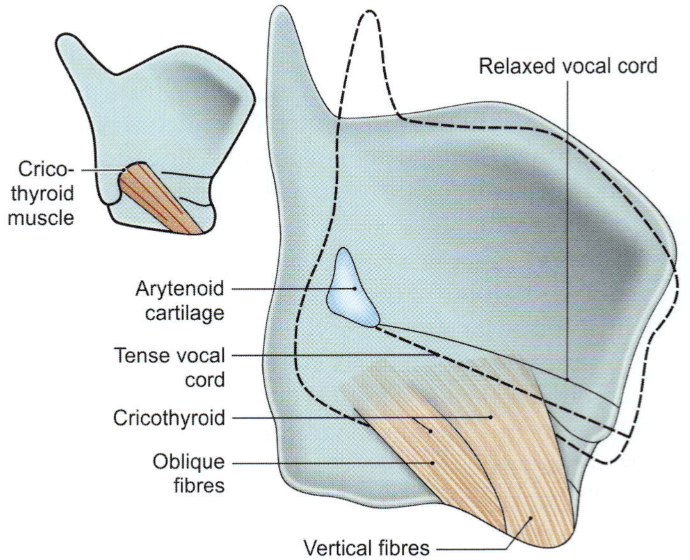

Fig. 24.9c: Cricothyroid muscle

ii. Transverse arytenoid
iii. Cricothyroids (tuning fork of larynx)
iv. Thyroarytenoids (Figs 24.11a and b).

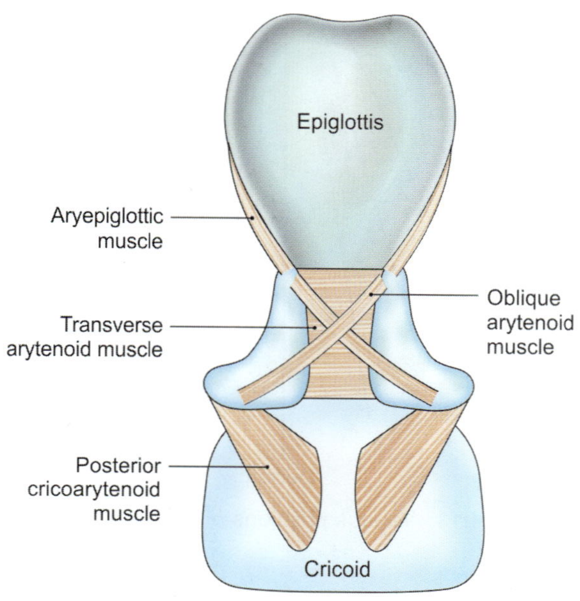

Fig. 24.10: Muscles of larynx: Posterior view

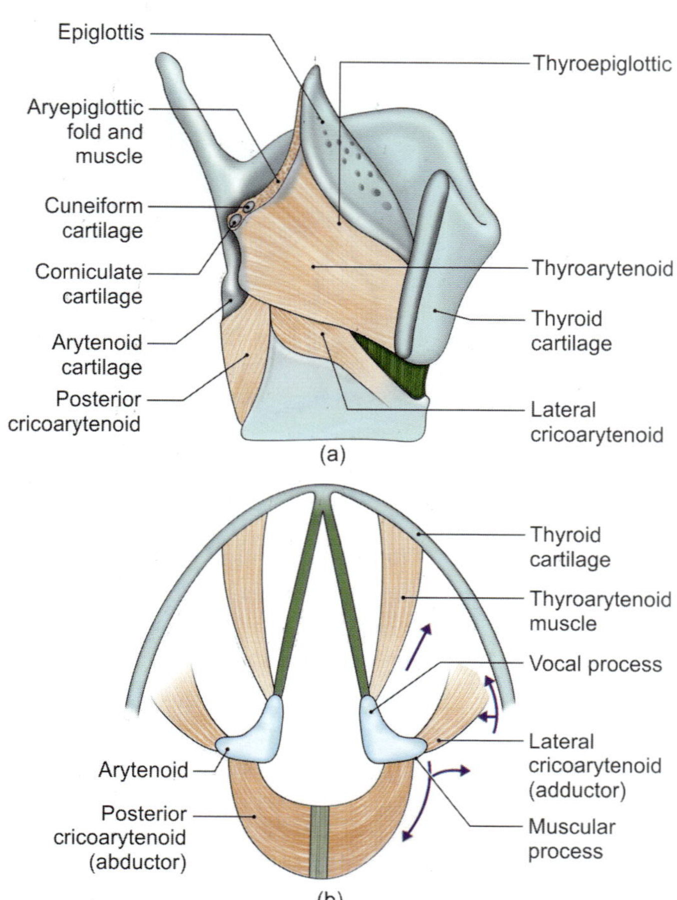

Figs 24.11a and b: Muscles of the larynx: (a) Lateral view; (b) Horizontal view

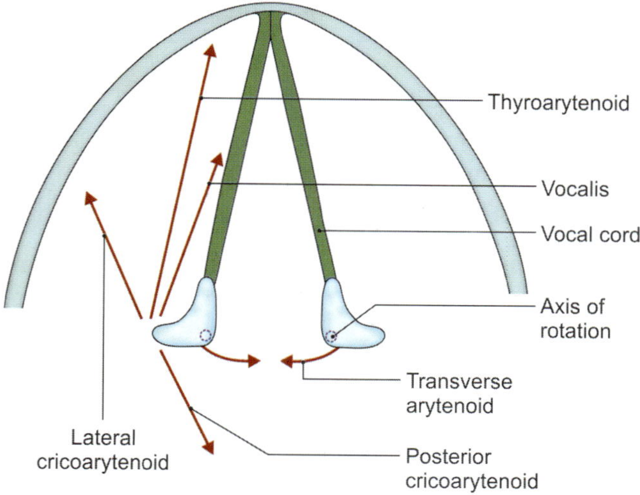

Fig. 24.12: Scheme to show the direction of pull of some intrinsic muscles of the larynx

c. Muscles which tense the vocal cords: Cricothyroids (Fig. 24.9c).
d. Muscles which relax the vocal cords:
   i. Thyroarytenoids (Fig. 24.12)
   ii. Vocalis.
e. Muscles which close the inlet of the larynx:
   i. Oblique arytenoids
   ii. Aryepiglottic (Fig. 24.11a).
f. Muscles which open the inlet of larynx: Thyroepiglotticus (Fig. 24.11b).

Arterial Supply and Venous Drainage

Up to the Vocal Folds

By the superior laryngeal artery, a branch of the superior thyroid artery. The superior laryngeal vein drains into the superior thyroid vein.

Below the Vocal Folds

By the inferior laryngeal artery, a branch of the inferior thyroid artery. The inferior laryngeal vein drains into the inferior thyroid vein.

Nerve Supply

Motor Nerves

Recurrent laryngeal nerve supplies posterior cricoarytenoid, lateral cricoarytenoid, transverse and oblique arytenoid, aryepiglottic, thyroarytenoid, thyroepiglottic muscles. It supplies all intrinsic muscles except cricothyroid.

External laryngeal nerve only supplies cricothyroid muscle.

Sensory Nerves

The internal laryngeal nerve supplies the mucous membrane up to the level of the vocal folds. The recurrent laryngeal nerve supplies it below the level of the vocal folds.

Lymphatic Drainage

Lymphatics from the part above the vocal folds drain along the superior thyroid vessels to the anterosuperior group of deep cervical nodes by piercing thyrohyoid membrane.

Those from the part below the vocal folds drain to the posteroinferior group of deep cervical nodes. A few of them drain into the prelaryngeal nodes by piercing cricothyroid. True vocal folds, i.e. glottis acts as watershed for lymphatics. It has 'no' lymphatics. Carcinoma of glottis carries best prognosis.

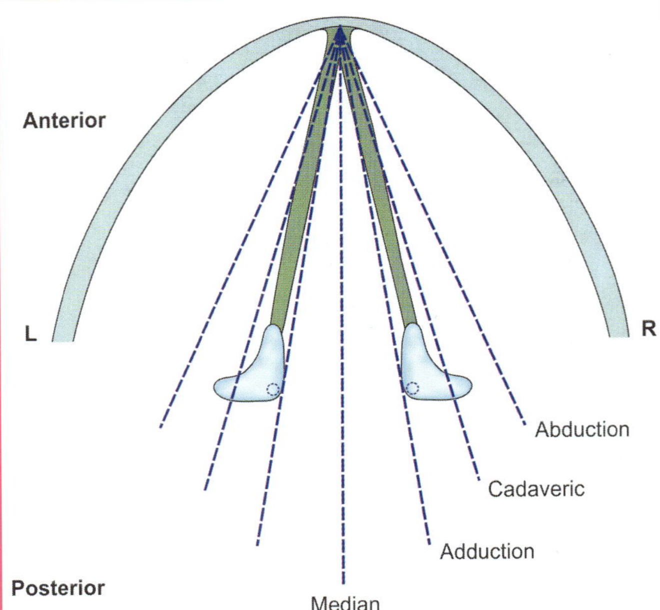

Fig. 24.13: Various positions of the vocal cords

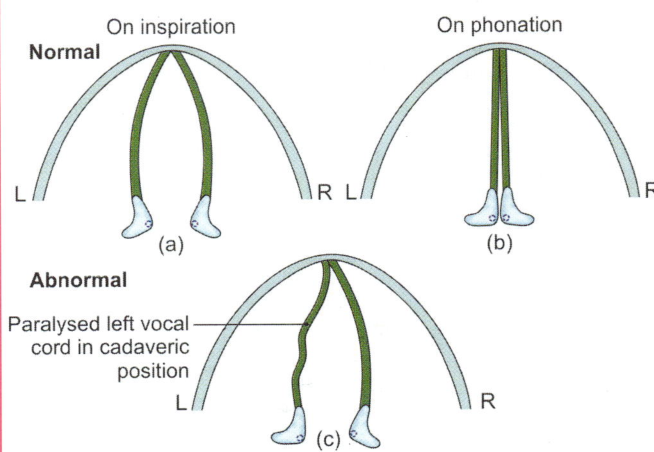

Figs 24.14a to c: Position of vocal cords: (a) Normal: Inspiration; (b) Normal: Phonation; (c) Abnormal conditions

CLINICAL ANATOMY

- When any foreign object enters the larynx severe protective coughing is excited to expel the object. However, damage to the internal laryngeal nerve produces anaesthesia of the mucous membrane in the supraglottic part of the larynx breaking the reflex arc so that foreign bodies can readily enter it.
- Damage to the external laryngeal nerve causes some weakness of phonation due to loss of the tightening effect of the cricothyroid on the vocal cord.
- When both recurrent laryngeal nerves are interrupted, the vocal cords lie in the cadaveric position in between abduction and adduction and phonation is completely lost. Deep breathing also becomes difficult through the partially opened glottis (Fig. 24.13).
- When only one recurrent laryngeal nerve is paralysed, the opposite vocal cord compensates for it and phonation is possible but there is hoarseness of voice. There is failure of forceful explosive part of voluntary and reflex coughing (Fig. 24.14c).
- Tumours in the piriform fossa cause dysphagia. These also cause referred pain in the ear. Pain of pharyngeal tumours may be referred to the ear, as X nerve carries sensation both from the pharynx and the external auditory meatus and the tympanic membrane.
- *Recurrent laryngeal nerve:* Mediastinal tumours may press on the left recurrent laryngeal nerve, as it is given off in the thorax. The pressure on the nerve may present as alteration in the voice. Right recurrent laryngeal nerve is given off in the neck, so it is not affected by mediastinal tumours.
- The larynx can be examined either directly through a laryngoscope or indirectly through a laryngeal mirror (indirect laryngoscopy) (Fig. 24.15).
- By laryngoscopy, one can inspect the base of the tongue, the valleculae, the epiglottis, the aryepiglottic folds, the piriform fossae, the vestibular folds, and the vocal folds.
- Tumours of the vocal cords can be diagnosed early, because there are changes in the voice. Tumours in subglottic area present late so are diagnosed late and have poor prognosis.

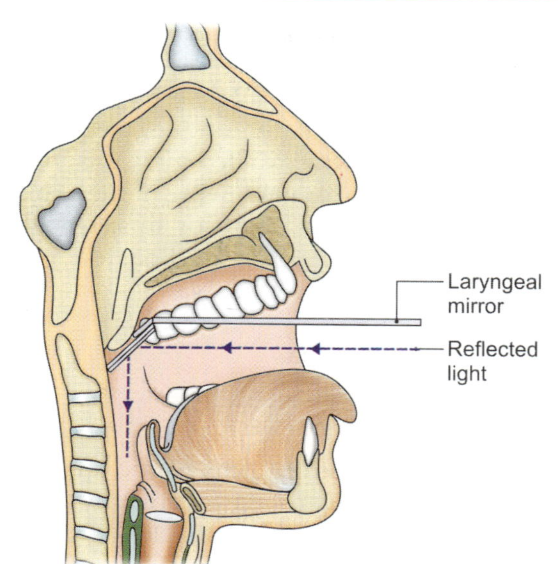

Fig. 24.15: Parts of larynx seen by indirect laryngoscopy

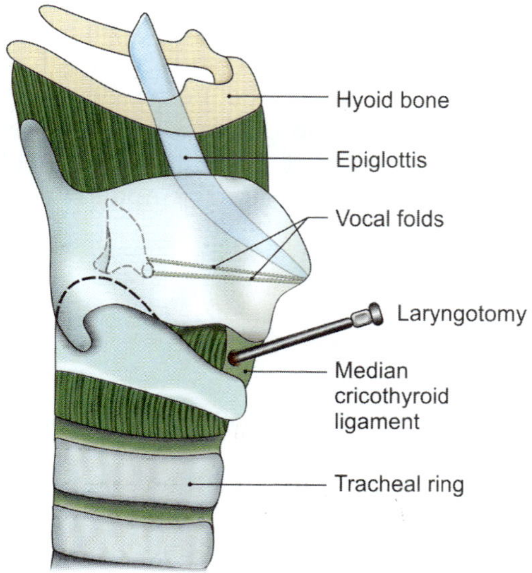

Fig. 24.16: Laryngotomy

- *Laryngotomy:* The needle is inserted in the midline of cricothyroid membrane, below the thyroid prominence. This is done as an emergency procedure (Fig. 24.16).
- Tracheostomy is a permanent procedure. Part of 2nd–4th rings of trachea are removed after incising the isthmus of the thyroid gland.
- If the patient is unconscious, one must remember—A: Airway, B: Breathing, C: Circulation in that order. For the patency of airway, pull the tongue out and also endotracheal tube needs to be passed. The tube should be passed between the right and left vocal cords down to the trachea.

MOVEMENTS OF VOCAL FOLDS

Movements of the vocal folds affect the shape and size of the rima glottidis.

1. During quiet breathing or condition of rest, the intermembranous part of the rima is triangular, and the intercartilaginous part is quadrangular (Fig. 24.17a).
2. During phonation or speech, the glottis is reduced to a chink by the adduction of the vocal folds (Figs 24.17b and 24.18).
3. During forced inspiration, both parts of the rima are triangular, so that the entire rima is lozenge-shaped; the vocal folds are fully abducted (Fig. 24.17c) (i.e. diamond-shaped glottis).
4. During whispering, the intermembranous part of the rima glottidis is closed, but the intercartilaginous part is widely open (Fig. 24.17d) (i.e. funnel-shaped glottis).

INFANT'S LARYNX

Cavity of infant's larynx is short and funnel-shaped.

- Size is one-third of an adult. Lumen is very narrow.
- Position is higher than in adult.

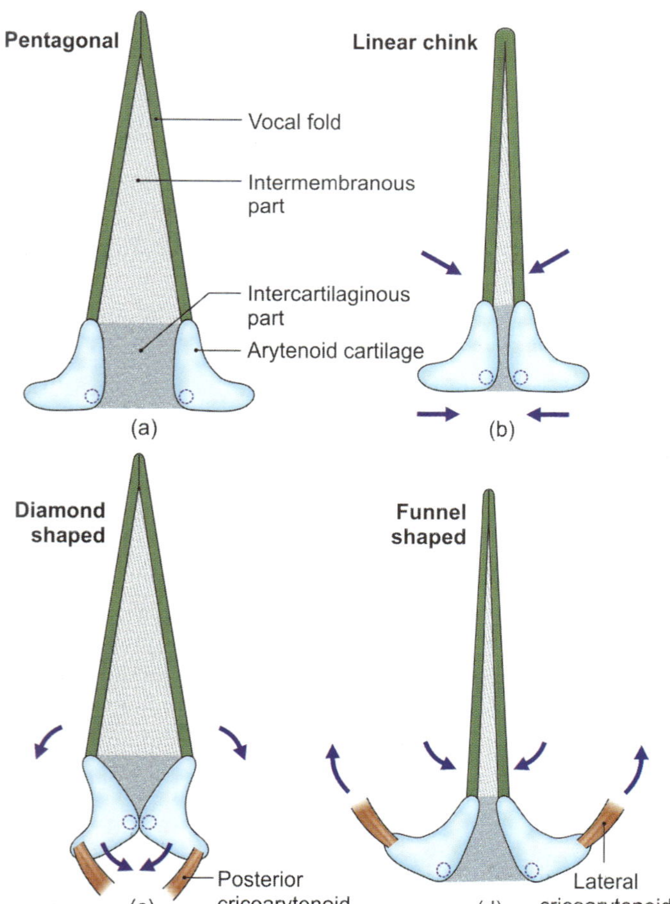

Figs 24.17a to d: Rima glottidis: (a) In quiet breathing; (b) In phonation or speech; (c) During forced inspiration; (d) During whispering

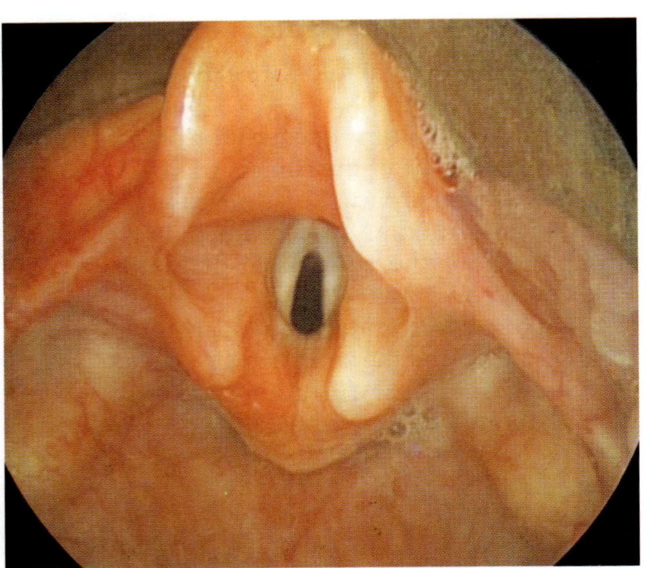

Fig. 24.18: Direct laryngoscopic view of vocal cords in adducted position

- Epiglottis lies at C2 and during elevation, it reaches C1, so that infant can use nasal airway for breathing while suckling.
- Laryngeal cartilages are softer, more pliable than in adult.
- Thyroid cartilage is shorter and broader.
- Vocal cords are only 4–4.5 mm long, shorter than in childhood and in adult.
- Supraglottic and subglottic mucosa are lax, swelling results in respiratory obstruction.
- One must be careful while giving anaesthesia to an infant (birth to one year).

MECHANISM OF SPEECH

The mechanism of speech involves the following four processes:
- Expired air from lungs
- Vibrators
- Resonators
- Articulators

Expired Air

As the air is forced out of lungs and larynx, it produces voice. Loudness or intensity of voice depends on the force of expiration of air.

Vibrators

The expired air causes vibrations of the vocal cords. Pitch of voice depends on the rate of vibration of vocal cords. Vowels are produced in the larynx. The air is not stopped by palate, tongue, teeth or lips.

Resonators

The column of air between vocal cords and nose and lips act as resonators. Quality of sound depends on resonators. One can make out change of quality of voice even on the telephone.

Articulators

These are formed by palate, tongue, teeth and lips. These narrow or stop the exhaled air. Consonants are produced by stoppage or narrowing of the expired air either by palate, tongue, teeth or lips. Consonants produced by lips are—Pa, Pha, Ba, Bha, Ma
Labiodental—Ta, Tha, Da, Dha, Na
Lingual—Cha, Ja, Jha
Palatal—Ka, Kha, Ga, Gha.

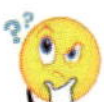

FACTS TO REMEMBER

- Only intrinsic muscle of larynx placed on the outer aspect of laryngeal cartilages is cricothyroid.
- Cricothyroid is the only muscle supplied by external laryngeal nerve.
- External laryngeal nerve runs with superior thyroid artery near the gland.
- Posterior cricoarytenoid is the only abductor of vocal cord and so it is a life-saving muscle.
- Piriform fossa is called smuggler's fossa as precious stones, etc. can be hidden here.
- The primary function of larynx is to protect the lower respiratory tract. Phonation has developed with evolution and is related to motor speech area of the cerebral cortex.

CLINICOANATOMICAL PROBLEM

Due to a severe infection of the voice box and with high temperature, a patient is not able to speak and breathe at all.
- Paralysis of which muscles causes extreme difficulty in breathing?
- Name the muscles of larynx and their actions.

Ans: Due to infection of the larynx, the branches of recurrent laryngeal nerve supplying posterior cricoarytenoid muscles are infected. Since this pair of muscle is the only abductor of vocal cord, the vocal cords get adducted, resulting in extreme difficulty in breathing. Tracheostomy is the main line of treatment, if infection is not controlled.

Movement of larynx	*Muscles*
Abduction of vocal cord	Posterior cricoarytenoid
Adduction of vocal cord	Lateral cricoarytenoid Transverse arytenoid Oblique arytenoid
Opening inlet of larynx	Thyroepiglottic
Closing inlet of larynx	Aryepiglottic
Tensor of vocal cord	Cricothyroid
Relaxor of vocal cord	Thyroarytenoid

FURTHER READING

- Moreau S, de Rugy MG, Babin E, et al. The recurrent laryngeal nerve: related vascular anatomy. Laryngoscope 1998; 108:1351–55.

  An explanation of the considerable variability in the perineural vasculature of the recurrent laryngeal nerve, which lies in close proximity to and is usually supplied by the posterior branch of the inferior thyroid artery.

- Aronson AE, Bless. Clinical Voice Disorders, 4th ed, New York: Thieme, 2009.

  A comprehensive summary of the organic disorders of voice due to laryngeal structural changes and neurological disease, as well as psychogenic voice disorders.

- Berkovitz BKB, Moxham BJ, Hickey S. The anatomy of the larynx. In: Ferlito A (ed). Diseases of the Larynx. London: Chapman & Hall; 2000; pp. 25–44.

  A description of all aspects of laryngeal anatomy, together with a very useful bibliography.

- Dickson DR, Maue-Dickson W. Anatomical and Physiological Bases of Speech, Boston: Little, Brown. 1982.

  Some highly detailed descriptions of the structure of the larynx.

- Welsh LW, Welsh II, Rizzo TA. Laryngeal spaces and lymphatics: Current anatomic concepts. Ann Otol Rhinol Laryngol Suppl 1983;105:19–31.

  A description of the 'tissue spaces' and lymphatic drainage of the larynx and their importance in determining the route of spread of tumours.

Frequently Asked Questions

1. Describe the intrinsic muscles of larynx. Add a note on their clinical importance.
2. Mention the structures attached to various parts of thyroid cartilage.
3. Write short notes on:
   a. Rima glottidis
   b. Epiglottis
   c. Cricoid cartilage
   d. Vocal folds
   e. Pyriform fossa

Multiple Choice Questions

1. Which histological type of cartilage is epiglottis?
   a. Fibrous
   b. Elastic
   c. Hyaline
   d. Fibroelastic
2. Which is the only abductor muscle of the vocal cord?
   a. Lateral cricoarytenoid
   b. Thyroarytenoid
   c. Posterior cricoarytenoid
   d. Thyroepiglottic
3. Recurrent laryngeal nerve supplies all muscles, *except:*
   a. Posterior cricoarytenoid
   b. Oblique arytenoids
   c. Lateral cricoarytenoid
   d. Cricothyroid
4. Angle of anterior borders of laminae of thyroid cartilage in adult male is:
   a. 90°
   b. 100°
   c. 80°
   d. 120°
5. Which of the following muscles is not inserted in the posterior border of thyroid cartilage?
   a. Palatopharyngeus
   b. Salpingopharyngeus
   c. Stylopharyngeus
   d. Levator veli palatini
6. Which muscle is not attached to cricoid cartilage?
   a. Cricothyroid
   b. Oblique arytenoid
   c. Lateral cricoarytenoid
   d. Posterior cricoarytenoid
7. Which of the following muscles is the 'safety' muscle of larynx?
   a. Lateral cricoarytenoid
   b. Posterior cricoarytenoid
   c. Oblique arytenoid
   d. Transverse arytenoids
8. Pain of pharyngeal tumours is referred to ear due to which of the following nerves?
   a. IX
   b. X
   c. V
   d. VII

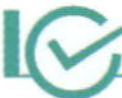

Answers

1. b **2.** c **3.** d **4.** a **5.** d **6.** b **7.** b **8.** b

VIVA VOCE

- How much is the angle of thyroid laminae in male and female?
- Name the muscles attached to the posterior border of thyroid cartilage.
- Name the paired and unpaired cartilages of the larynx.
- Name the laryngeal joints.
- Name the sensory nerves innervating the mucous membrane of larynx.
- Name the boundaries of piriform fossa. What is its importance?
- Where and why do the singer's nodules develop?
- Name the intrinsic muscles of larynx.
- Which muscles cause tension and relaxation of the vocal cords?
- Which is a life-saving muscle and why?
- Which muscles open/close the laryngeal inlet?
- Name the positions of vocal cords during quiet breathing, phonation, forced inspiration and whispering.
- Which is the only muscle supplied by external laryngeal nerve?
- Name the functions of larynx.
- What are the boundaries of inlet of larynx?

Larynx

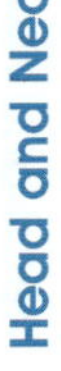

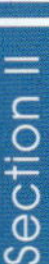

Chapter 25

Tongue

"Tongue is not steel, yet it cuts.
Taste makes waist."
—Anonymous

INTRODUCTION

The tongue is a muscular organ situated in the floor of the mouth. It is associated with the functions of (i) taste, (ii) speech, (iii) chewing, (iv) deglutition, and (v) cleansing of mouth.

Tongue comprises skeletal muscles which are voluntary. These voluntary muscles start behaving as involuntary in any classroom—funny?

Thanks to the taste buds that the multiple hotels, restaurants, fast food outlets, *chat–pakori* shops, etc. are flourishing. One need not be too fussy about the taste of the food. Nutritionally, it should be balanced and hygienic.

DISSECTION

In the sagittal section, identify fan-shaped genioglossus muscle. Cut the attachments of buccinator, superior constrictor muscles and the intervening pterygomandibular raphe and reflect these downwards exposing the lateral surface of the tongue. Look at the superior, inferior surfaces of your own tongue with the help of hand lens *(refer to BDC App)*.

PARTS OF TONGUE

The tongue has:

1 A root
2 A tip
3 A body, which has:
   a. A curved upper surface or dorsum (Fig. 25.1), and
   b. An inferior surface confined to the oral part only.

The *root* is attached to the styloid process and soft palate above, and to mandible and the hyoid bone below. Because of these attachments, we are not able to swallow the tongue itself. In between the mandible and hyoid bones, it is related to the geniohyoid and mylohyoid muscles.

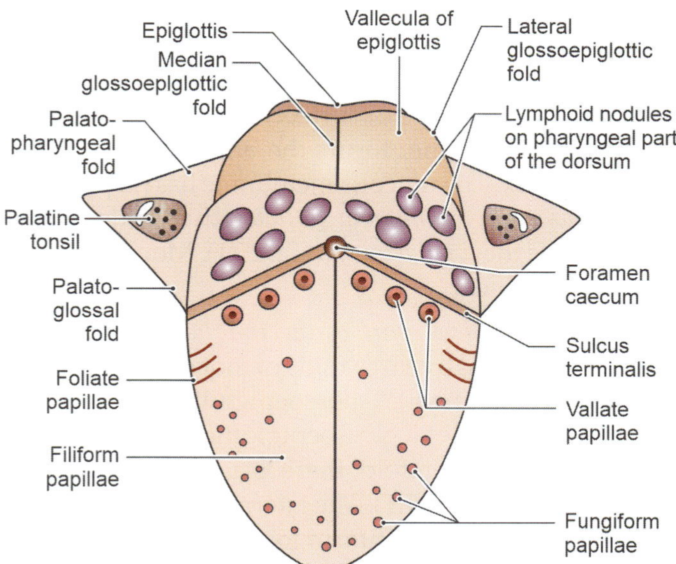

Fig. 25.1: The dorsum of the tongue, epiglottis and palatine tonsil

The *tip* of the tongue forms the anterior free end which, at rest, lies behind the upper incisor teeth.

The *dorsum* of the tongue (Fig. 25.1) is convex in all directions. It is divided into:

- An *oral part* or anterior two-thirds.
- A *pharyngeal part* or posterior one-third, by a faint V-shaped groove, the *sulcus terminalis.* The two limbs of the 'V' meet at a median pit, named the *foramen caecum.* They run laterally and forwards up to the palatoglossal arches. The foramen caecum represents the site from which the thyroid diverticulum grows down in the embryo. The oral and pharyngeal parts of the tongue differ in their development, topography, structure, and function (Table 25.3).
- Small posteriormost part

1 The *oral or papillary part of the tongue* is placed on the floor of the mouth. Its *margins* are free and in contact with the gums and teeth. Just in front of the palatoglossal arch, each margin shows 4 to 5 vertical folds, named the *foliate papillae*.

The *superior surface* of the oral part shows a median furrow and is covered with papillae which make it rough (Fig. 25.1).

The *inferior surface* is covered with a smooth mucous membrane, which shows a median fold called the *frenulum linguae.*

On either side of the frenulum, there is a prominence produced by the deep lingual veins. More laterally, there is a fold called the *plica fimbriata* that is directed forwards and medially towards the tip of the tongue (Fig. 25.2).

2 The *pharyngeal or lymphoid part of the tongue* lies behind the palatoglossal arches and the sulcus terminalis. Its posterior surface, sometimes called the base of the tongue, forms the anterior wall of the oropharynx. The mucous membrane has no papillae, but has many *lymphoid follicles* that collectively constitute the *lingual tonsil* (Fig. 25.1). Mucous glands are also present.

3 The *posteriormost part of the tongue* is connected to the epiglottis by three folds of mucous membrane. These are the median glossoepiglottic fold and the right and left lateral glossoepiglottic folds. On either side of the median fold, there is a depression called the *vallecula* (Fig. 25.1). The lateral folds separate the vallecula from the piriform fossa.

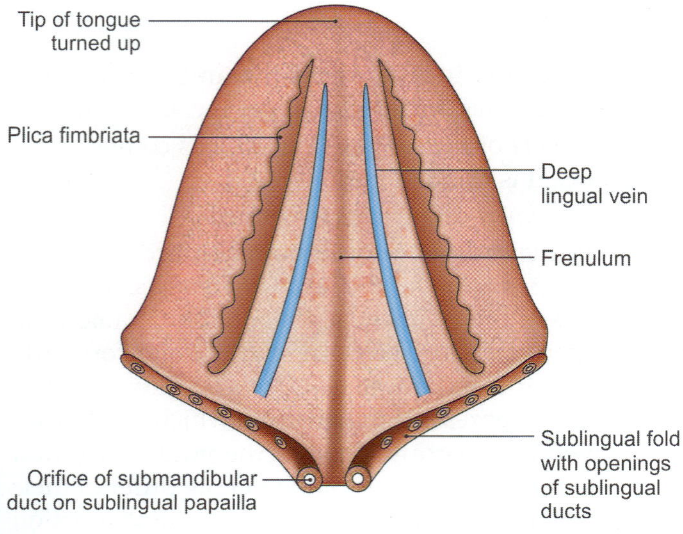

Fig. 25.2: The inferior surface of tongue and the floor of the mouth

CLINICAL ANATOMY

- Glossitis is usually a part of generalized ulceration of the mouth cavity or stomatitis. In certain anaemias, the tongue becomes smooth due to atrophy of the filiform papillae.
- The presence of a rich network of lymphatics and of loose areolar tissue in the substance of tongue is responsible for enormous swelling of tongue in *acute glossitis*. The tongue fills up the mouth cavity and then protrudes out of it.
- The undersurface of the tongue is a good site along with the bulbar conjunctiva for observation of jaundice.
- In unconscious patients, the tongue may fall back and obstruct the air passages. This can be prevented either by lying the patient on one side with head down (the 'tonsil position') or by keeping the tongue out mechanically.
- Lingual tonsil in the posterior one-third of the tongue forms part of Waldeyer's ring (*see* Fig. 22.13).

PAPILLAE OF THE TONGUE

These are projections of mucous membrane or corium which give the anterior two-thirds of the tongue, its characteristic roughness. These are of the following four types (Fig. 25.3).

1 *Vallate* or *circumvallate papillae:* They are large in size, 1–2 mm in diameter and are 8–12 in number. They are situated immediately in front of the sulcus terminalis. Each papilla is a cylindrical projection surrounded by a circular sulcus. The walls of the papilla have taste buds.

2 The *fungiform papillae* are numerous near the tip and margins of the tongue, but some of them are also scattered over the dorsum. These are smaller than the vallate papillae but larger than the filiform papillae. Each papilla consists of a narrow pedicle and a large rounded head. They are distinguished by their bright red colour (Fig. 25.3).

3 The *filiform papillae* or *conical papillae* cover the presulcal area of the dorsum of the tongue, and give it a characteristic velvety appearance. They are the smallest and most numerous of the lingual papillae. Each is pointed and covered with keratin; the apex is often split into filamentous processes.

4 *Foliate papillae* are present at the lateral border just in front of circumvallate papillae. They are leaf shaped.

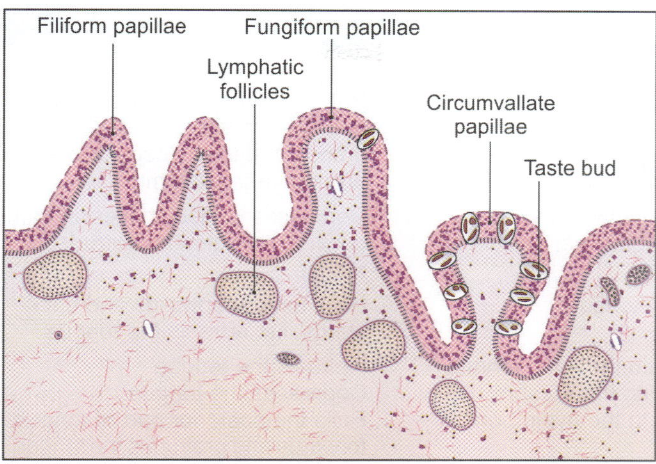

Fig. 25.3: Types of papillae and taste buds

MUSCLES OF THE TONGUE

A middle fibrous septum divides the tongue into right and left halves. Each half contains four intrinsic and four extrinsic muscles.

Intrinsic Muscles

They occupy the upper part of the tongue, and are attached to the submucous fibrous layer and to the median fibrous septum. They alter the shape of the tongue (Fig. 25.4).

1 *Superior longitudinal*: It arises from the fibrous tissue deep to the mucous membrane on the dorsum of the tongue and the midline lingual septum. They pass longitudinally back from the tip of the tongue to its root posteriorly. It inserts into the overlying mucous membrane. The superior longitudinal muscles act to elevate the tip and sides of the tongue superiorly. This shapes the tongue dorsum into a concavity and it shortens the tongue.

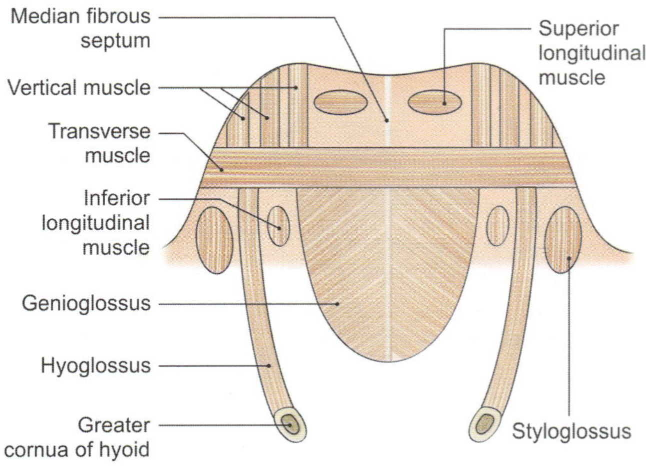

Fig. 25.4: Coronal section of the tongue showing arrangement of the intrinsic muscles and extrinsic muscles

2 *Inferior longitudinal*: It originates from the fibrous tissue beneath the mucous membrane stretching from tip of tongue longitudinally back to the root of the tongue and the hyoid bone. They insert into the mucous membrane of the tongue dorsum. It lies between the genioglossus and the hyoglossus.

The inferior longitudinal muscles act to curl the tip of the tongue inferiorly. This makes the dorsum of the tongue convex in shape and shortens the tongue.

3 *Transverse*: It lies as a sheet on either side of the midline in a plane that is deep to the superior longitudinal muscles but superficial to genioglossus.

They run transversely from their origin at the fibrous lingual septum to insert into the submucous fibrous tissue at the lateral margins of the tongue.

Contraction of the transverse muscles acts to narrow and increases the thickness of the tongue.

4 *Vertical*: It is found at the borders of the anterior part of the tongue. It makes the tongue broad.

Extrinsic Muscles

1 Genioglossus
2 Hyoglossus
3 Styloglossus
4 Palatoglossus

The *extrinsic muscles* connect the tongue to the mandible via genioglossus; to the hyoid bone through hyoglossus; to the styloid process via styloglossus, and the palate via palatoglossus. These are described in Table 25.1.

The actions of intrinsic and extrinsic muscles are mentioned in Table 25.2.

Arterial Supply

It is derived from the tortuous *lingual artery*, a branch of the external carotid artery. The root of the tongue is also supplied by the tonsillar artery, a branch of facial artery, and ascending pharyngeal branch of external carotid artery (Fig. 25.6). *See* Chapter 12 for the course and branches of the lingual artery.

Venous Drainage

1 *Deep lingual vein:* The chief vein of tongue, seen on the inferior surface of tongue near median plane.
2 *Venae comitantes*, accompany lingual artery. They are joined by dorsal lingual veins.
3 *Venae comitantes* accompanying the hypoglossal nerve.

These veins unite at the posterior border of the hyoglossus to form the lingual vein which ends in the internal jugular vein.

Table 25.1: Extrinsic muscles of tongue			
Muscle	*Origin*	*Insertion*	*Actions*
Palatoglossus (Fig. 25.6)	Oral surface of palatine aponeurosis	Descends in the palatoglossal arch to the side of tongue at the junction of oral and pharyngeal parts	Pulls up the root of tongue, approximates the palatoglossal arches and thus closes the oropharyngeal isthmus
Hyoglossus (Fig. 25.6)	Whole length of greater cornua and lateral part of hyoid bone	Side of tongue between styloglossus and inferior longitudinal muscle of tongue	Depresses tongue, makes dorsum convex, retracts the protruded tongue
Styloglossus (Fig. 25.6)	Tip and part of anterior surface of styloid process	Into the side of tongue	Pulls tongue upwards and backwards, i.e. retracts the tongue
Genioglossus Fan-shaped bulky muscle (Fig. 25.5)	Upper genial tubercle of mandible	Upper fibres into the tip of tongue Middle fibres into the dorsum Lower fibres into the hyoid bone	Retracts the tongue Depresses the tongue Pulls the posterior part of tongue forwards and protrudes the tongue. It is a *life-saving muscle*

Table 25.2: Summary of the actions of muscles	
Intrinsic muscles	*Actions*
Superior longitudinal	Shortens the tongue, makes its dorsum concave
Inferior longitudinal	Shortens the tongue, makes its dorsum convex
Transverse	Makes the tongue narrow and elongated
Vertical (Fig. 25.4)	Makes the tongue broad and flattened
Extrinsic muscles	*Actions*
Genioglossus (Fig. 25.5)	Protrudes the tongue
Hyoglossus (Fig. 25.6)	Depresses the tongue
Styloglossus (Fig. 25.6)	Retracts the tongue
Palatoglossus	Elevates the tongue

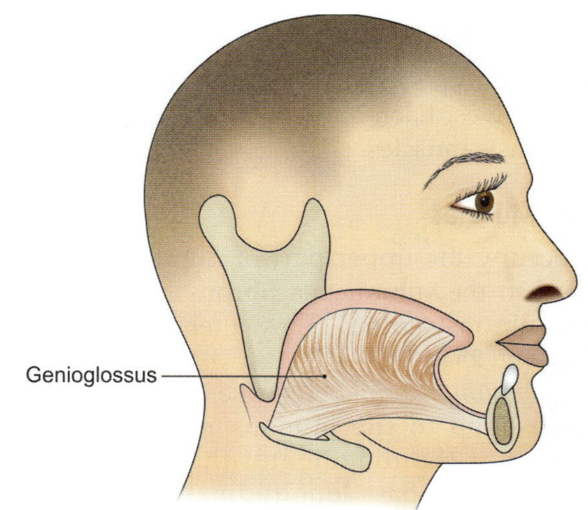

Fig. 25.5: Genioglossus

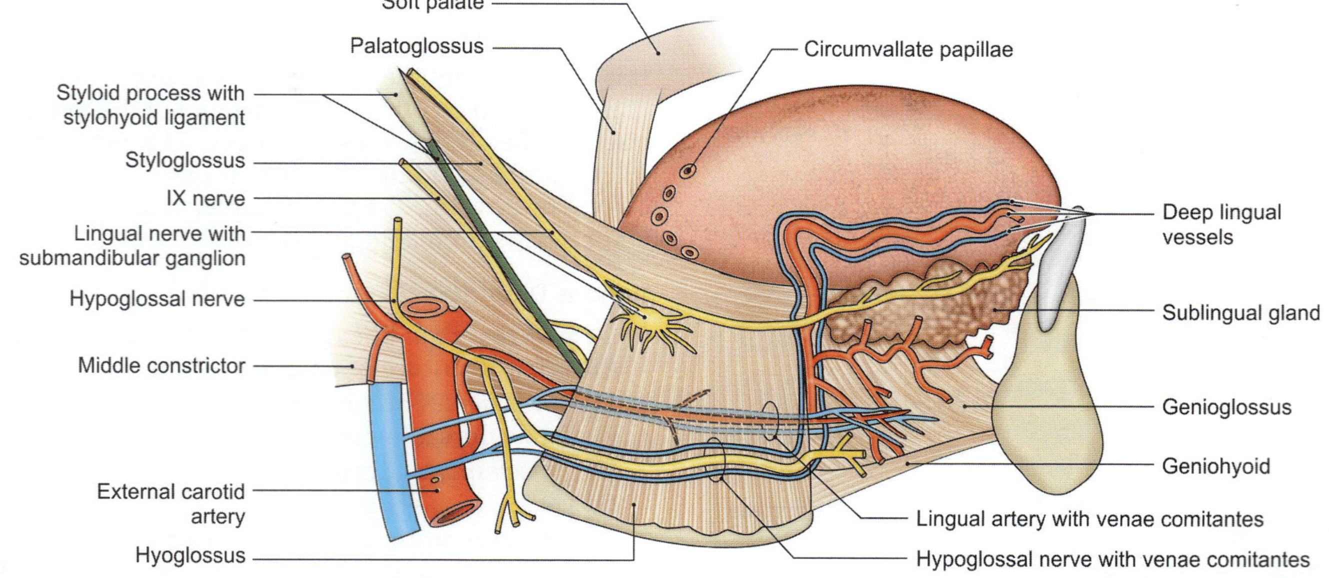

Fig. 25.6: Arterial supply and extrinsic muscles of the tongue

Lymphatic Drainage

1 The tip of the tongue drains bilaterally to the submental nodes (Figs 25.7a and b).
2 The right and left halves of the remaining part of the anterior two-thirds of the tongue drain unilaterally to the submandibular nodes. A few central lymphatics drain bilaterally to the deep cervical nodes (Fig. 25.7b).
3 The posteriormost part and posterior one-third of the tongue drain bilaterally into the upper deep cervical lymph nodes including jugulodigastric nodes.
4 The whole lymph finally drains to the *jugulo-omohyoid nodes. These are known as the lymph nodes of the tongue.*

Nerve Supply

Motor Nerves

All the intrinsic and extrinsic muscles, except the palatoglossus, are supplied by the hypoglossal nerve. The palatoglossus is supplied by the cranial root of the accessory nerve through the pharyngeal plexus.

So seven out of eight muscles are supplied by XII nerve (Fig. 25.8a).

Sensory Nerves

The lingual nerve is the nerve of general sensation and the chorda tympani is the nerve of taste for the anterior two-thirds of the tongue except vallate papillae (Fig. 25.8b).

The glossopharyngeal nerve is the nerve for both general sensation and taste for the posterior one-third of the tongue including the circumvallate papillae.

The posteriormost part of the tongue is supplied by the vagus nerve through the internal laryngeal branch (Table 25.3).

HYPOGLOSSAL NERVE—XII NERVE

Hypoglossal nerve is the nerve of muscles of the tongue.

It leaves the cranial cavity through anterior condylar/hypoglossal canal.

Course: Lies between internal jugular vein and internal carotid artery in front of vagus.

Lower down it curves forwards to cross both internal and external carotid arteries. It also crosses loop of lingual artery to lie on hyoglossus muscle. Finally it enters substance of tongue. It supplies 3 extrinsic muscles and all 4 intrinsic muscles of tongue.

CLINICAL ANATOMY

- Carcinoma of the tongue is quite common. The affected side of the tongue is removed surgically. All the deep cervical lymph nodes are also removed, i.e. block dissection of neck because recurrence of malignant disease occurs in lymph nodes. Carcinoma of the posterior one-third of the tongue is more dangerous due to bilateral lymphatic spread.

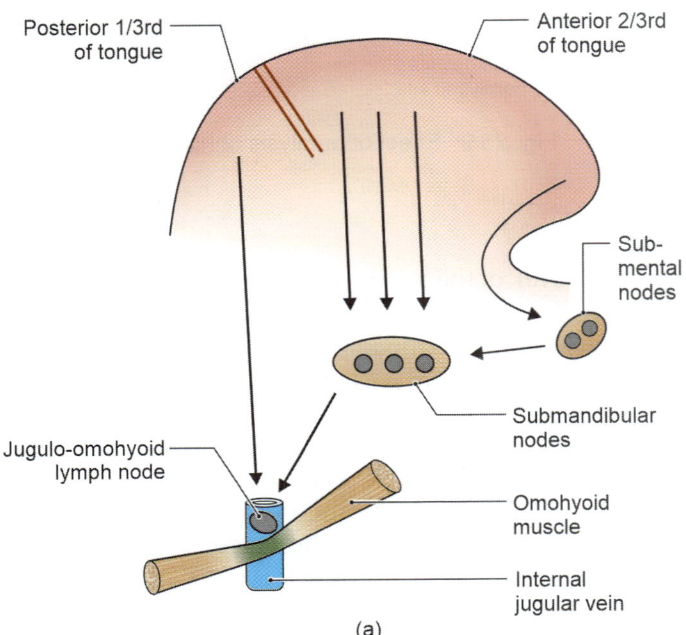

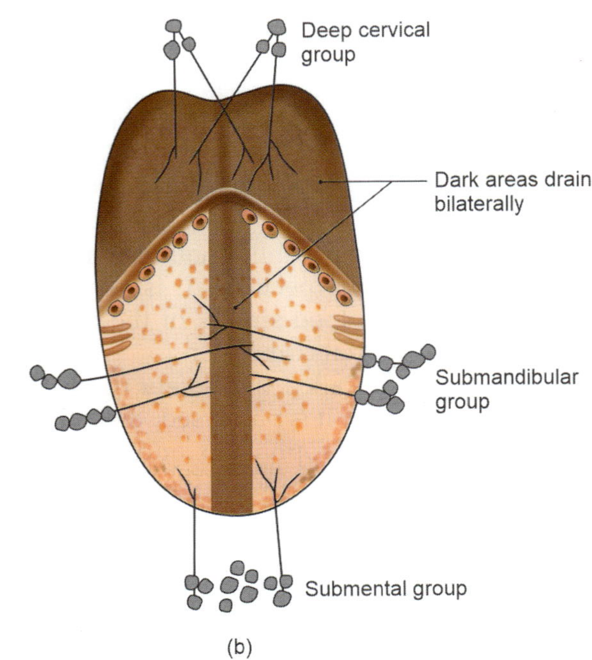

Figs 25.7a and b: Lymphatic drainage of tongue: (a) Lateral surface; (b) Dorsum, dark areas of tongue drain bilaterally

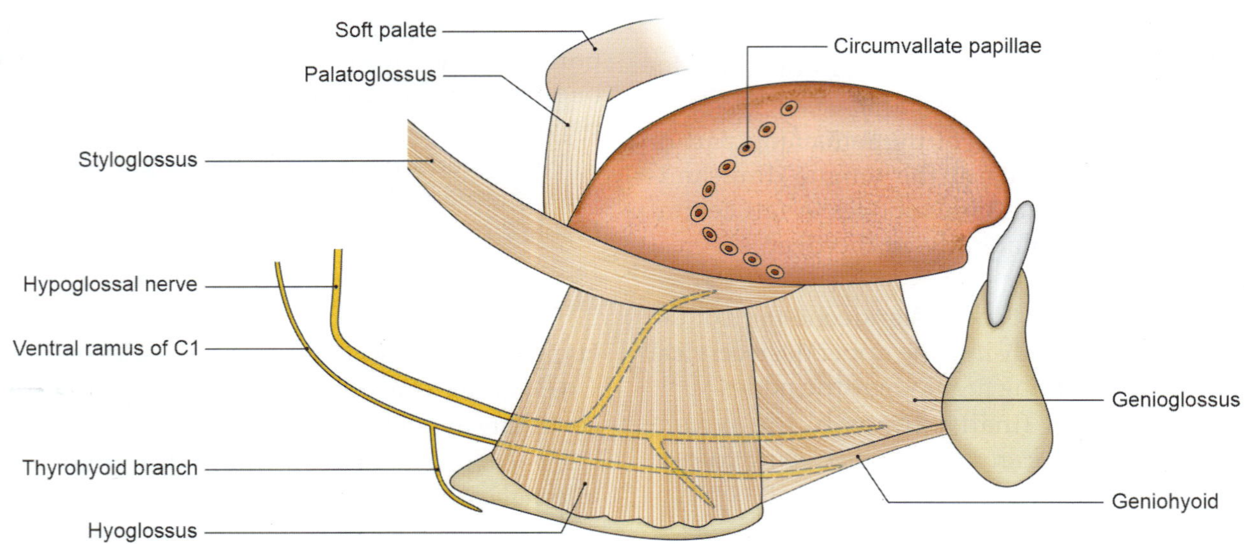

Fig. 25.8a: Hypoglossal nerve innervating three extrinsic muscles of the tongue

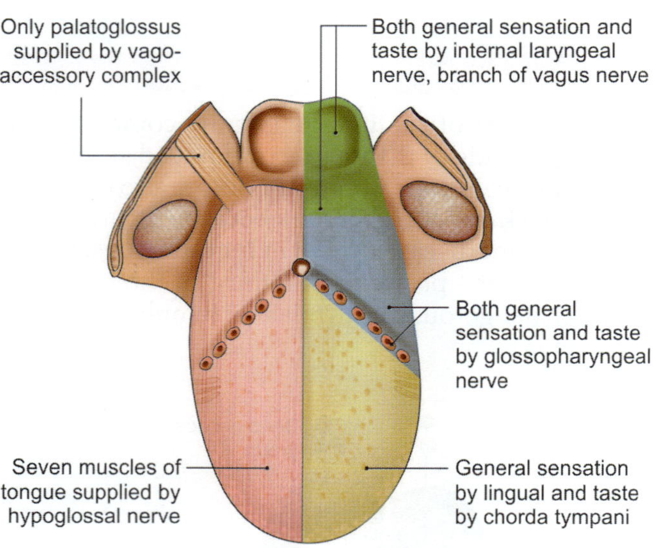

Fig. 25.8b: Nerve supply of tongue

- Sorbitrate is taken sublingually for immediate relief from angina pectoris. It is absorbed fast because of rich blood supply of the tongue and bypassing of portal circulation.
- Genioglossus is called the 'safety muscle of the tongue' because if it is paralysed, the tongue will fall back on the oropharynx and block the air passage. During anaesthesia, the tongue is pulled forwards to clear the air passage.
- Genioglossus is the only muscle of the tongue which protrudes it forwards. It is used for testing the integrity of hypoglossal nerve. If hypoglossal nerve of right side is paralysed, the tongue on protrusion will deviate to the right side. Normal left genioglossus will pull the base to left side and apex will get pushed to right side (apex and base lie at opposite ends) (Fig. 25.9).

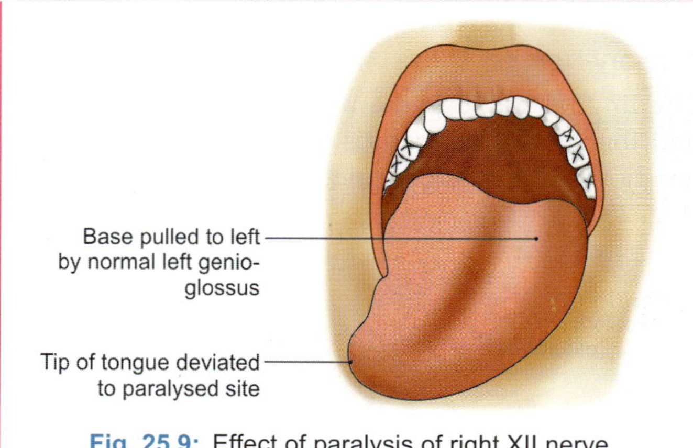

Fig. 25.9: Effect of paralysis of right XII nerve

HISTOLOGY

1 The bulk of the tongue is made up of striated muscles.
2 The *mucous membrane* consists of a layer of connective tissue (corium), lined by stratified squamous epithelium. On the oral part of the dorsum, it is thin, forms papillae (Fig. 25.3), and is adherent to the muscles. On the pharyngeal part of the dorsum, it is very rich in lymphoid follicles. On the inferior surface, it is thin and smooth. Numerous glands, both mucous and serous, lie deep to the mucous membrane.
3 *Taste buds* are most numerous on the sides of the circumvallate papillae, and on the walls of the surrounding sulci. Taste buds are numerous over the foliate papillae and over the posterior one-third

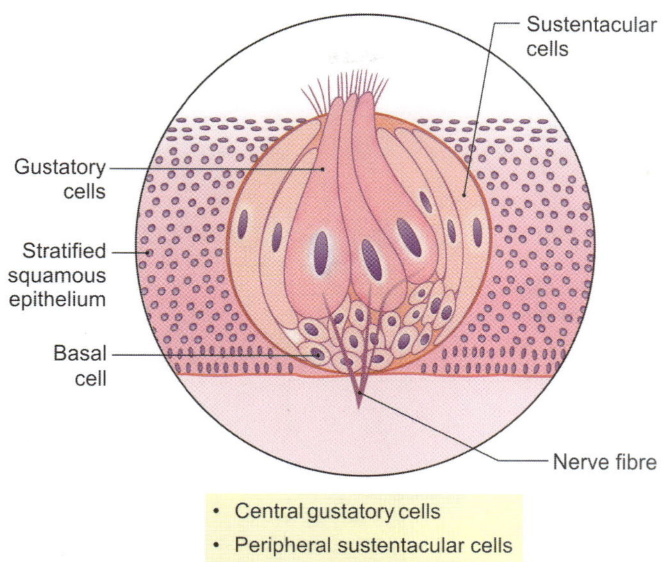

Fig. 25.10: Structure of taste bud

of the tongue; and sparsely distributed on the fungiform papillae, the soft palate, the epiglottis and the pharynx. There are no taste buds on the mid-dorsal region of the oral part of the tongue (Fig. 25.10).

Structure

There are two types of cells, the sustentacular or supporting cells and gustatory cells. The supporting cells are spindle-shaped while gustatory cells are long slender and centrally situated.

DEVELOPMENT OF TONGUE

Epithelium

1 *Anterior two-thirds:* From two lingual swellings, which arise from the first branchial arch (Fig. 25.11).

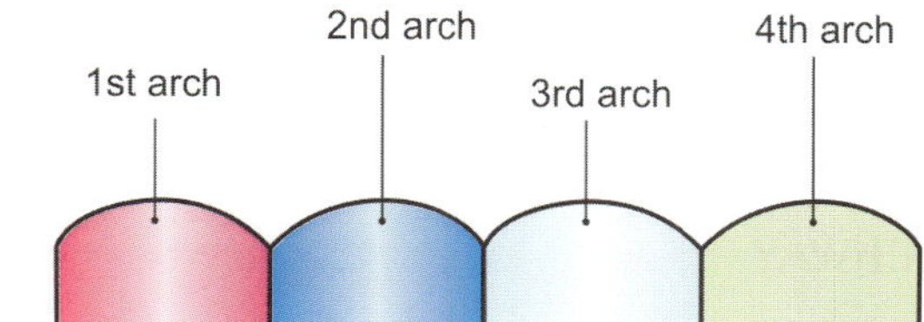

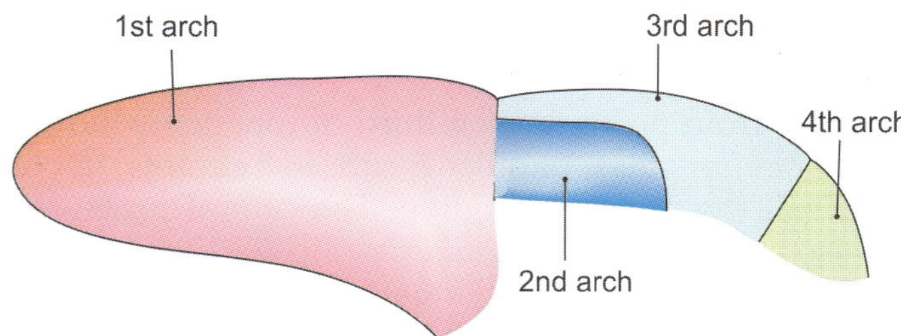

Fig. 25.11: Development of tongue

Therefore, it is supplied by lingual nerve (post-trematic) of 1st arch and chorda tympani (pre-trematic) of 2nd arch.

2 *Posterior one-third:* From cranial large part of the hypobranchial eminence, i.e. from the third arch. Therefore, it is supplied by the glossopharyngeal nerve (Table 25.3).

3 *Posteriormost part* from the fourth arch. This is supplied by the vagus nerve.

Table 25.3 shows the comparison of three parts of the tongue.

Muscles

The muscles develop from the occipital myotomes which are supplied by the hypoglossal nerve.

Table 25.3: Comparison of the parts of the tongue

	Anterior two-thirds	*Posterior one-third*	*Posteriormost part and vallecula*
Situation	Lies in mouth cavity	Oropharynx	Oropharynx
Structure	Contains papillae	Contains lymphoid tissue	—
Function	Chewing	Deglutition	Deglutition
Sensory nerve	Lingual (post-trematic branch of 1st arch)	Glossopharyngeal nerve of 3rd arch	Internal laryngeal branch of vagus (nerve of 4th arch)
Sensation of taste	Chorda tympani except circum-vallate papillae (pre-trematic branch of 2nd arch)	Glossopharyngeal including the vallate papillae	Internal laryngeal branch of vagus
Development of epithelium from endoderm	Lingual swellings of 1st arch. Tuberculum impar which soon disappears	Third arch which forms large ventral part of hypobranchial eminence	Fourth arch which forms small dorsal part of hypobranchial eminence

Muscles develop from occipital myotomes, so the cranial nerve XII (hypoglossal nerve) supplies all intrinsic and three extrinsic muscles. Only palatoglossus is supplied by cranial root of accessory through pharyngeal plexus and is developed from mesoderm of sixth arch

Connective Tissue

The connective tissue develops from the local mesenchyme.

TASTE PATHWAY

- The taste from anterior two-thirds of tongue, except from vallate papillae, is carried by *chorda tympani* branch of facial nerve till the geniculate ganglion. The central processes go to the *tractus solitarius* in the medulla.
- Taste from posterior one-third of tongue including the circumvallate papillae is carried by cranial nerve *IX* till the inferior ganglion. The central processes also reach the *tractus solitarius* (Fig. 25.12).
- Taste from posterior most part of tongue and epiglottis travels through internal laryngeal branch of *vagus* nerve till the inferior ganglion of vagus. These *central* processes also reach *tractus solitarius*.
- After a relay in tractus solitarius, the *solitariothalamic tract* is formed which becomes a part of *trigeminal lemniscus* and reaches posteroventromedial nucleus of thalamus of the opposite side. Another relay here takes them to *lowest part of postcentral gyrus*, which is the area for taste.

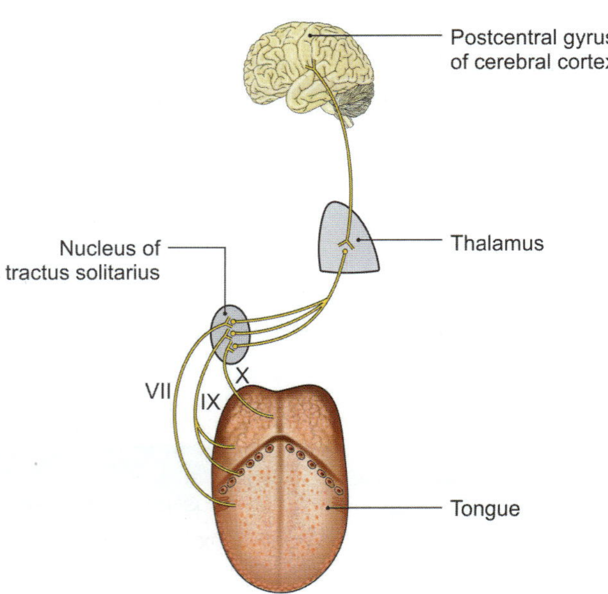

Fig. 25.12: Taste pathways

CLINICAL ANATOMY

- Injury to any part of the pathway causes abnormality in appreciation of taste.
- Referred pain is felt in the ear in diseases of posterior part of the tongue, as ninth and tenth nerves are common supply to both the regions. Other examples of referred pain are seen in Fig. 25.13.

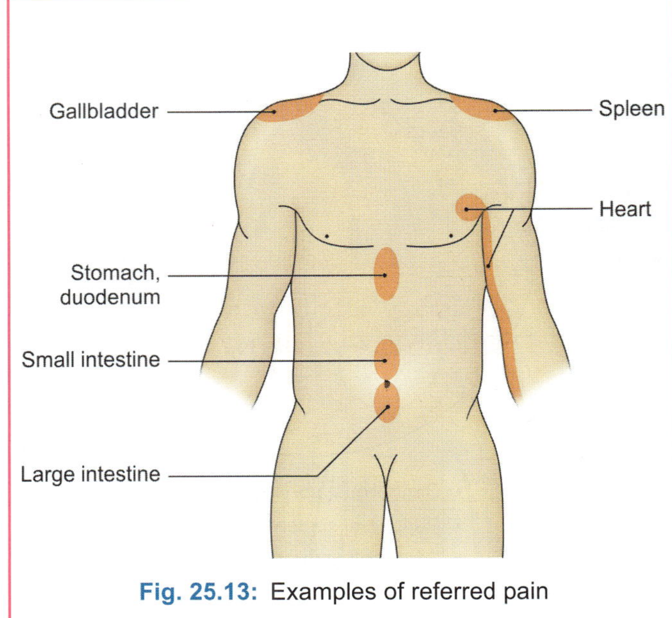

Fig. 25.13: Examples of referred pain

FACTS TO REMEMBER

- All 4 intrinsic muscles of tongue are supplied by XII nerve.
- Out of 4 extrinsic muscles of tongue, 3 are supplied by XII nerve. Only palatoglossus is supplied by vagoaccessory complex.
- Lingual artery is a tortuous artery as it moves up and down with movements of pharynx.
- Tongue is kept in position by its attachment to neighbouring structures through the 4 pairs of extrinsic muscles.
- Circumvallate papillae are only 10–12 in number, but have maximum number of taste buds. The taste from here is carried by IX nerve.
- Nerve supply correlates with development. Anterior two-thirds develop from 1st arch, the nerves being lingual and chorda tympani. Chorda tympani is pre-trematic branch of the 2nd arch.
- Posterior one-third develops from cranial part of 3rd arch. So it is supplied by IX nerve.
- Posteriormost part develops from 4th arch. So it is supplied by internal laryngeal branch of X nerve.
- Sorbitrate, the drug for prevention of angina, is taken sublingually as it reaches the blood very fast, bypassing the portal circulation.
- Genioglossus is the life-saving muscle as it protrudes the tongue forwards.

CLINICOANATOMICAL PROBLEM

A patient is diagnosed as 'medial medullary syndrome' on right side

- What is the effect on tongue?
- Name the nuclear column to which XII nerve belongs?
- Name the muscles of tongue.

Ans: In medial medullary syndrome, XII nerve, pyramidal fibres and medial lemniscus are damaged due to blockage of anterior spinal artery.

a. There is contralateral hemiplegia due to damage to pyramid of medulla oblongata.
b. Loss of sense of vibration and position due to damage to medial lemniscus.
c. Paralysis of muscles of tongue on the same side due to paralysis of XII nerve. The tip of tongue on protrusion will get protruded to the side of lesion. XII nerve belongs to general somatic efferent column (GSE).

Muscles of tongue are intrinsic and extrinsic:

Intrinsic muscle	Extrinsic muscle
Superior longitudinal	Genioglossus
Inferior longitudinal	Hyoglossus
Transverse	Palatoglossus
Vertical	Styloglossus

FURTHER READING

- Netter FH. Atlas of Human Anatomy. Los Angels: Icon Learning Systems, 1997.
- Whillis J. Movements of tongue in swallowing. Journal of Anatomy, 1996;80:115–16.

Frequently Asked Questions

1. Describe tongue under the following headings:
   a. Gross anatomy
   b. Dorsum of tongue
   c. Blood supply and nerve supply
   d. Lymphatic drainage
   e. Clinical anatomy
2. Describe the extrinsic and intrinsic muscles of tongue. Discuss their actions and importance of genioglossus muscle.
3. Write short notes on:
   a. Taste fibres from the tongue
   b. Sensory nerve supply
   c. Development of tongue

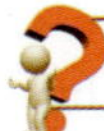

Multiple Choice Questions

1. Epithelium of tongue develops from all the following arches, *except:*
   a. 1st arch b. 2nd arch
   c. 3rd arch d. 4th arch
2. Muscles of tongue are mostly supplied by XII nerve, *except:*
   a. Genioglossus
   b. Palatoglossus
   c. Hyoglossus
   d. Styloglossus
3. Lymph from tongue drains into all the following lymph nodes, *except:*
   a. Submandibular b. Submental
   c. Deep cervical d. Preauricular
4. Taste from the tongue is carried by all nerves, *except:*
   a. VII b. IX
   c. X d. XI
5. Sensory fibres from tongue is carried by all nerves, *except:*
   a. V b. VIII
   c. IX d. X

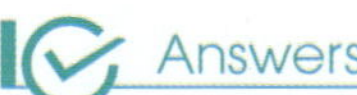

Answers

1. b **2.** b **3.** d **4.** d **5.** b

VIVA VOCE

- What are the parts of the tongue?
- Name the subdivisions of dorsum of tongue.
- How many types of papillae are there in the tongue? Which ones have the maximum number of taste buds?
- Name the extrinsic muscles of tongue with their nerve supply.
- Name the intrinsic muscles of tongue with their nerve supply.
- Which is the lymph node of the tongue?
- What is the importance of genioglossus muscle? What is its other name?
- How do the various parts of the tongue develop?
- Name the sensory and special sensory nerves of the various parts of the tongue.
- If right XII nerve is injured, which side will the tip of tongue deviate on protrusion and why?
- Trace the taste fibres from circumvallate papillae to the cerebrum.
- Which drug is put sublingually during angina pectoris and why?
- What is the clinical importance of colour and roughness of the tongue?

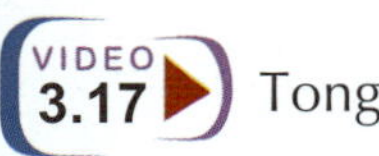

Tongue

Chapter

26

Ear

"Nature is wonderful. A million years ago SHE didn't know we are going to wear spectacles, yet look at the way she placed our ears. 'The ear is an engineering marvel'."

—Anonymous

INTRODUCTION

Tympanic membrane comprises all the three embryonic layers—outer layer is ectodermal, inner layer is endodermal while middle one is mesodermal in origin. The ossicles of the ear are the only bones fully formed at birth.

One hears with the ears. The centre for hearing is in the temporal lobe of brain above the ear. Reading aloud is a quicker way of memorising, as the ear, temporal lobes and motor speech area are also activated. The labyrinth is also supplied by an 'end artery' like the retina.

Noise pollution within the four walls of the homes from the music albums and advertisements emitted from the television sets cause a lot of damage to the cochlear nerves and temporal lobes, besides causing irritation, hypertension and obesity.

The ear is an organ of hearing. It is also concerned in maintaining the equilibrium of the body. It consists of three parts: The external ear, the middle ear and the internal ear. Tympanic membrane separates external ear from middle ear. Mastoid antrum lies in the petrous part of temporal bone. Mastoid air cells are situated in the mastoid process.

Features of the Temporal Bone

1 External auditory meatus is for air waves.

2 Internal auditory meatus is for passage of VII, VIII nerves and labyrinthine vessels.

3 Suprameatal triangle is the landmark for mastoid antrum. It is bounded by supramastoid crest, posterosuperior margin of external acoustic meatus and a tangent drawn from the crest to the margin. Mastoid antrum lies about 15 mm deep to the suprameatal triangle in adult (*see* Fig. 9.9b).

4 Tympanic canaliculus lies on the inferior surface of petrous temporal bone between carotid canal and jugular fossa.

5 Petrotympanic fissure gives passage to anterior tympanic artery, anterior ligament of malleus and chorda tympani nerve.

6 Stylomastoid foramen gives passage to posterior tympanic artery for middle ear and facial nerve.

7 Hiatus for greater petrosal nerve gives passage to nerve of the same name and a branch of middle meningeal artery.

8 Tegmen tympani on the anterior face of petrous temporal bone forms roof of the middle ear, mastoid antrum and canal for tensor tympani muscle.

9 The aqueduct of vestibule opens on posterior aspect of petrous temporal bone. It is plugged by ductus endolymphaticus.

10 Organ of Corti is the end organ for hearing, situated in the cochlear duct.

11 Crista is an end organ in the semicircular canal. These are kinetic balance receptors.

12 Macula are end organs in the utricle and saccule and are static balance receptors.

EXTERNAL EAR

The external ear consists of:

- The auricle or pinna
- The external acoustic meatus.

AURICLE/PINNA

The auricle is the part seen on the surface. The greater part of it is made up of a single crumpled plate of elastic cartilage which is lined on both sides by skin. It supports the spectacles. However, the lowest part of the auricle is soft and consists only of fibrofatty tissue covered by

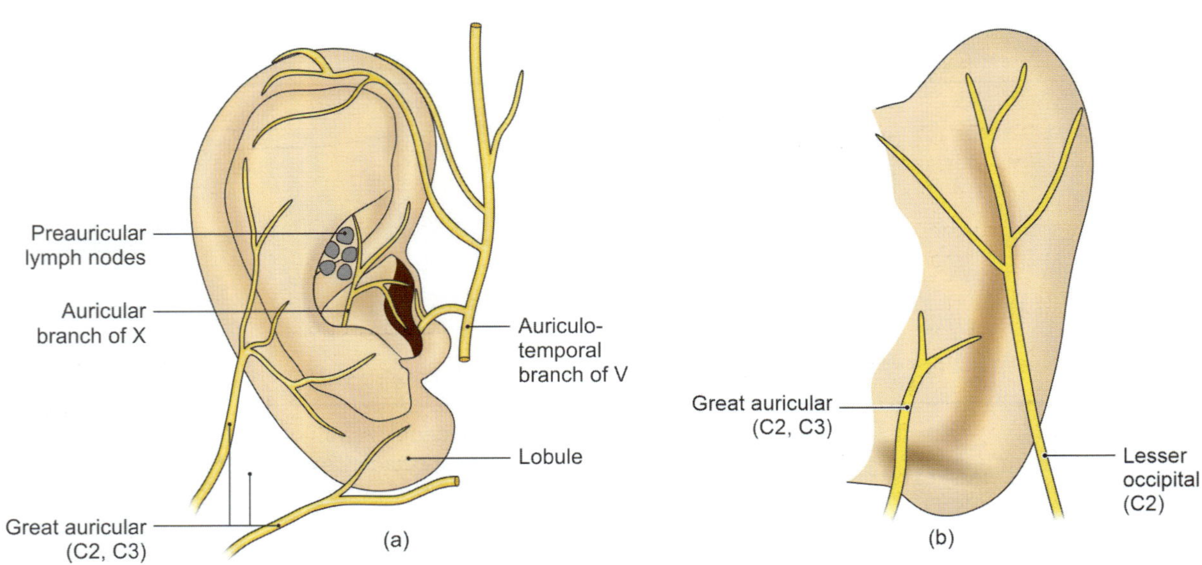

Figs 26.1a and b: Pinna of the ear: (a) Nerve supply and lymph nodes on the lateral surface, and (b) nerve supply on the medial surface

skin: This part is called the *lobule* for wearing the ear rings. The rest of the auricle is divided into a number of parts. These are helix, antihelix, concha, tragus, and scaphoid fossa (*see* Fig. 28.2). In particular, note the large depression called the *concha;* it leads into the external acoustic meatus.

In relation to the auricle, there are a number of muscles. These are all vestigeal in man. In lower animals, the *intrinsic* muscles alter the shape of the auricle, while the *extrinsic* muscles move the auricle as a whole.

Nerve Supply

The upper two-thirds of the lateral surface of the auricle are supplied by the auriculotemporal nerve; and the lower one-third by the great auricular nerve (Figs 26.1a and b). The upper two-thirds of the medial surface are supplied by the lesser occipital nerve; and the lower one-third by the great auricular nerve. The root of the auricle is supplied by the auricular branch of the vagus (Figs 26.1a and b). The auricular muscles are supplied through branches of the facial nerve.

Blood Supply

The blood supply of the auricle is derived from the posterior auricular and superficial temporal arteries (Fig. 26.2). The *lymphatics* drain into the preauricular, and postauricular lymph nodes (Figs 26.1a and b).

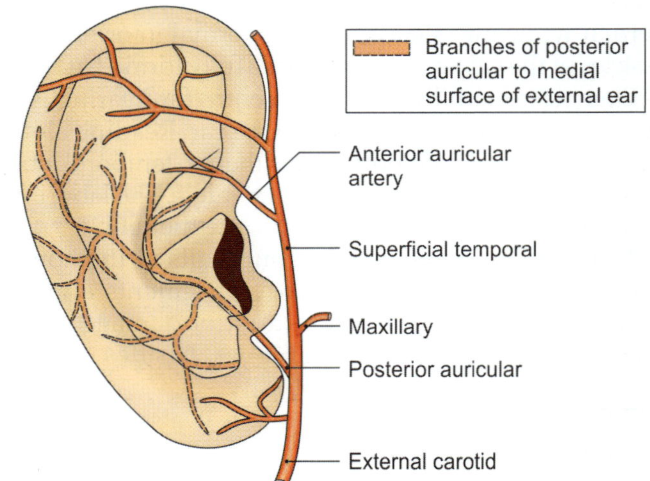

Fig. 26.2: Blood supply of the auricle

EXTERNAL ACOUSTIC MEATUS

Features

The external auditory meatus conducts sound waves from the concha to the tympanic membrane. The canal is S-shaped. Its outer part is directed medially, forwards and upwards. The middle part is directed medially, backwards and upwards. The inner part is directed medially, forwards and downwards. The meatus can be straightened for examination by pulling the auricle *upwards, backwards and slightly laterally.*

The meatus or canal is about 24 mm long, of which the medial two-thirds or 16 mm is bony, and the lateral one-third or 8 mm is cartilaginous. Due to the obliquity of the tympanic membrane, the anterior wall and floor are longer than the posterior wall and roof (Figs 26.3a and b).

The canal is oval in section. The greatest diameter is vertical at the lateral end, and anteroposterior at the medial end. The bony part is narrower than the cartilaginous part. The narrowest point, the *isthmus,* lies about 5 mm from the tympanic membrane.

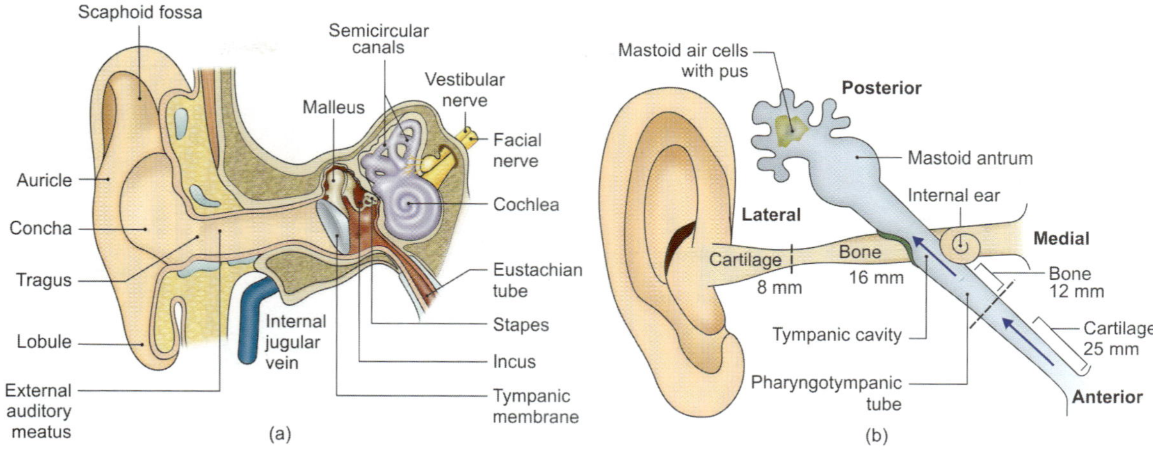

Figs 26.3a and b: (a) The normal ear, and (b) otitis media causing mastoid abscess

The *bony part* is formed by the tympanic plate of the temporal bone which is C-shaped in cross-section. The posterosuperior part of the plate is deficient. Here the wall of the meatus is formed by a part of the squamous temporal bone. The meatus is lined by thin skin, firmly adherent to the periosteum.

The *cartilaginous part* is also C-shaped in section; and the gap of the 'C' is filled with fibrous tissue. The lining skin is adherent to the perichondrium, and contains hairs, sebaceous glands, and ceruminous or wax glands. *Ceruminous glands* are modified sweat glands.

Blood Supply

The outer part of the canal is supplied by the superficial temporal and posterior auricular arteries, and the inner part, by the deep auricular branch of the maxillary artery.

Lymphatics

The lymphatics pass to preauricular, postauricular and superficial cervical lymph nodes.

Nerve Supply

The skin lining the anterior half of the meatus is supplied by the auriculotemporal nerve, and that lining the posterior half, by the auricular branch of the vagus.

DISSECTION

Expose the external auditory meatus by cutting the tragus of the auricle. Put a probe into the external auditory meatus and remove the anterior wall of cartilaginous and bony parts of the external auditory meatus with the scissors. Be slow and careful not to damage the tympanic membrane *(refer to BDC App)*.

TYMPANIC MEMBRANE

This is a thin, translucent partition between the external acoustic meatus and the middle ear. It forms the lateral wall of middle ear.

It is oval in shape, measuring 9 × 10 mm. It is placed obliquely at an angle of 55° with the floor of the meatus. It faces downwards, forwards and laterally (Figs 26.4a and b).

The membrane has outer and inner surfaces.

The outer surface of the membrane is lined by thin skin. It is concave.

The inner surface provides attachment to the handle of the malleus which extends up to its centre. The inner surface is convex. The point of maximum convexity lies at the tip of the handle of the malleus and is called the *umbo.*

The membrane is thickened at its circumference which is fixed to the tympanic sulcus of the temporal bone on the tympanic plate. Superiorly, the sulcus is deficient. Here the membrane is attached to the tympanic notch. From the ends of the notch, two bands, the anterior and posterior malleolar folds, are prolonged to the lateral process of the malleus.

While the greater part of the tympanic membrane is tightly stretched, and is, therefore, called the *pars tensa,* the part between the two malleolar folds is loose and is called the *pars flaccida*. The pars flaccida is crossed internally by the chorda tympani (Fig. 26.5). This part is more liable to rupture than the pars tensa.

The membrane is held tense by the inward pull of the tensor tympani muscle which is inserted into the upper end of the handle of the malleus.

Structure

The tympanic membrane is composed of the following three layers:

1 The *outer cuticular layer* of skin (Fig. 26.4a).
2 The *middle fibrous layer* made up of superficial radiating fibres and deep circular fibres. The circular fibres are minimal at the centre and maximal at the periphery (Fig. 26.4b). The fibrous layer is replaced by loose areolar tissue in the pars flaccida (Fig. 26.5).

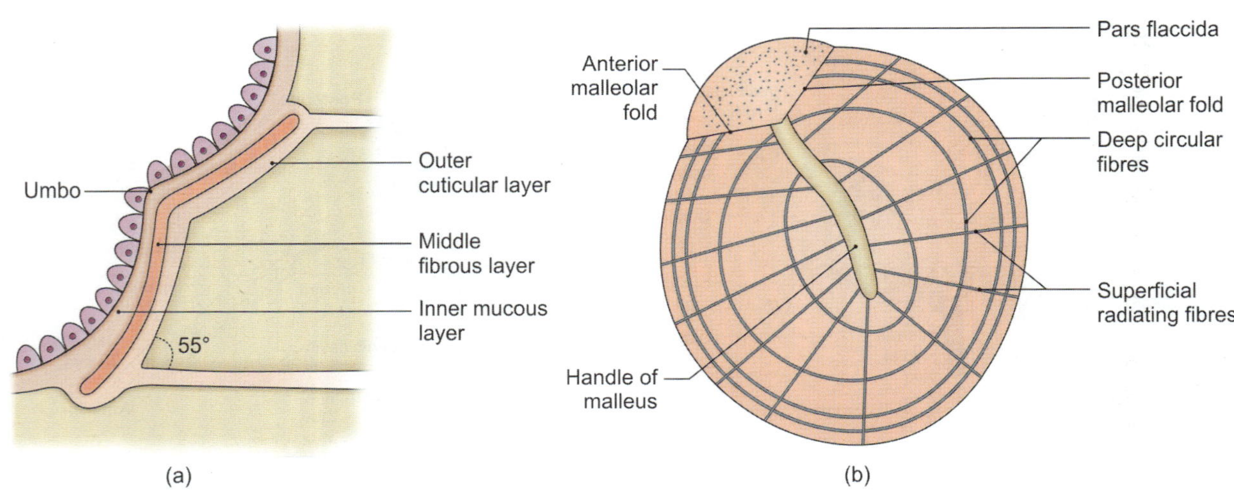

Figs 26.4a and b: (a) Tympanic membrane as seen in section; (b) Fibres of tympanic membrane

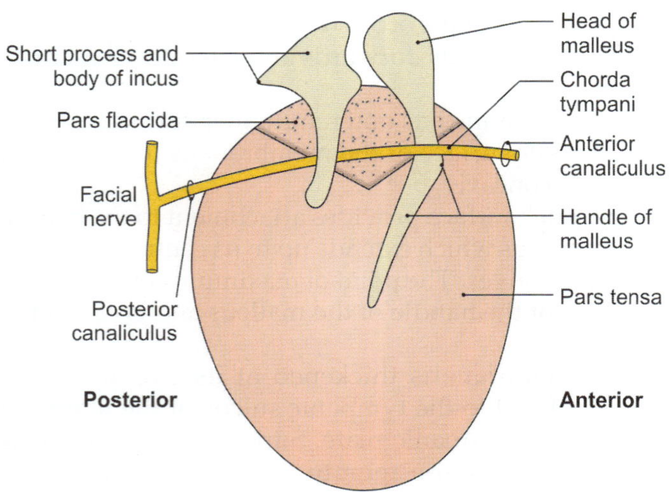

Fig. 26.5: Inner surface of the tympanic membrane

3 The *inner mucous layer* (Fig. 26.4a) is lined by a low ciliated columnar epithelium.

Blood Supply

1 The outer surface is supplied by the deep auricular branch of the maxillary artery.
2 The inner surface is supplied by the anterior tympanic branch of the maxillary artery (*see* Fig. 14.6) and by the posterior tympanic branch of the stylomastoid branch of the posterior auricular artery.

Venous Drainage

Veins from the outer surface drain into the external jugular vein. Those from the inner surface drain into the transverse sinus and into the venous plexus around the auditory tube.

Lymphatic Drainage

Lymphatics pass to the preauricular and retropharyngeal lymph nodes.

Nerve Supply

1 *Outer surface:* The anteroinferior part is supplied by the auriculotemporal nerve, and the posterosuperior part by the auricular branch of the vagus nerve with a communicating branch from facial nerve (Fig. 26.1).
2 *Inner surface:* This is supplied by the tympanic branch of the glossopharyngeal nerve through the tympanic plexus (Fig. 26.4a).

CLINICAL ANATOMY

- As already stated, for examination of the meatus and tympanic membrane, the auricle should be drawn upwards, backwards and slightly laterally. However, in infants, the auricle is drawn downwards and backwards because the canal is only cartilaginous and the outer surface of the tympanic membrane is directed mainly downwards (Fig. 26.6).
- Boils and other infections of the external auditory meatus cause a little swelling but are extremely painful, due to the fixity of the skin to the underlying bone and cartilage. Ear should be dried after head bath or swimming.
- Irritation of the auricular branch of the vagus in the external ear by ear wax or syringing may reflexly produce persistent cough called ear *cough*, vomiting or even death due to sudden cardiac inhibition. On the other hand, mild stimulation of this nerve may reflexly produce increased appetite.
- Accumulation of wax in the external acoustic meatus is often a source of excessive itching, although fungal infection and foreign bodies should be excluded. Troublesome impaction of large foreign bodies, like seeds, grains, insects, is common. Syringing is done to remove these (Fig. 26.7).

- Involvement of the ear in herpes zoster of the geniculate ganglion depends on the connection between the auricular branch of the vagus and the facial nerve within the petrous temporal bone.
- Small pieces of skin from the lobule of the pinna are commonly used for demonstration of lepra bacilli to confirm the diagnosis of leprosy.
- Pinna is used as grafting material.
- Hair on pinna in male represents Y-linked inheritance.
- A good number of ear traits follow mendelian inheritance.
- Infection of elastic cartilage may cause perichondritis.
- Bleeding within the auricle occurs between the perichondrium and auricular cartilage. If left untreated, fibrosis occurs as haematoma compromises blood supply to cartilage. Fibrosis leads to 'cauliflower ear'. It is usually seen in wrestlers.

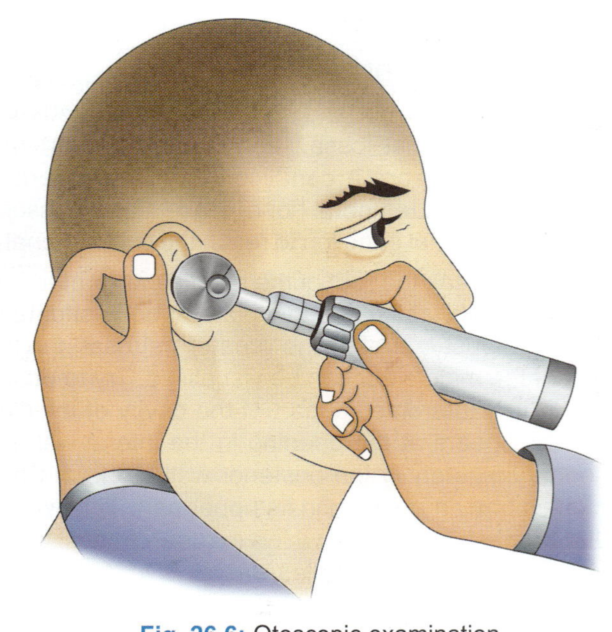

Fig. 26.6: Otoscopic examination

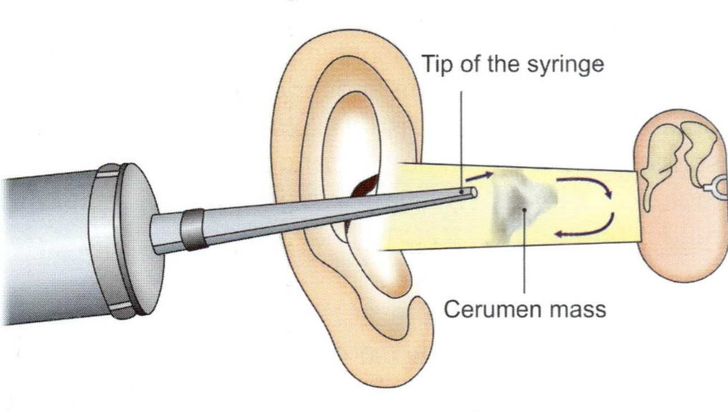

Fig. 26.7: Syringing of the ear

- Tympanic membrane is divided into an upper smaller sector, the pars flaccida bounded by anterior and posterior malleolar folds and a larger sector, the pars tensa. Behind pars flaccida lies the chorda tympani, so disease in pars flaccida should be treated carefully (Fig. 26.8).
- When the tympanic membrane is illuminated for examination, the concavity of the membrane produces a 'cone of light' over the *anteroinferior quadrant* which is the farthest or deepest quadrant with its apex at the umbo (Fig. 26.9). Through the membrane, one can see the underlying handle of the malleus and the long process of the incus.
- The membrane is sometimes incised to drain pus present in the middle ear. The procedure is called

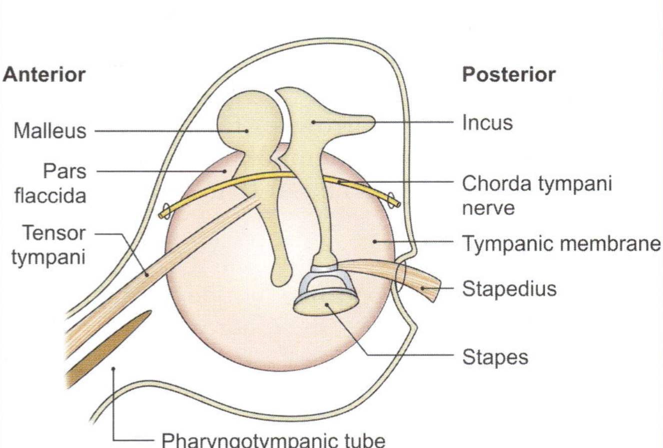

Fig. 26.8: Care to be taken in disease of pars flaccida

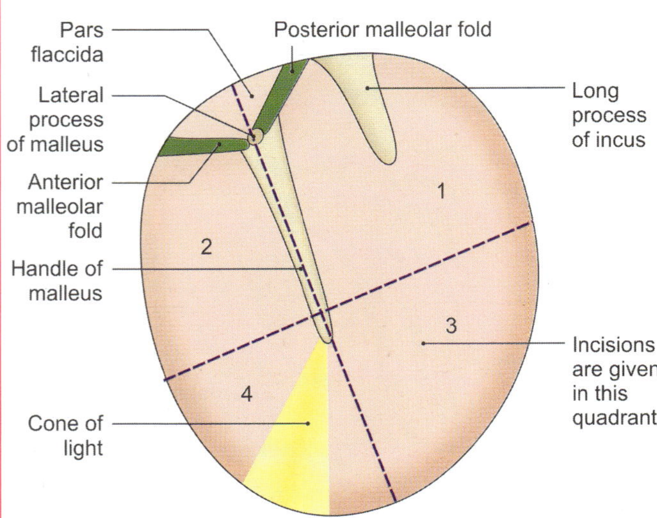

Fig. 26.9: The left tympanic membrane seen through the external acoustic meatus. (1) Posterosuperior quadrant; (2) Anterosuperior quadrant; (3) Posteroinferior quadrant; (4) Anteroinferior quadrant

myringotomy (Fig. 26.9). The incision for myringotomy is usually made in the posteroinferior quadrant of the membrane where the bulge is most prominent. In giving an incision, it has to be remembered that the chorda tympani nerve runs downwards and forwards across the inner surface of the membrane, lateral to the long process of the incus, but medial to the neck of the malleus. If the nerve is injured, taste from most of anterior two-thirds of tongue is not perceived. Also salivation from submandibular and sublingual glands gets affected.

MIDDLE EAR

Features

The middle ear is also called the tympanic cavity, or tympanum.

The middle ear is a narrow air-filled space situated in the petrous part of the temporal bone between the external ear and the internal ear (Fig. 26.10).

Shape and Size

The middle ear is shaped like a cube. Its lateral and medial walls are large, but the other walls are narrow, because the cube is compressed from side-to-side. Its vertical and anteroposterior diameters are both about 15 mm. When seen in coronal section the cavity of the middle ear is biconcave, as the medial and lateral walls are closest to each other in the centre. The distances separating them are 6 mm near the roof, 2 mm in the centre, and 4 mm near the floor (Fig. 26.11).

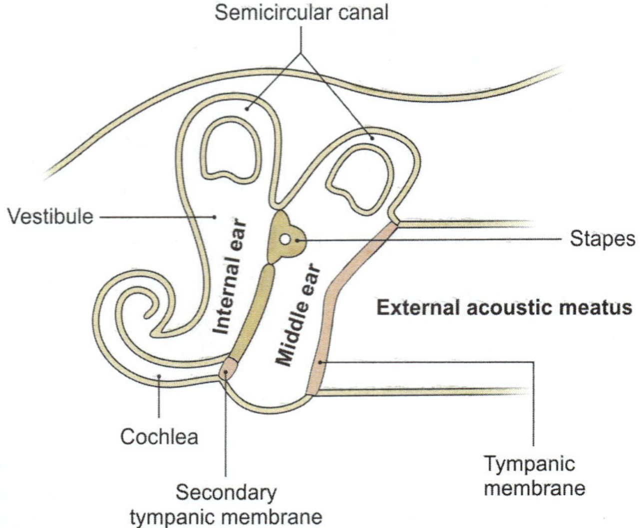

Fig. 26.10: Scheme to show the three parts of the ear

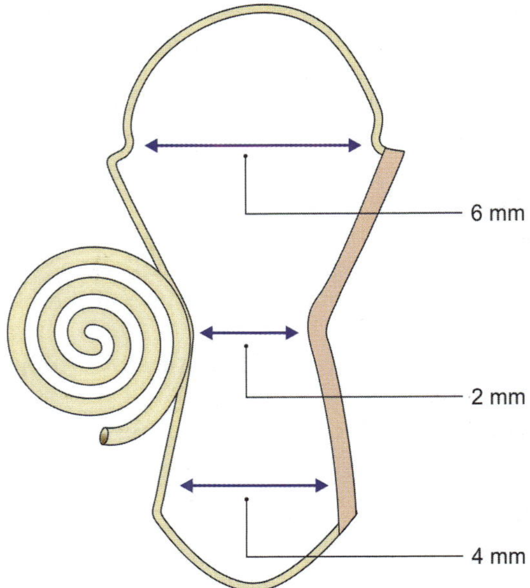

Fig. 26.11: Measurements

DISSECTION

Remove the dura mater and endosteum from the floor of the middle cranial fossa. Identify greater petrosal nerve emerging from a canaliculus on the anterior surface of petrous temporal bone. Trace it as it passes inferior to trigeminal ganglion to reach the carotid canal.

Carefully break the roof of the middle ear formed by tegmen tympani which is a thin plate of bone situated parallel and just lateral to the greater petrosal nerve. Cavity of the middle ear can be visualised. Try to put a probe in the anteromedial part of the cavity of middle ear till it appears at the opening in the lateral wall of nasopharynx. Identify the posterior wall of the middle ear which has an opening in its upper part. This is the aditus to mastoid antrum, which in turn, connects the cavity to the mastoid air cells *(refer to BDC App)*.

Ear ossicles

Identify the bony ossicles. Locate the tendon of tensor tympani muscle passing from the malleus towards the medial wall of the cavity where it gets continuous with the muscle. Trace the tensor tympani muscle traversing in a semicanal above the auditory tube. Break one wall of the pyramid to visualise the stapedius muscle. Just superior to the attachment of tendon of tensor tympani, look for chorda tympani traversing the tympanic membrane.

Parts

The cavity of the middle ear can be subdivided into the tympanic cavity proper which is opposite the tympanic membrane; and the epitympanic recess which lies above the level of the tympanic membrane.

Communications

The middle ear communicates anteriorly with the nasopharynx through the auditory tube, and posteriorly with the mastoid antrum and mastoid air cells through the aditus to the mastoid antrum (Fig. 26.12a).

The middle ear is likened to a pistol in the sloping course of the aditus to the epitympanic recess and the auditory tube (Fig. 26.12a). The trigger of pistol is tympanic cavity. Outlet is auditory tube. Handle is aditus to mastoid antrum and mastoid air cells (Fig. 26.12b).

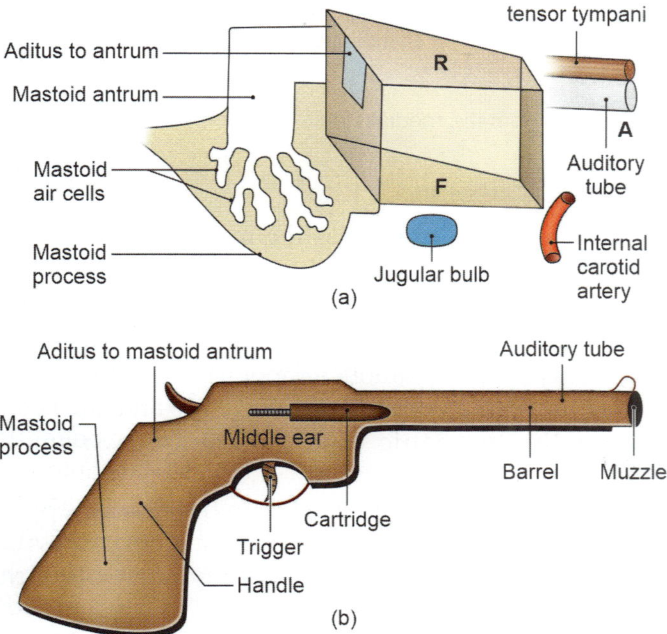

Figs 26.12a and b: (a) Scheme to show some relationships of the middle ear cavity; (b) Note that the cavity resembles a pistol

The mucous membrane lining the middle ear cavity invests all the contents and forms several vascular folds which project into the cavity. This gives the cavity, a honeycombed appearance.

Boundaries

Roof or Tegmental Wall

1 The roof separates the middle ear from the middle cranial fossa. It is formed by a thin plate of bone called the *tegmen tympani*. This plate is prolonged forwards as the roof of the canal for the tensor tympani (Fig. 26.13).

2 In young children, the roof presents a gap at the unossified petrosquamous suture where the middle ear is in direct contact with the meninges. In adults, the suture is ossified and transmits a vein from the middle ear to the superior petrosal sinus.

Floor or Jugular Wall

The floor is formed by a thin plate of bone which separates the middle ear from the superior bulb of the internal jugular vein. This plate is a part of the temporal bone (Fig. 26.13).

Near the medial wall, the floor presents the tympanic canaliculus which transmits the tympanic branch of the glossopharyngeal nerve to the medial wall of the middle ear.

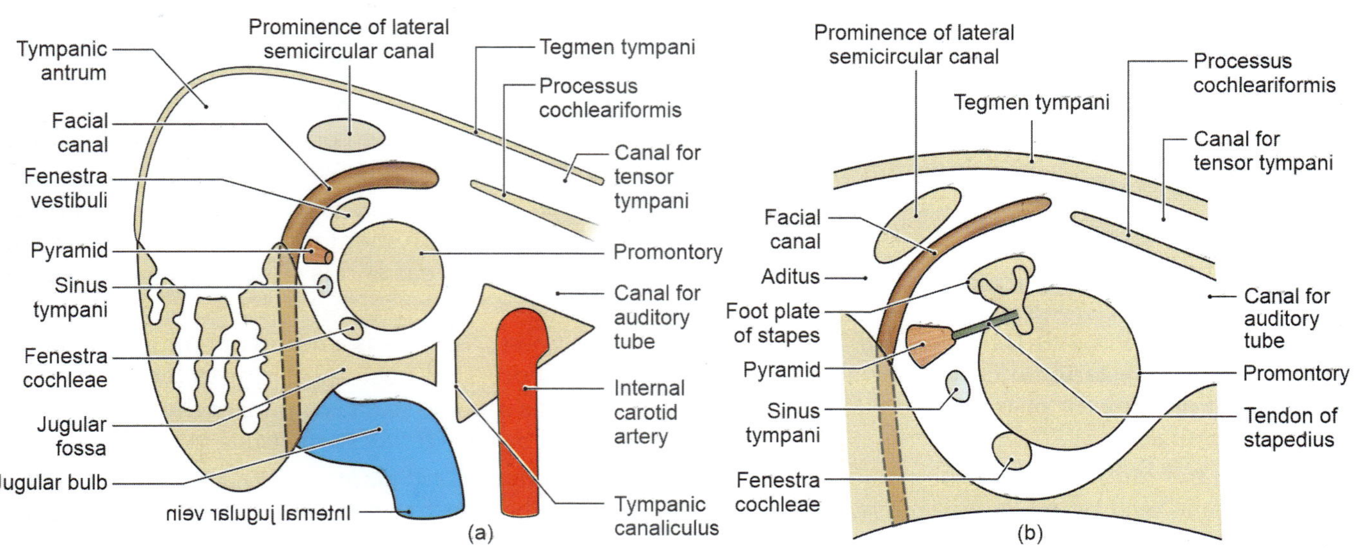

Fig. 26.13: Scheme to show the landmarks on the medial wall of the middle ear. Some related structures are also shown

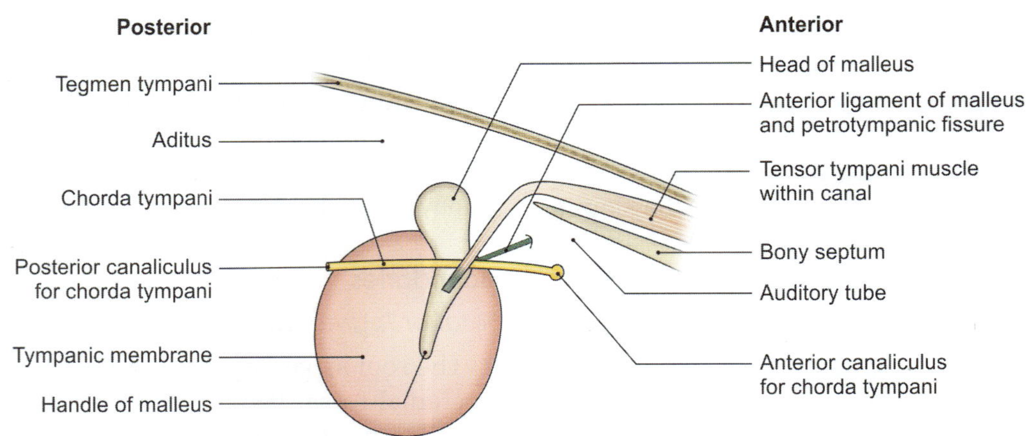

Fig. 26.14: Lateral wall of the middle ear viewed from the medial side

Anterior or Carotid Wall

The anterior wall is narrow due to the approximation of the medial and lateral walls, and because of descent of the roof.

The uppermost part of the anterior wall bears the opening of the canal for the tensor tympani.

The middle part has the opening of the auditory tube.

The inferior part of the wall is formed by a thin plate of bone which forms the posterior wall of the carotid canal. The plate separates the middle ear from the internal carotid artery. This plate of bone is perforated by the superior and inferior sympathetic caroticotympanic nerves and the tympanic branch of the internal carotid artery (Fig. 26.14).

The bony septum between the canals for the tensor tympani and for the auditory tube is continued posteriorly on the medial wall as a curved lamina called the *processus cochleariformis.* Its posterior end forms a pulley around which the tendon of the tensor tympani turns laterally to reach the upper part of the handle of the malleus.

Posterior or Mastoid Wall

The posterior wall presents these features from above downwards.

1 Superiorly, there is an opening or *aditus* through which the epitympanic recess communicates with the mastoid or tympanic antrum (Figs 26.12a and 26.13).
2 The *fossa incudis* is a depression which lodges the short process of the incus.
3 A conical projection, called the *pyramid,* lies near the junction of the posterior and medial walls. It has an opening at its apex for passage of the tendon of the stapedius muscle.
4 Lateral to pyramid and near the posterior edge of the tympanic membrane, is the *posterior canaliculus for the chorda tympani* through which the nerve enters the middle ear cavity (Fig. 26.14).

Lateral or Membranous Wall

1 The lateral wall separates the middle ear from the external acoustic meatus. It is formed:
   a. Mainly by the tympanic membrane along with the tympanic ring and sulcus (described earlier).
   b. Partly by the squamous temporal bone, in the region of the epitympanic recess (Figs 26.13 and 26.5).
2 Near the tympanic notch, there are two small apertures.
   a. The *petrotympanic fissure* lies in front of the upper end of the bony rim. It lodges the anterior process of the malleus and transmits the tympanic branch of the maxillary artery.
   b. The *anterior canaliculus for the chorda tympani* nerve lies either in the fissure or just in front of it. The nerve leaves the middle ear through this canaliculus to emerge at the base of the skull (Figs 26.5 and 26.14).

Medial or Labyrinthine Wall

The medial wall separates the middle ear from the internal ear. It presents the following features.

1 The *promontory* is a rounded bulging produced by the first turn of the cochlea. It is grooved by the tympanic plexus (Fig. 26.13).
2 The *fenestra vestibuli* is an oval opening posterosuperior to the promontory. It leads into the vestibule of the internal ear and is closed by the foot-plate of the stapes.
3 The *fenestra cochleae* is a round opening at the bottom of a depression posteroinferior to the promontory. It opens into the scala tympani of the cochlea, and is closed by the *secondary tympanic membrane.*
4 The *prominence of the facial canal* runs backwards just above the fenestra vestibuli, to reach the lower margin of the aditus. The canal then descends behind the posterior wall to end at the stylomastoid foramen.

5 Prominence of lateral semicircular canal above the facial canal.
6 The *sinus tympani* is a depression behind the promontory, opposite the ampulla of the posterior semicircular canal.

Contents

The middle ear contains the following.

1 Three small bones or ossicles, namely the malleus, the incus and the stapes. The upper half of the malleus, and the greater part of the incus lie in the epitympanic recess.
2 Joints between the ear ossicles.
3 Two muscles—the tensor tympani and the stapedius.
4 Vessels supplying and draining the middle ear.
5 Nerves—chorda tympani and tympanic plexus.
6 Air.

Ear Ossicles

Malleus

The malleus (Latin *hammer*) is so-called because it resembles a hammer. It is the largest, and the most laterally placed ossicle. It has the following parts:

1 The rounded *head* lies in the epitympanic recess. It articulates posteriorly with the body of the incus. It provides attachment to the superior and lateral ligaments (Fig. 26.5).
2 The *neck* lies against the pars flaccida and is related medially to the chorda tympani nerve (Fig. 26.14).
3 The *anterior process* is connected to the petrotympanic fissure by the anterior ligament.
4 The *lateral process* projects from the upper end of the handle and provides attachment to the malleolar folds.
5 The *handle* extends downwards, backwards and medially, and is attached to the upper half of the tympanic membrane (Figs 26.4b and 26.14).

Incus or Anvil

It is so-called because it resembles an anvil, used by blacksmiths. It resembles a molar tooth and has the following parts:

1 The *body* is large and bears an articular surface that is directed forwards. It articulates with the head of the malleus.
2 The *long process* projects downwards just behind and parallel with the handle of the malleus. Its tip bears a lentiform nodule directed medially which articulates with the head of the stapes (Figs 26.9 and 26.15).

Stapes

This bone is so-called because it is shaped like a stirrup. It is the smallest, and the most medially placed ossicle of the ear (Fig. 26.15).

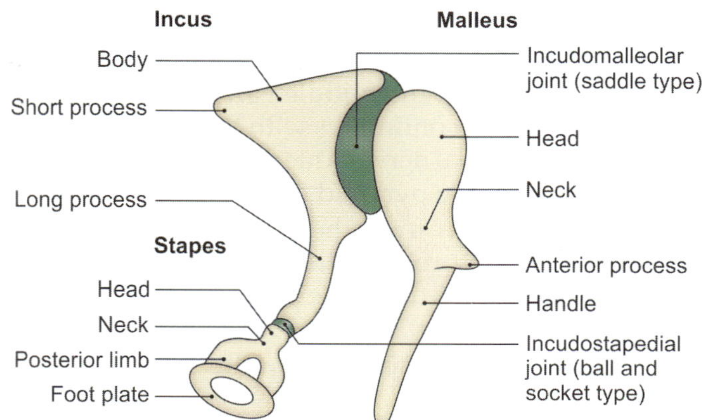

Fig. 26.15: Ossicles of the left ear, seen from the medial side

It has the following parts:

a. The small *head* has a concave facet which articulates with the lentiform nodule of the incus.
b. The narrow *neck* provides insertion, posteriorly, to the thin tendon of the stapedius.
c. *Two limbs* or crura; anterior, the shorter and less curved; and posterior, the longer which diverge from the neck and are attached to the footplate.
d. The *footplate,* a *footpiece* or *base,* is oval in shape, and fits into the fenestra vestibuli.

Joints of the Ossicles

1 The *incudomalleolar joint* is a saddle joint.
2 The *incudostapedial joint* is a ball and socket joint. Both of them are synovial joints. They are surrounded by capsular ligaments. Accessory ligaments are three for the malleus, and one each for the incus and the stapes which stabilize the ossicles. All ligaments are extremely elastic (Fig. 26.15).

Muscles of the Middle Ear

There are two muscles—the tensor tympani and the stapedius. Both act simultaneously to damp down the intensity of high-pitched sound waves and thus protect the internal ear (Fig. 26.8).

The *tensor tympani* lies in a bony canal that opens at its lateral end on the anterior wall of the middle ear, and at the medial end on the base of the skull. The auditory tube lies just below this canal.

The muscle arises from the walls of the canal in which it lies. Some fibres arise from the cartilaginous part of the auditory tube and some from the base of the skull.

The muscle ends in a tendon which reaches the medial wall of the middle ear and bends sharply around the processus cochleariformis. It then passes laterally across the tympanic cavity to be inserted into the handle of the malleus.

The tensor tympani is supplied by the *mandibular nerve*. The fibres pass through the nerve to the medial pterygoid, and through the otic ganglion, without any relay.

It develops from the *mesoderm of first branchial arch.*

The *stapedius* lies in a bony canal that is related to the posterior wall of the middle ear. Posteriorly, and below, this canal is continuous with the vertical part of the canal for the facial nerve. Anteriorly, the canal opens on the summit of the pyramid.

The muscle arises from the walls of this canal. Its tendon emerges through the pyramid and passes forwards to be inserted into the posterior surface of the neck of the stapes.

The stapedius is supplied by the *facial nerve.* It develops from the *mesoderm of the second branchial arch.*

Arterial Supply

The main arteries of the middle ear are as follows.

1 The anterior tympanic branch of the maxillary artery which enters the middle ear through the petro-tympanic fissure.
2 The posterior tympanic branch of the stylomastoid branch of the posterior auricular artery which enters through the stylomastoid foramen.
3 Petrosal and superior tympanic branches of middle meningeal artery.
4 Branches of ascending pharyngeal artery.
5 Tympanic branches of internal carotid artery.

Venous Drainage

Veins from the middle ear drain into the superior petrosal sinus and the pterygoid plexus of the veins.

Lymphatic Drainage

Lymphatics pass to the preauricular and retro-pharyngeal lymph nodes.

Nerve Supply

The nerve supply is derived from the tympanic plexus which lies over the promontory. The plexus is formed by the following.

1 The tympanic branch of the glossopharyngeal nerve. Its fibres are distributed to the mucous membrane of the middle ear, the auditory tube, the mastoid antrum and air cells. It also gives off the lesser petrosal nerve.
2 The superior and inferior caroticotympanic nerves arise from the sympathetic plexus around the internal carotid artery. These fibres are vasomotor to the mucous membrane.

FUNCTIONS OF THE MIDDLE EAR

1 It transmits sound waves from the external ear to the internal ear through the chain of ear ossicles, and thus transforms the air-borne vibrations from the tympanic membrane to liquid-borne vibrations in the internal ear.
2 The intensity of the sound waves is increased ten times by the ossicles. It may be noted that the frequency of sound does not change.

TYMPANIC OR MASTOID ANTRUM

Features

Mastoid antrum is a small, circular, air-filled space situated in the posterior part of the petrous temporal bone. It is of adult size at birth, size of a small pea, or 1 cm in diameter and has a capacity of about one milliliter (Fig. 26.13).

Boundaries

1 *Superiorly:* Tegmen tympani, and beyond it the temporal lobe of the cerebrum.
2 *Inferiorly:* Mastoid process containing the mastoid air cells.
3 *Anteriorly:* It communicates with the epitympanic recess through the aditus. The aditus is related medially to the ampullae of the superior and lateral semicircular canals, and posterosuperiorly to the facial canal.
4 *Posteriorly:* It is separated by a thin plate of bone from the sigmoid sinus. Beyond the sinus there is the cerebellum.
5 *Medially:* Petrous temporal bone.
6 *Laterally:* It is bounded by part of the squamous temporal bone. This part corresponds to the *suprameatal triangle* seen on the surface of the bone. This wall is 2 mm thick at birth, but increases in thickness at the rate of about 1 mm per year up to a maximum of about 12 to 15 mm.

DISSECTION

Clean the mastoid temporal bone off all the muscles and identify suprameatal triangle and supramastoid crest. Use a fine chisel to remove the bone of the triangle till the mastoid antrum is reached. Examine the extent of mastoid air cells.

Remove the posterior and superior walls of external auditory meatus till the level of the roof of mastoid antrum. Identify the chorda tympani nerve at the posterosuperior margin of tympanic membrane.

Look for arcuate eminence on the anterior face of petrous temporal bone. Identify internal acoustic meatus on the posterior face of petrous temporal bone, with the nerves in it. Try to break off the superior part of petrous temporal bone above the internal acoustic meatus. Identify the facial nerve as it passes towards the aditus. Identify the sharp bend of the facial nerve with the geniculate ganglion.

Identify the facial nerve turning posteriorly into the medial wall. Trace it above the fenestra vestibuli till it turns inferiorly in the medial wall of aditus.

Identify facial nerve at the stylomastoid foramen. Try to break the bone vertically along the lateral edge of the foramen to expose the whole of facial nerve canal. Facial nerve is described in detail in *Chapter 4, BD Chaurasia's Human Anatomy, Voulme 4*. Learn it from there.

Break off more of the superior surface of the petrous temporal bone. Remove the bone gently. Examine the holes in the bone produced by semicircular canals and look for the semicircular ducts lying within these canals. Note the branches of vestibulocochlear nerve entering the bone at the lateral end of the meatus. Study the internal ear from the models in the museum.

Mastoid Air Cells

Mastoid air cells are a series of intercommunicating spaces of variable size present within the mastoid process. Their number varies considerably. Sometimes there are just a few, and are confined to the upper part of the mastoid process. Occasionally, they may extend beyond the mastoid process into the squamous or petrous parts of the temporal bone (Fig. 26.12a).

Vessels, Lymphatics and Nerves

The mastoid antrum and air cells are supplied by the *posterior tympanic artery* derived from the stylomastoid branch of the posterior auricular artery. The *veins* drain into the mastoid emissary vein, the posterior auricular vein and the sigmoid sinus.

Lymphatics pass to the postauricular and upper deep cervical lymph nodes.

Nerves are derived from the tympanic plexus formed by the glossopharyngeal nerve and from the meningeal branch of the mandibular nerve.

CLINICAL ANATOMY

- Fracture of the middle cranial fossa breaks the roof of the middle ear, ruptures the tympanic membrane, and thus causes bleeding through the ear along with discharge of CSF.
- Throat infections commonly spread to the middle ear through the auditory tube and cause otitis media. The pus from the middle ear may take one of the following courses:
  a. It may be discharged into the external ear following rupture of the tympanic membrane.
  b. It may erode the roof and spread upwards, causing meningitis and brain abscess.
  c. It may erode the floor and spread downwards, causing thrombosis of the sigmoid sinus and the internal jugular vein (Fig. 26.16).
  d. It may spread backwards, causing mastoid abscess (Fig. 26.3).

  Chronic otitis media and mastoid abscess are responsible for persistent discharge of pus through the ear. Otitis media is more common in children than in adults.
- Inflammation of the auditory tube (eustachian catarrh) is often secondary to an attack of common cold. This causes pain in the ear which is aggravated by swallowing, due to blockage of the tube. Pain is relieved by installation of decongestant drops in the nose which helps to open the ostium.
- *Otosclerosis:* Sometimes bony fusion takes place between the foot plate of the stapes and the margins of the fenestra vestibuli. This leads to deafness. The condition may be surgically corrected by putting a prosthesis (Figs 26.17a and b).
- Mastoid abscess is secondary to otitis media. It is difficult to treat. A proper drainage of pus from the mastoid requires an operation through the suprameatal triangle. The facial nerve should not be injured during this operation (Fig. 26.18).
- Infection from the mastoid antrum and air cells can spread to any of the structures related to them including the temporal lobe of the cerebrum, the cerebellum, and the sigmoid sinus.
- The ear on infected side is displaced laterally and can be appreciated from the back.
- *Hyperacusis:* Due to paralysis of stapedius muscle, movements of stapes are dampened; so sounds get distorted and get too high in volume. This is called hyperacusis.

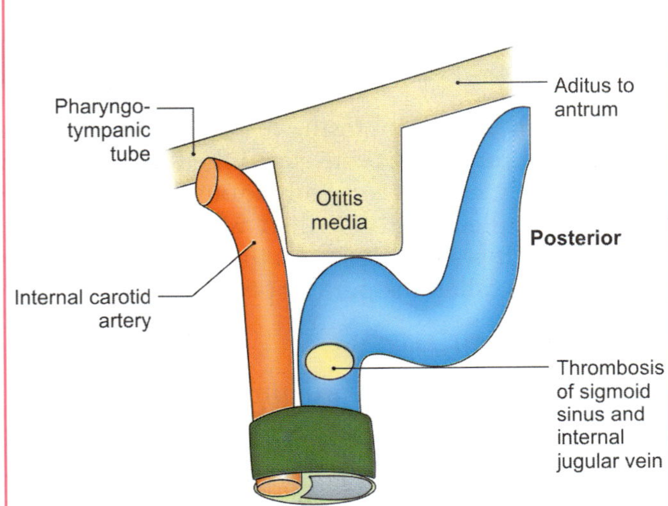

Fig. 26.16: Otitis media causing thrombosis of the sigmoid sinus and the internal jugular vein

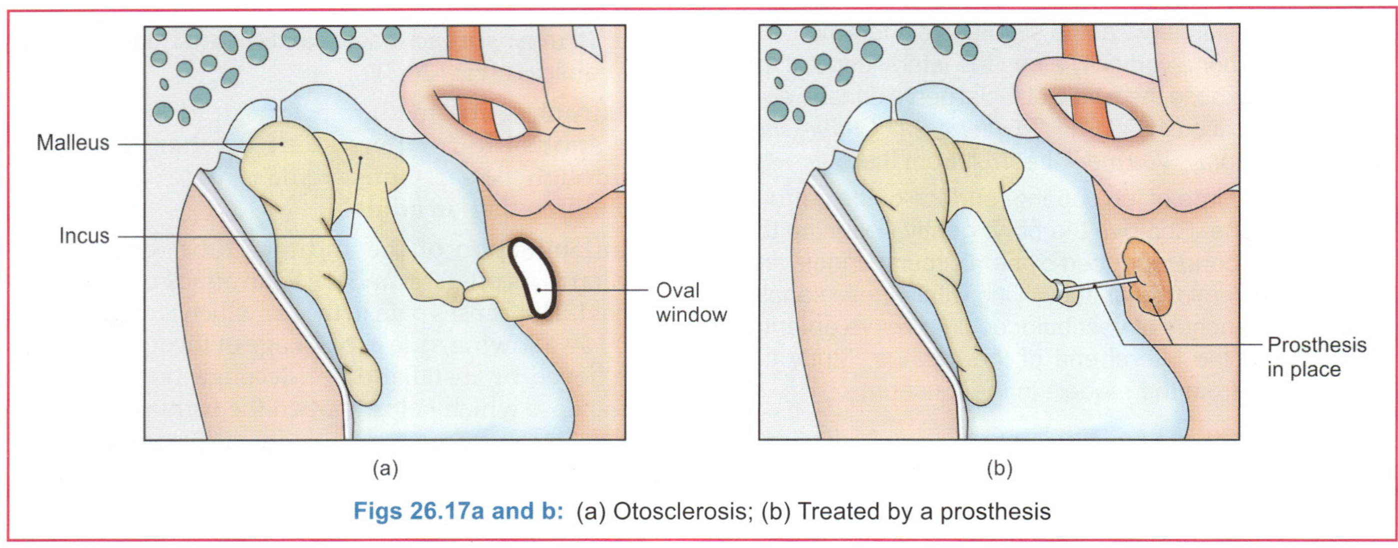

Figs 26.17a and b: (a) Otosclerosis; (b) Treated by a prosthesis

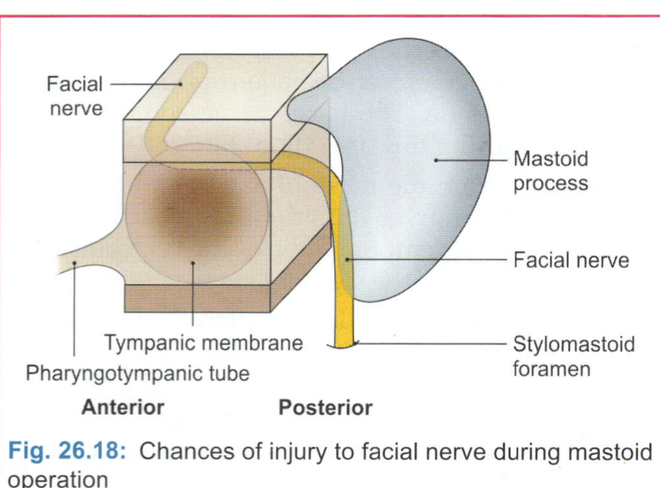

Fig. 26.18: Chances of injury to facial nerve during mastoid operation

INTERNAL EAR

The internal ear, or labyrinth, lies in the petrous part of the temporal bone. It consists of the bony labyrinth within which there is a membranous labyrinth. The membranous labyrinth is filled with a fluid called endolymph. It is separated from the bony labyrinth by another fluid called the perilymph.

BONY LABYRINTH

The bony labyrinth consists of three parts:

- Cochlea, anteriorly (Fig. 26.19a).
- Vestibule, in the middle.
- Semicircular canals, posteriorly (Fig. 26.19).

Cochlea

The bony cochlea resembles the shell of a common snail. It forms the anterior part of the labyrinth. It has a conical central axis known as the *modiolus* around which the cochlear canal makes two and three quarter turns.

The modiolus is directed forwards and laterally. Its apex points towards the anterosuperior part of the medial wall of the middle ear and the base towards the fundus of the internal acoustic meatus.

A spiral ridge of the bone, the *spiral lamina,* projects from the modiolus and partially divides the cochlear canal into the scala vestibuli above, and the scala tympani below. These relationships apply to the lowest part or basal turn of the cochlea. The division between the two passages is completed by the basilar membrane. The scala vestibuli communicates with the scala tympani at the apex of the cochlea by a small opening, called the *helicotrema*.

Vestibule

This is the central part of the bony labyrinth. It lies medial to the middle ear cavity. Its lateral wall opens into the middle ear at the fenestra vestibuli which is closed by the footplate of the stapes.

Three semicircular canals open into its posterior wall. The medial wall is related to the internal acoustic meatus, and presents the *spherical recess* in front, and the *elliptical recess* behind. The two recesses are separated by a *vestibular crest* which splits inferiorly to enclose the *cochlear recess* (Fig. 26.19).

Just below the elliptical recess, there is the opening of a diverticulum, the aqueduct of the vestibule which opens at a narrow fissure on the posterior aspect of the petrous temporal bone, posterolateral to the internal acoustic meatus. It is plugged in life by the ductus endolymphaticus and a vein; no perilymph escapes through it.

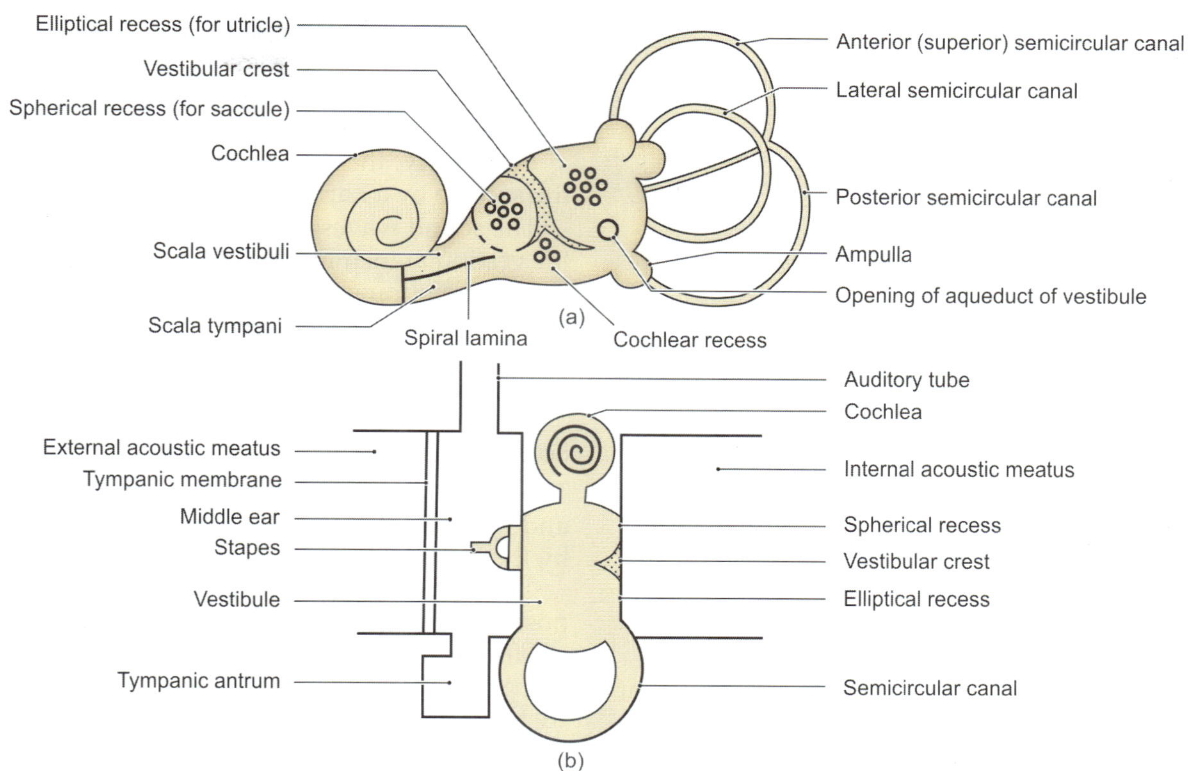

Figs 26.19a and b: (a) Scheme to show some features of the bony labyrinth (seen from the lateral side); (b) Schematic diagram

Semicircular Canals

There are three bony semicircular canals: (1) An anterior or superior, (2) posterior, and (3) lateral; each has two ends. They lie posterosuperior to the vestibule, and are set at right angles to each other. Each canal describes two-thirds of a circle, and is dilated at one end to form the *ampulla*. *These three* canals open into the vestibule by *five* openings.

The *anterior* or *superior semicircular canal* lies in a vertical plane at right angles to the long axis of the petrous temporal bone. It is convex upwards. Its position is indicated by the arcuate eminence seen on the anterior surface of the petrous temporal bone. Its ampulla is situated anterolaterally. Its posterior end unites with the upper end of the posterior canal to form the *crus commune* which opens into the medial wall of the vestibule.

The *posterior semicircular canal* also lies in a vertical plane parallel to the long axis of the petrous temporal bone. It is convex backwards. Its ampulla lies at its lower end. The upper end joins the anterior canal to form the crus commune.

The *lateral semicircular canal* lies in the horizontal plane with its convexity directed posterolaterally. The ampulla lies anteriorly, close to the ampulla of the anterior canal.

Note that the lateral semicircular canals of the two sides lie in the same plane. The anterior canal of one side lies in the plane of the posterior canal of the other side (Figs 26.19 and 26.20).

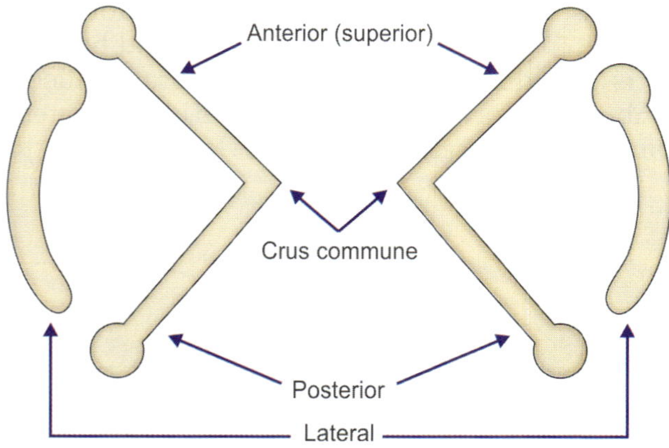

Fig. 26.20: The semicircular canals

MEMBRANOUS LABYRINTH

It is in the form of a complicated, but continuous closed cavity filled with endolymph. The epithelium of the membranous labyrinth is specialized to form receptors for sound, i.e. organ of Corti; for static balance, the maculae; and for kinetic balance, the cristae.

Like the bony labyrinth, the membranous labyrinth also consists of three main parts:

a. The spiral duct of the cochlea or organ of Corti, anteriorly.

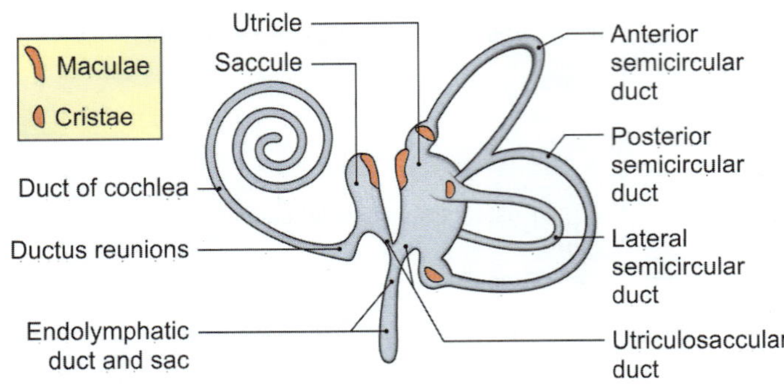

Fig. 26.21: Parts of the membranous labyrinth (as seen from the lateral side)

b. The utricle and saccule with maculae, the organs of static balance, within the vestibule.
c. The semicircular ducts with cristae, the organs of kinetic balance, posteriorly (Fig. 26.21).

Duct of the Cochlea or the Scala Media

The spiral duct occupies the middle part of the cochlear canal between the scala vestibuli and the scala tympani. It is triangular in cross-section. The floor is formed by the *basilar membrane;* the roof by the *vestibular* or *Reissner's membrane;* and the outer wall by the bony wall of the cochlea. The basilar membrane supports the spiral *organ of Corti* which is the end organ for hearing (Fig. 26.22). It comprises rods of Corti and hair cells. Hair is embedded in a gelatinous membrane called the membrana tectoria. The organ of Corti is innervated by peripheral processes of bipolar cells located in the *spiral ganglion*. This ganglion is located in the spiral canal present within the modiolus at the base of the spiral lamina. The central processes of the ganglion cells form the cochlear nerve.

Posteriorly, the duct of the cochlea is connected to the saccule by a narrow *ductus reunions.*

The sound waves reaching the endolymph through the vestibular membrane make appropriate parts of the basilar membrane vibrate, so that different parts of the organ of Corti are stimulated by different frequencies of sound. The loudness of the sound depends on the amplitude of vibration.

Saccule and Utricle

The *saccule* lies in the anteroinferior part of the vestibule, and is connected to the basal turn of the cochlear duct by the ductus reunions.

The *utricle* is larger than the saccule and lies in the posterosuperior part of the vestibule. It receives *the ends of three* semicircular ducts through *five openings*. The duct of the saccule unites with the duct of the utricle to form the *ductus endolymphaticus*. The ductus endolymphaticus ends in a dilatation, the saccus endolymphaticus. The ductus and saccus occupy the aqueduct of the vestibule.

The medial walls of the saccule and utricle are thickened to form a *macula* in each chamber. The maculae are end organs that give information about the position of the head. They are static balance receptors. They are supplied by peripheral processes of neurons in the vestibular ganglion.

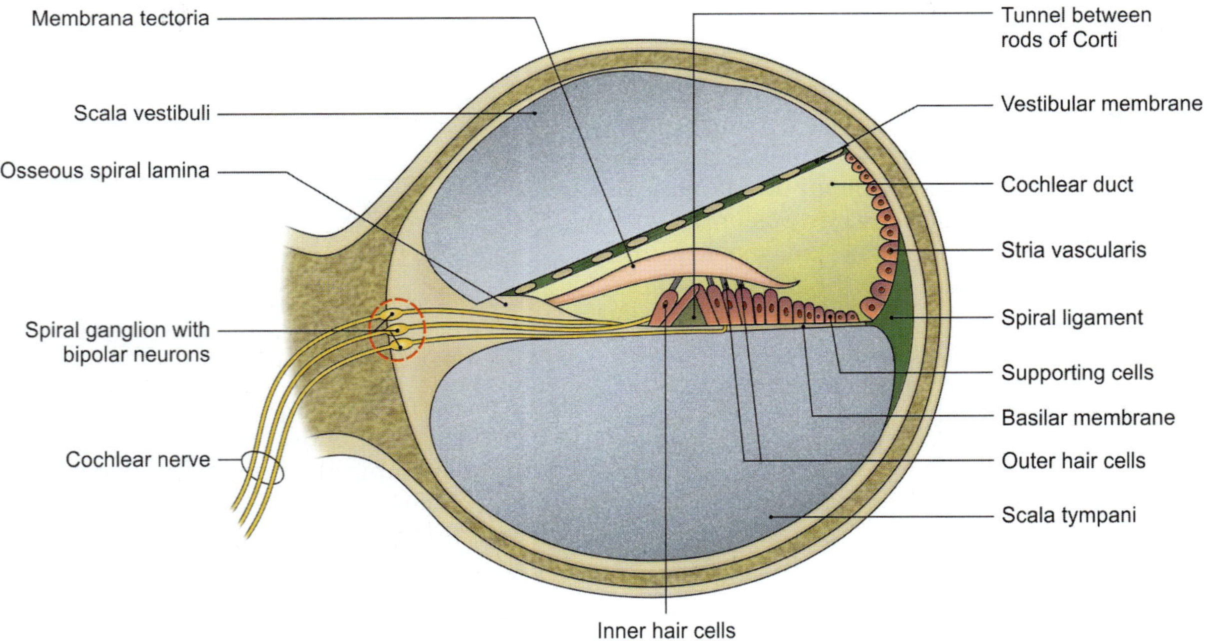

Fig. 26.22: Schematic section through one turn of the cochlea

Saccule gets stimulated by vertical linear motions, e.g. going in 'lift'. Utricle gets stimulated by horizontal linear motion, e.g. going in car.

Semicircular Ducts

The three semicircular ducts lie within the corresponding bony canals. Each duct has an ampulla corresponding to that of the bony canal. In each ampulla, there is an end organ called the ampullary crest or *crista* or cupola (Fig. 26.21). Cristae respond to pressure changes in the endolymph caused by movements of the head.

Blood Supply of Labyrinth

The arterial supply is derived mainly from the labyrinthine branch of the basilar artery which accompanies the vestibulocochlear nerve; and partly from the stylomastoid branch of the posterior auricular artery.

The labyrinthine vein drains into the superior petrosal sinus or the transverse sinus. Other inconstant veins emerge at different points and open separately into the superior and inferior petrosal sinuses and the internal jugular vein.

VESTIBULOCOCHLEAR NERVE

Cochlear Pathway

Vestibulocochlear nerve comprises hearing and vestibular parts. The first neurons of the pathway are located in the spiral ganglion. They are bipolar. Their peripheral processes innervate the spiral organ of Corti, while central processes form the cochlear nerve. This nerve terminates in the dorsal and ventral cochlear nuclei. From cochlear nuclei, fibres travel through pons, midbrain, thalamus and internal capsule to reach auditory area in temporal pole (Fig. 26.23).

Vestibular Pathway

The vestibular receptors are the maculae of the saccule and utricle (for static balance) and in the crista of the ampullaris of semicircular ducts (for kinetic balance). Fibres from cristae of anterior and lateral semicircular canals and some fibres from the two maculae lie in superior vestibular area of internal acoustic meatus.

Fibres of crista of posterior semicircular canal lie in foramen singulare.

Most of the fibres from maculae of utricle and saccule lie in inferior vestibular area (Fig. 26.23).

These three nerve divisions are peripheral processes of bipolar neurons of the vestibular ganglion. This ganglion is situated in the internal acoustic meatus. The central processes arising from the neurons of the ganglion form the vestibular nerve which ends in the vestibular nuclei.

These nuclei send fibres:

a. To the archicerebellum through the inferior cerebellar peduncle.
b. To the motor nuclei of the brainstem (chiefly of the III, IV, VI and XI nerves)

Through the vestibular pathway, the impulses arising in the labyrinth can influence the movements of the eyes, the head, the neck and the trunk.

Facial nerve: Facial nerve enters the petrous temporal bone through internal acoustic meatus. It travels in relation to internal ear and middle ear and exits through stylomastoid foramen. The course and branches of this part are given in section of brain, Chapter 32.

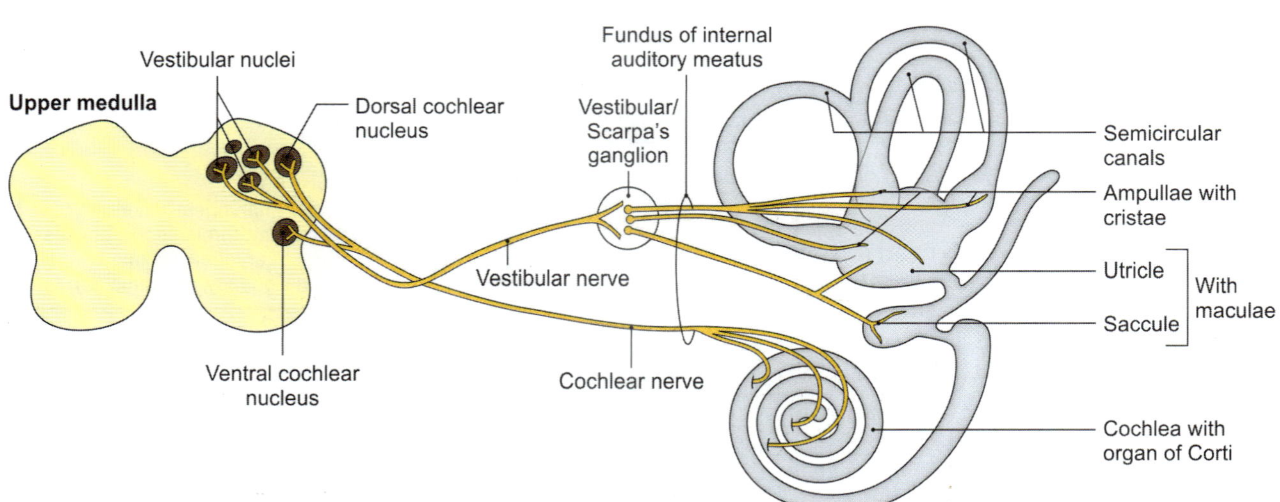

Fig. 26.23: Course of vestibulocochlear nerve

CLINICAL ANATOMY

- Endolymph is produced by striae vascularis. This process requires melanocytes. The disorders of melanocytes, i.e. albinism, are associated with deafness.
- Acoustic neuroma is a tumour of Schwann cells of VIII nerve. If neuroma extends into internal auditory meatus, VII nerve will get pressed. There will be VIII nerve paralysis and VII nerve paralysis as well.
- Reasons of earache are depicted in Flowchart 26.1.

DEVELOPMENT

1. *External auditory meatus:* Dorsal part of 1st ectodermal cleft.
2. *Auricle:* Tubercles appearing on 1st and 2nd branchial arches around the opening of external auditory meatus.
3. *Middle ear cavity and auditory tube:* Tubotympanic recess (*see* Tables A.6 and A.7 in Appendix).
4. *Ossicles*
   a. *Malleus and incus:* From *1st arch cartilage.*
   b. *Stapes:* From *2nd arch cartilage* (*see* Table A.5 in Appendix).
5. *Muscles*
   a. *Tensor tympani:* From *1st pharyngeal arch mesoderm.*
   b. *Stapedius:* From *2nd pharyngeal arch mesoderm.*
6. Membranous labyrinth from ectodermal vesicle on each side of hindbrain vesicle. Organ of Corti—ectodermal.

Molecular Regulation

The proteins WNT and bone morphogenetic protein (BMP) of surrounding region are important for the formation of otic placode.

Retinoic acid plays an important role in the anteroposterior differentiation of otic vesicle.

WNT and SHH are required for the formation of semicircular canals and cochlear duct.

Defects in Noggin and PAX2 genes result in sensory neural deafness that plays a role in formation of cochlea.

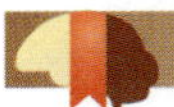

Mnemonics

Ear: Bones of middle ear MISs

M–Malleus
I–Incus
Ss–Stapes

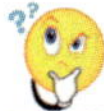

FACTS TO REMEMBER

- Tympanic membrane develops from ectoderm, mesoderm and endoderm.
- Outer aspect of tympanic membrane is supplied by part of V and X nerves.
- Syringing the ear may cause slowing of the heart rate and feeling of nausea.
- Malleus and incus develop from 1st pharyngeal arch, while stapedius develops from second pharyngeal arch.
- Tensor tympani develops from 1st arch and is supplied by V3, while stapedius develops from 2nd arch and is supplied by VII nerve.

Flowchart 26.1: Reasons of earache

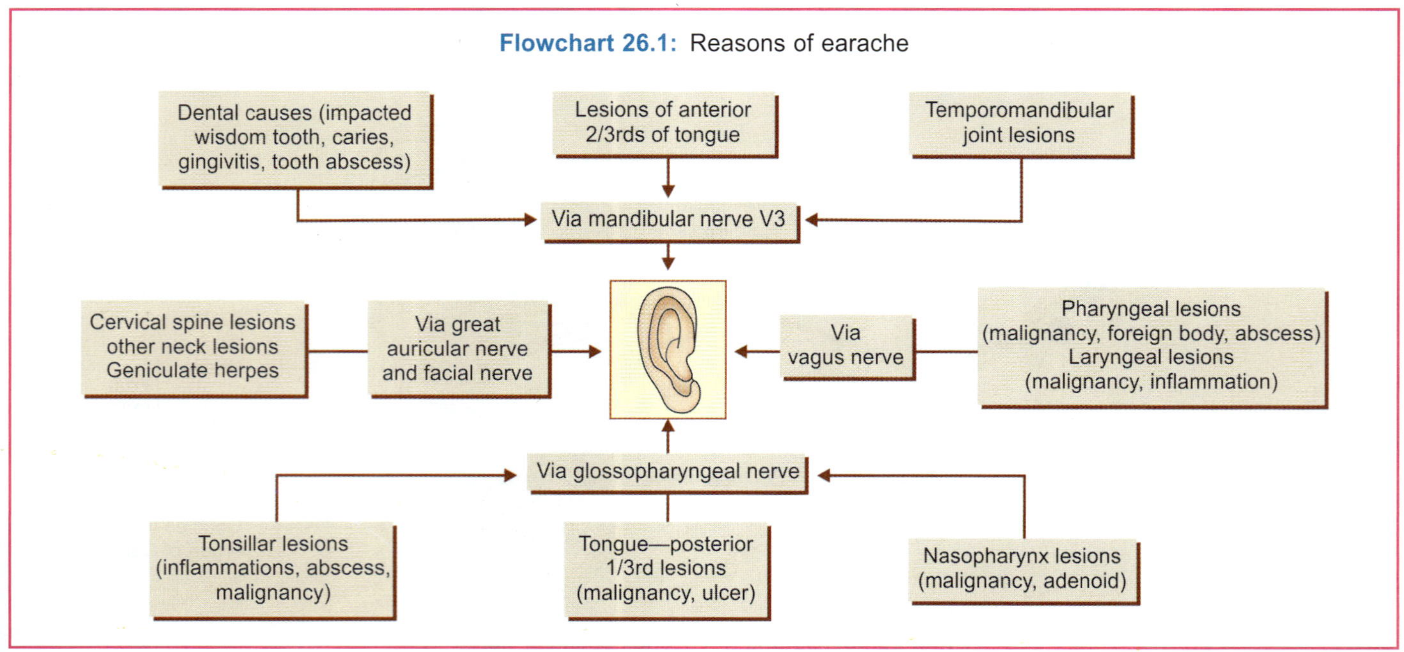

- Suprameatal triangle (Macewen's triangle) demarcates the position of mastoid antrum at a depth of 12–13 mm in adult.
- Eustachian tube equalizes the pressure on both sides of the tympanic membrane. This tube connects the nasopharynx to the anterior wall of middle ear.
- Malleus, incus and stapes are *bone within bone*, as these 3 bony ossicles lie within the petrous temporal bone.
- There are 2 synovial joints between these three bony ossicles, which are fully developed at birth.
- Ear is an engineering marvel.
- One may slowly become deaf to soft sounds, if one is continuously exposed to a lot of loud sounds.

CLINICOANATOMICAL PROBLEM

A young boy has only deformity of the auricle/pinna. No treatment is done and he is fine in studies, games, etc.

- What are the uses of the auricle?
- Name its nerve supply.

Ans: There is hardly any medical use of the pinna in human. It is mainly cosmetic. However, there are other uses. These are:

- Lobule, the lowest part of auricle is used for wearing ear rings of different shape, size, colour and quality.
- It is used for supporting glasses. Nature knew million of years ago that human would need glasses, and the auricles were not removed.
- A small bit of skin is taken to examine lepra bacilli
- Hairy pinna is the only symptom of Y chromosome
- Pinna used to be pulled as a part of punishment for disobedience.

Nerve supply: Medial surface in its upper two-thirds part is supplied by lesser occipital and in its lower one-third part by great auricular. Lateral surface in its upper two-thirds part is supplied by auriculotemporal nerve and in its lower one-third part by great auricular again.

FURTHER READING

- Allam AF. Pneumatization of the temporal bone: Ann Otol Rhino Laryngol 1969;78:49–64.
- Anderson SD. The Intratympanic muscles. In: Hinchcliffe R (ed). Scientific Foundations of Otolaryngology. London: Heinemann; 1976; pp. 257–80.
- Duman D, Tekin M. Autosomal recessive nonsyndromic deafness genes: A review. Front Biosci 2013;17:2213–36.

  A review that summarizes genes and mutations reported in families with ARNSHL. Mutations in GJB2, encoding connexin 26, make this gene the most common cause of hearing loss in many populations. Other relatively common deafness genes include SLC26A4, MYO15A, OTOF, TMC1, CDH23 and TMPRSS3.
- Fettiplace R. Hackney CM. The sensory and motor roles of auditory hair cells. Nat Rev Neurosci 2006;7:19–29.

  A description of proteins involved in the sensory and motor functions of auditory hair cells, with evidence for each force generator.
- Proctor B, Nager GT. The facial canal: Normal anatomy, variations and anomalis. Ann Rhinol Laryngol 1982;91:33–61.

  A detailed anatomical description, emphasising the relations of the facial canal to adjacent structures and variations in the course of the canal.

NOISE POLLUTION

"Noise pollution leads to mind body suffering
Plug the ears, decrease volume, seek policing

Sweet soft "lecture" induces happy sleeping
Loud prolonged noise causes auditory crippling

One should not even mind job changing
But do not, at any cost lose your hearing

Lest one's very dear cell phone
One would not be hearing"

Frequently Asked Questions

1. Discuss the middle ear under the following headings.
   a. Walls
   b. Ossicles
   c. Muscles
   d. Clinical anatomy
2. Write short notes on:
   a. Tympanic membrane
   b. Contents of middle ear
   c. Chorda tympani nerve
   d. Parts of internal ear
   e. Cochlear duct

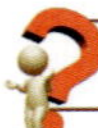

Multiple Choice Questions

1. Tegmen tympani forms the roof of the following, *except:*
   a. Mastoid antrum
   b. Tympanic cavity
   c. Canal for tensor tympani
   d. Internal auditory meatus
2. Which nerve supplies stapedius muscle?
   a. Oculomotor
   b. Trochlear
   c. Trigeminal
   d. Facial
3. By how many openings do the semicircular canals open in the vestibule?
   a. 3
   b. 5
   c. 4
   d. 2
4. Which of the following nerves supplies the outer aspect of the tympanic membrane?
   a. Auricular branch of vagus
   b. Greater occipital
   c. Lesser occipital
   d. Anterior ethmoidal
5. Which of the following nerves supplies middle ear cavity?
   a. Facial
   b. Trigeminal
   c. Glossopharyngeal
   d. Vagus
6. Derivatives of all the germ layers; ectoderm, mesoderm and endoderm are present in:
   a. Heart
   b. Tympanic membrane
   c. Cornea
   d. Urachus

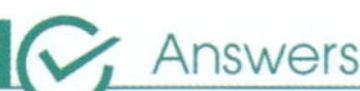

1. d **2.** d **3.** b **4.** a **5.** c **6.** b

VIVA VOCE

- What is type of cartilage present in the auricle/ pinna?
- What is the nerve supply of tympanic membrane on both its surfaces?
- Name the bony ossicles and the types of joints formed between them.
- Name the muscles of the middle ear with their nerve supply.
- Which embryonic layers form the tympanic membrane?
- How can syringing of the ear cause nausea and bradycardia?
- Name the walls of the middle ear.
- Which structures form posterior wall of the middle ear?
- Which structures form the medial wall of the middle ear?
- Which two tubes lie in the anterior wall of the middle ear?
- How many semicircular canals (bony and membranous) are there in internal ear?
- How many cristae are there in three membranous semi-circular canals?
- What is the receptor in saccule and utricle?
- Which is the end organ for hearing?
- How do auditory tube and middle ear cavity develop?
- Which embryonic layer gives rise to the membranous labyrinth?
- Enumerate the reasons for 'earache'.
- How does one mark the suprameatal triangle? What is its importance?
- Enumerate the complications of otitis media.
- What are the parts of the tympanic membrane?

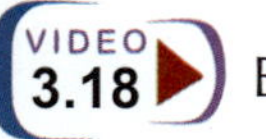

Ear

Chapter 27

Eyeball

"Our eyes are placed in front because it is more important to look ahead than look back."
—Anonymous

INTRODUCTION

Sense of sight perceived through retina of the eyeball is one of the five special senses. Its importance is obvious in the varied ways of natural protection. Bony orbit, projecting nose and various coats protect the precious retina. Each and every component of its three coats is assisting the retina to focus the light properly. A lot of advances have been made in correcting the defects of the eye. Eyes can be donated at the time of death, and a 'will' can be prepared accordingly.

About 75% of afferents reach the brain through the eyes. Adequate rest to eye muscles is important. A good place for rest could be the 'classroom' where palpebral part of orbicularis oculi closes the eyes gently.

The eyeball is the organ of sight. The camera closely resembles the eyeball in its structure. It is almost spherical in shape and has a diameter of about 2.5 cm. Eyeball is made up of three concentric coats. The outer or *fibrous coat* comprises the sclera and cornea. The middle or *vascular coat* also called the uveal tract consists of the choroid, the ciliary body and the iris. The inner or *nervous coat* is the retina (Fig. 27.1).

Light entering the eyeball passes through several *refracting media*. From before backwards, these are the cornea, the aqueous humour, the lens and the vitreous body.

OUTER COAT

SCLERA

The sclera (*skleros* = hard) is opaque and forms the posterior five-sixths of the eyeball. It is composed of dense fibrous tissue which is firm and maintains the shape of the eyeball. It is thickest behind, near the

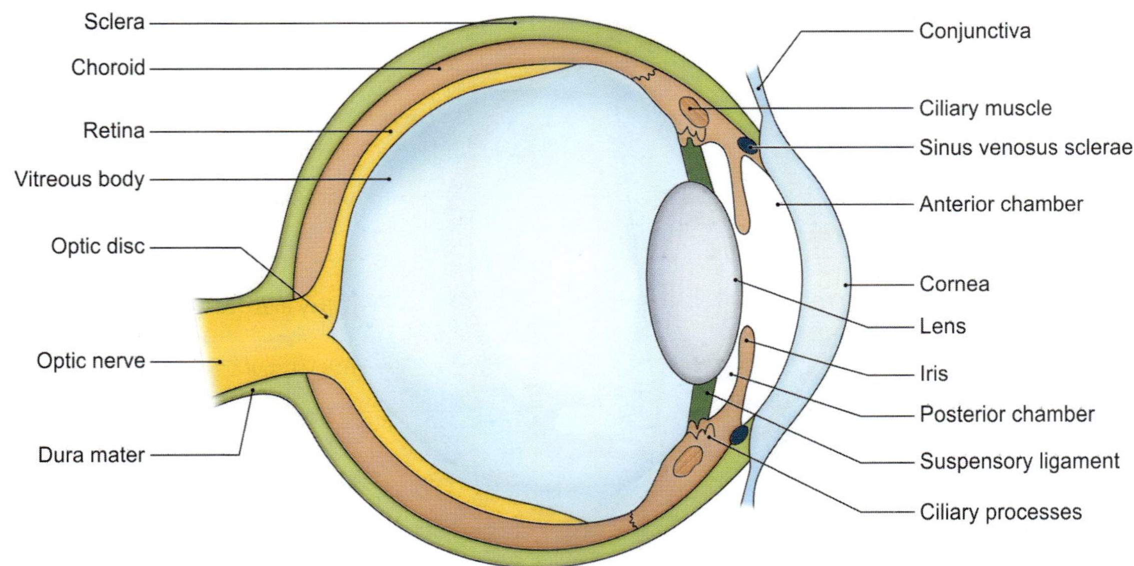

Fig. 27.1: Sagittal section through the eyeball

entrance of the optic nerve, and thinnest about 6 mm behind the sclerocorneal junction where the recti muscles are inserted. However, it is weakest at the entrance of the optic nerve. Here the sclera shows numerous perforations for passage of fibres of the optic nerve. Because of its sieve-like appearance, this region is called the *lamina cribrosa* (*crib* = sieve).

The *outer surface* of the sclera is white and smooth, it is covered by Tenon's capsule (*see* Fig. 21.3). Its anterior part is covered by conjunctiva through which it can be seen as the white of the eye. The *inner surface* is brown and grooved for the ciliary nerves and vessels. It is separated from the choroid by the *perichoroidal space* which contains a delicate cellular tissue, termed the *suprachoroidal lamina* or *lamina fusca of the sclera.*

The sclera is continuous anteriorly with the cornea at the *sclerocorneal junction or limbus* (Fig. 27.1). The deep part of the limbus contains a circular canal, known as the *sinus venosus sclerae or the canal of Schlemm.* The aqueous humour drains into the anterior scleral or ciliary veins through this sinus.

The sclera is fused posteriorly with the *dural sheath of the optic nerve.* It provides insertion to the extrinsic muscles of the eyeball: The recti in front of the equator, and the oblique muscles behind the equator.

The sclera is pierced by a number of structures:

a. The *optic nerve* pierces it a little inferomedial to the posterior pole of the eyeball.
b. The *ciliary nerves and arteries* pierce it around the entrance of the optic nerve.
c. The *anterior ciliary arteries,* derived from muscular arteries to the recti, pierce it near the limbus.

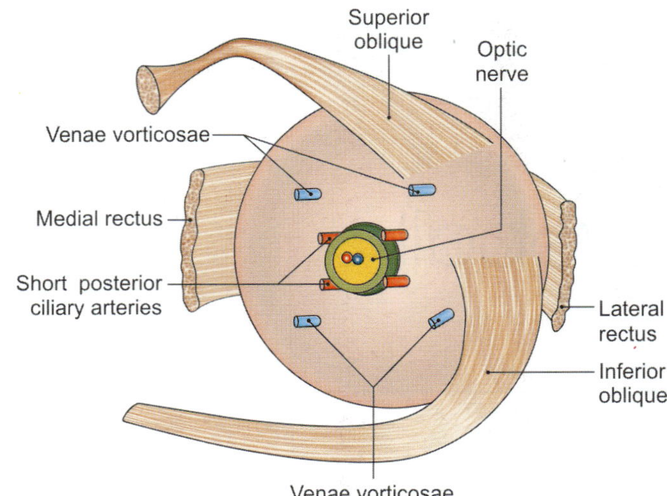

Fig. 27.2: Structures piercing the posterior aspect of the eyeball

d. Four *venae vorticosae* or the choroid veins pass out through the sclera just behind the equator (Figs 27.2 and 27.3).

The sclera is almost avascular. However, the loose connective tissue between the conjunctiva and sclera called as the *episclera* is vascular.

DISSECTION

Use the fresh eyeball of the goats for this dissection. Clean the eyeball by removing all the tissues from its surface. Cut through the fascial sheath around the margin of the cornea. Clean and identify the nerve with posterior ciliary arteries and ciliary nerves close to the posterior

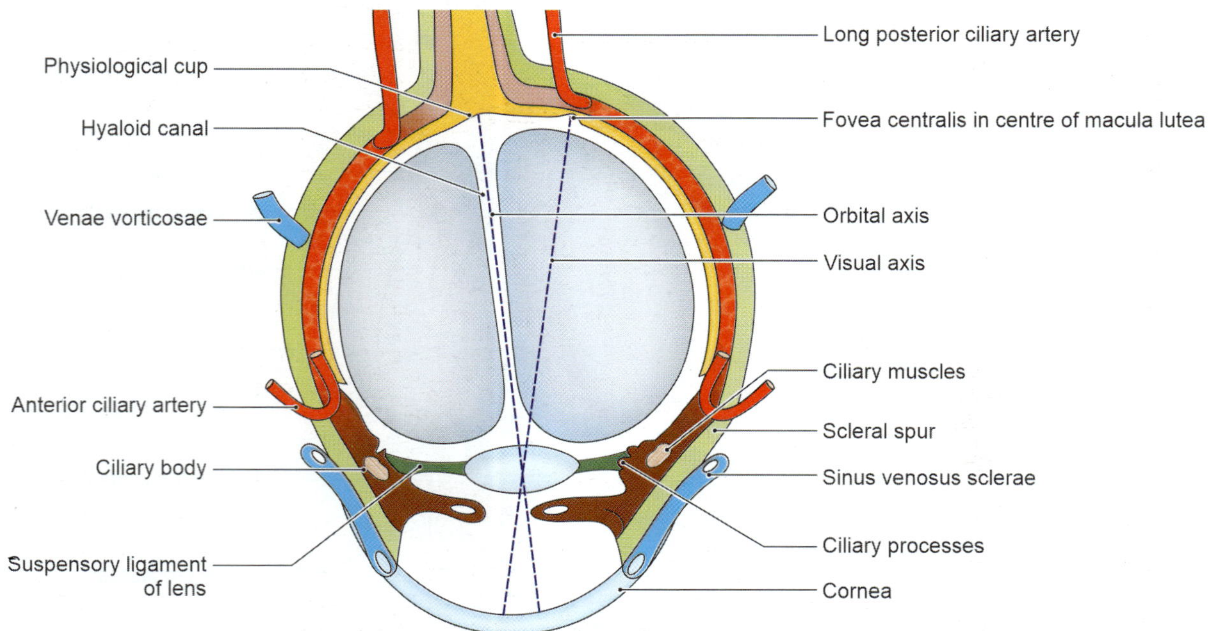

Fig. 27.3: Structures piercing the eyeball seen in a sagittal section

pole of the eyeball. Identify venae vorticosae piercing the sclera just behind the equator *(refer to BDC App)*.

Incise only the sclera at the equator and then cut through it all around and carefully strip it off from the choroid. Anteriorly, the ciliary muscles are attached to the sclera, offering some resistance. As the sclera is steadily separated, the aqueous humour will escape from the anterior chamber of the eye. On dividing the optic nerve fibres, the posterior part of sclera can be removed.

CORNEA

Features

The cornea is transparent. It replaces the sclera over the anterior one-sixth of the eyeball. Its junction with the sclera is called the *sclerocorneal junction or limbus.*

The cornea is more convex than the sclera, but the curvature diminishes with age. It is separated from the iris by a space called the *anterior chamber of the eye*.

The cornea is avascular and is nourished by lymph which circulates in the numerous corneal spaces and by the lacrimal fluid.

It is supplied by branches of the ophthalmic nerve and the short ciliary nerves (through the ciliary ganglion). Pain is the only sensation aroused from the cornea.

DISSECTION

Identify the cornea. Make an incision around the corneoscleral junction and remove the cornea so that the iris is exposed for examination. Identify the middle coat comprising choroid, ciliary body and iris deep to the sclera. Lateral to iris is the ciliary body with ciliary muscles and ciliary processes.

Strip off the iris, ciliary processes, anterior part of choroid. Remove the lens and put it in water. As the lens is removed, the vitreous body also escapes. Only the posterior part of choroid and subjacent retina is left.

Histology/Microanatomy

Structurally, the cornea consists of these layers, from before backwards:

1 *Corneal epithelium* (stratified squamous non-keratinized type) (Fig. 27.4)
2 *Bowman's membrane* or anterior elastic lamina
3 The *substantia propria*
4 *Descemet's membrane* or posterior elastic lamina
5 Simple squamous *mesothelium*.

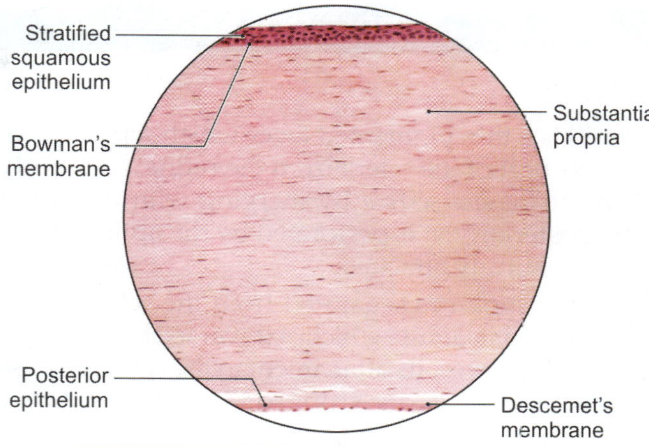

- Stratified squamous epithelium
- Substantia propria is thick
- Descemet's membrane next to posterior epithelium

Fig. 27.4: Histology of cornea

CLINICAL ANATOMY

- Cornea can be grafted from one person to the other, as it is avascular.
- Injury to cornea may cause opacities. These opacities may interfere with vision.
- Eye is a very sensitive organ and even a dust particle gives rise to pain.
- Bulbar conjunctiva is vascular. Inflammation of the conjunctiva leads to conjunctivitis. The look of palpebral conjunctiva is used to judge haemoglobin level.
- The anteroposterior diameter of the eyeball and shape and curvature of the cornea determine the focal point. Changes in these result in myopia or short-sightedness, hypermetropia or long-sightedness (Fig. 27.5).

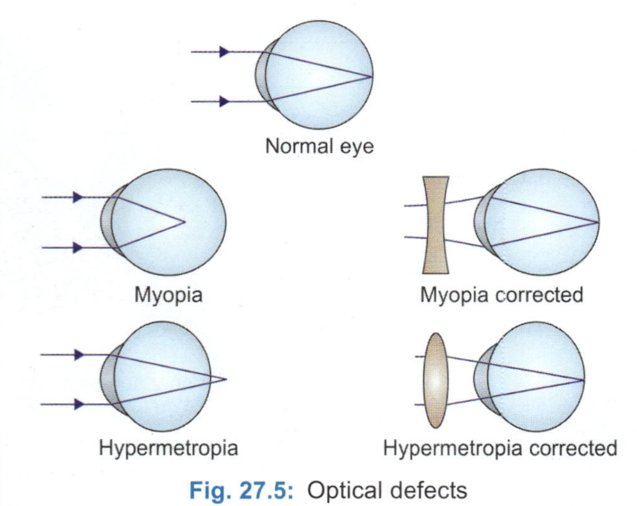

Fig. 27.5: Optical defects

MIDDLE COAT

CHOROID

Choroid is a thin pigmented layer which separates the posterior part of the sclera from the retina. Anteriorly, it ends at the *ora serrata* by merging with the ciliary body. Posteriorly, it is perforated by the optic nerve to which it is firmly attached.

Its *outer surface* is separated from the sclera by the suprachoroidal lamina which is traversed by the ciliary vessels and nerves. Its attachment to the sclera is loose, so that it can be easily stripped. The *inner surface* is firmly united to the retina.

Structurally, it consists of:

a. *Suprachoroid lamina*
b. *Vascular lamina*
c. The *choriocapillary lamina*
d. The inner *basal lamina* or membrane of Bruch.

CILIARY BODY

Ciliary body is a thickened part of the uveal tract lying just posterior to the corneal limbus. It is continuous anteriorly with the iris and posteriorly with the choroid. It suspends the lens and helps it in accommodation for near vision.

1 The ciliary body is triangular in cross-section. It is thick in front and thin behind (Fig. 27.6). The scleral surface of this body contains the ciliary muscle. The posterior part of the vitreous surface is smooth and black (pars plana). The anterior part is ridged anteriorly (pars plicata) to form about 70 ciliary processes. The central ends of the processes are free and rounded.
2 Ciliary zonule is thickened vitreous membrane fitted to the posterior surfaces of ciliary processes (Fig. 27.7). The posterior layer lines hyaloid fossa and anterior thick layer form the suspensory ligament of lens (Fig. 27.6).
3 The *ciliary muscle* (Fig. 27.6) is a ring of unstriped muscle which are longitudinal or meridional, radial and circular. The longitudinal or meridional *fibres* arise from a projection of sclera or scleral spur near the limbus. They radiate backwards to the suprachoroidal lamina. The radial fibres are obliquely placed and get continuous with the circular fibres.

   The *circular fibres* lie within the anterior part of the ciliary body and are nearest to the lens. The contraction of *all the parts* relaxes the suspensory ligament so that the lens becomes more convex (Fig. 27.6). All parts of the muscle are supplied by parasympathetic nerves. The pathway involves the Edinger-Westphal nucleus, oculomotor nerve and the ciliary ganglion (*see* Flowchart A.4 in Appendix).

IRIS

1 This is the anterior part of the uveal tract. It forms a circular curtain with an opening in the centre, called the *pupil*. By adjusting the size of the pupil, it controls the amount of light entering the eye, and thus behaves like an adjustable diaphragm (Fig. 27.3).
2 It is placed vertically between the cornea and the lens, thus divides the anterior segment of the eye into anterior and posterior chambers, *both containing aqueous humour*. Its *peripheral margin* is attached to the middle of the anterior surface of the ciliary body and is separated from the cornea by the iridocorneal

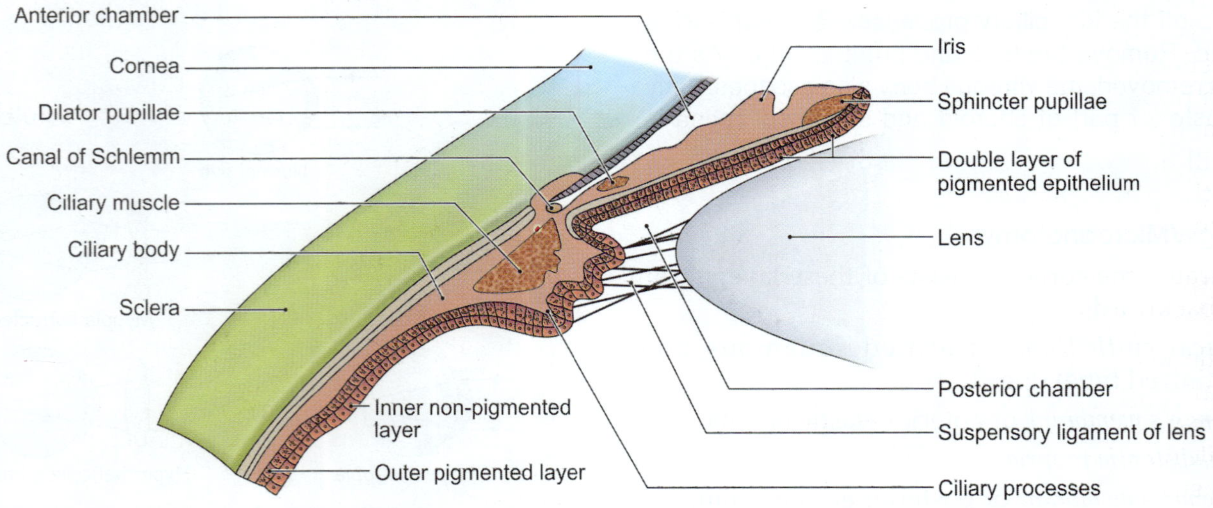

Fig. 27.6: Components of ciliary body and iris (sclerocorneal junction)

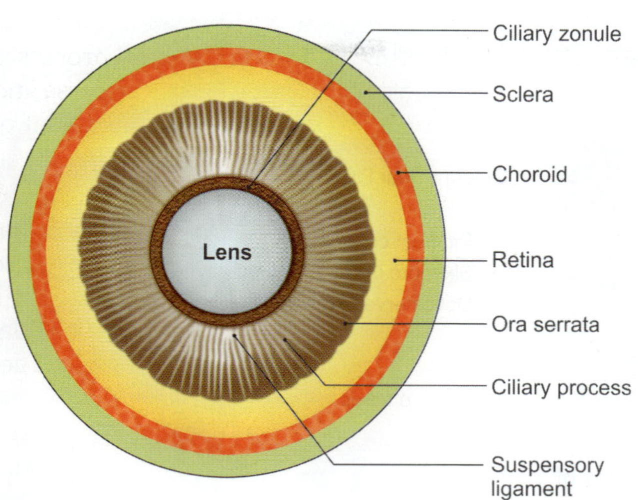

Fig. 27.7: Anterior part of the inner aspect of the eyeball seen after vitreous has been removed

angle or angle of the anterior chamber. The *central free margin* forming the boundary of the pupil rests against the lens (Fig. 27.1).

3 The anterior surface of the iris is covered by a single layer of mesothelium, and the posterior surface by a double layer of deeply pigmented cells which are continuous with those of the ciliary body (Fig. 27.6). The main bulk of the iris is formed by stroma made up of blood vessels and loose connective tissue in which there are pigment cells. The long posterior and the anterior ciliary arteries join to form the *major arterial circle* at the periphery of the iris. From this circle, vessels converge towards the free margin of the iris and join together to form the *minor arterial circle* of the iris (*see* Fig. 21.10).
The colour of the iris is determined by the number of pigment cells in its connective tissue. If the pigment cells are absent, the iris is blue in colour due to the diffusion of light in front of the black posterior surface.

4 The iris contains a well-developed ring of muscle called the *sphincter pupillae* which lies near the margin of the pupil. Its nerve supply (parasympathetic) is similar to that of the ciliary muscle. The *dilator pupillae* is an ill-defined sheet of radial muscle fibres placed near the posterior surface of the iris. It is supplied by sympathetic nerves (Fig. 27.6).

CLINICAL ANATOMY

- While looking at infinite far, the light rays run parallel; ciliary muscle is relaxed, suspensory ligament is tense and lens is flat (Fig. 27.8a).
- While reading a book, the ciliary muscles contract and suspensory ligament is relaxed making the lens more convex (Fig. 27.8b).

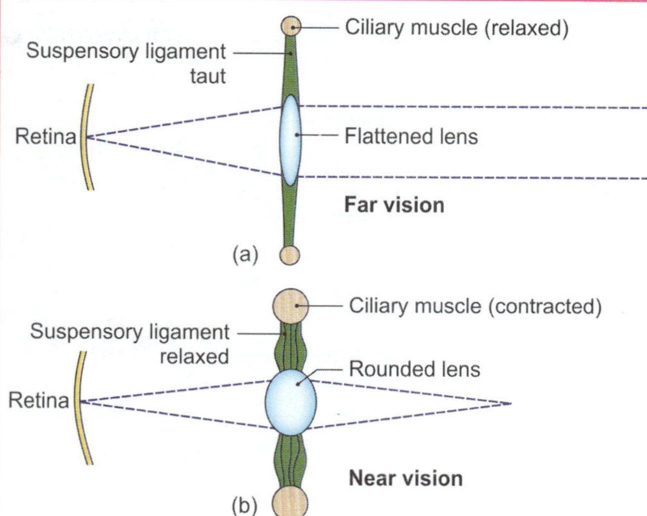

Figs 27.8a and b: (a) Relaxed ciliary muscles with flattened lens; (b) Contracted ciliary muscles with round lens

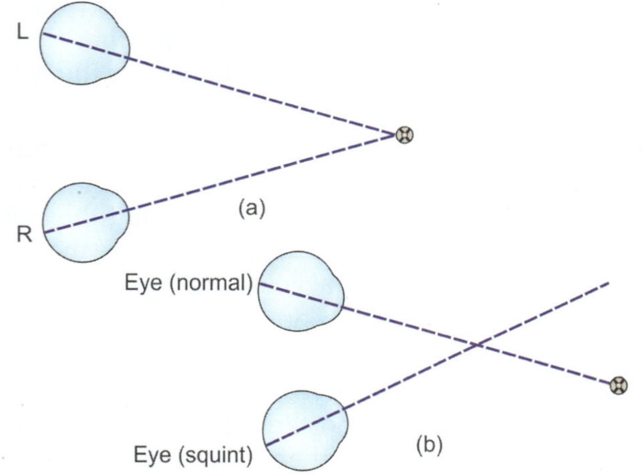

Figs 27.9a and b: (a) Normal eyes; (b) In squinting eyes

- Human vision is coloured, binocular and three-dimensional. Normally, right and left eyes are focused on one object (Fig. 27.9a). In squinting, fixing eye (F) focuses on the object, but the squinting eye (S) is 'turned inwards' resulting in a convergent squint (Fig. 27.9b).

INNER COAT/RETINA

1 This is the thin, delicate inner layer of the eyeball. It is continuous posteriorly with the optic nerve. The outer surface of the retina (formed by pigment cells) is attached to the choroid, while the inner surface is in contact with the hyaloid membrane (of the vitreous). Opposite the entrance of the optic nerve (infero-medial to the posterior pole), there is a circular area known as the *optic disc.* It is 1.5 mm in diameter.

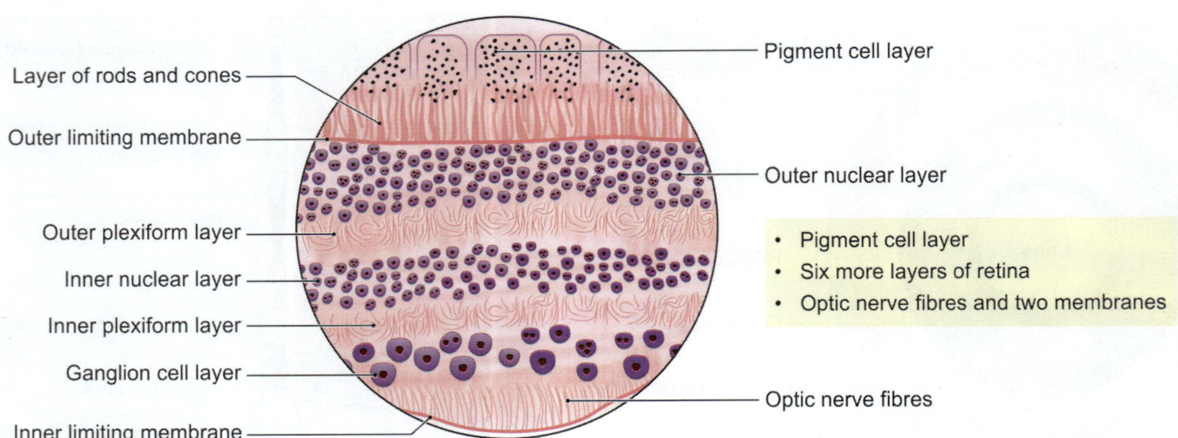

Fig. 27.10: Histological layers of the retina

2 The retina diminishes in thickness from behind forwards and is divided into optic, ciliary and iridial parts. The *optic part of the retina* contains nervous tissue and is sensitive to light. It extends from the optic disc to the posterior end of the ciliary body. The anterior margin of the optic part of the retina forms a wavy line called the ora serrata (Fig. 27.1).

Beyond the ora serrata, the retina is continued forwards as a thin, non-nervous insensitive layer that covers the ciliary body and iris, forming the *ciliary and iridial parts of the retina*. These parts are made up of two layers of epithelial cells (Fig. 27.6).

3 The depressed area of the optic disc is called the *physiological cup* (Fig. 27.3). It contains no rods or cones and is, therefore, insensitive to light, i.e. it is the *physiological blind spot*. At the posterior pole of the eye 3 mm lateral to the optic disc, there is another depression of similar size, called the *macula lutea*. It is avascular and yellow in colour. The centre of the macula is further depressed to form the *fovea centralis*. This is the thinnest part of the retina. It contains cones only, and is the site of maximum acuity of vision (Fig. 27.3).

4 The rods and cones are the light receptors of the eye. The *rods* contain a pigment called *visual purple*. They can respond to dim light (*scotopic vision*). The periphery of the retina contains only rods, but the fovea has none at all. The *cones* respond only to bright light (*photopic vision*) and are sensitive to colour. The fovea centralis has only cones. Their number diminishes towards the periphery of the retina.

5 The retina is composed of ten layers (Fig. 27.10):
   a. The outer pigmented layer
   b. Layer of rods and cones
   c. External limiting membrane
   d. Outer nuclear layer
   e. Outer plexiform layer
   f. Inner nuclear layer (bipolar cells)
   g. Inner plexiform layer
   h. Ganglion cell layer
   i. Nerve fibre layer
   j. The internal limiting membrane.

6 The retina is supplied by the *central artery*. This is an end artery. In the optic disc, it divides into an upper and a lower branch, each giving off nasal and temporal branches. The artery supplies the deeper layers of the retina up to the bipolar cells. The rods and cones are supplied by diffusion from the capillaries of the choroid. The retinal veins run with the arteries (Fig. 27.11).

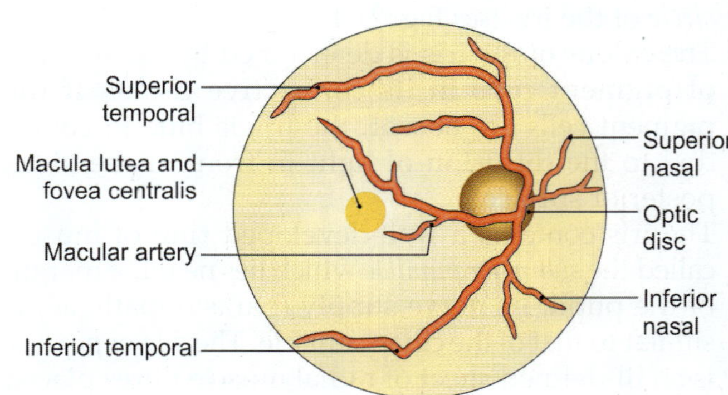

Fig. 27.11: Distribution of central artery of the retina

CLINICAL ANATOMY

Retinal detachment occurs between outer single pigmented layer and inner nine nervous layers. Actually, it is an inter-retinal detachment. Silicone sponge is put over the detached retina, which is kept in position by a 'band' (Figs 27.12a and b).

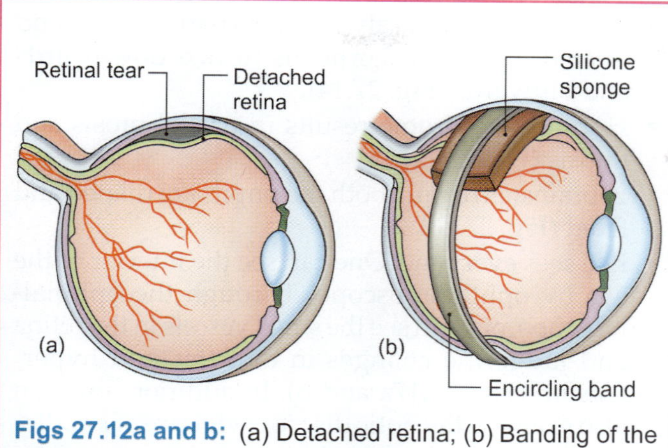

Figs 27.12a and b: (a) Detached retina; (b) Banding of the retina

AQUEOUS HUMOUR

This is a clear fluid which fills the space between the cornea in front and the lens behind the anterior segment. This space is divided by the iris into anterior and posterior chambers which freely communicate with each other through the pupil.

The aqueous humour is secreted into the posterior chamber from the capillaries in the ciliary processes. It passes into the anterior chamber through the pupil. From the anterior chamber, it is drained into the anterior ciliary veins through the spaces of the iridocorneal angle or angle of anterior chamber (located between the fibres of the ligamentum pectinatum) and the canal of Schlemm (Figs 27.3 and 27.6).

Interference with the drainage of the aqueous humour into the canal of Schlemm results in an increase of intraocular pressure (glaucoma). This produces cupping of the optic disc and pressure atrophy of the retina causing blindness.

The intraocular pressure is due chiefly to the aqueous humour which maintains the constancy of the optical dimensions of the eyeball. The aqueous is rich in ascorbic acid, glucose and amino acids, and nourishes the avascular tissues of the cornea and lens.

CLINICAL ANATOMY

Over production of aqueous humour or lack of its drainage or combination of both raise the intraocular pressure. The condition is called glaucoma. It must be treated urgently.

LENS

Features

The lens is a transparent biconvex structure which is placed between the anterior and posterior segments of the eye. It is circular in outline and has a diameter of 1 cm. The central points of the anterior and posterior surfaces are called the anterior and posterior *poles* (Fig. 27.13). The line connecting the poles constitutes the *axis* of the lens, while the marginal circumference is termed the *equator*. The chief advantage of the lens is that it can vary its dioptric power. It contributes about 15 dioptres to the total of 58 dioptric power of the eye. A dioptre is the inverse of the focal length in meters. A lens having a focal length of half meter has a power of two dioptres.

The posterior surface of the lens is more convex than the anterior. The anterior surface is kept flattened by the tension of the suspensory ligament. When the ligament is relaxed by contraction of the ciliary muscle, the anterior surface becomes more convex due to elasticity of the lens substance.

The lens is enclosed in a transparent, structureless elastic *capsule* which is thickest anteriorly near the circumference. Deep to capsule, the anterior surface of the lens is covered by a *capsular epithelium.* At the centre of the anterior surface, the epithelium is made up of a single layer of cubical cells, but at the periphery, the cells elongate to produce the *fibres* of the lens. The fibres are concentrically arranged to form the lens substance. The centre (nucleus) of the lens is firm (and consists of the oldest fibres), whereas the periphery (cortex) is soft

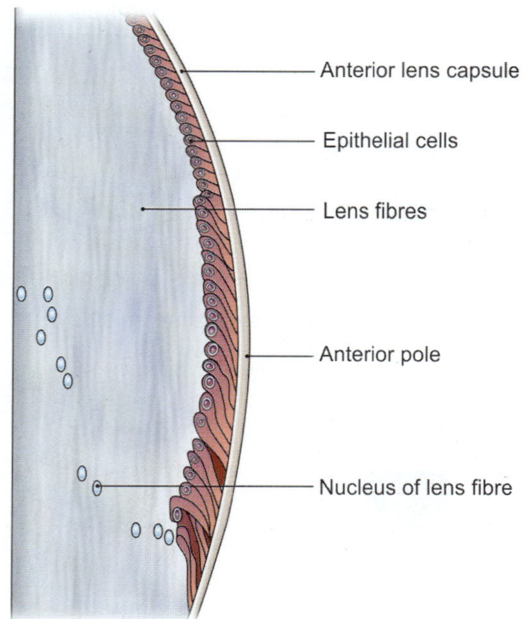

Fig. 27.13: The lens

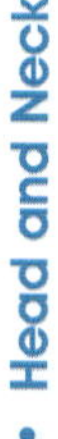

and is made up of more recently formed fibres (Fig. 27.13).

The *suspensory ligament of the lens* (or the zonule of Zinn) retains the lens in position and its tension keeps the anterior surface of the lens flattened. The ligament is made up of a series of fibres which are attached peripherally to the ciliary processes, to the furrows between the ciliary processes, and to the ora serrata. Centrally, the fibres are attached to the lens, mostly in front, and a few behind the equator (Fig. 27.5).

DISSECTION

Give an incision in the anterior surface of lens and with a little pressure of fingers and thumb press the body of lens outside from the capsule.

CLINICAL ANATOMY

- Lens becomes opaque with increasing age (cataract). Since the opacities cause difficulty in vision, lens has to be replaced.
- The central artery of retina is an end-artery. Blockage of the artery leads to sudden blindness.
- Left third nerve paralysis causes partial ptosis and dilated pupil. The cornea is turned downwards and outwards (Fig. 27.14).
- Horner's syndrome results in partial ptosis and miosis (Fig. 27.15).
- In brainstem death, both the pupils are dilated and fixed (Fig. 27.16).
- Eye sees everyone. One can see the interior of the eye by ophthalmoscope. Through the ophthalmoscope, one can see the small vessels in the retina and judge the changes in diabetes and hypertension (Figs 27.17a and b). In addition, one can also examine the optic disc for evidence of papilloedema, caused by raised intracranial pressure.

VITREOUS BODY

It is a colourless, jelly-like transparent mass which fills the posterior segment (posterior four-fifths) of the eyeball. It is enclosed in a delicate homogeneous *hyaloid membrane*. Behind, it is attached to the optic disc, and in front to the ora serrata; in between it is free and lies in contact with the retina. The anterior surface of the

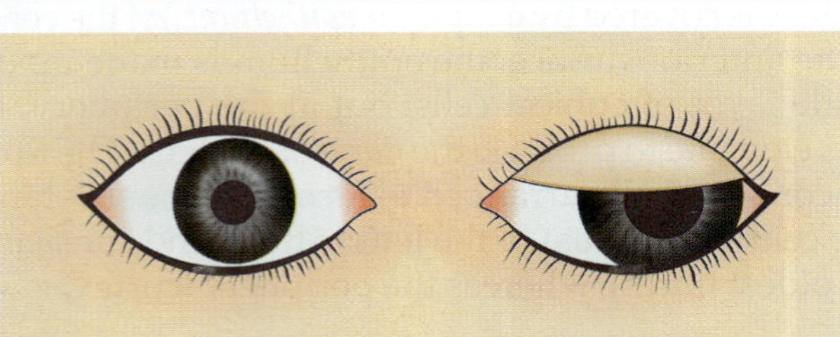

Fig. 27.14: Left third nerve paralysis

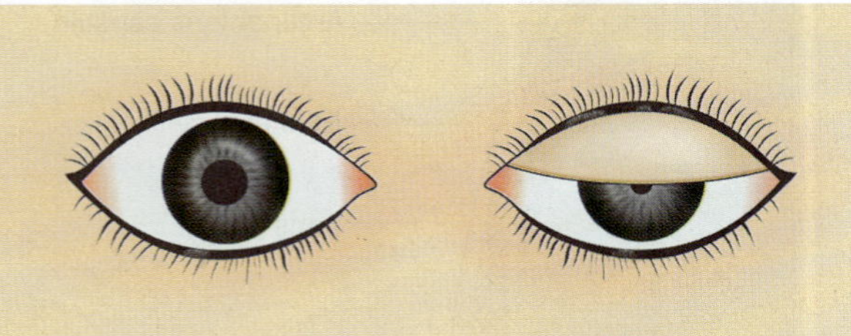

Fig. 27.15: Horner's syndrome in left eye

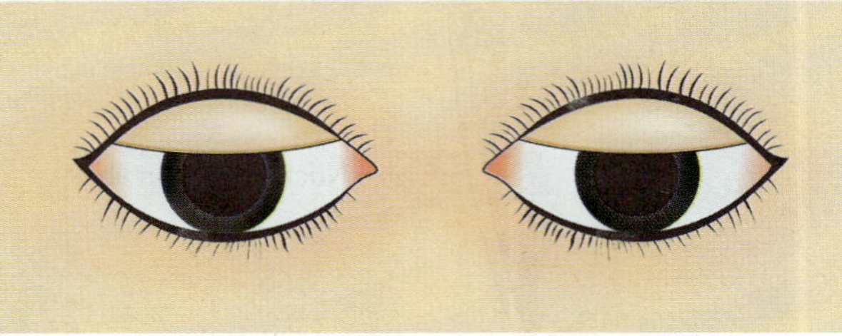

Fig. 27.16: Brainstem death

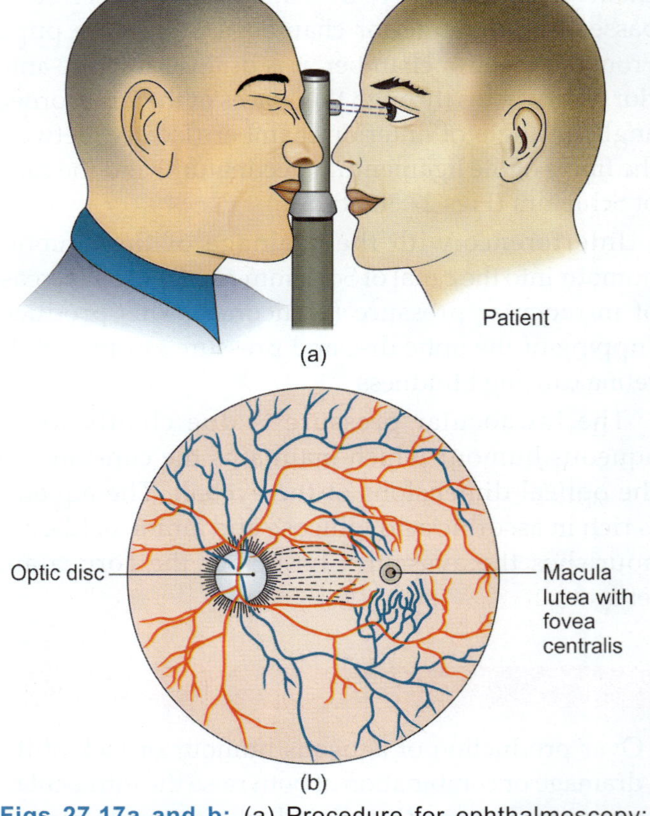

Figs 27.17a and b: (a) Procedure for ophthalmoscopy; (b) Retina as seen by ophthalmoscope

vitreous body is indented by the lens and ciliary processes (Fig. 27.1).

DEVELOPMENT

Optic vesicle forms optic cup. It is an outpouching from the *forebrain* vesicle.

Lens from *lens placode (ectodermal)*

Retina—pigment layer from the *outer layer of optic cup;* nervous layers from the *inner layer of optic cup.*

Choroid, sclera—*mesoderm*

Cornea—*surface ectoderm forms the epithelium, other layers develop from mesoderm.*

Molecular Regulation

The proteins WNT, BMP, TGF-β and FGF (fibroblast growth factor) are responsible for optic vesicle and PAX6 for lens vesicle differentiation.

Inhibition of sonic hedgehog (SHH) and expansion of PAX2 expression causes failure of separation of eyes resulting in cyclops. Overexpression of SHH causes loss of eye structures.

Vitamin A deficiency during embryonic development can result in anterior segment defects (of cornea and eyelid).

FACTS TO REMEMBER

- Cornea is used for grafting or transplantation.
- Sclera is pierced by number of structures including the optic nerve.
- Choroid contains big capillaries. These nourish the layer of rods and cones of retina by diffusion.
- Ciliary body contains ciliary muscles supplied by short ciliary nerves. These contract to relax the suspensory ligament of lens, so that the anterior surface of lens can become more convex for accommodation.
- Iris contains a weak dilator pupillae at the periphery, supplied by sympathetic fibres. It also contains a strong constrictor or sphincter pupillae near the pupillary margin. This is supplied by parasympathetic fibres relayed through ciliary ganglion.
- Central artery of retina is an 'end artery'
- Through dilated pupil, one can see the state of blood vessels of the retina.

CLINICOANATOMICAL PROBLEM

A patient was diagnosed as a case of 'retinal detachment'.

- Is retinal detachment, detachment of retina from the choroid?
- Name the layers of retina with its blood supply.

Ans: The retinal detachment is actually an inter-retinal detachment. The outer pigmented layer stays with choroid, while the inner nine layers get detached and cause the problem. The outer layer is developed from the outer layer of optic cup whereas the inner layers arise from the inner layer of optic cup. The blood supply of the outer five layers is from choroidal arteries whereas those of the inner nervous layers is by the 'central artery of retina', which is an absolute end-artery. The layers of retina (Fig. 27.10) are:

1. Outer pigmented layer
2. Layer of rods and cones
3. External limiting membrane
4. Outer nuclear layer
5. Outer plexiform layer
6. Bipolar cell layer
7. Inner plexiform layer
8. Ganglionic cell layer
9. Layer of optic nerve fibres
10. Inner limiting membrane

FURTHER READING

- O'Rahilly R. The timing and sequence of events in the development of the human eye and ear during the embryonic period proper. Anat Embryol Berl 1983;168:87–99.

  This paper presents the stages of human ear development.
- Kolb H, Linberg KA, Fisher SK. Neurons of the human retina—a Golgi study. J Comp Neurol 1992;318:147–87.

  The most comprehensive description of the morphology of neural cell types in the human retina.
- Tabinda Hasan, Satyam Khare, Shilpi Jain, Puneet Gupta, Sanjay Sharma. Retinal Vasculature—an imaging based morphological study. Journal of the Anatomical Society of India, 2013;62:146–56.

Frequently Asked Questions

1. Write short notes/enumerate:
   a. Cornea
   b. Choroid
   c. Structures piercing the sclera
   d. Layers of retina
   e. Ciliary muscles
   f. Lens
   g. Aqueous humour

Multiple Choice Questions

1. Which of the following muscles does not develop from mesoderm?
   a. Muscles of heart
   b. Muscles of iris
   c. Deltoid
   d. Superior rectus
2. Which of the following nerves supplies the cornea?
   a. Supraorbital
   b. Nasociliary
   c. Lacrimal
   d. Infraorbital
3. Parasympathetic fibres supply all the following muscles, *except:*
   a. Constrictor pupillae
   b. Dilator pupillae
   c. Radial fibres of ciliaris muscle
   d. Circular fibres of ciliaris muscle
4. Retina consists which of the following number of layers?
   a. Eight
   b. Ten
   c. Nine
   d. Eleven
5. One of the following symptoms is not seen in Horner's syndrome:
   a. Partial ptosis
   b. Miosis
   c. Anhydrosis
   d. Exophthalmos

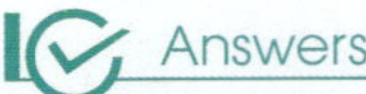

Answers

1. b **2.** b **3.** b **4.** b **5.** d

VIVA VOCE

- Name the layers of the eyeball.
- Enumerate the structures piercing the sclera.
- Name the histological layers of the cornea.
- What is myopia? How is it corrected?
- Name the muscles present in the ciliary body.
- What is the action and nerve supply of ciliary muscles?
- Name the muscles present in the iris. Which nerves supply these muscles?
- What are the layers of retina?
- Why is optic disc called the 'blind spot'?
- Trace the secretion, circulation and absorption of aqueous humour.
- What are the results of Horner's syndrome?
- How does lens develop?
- How does retina develop?
- How does cornea develop?
- Where does retinal detachment occur?
- Why do cataract and glaucoma develop?

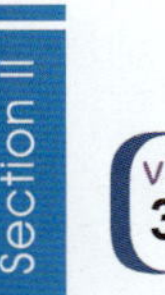

Eyeball

Chapter 28

Surface Marking and Radiological Anatomy

"Prayer does not change God, it changes us."
—B. Graham

INTRODUCTION

The bony and soft tissue landmarks on the head, face and neck help in surface marking of various structures. These landmarks are of immense value to the clinician for locating the part to be examined or to be operated.

SURFACE LANDMARKS

LANDMARKS ON THE FACE

Some important named features to be identified on the living face have been described in Chapter 10. Other landmarks are as follows.

1 The *supraorbital margin* lies beneath the upper margin of the eyebrow. The *supraorbital notch* (Fig. 28.1) is palpable at the junction of the medial one-third with the lateral two-thirds of the supraorbital margin (except in those cases in which the notch is converted into a foramen). A vertical line drawn from the supraorbital notch to the base of the mandible, passing midway between the lower two premolar teeth, crosses the infraorbital foramen 5 mm below the infraorbital margin, and the mental foramen midway between the upper and lower borders of the mandible (Fig. 28.1).

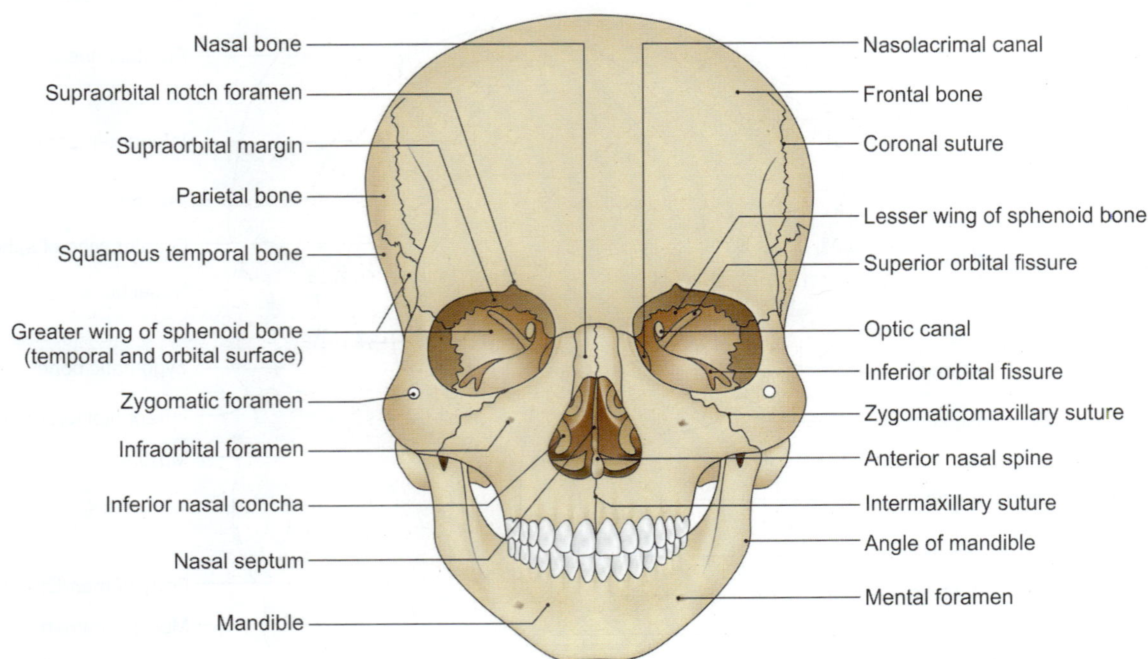

Fig. 28.1: Foramina in norma frontalis

2 The *superciliary arch* is a curved bony ridge situated immediately above the medial part of each supraorbital margin. The *glabella* is the median elevation connecting the two superciliary arches and corresponds to the elevation between the two eyebrows.
3 The *nasion* is the point where the internasal and frontonasal sutures meet. It lies a little above the floor of the depression at the root of the nose, below the glabella (Fig. 28.1).

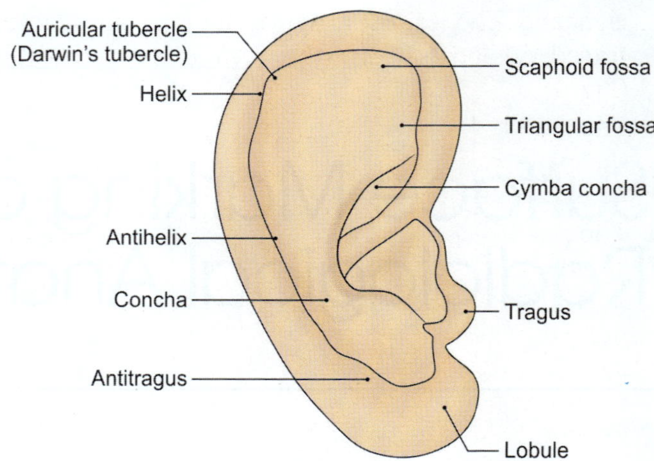

Fig. 28.2: Named features on the pinna

LANDMARKS ON THE LATERAL SIDE OF THE HEAD

The external ear or pinna is a prominent feature on the lateral aspect of the head. The named features on the pinna are shown in Fig. 28.2. Other landmarks on the lateral side of the head are as follows.

1 The *zygomatic bone* forms the prominence of the cheek at the inferolateral corner of the orbit. The *zygomatic arch* bridges the gap between the eye and the ear. It is formed anteriorly by the temporal process of the zygomatic bone, and posteriorly by the zygomatic process (zygoma) of the temporal bone. The *preauricular point* lies on the posterior root of the zygoma immediately in front of the upper part of the tragus (Fig. 28.3).
2 The head of the mandible lies in front of the tragus. It is felt best during movements of the lower jaw. The *coronoid process* of the mandible can be felt below the lowest part of the zygomatic bone when the mouth is opened. The process can be traced downwards into the anterior border of the *ramus* of the mandible. The posterior border of the ramus, though masked by parotid gland, can be felt through the skin. The outer surface of the ramus is covered by the masseter which can be felt when the teeth are

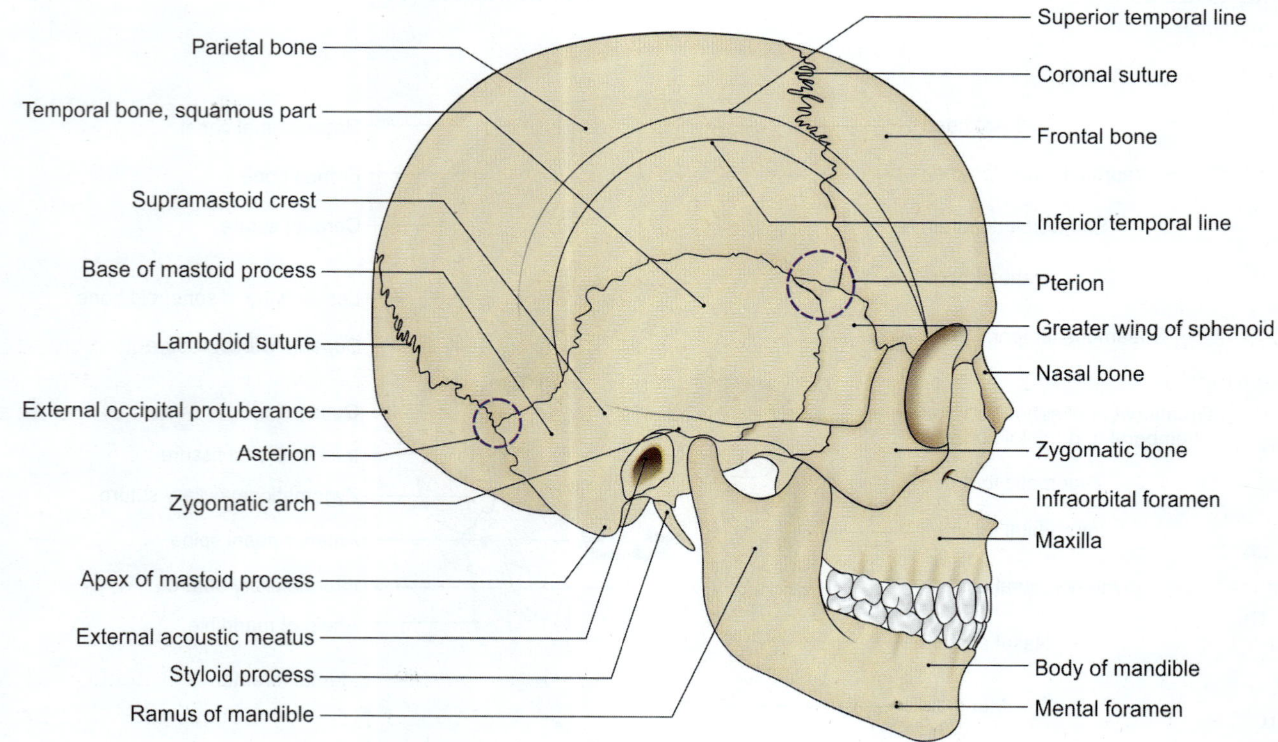

Fig. 28.3: Parts of mandible seen in norma lateralis

clenched. The lower border of the mandible can be traced posteriorly into the *angle* of the mandible (Fig. 28.3).

3 The *parietal eminence* is the most prominent part of the parietal bone, situated far above and a little behind the auricle.

4 The *mastoid process* is a large bony prominence situated behind the lower part of the auricle. The *supramastoid crest*, about 2.5 cm long, begins immediately above the external acoustic meatus and soon curves upwards and backwards. The crest is continuous anteriorly with the posterior root of the zygoma, and posterosuperiorly with the temporal line (Fig. 28.3).

5 The inferior *temporal line* forms the upper boundary of the temporal fossa which is filled up by the temporalis muscle. The upper margin of the contracting temporalis helps in defining this line which begins at the zygomatic process of the frontal bone, arches posterosuperiorly across the coronal suture, passes a little below the parietal eminence, and turns downwards to become continuous with the supramastoid crest. The area of the temporal fossa on the side of the head, above the zygomatic arch, is called the *temple* or temporal region.

6 The *pterion* is the area in the temporal fossa where four bones (frontal, parietal, temporal and sphenoid) adjoin each other across an H-shaped suture. The centre of the pterion is marked by a point 4 cm above the midpoint of the zygomatic arch, falling 3.5 cm behind the frontozygomatic suture. Deep to the pterion lie the anterior branch of the middle meningeal artery, the middle meningeal vein, and deeper still the stem of the lateral sulcus of the cerebral hemisphere (at the *Sylvian point*) dividing into three rami. The pterion is a common site for trephining (making a hole in the skull) during operation (Fig. 28.4). Surface marking of middle meningeal artery is given later.

7 The junction of the back of the head with the neck is indicated by the external occipital protuberance and the superior nuchal lines. The *external occipital protuberance* is a bony projection felt in the median plane on the back of the head at the upper end of the nuchal furrow. The *superior nuchal lines* are indistinct curved ridges which extend from the protuberance to the mastoid processes. The back of the head is called the *occiput*. The most prominent median point situated on the external occipital protuberance is known as the *inion*. However, the posterior most point on the occiput lies a little above the protuberance (Fig. 28.5).

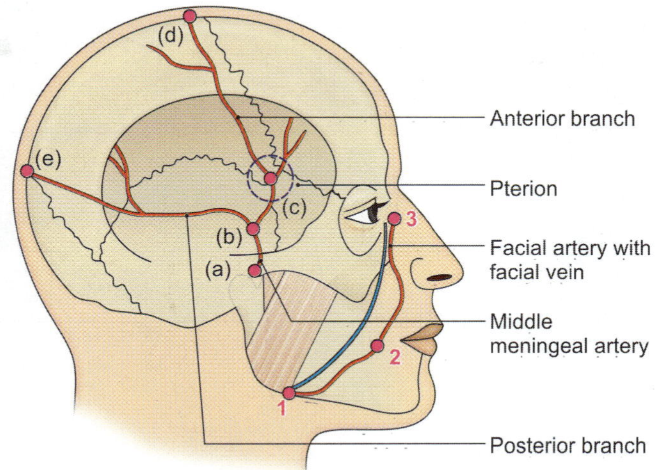

Fig. 28.4: Middle meningeal artery (a–e) and facial artery (1–3) with facial vein

LANDMARKS ON THE SIDE OF THE NECK

1 The *sternocleidomastoid muscle* is seen prominently when the face is turned to the opposite side. The ridge raised by the muscle extends from the sternum to the mastoid process (Fig. 28.6).

2 The *external jugular vein* crosses the sternocleidomastoid obliquely, running downwards and backwards from near the auricle to the clavicle. It is better seen in old age (Fig. 28.7).

3 The *greater supraclavicular fossa* lies above and behind the middle one-third of the clavicle. It overlies the cervical part of the brachial plexus and the third part of the subclavian artery (Fig. 28.6).

4 The *lesser supraclavicular fossa* is a small depression between the sternal and clavicular parts of the sternocleidomastoid. It overlies the internal jugular vein.

5 The *mastoid process* is a large bony projection behind the auricle (concha) (Fig. 28.6).

6 The *transverse process of the atlas vertebra* can be felt on deep pressure midway between the angle of the mandible and the mastoid process, immediately anteroinferior to the tip of the mastoid process. The *fourth cervical transverse process* is just palpable at the level of the upper border of the thyroid cartilage; and the *sixth cervical transverse process* at the level of the cricoid cartilage. The anterior tubercle of the *transverse process of the sixth cervical vertebra* is the largest of all such processes and is called the *carotid tubercle* (of Chassaignac). The common carotid artery can be best pressed against this tubercle, deep to the anterior border of the sternocleidomastoid muscle.

7 The *anterior border of the trapezius muscle* becomes prominent on elevation of the shoulder against resistance (Fig. 28.6).

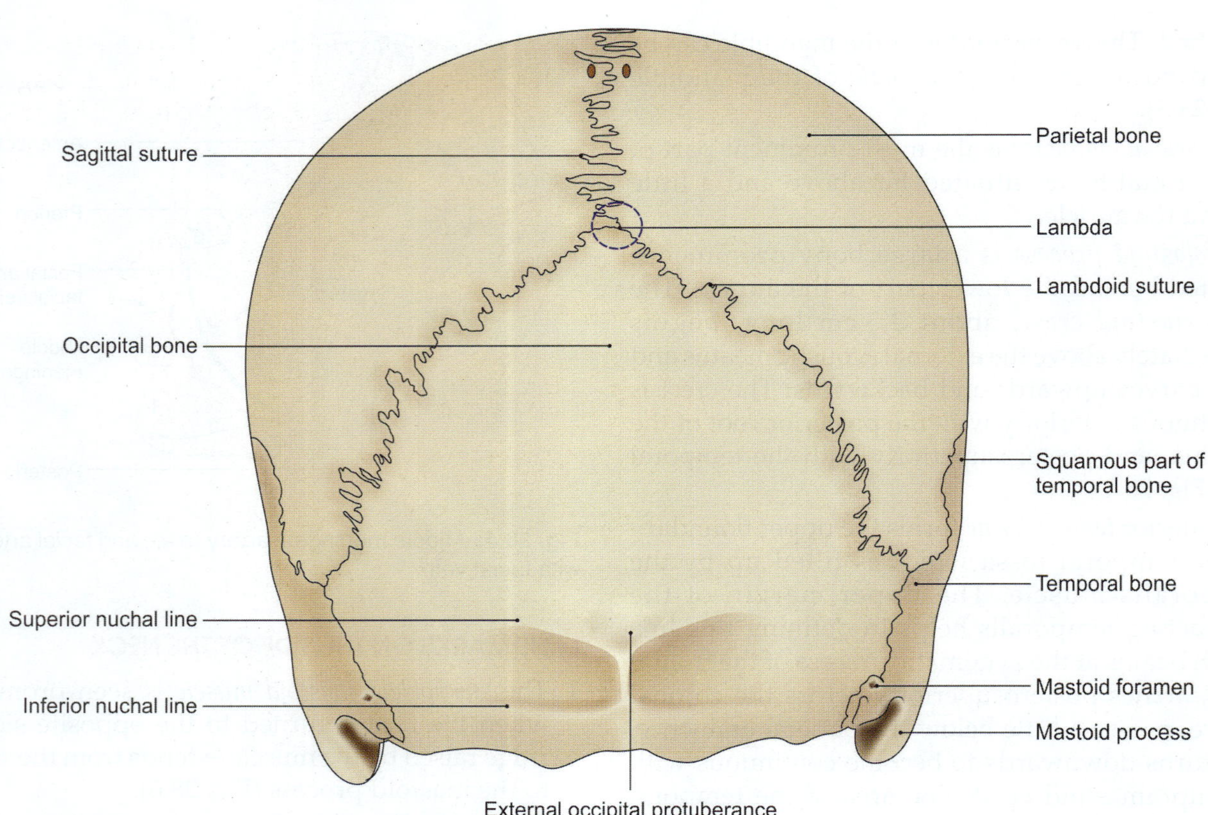

Fig. 28.5: Structures felt in norma occipitalis

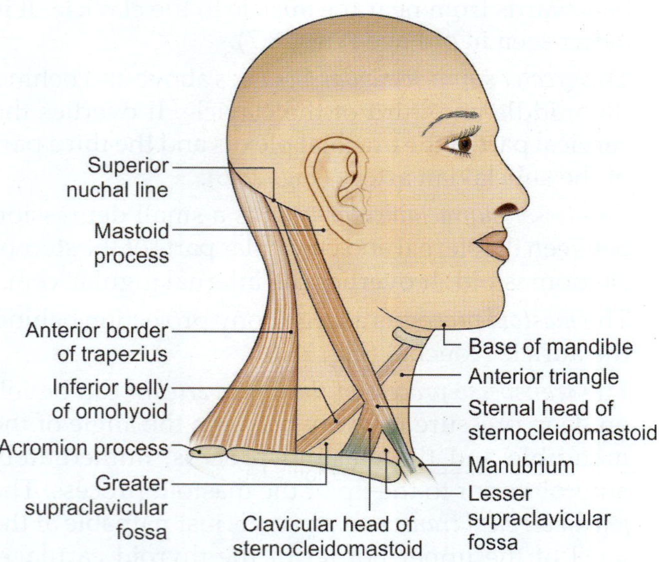

Fig. 28.6: Muscles: Sternocleidomastoid, trapezius and inferior belly of omohyoid

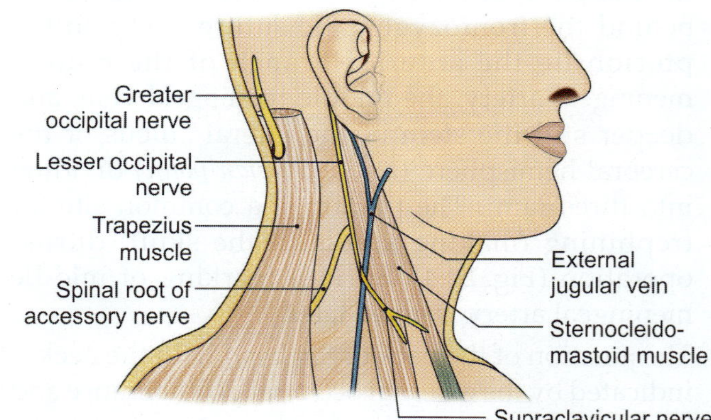

Fig. 28.7: External jugular vein and cutaneous nerves

LANDMARKS ON THE ANTERIOR ASPECT OF THE NECK

1 The *mandible* forms the lower jaw. The lower border of its horseshoe-shaped body is known as the *base of the mandible* (Fig. 28.8). Anteriorly, this base forms the *chin*, and posteriorly it can be traced to the *angle of the mandible*. Numerous structures are attached to mandible.

2 The body of the U-shaped *hyoid bone* can be felt in the median plane just below and behind the chin, at the junction of the neck with the floor of the mouth. On each side, the body of hyoid bone is continuous posteriorly with the *greater cornua* which is overlapped in its posterior part by the sternocleidomastoid muscle (Fig. 28.9).

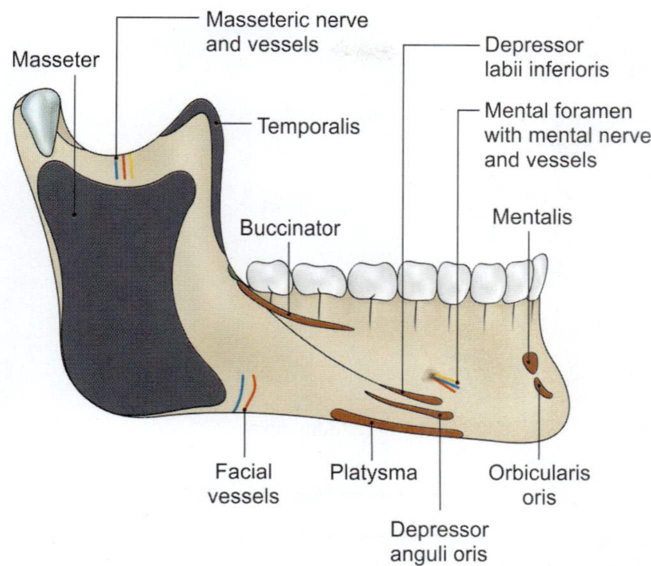

Fig. 28.8: Attachments on the mandible

3 The *thyroid cartilage* of the larynx forms a sharp protuberance in the median plane just below the hyoid bone. This protuberance is called the *laryngeal prominence or Adam's apple.* It is more prominent in males than in females (Fig. 28.10).
4 The rounded arch of the *cricoid cartilage* lies below the thyroid cartilage at the upper end of the trachea (Fig. 28.10).
5 The trachea runs downwards and backwards from the cricoid cartilage. It is identified by its cartilaginous rings. However, it is partially masked by the *isthmus of the thyroid gland* which lies against the second to fourth tracheal rings. The trachea is commonly palpated in the *suprasternal notch* which lies between the tendinous heads of origin of the right and left sternocleidomastoid muscles. In certain diseases, the trachea may shift to one side from the median plane. This indicates a shift in the mediastinum (Fig. 28.10).

OTHER IMPORTANT LANDMARKS

1 The *frontozygomatic suture* can be felt as a slight depression in the upper part of the lateral orbital margin.
2 The *marginal tubercle* lies a short distance below the frontozygomatic suture along the posterior border of the frontal process of the zygomatic bone.
3 The *Frankfurt's plane* is represented by a horizontal line joining the infraorbital margin to the centre of the external acoustic meatus. Posteriorly, the line passes through a point just below the external occipital protuberance (*see* Fig. 9.1).
4 The *jugal point* is the anterior end of the upper border of the zygomatic arch where it meets the frontal process of the zygomatic bone.
5 The *mandibular notch* is represented by a curved line concave upwards, extending from the head of the mandible to the anterior end of the zygomatic arch. The notch is 1–2 cm deep (Fig. 28.8).

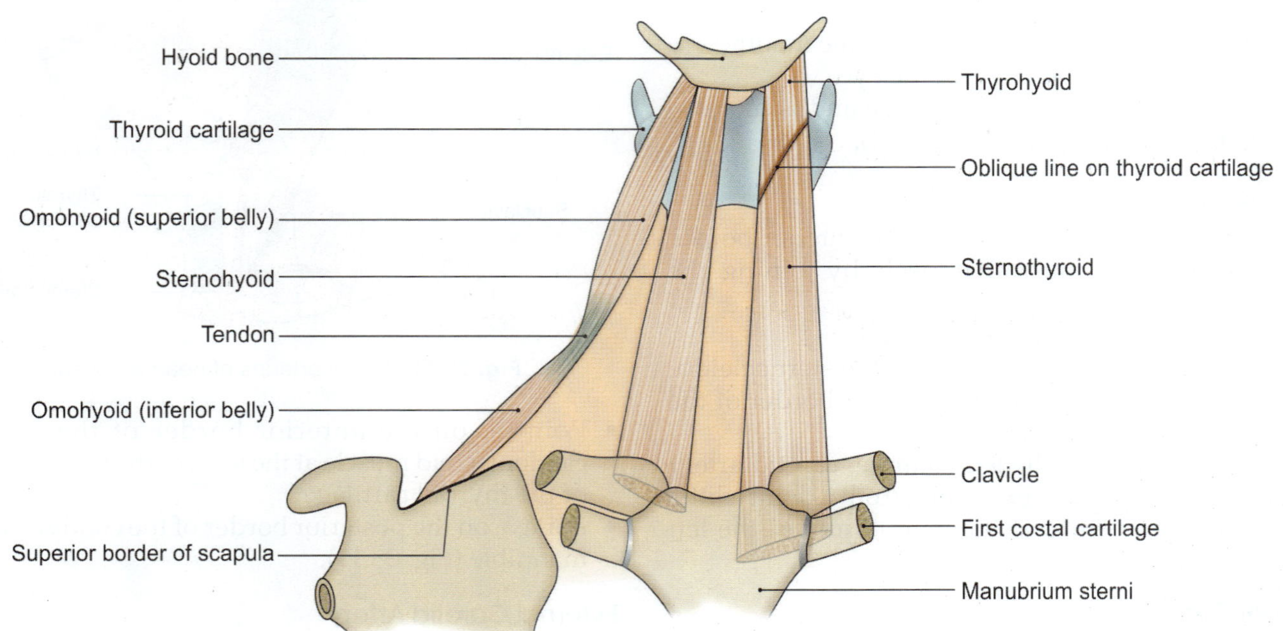

Fig. 28.9: Attachments on hyoid bone and thyroid cartilage

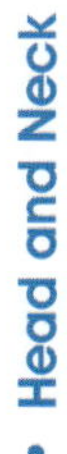

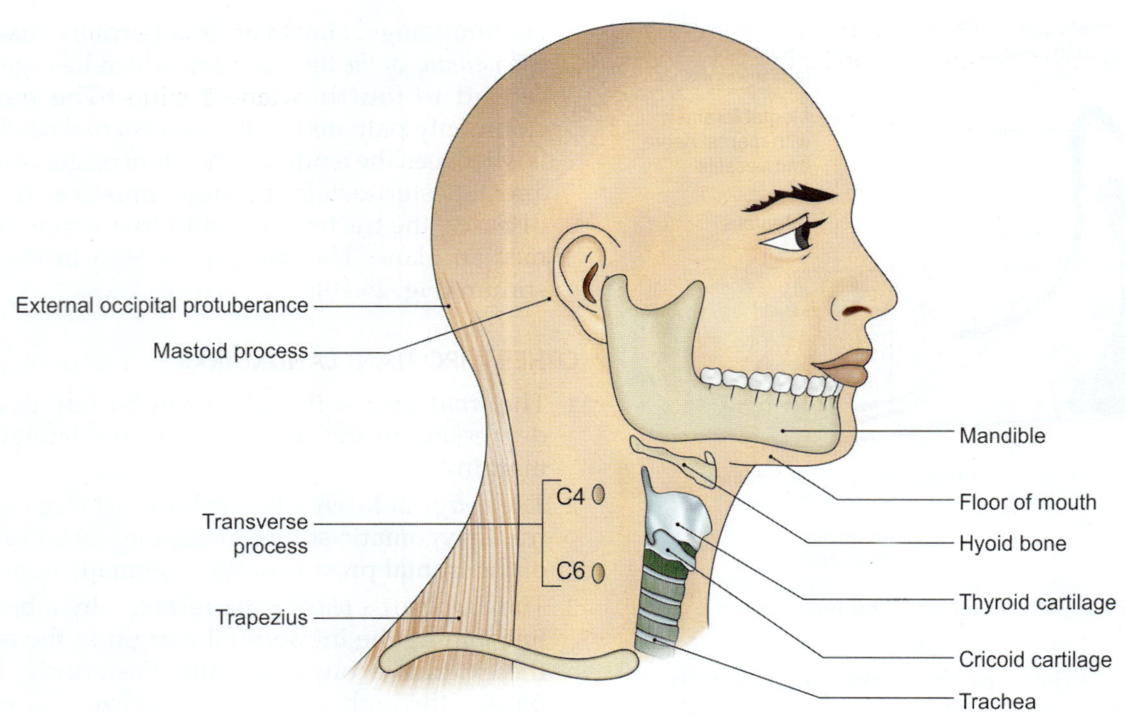

Fig. 28.10: Landmarks on anterior aspect of neck

SURFACE MARKING OF VARIOUS STRUCTURES

ARTERIES

Facial Artery

It is marked on the face by joining these three points (Fig. 28.4).

- Point 1, on the base of the mandible at the anterior border of the masseter muscle.
- Point 2, 1.2 cm lateral to the angle of the mouth.
- Point 3, at the medial angle of the eye.

The artery is tortuous in its course and is more so between the first two points (Fig. 28.4).

Common Carotid Artery

It is marked by a broadline along the anterior border of the sternocleidomastoid muscle by joining the following two points (Fig. 28.11).

- Point 1, on the sternoclavicular joint.
- Point 2, on the anterior border of the sternocleidomastoid muscle at the level of upper border of the thyroid cartilage (Fig. 28.11).

The thoracic part of the left common carotid artery is marked by a broadline extending from a point a little to the left of the centre of the manubrium to the left sternoclavicular joint.

Internal Carotid Artery

It is marked by a broadline joining these two points (Fig. 28.11).

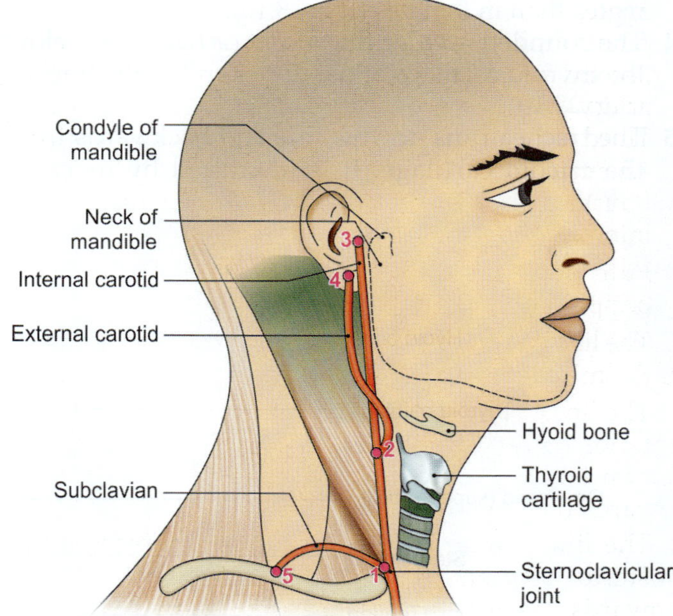

Fig. 28.11: Some arteries of head and neck

- Point 2, on the anterior border of the sternocleidomastoid muscle at the level of the upper border of the thyroid cartilage.
- Point 3, on the posterior border of the condyle of the mandible (Fig. 28.11).

External Carotid Artery

The artery is marked by joining these two points (Fig. 28.11).

- Point 2, on the anterior border of the sternocleidomastoid muscle at the level of the upper border of the thyroid cartilage.
- Point 4, on the posterior border of the neck of the mandible.

The artery is slightly convex forwards in its lower half and slightly concave forwards in its upper half (Fig. 28.11).

Subclavian Artery

It is marked by a broad curved line, convex upwards, by joining these two points (Fig. 28.11).

- Point 1, on the sternoclavicular joint.
- Point 5, at the middle of the lower border of the clavicle (Fig. 28.11).

The artery rises about 2 cm above the clavicle.

The thoracic part of the left subclavian artery is marked by a broad vertical line along the left border of the manubrium a little to the left of the left common carotid artery.

Middle Meningeal Artery

It is marked by joining these points.

- First point (a), immediately above the middle of the zygoma. The artery enters the skull opposite this point (Fig. 28.4).
- Second point (b), 2 cm above the first point. The artery divides deep to this point.
- Third point (c) (centre of pterion), 3.5 cm behind and 1.5 cm above the frontozygomatic suture.
- Fourth point (d), midway between the nasion and inion.
- Fifth point (e) (lambda), 6 cm above the external occipital protuberance.

The line joining points (a) and (b) represents the stem of the middle meningeal artery inside the skull.

The line joining points (b), (c) and (d) represents the anterior (frontal) branch. It first runs upwards and forwards (b), (c) and then upwards and backwards, towards the point (d).

The line joining points (b) and (e) represents the posterior (parietal) branch. It runs backwards and upwards, towards the point (e) (Fig. 28.4).

VEINS/SINUSES

Facial Vein

It is represented by a line drawn just behind the facial artery (Fig. 28.4).

External Jugular Vein

The vein is usually visible through the skin and can be made more prominent by blowing with the mouth and nostrils closed (Fig. 28.12).

It can be marked, if not visible, by joining these points (Fig. 28.12).

- Point 1, a little below and behind the angle of the mandible.
- Point 2, on the clavicle just lateral to the posterior border of the sternocleidomastoid (Fig. 28.12).

Internal Jugular Vein

Internal jugular vein is marked by a broadline by joining these two points (Fig. 28.12).

- Point 3, on the neck medial to the lobule of the ear.
- Point 4, at the medial end of the clavicle (Fig. 28.12).

The lower bulb of the vein lies beneath the lesser supraclavicular fossa between the sternal and clavicular heads of the sternocleidomastoid muscle.

Subclavian Vein

Subclavian vein is represented by a broadline along the clavicle extending from a little medial to its midpoint to the medial end of the bone.

Superior Sagittal Sinus

Superior sagittal sinus is marked by two lines (diverging posteriorly) joining these two points (Fig. 28.13).

- One point (1), at the glabella.
- Two points (2), at the inion, situated side by side, 1.2 cm apart (Fig. 28.13).

Transverse Sinus

Transverse sinus is marked by two parallel lines, 1.2 cm apart extending between the following points (Fig. 28.13).

- Two points (2), at the inion, situated one above the other and 1.2 cm apart.

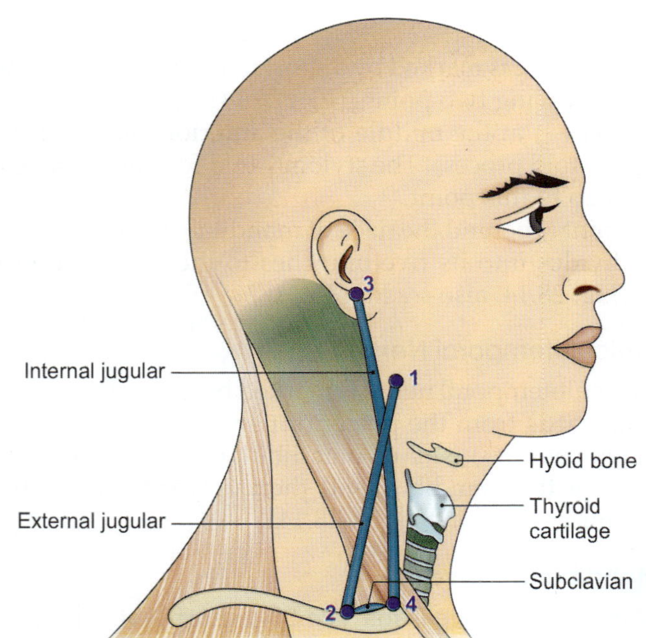

Fig. 28.12: Internal and external jugular veins

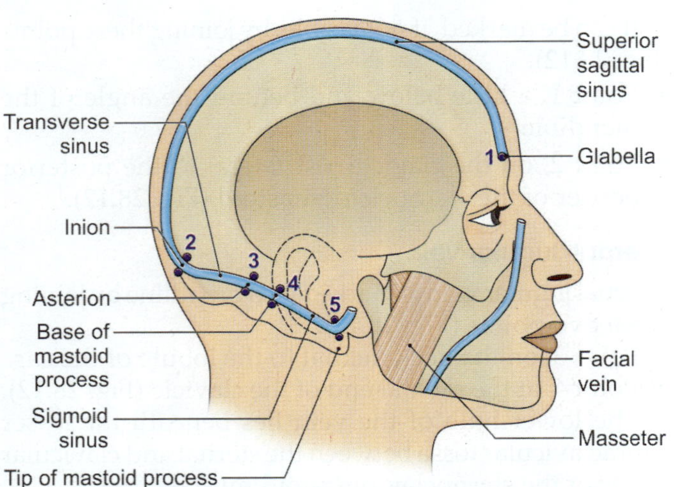

Fig. 28.13: Superior sagittal, transverse and sigmoid sinuses

- Two points (3), at asterion 3.75 cm behind external auditory meatus and 1.25 cm above this point (Fig. 28.13).
- Two points (4), at the base of the mastoid process, situated one in front of the other and 1.2 cm apart.

Sigmoid Sinus

Sigmoid sinus is marked by two parallel lines situated 1.2 cm apart and extending between the following two points (Fig. 28.13):

- Two points (4), at the base of the mastoid process, situated one in front of the other and 1.2 cm apart.
- Two similar points (5), near the posterior border and 1.2 cm above the tip of mastoid process.

NERVES

Facial Nerve

Facial nerve is marked by a short horizontal line joining the following two points (Fig. 28.14).

- Point 1, at the middle of the anterior border of the mastoid process. The stylomastoid foramen lies 2 cm deep to this point.
- Point 2, behind the neck of mandible. Here the nerve divides into its five branches to the facial muscles (Fig. 28.14, also *see* Fig. 13.3).

Auriculotemporal Nerve

Auriculotemporal nerve is marked by a line drawn first backwards from the posterior part of the mandibular notch (point 3) (site of mandibular nerve) across the neck of the mandible, and then upwards across the preauricular point 4 (Fig. 28.14).

Mandibular Nerve

Mandibular nerve is marked by a short vertical line in the posterior part of the mandibular notch just in front of the head of the mandible.

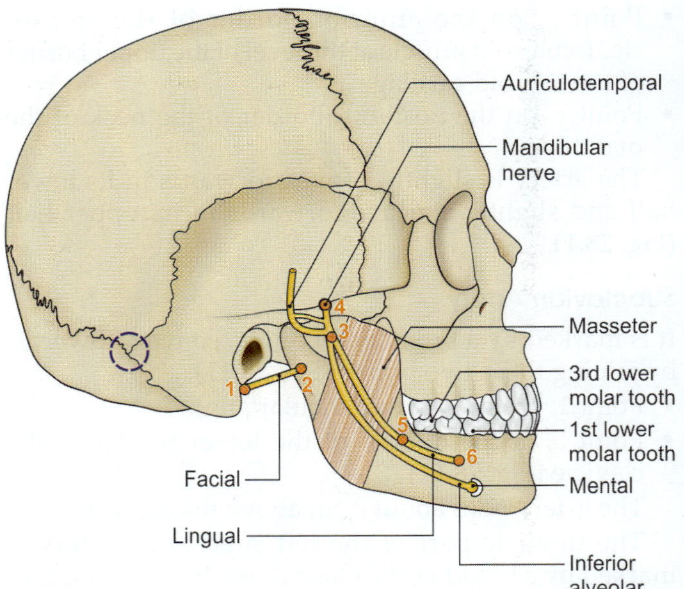

Fig. 28.14: Position of facial and some branches of mandibular nerves

Lingual and Inferior Alveolar Nerves

Lingual nerve is marked by a curved line running downwards and forwards by joining these points (Fig. 28.14).

- Point 3, on the posterior part of the mandibular notch, in line with the mandibular nerve.
- Point 5, a little below and behind the last lower molar tooth.
- Point 6, opposite the first lower molar tooth.

The concavity in the course of the nerve is more marked between the 5 and 6 points and is directed upwards.

Inferior alveolar nerve lies a little below and parallel to the lingual nerve.

Glossopharyngeal Nerve

Glossopharyngeal nerve is marked by joining the following points (Fig. 28.15).

- Point 1, on the anteroinferior part of the tragus.
- Point 2, anterosuperior to the angle of the mandible.

From 2nd point, the nerve runs forwards for a short distance above the lower border of the mandible. The nerve describes a gentle curve in its course (Fig. 28.15).

Vagus Nerve

The nerve runs along the medial side of the internal jugular vagus vein. It is marked by joining these two points (Fig. 28.15).

- Point 1, at the anteroinferior part of the tragus.
- Point 3, at the medial end of the clavicle (Fig. 28.15).

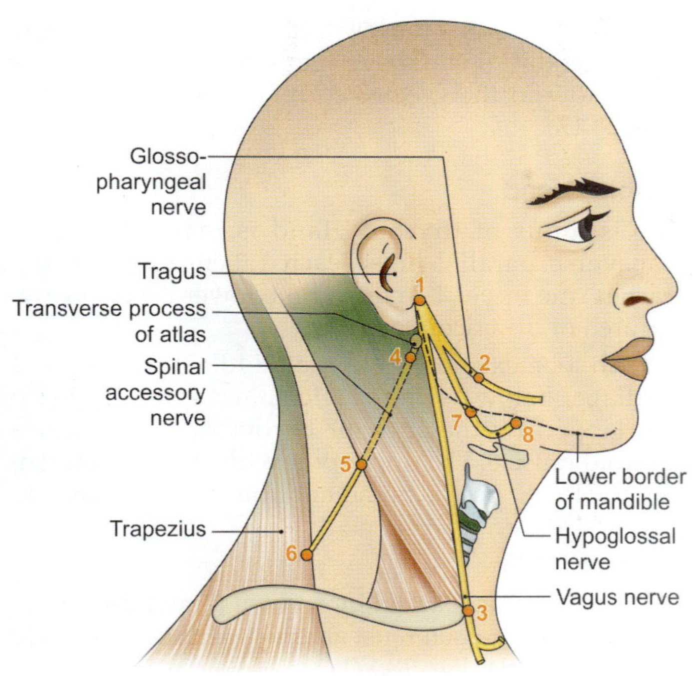

Fig. 28.15: Position of last four cranial nerves

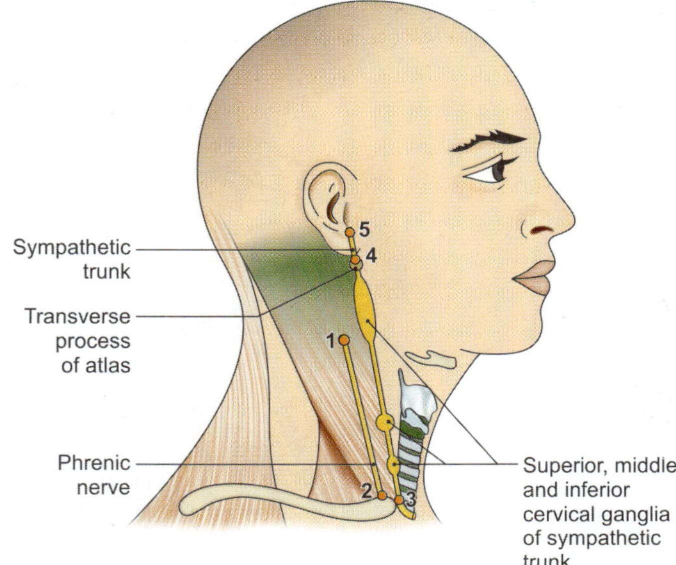

Fig. 28.16: Position of phrenic nerve and sympathetic trunk

Accessory Nerve (Spinal Part)

Accessory nerve (spinal part) is marked by joining the following four points (Fig. 28.15).

- Point 1, at the anteroinferior part of the tragus.
- Point 4, at the tip of the transverse process of the atlas.
- Point 5, at the middle of the posterior border of the sternocleidomastoid muscle.
- Point 6, on the anterior border of the trapezius 6 cm above the clavicle (Fig. 28.15).

Hypoglossal Nerve

Hypoglossal nerve is marked by joining these points (Fig. 28.15).

- Point 1, at the anteroinferior part of the tragus.
- Point 7, posterosuperior to the tip of the greater cornua of the hyoid bone.
- Point 8, midway between the angle of the mandible and the symphysis menti.

The nerve describes a gentle curve in its course (Fig. 28.15).

Phrenic Nerve

Phrenic nerve is marked by a line joining the following points (Fig. 28.16).

- Point 1, on the side of the neck at the level of the upper border of the thyroid cartilage and 3.5 cm from the median plane.
- Point 2, at the medial end of the clavicle (Fig. 28.16).

Cervical Sympathetic Chain

Cervical sympathetic chain is marked by a line joining the following points (Fig. 28.16).

- Point 3, at the sternoclavicular joint.
- Point 5, at the posterior border of the condyle of the mandible.

The *superior cervical ganglion* extends from the transverse process of the atlas (point 4) to the tip of the greater cornua of the hyoid bone. The *middle cervical ganglion* lies at the level of the cricoid cartilage, and the *inferior cervical ganglion*, at a point 3 cm above the sternoclavicular joint (Fig. 28.16).

Trigeminal Ganglion

Trigeminal ganglion lies a little in front of the preauricular point at a depth of about 4.5 cm.

GLANDS

Parotid Gland

Parotid gland is marked by joining these four points with each other (Fig. 28.17).

- The first point (a), at the upper border of the head of the mandible.
- The second point (b), just above the centre of the masseter muscle.
- The third point (c), posteroinferior to the angle of the mandible.
- The fourth point (d), on the upper part of the anterior border of the mastoid process.

The anterior border of the gland is obtained by joining the points (a), (b), (c); the posterior border, by joining the points (c), (d); and the superior curved border with its concavity directed upwards and

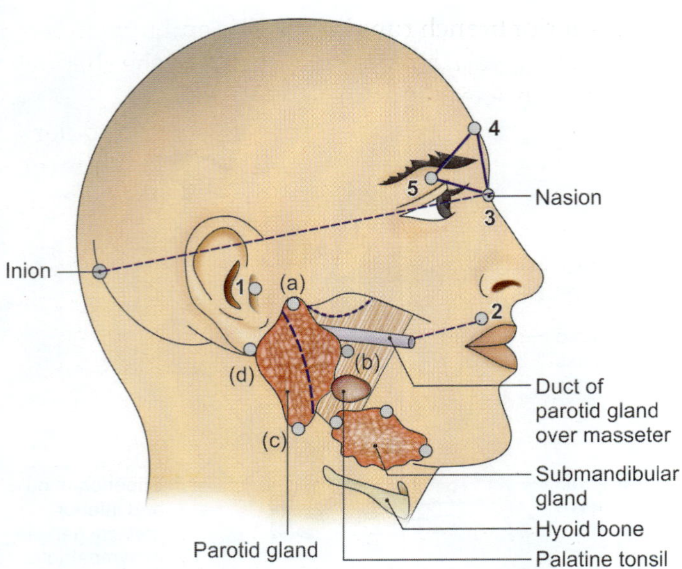

Fig. 28.17: Position of parotid gland with its duct, submandibular gland, palatine tonsil and frontal sinus

backwards, by joining the points (a), (d) across the lobule of the ear (Fig. 28.17).

Parotid Duct

To mark this duct, first draw a line joining these two points (Fig. 28.17).

- First point 1, at the lower border of the tragus.
- Second point 2, midway between the ala of the nose and the red margin of the upper lip.

The middle-third of this line represents the parotid duct (Fig. 28.17).

Submandibular Gland

The submandibular salivary gland is marked by an oval area over the posterior half of the base of the mandible, including the lower border of the ramus. The area extends 1.5 cm above the base of the mandible, and below to the greater cornua of the hyoid bone (Fig. 28.17).

Thyroid Gland

The isthmus of thyroid gland is marked by two transverse parallel lines (each 1.2 cm long) on the trachea, the upper 1.2 cm and the lower 2.5 cm below the arch of the cricoid cartilage.

Each lobe extends up to the middle of the thyroid cartilage, below to the clavicle, and laterally to be overlapped by the anterior border of sternocleidomastoid muscle. The upper pole of the lobe is pointed, and the lower pole is broad and rounded (Fig. 28.18).

Palatine Tonsil

Palatine tonsil is marked by an oval (almond-shaped) area over the masseter just anterosuperior to the angle of the mandible (Fig. 28.17).

PARANASAL SINUSES

Frontal Sinus

Frontal sinus is marked by a triangular area formed by joining these three points (Fig. 28.17).

- The point 3, at the nasion.
- The point 4, 2.5 cm above the nasion.
- The point 5, at the junction of medial one-third and lateral two-thirds of the supraorbital margin, i.e. at the supraorbital notch.

Maxillary Sinus

The roof of maxillary sinus is represented by the inferior orbital margin; the floor, by the alveolus of the maxilla; the base, by the lateral wall of the nose. The apex lies on the zygomatic process of the maxilla.

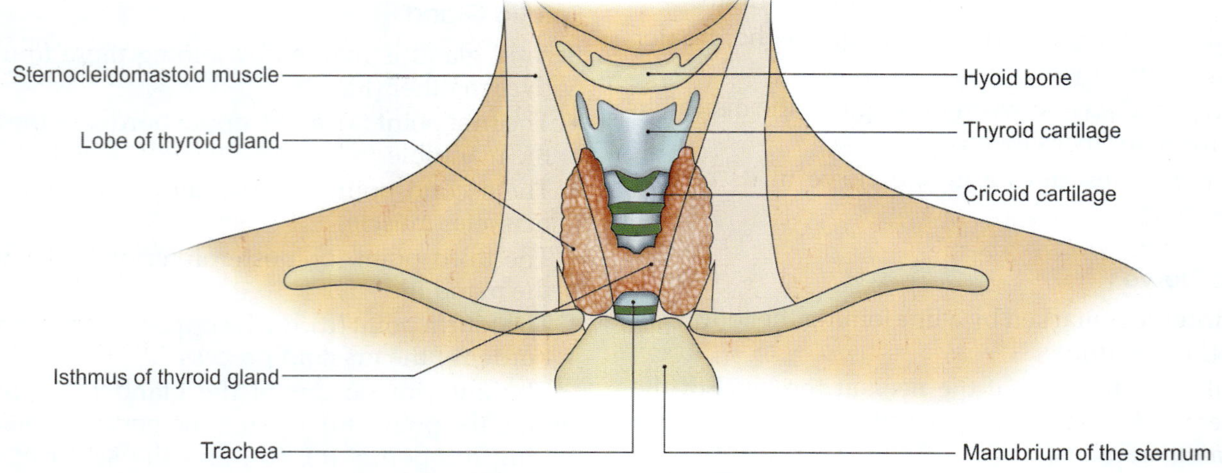

Fig. 28.18: Thyroid gland

RADIOLOGICAL ANATOMY

In routine clinical practice, the following X-ray pictures of the skull are commonly used.

1 Lateral view for general survey of the skull including cervical vertebrae.
2 A special posteroanterior view (in Water's position) to study the paranasal sinuses.

LATERAL VIEW OF SKULL (PLAIN SKIAGRAM)

The radiogram is studied systematically as described here.

Cranial Vault

1 *Shape and size:* It is important to be familiar with the normal shape and size of the skull so that abnormalities, like oxycephaly (a type of craniostenosis), hydrocephalus, microcephaly, etc. may be diagnosed.

2 *Structure of cranial bones:* The bones are unilamellar during the first three years of life. Two tables separated by diploe appear during the fourth year, and the differentiation reaches its maximum by about 35 years when diploic veins produce characteristic markings in radiograms. The sites of the external occipital protuberance and frontal bone are normally thicker than the rest of the skull. The squamous temporal and the upper part of the occipital bone are thin.
Generalized thickened bones are found in Paget's disease. Thalassaemia, a congenital haemolytic anaemia, is associated with thickening and a characteristic sunray appearance of the skull bones. A localised hyperostosis may be seen over a meningioma. In multiple myeloma and secondary carcinomatous deposits, the skull presents large punched out areas. Fractures are more extensive in the inner table than in the outer table.

3 *Sutures:* The coronal and lambdoid sutures are usually visible clearly. The coronal suture runs downwards and forwards in front of the central sulcus of the brain. The lambdoid suture traverses the posteriormost part of the skull.
Obliteration of sutures begins first on the inner surface (between 30 and 40 years) and then on the outer surface (between 40 and 50 years). Usually, the lower part of the coronal suture is obliterated first, followed by the posterior part of the sagittal suture. Premature closure of sutures occurs in craniostenosis, a hereditary disease. Sutures are opened up in children by an increase in intracranial pressure.

4 *Vascular markings*
   a. *Middle meningeal vessels:* The anterior branch runs about 1 cm behind the coronal suture. The posterior branch runs backwards and upwards at a lower level across the upper part of the shadow of the auricle.
   b. The *transverse sinus* may be seen as a curved dark shadow, convex upwards, extending from the internal occipital protuberance to the petrous temporal.
   c. The *diploic venous markings* are seen as irregularly anastomosing, worm-like shadows produced by the frontal, anterior temporal, posterior temporal and occipital diploic veins. These markings become more prominent in raised intracranial pressure.

5 *Cerebral moulding,* indicating normal impressions of cerebral gyri, can be seen. In raised intracranial tension, the impressions become more pronounced and produce a characteristic *silver beaten* (or *copper beaten) appearance* of the skull.

6 *Arachnoid granulations* may indent the parasagittal area of the skull to such an extent as to simulate erosion by a meningioma.

7 *Normal intracranial calcifications*
   a. Pineal concretions (brain sand) appear by the age of 17 years. The pineal body is located 2.5 cm above and 1.2 cm behind the external acoustic meatus. When visible it serves as an important radiological landmark.
   b. Other structures which may become calcified include the choroid plexuses, arachnoid granulations, falx cerebri, and other dural folds.

8 *The auricle:* The curved margin of the auricle is seen above the petrous temporal.

9 The *frontal sinus* produces a dark shadow in the anteroinferior part of the skull vault.

Base of Skull

1 The *floor of the anterior cranial fossa* slopes backwards and downwards. The shadows of the two sides are often seen situated one above the other. The surface is irregular due to gyral markings. It also forms the roof of the orbit (Fig. 28.19).

2 The *hypophyseal fossa* represents the middle cranial fossa in this view. It is overhung anteriorly by the anterior clinoid process (directed posteriorly), and posteriorly by the posterior clinoid process. It measures 8 mm vertically and 14 mm anteroposteriorly. The interclinoid distance is not more than 4 mm. The fossa is enlarged in cases of pituitary tumours, arising particularly from acidophil or chromophobe cells.

3 The *sphenoidal air sinus* lies anteroinferior to the hypophyseal fossa. The shadows of the orbit, the

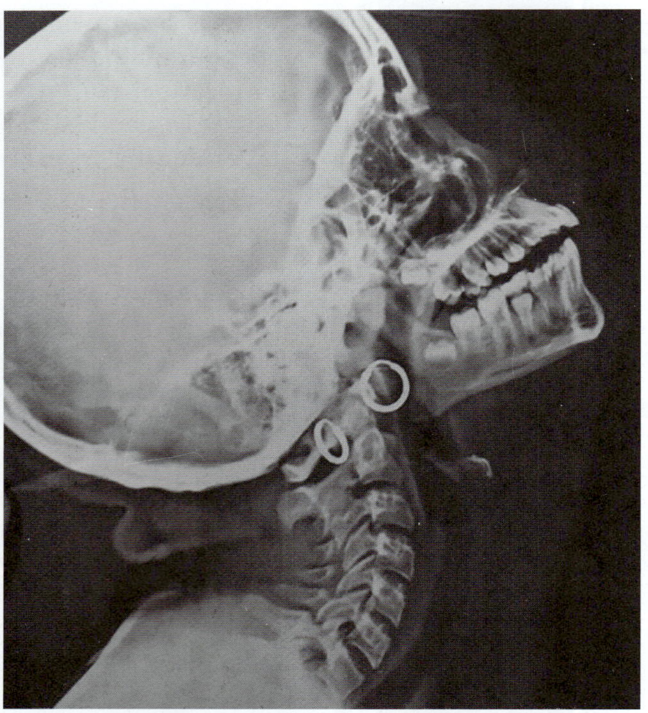

Fig. 28.19: Lateral view of the skull and cervical vertebrae

nasal cavities, and the ethmoidal and maxillary sinuses lie superimposed on one another, below the anterior cranial fossa.

4 The *petrous part of the temporal bone* produces a dense irregular shadow posteroinferior to the hypophyseal fossa. Within this shadow, there are two dark areas representing the external acoustic meatuses of the two sides; each shadow lies immediately behind the head of the mandible of that side. Similar dark shadows of the internal acoustic meatuses may also be seen. The posterior part of the dense shadow merges with the mastoid air cells producing a honeycomb appearance.

5 In addition to the features mentioned above, the *mandible* lies anteriorly forming the lower part of the facial skeleton. The *upper cervical vertebrae* lie posteriorly and are seen as a pillar supporting the skull.

Cervical Vertebrae

The cervical vertebrae can be visualised in lateral view of the neck. In this view, the body of cervical vertebrae, intervertebral discs, pedicles, spines, the adjacent inferior articular and superior articular processes and intervertebral foramen are visualised (Fig. 28.19).

SPECIAL PA VIEW OF SKULL FOR PARANASAL SINUSES

This picture is taken with the head extended in such a way that the chin rests against the film and the nose is raised from it (Water's position). This view shows the frontal and maxillary sinuses clearly (Fig. 28.20).

The frontal sinuses are seen immediately above the nose and medial parts of the orbits. The nasal cavities are flanked on each side by the orbits above, and the maxillary sinuses below. The normal sinuses are clear and radiolucent, i.e. they appear dark. If a sinus is infected, the shadow is either hazy or radio-opaque.

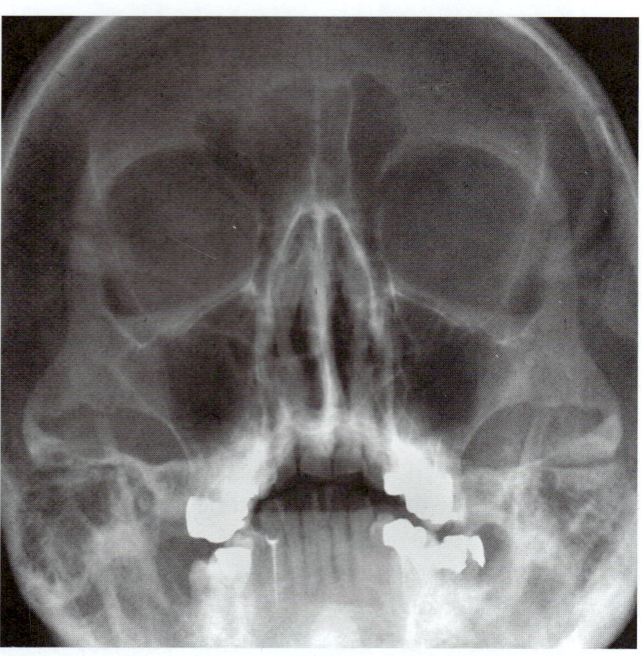

Fig. 28.20: X-ray of skull showing paranasal sinuses

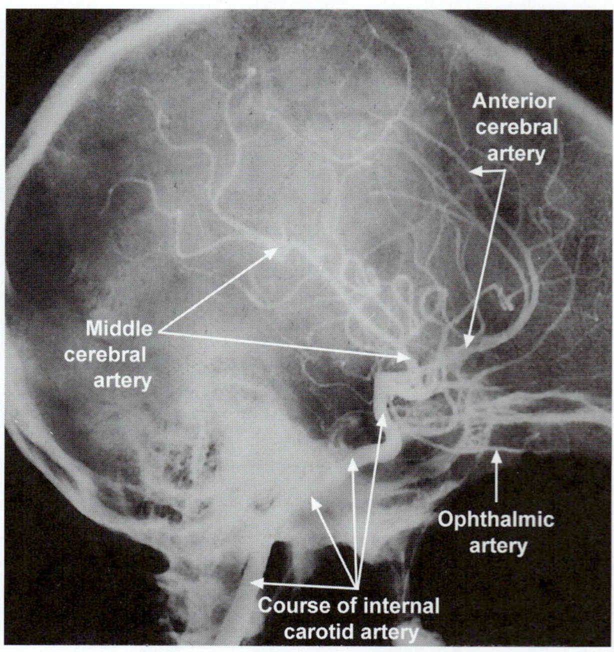

Fig. 28.21: Carotid angiogram

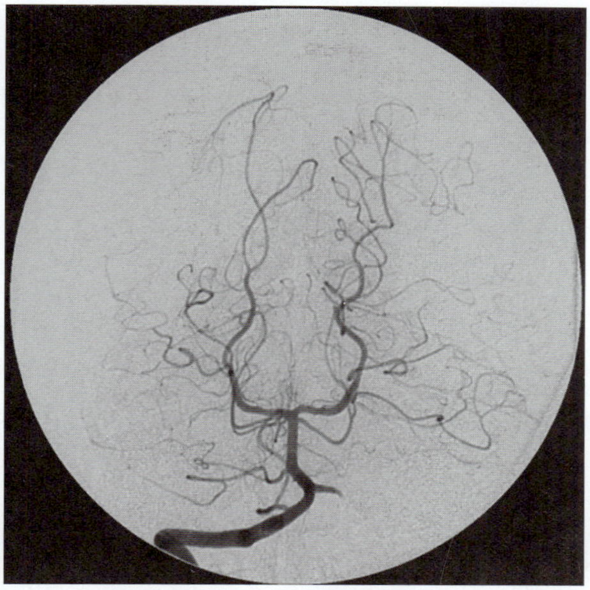

Fig. 28.22: Vertebral angiogram

Carotid Angiogram

Carotid angiogram lateral view. A radio-opaque dye was injected into the carotid artery just before the radiograph was taken (Fig. 28.21). Internal carotid artery is seen to give an ophthalmic branch and then ends by dividing into a smaller anterior cerebral and a larger middle cerebral arteries.

Vertebral Angiogram

Figure 28.22 shows single basilar artery formed by union of 2 vertebral arteries. Basilar artery ends by dividing into 2 posterior cerebral arteries.

FURTHER READING

- Abrahams PH, Meminn RMH, Hutchings RT, et al. Mcminns color atlas of human anatomy (5th edition). Philadelphia: Mosby 2003.
- A Halim. Surface and Radiological Anatomy, 3ed. CBS Publishers and Distributors Pvt Ltd.

Appendix

Parasympathetic Ganglia, Arteries, Pharyngeal Arches and Clinical Terms

"What matters is not to add years to your life but life to your years."
—Alexis Carrel

INTRODUCTION

The appendix contains upper cervical nerves, and sympathetic trunk of the neck in Table A.1.

The four parasympathetic ganglia are shown in Flowcharts A.1 to A.4 and Table A.2.

Summary of the arteries is depicted in Tables A.3 to A.5.

The pharyngeal arches, pouches and clefts are shown in Tables A.6 to A.8. It also includes the Clinical Terms.

CERVICAL PLEXUS

Ventral rami of C1–C4 form the cervical plexus. C1 runs along hypoglossal and supplies geniohyoid and thyrohyoid. It also gives superior limb of ansa cervicalis, which supplies superior belly of omohyoid and joins with inferior limb to form ansa. Inferior limb of ansa cervicalis is formed by ventral rami of C2, C3. Branches from ansa supply sternohyoid, sternothyroid, and inferior belly of omohyoid. Cervical plexus also gives four cutaneous branches—lesser occipital (C2), great auricular (C2, C3), supraclavicular (C3, C4) and transverse or anterior nerve of neck (C2, C3) (*see* Figs 11.6 and 17.8).

PHRENIC NERVE

Phrenic nerve arises primarily from ventral rami of C4 with small contributions from C3 and C5 nerve roots or through nerve to subclavius. It is the only motor supply to its own half of diaphragm and sensory to mediastinal pleura, peritoneum and fibrous pericardium. Inflammation of peritoneum under diaphragm causes referred pain in the area of supraclavicular nerves supply, especially tip of the shoulders as their root value is also ventral rami of C3 and C4 (*see* Fig. 17. 9).

SYMPATHETIC TRUNK

Branches of cervical sympathetic ganglia of sympathetic trunk are given in Table A.1.

PARASYMPATHETIC GANGLIA (TABLE A.2)

SUBMANDIBULAR GANGLION

Situation (Fig. A.1)

The submandibular ganglion lies superficial to hyoglossus muscle in the submandibular region. Functionally, submandibular ganglion is connected to

Table A.1: Branches of cervical sympathetic ganglia

	Superior cervical ganglion	*Middle cervical ganglion*	*Inferior cervical ganglion*
Arterial branches	i. Along internal carotid artery as internal carotid nerve ii. Along common carotid and external carotid arteries	Along inferior thyroid artery	Along subclavian and vertebral arteries
Grey rami communicantes along cervical and cranial nerves	Along 1–4 cervical nerves Along cranial nerves IX, X, XI and XII	Along 5 and 6 cervical nerves –	Along 7 and 8 cervical nerves –
Visceral branches	Pharynx, cardiac	Thyroid, cardiac	Cardiac

Flowchart A.1: Connections of submandibular ganglion

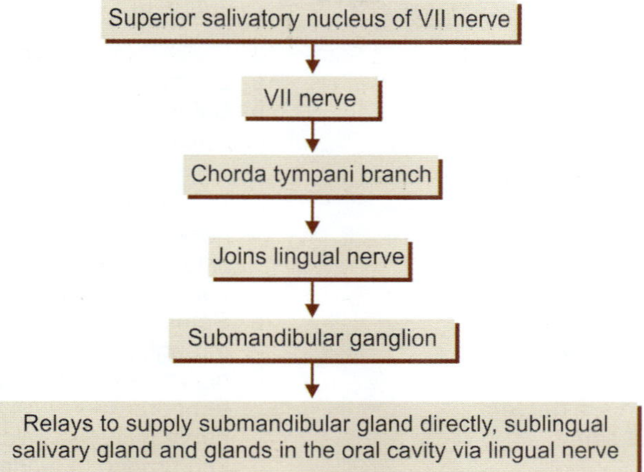

Flowchart A.2: Connections of pterygopalatine ganglion

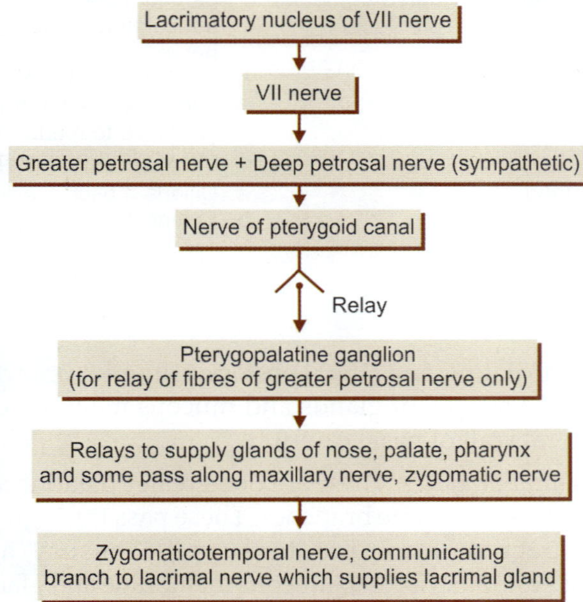

Flowchart A.3: Connections of otic ganglion

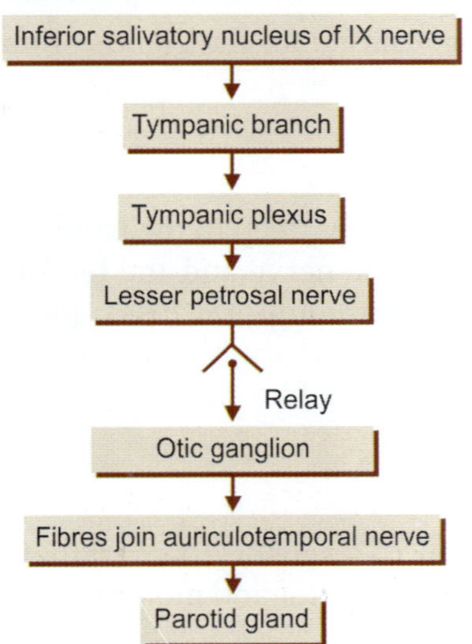

Flowchart A.4: Connections of ciliary ganglion

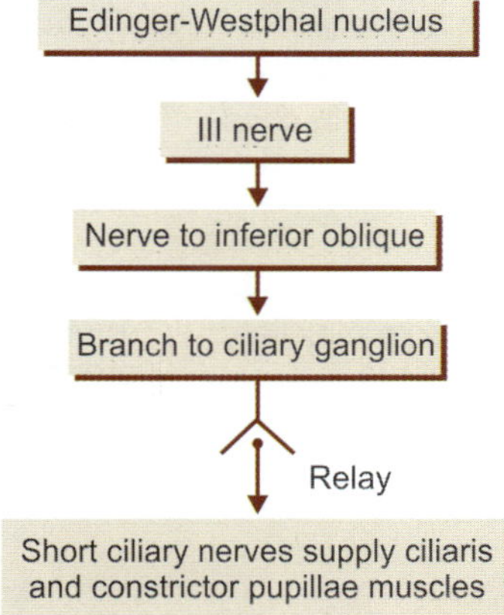

facial nerve, while topographically it is connected to lingual branch of mandibular nerve (*see* Fig. 15.9).

Roots

The ganglion has sensory, sympathetic and secretomotor or parasympathetic roots.

1. Sensory root is from the lingual nerve. It is suspended by two roots of lingual nerve.
2. Sympathetic root is from the sympathetic plexus around the facial artery. This plexus contains postganglionic fibres from the superior cervical ganglion of sympathetic trunk. These fibres pass express through the ganglion and are vasomotor to the gland.
3. Secretomotor root is from superior salivatory nucleus through nervus intermedius via chorda tympani which is a branch of cranial nerve VII. Chorda tympani joins lingual nerve. The parasympathetic fibres get relayed in the submandibular ganglion (Flowchart A.1).

Branches

The ganglion gives direct branches to the submandibular salivary gland.

Some postganglionic fibres reach the lingual nerve to be distributed to sublingual salivary gland and glands in the oral cavity.

PTERYGOPALATINE GANGLION

Situation

Pterygopalatine or sphenopalatine is the largest parasympathetic ganglion, suspended by two roots of maxillary nerve. Functionally, it is related to cranial nerve VII. It is called the ganglion of 'hay fever'.

Roots

The ganglion has sensory, sympathetic and secretomotor or parasympathetic roots.

1. Sensory root is from maxillary nerve. The ganglion is suspended by 2 roots of maxillary nerve.

Table A.2: Connections of parasympathetic ganglia (Fig. A.1)

Ganglia	*Sensory root*	*Sympathetic root*	*Secretomotor root/ parasympathetic root*	*Motor root*	*Distribution*
Submandibular (Fig. A.1)	Two branches from lingual nerve	Branch from plexus around facial artery	Superior salivatory nucleus → facial nerve → chorda tympani (joins the lingual nerve)	— —	a. Submandibular b. Sublingual c. Anterior lingual glands
Pterygopalatine (Fig. A.1)	Two branches from maxillary nerve	Deep petrosal from plexus around internal carotid artery	Superior salivatory nucleus, and lacrimatory nucleus → nervus intermedius → facial nerve → geniculate ganglion → greater petrosal nerve + deep petrosal nerve = nerve of pterygoid canal	—	a. Mucous glands of nose, paranasal sinuses, palate, nasopharynx b. Some fibres pass through zygomatic nerve → zygomatico-temporal nerve → communicating branch to lacrimal nerve → lacrimal gland
Otic (Flowchart A.3)	Branch from auriculotemporal nerve	Plexus along middle meningeal artery	Inferior salivatory nucleus → glosso-pharyngeal nerve → tympanic branch → tympanic plexus → lesser petrosal nerve	Branch from nerve to medial pterygoid	a. Secretomotor to parotid gland via auriculotemporal nerve b. Tensor veli palatini and tensor tympani via nerve to med. pterygoid (unrelayed)
Ciliary (Flowchart A.4)	From nasociliary nerve	Plexus along ophthalmic artery	Edinger-Westphal nucleus → oculomotor nerve → nerve to inferior oblique	—	a. Ciliaris muscles b. Sphincter pupillae

2 Sympathetic root is from postganglionic plexus around internal carotid artery. The nerve is called deep petrosal. It unites with greater petrosal to form the nerve of pterygoid canal. The fibres of deep petrosal do not relay in the ganglion (Fig. 23.18).

3 Secretomotor or parasympathetic root is from greater petrosal nerve which arises from geniculate ganglion of cranial nerve VII. These fibres relay in the ganglion (Flowchart A.2).

Branches

The ganglion gives number of branches. These are:

1 *For lacrimal gland:* The postganglionic fibres pass through zygomatic branch of maxillary nerve. These fibres hitch hike through zygomaticotemporal nerve into the communicating branch between zygomaticotemporal and lacrimal nerves, then to the lacrimal nerve for supplying the lacrimal gland.

2 *Nasopalatine nerve:* This nerve runs on the nasal septum and ends in the anterior part of hard palate. It supplies secretomotor fibres to both nasal and palatal glands.

3 *Nasal branches:* These are medial, posterior, superior branches for the supply of glands and mucous membrane of nasal septum; the largest is named nasopalatine; and lateral posterior superior branches for the supply of glands and mucous membrane of lateral wall of nasal cavity.

4 *Palatine branches:* These are one greater palatine and 2–3 lesser palatine branches. These pass through the respective foramina to supply sensory and secretomotor fibres to mucous membrane and glands of soft palate and hard palate (Fig. 23.18).

5 *Orbital branches* for the orbital periosteum.

6 *Pharyngeal branches* for the glands of pharynx.

OTIC GANGLION

Situation

The otic ganglion lies deep to the trunk of mandibular nerve, between the nerve and the tensor veli palatini muscle in the infratemporal fossa, just distal to the foramen ovale. Topographically, it is connected to mandibular nerve, while functionally it is related to cranial nerve IX.

Roots

This ganglion has sensory, sympathetic, parasympathetic or secretomotor and motor roots (*see* Figs 14.17 and 14.18).

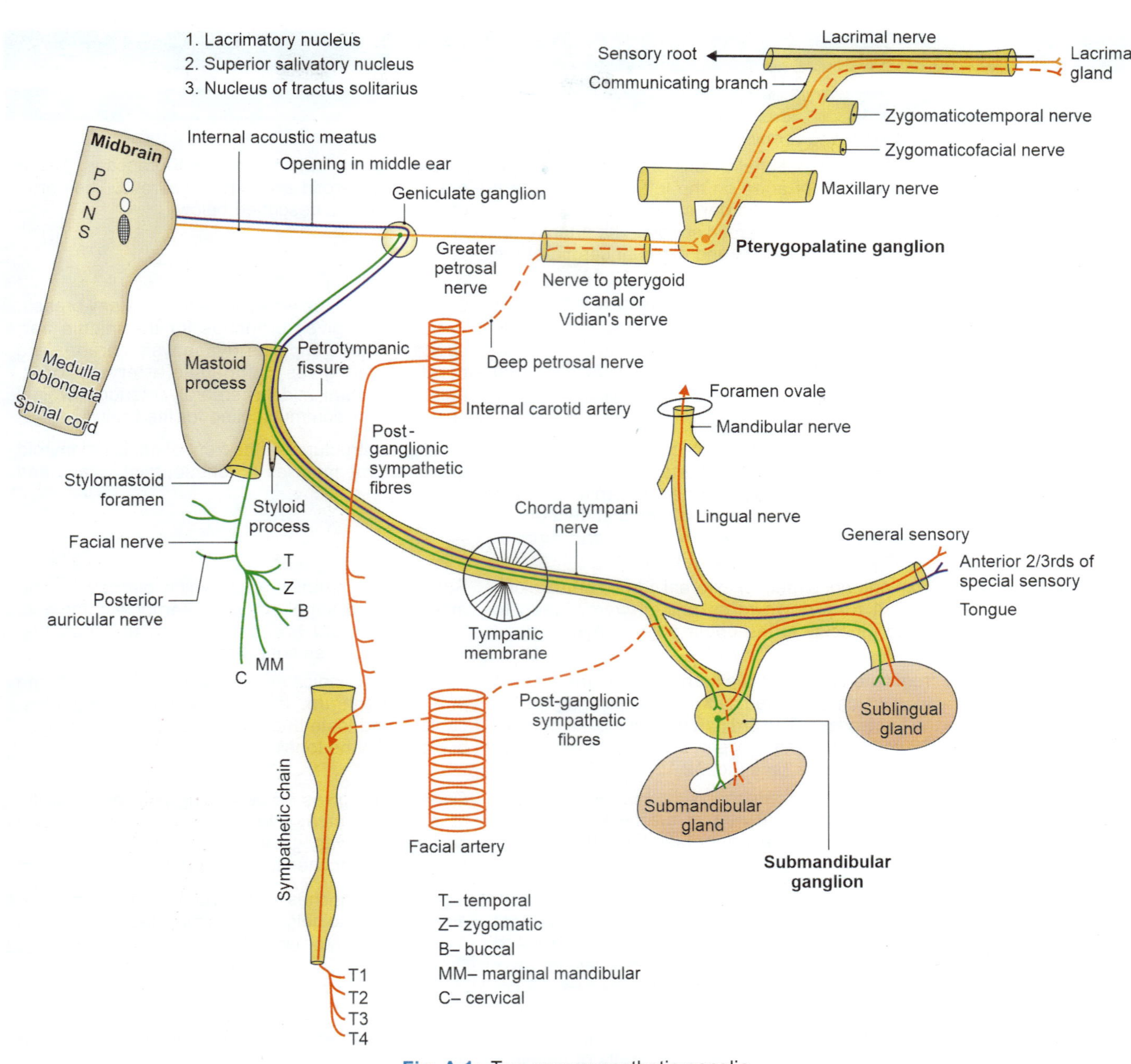

Fig. A.1: Two parasympathetic ganglia

1 Sensory root is by the auriculotemporal nerve.
2 Sympathetic root is by the sympathetic plexus around middle meningeal artery.
3 Secretomotor root is by the lesser petrosal nerve from the tympanic plexus formed by tympanic branch of cranial nerve IX. Fibres of lesser petrosal nerve relay in the otic ganglion. Postganglionic fibres reach the parotid gland through auriculotemporal nerve (Flowchart A.3).
4 Motor root is by a branch from nerve to medial pterygoid. This branch passes unrelayed through the ganglion and divides into two branches to supply tensor veli palatini and tensor tympani.

Branches

The postganglionic branches of the ganglion pass through auriculotemporal nerve to supply the parotid gland.

The motor branches supply the two muscles—tensor veli palatini and tensor tympani.

CILIARY GANGLION

Situation

The ciliary ganglion is very small ganglion present in the orbit. Topographically, the ganglion is related to nasociliary nerve, branch of ophthalmic division of

ARTERIES OF HEAD AND NECK

Table A.3: Common carotid artery

Artery	*Beginning, course and termination*	*Area of distribution*
Common carotid	It is a branch of brachiocephalic trunk on right side and a direct branch of arch of aorta on the left side. The artery runs upwards along medial border of sternocleidomastoid muscle enclosed within the carotid sheath. The artery ends by dividing into internal carotid and external carotid at the upper border of thyroid cartilage (*see* Fig. 12.14)	This artery has only two terminal branches. These are internal carotid and external carotid. Their area of distribution is described below.
Internal carotid	It is a terminal branch of common carotid artery. It first runs through the neck (cervical part), then passes through the petrous bone (petrous part), then courses through the sinus (cavernous part) and lastly lies in relation to the brain (cerebral part)	Cervical part of the artery does not give any branch. Petrous part gives branches for the middle ear; cavernous part supplies hypophysis cerebri. The cerebral part gives ophthalmic artery for orbit, anterior cerebral, middle cerebral, anterior choroidal and posterior communicating for the brain
External carotid	It is one of the terminal branches of common carotid artery and lies anterior to internal carotid artery. External carotid artery starts at the level of upper border of thyroid cartilage, runs upwards and laterally to terminate behind the neck of mandible by dividing into larger maxillary and smaller superficial temporal branches (*see* Fig. 12.13)	It supplies structures in the front of neck, i.e. thyroid gland, larynx, muscles of tongue, face, scalp, and ear
Superior thyroid	It arises from anterior aspect of external carotid artery close to its origin. It runs downwards and forwards deep to the infrahyoid muscles to the upper pole of thyroid gland (*see* Fig. 14.6)	Superior laryngeal branch which pierces thyroid membrane to supply larynx. Sternocleidomastoid and cricothyroid branches are to the muscles. Terminal branches supply the thyroid gland
Lingual	It arises from anterior aspect of external carotid artery forms a typical loop which is crossed by XII nerve. Its 2nd part lies deep to the hyoglossus. The 3rd part runs along the anterior border of hyoglossus and 4th part runs forwards on the under surface of tongue (*see* Fig. 12.15)	As the name indicates, it is the chief artery of the muscular tongue. It supplies various muscles, papillae and taste buds of the tongue. It also gives branches to the tonsil
Facial	This tortuous artery from anterior side also arises a little higher than lingual artery. It runs in the neck as cervical part and in the face as facial artery (*see* Fig. 10.17)	Cervical part gives off ascending palatine, tonsillar, glandular branches for the submandibular and sublingual salivary glands. The facial part lies on the face giving branches to muscles of face and its skin
Occipital	It arises form the posterior aspect of external carotid artery and runs upwards along the lower border of posterior belly of digastric muscle. Then it runs deep to mastoid process and the muscles attached to it. The artery then crosses the apex of suboccipital triangle and then it pierces trapezius 2.5 cm from midline to supply the layers of scalp (*see* Fig. 12.14)	It gives two branches to sternocleidomastoid muscle, and branches to neighbouring muscles. It also gives a meningeal and mastoid branch
Posterior auricular	It arises from posterior aspect of external carotid artery, it runs along the upper border of posterior belly of digastric muscle to reach the back of auricle	It gives branches to scalp. Its stylomastoid branch enters the foramen of the same name to supply mastoid antrum, nerve air cells and the facial
Ascending pharyngeal	It arises from the medial side of external carotid artery, close to its origin. It runs upwards and between pharynx and tonsil on medial side and medial wall of middle ear on the lateral side (*see* Fig. 12.13)	It gives branches to tonsil, pharynx and a few meningeal branches
Superficial temporal	It is the smaller terminal branch of external carotid artery. It begins behind the neck of the mandible, runs upwards and crosses the preauricular point, where its pulsations can be felt. 5 cm above the preauricular point it ends by dividing into anterior and posterior branches (*see* Fig. 10.5)	Its two terminal branches supply layers of scalp and superficial temporal region. It also supplies parotid gland, facial muscles and temporalis muscle
Maxillary	It is the larger terminal branch of external carotid artery. It is given off behind the neck of the mandible. Its course is divided into 1st, 2nd and 3rd parts according to its relations with lateral pterygoid muscle. 1st part lies below the lateral pterygoid, 2nd part lies on the lower head of lateral pterygoid and 3rd part lies between the two heads	Branches of—1st part: Deep auricular, anterior tympanic, middle meningeal and inferior alveolar. 2nd part: Muscular branches to medial pterygoid, masseter, temporalis and lateral pterygoid 3rd part: Posterior superior alveolar, infraorbital, greater palatine and sphenopalatine branches, pharyngeal and artery of pterygoid canal

Table A.4: Maxillary artery

Branches	*Foramina transmitting*	*Distribution*
A. Of first part (*see* Fig. 14.6)		
1. Deep auricular	Foramen in the floor (cartilage or bone) of external acoustic meatus	Skin of external acoustic meatus, and outer surface of tympanic membrane
2. Anterior tympanic	Petrotympanic fissure	Inner surface of tympanic membrane
3. Middle meningeal	Foramen spinosum	Supplies more of bone and less of meninges; also V and VII nerves, middle ear and tensor tympani
4. Accessory meningeal	Foramen ovale	Main distribution is extracranial to pterygoids
5. Inferior alveolar	Mandibular foramen	Lower teeth and mylohyoid muscle
B. Of second part		
1. Masseteric	—	Masseter
2. Deep temporal (anterior)	—	Temporalis
3. Deep temporal (posterior)	—	Temporalis
4. Pterygoid	—	Lateral and medial pterygoids
5. Buccal	—	Skin of cheek
C. Of third part (*see* Fig. 14.7)		
1. Posterior superior alveolar	Alveolar canals in body of maxilla	Upper molar and premolar teeth and gums; maxillary sinus
2. Infraorbital	Inferior orbital fissure	Lower orbital muscles, lacrimal sac, maxillary sinus, upper incisor and canine teeth
3. Greater palatine	Greater palatine canal	Soft palate, tonsil, palatine glands and mucosa; upper gums
4. Pharyngeal	Pharyngeal (palatinovaginal) canal	Roof of nose and pharynx, auditory tube, sphenoidal sinus
5. Artery of pterygoid canal	Pterygoid canal	Auditory tube, upper pharynx, and middle ear
6. Sphenopalatine (terminal part)	Sphenopalatine foramen	Lateral and medial walls of nose and various air sinuses

Table A.5: Subclavian artery

Course	*Branches and area of distribution*
It is the chief artery of the upper limb. It also supplies part of neck and brain. On the right side, subclavian artery is a branch of the brachiocephalic trunk. On the left side, it is a direct branch of arch of aorta. The artery on either side ascends and enters the neck posterior to the sternoclavicular joint. The arteries of two sides have similar course. The artery arches from the sternoclavicular joint to the outer border of the first rib where it continues as the axillary artery. It is divided into three parts by the crossing of scalenus anterior muscle (*see* Figs 16.19 and 16.20)	Branches of 1st part: • Vertebral artery is the largest branch. It supplies the brain. The artery passes through foramina transversaria of C6–C1 vertebrae, then it courses through suboccipital triangle to enter cranial cavity • Internal thoracic artery runs downwards and medially to enter thorax by passing behind first costal cartilage. It runs vertically 2 cm, on lateral side of sternum till 6th intercostal space to divide into musculophrenic and superior epigastric branches • Thyrocervical trunk is a short wide vessel which gives suprascapular, transverse cervical and important inferior thyroid branch. Inferior thyroid artery gives glandular branches to thyroid and parathyroid glands. In addition, this artery gives inferior laryngeal branch for the supply of mucous membrane of larynx • Costocervical trunk arises from 2nd part of subclavian artery on right side and from 1st part on left side. It ends by dividing into superior intercostal and deep cervical branches • 3rd part may give dorsal scapular branch

PHARYNGEAL APPARATUS

Table A.6: Structures derived from skeletal and muscular components of pharyngeal arches

Pharyngeal arch	*Nerve of the arch*	*Muscles derived*	*Skeletal and ligamentous structures derived*
First (mandibular) arch (I) Meckel's cartilages	Trigeminal: Maxillary and mandibular divisions of trigeminal–post-trematic (V cranial nerve) Chorda tympani–pre-trematic	Muscles of mastication (temporalis, masseter, medial and lateral pterygoids) Mylohyoid Anterior belly of digastric tensor tympani Tensor veli palatini	Premaxilla, maxilla zygomatic, part of temporal, Meckel's cartilage Malleus Incus Anterior ligament of malleus Sphenomandibular ligament Spine of sphenoid Most of the mandible Genial tubercles
Second (hyoid) arch (II) Reichert's cartilage	Facial (VII cranial nerve)	Muscles of facial expression (buccinator, auricularis, frontalis, platysma, orbicularis oris, and orbicularis oculi) Posterior belly of digastric Stylohyoid, stapedius	Stapes Styloid process Lesser cornua of hyoid Upper part of body of hyoid Stylohyoid ligament
Third (III)	Glossopharyngeal (IX cranial nerve)	Stylopharyngeus	Greater cornua of hyoid Lower part of body of hyoid bone
Fourth (IV)	Superior laryngeal branch of vagus	Cricothyroid Levator veli palatini Striated muscles of oesophagus Constrictors of pharynx	Thyroid cartilage Corniculate cartilage Cuneiform cartilage
Sixth (VI)	Recurrent laryngeal branch of vagus (X cranial nerve)	Intrinsic muscles of larynx	Cricoid cartilage Arytenoid cartilage

By intramembranous ossification of mesenchyme of I arch, maxilla, zygomatic, squamous part of temporal are developed.

Table A.7: Derivatives of endodermal pouches

Pharyngeal pouch	*Derivatives*
Dorsal ends of I and II pouches form tubotympanic recess	Proximal part of tubotympanic recess gives rise to auditory tube Distal part gives rise to tympanic cavity and mastoid antrum Mastoid cells develop at about 2 years of age
Ventral part of II pharyngeal pouch	Epithelium covering the palatine tonsil and tonsillar fossa Lymphoid tissue is mesodermal in origin
III pharyngeal pouch	Thymus and inferior parathyroid gland or parathyroid III. Thymic epithelial reticular cells and Hassall's corpuscles are endodermal. Lymphocytes are derived from haemopoietic stem cells during 12th week
IV pharyngeal pouch	Superior parathyroid or parathyroid IV
V pharyngeal pouch (ultimobranchial body)	Parafollicular or 'C' cells of the thyroid gland

Table A.8: Derivatives of ectodermal clefts

Pharyngeal cleft	*Derivatives*
Dorsal part of I ectodermal cleft	Epithelium of external auditory meatus.
Auricle	Six auricular hillocks; three from I arch and three from II arch
Rest of ectodermal clefts	Obliterated by the overgrowth of II pharyngeal arch. The closing membrane of the first cleft is the tympanic membrane.

trigeminal nerve, but functionally it is related to oculomotor nerve. This ganglion gets parasympathetic fibres (Flowchart A.4).

Roots

It has three roots—the sensory, sympathetic and parasympathetic. Only the parasympathetic root fibres relay to supply the intraocular muscles.

1 Sensory root is from the long ciliary nerve.
2 Sympathetic root is by the long ciliary nerve from plexus around ophthalmic artery (Fig. 21.11).
3 Parasympathetic root is from a branch to inferior oblique muscle. These fibres arise from Edinger-Westphal nucleus, join oculomotor nerve and leave it via the nerve to inferior oblique, to be relayed in the ciliary ganglion (Flowchart A.5).

Branches

The ganglion gives 10–12 short ciliary nerves containing postganglionic fibres for the supply of constrictor or sphincter pupillae for narrowing the size of pupil and ciliaris muscle for increasing the curvature of anterior surface of lens required during accommodation of the eye.

MOLECULAR REGULATION OF PHARYNGEAL ARCHES

Neural crest cells arise from caudal midbrain and from rhombomeres—the segments in the hindbrain.

Pharyngeal pouch endoderm expresses genes which regulate the patterning of the skeletal parts in the pharyngeal arches.

The mechanism of epithelial–mesenchymal interaction with endoderm of the pouches send signals to the mesenchyme. Mesenchymal gene expression is determined by OTX2 and HOX genes carried by pharyngeal arches by migrating neural crest cells.

CLINICAL TERMS

Anaesthetist's arteries: These are the arteries used by the anaesthetists who are sitting at the head end of the patient being operated:

- The superficial temporal artery as it crosses the root of zygoma in front of ear (*see* Fig. 13.3a).
- Facial artery at the anteroinferior angle of masseter muscle (*see* Fig. 10.17).
- Common carotid at the anterior border of sternocleidomastoid.

Hilton's method of draining parotid gland abscess: The incision given to drain parotid abscess is the horizontal incision or by making many holes. This incision does not endanger the various branches of facial nerve, coursing through the gland (*see* Fig. 13.8).

Frey's syndrome: The sign of Frey's syndrome is the appearance of perspiration on the face while the patient eats food. In certain healing of wounds, the auriculotemporal nerve and great auricular nerves may join with each other. When the person eats food, instead of saliva, sweat appears on the face.

Waldeyer's ring: It is the ring of lymphoid tissue present at the oropharyngeal junction. Its components are lingual tonsils anteriorly, palatine tonsils laterally, tubal tonsils above and laterally and pharyngeal tonsils posteriorly (*see* Fig. 22.13).

Killian's dehiscence: It is a potential gap between upper thyropharyngeus and lower cricopharyngeus parts of inferior constrictor muscle. Thyropharyngeus is the propulsive part of the muscle, supplied by recurrent laryngeal nerve, while cricopharyngeus is the sphincteric part, supplied by external laryngeal nerve. If there is incoordination between these two parts, bolus of food is pushed backwards in region of Killian's dehiscence, producing pharyngeal pouch or diverticula (*see* Fig. 22.22).

Safety muscle of larynx: Posterior cricoarytenoid muscles are the only abductors of vocal cords. The paralysis of both these muscles causes unopposed adduction of vocal cords, with severe dyspnoea. So posterior cricoarytenoid is the life-saving muscle (*see* Figs 24.10, 24.11b).

Singer's nodules: These are little swellings on the vocal cords at the junction of anterior one-third and posterior two-thirds of vocal cords. During phonation, the cords come close together, and there is slight friction as well. If friction is more and continuous, there is some inflammation with thickening of vocal cords, leading to Singer's or Teacher's nodules.

Tongue is pulled out during anaesthesia: Genioglossus muscles are responsible for protrusion of tongue. If these muscles are paralysed, the tongue falls back upon itself and blocks the airway. So tongue is pulled out during anaesthesia to keep there air passage clean (see Fig. 25.5).

Passavant's ridge: The horizontal fibres of right and left palatopharyngeus muscles form a Passavant's fold at the junction of nasopharynx and oropharynx. During swallowing, palatopharyngeus muscles form a ridge, which closes nasopharynx from oropharynx, so that bolus of food passes, through oropharynx only. In paralysis of these muscles, there is nasal regurgitation.

Ludwig's angina: When there is cellulitis of floor of the mouth, due to infected teeth, the condition is known as Ludwig's angina. The tongue is pushed upwards and mylohyoid is pushed downwards. This cellulitis may spread backwards to cause oedema of larynx and asphyxia.

Little's area of nose: This is the area in the antero-inferior part of nasal septum. Four arteries take part in Kiesselbach's plexus formed by:

Septal branch of superior labial from facial artery, terminal part of sphenopalatine artery:

- Anterior ethmoidal artery,
- Greater palatine artery.

  Picking of the nose may give rise to nasal bleeding or epistaxis (*see* Fig. 23.5).

Syringing of ear causes decreased heart rate: The external auditory meatus is supplied by auricular branch of vagus. Vagus also supplies the heart with cardio-inhibitory fibres. During syringing of the ear, vagus nerve is stimulated which causes bradycardia (*see* Fig. 26.7).

Nerve of near vision: Oculomotor nerve is the nerve of close vision. It supplies medial rectus, superior and inferior recti. The sphincter pupillae and ciliaris muscles are supplied by parasympathetic fibres via III nerve. It also supplies levator palpebrae superiors which opens the eye.

Injury to spine of sphenoid: Chorda tympani nerve is related on the medial side of spine of sphenoid, while auriculotemporal nerve is related on the lateral side. Chorda tympani gives secretomotor fibres to submandibular and sublingual salivary glands, whereas auriculotemporal gives secretomotor fibres to the parotid gland. So injury to spine of sphenoid may injure both these nerves affecting the secretion from all three salivary glands (*see* Fig. 14.11a).

Extradural haemorrhage: There is collection of blood due to rupture of middle meningeal vessels in the space between skull and the endosteum. It may press upon the motor area of brain. Blood has to be drained out from the point called 'pterion' (*see* Fig. 9.10).

Loss of corneal blink reflex: In case of injury to ophthalmic nerve, there is loss of corneal blink reflex as the afferent part of reflex arc is damaged.

Loss of sneeze reflex: In injury to maxillary nerve, the sneeze reflex is lost, as afferent loop of the reflex arc formed by the maxillary nerve is damaged.

Loss of jaw jerk reflex: The afferent and efferent limbs of the reflex arc are by V nerve. Damage to mandibular nerve causes loss of jaw jerk reflex.

SPOTS

1. a. Identify the foramen.
   b. Name the structures passing through it.

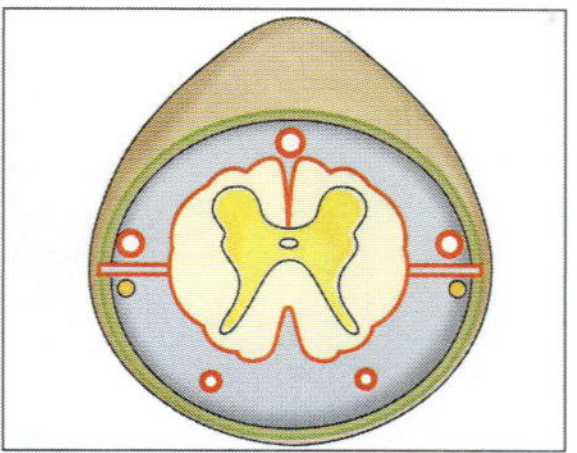

2. a. Identify the foramen.
   b. Name the structures passing through it.

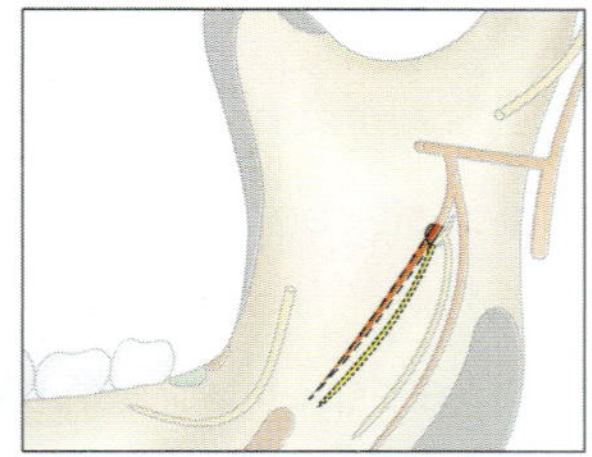

3. a. Identify the muscle.
   b. Name its parts.

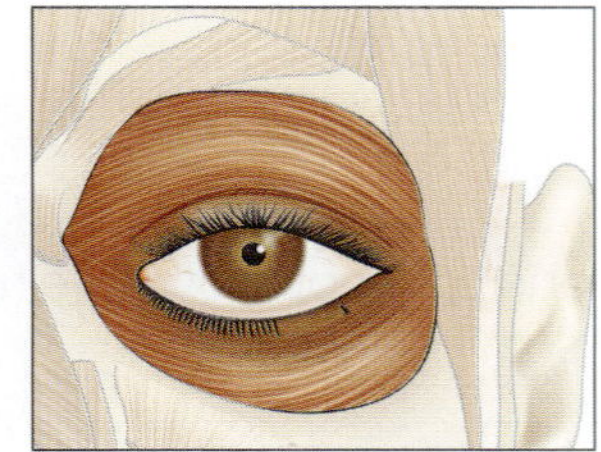

4. a. Identify the arrow marked circled structure.
   b. What are types of fibres carried by it?

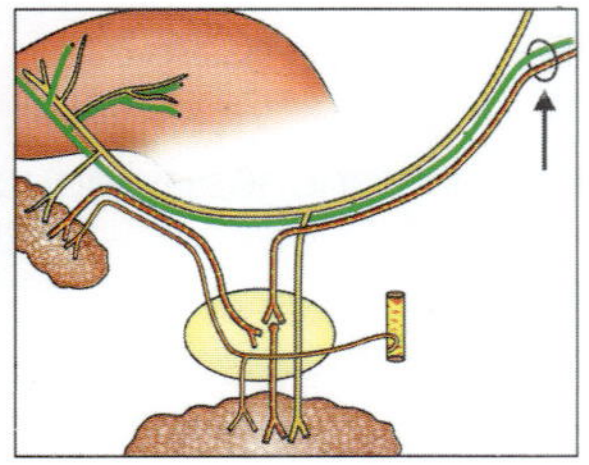

5. a. Identify the highlighted structure.
   b. Trace its secretomotor fibres.

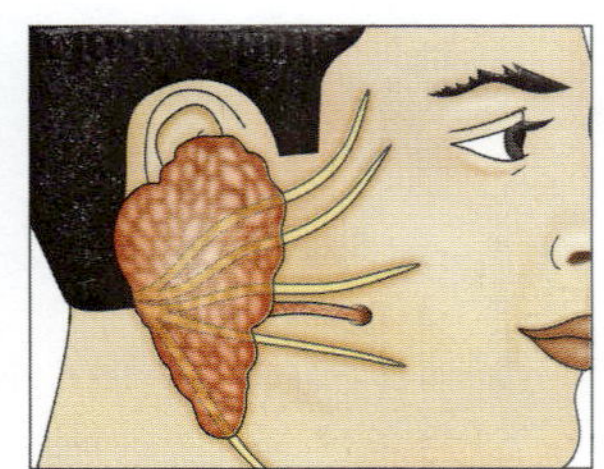

6. a. Identify the structure.
   b. Name its branches in order.

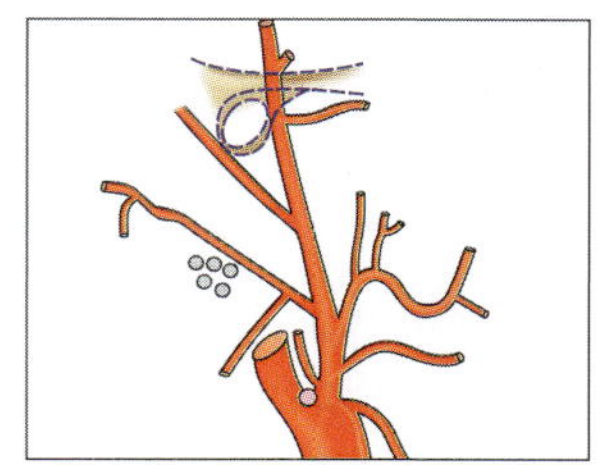

7. a. Identify the marked area.
   b. Name the vessels present here.

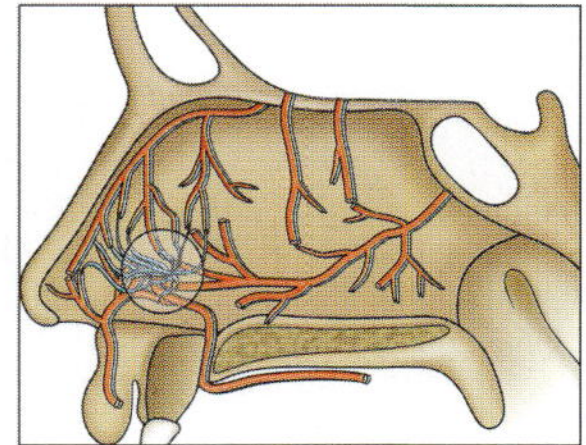

8. a. Identify the structure.
   b. Name its extrinsic muscles with their nerve supply.

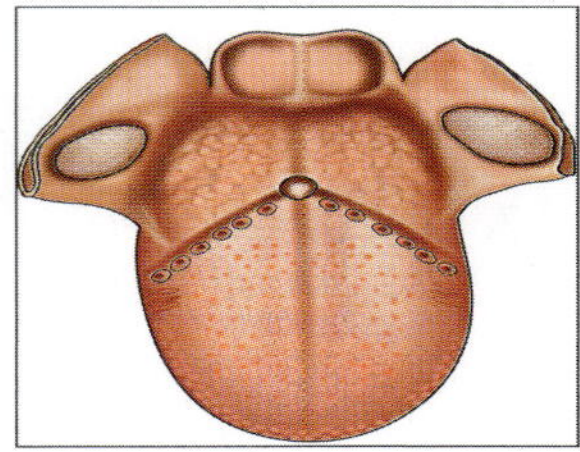

9. a. Identify the highlighted muscle.
   b. What is its action?

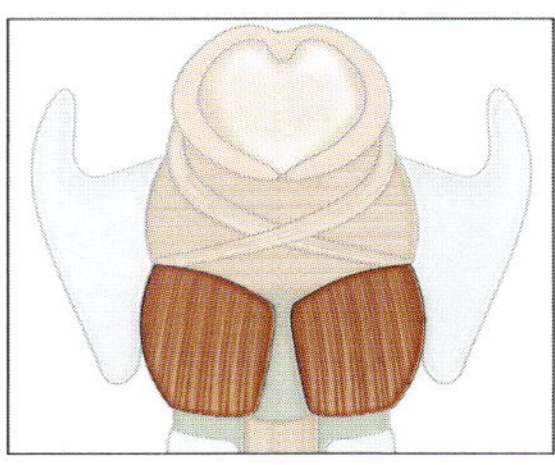

10. a. Identify the organ.
    b. Name the arteries supplying it.

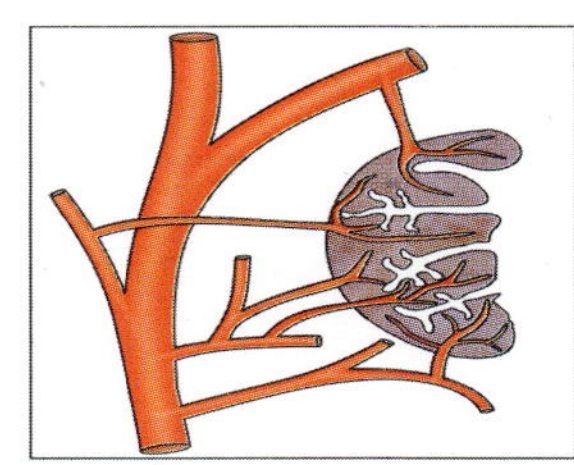

ANSWERS OF SPOTS

1. a. Foramen magnum
   b. Lowest part of medulla oblongata
   Three meninges
   One anterior spinal artery
   Two posterior spinal arteries
   Two vertebral arteries
   Spinal root of XI

2. a. Mandibular canal
   b. Inferior alveolar artery and nerve

3. a. Orbicularis oculi
   b. Orbital part, palpebral part and lacrimal part

4. a. Chorda tympani nerve
   b. General visceral efferent (GVE) fibres and special visceral afferent (Sp. VA) fibres

5. a. Parotid gland
   b. Inferior salivatory nucleus → IX nerve → tympanic plexus → lesser petrosal nerve → otic ganglion → postganglionic fibres join auriculotemporal nerve → parotid gland

6. a. External carotid artery.
   b. Anterior: Superior thyroid, lingual and facial
   Medial: Ascending pharyngeal
   Posterior: Occipital and posterior auricular
   Terminal: Superficial temporal and maxillary

7. a. Little's area
   b. Superior labial, greater palatine, anterior ethmoidal and sphenopalatine veins and capillaries.

8. a. Tongue
   b. Palatoglossus, hyoglossus, styloglossus, genioglossus
   Palatoglossus is supplied by vagoaccessory complex, other three are supplied by hypoglossal nerve.

9. a. Posterior cricoarytenoid muscle
   b. Only abductor of the vocal cords

10. a. Palatine tonsil
    b. Ascending palatine, ascending pharyngeal, dorsal lingual branches of lingual and greater palatine branch of maxillary artery.

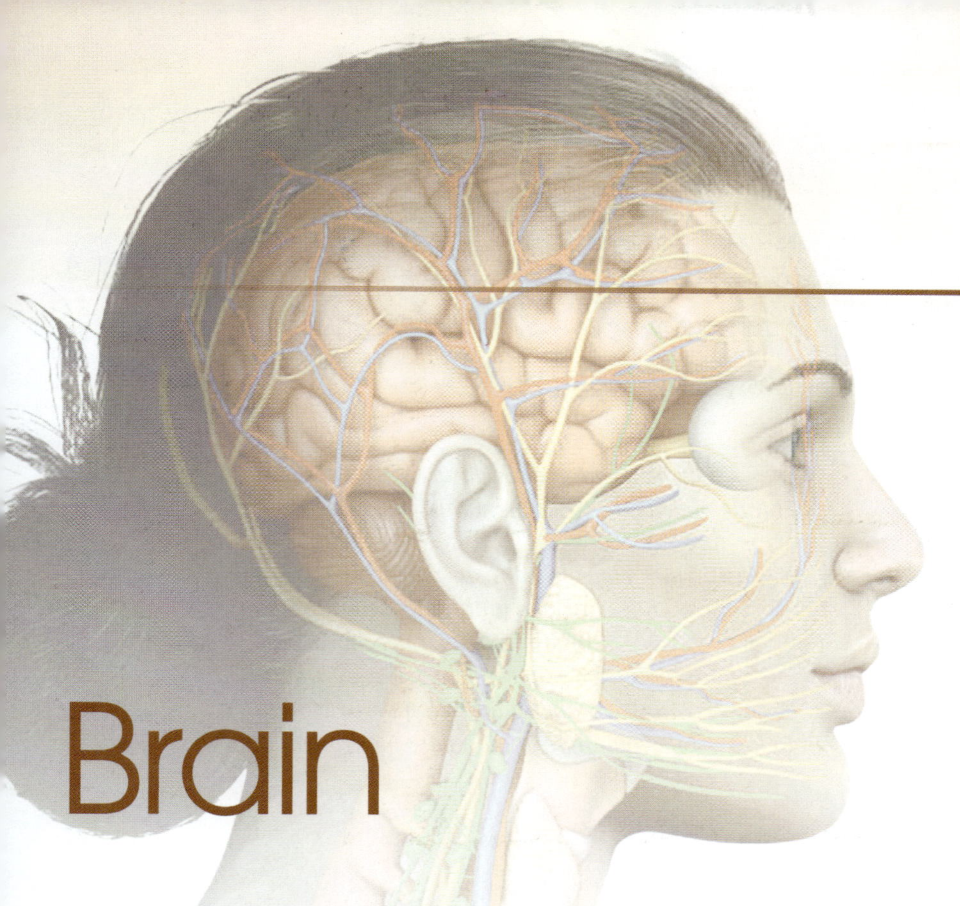

Section
III

Brain

Anatomy Made Easy

Ichak dana, bichak dana, dane uper dana
Hands naache, feet naache, brain hai khushnama
Ichak dana
Seventh ka nucleus ghoom kar aaye fifth ke pass,
nucleus ambiguus laterally jaye
Spinal accessory neeche ko aaye,
motor sensory pass ho jaye,
kaisa aashikana—ichak dana
Bolo kya—Neurobiotaxis, bolo kya—Neurobiotaxis

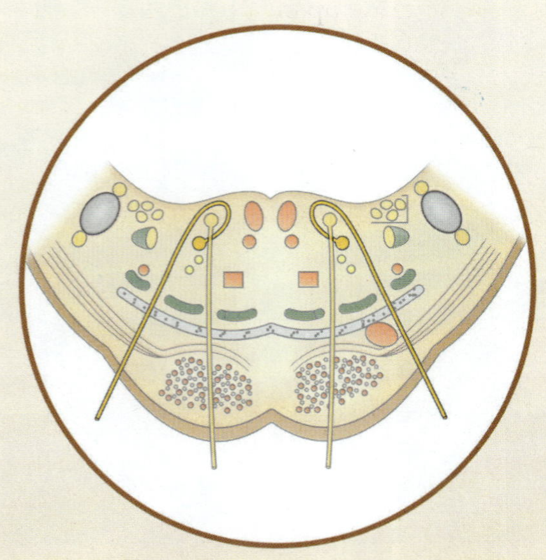

Introduction

Chapter 29

"On earth there is nothing great but man. In man there is nothing greater than mind."
—Anonymous

Nervous system is the chief controlling and coordinating system of the body. It adjusts the body to the surroundings and regulates all bodily activities both voluntary and involuntary.

Average weight of adult brain in air is 1500 grams. Since brain floats in cerebrospinal fluid, it only weighs 50 grams which is comfortable.

There are about 200 billion neurons in an adult brain (very rich).

DIVISIONS OF NERVOUS SYSTEM

Anatomical

It is divided into:

a. Central nervous system (CNS) comprises brain and spinal cord. CNS is the seat of learning, memory, intelligence and emotions.
b. Peripheral nervous system (PNS) includes 12 pairs of cranial nerves and 31 pairs of spinal nerves. These provide afferent impulses to CNS and carries efferent impulses to muscles, glands and blood vessels.

Functional

Nervous system functionally has two components:

a. Afferent component provides sensory information to CNS.
b. Efferent component carries motor information to muscles, glands, blood vessels and heart via:
   - Somatic nervous system for the control of skeletal muscles.
   - Autonomic nervous system for control of heart, smooth muscle of the organs, glands and blood vessels.

CELLULAR ARCHITECTURE

The nervous tissue is made up of:

a. Nerve cells or neurons (Fig. 29.1).
b. Neuroglial cells (neuroglia), forming the supporting (connective) tissue of the CNS.

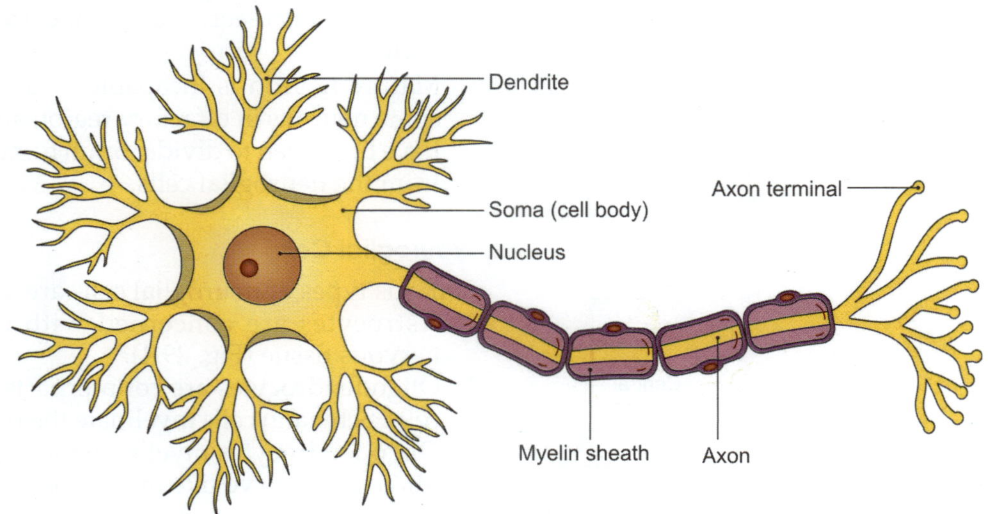

Fig. 29.1: Structure of a neuron

Neuron

Each neuron is made up of the following.

a. *Cell body:* Collectively, they form grey matter and the nuclei in the CNS, and ganglia in the peripheral nervous system.

b. *Numerous cell processes of two varieties:*
   i. Dendrites are many, short, richly branched and often varicose (Fig. 29.2).
   ii. The axon is a single elongated process. Collectively the axons form tracts (white matter) in the CNS, and nerves in the peripheral nervous system. The branches of axons often arise at right angles and are called the collaterals.

Functionally, each neuron is specialized for **sensitivity** and **conductivity**. The impulses can flow in them with great rapidity, in some cases about 125 metres per second. A neuron shows *dynamic polarity* in its processes. The impulse flows towards the cell body in the dendrites, and away from the cell body in the axon.

The neurons are connected to one another by their processes, forming long chains along which the impulses are conducted. The site of contact (contiguity without continuity) between the nerve cells in known as 'synapse' (Fig. 29.3).

Classification of Neurons

A. *According to the number of their processes, into four types.*
   a. *Multipolar neurons.* Most of the neurons in man are multipolar, e.g. all motor and internuncial neurons (Fig. 29.2).

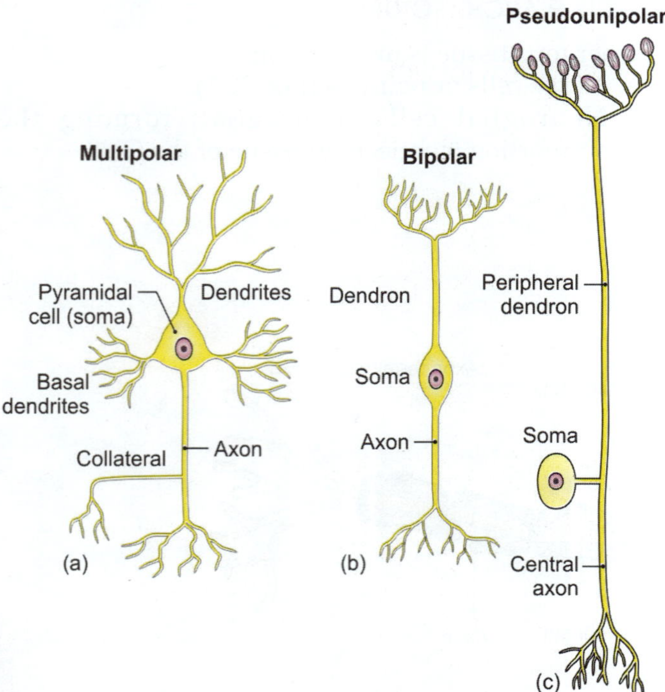

Figs 29.2a to c: Types of neuron

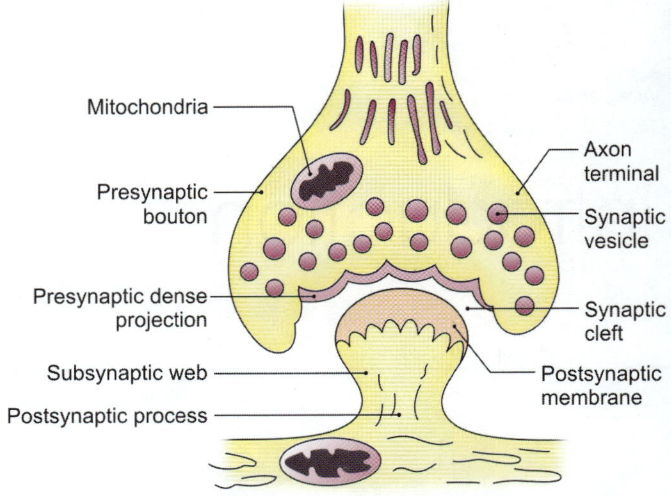

Fig. 29.3: Typical synapse seen with electron microscope

   b. *Bipolar neurons* are confined to the first neuron of the retina, ganglia of eighth cranial nerve, and the olfactory mucosa.
   c. *Pseudounipolar neurons* are actually unipolar to begin with but become bipolar functionally and are found in dorsal nerve root ganglia and sensory ganglia of the cranial nerves (Fig. 29.2).
   d. *Unipolar neurons* are present in the mesencephalic nucleus of trigeminal nerve and also occur during foetal life. These cells are more common in lower vertebrates.

B. *According to length of axon:*

Golgi Type I: These neurons have long axons and numerous short dendrites. These are seen in pyramidal cells of cerebral cortex, Purkinje cells of cerebellum and anterior horn cells of spinal cord.

Golgi Type II: These are neurons with small axons, and establish synapses with neighbouring neurons. These are also seen in cerebral cortex and cerebellar cortex.

Mature neuron is incapable of dividing. Recently, some neurons in olfactory region and hippocampus have been seen to divide. Brain tumours arise chiefly from the neuroglial cells.

Neuroglial Cells

Various types of neuroglial cells are as follows:

a. Astrocytes are concerned with nutrition of the nervous tissue (Fig. 29.4).
b. Oligodendrocytes are counterparts of the Schwann cells. Schwann cells myelinate the peripheral nerves. Oligodendrocytes myelinate the tracts.
c. Microglia behave like macrophages of the CNS.
d. Ependymal cells are columnar cells lining the cavities of the CNS. These secrete cerebrospinal fluid.

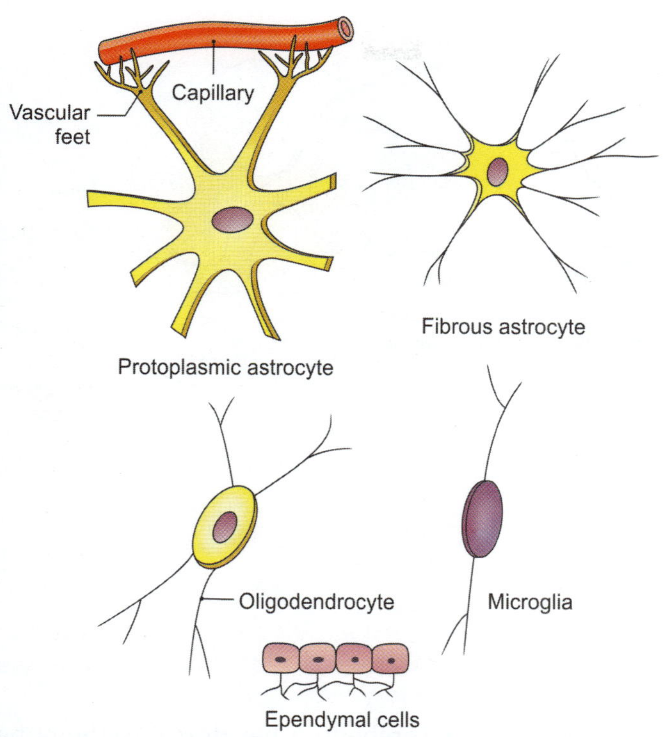

Fig. 29.4: Types of neuroglia

Reflex Arc

A reflex arc is the functional unit of the nervous system. In its simplest form, (monosynaptic reflex arc) it consists of

a. A receptor, e.g. the skin.
b. The sensory neuron.
c. The motor neuron.
d. The effector, e.g. the muscle.

Reflex action is chief function of spinal cord. Knee jerk is a monosynaptic reflex arc (Fig. 29.5). Some common reflex arcs are put in Table 29.1.

PARTS OF THE NERVOUS SYSTEM

Central Nervous System (CNS)

1 *Brain.* Occupies cranial cavity.
2 *Spinal cord.* Occupies upper two-thirds of the vertebral canal.

Peripheral Nervous System

1 Somatic (cerebrospinal) nervous system. It is made up of 12 pairs of cranial nerves and 31 pairs of spinal nerves. Its efferent fibres reach the effectors without interruption.
2 Autonomic (splanchnic) nervous system. It consists of sympathetic and parasympathetic systems. Its efferent fibres first relay in a ganglion, and then the postganglionic fibres pass to the effectors.

The central nervous system includes:

1 *The spinal cord:* It extends from the base of the skull to the first lumbar vertebra. The spinal cord receives sensory information from the skin, joints, and muscles of the trunk and limbs, and contains the motor neurons responsible for both voluntary and reflex movements. It also receives sensory information from the internal organs and control many visceral functions. Within the spinal cord there is an orderly arrangement of sensory cell groups that receive input from the periphery and motor cell groups that control specific muscle groups. In addition, the spinal cord contains ascending pathway through which sensory information reaches the brain and descending pathways that relay motor command from the brain to motor neurons.
2 *Brain stem:* It includes
   a. The medulla—this is the direct rostral extension of the cord. It participates in regulating blood

Table 29.1: Some common reflexes

Name of reflex	*Way of eliciting*	*Result*	*Comment*
Biceps jerk	Striking biceps tendon	Flexion of the elbow joint	C5, C6 segments intact Tendon jerks may be exaggerated in upper motor neuron lesion or lost in lower motor neuron lesion
Triceps jerk	Striking triceps tendon	Extension of the elbow joint	C7, C8, segments intact
Knee jerk (Fig. 29.5)	Striking the ligamentum patellae	Extension of the knee joint	L3, L4 segments of spinal cord intact
Ankle jerk	Striking tendocalcaneus	Plantar flexion of the ankle joint	S1, S2 segments intact
Abdominal reflex	Striking a quadrant of abdomen	Contraction of abdominal muscles	Positive reflex indicates normal pyramidal tract with T7–T12 nerves intact
Plantar reflex	Scratching the sole of foot from lateral side towards big toe	Plantar flexion of the great toe and other toes	A normal plantar response indicates intact pyramidal tract
Babinski's sign (Fig. 29.6)	Same as in plantar reflex	Dorsiflexion of the great toe and fanning of other toes	Babinski's sign indicates pyramidal tract injury, except in infants

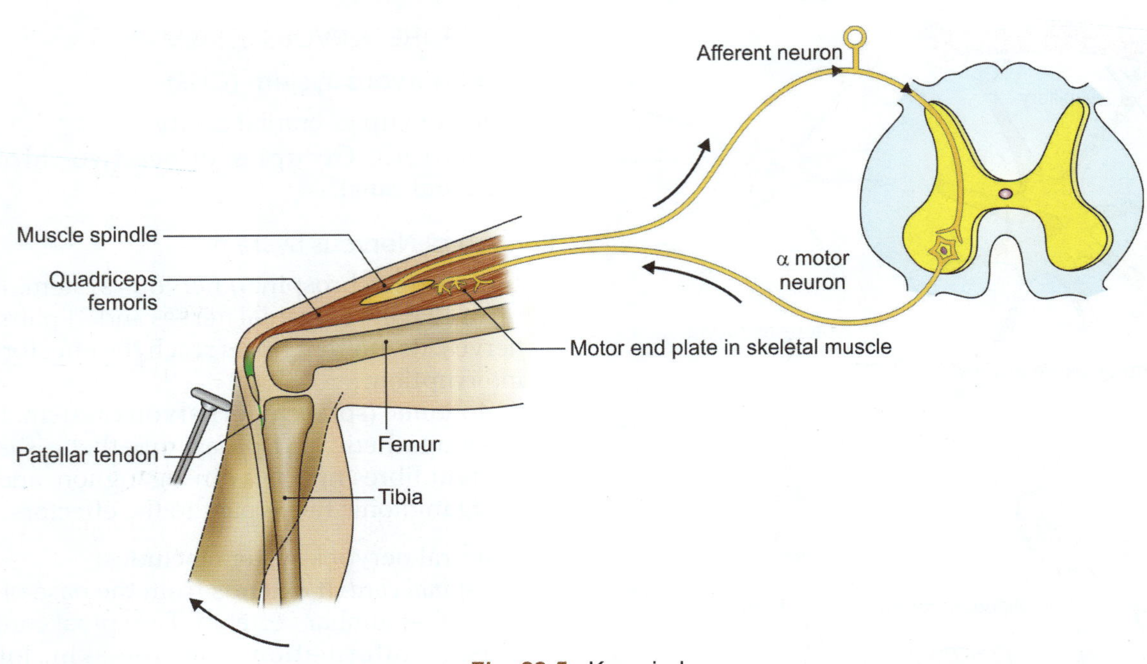

Fig. 29.5: Knee jerk

pressure and respiration control. It resembles the spinal cord in both organization and function.

b. The pons—it lies rostral to the medulla and contains a large number of neurons that relay information from the cerebral hemispheres to the cerebellum.

c. The midbrain—this is the smallest brain stem component which lies rostral to the pons. The midbrain contains essential relay nuclei of the auditory and visual system. Several regions of this structure play and important role in the direct control of eye movement, whereas others are involved in motor control of skeletal muscles.

3 *Cerebellum:* The cerebellum lies dorsal to the pons and medulla. It has a corrugated surface. The cerebellum receives somatosensory imput from the spinal cord, motor information from the cerebral cortex and balance information from the vestibular organs of the inner ear. The cerebellum integrates this information and coordinates the planning, timing and patterning of skeletal muscle contractions during movement. The cerebellum plays a major role in the control of posture, head and eye movements.

The main parts and their subdivisions are shown in Table 29.2 and Fig. 29.7.

Table 29.2: Parts of brain

Parts	*Subdivisions*	*Cavity*
1. Forebrain (prosencephalon)	A. Telencephalon (cerebrum), made up of two cerebral hemispheres and the median part in front of the interventricular foramen	Lateral ventricle
	B. Diencephalon (thalamencephalon), hidden by the cerebrum, consists of : (a) Thalamus (b) Hypothalamus (c) Metathalamus, including the medial and lateral geniculate bodies, and (d) Epithalamus, including the pineal body, habenular trigone and posterior commissure (e) Subthalamus	Third ventricle
2. Midbrain (mesencephalon)	Crus cerebri, substantia nigra, tegmentum, and tectum, from before backwards	Cerebral aqueduct
3. Hindbrain (rhombencephalon)	A. Metencephalon, made up of pons and cerebellum B. Myelencephalon or medulla oblongata	Fourth ventricle

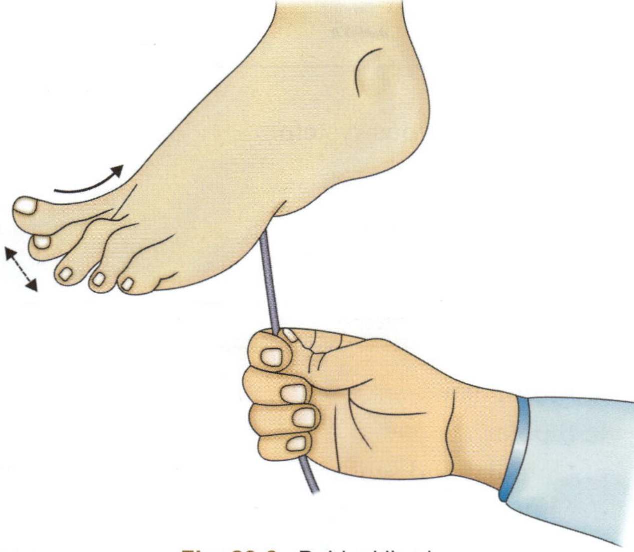

Fig. 29.6: Babinski's sign

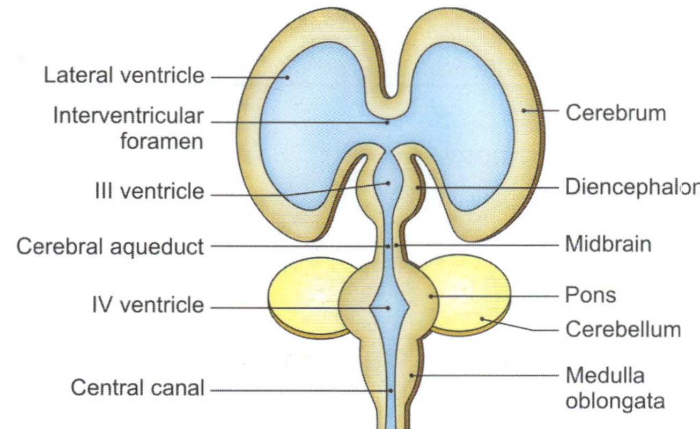

Fig. 29.7: Parts of brain

4 *The diencephalon:* It includes the thalamus and hypothalamus. It is present between the cerebral hemispheres and the midbrain. The thalamus receives almost all sensory and motor information going to the cerebral cortex except smell. It regulates levels of awareness and some emotional aspects of sensory experiences. The hypothalamus lies ventral to the thalamus and regulates autonomic activity and the hormonal secretion by the pituitary gland.

5 *The cerebral hemispheres:* The largest region of the brain. It consists of the cerebral cortex/grey mater and the fibres which form white matter with deeply located nuclei: the basal ganglia, the hippocampal formation and the amygdala. The cerebral hemispheres are cognition, emotion, memory and high motor functions.

The brainstem includes the midbrain, pons and medulla. Hindbrain includes pons, medulla and cerebellum.

CLINICAL ANATOMY

- If a nerve (axons) is injured or cut, a series of degenerative and then regenerative changes follow. The degenerative changes occur in:
  a. *Cell body:* It undergoes chromatolysis. Nissl granules disappear; cell becomes swollen and rounded; and the nucleus is pushed to the periphery.
  b. *The proximal part of the cut fibre:* So long the mother cell is intact, it survives, and only a part near the cut end degenerates in a way similar to the distal part.
  c. *The distal part of the cut fibre:* It degenerates completely. Axis cylinder becomes fragmented; myelin sheath breaks up into fat droplets, and the nuclei of Schwann cells multiply and fill up the neurilemmal tube. During regeneration, the tip of the axon still connected with the cell body begins to grow through the neurilemmal tube. The rate of growth is about 1–2 mm per day in man. Myelin sheath is reformed. Restoration of function may be considerable but rarely complete. The role of neurilemmal tube as a guiding factor to the regenerating proximal axon is considered to be of paramount importance.

Thus a nerve can regenerate because it has a neurilemmal sheath. A tract cannot regenerate because it has no such sheath. However, a tract after demyelination can remyelinate, as is seen in demyelinating diseases.

FACTS TO REMEMBER

- Neurons in human brain are about 180–200 billion.
- Mature neurons do not divide after birth except in olfactory region and in hippocampus.
- If neurons divide one will have fleeting (short time) memory.
- Impulse travels from dendrite to cell body and then into axon.
- Contact between neurons is by contiguity (like hand shake) and not by continuity.
- Human has the largest cerebrum so far.
- Ependymal cells are responsible for the formation of cerebrospinal fluid. Astrocytes form the blood–brain barrier.

Frequently Asked Questions

1. Write short notes on:
   a. Synapse
   b. Neuroglial cells
   c. Parts of nervous system
   d. Reflex arc
   e. Babinski's sign

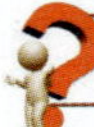

Multiple Choice Questions

1. Branched nerve fibre that convey impulses towards cell body of a neuron is called:
   a. Axon b. Dendrites
   c. Axon collaterals d. Axon terminals
2. Myelin sheath on peripheral nerves is contributed by:
   a. Axon itself
   b. Secretory vesicles
   c. Schwann cells
   d. Cell bodies of neuron
3. A neuron with many dendrites arising from cell body and carrying impulses away from the neuron via the axon is:
   a. Multipolar
   b. Bipolar
   c. Unipolar and sensory
   d. Multipolar and motor
4. The grey appearance of spinal grey matter is due to
   a. Neuronal body b. Neuroglia
   c. Neurites d. Blood vessels
5. Three parts of hindbrain are:
   a. Cerebrum, pons, cerebellum
   b. Pons, medulla oblongata, cerebellum
   c. Pons, midbrain, cerebellum
   d. Thalamus, pons, cerebellum

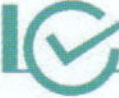

Answers

1. b **2.** c **3.** d **4.** a **5.** b

Chapter 30

Meninges of the Brain and Cerebrospinal Fluid

"Great minds think alike."
—Anonymous

INTRODUCTION

The brain is a very important but delicate organ. It is protected by the following coverings.

1 Bony covering of the cranium.
2 Three membranous coverings (meninges)
  a. The outer dura mater (pachymeninx).
  b. The middle arachnoid mater.
  c. The inner pia mater. The arachnoid and pia are together known as the leptomeninges.
3 The cerebrospinal fluid fills the space between the arachnoid and the pia maters (subarachnoid space) and acts as a water cushion.

DURA MATER

The cerebral dura mater has been studied in detail with the head and neck in Chapter 20. However, it may be recapitulated that it is made up of two layers, an outer endosteal layer and an inner meningeal layer, enclosing the cranial venous sinuses between the two. The meningeal layer forms four folds which divide the cranial cavity into intercommunicating compartments for different parts of the brain (Fig. 30.1 and Table 30.1).

ARACHNOID MATER

The arachnoid mater is a thin transparent membrane that loosely surrounds the brain *without* dipping into its sulci.

Prolongations

1 It provides sheaths for the cranial nerves as far as their exit from the skull.
2 Arachnoid villi are small, finger-like processes of arachnoid tissue, projecting into the cranial venous sinuses. They absorb CSF.

PIA MATER

The pia mater is a thin vascular membrane which closely invests the brain, dipping into various sulci.

Prolongations

1 It provides sheaths for the cranial nerves.

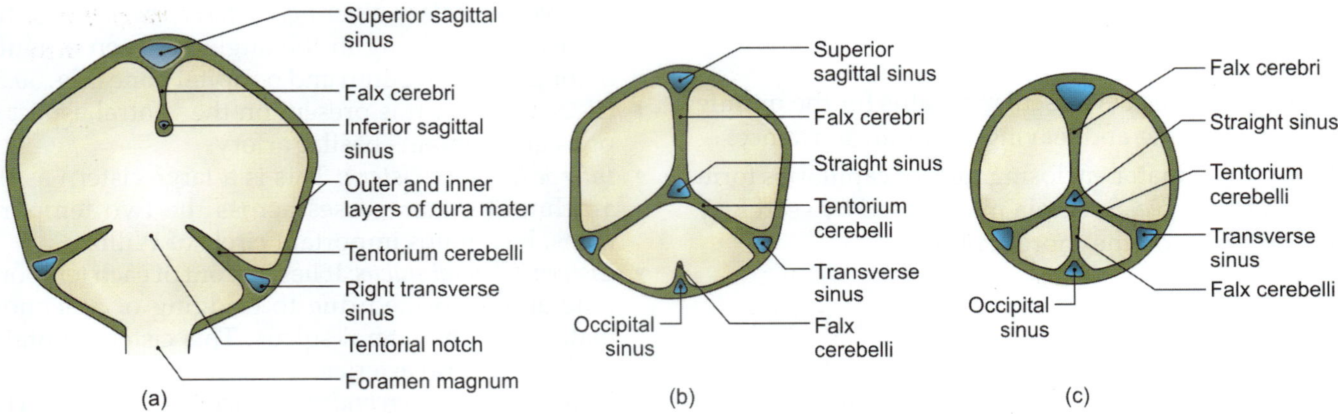

Figs 30.1a to c: Coronal sections through the posterior cranial fossa showing folds of dura mater and the venous sinuses enclosed in them. (a) Section through the tentorial notch (anterior part of the fossa); (b) Section through the middle part of the fossa, and (c) Section through the posterior-most part

Table 30.1: The meningeal layer sends inwards following folds of dura mater

Folds	*Shape*	*Attachments*	*Venous sinuses enclosed*
Falx cerebri (Fig. 30.2)	Sickle-shaped, separates the right from left cerebral hemisphere	Superior, convex margins are attached to sides of the groove lodging the superior sagittal sinus. Inferior concave margin is free Anterior attachment to crista galli, posterior to upper surface of tentorium cerebelli	Superior sagittal sinus Inferior sagittal sinus Straight sinus
Tentorium cerebelli (Fig. 30.3)	Tent-shaped, separates the cerebral hemispheres from hindbrain and lower part of mid-brain Lifts off the weight of occipital lobes from the cerebellum	Has a free anterior margin. Its ends are attached to anterior clinoid processes. Rest is free and concave. Posterior margin is attached to the lips of groove containing transverse sinuses, superior petrosal sinuses and to posterior clinoid processes	Transverse sinuses, superior petrosal sinuses
Falx cerebelli	Small sickle-shaped fold partly separating two cerebellar hemispheres	Base is attached to posterior part of inferior surface of tentorium cerebelli Apex reaches till foramen magnum	Occipital sinus
Diaphragma sellae (Fig. 30.4)	Small horizontal fold	Anterior attachment is to tuberculum sellae Posterior attachment is to dorsum sellae; laterally continuous with dura mater of middle cranial fossa	Anterior and posterior intercavernous sinuses

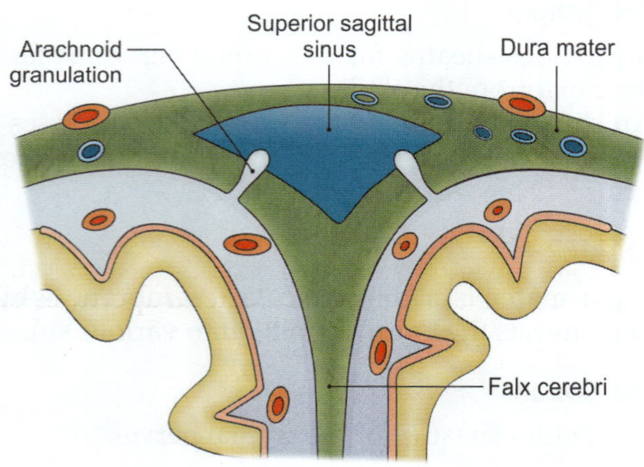

Fig. 30.2: Falx cerebri

2 It also provides perivascular sheaths for the minute vessels entering and leaving the brain substance.

3 Folds of pia mater enclosing tufts of capillaries form the *telachoroidea.* Such pia mater lined by secretory ependyma form the choroid plexus.

EXTRADURAL (EPIDURAL) AND SUBDURAL SPACES

The extradural or epidural space is a potential space between the inner aspect of skull bone and the endosteal layer of dura mater.

The subdural space is also a potential space between the dura and arachnoid maters.

SUBARACHNOID SPACE

This is the space between the arachnoid and the pia maters. It is traversed by a network of arachnoid trabeculae which give it a sponge-like appearance.

The subarachnoid space contains CSF, and large vessels of the brain. Cranial nerves pass through the space.

Larger arteries lie in subarachnoid space. Smaller ones carry sheaths of pia and arachnoid mater.

Cisterns

At the base of the brain and around the brainstem, the subarachnoid space forms intercommunicating pools, called *cisterns.* The subarachnoid cisterns are as follows.

- *Cerebellomedullary cistern or cisterna magna:* It is the largest cistern lying in the angle between medulla oblongata, cerebellum and occipital bone (Fig. 30.5).
- *Cisterna pontis:* It is present on the ventral aspect of pons and contains basilar artery.
- *Interpeduncular cistern:* This is a large cistern as the arachnoid mater passes across the two temporal lobes. It contains important circle of Willis.
- *Cistern of lateral sulcus:* It lies in front of each temporal pole and is formed due to bridging of arachnoid mater over the lateral sulcus. This cistern contains middle cerebral arteries.
- *Cistern of great cerebral vein (cisterna ambiens):* This cistern lies in the space between splenium of corpus callosum and superior surface of cerebellum (Fig. 30.5).

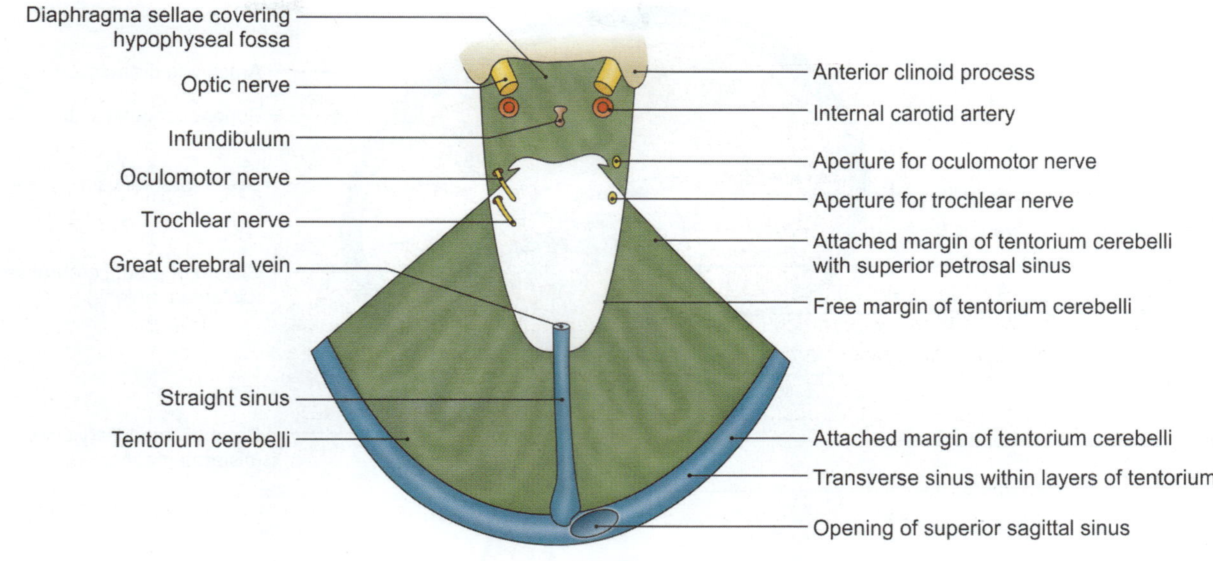

Fig. 30.3: Tentorium cerebelli

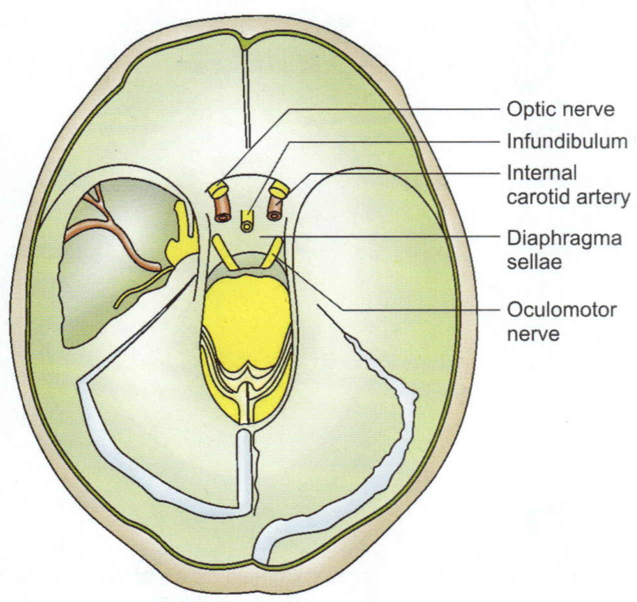

Fig. 30.4: Diaphragma sellae

Communications

The subarachnoid space communicates with the ventricular system of the brain at:

a. A median foramen (of Magendie).
b. Two lateral foramina (of Luschka), situated in the roof of the fourth ventricle. The CSF passes through these foramina from the fourth ventricle to the subarachnoid space.

CEREBROSPINAL FLUID (CSF)

The cerebrospinal fluid is a modified tissue fluid. It is contained in the ventricular system of the brain and in the subarachnoid space around the brain and spinal cord. CSF replaces lymph in the CNS (Fig. 30.6).

Formation

The bulk of the CSF is formed by the choroid plexuses of the lateral ventricles.

The total quantity of CSF is about 150 ml. The normal pressure of CSF is 60 to 100 mm of CSF (or of water).

Circulation

CSF passes from each lateral ventricle to the third ventricle through the interventricular foramen (of Monro). From the third ventricle, it passes to the fourth ventricle through the cerebral aqueduct. From the fourth ventricle, the CSF passes to the subarachnoid space through the median and lateral apertures of the fourth ventricle (Flowchart 30.1).

Absorption

CSF is absorbed chiefly through the arachnoid villi and granulations, and is thus drained into the cranial venous sinuses.

Functions of CSF

1 CSF decreases the sudden pressure or forces on delicate nervous tissue.
2 CSF nourishes nervous tissue. Only CSF comes in contact with neurons. Even blood cannot directly come in contact with neurons. It provides nourishment and returns products of metabolism to the venous sinuses.
3 Neurons cannot live without glucose and oxygen for more than 3–4 minutes. These are constantly provided by CSF.
4 Pineal gland secretions reach pituitary gland via CSF.

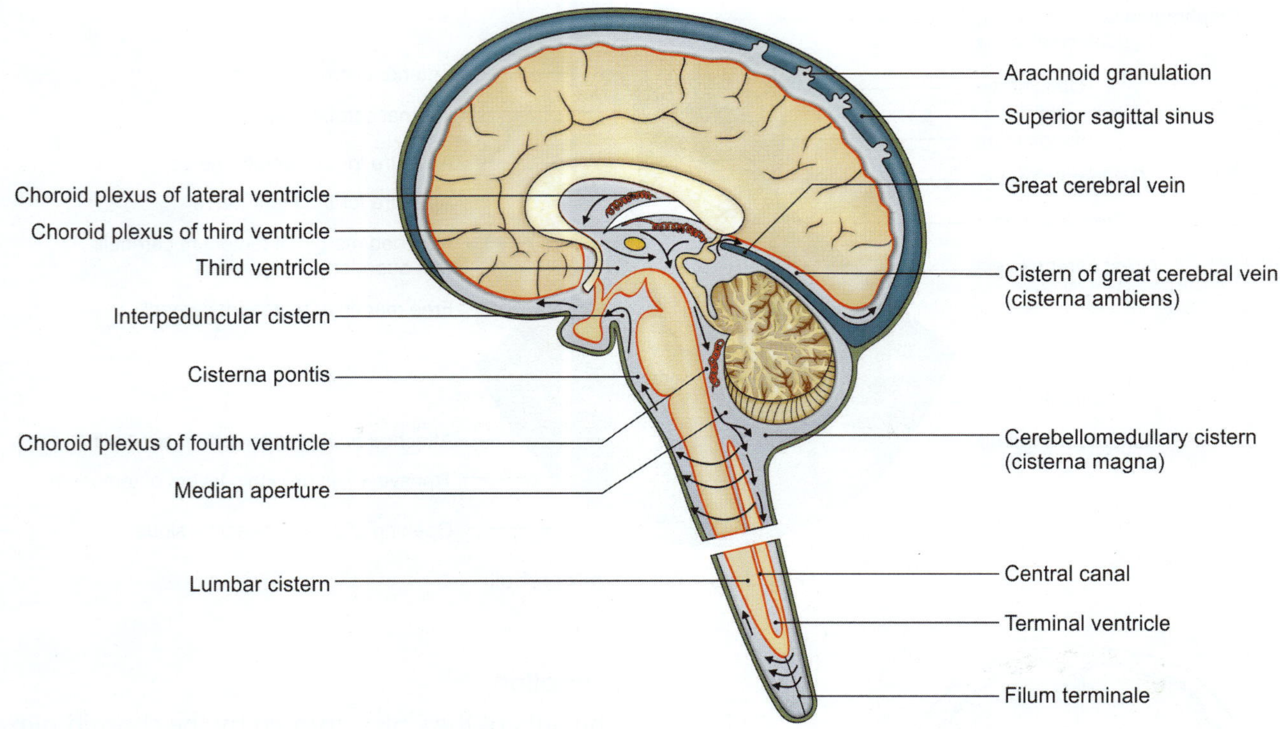

Fig. 30.5: Subarachnoid cisterns

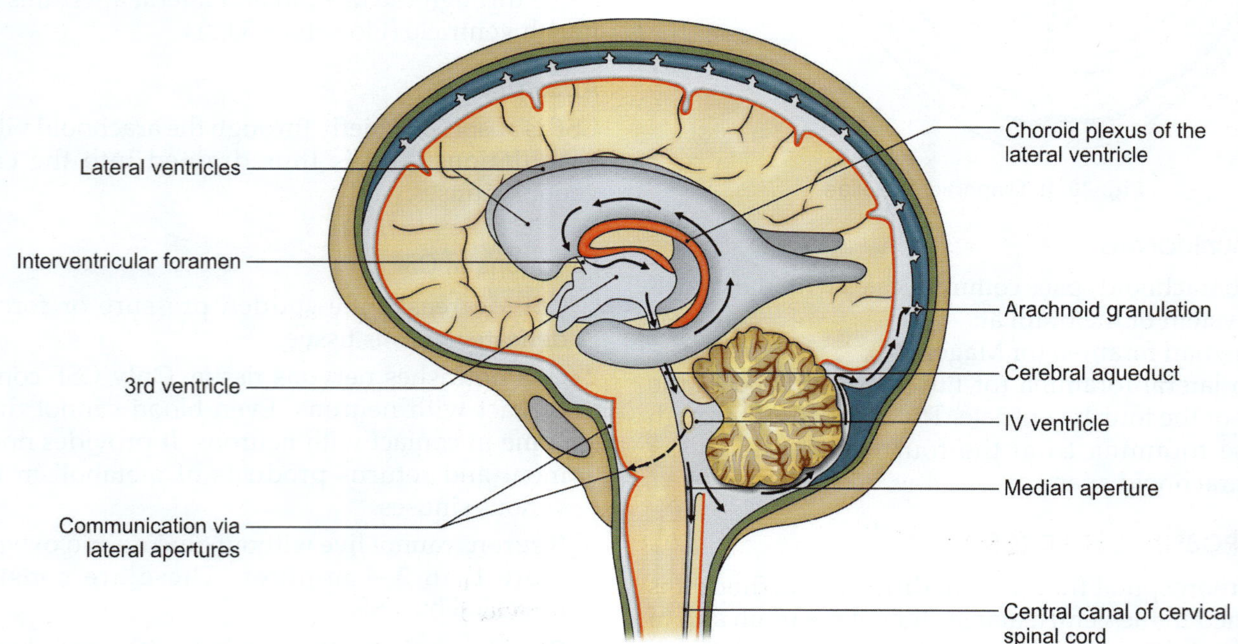

Fig. 30.6: Formation, circulation and absorption of CSF

Flowchart 30.1: Cerebrospinal fluid (CSF)

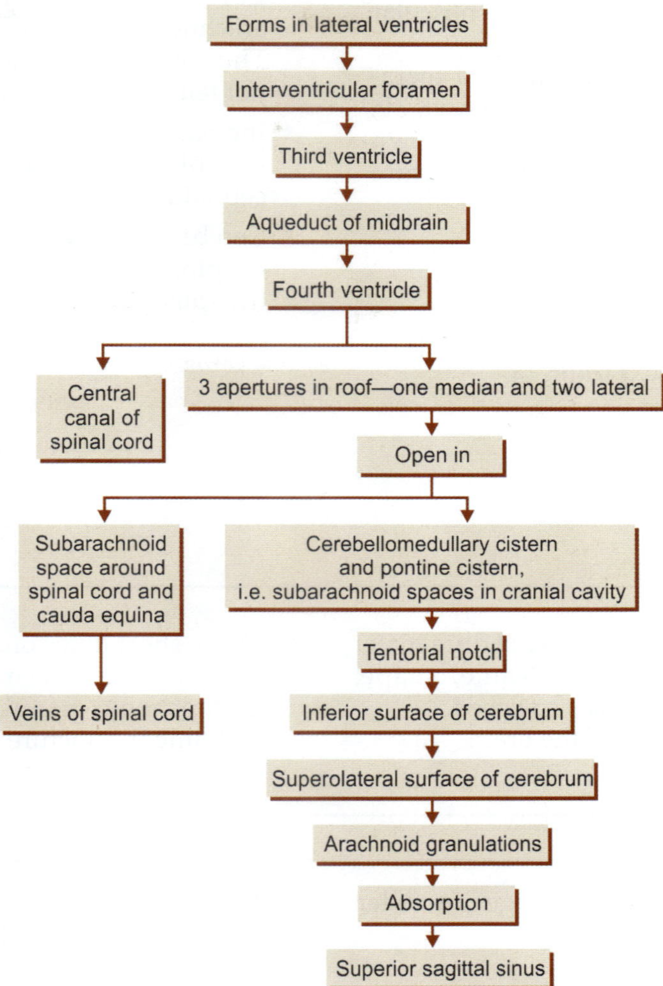

5 A major function of CSF is to cushion the brain within its solid vault. The brain and CSF have approximately the same specific gravity, so that the brain simply floats in the fluid. So a blow to the head moves the entire brain simultaneously, causing no one portion of the brain to be contorted by the blow.

CLINICAL ANATOMY

- CSF can be obtained by
  (a) Lumbar puncture;
  (b) Cisternal puncture; or
  (c) Ventricular puncture.
  Lumbar puncture is the easiest method and is commonly used.
  It is done by passing a needle in the interspace between the third and fourth lumbar spines.
- Biochemical analysis of CSF is of diagnostic value in various diseases.
- Obstruction to the flow of CSF in the ventricular system of the brain leads to *hydrocephalus* in children, and raised intracranial pressure in adults.
- *Hydrocephalus:* It is the dilatation of the ventricular system and occurs due to obstruction of CSF circulation. It may be of the following types:
  a. *Communicating:* If the obstruction is outside the ventricular system, usually in the subarachnoid space or arachnoid granulations, it is termed as communicating. This occurs due to fibrosis following meningitis. It is also called external hydrocephalus.

  Clinical features are:
  - Head size is rather large.
  - Tense anterior fontanelle
  - Dilated veins over thin scalp.

  b. *Non-communicating:* If the obstruction is within the ventricular system. It is called non-communicating or internal hydrocephalus. This is usually caused by a tumour or inflammation

(Figs 22.6a and b). A shunt procedure is employed to divert the CSF from the ventricular system into the peritoneal cavity.
- Drainage of CSF at regular intervals is of therapeutic value in meningitis. Certain intractable headaches of unknown aetiology are also known to have been cured by a mere lumbar puncture with drainage of CSF.

FACTS TO REMEMBER

- Cisterns contain increased amount of CSF to protect the big veins, circle of Willis etc.
- CSF is present outside the brain in the subarachnoid space; within the brain in its ventricles. Thus the brain is floating in CSF and its weight is not felt by the person.
- Increased formation or decreased absorption or any obstruction in its flow leads to hydrocephalus.
- Cerebrospinal fluid is present in the central canal of spinal cord and in subarachnoid space around the spinal cord.

Frequently Asked Questions

1. Describe the folds of meningeal layer of dura mater under the following headings: Name, shape, attachments, and venous sinuses enclosed.
2. Describe the various cisterns of the brain.
3. Write short notes on:
   a. Formation and circulation of CSF
   b. Arachnoid granulations
   c. Lumbar puncture

Multiple Choice Questions

1. Which sequence lists cranial meninges in order from superficial to deep?
   a. Pia, arachnoid, dura
   b. Dura, pia, arachnoid
   c. Dura, arachnoid, pia
   d. Arachnoid, dura, pia
2. In region where two layers of dura mater separate, the gap between them contains:
   a. Dural venous sinus b. Epidural veins
   c. Subdural fluid d. Subarachnoid fluid
3. Largest of cranial dural partition is:
   a. Sella turcica
   b. Falx cerebri
   c. Tentorium cerebelli
   d. Falx cerebelli
4. Dura and arachnoid extend up to the lower border of which vertebra?
   a. 2nd lumbar b. 3rd lumbar
   c. 2nd sacral d. 5th sacral
5. CSF perform which of following functions?
   a. Provide buoyancy for brain
   b. Cushion neural structure from sudden jerks
   c. Deliver nutrition and chemical messengers
   d. All of above

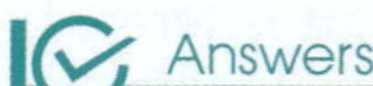

Answers

1. c **2.** a **3.** b **4.** c **5.** d

VIVA VOCE

- Name the meninges of the cranial cavity.
- What venous sinuses lie at the attachments of the tentorium cerebelli?
- How is CSF absorbed?
- Name the cisterns of the brain. Enumerate their contents as well.
- What is the function of diaphragma sellae?
- What artery lies in extradural space?
- What is extradural haematoma?
- Why do we not feel the weight of brain?
- What is function of arachnoid granulations?
- Enumerate the functions of CSF.

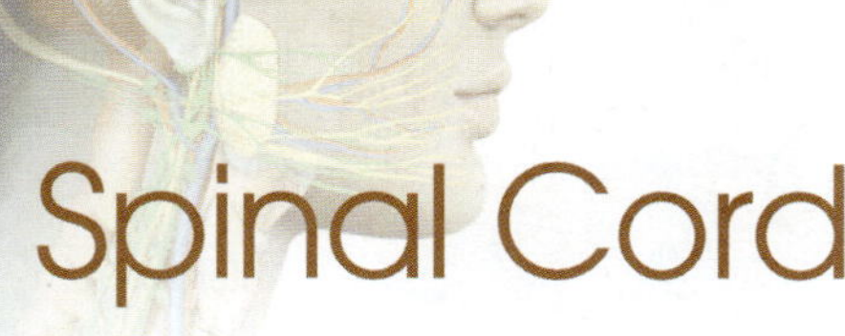

Chapter
31

Spinal Cord

"Learning makes a human fit company for himself."
—Anonymous

INTRODUCTION

The spinal cord is the long cylindrical lower part of central nervous system. It occupies upper two-thirds of vertebral canal. It gives rise to 31 pairs of spinal nerves and retains the basic structural pattern (Fig. 31.1).

Length: It is 18 inches or 45 cm in an adult male.

Extent: It extends from upper border of atlas vertebra to the lower border of first lumbar vertebra in an adult.

As the spinal cord is much shorter than the length of the vertebral column, the spinal segments do not lie opposite the corresponding vertebrae. The level of spinal segment with their vertebral level is shown in Table 31.1.

The spinal cord extends up to the level of first lumbar vertebra as conus medullaris. Below the level of conus medullaris only pia mater is continued as a thin fibrous cord, the filum terminale. The filum terminale is 20 cm long and after leaving through sacral hiatus ends by getting attached to the periosteum of dorsal surface of first segment of coccyx.

The dura and arachnoid along with subarachnoid space containing CSF extend up to 2nd sacral vertebra.

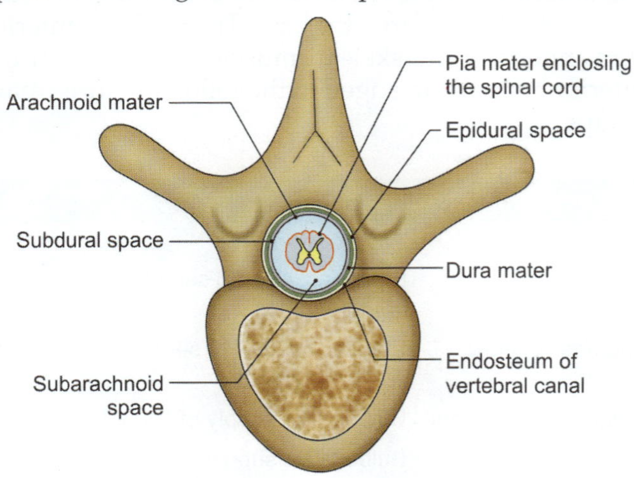

Fig. 31.1: Spinal cord with its meninges

Table 31.1: Level of spinal segment and vertebral levels

Spinal segment	*Vertebral level*
C1–C3	C1–C3
C4–C8	C4–C7
T1–T6	T1–T4
T7–T12	T5–T9
L1–L5	T10–T11
S1–S5 and Co1	T12–L1

Between the lower border of L1 and S2 vertebrae, the subarachnoid space contains 40 spinal nerve roots of L2–L5, S1-S5 and Co1 which constitute the cauda equina.

It is due to this feature that lumbar puncture is done below L2 vertebra without any danger to spinal cord.

Enlargements

Spinal cord presents cervical enlargement for supply of upper limb muscles. This extends from C4 to T2 spinal segments with maximum diameter of 38 mm at the level of C6 segment (Fig. 31.2).

Another enlargement is the lumbar enlargement for supply of muscles of lower limb. It extends from level of L2 to S3 segments. Its maximum diameter 35 mm is at the level of S1 segment.

External Features of Spinal Cord

Anteriorly, the spinal cord reveals a deep anterior median fissure. Posterior median sulcus is a thin longitudinal groove from which a septum runs in the depth of spinal cord (Fig. 31.3).

Internal Structure

White matter, i.e. nerve fibres lie outside and grey matter lies inside. In the centre of grey matter is the central canal containing CSF (Fig. 31.3). The grey matter

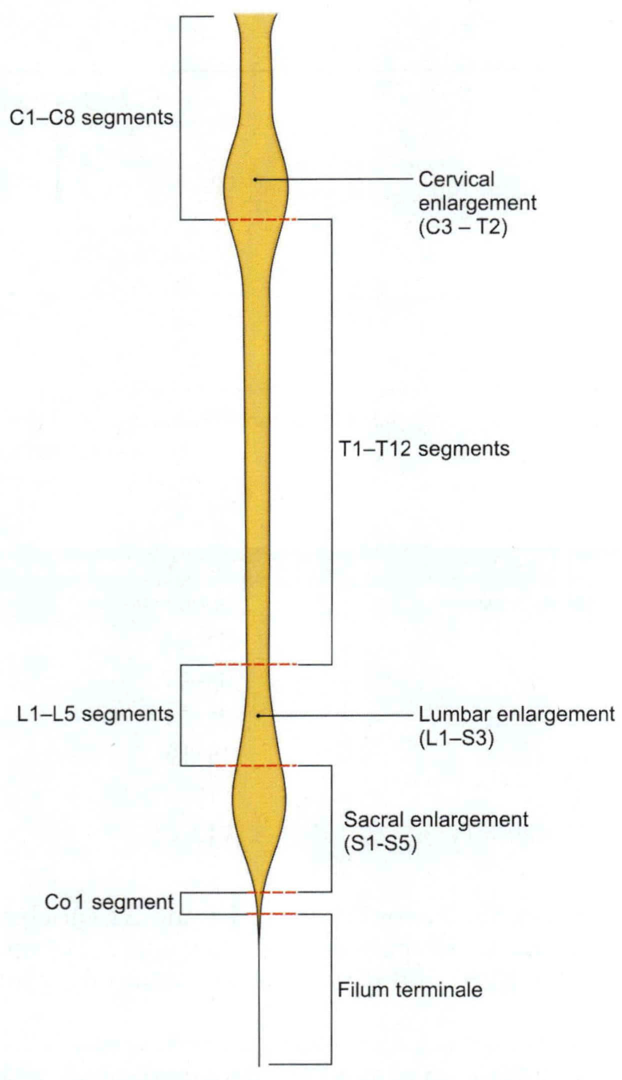

Fig. 31.2: Segmental levels of spinal cord with vertebral level including the enlargements of spinal cord

is in the form of "H" with a grey commissure joining the grey matter of right and left sides.

Grey matter comprises one posterior horn and one anterior horn on each side in the entire extent of the cord. Only in T1–L2 and S2–S4 segments, there is an additional lateral horn for the supply of the viscera. This is part of autonomic nervous system.

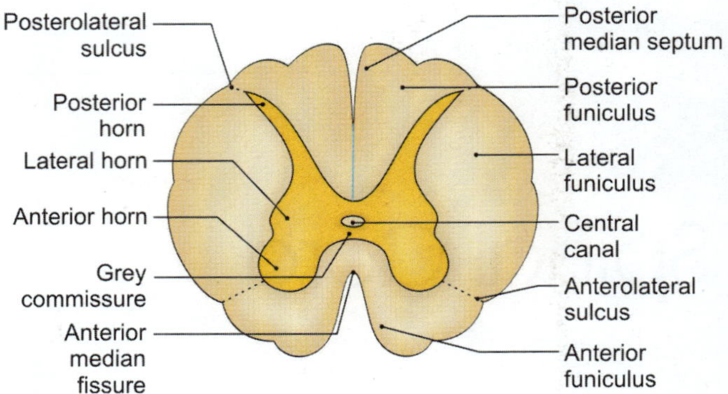

Fig. 31.3: Transverse section of thoracic segment of spinal cord

Shape and size of the horns differ in different segments due to functional reasons. These are placed in Table 31.2.

SPINAL NERVES

Spinal nerves arise in pairs, 8 cervical, 12 thoracic, 5 lumbar, 5 sacral, 1 coccygeal (Fig. 31.4). Each spinal nerve arises by a series of dorsal and ventral nerve rootlets. These rootlets unite in or near the intervertebral foramen to form the spinal nerve (Fig. 31.5).

Spinal Segment

Segment or part of spinal cord to which a pair of dorsal nerve roots, right and left and a pair of ventral nerve roots is attached is called a spinal segment.

NUCLEI OF SPINAL CORD

The grey matter of spinal cord is arranged in three horns. Anterior is motor, lateral being visceral efferent and afferent in function, and posterior is sensory in function.

Nuclei in Anterior Grey Column or Horn

The anterior horn is divided into a ventral part—the head and a dorsal part—the base. The nuclei in anterior horn innervate the skeletal muscles. The cells in the anterior horn are arranged in the following three main groups.

Table 31.2: Shape of horns in different segments of spinal cord

Segments of spinal cord	*Posterior horn*	*Lateral horn*	*Anterior horn*
Cervical, oval shape	Slender	Absent	Broad in C4 to C8 segments for supply of upper limbs
Thoracic, circular shape	Slender	Present for thoracolumbar outflow	Slender in T3–T12 segments, broad in T1–T2 segments
Lumbar, circular shape	Bulbous	Present only in lumbar 1–2 segments	Bulbous for supply of lower limbs
Sacral, circular but smaller	Thick	Present in sacral 2–4 segments for sacral outflow	Bulbous for supply of lower limbs

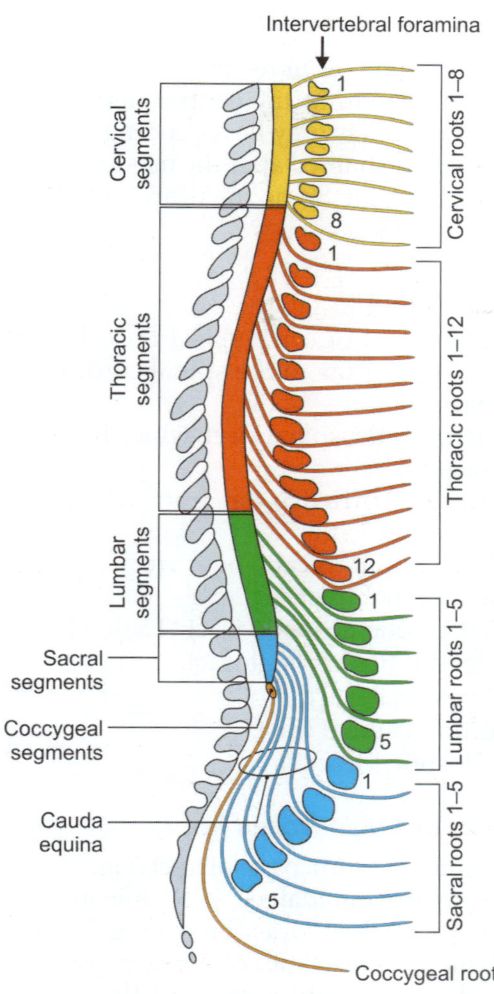

Fig. 31.4: Spinal cord with its 31 pairs of spinal nerves

a. *Medial group:* It is present throughout the entire extent of spinal cord and innervates the axial muscles of the body (Fig. 31.6).
b. *Lateral group:* Present only in the cervical and lumbar enlargements and supplies musculature of limbs.
c. *Central group:* Only in upper cervical segments as phrenic nerve nucleus and nucleus of spinal root of accessory nerve.

Nuclei in Lateral Horn

Nuclei in lateral horn are as follows:

a. *Intermediolateral nucleus:* This acts as both efferent and afferent nuclear columns. This nucleus is seen at two levels.
   i. From T1 to L2 segments, giving rise to preganglionic sympathetic fibres (thoracolumbar outflow).
   ii. From S2 to S4 segments, giving rise to preganglionic parasympathetic fibres chiefly for the pelvic viscera.

   At these two levels, the intermediolateral cell column receives visceral afferent fibres.
b. *Intermediomedial nucleus:* This is mostly internuncial neuronal column.

Nuclei in Posterior Grey Column

Afferent Nuclear Group Column

The four main afferent nuclei are seen in this are:

i. *Posteromarginal nucleus:* Thin layer of neurons caps the posterior horn. It receives some of incoming dorsal root fibres.

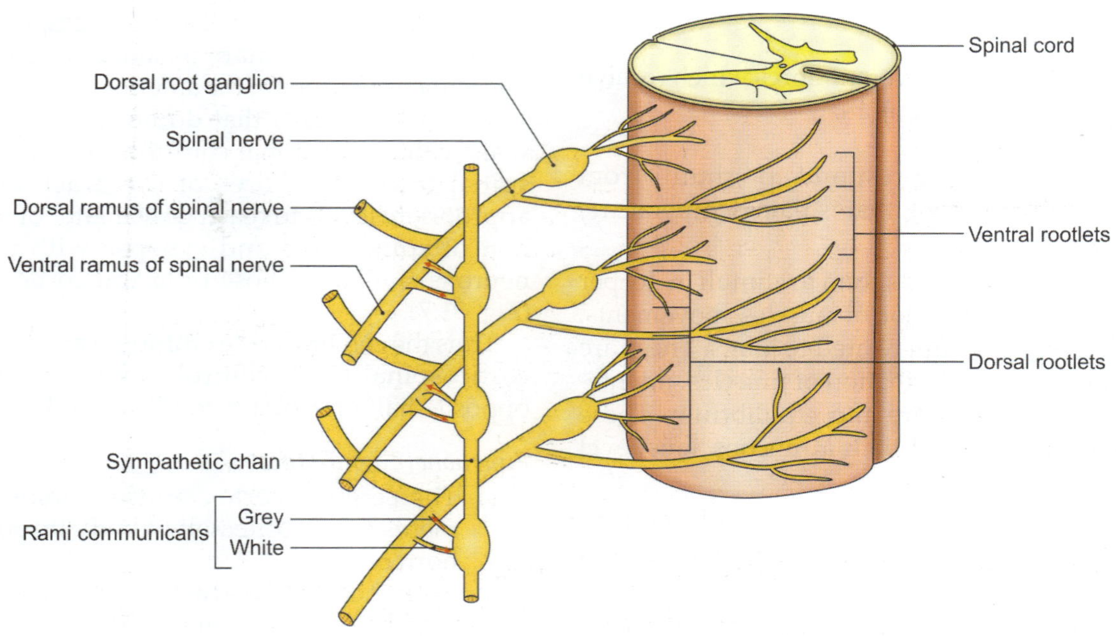

Fig. 31.5: Typical spinal nerve with sympathetic trunk

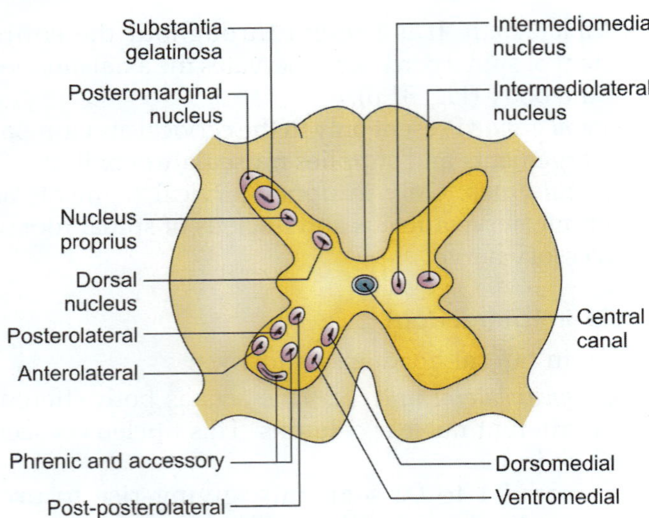

Fig. 31.6: Cell groups in spinal cord

ii. *Substantia gelatinosa:* This is found at the tip of posterior horn through the entire extent of spinal cord. It acts as a relay station for pain and temperature fibres. Its axons give rise to the lateral spinothalamic tract.

iii. *Nucleus proprius:* It lies subjacent to the substantia gelatinosa (Fig. 31.6).

iv. *Nucleus dorsalis* also known as thoracic nucleus at the medial part of base of posterior horn extending from C8 to L3 segments. It is a relay nuclear column for reflex or unconscious proprioceptive impulses to the cerebellum and its axons give rise to the posterior spinocerebellar tract.

SENSORY RECEPTORS

The peripheral endings of afferent fibres which receive impulses are known as receptors.

Functional classification:

i. *Exteroceptors:* These respond to stimuli from external environment, that is pain, temperature, touch and pressure.

ii. *Proprioceptors:* These respond to stimuli in deeper tissues that is contraction of muscles, movements, position and pressure related to joints. These are responsible for coordination of muscles, maintenance of body posture and equilibrium. These actions are perceived both at unconscious level and at conscious level.

iii. *Interoceptors/enteroceptors:* These include receptor end-organs in the walls of viscera, glands and blood vessels.

iv. *Special sense receptors:* These are concerned with vision, hearing, smell, balance and taste.

TRACTS OF THE SPINAL CORD

A collection of nerve fibres that connects two masses of grey matter within the central nervous system is called a tract. Tracts may be ascending or descending. They are usually named after the masses of grey matter connected by them. Some tracts are called fasciculi or lemnisci.

Descending Tracts

A. The pyramidal or *corticospinal tract* descends from the cerebral cortex to the spinal cord. It consists of two parts:
   1. Lateral corticospinal tract, which lies in the lateral funiculus.
   2. Anterior corticospinal tract which lies in the anterior funiculus.

B. Extrapyramidal tracts. These are:
   1. Rubrospinal tract.
   2. Medial reticulospinal tract (Table 31.3).
   3. Lateral reticulospinal tract.
   4. Olivospinal tract.
   5. Vestibulospinal tract.
   6. Tectospinal tract.

Pyramidal or Corticospinal Tract

The pyramidal or corticospinal tract (Fig. 31.7) is formed by the axons of pyramidal cells predominantly lying in the motor area of cerebral cortex. From here, the fibres course through the posterior limb of internal capsule, midbrain, pons and medulla oblongata. At the lower level of medulla oblongata, 80% of fibres cross to the opposite side. This is known as pyramidal decussation. The fibres that have crossed enter lateral column of white matter of spinal cord and descend as lateral corticospinal tract. Most of these fibres terminate by synapsing through the internuncial neurons at the anterior horn cells.

The 20% of fibres that do not cross enter anterior white column of spinal cord to form anterior corticospinal tract. The fibres of this tract also cross at appropriate levels to reach grey matter of the opposite half of spinal cord and synapse with internuncial neurons similar to those of lateral corticospinal tract (Fig. 31.7).

Thus the cerebral cortex through lateral and anterior corticospinal tracts controls anterior horns cells of opposite half of spinal cord (Table 31.3).

Functional Significance

i. The cerebral cortex controls voluntary movements of opposite half of body through anterior horn cells.

ii. Influence of this tract is supposed to be facilitatory for flexors and inhibitory for extensors. Extrapyramidal tracts are show in Table 31.3.

Table 31.3: The descending tracts

Name	*Function*	*Crossed uncrossed*	*Beginning*	*Termination*
Pyramidal tracts				
A1. Lateral corticospinal	Main motor tract for skillful voluntary movements	Crossed in medulla	Motor area of cortex area number 4,6	Anterior grey column cells alpha motor neurons
A2. Anterior corticospinal	Facilitates flexors	Crosses in corresponding spinal segement	Motor area of cortex area number 4,6	Anterior grey column cells alpha motor neurons
Extrapyramidal tracts				
B1. Rubrospinal	Efferent pathway for cerebellum and corpus striatum	Crossed	Red nucleus of midbrain	Anterior grey column cells
B2. Medial reticulospinal	Extrapyramidal tract Facilitates extensors	Uncrossed	Reticular formation of grey matter of pons	Anterior grey column cells (interneurons)
B3. Lateral reticulospinal	Extrapyramidal tract Facilitates flexors	Uncrossed and crossed	Reticular formation of grey matter of medulla oblongata	Anterior grey column cells (interneurons)
B4. Olivospinal (Fig. 31.8)	Extrapyramidal tract	Uncrossed	Inferior olivary nucleus	Anterior grey column cells
B5. Lateral vestibulospinal	Efferent pathway for equilibratory control	Uncrossed	Lateral vestibular nucleus	Anterior grey column cells
B6. Tectospinal	Efferent pathway for visual reflexes	Crossed	Superior colliculus	Anterior grey column cells

Ascending Tracts

1. Lateral spinothalamic tract (Fig. 31.9)
2. Anterior spinothalamic tract
3. Fasciculus gracilis (medially)
4. Fasciculus cuneatus (laterally)
5. Dorsal or posterior spinocerebellar tract
6. Ventral or anterior spinocerebellar tract
7. Spino-olivary tract
8. Spinotectal tract.

For the sensory pathways, the first neuron fibres always start in the dorsal root ganglia which has pseudounipolar cells. The peripheral process of these cells form the sensory fibres of peripheral nerves. The central process of the neurons in the dorsal root ganglia enter the spinal cord through dorsal nerve root and terminate either by synapsing with cells in posterior grey column of spinal cord or at higher level in the medulla oblongata with the cells of nucleus gracilis and nucleus cuneatus.

After relay in the nuclei, second neuron fibres start and ascend to either thalamus or cerebellum. The cerebellum finally recieves second neurons fibres, whereas from the thalamus relayed third neuron fibres are projected to the sensory areas in the cerebral cortex (Table 31.4).

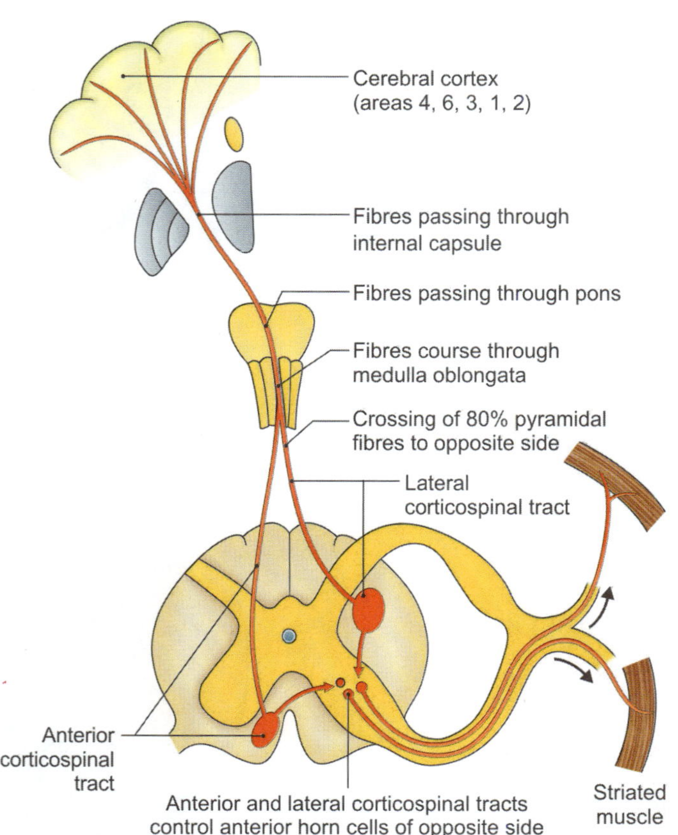

Fig. 31.7: Course of corticospinal fibres

Fine touch, pressure, vibration, movement, position
C
Th
L
S
Fasciculus gracilis
Fasciculus cuneatus
Posterolateral tract
Posterior spinocerebellar tract
Lateral spinothalamic tract
Anterior spinocerebellar tract
Spino-olivary tract
Anterior spinothalamic tract
Medial reticulospinal
Lateral corticospinal tract
Rubrospinal tract
Lateral reticulospinal
Intersegmental tract
Anterior corticospinal tract
Olivospinal tract
Vestibulospinal tract
Tectospinal tract
C-Cervical
Th-Thoracic
L-Lumbar
S-Sacral
Pain
Temp
Touch
Pressure

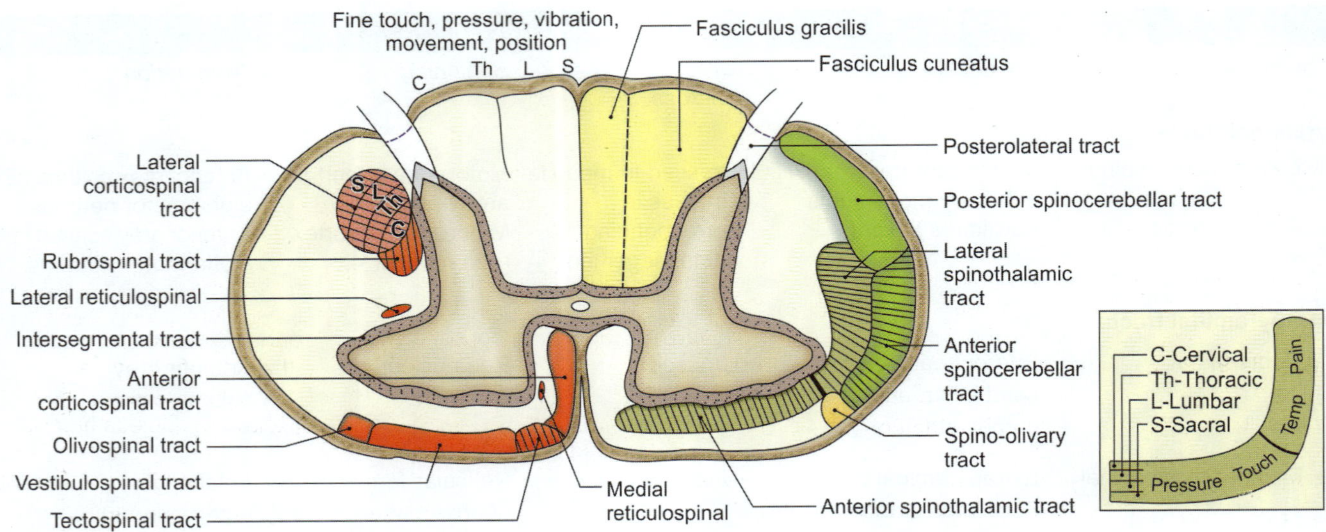

Fig. 31.8: Location of descending tracts in spinal cord (shown only on one side)

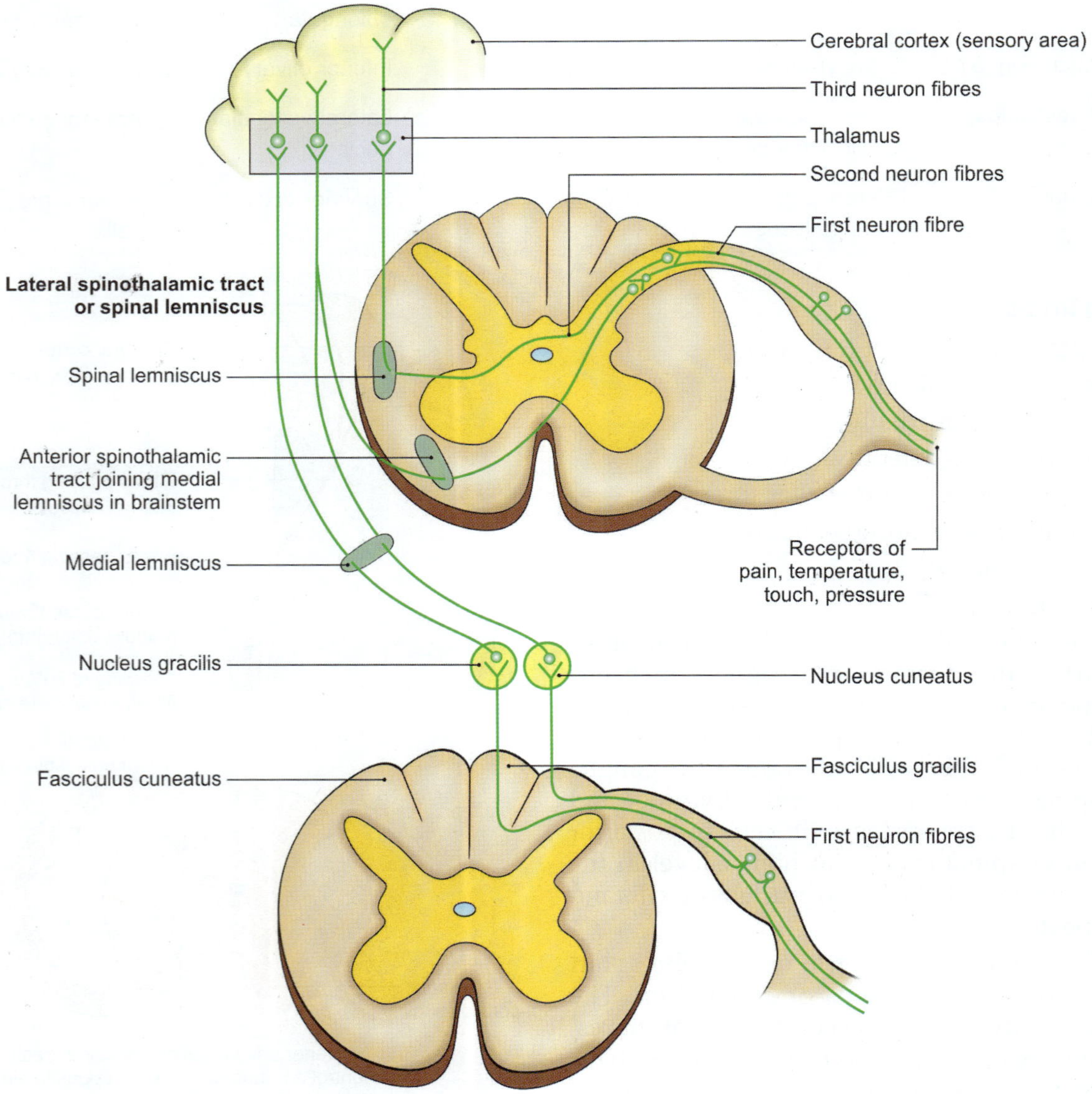

Cerebral cortex (sensory area)
Third neuron fibres
Thalamus
Second neuron fibres
First neuron fibre
Lateral spinothalamic tract or spinal lemniscus
Spinal lemniscus
Anterior spinothalamic tract joining medial lemniscus in brainstem
Medial lemniscus
Receptors of pain, temperature, touch, pressure
Nucleus gracilis
Nucleus cuneatus
Fasciculus cuneatus
Fasciculus gracilis
First neuron fibres

Fig. 31.9: Pathway of posterior funiculus tracts and anterior with lateral spinothalamic tracts

Table 31.4: The ascending tracts of the spinal cord

Name	*Function*	*Crossed/ uncrossed*	*Beginning*	*Termination*
1. Lateral spinothalamic (axons of 2nd order neurons) (Fig. 31.9)	Pain and temperature from opposite half of body	Crosses to opposite side in the same spinal segment	Substantia gelatinosa of posterior grey column	Forms spinal lemniscus in medulla, reaches postero-lateral ventral nucleus of thalamus for another relay and ends in areas 3, 1, 2
2. Anterior spinothalamic (axons of 2nd order neurons) (Fig. 31.9)	Touch (crude) and pressure from opposite half of body	Ascends to 2–3 spinal segments to cross to opposite side	Posterior grey column of opposite side	Joins spinal lemniscus in brainstem reaches postero-lateral ventral nucleus of thalamus for another relay and ends in areas 3, 1, 2
3. Fasciculus gracilis (axons of 1st order sensory neurons) (Fig. 31.9)	Conscious proprioception Discriminatory touch Vibratory sense Stereognosis	Uncrossed in spinal cord, crosses in medulla oblongatea	Dorsal root ganglion cells	Relays in nucleus gracilis, 2nd order fibres cross to form medial lemniscus which reaches posterolateral ventral nucleus of thalamus for another relay and ends in areas 3, 1, 2
4. Fasciculus cuneatus (axons of 1st order sensory neurons) (Fig. 31.9)	Same as above	Same as above	Same as above	Relays in nucleus cuneatus, rest is same as above
5. Posterior spinocerebellar (axons of 2nd order neurons) (Fig. 31.10)	Unconscious proprioception from individual muscles of lower limb	Uncrossed	Thoracic nucleus of posterior grey column	Vermis of cerebellum (via inferior cerebellar peduncle)
6. Anterior spinocerebellar (axons of 2nd order neurons) (Fig. 31.11)	Unconscious proprioception from lower limb as a whole	Crosses twice, once in spinal cord and recrosses in midbrain	Posterior grey column same side	Vermis of cerebellum (via superior cerebellar peduncle) via re-crossing
7. Spino-olivary (axons of 2nd order neurons)	Proprioceptive sense	Uncrossed	Posterior grey column	Dorsal and medial accessory olivary nuclei
8. Spinotectal (axons of 2nd order neurons)	Afferent limb of reflex movements of eyes and head towards source of stimulation	Crossed	Posterior grey column of opposite side	Tectum or superior colliculus of midbrain

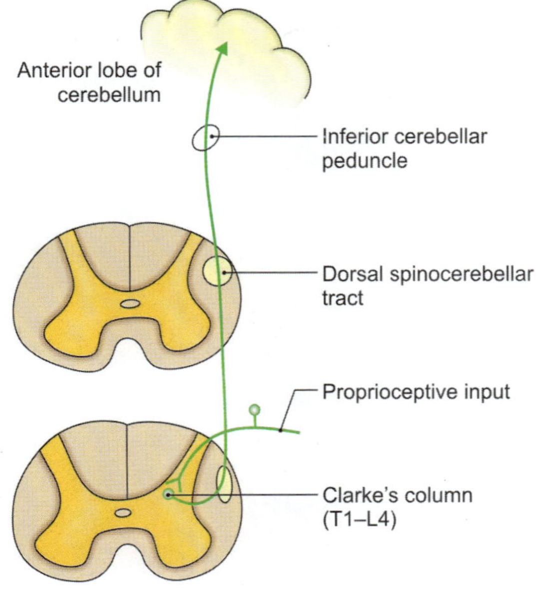

Fig. 31.10: Pathway of posterior spinocerebellar tract

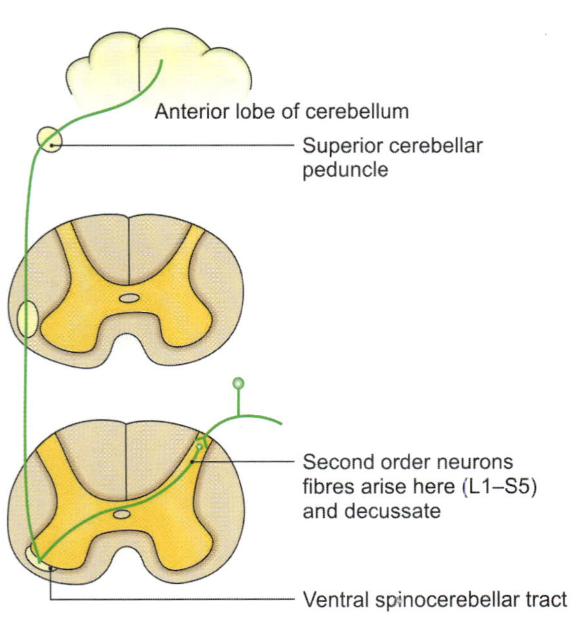

Fig. 31.11: Pathway of anterior spinocerebellar tract

Table 31.5: Comparison between lower motor neuron (LMN) and upper motor neuron (UMN) paralysis

LMN paralysis	*UMN paralysis*
Muscle tone abolished	Muscle tone increased
Leads to flaccid paralysis	Leads to spastic paralysis
Muscles atrophy later	No atrophy of muscles
Reaction of degeneration seen	Reaction of degeneration not seen
Tendon reflexes absent	Tendon reflexes exaggerated
Limited damage	Extensive damage
Ipsilateral	Mostly contralateral

CLINICAL ANATOMY

- *Syringomyelia:* There is formation of cavities around the central canal usually in the lower cervical region. Its features are:
  a. Bilateral loss of pain and temperature occurs due to injury to the decussating fibres of lateral spinothalamic fibres.
  b. Bilateral loss of touch occurs due to injury to anterior spinothalamic tract.

  As the decussation of lateral and anterior spinothalamic tracts occurs at different levels, there is dissociated sensory loss.

  As this disease occurs in lower cervical and upper thoracic regions there is problem in both the upper limbs and front of chest.

  Syringomyelia disrupts the crossing fibres of anterolateral system. The medial lemniscal system is spared.
- *Tabes dorsalis*: It occurs during tertiary stage of syphilis. There is degenerative lesions of dorsal nerve roots and of posterior white columns. Its feature is severe pain in lower limbs, as the disease occurs in lower thoracic and lumbosacral segments, lower limbs are affected.
- *Poliomyelitis:* It is a viral disease which involves anterior horn cells leading to flaccid paralysis of the affected segments. It is a lower motor neuron paralysis.

FACTS TO REMEMBER

- Spinal cord shows cervical enlargement for the supply of upper limb muscles. It also shows lumbosacral enlargement for the supply of lower limb muscles.
- Spinal cord in adult is much shorter than the vertebral canal. The cord ends at the lower border of lumbar one vertebra.
- Lateral horn is only present in T1–L2 and S2–S4 segments of spinal cord.
- Sympathetic fibres (white ramus communicans) start from lateral horn → ventral root → trunk of spinal nerve → ventral primary ramus → sympathetic ganglion (Fig. 31.8).
- The sympathetic ganglion gives grey ramus communicans (grc), after receiving and relaying the white ramus communicans (wrc).
- Corticospinal fibres cross to the opposite side; 80% cross in pyramidal decussation, rest 20% cross in the spinal cord gradually.
- Poliomyelitis virus affects the neurons of anterior horn cells of the spinal cord. Polio drops as a vaccine has finished the dreadful disease.

Frequently Asked Questions

1. Describe the ascending tracts of spinal cord.
2. Describe the descending tracts of spinal cord.
3. Write short notes on:
   a. Sensory receptors
   b. Nuclei in posterior grey column
   c. Syringomyelia
   d. Differences between upper motor neuron and lower motor neuron paralyses

Multiple Choice Questions

1. In spinal cord, myelin sheath is formed by:
   a. Schwann cells
   b. Oligodendrocytes
   c. Astrocytes
   d. Microglia
2. Medial lemniscus carries:
   a. Pain and temperature sensation from trunk and limbs
   b. Proprioceptive sensations from trunk and limbs
   c. Proprioceptive sensation from head
   d. Auditory sensation
3. Regarding spinal cord, the following are true *except:*
   a. It has cervical and lumbar enlargements
   b. It ends at lower border of 3rd lumbar vertebra
   c. It is traversed by the central canal
   d. It begins at level of foramen magnum as a continuation of medulla oblongata
4. Regarding corticospinal tract all of the following are true *except:*
   a. Most of fibres decussate at lower end of medulla oblongata
   b. It arises from motor area of cerebral cortex
   c. It ends in anterior horn cells
   d. Its lesion at level of pons produces paralysis of ipsilateral side
5. Injury of lateral spinothalamic tract results in:
   a. Ipsilateral loss of pain and temperature
   b. Contralateral loss of touch and pressure
   c. Contralateral loss of pain and temperature
   d. None of above

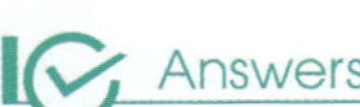

Answers

1. b **2.** b **3.** b **4.** d **5.** c

VIVA VOCE

- Name the meninges present in brain.
- Where does spinal cord end in an adult and in a child?
- Is there a real ascent of spinal cord?
- What is vertebral level of C1–C8 spinal nerves.
- Where does spinal segments S1–S5 and Co 1 lie in relation to the vertebrae.
- How and why is cauda equina formed?
- Which segments of spinal cord have the lateral horns? Where do these lie in relation to vertebral levels?
- Where are the enlargements in the spinal cord and why?
- Name the functional sensory receptors.
- Name the pyramidal tracts.
- Name the extrapyramidal tracts.
- Name the ascending tracts of spinal cord.

Chapter

32

Cranial Nerves

"Difficult does not mean impossible, it simply means you have to work hard."
—Anonymous

The 12 pairs of cranial nerves supply muscles of eyeball, face, palate, pharynx, larynx, tongue and two large muscles of neck. Besides these are afferent to special senses like smell, sight, hearing, taste and touch. Some nerves form the afferent loop and others form the efferent loop of the reflex arc. Optic nerve is afferent from eye while III, IV and VI are efferent to the eye muscles. Statoacoustic nerve is afferent for hearing and balance while spinal root accessory acts as its efferent component for turning the face to the side from where sound is heard. VII, IX and X are carrying sensation of taste from tongue and efferent component is XII nerve for movements of tongue and nucleus ambiguus which gives fibres to IX, X, and cranial root of XI for the muscles of palate, pharynx and larynx.

Olfactory takes the sense of smell and stimulates dorsal nucleus of vagus for enhanced secretion, if the smell is good. CN V, the largest cranial nerve, is mainly sensory to the face. The motor nerve of face is VII nerve. To come close to V nerve nucleus, VII nucleus winds around VI nucleus so that a reflex arc can be mediated between the afferent and efferent loops of the arc.

CRANIAL NERVES

There are 12 pairs of cranial nerves. Each cranial nerve has a number and a name as follows.

		Mnemonic	*Mnemonic*
I	Olfactory	oh,	oh,
II	Optic	oh,	oh,
III	Oculomotor	oh,	oh,
IV	Trochlear	try,	to
V	Trigeminal	try,	touch
VI	Abducent	again	and
VII	Facial	failure,	feel
VIII	Vestibulocochlear (or statoacoustic)	victory	very
IX	Glossopharyngeal	give	giant
X	Vagus	value	volcano
XI	Accessory	and	ahh
XII	Hypoglossal	happiness	hot

Out of these, the I and II nerves are attached to the forebrain; the III and IV to the midbrain; the V, VI, VII and VIII to the pons; and the IX, X, XI, and XII to the medulla (Fig. 32.1).

The olfactory, optic nerves have no nuclei. The nuclei connected to the remaining nerves are as follows. Note that several cranial nerves are connected to more than one nucleus; and that some nuclei contribute fibres to more than one nerve.

EMBRYOLOGY

During early stages of development, the wall of the neural tube is made up of three layers:

a. The inner ependymal layer.
b. The middle mantle layer.
c. The outer marginal layer.

The mantle layer represents grey matter and the marginal layer, the white matter.

Soon the mantle layer differentiates into a dorsal alar lamina (sensory) and a ventral basal lamina (motor), the two are partially separated internally by the sulcus limitans.

In the spinal cord, though grey matter forms a compact fluted column in the centre, it shows differentiation into two somatic and two visceral functional columns. The somatic columns are the general somatic efferent (motor or anterior horn) and the general somatic afferent (sensory or posterior horn); they supply structures derived from somites. The visceral columns are the general visceral efferent (motor) and the general visceral afferent (sensory); these are autonomic columns and supply the viscera, vessels and glands.

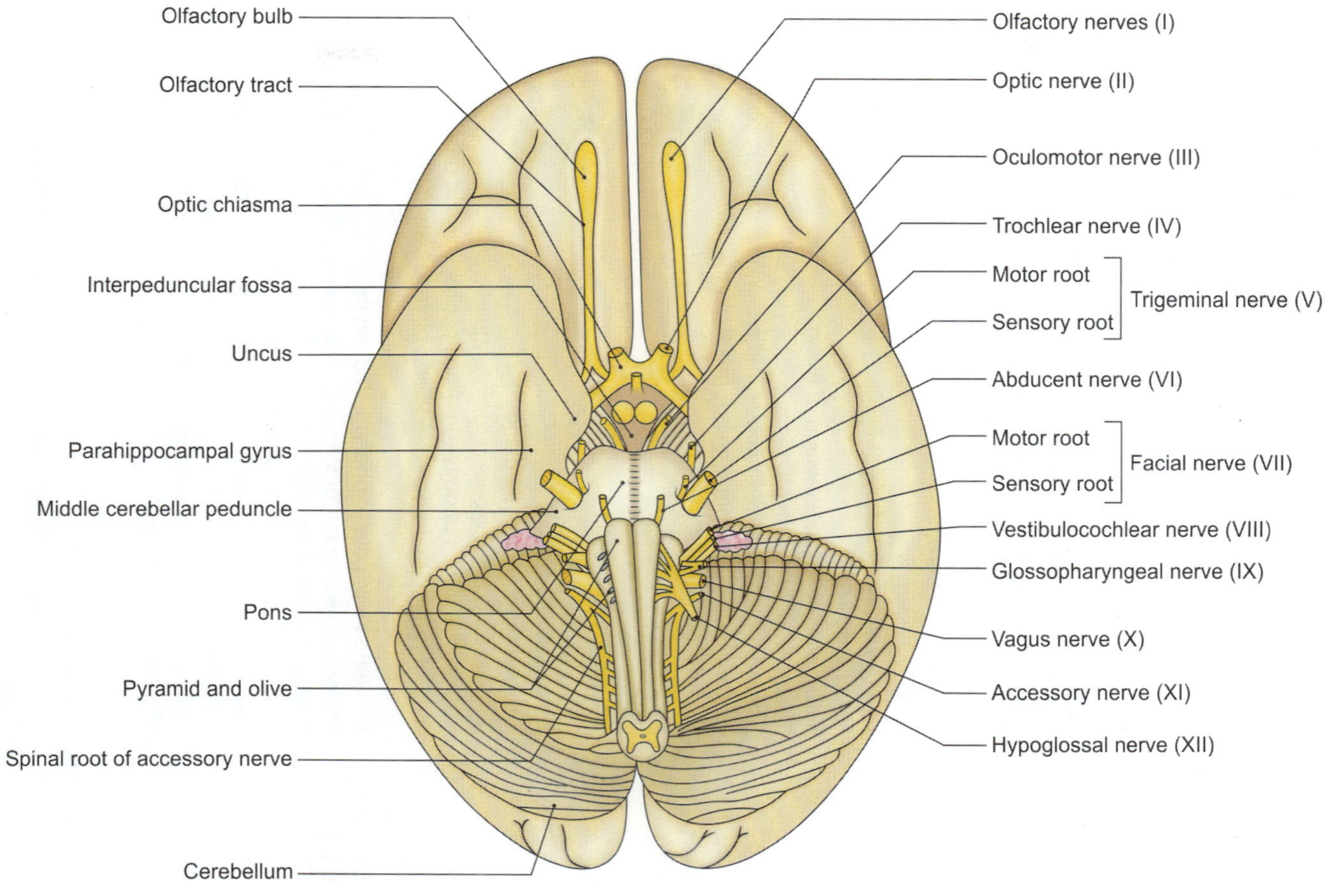

Fig. 32.1: Attachment of cranial nerves to the base of brain

In the brainstem, particularly hindbrain, the alar and basal laminae come to lie in the same ventral plane because of stretching of the roof plate (dorsal wall) of neural tube by pontine flexure. Further, the grey matter forms separate longitudinal functional columns, where the motor columns (from basal lamina) are medial and the sensory columns (from alar lamina) lateral in position.

In addition to the four functional columns differentiated in the spinal cord, there appear two more columns (a motor and a sensory) for the branchial apparatus of the head region, namely the special visceral (branchial) efferent and the special visceral afferent; and one column more for the special senses, namely the special somatic afferent. Thus a total of seven columns (3 motor and 4 sensory) are formed. Each column, in its turn, breaks up into smaller fragments to form nuclei of the cranial nerves (Fig. 32.2).

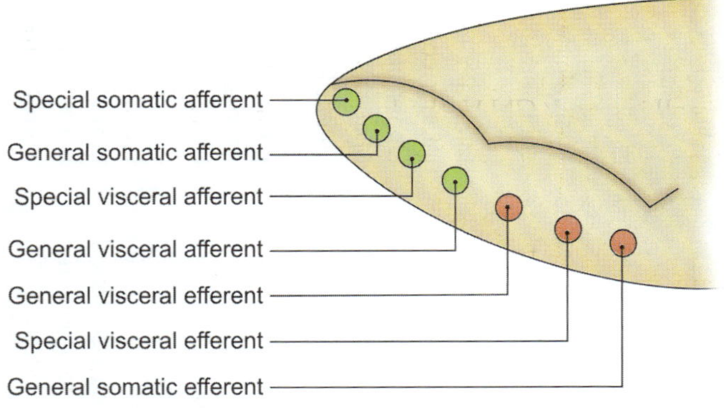

Fig. 32.2: Transverse section of the hindbrain of an embryo showing the arrangement of functional/nuclear columns of cranial nerve nuclei

Nuclei

The details of the nuclei of cranial nerves are summarized in Table 32.1.

General Somatic Efferent Nuclei (GSE)

These nuclei supply skeletal muscle of somatic origin.

1. The *oculomotor nucleus* is situated in the midbrain at the level of the superior colliculus. Its fibres enter the oculomotor nerve and supply five extrinsic muscles of the eyeball except the lateral rectus and the superior oblique.
2. The *trochlear nucleus* is situated in the midbrain at the level of the inferior colliculus. It supplies the superior oblique muscle through the trochlear nerve.

Table 32.1: Nuclei of the cranial nerves

Nerves	*Nuclei*	*Location*	*Functions***	*Function of the nerve component*
I	—	—		Smell
II	—	—		Sight
III	Oculomotor nucleus	Midbrain, level of superior colliculus	GSE	Movements of eyeball
			GVE	Contraction of pupil, accommodation
			GSA*	Proprioceptive
IV	Trochlear nucleus	Midbrain, level of inferior colliculus	GSE	Movement of eyeball (superior oblique)
			GSA*	Proprioceptive
V	1. Motor nucleus	Upper pons	BE/SVE	Movement of mandible
	2. Mesencephalic nucleus	Midbrain	GSA	Proprioceptive, muscles of mastication, face and eye
	3. Superior sensory nucleus	Upper pons	GSA	Touch and pressure from skin and mucous membrane of facial region
	4. Spinal nucleus	From upper pons to C2 segment of spinal cord	GSA	Pain and temperature of face
VI	Abducent nucleus	Lower pons	GSE	Lateral movement of eyeball
			GSA*	Proprioceptive
VII	1. Motor nucleus	Lower pons	BE/SVE	Facial expressions, elevation of hyoid
	2. Nucleus of tractus solitarius	Lower pons	SVA	Taste, anterior two-thirds tongue
	3. Superior salivatory nucleus	Lower pons	GVE	Secretomotor to submandibular and sublingual salivary glands
	4. Lacrimatory nucleus	Lower pons	GVE	Secretomotor to lacrimal gland, nasal glands, etc.
			GSA	Proprioceptive
VIII Cochlear	Two cochlear nuclei—dorsal and ventral	Junction of medulla and pons	SSA	Hearing
Vestibular	Four vestibular nuclei—superior, spinal, medial and lateral	,,	SSA	Equilibrium of head
IX	1. Nucleus ambiguus	Medulla	BE/SVE	Elevation of larynx
	2. Inferior salivatory nucleus	,,	GVE	Secretomotor to parotid gland
	3. Nucleus of tractus solitarius	,,	SVA	Taste from posterior one-third of tongue
			GVA* GSA*	Sensations from mucous membrane of pharynx and posterior one-third of tongue go to dorsal nucleus of vagus and spinal nucleus of V nerve
X and cranial part of XI	1. Nucleus ambiguus	Medulla	BE/SVE	Movements of palate, pharynx and larynx
	2. Dorsal nucleus of vagus	,,	GVE	Motor and secretomotor to bronchial tree and gut; inhibitory to heart
			GVA	Sensations from viscera
	3. Nucleus of tractus solitarius	,,	SVA	Taste from posterior most part of tongue and epiglottis
			GSA*	Sensations from the skin of external ear go to the spinal nucleus of V nerve
Spinal part of XI	Spinal nucleus of accessory nerve	Spinal cord, CI-5	BE/SVE	Sternocleidomastoid and trapezius
XII	Hypoglossal nucleus	Medulla	GSE	Movements of tongue
			GSA	Proprioceptive

* These components do not have corresponding nuclei and terminate in the nuclei of different nerves.

** Functional components: GSE = general somatic efferent; BE = branchial efferent; GVE = general visceral efferent; GVA = general visceral afferent; SVA = special visceral afferent; GSA = general somatic afferent; SSA = special somatic afferent.

3 The *abducent nucleus* is situated in the lower part of the pons. It supplies the lateral rectus muscle through the abducent nerve.
4 The *hypoglossal nucleus* lies in the medulla. It is elongated and extends into both the open and closed parts of the medulla. It supplies most of the muscles of the tongue through the hypoglossal nerve.

Special Visceral Efferent/Branchial Efferent Nuclei

These nuclei supply striated muscle derived from the branchial arches.

1 The *motor nucleus of the trigeminal nerve* lies in the upper part of the pons. It supplies the muscles of mastication through the mandibular nerve.
2 The *nucleus of the facial nerve* lies in the lower part of the pons. It supplies the various muscles innervated by the facial nerve.
3 The *nucleus ambiguus* lies in the medulla. It forms an elongated column lying in both the open and closed parts of the medulla. It supplies:
   a. The stylopharyngeus muscle through the glossopharyngeal nerve; and
   b. The muscles of the pharynx, the soft palate and the larynx through the vagus and the cranial part of the accessory nerve (Fig. 32.3).

General Visceral Efferent Nuclei

These nuclei give origin to preganglionic neurons that relay in a peripheral autonomic ganglion. Postganglionic fibres arising in the ganglion supply smooth muscle or glands.

1 The *Edinger-Westphal nucleus* lies in the midbrain in close relation to the oculomotor nucleus. Its fibres pass through the oculomotor nerve to the ciliary ganglion to supply the sphincter pupillae and the ciliaris muscles.
2 The *lacrimatory nucleus* lies near the salivatory nuclei (in the lower pons). It gives off fibres that pass through the facial nerve and its branch the greater petrosal nerve to relay in the pterygopalatine ganglion and supply the lacrimal, nasal and palatal glands.

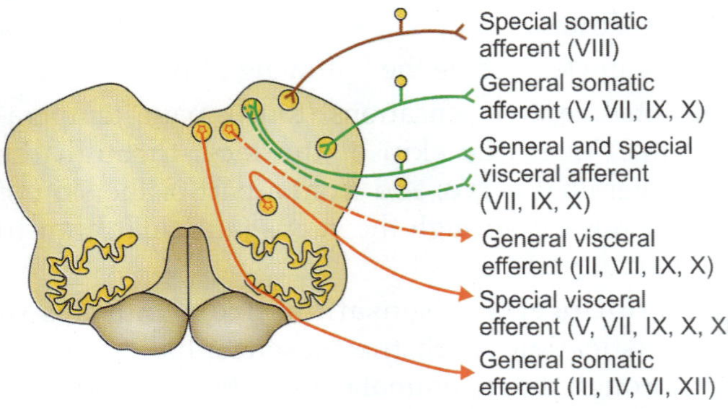

Fig. 32.3: Transverse section of medulla oblongata showing the position of cranial nerve nuclear columns

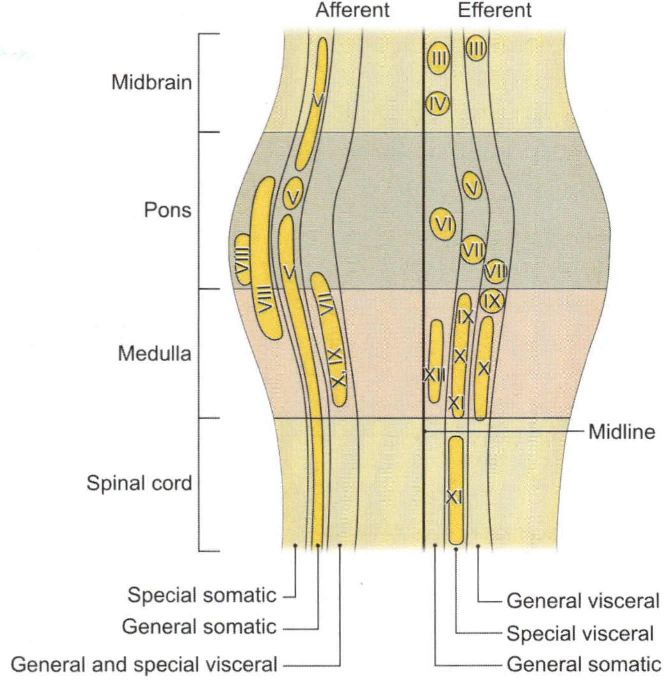

Fig. 32.4a: Position of cranial nerve nuclear columns in brainstem

3 The *superior salivatory nucleus* lies in the lower part of the pons. It sends fibres through the facial nerve and its chorda tympani branch to the submandibular ganglion for supply of the submandibular and sublingual salivary glands.
4 The *inferior salivatory nucleus* lies in the lower part of the pons just below the superior nucleus. It sends fibres through the glossopharyngeal nerve to the otic ganglion for supply of the parotid gland (Fig. 32.4).
5 The *dorsal nucleus of the vagus* is a long column extending into the open and closed parts of the medulla. It gives off fibres that pass through the vagus nerve to be distributed to thoracic and abdominal viscera. (The ganglia concerned are present in the walls of the viscera supplied.)

General Visceral Afferent Nucleus and Special Visceral Afferent Nucleus (Table 32.1)

The only nucleus in this category is the *nucleus of solitary tract* or tractus solitarius. It lies in the medulla and extends into both its closed and open parts.

It receives *general visceral sensations* as follows:

i. Through the glossopharyngeal nerve, from the tonsil, pharynx, the posterior part of the tongue, carotid body and carotid sinus.
ii. Through the vagus nerve, from the pharynx, the larynx, the trachea, the oesophagus and other thoracic and abdominal viscera.

It also receives *sensations of taste* (special visceral afferent) as follows.

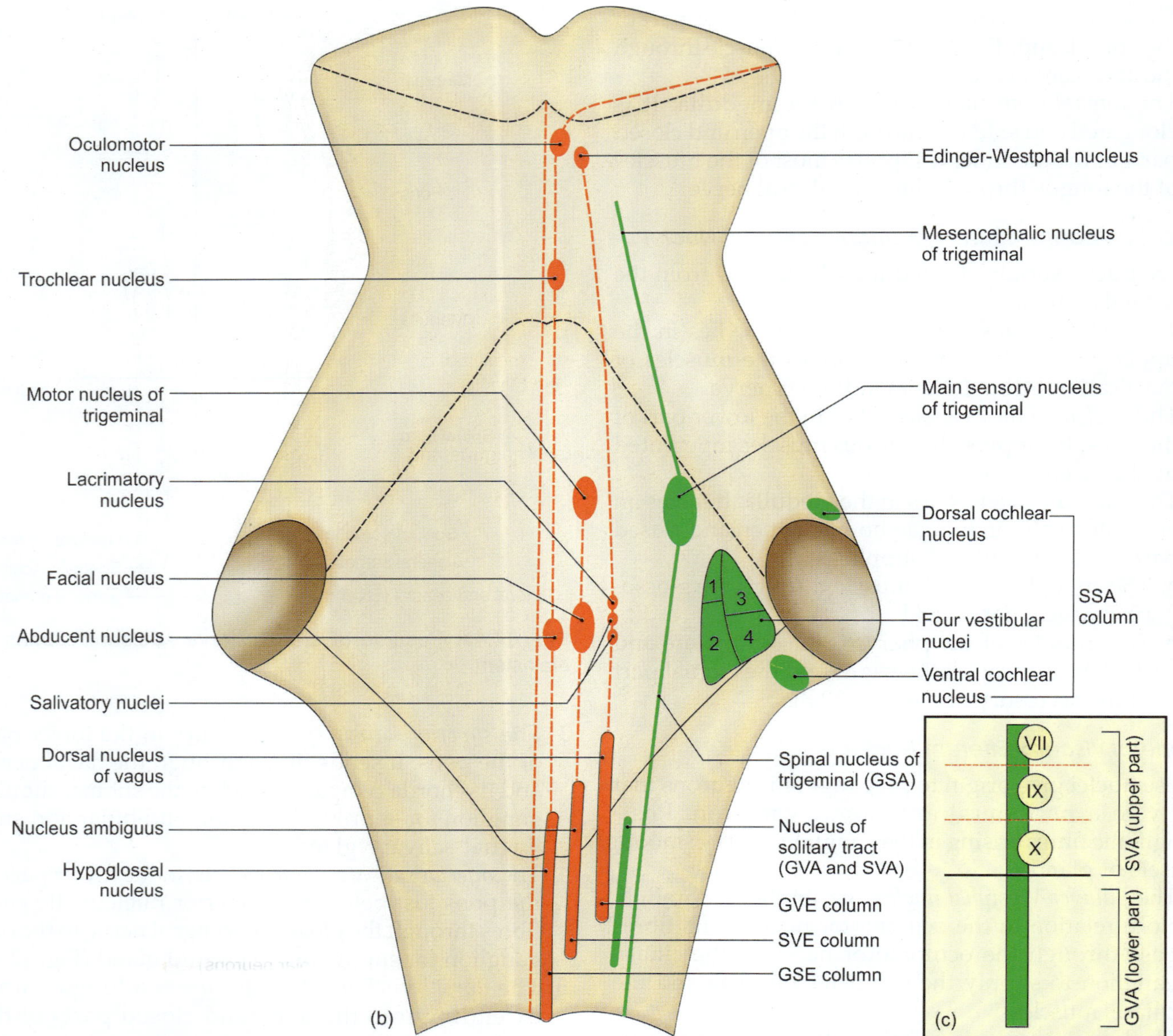

Figs 32.4b and c: (b) Scheme to show the cranial nerve nuclei as projected on to the posterior surface of the brainstem. Vestibular nuclei: 1. Superior; 2. medial; 3. lateral, 4. spinal, (c) GVA and SVA nuclei

a. From the anterior two-thirds of the tongue, and the palate except circumvallate papillae through the facial nerve.
b. From the posterior one-third of the tongue through the glossopharyngeal nerve, including the circumvallate papillae.
c. From the posterior most part of the tongue and from the epiglottis through the vagus nerve.

General Somatic Afferent Nuclei

These are all related to the trigeminal nerve.

1 The *main or superior sensory nucleus of the trigeminal nerve* lies in the upper part of the pons (Fig. 32.1).

2 The *spinal nucleus of the trigeminal nerve* descends from the main nucleus into the medulla. It reaches the upper two segments of the spinal cord.

3 The *mesencephalic nucleus of the trigeminal nerve* extends upwards from the main sensory nucleus into the midbrain.

These nuclei receive the following fibres:

a. Exteroceptive sensations (touch, pain, temperature) from the skin of the face, through the trigeminal nerve; and from a part of the skin of the auricle through the vagus (auricular branch) nerve.
b. Proprioceptive sensations from muscles of mastication reach the mesencephalic nucleus through the trigeminal nerve. The nucleus is also believed to receive proprioceptive fibres from the ocular, facial and lingual muscles.

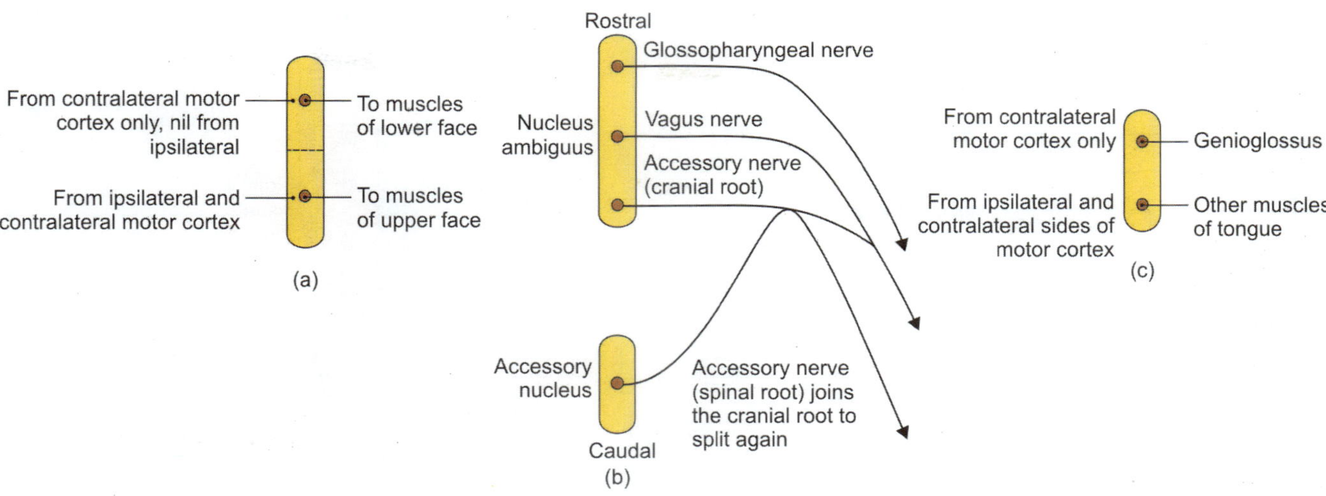

Figs 32.5a to c: (a) Nucleus of facial nerve, (b) nucleus ambiguus and (c) nucleus of hypoglossal nerve

Special Somatic Afferent Nuclei

1 The *cochlear nuclei* (dorsal and ventral) that receive impulses of hearing through the cochlear nerve.
2 The *vestibular nuclei* (superior, spinal, medial and lateral) that receive fibres from the semicircular canals, the utricle and the saccule through the vestibular nerves (Table 32.1).

Special Features

Muscles of facial expression of lower face are supplied only from contralateral motor cortex.

The muscles of upper face are supplied both from ipsilateral and contralateral motor cortex (Fig. 32.5a).

Cranial part of nucleus ambiguus gives fibres to IX, X and cranial root of XI nerve. The caudal part of this nucleus gives fibres to spinal root of XI nerve (Fig. 32.5b).

The genioglossus muscle of the tongue receives fibres from contralateral motor cortex only. Rest of the muscles of the tongue receive from both ipsilateral and contralateral motor cortex (Fig. 32.5c).

FIRST CRANIAL NERVE

OLFACTORY (SMELL) PATHWAY

Receptors and the First Neuron

a. The *olfactory cells* (16–20 million in man) are bipolar neurons. They lie in the olfactory part of the nasal mucosa, and serve both as receptors as well as the first neurons in the olfactory pathway.
b. The *olfactory* nerve rootlets about 20 in number, represent central processes of the olfactory cells.

Second Neuron

The mitral and tufted cells in the olfactory bulb give off fibres that form the *olfactory tract* and reach the primary olfactory areas.

Third Neuron

These are located in the primary olfactory cortex which includes the anterior perforated substance, and several small masses of grey matter around it.

Fourth Neuron

Fibres arising in the primary olfactory cortex go to the secondary olfactory cortex (or entorhinal area) located in the uncus and anterior part of the parahippocampal gyrus. Smell is perceived in both the primary and secondary olfactory areas (Fig. 32.6).

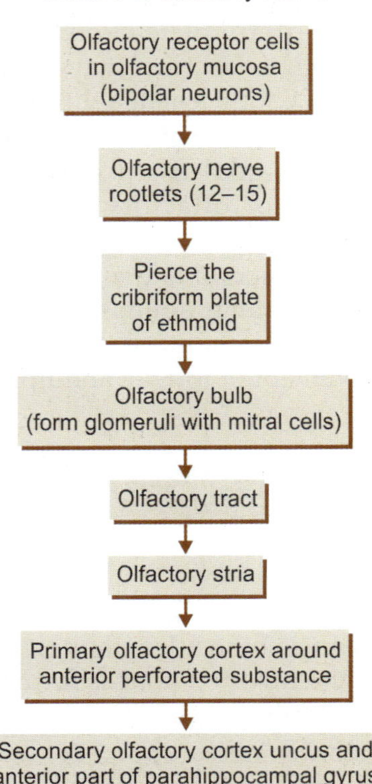

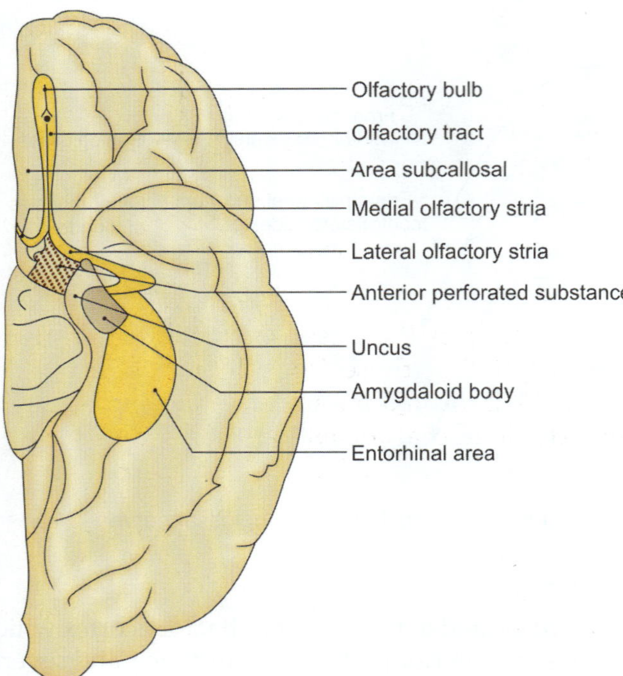

Fig. 32.6: Inferior view of brain showing olfactory areas

CLINICAL ANATOMY

- *Anosmia:* Loss of olfactory fibres with ageing.
- Sense of smell is tested separately in each nostril.
- Allergic rhinitis causes temporary olfactory impairment.
- *Head injury:* Olfactory bulbs may be torn away from olfactory nerves as these pass through fractured cribriform plate of ethmoid leading to anosmia. Such a fracture may also cause CSF rhinorrhoea, i.e. CSF leakage through the nose.
- Abscess of frontal lobe of brain or meningioma in the anterior cranial fossa may press on the olfactory bulb or olfactory tract resulting in anosmia.
- *Uncinate fits:* Lesion of lateral olfactory area may cause temporal lobe epilepsy or uncinate fits. These fits are of imaginary disagreeable odours with involvement of tongue and lips.

SECOND CRANIAL NERVE

OPTIC NERVE

Optic nerve is the nerve of sight which is a special sense.

Human vision is binocular, though one sees with both the eyes, the inverted images formed are seen as one and straight only (Fig. 32.7).

Human vision is stereoscopic, i.e. one see height, width and thickness of the object.

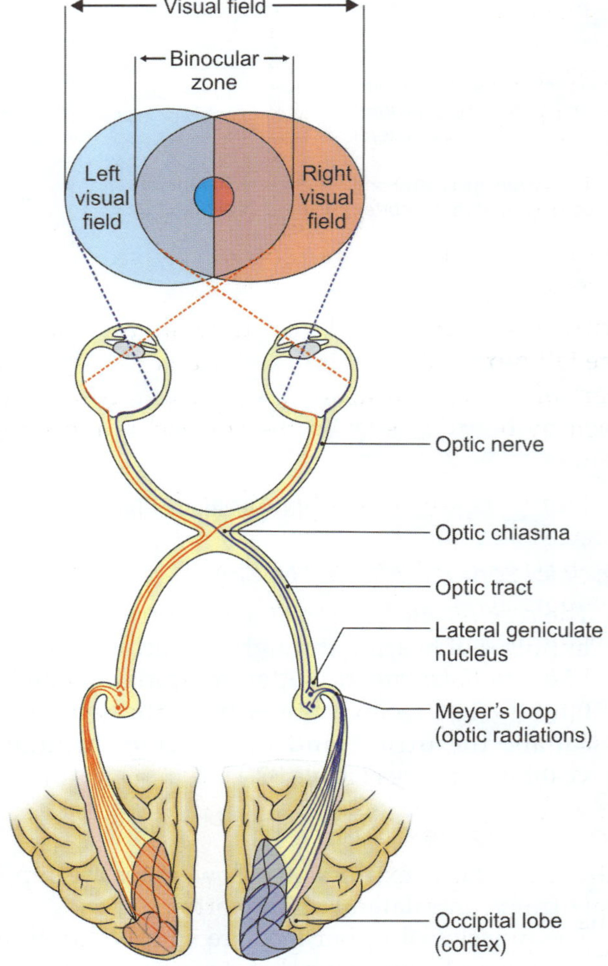

Fig. 32.7: Visual pathways

Human vision is coloured, one sees different colours put up by nature.

When one looks at an object, both eyes are focused on it. Right eye sees a little additional of right side whereas left eye sees a little additional of left side of the object. These visions are monocular visions. Main part is the binocular vision.

Field of Vision

There is a temporal field of vision and a nasal field of vision.

Field of vision are also upper and lower. So there are four fields on each side—upper temporal, lower temporal, upper nasal and lower nasal.

Most importantly, there is a macular vision which is the most acute or sharp and coloured vision. Nasal fields are smaller than the temporal fields.

Larger right temporal and smaller right nasal fields of vision fuse to form right part of binocular field.

Left halves of field of vision, i.e. larger temporal half and smaller nasal half of left field of vision form left half of binocular field.

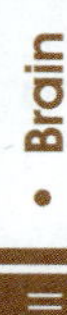

Retina: In human, the eyeballs are placed medially, with the nose intervening. Retina is also divided into temporal and nasal parts and each is further subdivided into upper and lower parts. Macula lutea lies in the centre of the posterior part of the retina.

Light rays travel in a straight line. Temporal field is seen by nasal hemiretina and vice versa. Both these hemiretinae include half part of macula each.

The small right monocular field is seen by the anterior part of the right nasal hemiretina. Similarly, the left monocular field is appreciated by the anterior part of the left nasal hemiretina. Binocular field is seen by both the eyes in the corresponding parts of retina.

Fibres from the nasal parts of the two retinae decussate to form the optic chiasma and travel to the contralateral side in the optic tract. Fibres from the temporal hemiretinae continue ipsilaterally in the optic tract.

Right optic tract carries the fibres of the right temporal hemiretina and the left nasal hemiretina and vice versa. Macular fibres lie in the central part of optic tract, upper retinal fibres project downwards and lower retinal fibres project upwards.

VISUAL (OPTIC) PATHWAY

The visual pathways include structures which are concerned with the reception, transmission and perception of visual impulses. However, certain structures concerned with visual reflexes may also be conveniently mentioned here.

Structures in Visual Pathway

1. Retina
2. Optic nerve
3. Optic chiasma
4. Optic tract, with its lateral and medial roots
5. Lateral geniculate body
6. Optic radiation
7. Visual area in the cortex.

Structures Concerned with Visual Reflexes

1. Pretectal nucleus
2. Oculomotor nucleus and nerve with ciliary ganglion
3. Frontal eye field of cerebral cortex
4. Superior colliculus with tectobulbar and tectospinal tracts.

Retina

It is described in Chapter 27.

Optic Nerve

Optic nerve is made up of axons of ganglion cells of the retina. In a strict sense, the optic nerve is not a peripheral nerve because its fibres have no neurilemmal sheaths. It is a tract. Its fibres have no power of regeneration. The nerve is described in Chapter 21.

Optic Chiasma

In the chiasma, the nasal fibres (i.e. fibres of the optic nerve arising in the nasal, or medial half of the retina) including those from the nasal half of the macula, cross the midline and enter the opposite optic tract. The temporal (or lateral) fibres pass through the chiasma to enter the optic tract of the same side (Fig. 32.7).

Optic Tract

Each optic tract winds round the cerebral peduncle of the midbrain. Near the lateral geniculate body, it divides into lateral and medial roots. The lateral root is thick and terminates in the lateral geniculate body. A few of its fibres pass to the superior colliculus, the pretectal nucleus and the hypothalamus. The medial root is believed to contain the supraoptic commissural fibres.

Each optic tract contains temporal fibres of retina of the same side and nasal fibres of the opposite side.

Lateral Geniculate Body

Lateral geniculate body receives the lateral root of the optic tract. Medially, it is connected to the superior colliculus, and laterally, it gives rise to the optic radiation.

The cells in this body are arranged in six layers. Layers 2, 3, 5 receive ipsilateral fibres, and layers 1, 4, 6 receive contralateral fibres.

Optic Radiation (Geniculocalcarine Tract)

Optic radiation begins from the lateral geniculate body, passes through the retrolentiform part of internal capsule, and ends in the visual cortex (Fig. 32.7).

Visual Cortex

The optic radiation in the striate area (area 17) where the colour, size, shape, motion, illumination and transparency are appreciated separately. Objects are identified by integration of these perceptions with past experience stored in the parastriate and peristriate areas (areas 18, 19).

The area of the visual cortex that receives impulses from the macula is relatively much larger than the part related to the rest of the retina.

Course of optic nerve

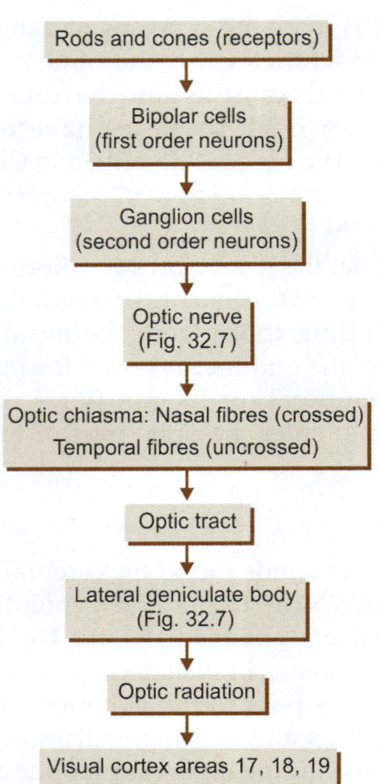

Reflexes

Pupillary light reflex—left eye and consensual light reflex—right eye (Fig. 32.8).

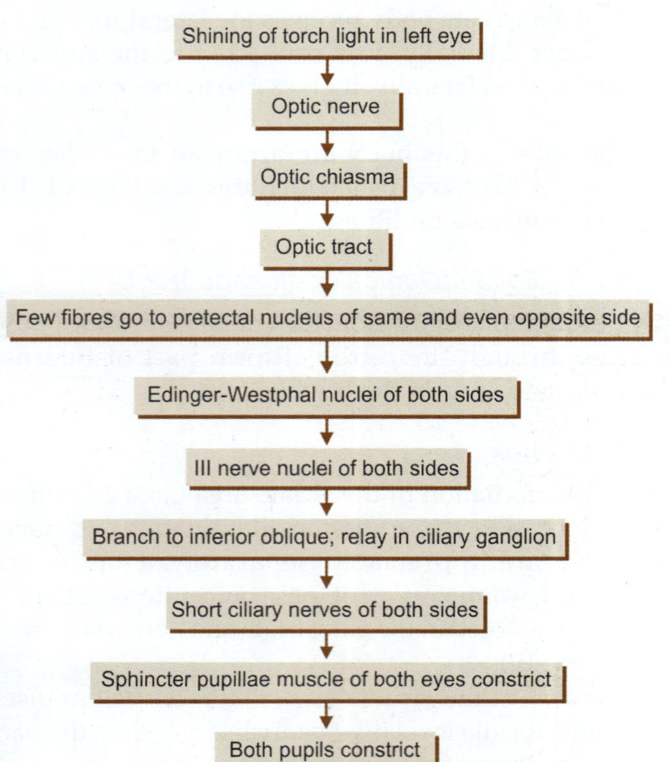

Accommodation reflex (Fig. 32.9)

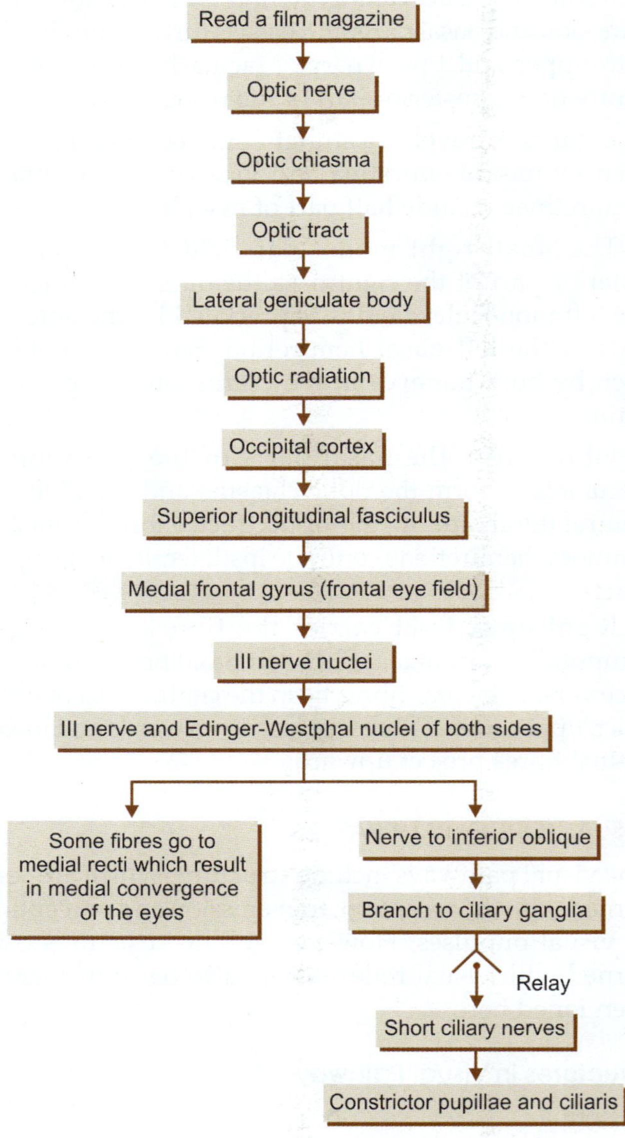

CLINICAL ANATOMY

- Lesion in retina leads to scotoma, that is certain points may become blind spots.
- Optic nerve damage results in complete blindness of that eye.
- *Optic neuritis:* Lesion of optic nerve that results in decrease of visual acuity. Optic disc appears pale and smaller. Methyl alcohol is a usual toxic chemical leading to blindness.
- Complete destruction of optic tract, lateral geniculate body, optic radiation or visual cortex of one side results in loss of the opposite half of field of vision.
- A lesion on the right side leads to left homonymous hemianopia.

Fig. 32.8: Pupillary light and consensual light reflex

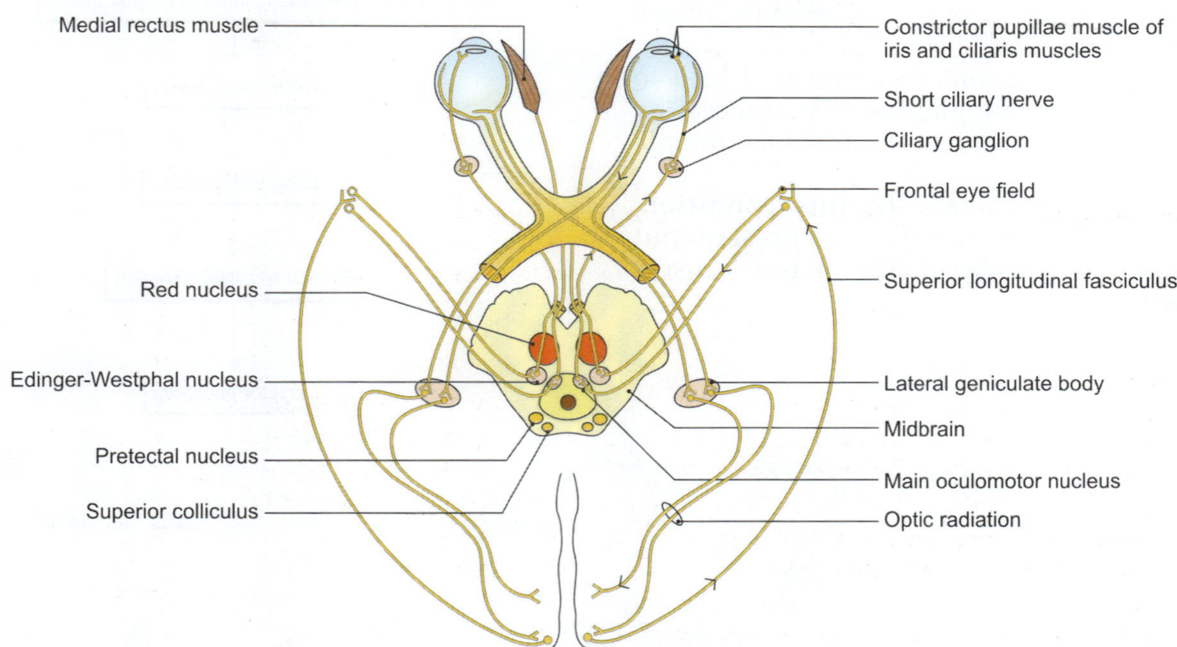

Fig. 32.9: Accommodation reflex

Corneal/conjunctival reflex (Fig. 32.10)

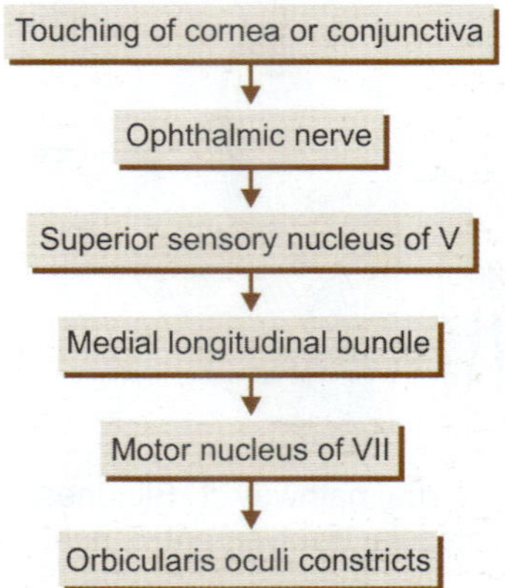

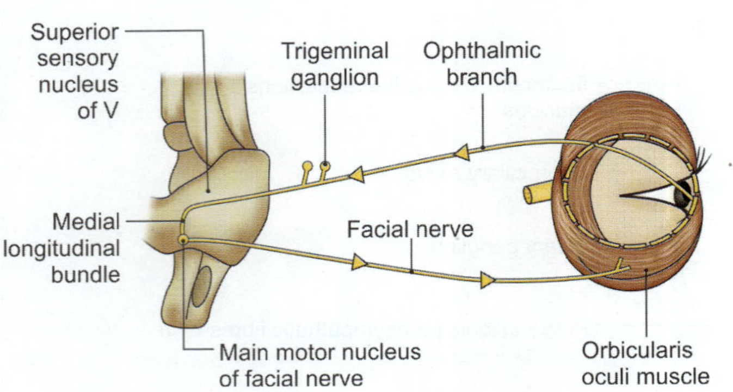

Fig. 32.10: Corneal/conjunctival reflex

- *Papilloedema:* Results due to increased intracranial pressure. It leads to swelling of optic disc due to blockage of tributaries of the retinal veins.
- Optic chiasma lesion, if central will lead to bitemporal hemianopia; but if peripheral on both sides, will lead to binasal hemianopia (Fig. 32.11).
- *Argyll-Robertson pupil:* In this condition, the accommodation reflex is present but the light reflex is absent. The pretectal area is affected.

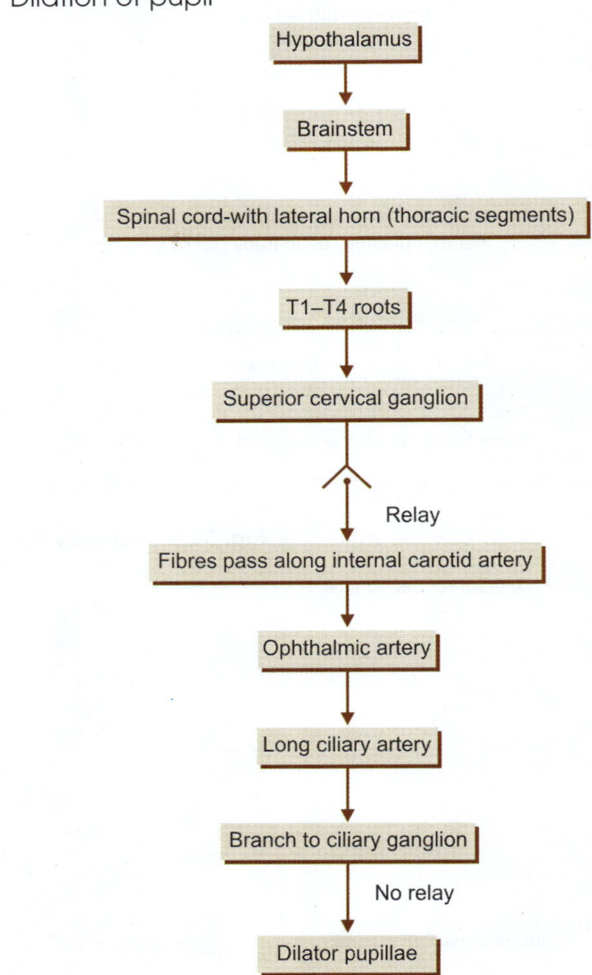

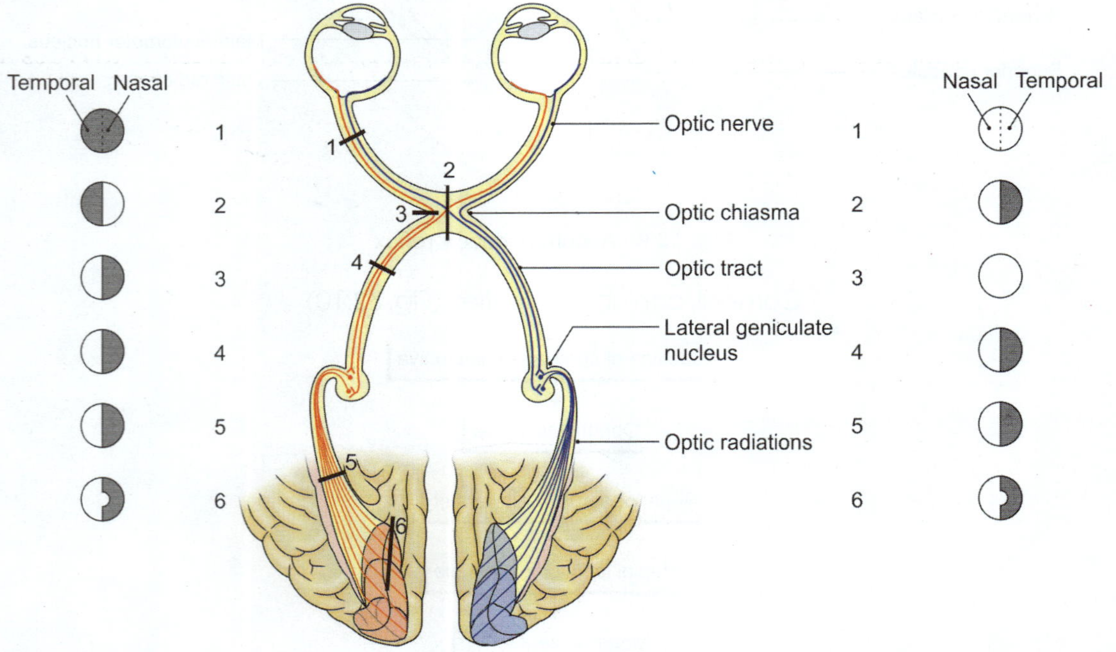

Fig. 32.11: Field defects associated with lesion of visual pathway. 1. Blindness of left eye, 2. bitemporal hemianopia, 3. left nasal hemianopia, 4. right homonymous hemianopia with macular involvement, 5. right homonymous hemianopia, and 6. right homonymous hemianopia with macular sparing

THIRD CRANIAL NERVE

Oculomotor Nerve

This is the third cranial nerve. It is distributed to the extraocular as well as the intraocular muscles. Since it is a somatic motor nerve, it is in series with the IV, VI and XII cranial nerves, and also with the ventral root of spinal nerves.

Functional Components

1. General somatic efferent, for movements of the eyeball (Fig. 32.12).
2. General visceral efferent or parasympathetic, for contraction of pupil and accommodation.
3. General somatic afferent column carries proprioceptive fibres from the extraocular muscles to mesencephalic nucleus of V.

Nucleus

The oculomotor nucleus is situated in the ventromedial part of central grey matter of midbrain at the level of superior colliculus. The fibres for the constrictor pupillae and for the ciliaris arise from the Edinger-Westphal nucleus which forms part of the oculomotor nuclear complex.

Ventrolaterally, it is closely related to the medial longitudinal bundle.

Course and Distribution

1. In their *intraneural course,* the fibres arise from the nucleus and pass ventrally through the tegmentum, red nucleus and substantia nigra.
2. *At the base of the brain,* the nerve is attached to the oculomotor sulcus on the medial side of the crus cerebri (Fig. 32.12).
3. The nerve passes between the superior cerebellar and posterior cerebral arteries, and runs forwards in the interpeduncular cistern, on the lateral side of posterior communicating artery to reach the cavernous sinus (Fig. 32.13).
4. The nerve *enters the cavernous sinus* (Fig. 32.14) by piercing the posterior part of its roof on the lateral side of the posterior clinoid process. It descends to the lateral wall of the sinus where it lies above the trochlear nerve. In the anterior part of the sinus, the nerve divides into upper and lower divisions.
5. The two divisions of the nerve *enter the orbit* through the middle part of the superior orbital fissure. In the fissure, the nasociliary nerve lies in between the two divisions while the abducent nerve lies inferolateral to them (*see* Fig. 21.4).
6. *In the orbit,* the smaller upper division ascends on the lateral side of optic nerve, and supplies the superior rectus and part of the levator palpebrae superioris.

   The larger, lower, division divides into three branches—the medial rectus, the inferior rectus and the inferior oblique. The nerve to the inferior oblique is the longest of these. It gives off the motor root to

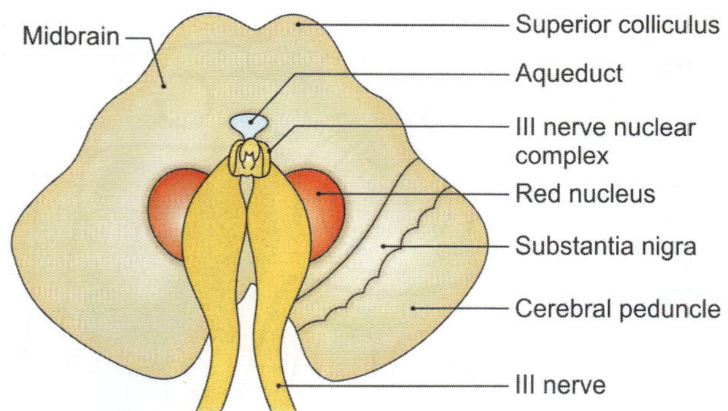

Fig. 32.12: Third cranial nerve and its nucleus

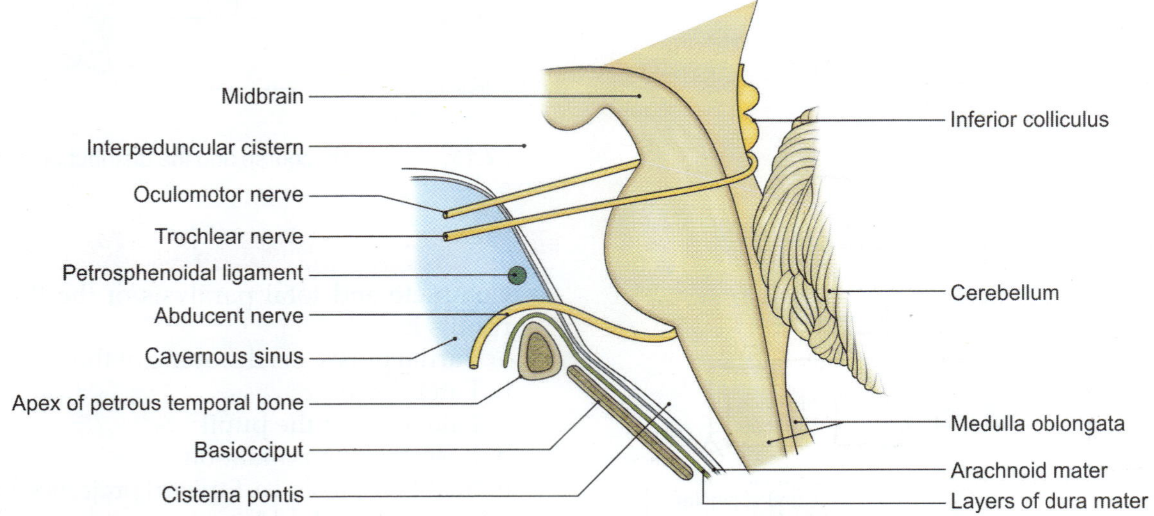

Fig. 32.13: Scheme to show the precavernous courses of the third, fourth and sixth cranial nerves

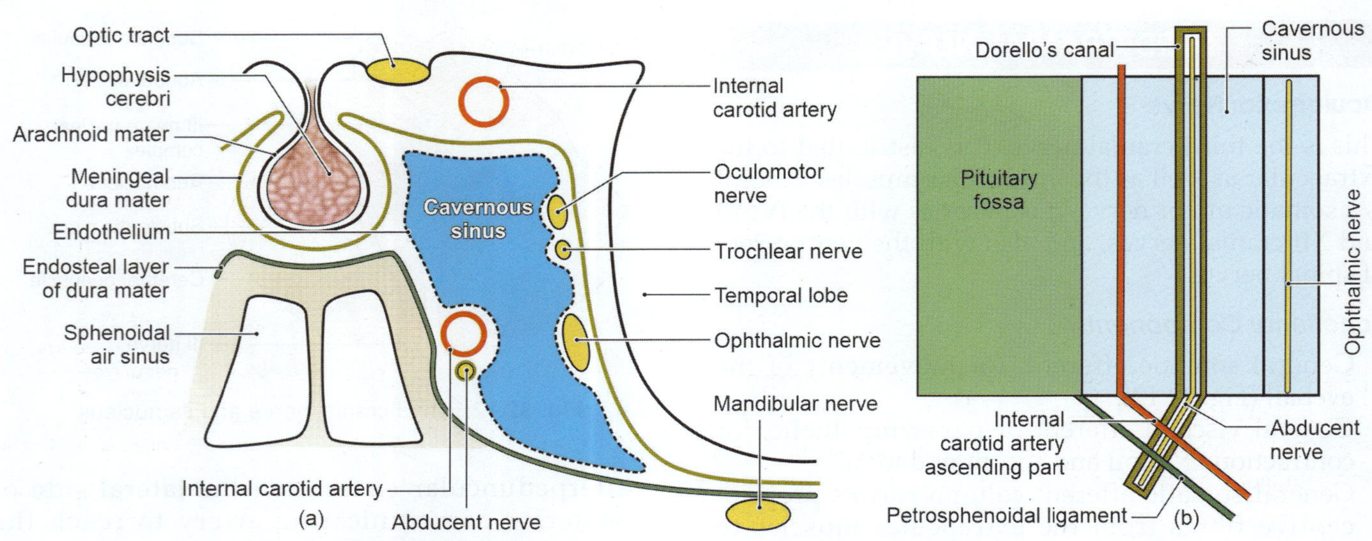

Fig. 32.14: Course of III, IV, V and VI nerves in the cavernous sinus (*Courtesy:* Dr SN Kazi)

the ciliary ganglion and then supplies the inferior oblique muscle (Fig. 32.15).

All branches enter the muscles on their ocular surfaces except that for the inferior oblique which enters its posterior border.

Figures 21.7a to c show the actions of the extraocular muscles.

Course of oculomotor nerve

Nuclear columns
1. General somatic efferent: Oculomotor nucleus
2. General visceral efferent (GVE): Edinger-Westphal nucleus
3. General somatic afferent: Mesencephalic nuclues

↓

Emerges on medial side of cerebral peduncle of midbrain (Fig. 32.12)

↓

Between posterior cerebral and superior cerebellar arteries

↓

Pierces dura mater and enters lateral wall of cavernous sinus (Fig. 32.14)

↓

Passes through the common tendinous ring and superior orbital fissure

↓

Divides into two divisions (Fig. 32.15)

- Upper division → Part of levator palpebrae superioris and superior rectus
- Lower division → Medial rectus; Inferior rectus; Inferior oblique; GVE → Ciliary ganglion → Ciliaris and sphincter pupillae for accomodation

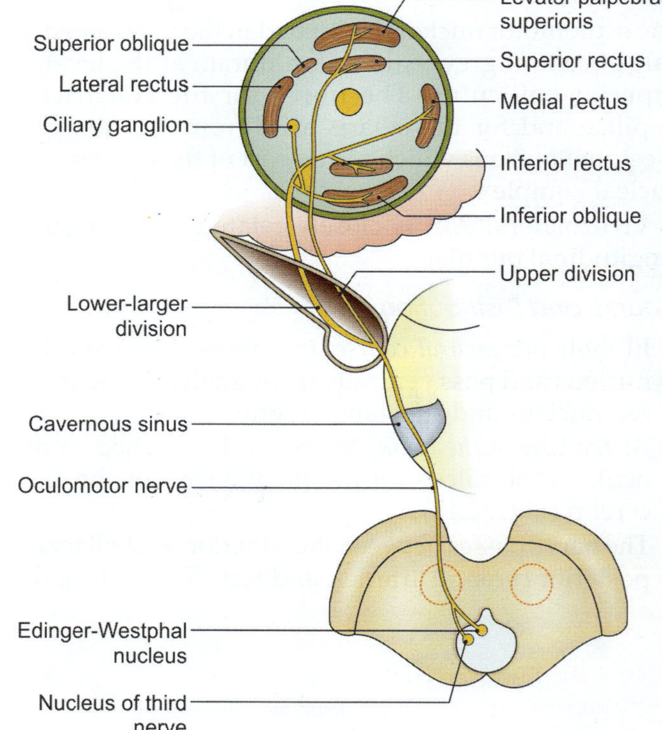

Fig. 32.15: The origin, course and the distribution of oculomotor nerve

CLINICAL ANATOMY

- Complete and total paralysis of the third nerve results in:
  a. Partial ptosis, i.e. drooping of the upper eyelid.
  b. Lateral squint
  c. Dilatation of the pupil
  d. Loss of accommodation
  e. Slight proptosis, i.e. forward projection of the eye
  f. Diplopia or double vision.

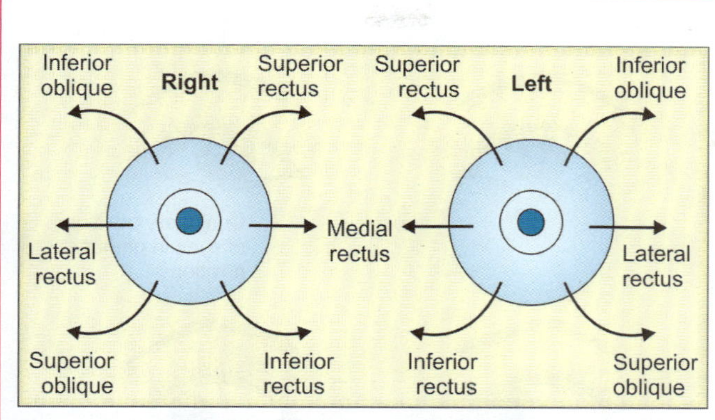

Fig. 32.16: Action of individual extraocular muscle. Arrows indicate direction of movement

- Parital ptosis or drooping of upper eyelid due to paralysis of voluntary part of levator palpebrae superioris muscle.
- Pupillary light reflex in affected eye is absent.
- Dilatation of pupil due to paralysis of parasympathetic fibres to sphincter pupillae muscle.
- Eyeball gets turned downwards and laterally due to unopposed action of lateral rectus and superior oblique muscles.
- Loss of accommodation due to paralysis of ciliary muscles.
- Pupil dilates and becomes fixed to light.
- *Aneurysm of posterior cerebral or superior cerebellar artery:* Aneurysm of any of these two arteries may compress III nerve as it passes between them.

FOURTH CRANIAL NERVE

TROCHLEAR NERVE

This is the fourth cranial nerve. It supplies only the superior oblique muscle of the eyeball (Fig. 32.16).

Functional Components

1. General somatic efferent, for lateral movement of the eyeball.
2. The general somatic afferent, for proprioceptive impulses from the muscle to the mesencephalic nucleus of V nerve.

Nucleus

The trochlear nucleus is situated in the ventromedial part of the central grey matter of midbrain at the level of inferior colliculus. Ventrally, it is closely related to the medial longitudinal bundle (Fig. 32.17).

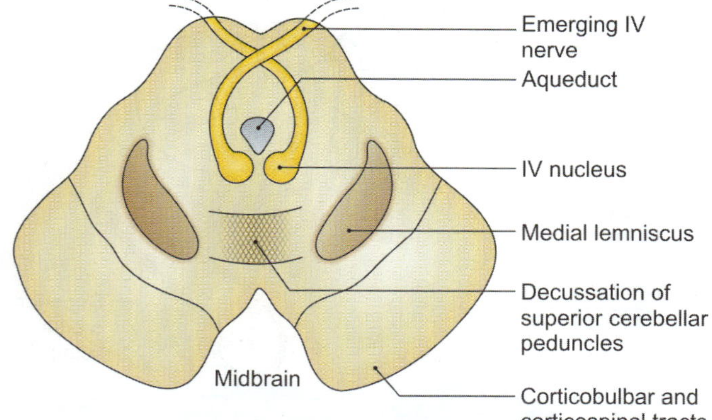

Fig. 32.17: Emerging fibres of trochlear nerves with their nuclei

Course and Distribution

1. In its *intraneural course,* the nerve runs dorsally round the central grey matter to reach the upper part of the superior or anterior medullary velum where it decussates with the opposite nerve to emerge on the opposite side.
2. *Surface attachment.* Trochlear nerve is attached to the superior medullary velum one on each side of the frenulum veli just below the inferior colliculus. It is the only cranial nerve which emerges on the dorsal aspect of the brainstem (Fig. 32.1).
3. The nerve winds round the superior cerebellar peduncle and the cerebral peduncle just above the pons. It passes between the posterior cerebral and superior cerebellar arteries to appear ventrally between the temporal lobe and upper border of pons.
4. The nerve *enters the cavernous sinus* by piercing the posterior corner of its roof. Next it runs forwards in the lateral wall of cavernous sinus between the oculomotor and ophthalmic nerves. In the anterior part of sinus, it crosses over the oculomotor nerve.
5. Trochlear nerve *enters the orbit* through the lateral part of the superior orbital fissure.
6. *In the orbit,* it passes medially, above the origin of levator palpebrae superioris and ends by supplying the superior oblique muscle on its orbital surface (Fig. 32.18).

CLINICAL ANATOMY

- When trochlear nerve is damaged, diplopia occurs on looking downwards; vision is single so long as the eyes look above the horizontal plane.
- Paralysis of the trochlear nerve results in:
  a. Defective depression of the adducted eye.
  b. Diplopia (Fig. 32.19).

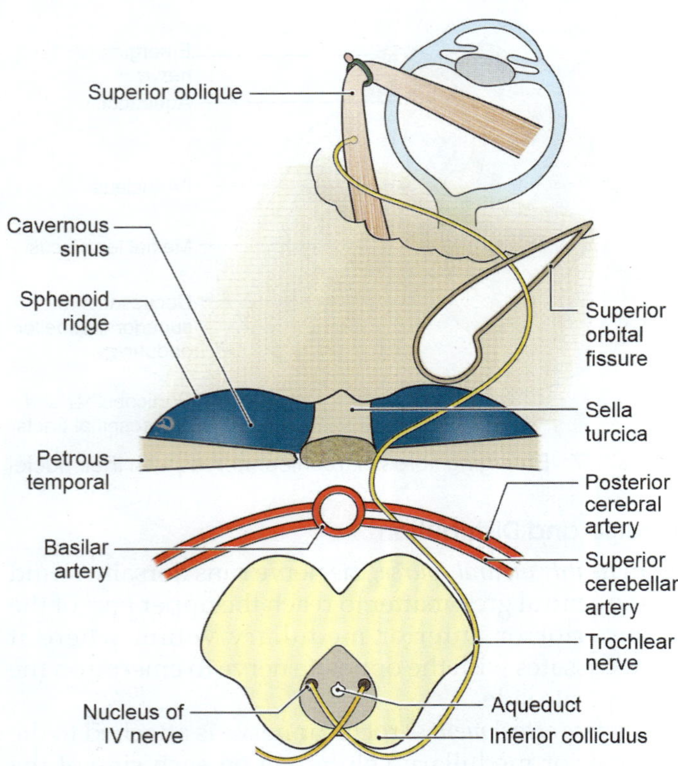

Fig. 32.18: The origin, course and the distribution of the trochlear nerve

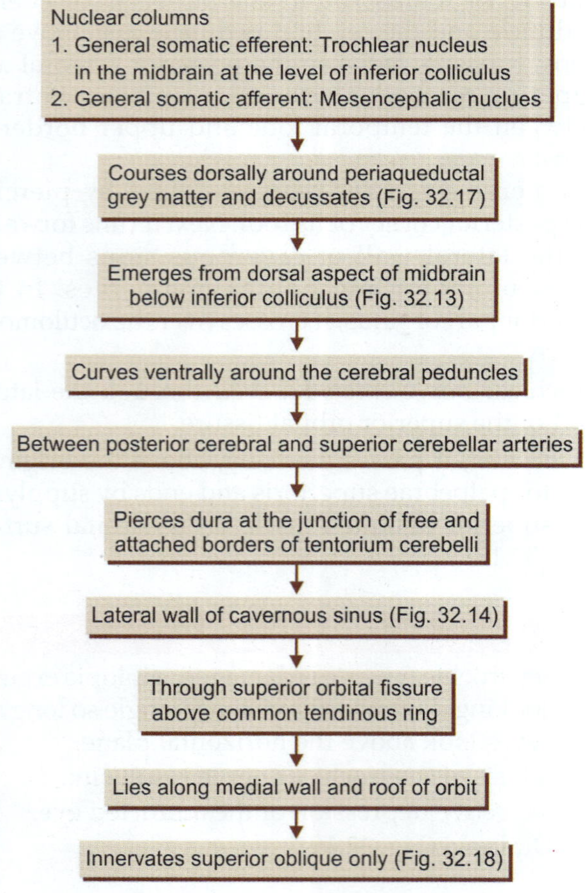

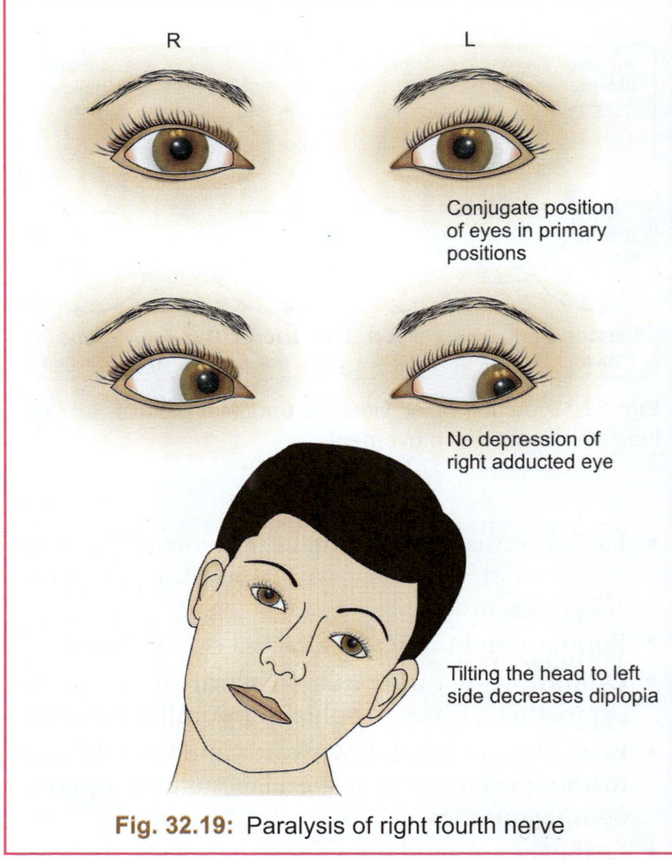

Fig. 32.19: Paralysis of right fourth nerve

SIXTH CRANIAL NERVE

ABDUCENT NERVE

It is the sixth cranial nerve which supplies the lateral rectus muscle of the eyeball (Fig. 32.20). One nerve fibre supplies only six to ten muscle fibres.

Functional Components

1 General somatic efferent, for lateral movement of the eyeball.
2 The general somatic afferent, for proprioceptive impulses from the muscle to the mesencephalic nucleus of V nerve.

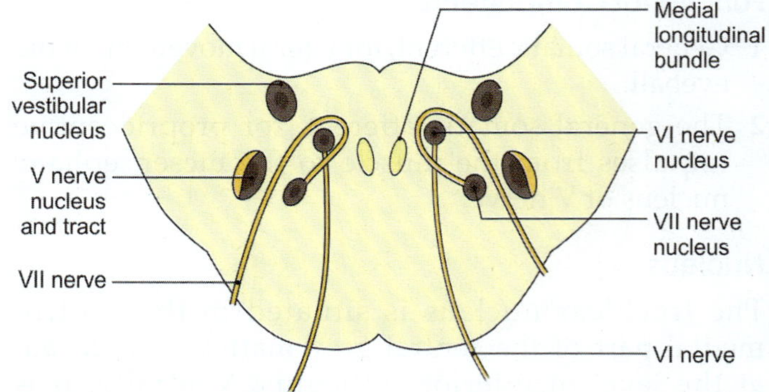

Fig. 32.20: VI nerve with its nucleus. It includes unusual course of VII nerve

Nucleus

Abducent nucleus is situated in the upper part of the floor of fourth ventricle in the lower pons, beneath the facial colliculus. Ventromedially, it is closely related to the medial longitudinal bundle.

Course and Distribution

1 In their *intraneural course,* the fibres of the VI nerve run ventrally and downwards through the trapezoid body, medial lemniscus and basilar part of pons to reach the lower border of the pons.
2 The nerve is attached to the lower border of the pons, opposite the upper end of the pyramid of the medulla (Fig. 32.1).
3 The nerve then runs upwards, forwards and laterally through the cisterna pontis and usually dorsal to the anterior inferior cerebellar artery to reach the cavernous sinus.
4 Abducent nerve enters the cavernous sinus by passing inferior to the petrosphenoidal ligament within a dural tunnel (Dorello's canal) just posterior to the short ascending portion of the cavernous carotid artery, and then runs on the inferolateral side of the horizontal portion of the cavernous carotid artery, just medial to the ophthalmic nerve at the lateral wall of the sinus, known as infratrochelear or Parkinson's triangle. It gives access to the horizontal portion of the cavernous carotid artery and the abducent nerve (Fig. 20.6b).
5 The abducent nerve *enters the orbit* through the middle part of the superior orbital fissure. Here it lies inferolateral to the oculomotor and nasociliary nerves (Fig. 32.21).

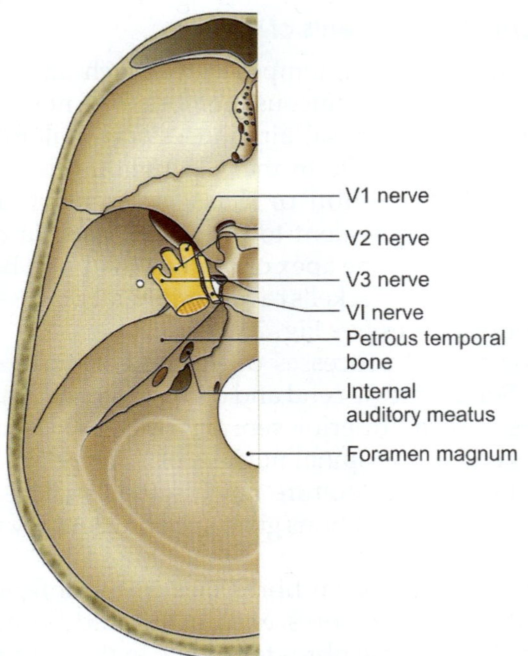

Fig. 32.21: V1 nerve about to enter the superior orbital fissure

6 *In the orbit,* the nerve ends by supplying only the lateral rectus muscle. It enters the ocular surface of the muscle (Fig. 32.22).

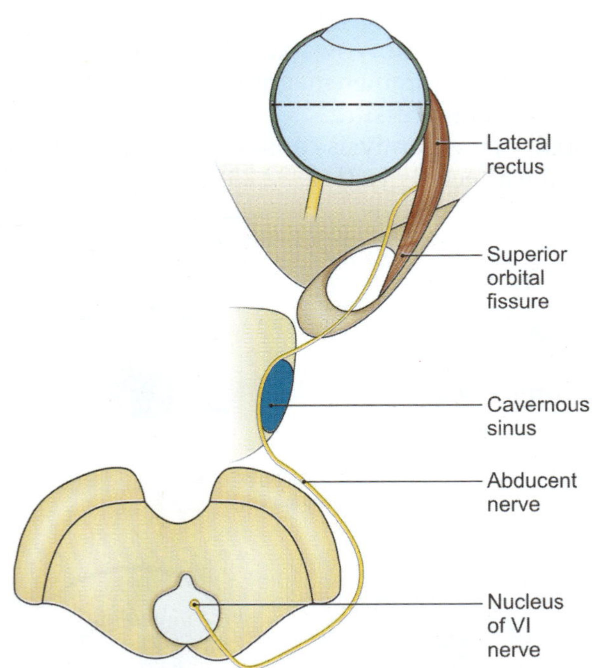

Fig. 32.22: The origin, course and distribution of the abducent nerve

Course of abducent nerve

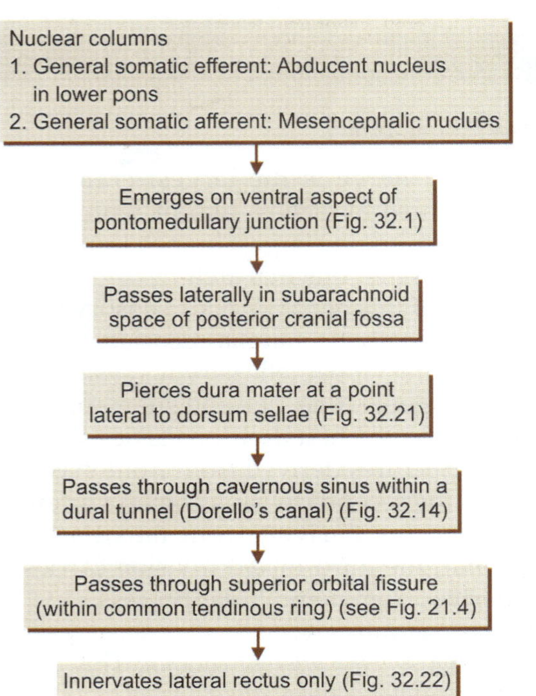

CLINICAL ANATOMY

- Sixth nerve paralysis is one of the commonest false localizing signs in cases with raised intracranial pressure. Its susceptibility to such damage is due to its long course in the cisterna pontis, to its sharp bend over the superior border of petrous temporal bone and the downward shift of the brainstem towards the foramen magnum produced by raised intracranial pressure.
- Sixth nerve paralysis causes failure of abduction of the affected eye (Fig. 32.23).

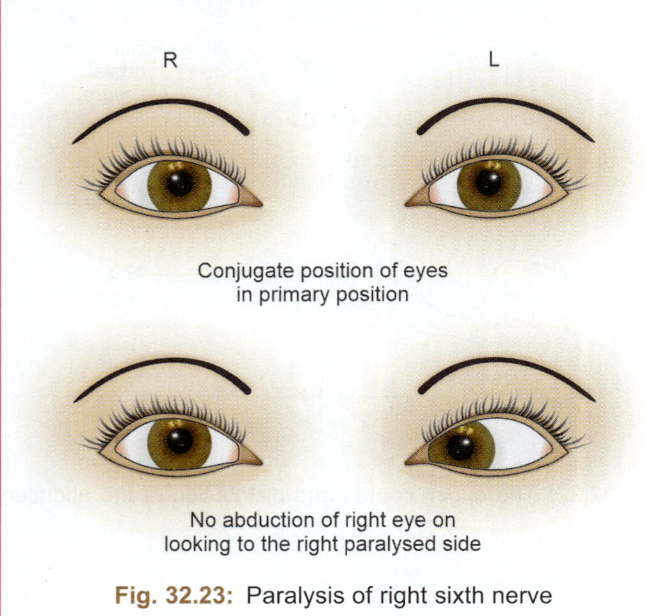

Fig. 32.23: Paralysis of right sixth nerve

FIFTH CRANIAL NERVE

TRIGEMINAL NERVE

Fifth cranial nerve is the largest cranial nerve. It comprises three branches, two of which are purely sensory and third, the largest branch is mixed nerve. It is the nerve of first brachial arch.

Branches of this nerve provide sensory fibres to the four parasympathetic ganglia associated with cranial outflow of parasympathetic nervous system. These are ciliary, pterygopalatine, otic and submandibular.

Ophthalmic, the first division carries sensory fibres from the structures derived from frontonasal process. Maxillary, the second division conveys afferent fibres from structures derived from maxillary process. Mandibular, the third mixed division carries sensory fibres derives from mandibular process.

Nuclear columns are:

i. *General somatic afferent column:* This column has three nuclei. These are:

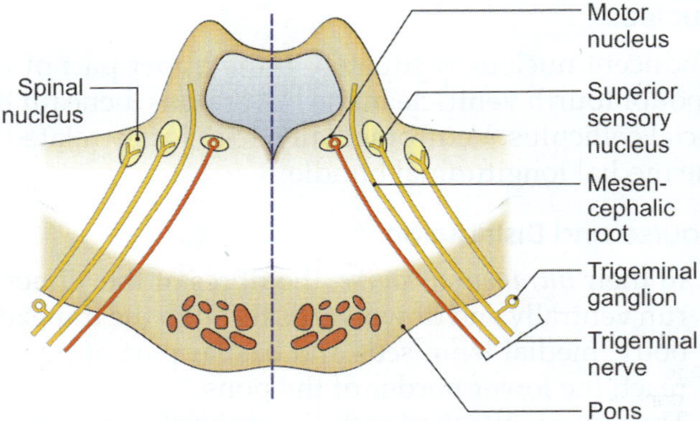

Fig. 32.24: Nuclei of trigeminal nerve at level of upper pons

- *Spinal nucleus of V nerve:* It takes pain and temperature sensations from most of the face area which relay here. The crossed fibres are called trigeminal lemniscus which go to ventroposteromedial nucleus of thalamus for another relay, to finally terminate in lower part of postcentral gyrus (Fig. 32.24).
- *Superior sensory nucleus of V nerve:* Fibres carrying touch and pressure relay in this nucleus. Remaining path is same as of spinal nucleus.
- *Mesencephalic nucleus:* This nucleus extends from pons till the midbrain. It receives proprioceptive impulses from muscles of mastication, extraocular muscles, temporomandibular joint and teeth.

ii. *Branchial efferent column:* The nucleus of V nerve is situated at the level of upper pons. The fibres of the motor nucleus supply eight muscles derived from first branchial arch.

Sensory Components of V Nerve

Sensations of pain, temperature, touch and pressure from skin of face, mucous membrane of nose, most of the tongue, paranasal air sinuses travel along axons. Their cell bodies lie in the V ganglion (Fig. 32.28) or semilunar ganglion or Gasserian ganglion. This ganglion is equivalent to the spinal ganglia of other nerves. It lies at the apex of petrous temporal bone in a dural cave, the Meckel's cave. Peripheral processes form the three nerves (*see* Fig. 20.3).

The central processes of V ganglion form sensory root. Some fibres ascend and other descend. Ascending fibres end in superior sensory nucleus. Descending fibres end in the spinal nucleus of V nerve.

Pain and temperature reach spinal nucleus. Touch and pressure sensations go to superior sensory nucleus (Fig. 32.25).

Ophthalmic nerve fibres end in the inferior part, maxillary nerve fibres end in the middle part and mandibular nerve fibres terminate in the upper part of spinal nucleus.

Fig. 32.25: Trigeminal ganglia and three of its branches

According to another view, the ophthalmic fibres lie in the median part, maxillary fibres in the medial part and the mandibular fibres in the lateral part of the nucleus.

Proprioceptive fibres from muscles of mastication, extraocular muscles and facial muscles bypass V ganglion to reach unipolar cells of mesencephalic nucleus.

Axons of neurons of spinal nucleus, superior sensory nucleus and central processes of cells of mesencephalic nucleus cross to the opposite side and ascend as trigeminal lemniscus. The lemniscus ends in the ventral posteromedial nucleus of thalamus, where these fibres relay. The third neuron fibres end in areas 3, 1 and 2 of cerebral cortex.

Motor Component

The motor nucleus receives impulses from the right and left cerebral hemispheres, red nucleus and mesencephalic nucleus. Fibres of motor root supply four muscles of mastication (Fig. 32.27) and four other muscles. These are tensor veli palatini, tensor tympani, mylohyoid and anterior belly of digastric.

Cranial nerve V/trigeminal nerve comprises three branches, ophthalmic V1, maxillary V2 and mandibular V3 (Fig. 32.26).

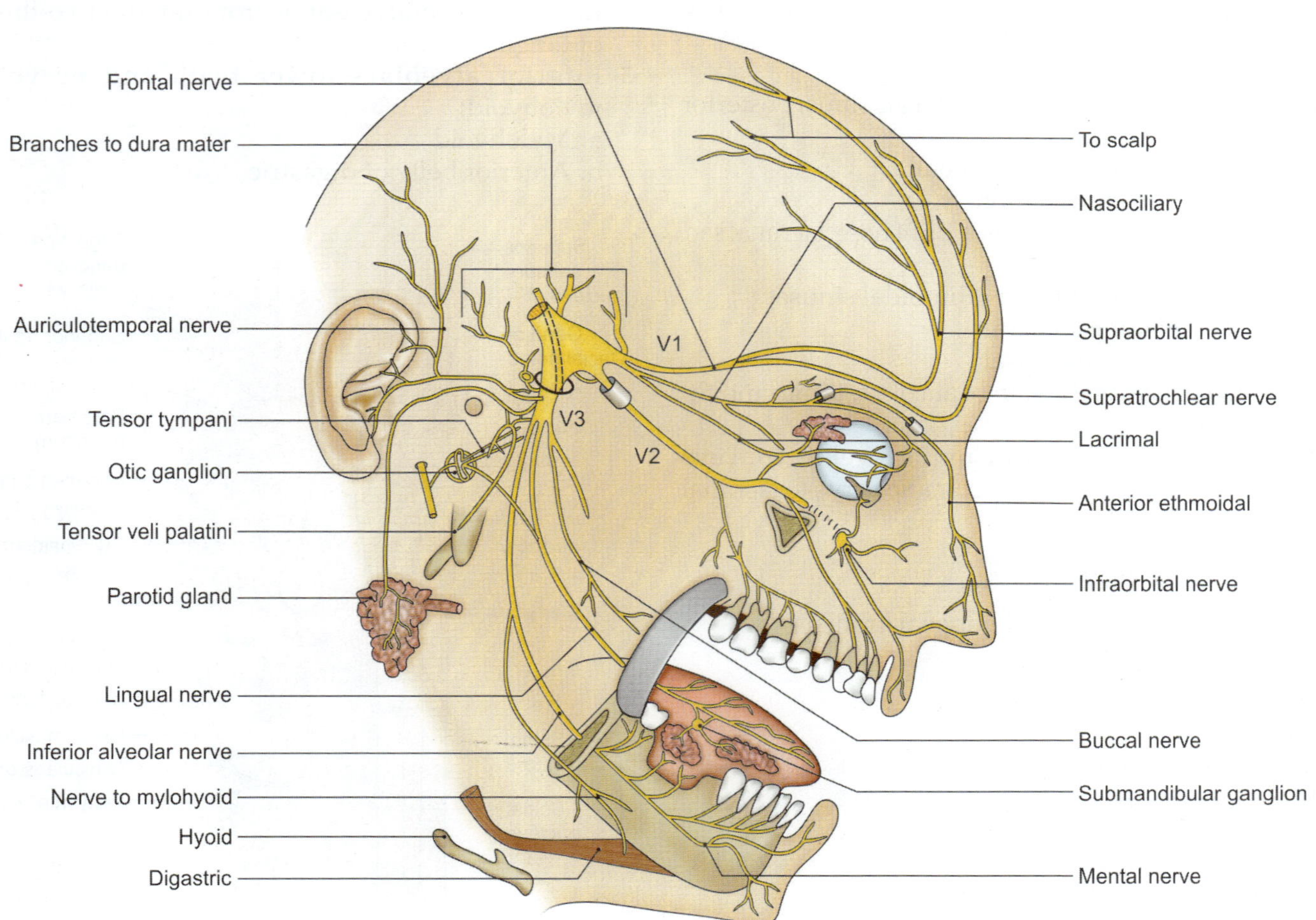

Fig. 32.26: Distribution of three branches of trigeminal nerve

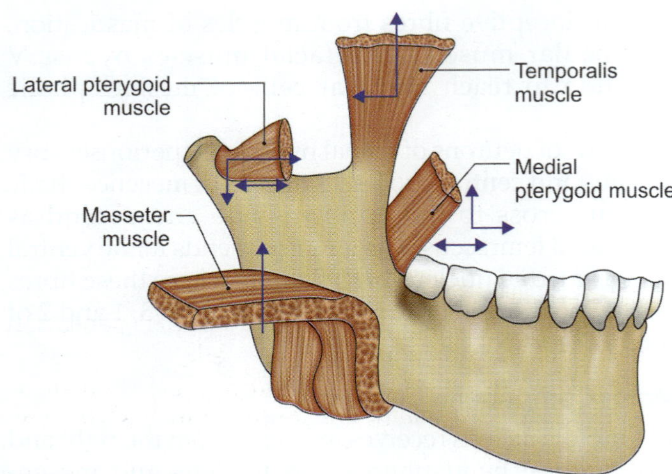

Fig. 32.27: Distribution of mandibular nerve to muscles of mastication. Arrows show direction of movement at temporomandibular joint

Ophthalmic Nerve (V1)

Ophthalmic nerve is sensory. Its branches are:

1 ***Frontal***
   a. *Supratrochlear:* Upper eyelid, conjunctiva, lower part of forehead.
   b. *Supraorbital:* Frontal air sinus, upper eyelid, forehead, scalp till vertex.

2 ***Nasociliary***
   a. *Posterior ethmoidal:* Sphenoidal air sinus, posterior ethmoidal air sinuses.
   b. *Long ciliary:* Sensory to eyeball.
   c. Nerve to ciliary ganglion.
   d. *Infratrochlear:* Both eyelids, side of nose, lacrimal sac.
   e. *Anterior ethmoidal:*
      1. Middle and anterior ethmoidal sinuses
      2. Medial internal nasal
      3. Lateral internal nasal
      4. External nasal—skin of ala of vestibule and tip of nose.

3 ***Lacrimal:*** Lateral part of upper eyelid; conveys secretomotor fibres from zygomatic nerve to lacrimal gland (Fig. 32.26).

Maxillary Nerve (V2)

In Middle Cranial Fossa: Meningeal branch

In Pterygopalatine Fossa:

1 Ganglionic branches
2 Zygomatic:
   a. Zygomaticotemporal
   b. Zygomaticofacial
3 Posterior superior alveolar

In Infraorbital Canal: **Infraorbital**

1 Middle superior alveolar
2 Anterior superior alveolar

On Face: Terminal

a. Palpebral
b. Labial
c. Nasal

Mandibular Nerve (V3)

Trunk (Fig. 32.28)

1 Meningeal
2 Nerve to medial pterygoid
   a. Tensor veli palatini
   b. Tensor tympani
   c. Medial pterygoid.

Anterior Division

1 Deep temporal (Fig. 32.27)
2 Lateral pterygoid
3 Masseteric
4 Buccal—skin of cheek (Fig. 32.26).

Posterior Division

1 Auriculotemporal (Fig. 32.26):
   a. Auricular
   b. Superficial temporal
   c. Articular to temporomandibular joint
   d. Secretomotor to parotid gland.
2 Lingual—general sensation from anterior two-thirds of tongue.
3 Inferior alveolar—lower teeth and nerve to mylohyoid:
   a. Mylohyoid
   b. Anterior belly of digastric.

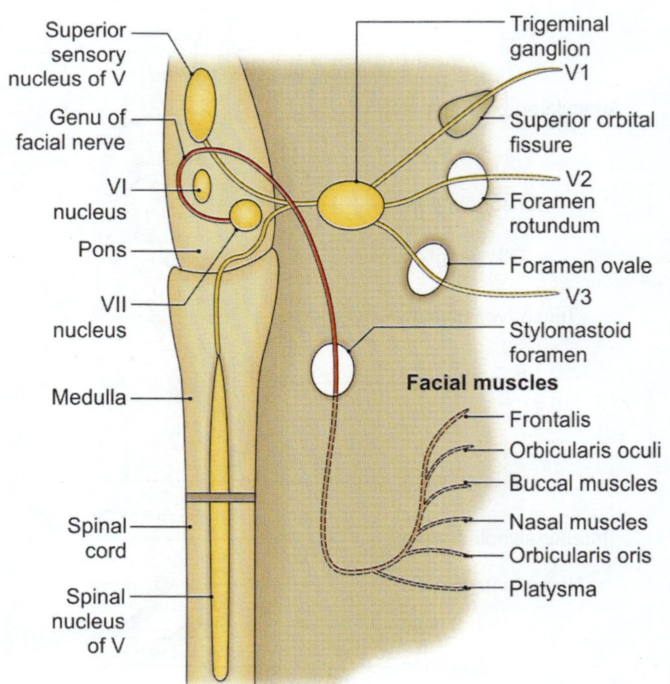

Fig. 32.28: Sensory input of trigeminal (yellow) and motor output of facial nerve (red)

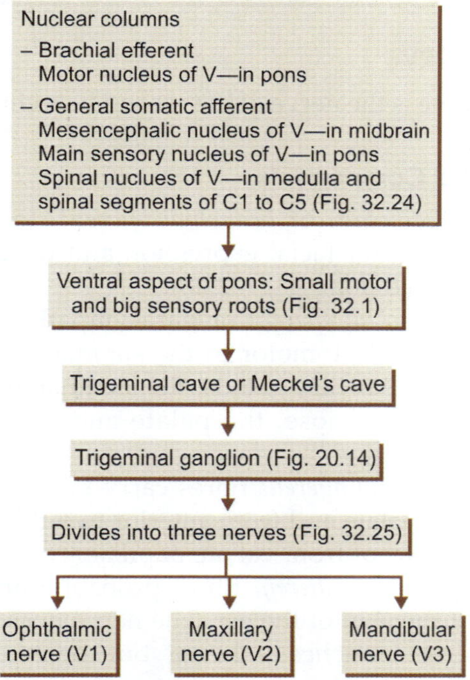

CLINICAL ANATOMY

- Fifth cranial nerve subserves sensation from face and neighbouring areas. It also innervates the muscles of mastication (Fig. 32.29).
- Proprioceptive fibres terminate in mesencephalic nucleus.

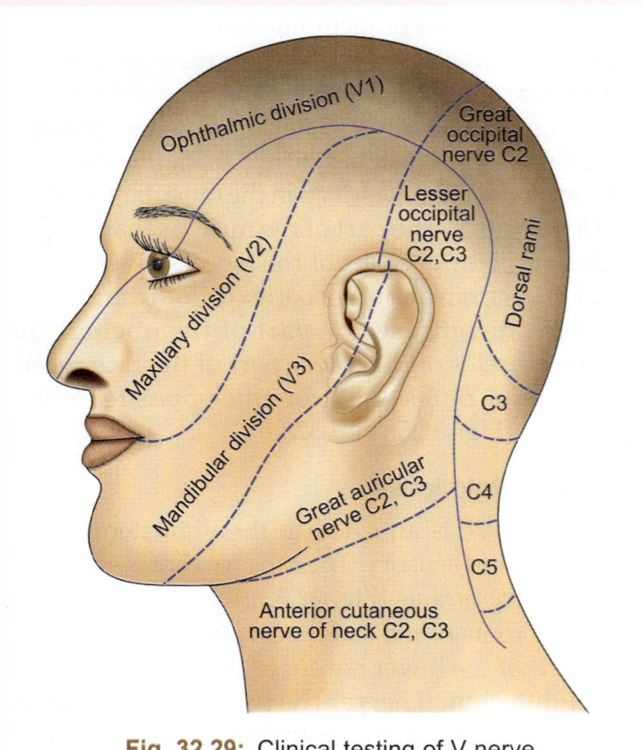

Fig. 32.29: Clinical testing of V nerve

- Light touch fibres end in the main sensory or superior sensory nucleus.
- Pain and temperature fibres terminate in nucleus of spinal tract of trigeminal.
- Motor fibres begin from the motor nucleus of trigeminal.
- The separate location of main sensory nucleus and spinal nucleus account for dissociated sensory loss, i.e. low pontine or medullary lesion will result in loss of pain and temperature sensation while light sensation is preserved.
- Low pontine, medullary and cervical lesions produce a characteristic 'onion skin' distribution of pin prick and temperature loss.
- An ascending lesion spares the muzzle area till last (openings of nose and mouth).
- Test pin prick, temperature and light touch over each side of the whole face.
- The sensations in three branches of V nerve can tested clinically (Fig. 32.29).
- Brainstem lesion results in 'onion skin' pattern as shown in Fig. 32.30.
- *Motor examination:* Look for wasting or thinning of temporalis muscle. There may be 'hollowing out' of the temporal fossa.
- Ask the patient to press upper and lower teeth together and feel for temporalis and masseter muscles.
- Ask patient to open the mouth. If pterygoid muscles are weak, the jaw would deviate to weak side as the normal muscles will push the jaw to the weak side.
- In injury to:
  Ophthalmic nerve: There is loss of corneal blink reflex. This reflex is mediated by V1 which is afferent pathway and VII nerve which subserves as efferent pathway (Fig. 32.31).
  Maxillary nerve: There is loss of sneeze reflex. This branch is the afferent path of sneeze reflex.
  Mandibular nerve: There is loss of jaw jerk reflex (Fig. 32.32).
- *Trigeminal neuralgia:* The principal disease affecting sensory root of V nerve is characterized by attacks of severe pain in the area of distribution of maxillary or mandibular divisions. Maxillary nerve is most frequently involved.
- The trigeminal ganglion harbours the herpes zoster virus causing shingles in the distribution of the nerve.
- Flaccid paralysis of muscles of mastication in injury of mandibular nerve leading to decrease strength of bite.
- Hypoacusis, i.e. partial deafness to low pitched sounds due to paralysis of tensor tympani muscle.

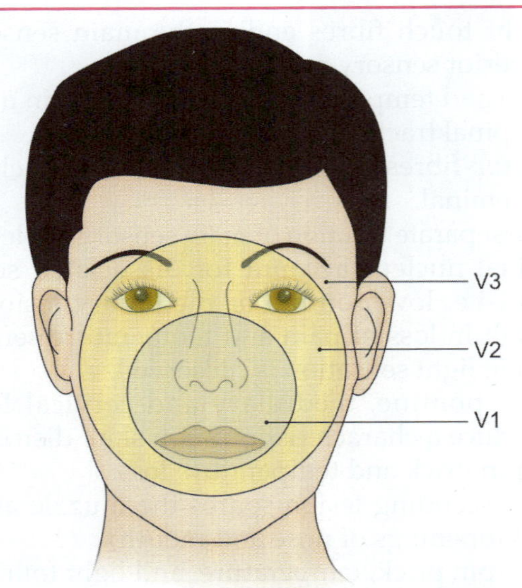

Fig. 32.30: Brainstem lesion of V nerve

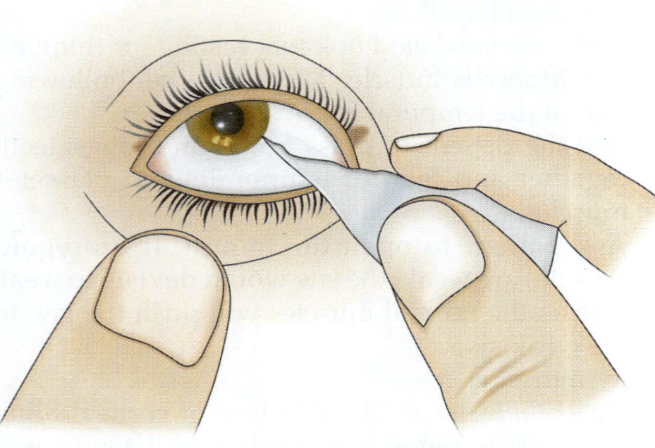

Fig. 32.31: Testing the corneal blink reflex

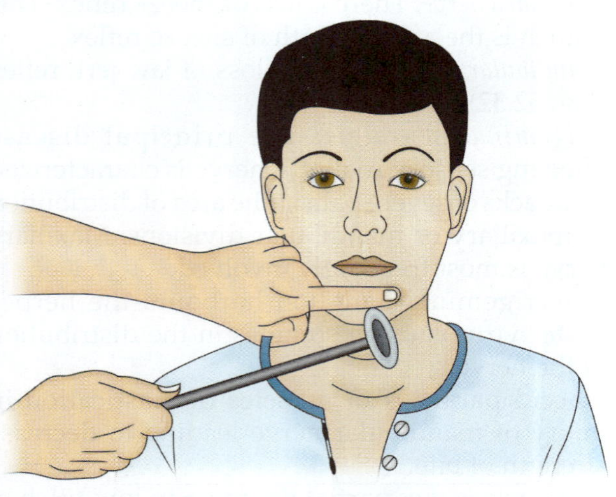

Fig. 32.32: Elicitation of jaw jerk reflex

SEVENTH CRANIAL NERVE

FACIAL NERVE

Facial nerve is the nerve of the second branchial arch.

Functional Components

1. Special visceral or *branchial efferent,* to muscles responsible for facial expression and for elevation of the hyoid bone (Fig. 32.28).
2. *General visceral efferent* or parasympathetic. These fibres are secretomotor to the submandibular and sublingual salivary glands, the lacrimal gland, and glands of the nose, the palate and the pharynx (Fig. 32.3).
3. *Special visceral afferent* fibres carry taste sensations from the palate and from anterior two-thirds of the tongue except from vallate papillae.
4. *General somatic afferent* fibres probably innervate a part of the skin of the ear. The nerve does not give any direct branches to the ear, but some fibres may reach it through communications with the vagus nerve. Proprioceptive impulses from muscles of the face travel through branches of the trigeminal nerve to reach the mesencephalic nucleus of the nerve.

Nuclei

The fibres of the nerve are connected to four nuclei situated in the lower pons.

1. Motor nucleus or branchiomotor.
2. Superior salivatory nucleus or parasympathetic.
3. Lacrimatory nucleus is also parasympathetic.
4. Nucleus of the tractus solitarius which is gustatory and also receives afferent fibres from the glands.

The motor nucleus lies deep in the reticular formation of the lower pons. The part of the nucleus that supplies muscles of the upper part of the face receives cortico-nuclear fibres from the motor cortex of both the right and left sides. In contrast, the part of the nucleus that supplies muscles of the lower part of the face receive corticonuclear fibres only from the opposite cerebral hemisphere (Figs 32.5a and 32.28).

Course and Relations

The facial nerve is attached to the brainstem by two roots, motor and sensory. The sensory root is also called the *nervus intermedius* (Fig. 32.33).

The two roots of the facial nerve are attached to the lateral part of the lower border of the pons just medial to the eighth cranial nerve. The two roots run laterally and forwards, with the eighth nerve to reach the internal acoustic meatus.

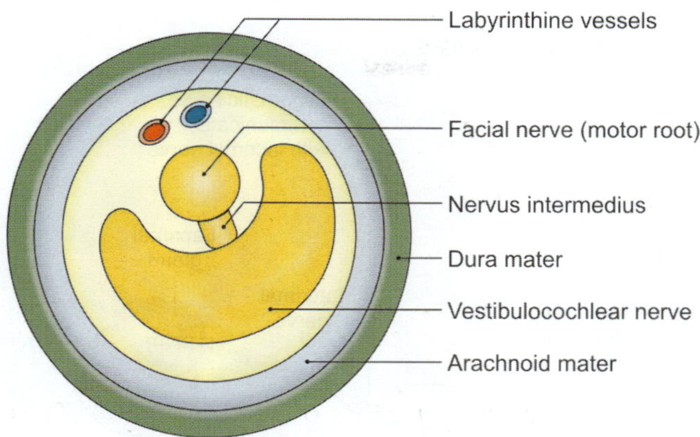

Fig. 32.33: Structures in the left internal acoustic meatus

In the meatus, the motor root lies in a groove on the eighth nerve, with the sensory root intervening. Here the seventh and eighth nerves are accompanied by the labyrinthine vessels. At the bottom or fundus of the meatus, the two roots, sensory and motor, fuse to form a single trunk, which lies in the facial canal of petrous temporal bone (Fig. 32.34).

Within the canal, the course of the nerve can be divided into three parts by two bends (Fig. 32.35).

The first part is directed laterally above the vestibule; the second part runs backwards in relation to the medial wall of the middle ear, above the promontory. The third part is directed vertically downwards behind the promontory.

The first bend at the junction of the first and second parts is sharp. It lies over the anterosuperior part of the promontory, and is also called the *genu*. The geniculate ganglion of the nerve is so called because it lies on the genu. The second bend is gradual, and lies between the promontory and the aditus to the mastoid antrum.

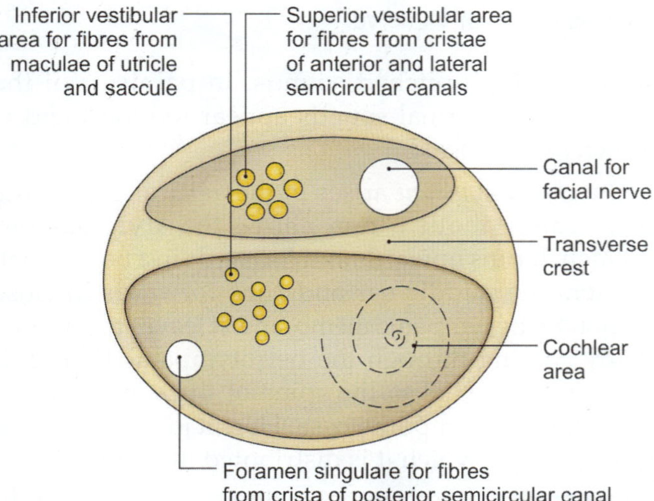

Fig. 32.34: Some features seen on the fundus of the left internal acoustic meatus

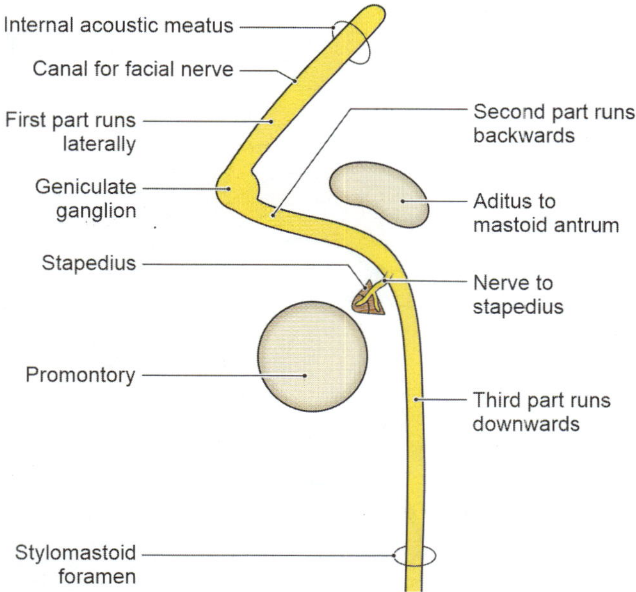

Fig. 32.35: Course of facial nerve

The facial nerve leaves the skull by passing through the stylomastoid foramen.

In its *extracranial course,* the facial nerve crosses the lateral side of the base of the styloid process. It enters the posteromedial surface of the parotid gland, runs forwards through the gland crossing the retromandibular vein and the external carotid artery. Behind the neck of the mandible, it divides into its five terminal branches which emerge along the anterior border of the parotid gland.

Branches and Distribution

A. Within the facial canal:
   1. Greater petrosal nerve
   2. The nerve to the stapedius
   3. The chorda tympani (Fig. 32.36).

B. At its exit from the stylomastoid foramen:
   1. Posterior auricular
   2. Digastric
   3. Stylohyoid.

C. Terminal branches within the parotid gland:
   1. Temporal (Fig. 32.36).
   2. Zygomatic
   3. Buccal
   4. Marginal mandibular
   5. Cervical.

D. Communicating branches with adjacent cranial and spinal nerves.

Greater petrosal nerve—course has been traced in Flowchart 32.1.

The *nerve to the stapedius* arises opposite the pyramid of the middle ear, and supplies the stapedius muscle. The muscle dampens excessive vibrations of the stapes

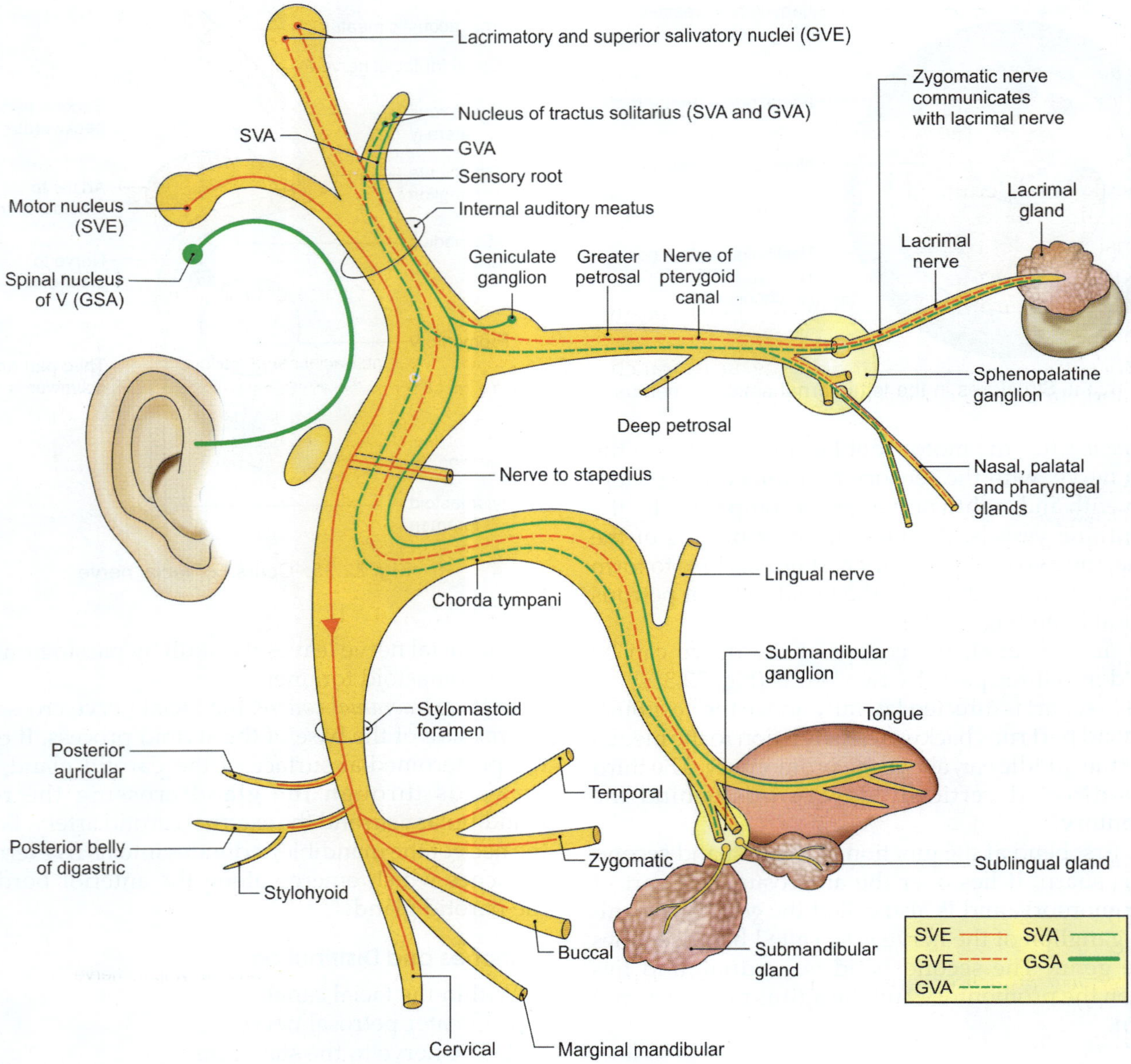

Fig. 32.36: Distribution of functional components of VII nerve

Flowchart 32.1: Tracing nerve supply of lacrimal gland

Greater petrosal nerve
↓
Deep petrosal nerve
↓
Nerve of pterygoid canal
↓
Relay
↓
Postganglionic for lacrimal gland join zygomatic nerve
↓
Pass through communicating branch
↓
Lacrimal nerve
↓
Lacrimal gland

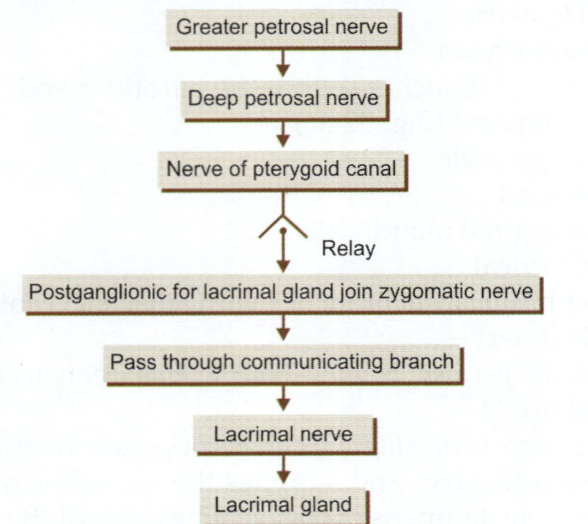

caused by high-pitched sounds. In paralysis of the muscle, even normal sounds appear too loud and is known as *hyperacusis*.

The *chorda tympani* arises in the vertical part of the facial canal about 6 mm above the stylomastoid foramen. It runs upwards and forwards in a bony canal. It enters the middle ear and runs forwards in close relation to the tympanic membrane. It leaves the middle ear by passing through the petrotympanic fissure. It then passes medial to the spine of the sphenoid and enters the infratemporal fossa. Here it joins the lingual nerve through which it is distributed. It carries:

a. Preganglionic secretomotor fibres to the submandibular ganglion for supply of the sub-mandibular and sublingual salivary glands.

b. Taste fibres from the anterior two-thirds of the tongue except circumvallate papillae.

The *posterior auricular nerve* arises just below the stylomastoid foramen. It ascends between the mastoid process and the external acoustic meatus, and supplies:

a. Auricularis posterior
b. Occipitalis
c. Intrinsic muscles on the back of auricle.

The *digastric branch* arises close to the previous nerve. It is short and supplies the posterior belly of the digastric.

The *stylohyoid branch* arises with the digastric branch, is long and supplies the stylohyoid muscle.

The *temporal branches* cross the zygomatic arch and supply:

a. Auricularis anterior
b. Auricularis superior
c. Intrinsic muscles on the lateral side of the ear
d. Frontalis
e. Orbicularis oculi
f. Corrugator supercilii.

The *zygomatic branches* run across the zygomatic bone and supply the orbicularis oculi.

The *buccal branches* are two in number. The upper buccal branch runs above the parotid duct and the lower buccal branch below the duct. They supply muscles in that vicinity especially the buccinator.

The *marginal mandibular branch* runs below the angle of the mandible deep to the platysma. It crosses the body of the mandible and supplies muscles of the lower lip and chin (*see* Fig. 10.18).

The *cervical branch* emerges from the apex of the parotid gland, and runs downwards and forwards in the neck to supply the platysma (*see* Fig. 10.12a).

Communicating branches. For effective coordination between the movements of the muscles of the first, second and third branchial arches, the motor nerves of the three arches communicate with each other. The facial nerve also communicates with the sensory nerves distributed over its motor territory.

Ganglia

The ganglia associated with the facial nerve are as follows.

1 The geniculate ganglion is located on the first bend of the facial nerve, in relation to the medial wall of the middle ear. It is a *sensory ganglion.* The taste fibres present in the nerve are peripheral processes of pseudounipolar neurons present in the geniculate ganglion.

2 The submandibular ganglion is a *parasympathetic ganglion* for relay of secretomotor fibres to the submandibular and sublingual glands. The preganglionic fibres come from the chorda tympani nerve. It is described in Chapter 23 (*see* Fig. 23.10) and in Table 32.2.

3 The pterygopalatine ganglion is also a parasympathetic ganglion. Secretomotor fibres meant for the lacrimal gland relay in this ganglion. The fibres reach the ganglion from the nerve to the pterygoid canal. It is described in Chapter 23 and in Table 32.2.

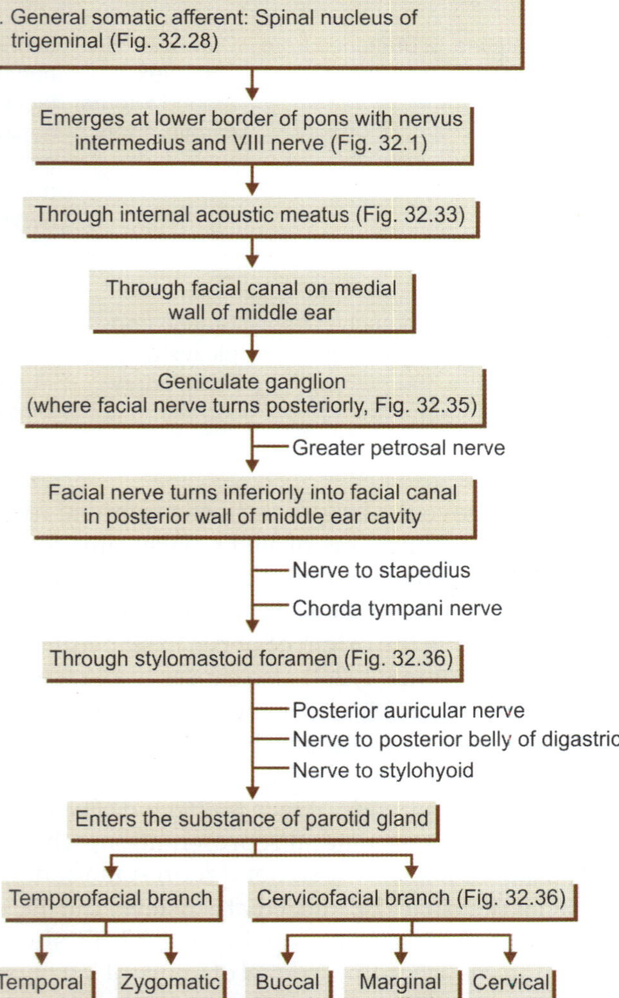

CLINICAL ANATOMY

- *Bells's palsy:* Sudden paralysis of facial nerve at the stylomastoid foramen. Result is asymmetry of corner of mouth, inability to close the eye, disappearance of nasolabial fold and loss of wrinkling of skin of forehead on the same side.

Table 32.2: Connections of parasympathetic ganglia

Ganglia	*Sensory root*	*Sympathetic root*	*Secretomotor root*	*Motor root*	*Distribution*
Ciliary (*see* Fig. 21.11)	From nasociliary nerve	Plexus along ophthalmic artery	—	Edinger-Westphal nucleus → oculomotor nerve → nerve to inferior oblique	Ciliaris muscles Sphincter pupillae
Otic (*see* Fig. 14.17)	Branch from auriculotemporal nerve	Plexus along middle meningeal artery	Inferior salivatory nucleus → glosso-pharyngeal nerve → tympanic branch → tympanic plexus → lesser petrosal nerve	Branch from nerve to medial pterygoid	Secretomotor to parotid gland via auriculotemporal nerve Tensor veli palatini and tensor tympani via nerve to medial pterygoid (unrelayed)
Pterygopalatine (*see* Fig. 23.17)	2 branches from maxillary nerve	Deep petrosal from plexus around internal carotid artery	Lacrimatory nucleus → nervus intermedius → facial nerve → geniculate ganglion → greater petrosal nerve + deep petrosal nerve = nerve of pterygoid canal	—	Mucous glands of nose, paranasal sinuses, palate, nasopharynx Some fibres pass through zygomatic nerve—zygomaticotemporal nerve—communicating branch to lacrimal nerve—lacrimal gland
Submandibular (*see* Fig. 15.9)	2 branches from lingual nerve	Branch from plexus around facial artery	Superior salivatory nucleus → facial nerve → chorda tympani-joins the lingual nerve	—	Submandibular, Sublingual and Anterior lingual glands

- Lesion above the origin of chorda tympani nerve will show symptoms of Bell's palsy plus loss of taste from anterior two-thirds of tongue except vallate papillae (Fig. 32.37).
- Lesion above the origin of nerve to stapedius will cause symptoms 1, 2. It also causes hyperacusis.
- Lesions 1, 2 and 3 are lower motor neuron type. Upper motor neuron paralysis will not affect the upper part of face, i.e. orbicularis oculi, only lower half of opposite side of face is affected. The upper half of face has bilateral representation, whereas lower half has only ipsilateral representation.
- Facial nerve can be injured at any level during its course. Accompanying Figure 32.37 shows symptoms according to level of injury of VII nerve. Lower motor neuron paralysis of VII nerve causes paralysis of ipsilateral half of face, i.e. both upper quadrant and lower quadrant of same side as the injury. Upper motor neuron paralysis of VII nerve results in paralysis of contralateral lower quadrant of face only.
- For clinical testing of the facial nerve, and for different types of facial paralysis—infranuclear (*see* Fig. 10.31) and for supranuclear (*see* Fig. 10.32).
- *Facial nerve palsy in newborn:* The mastoid process is absent in newborn and stylomastoid foramen is superficial. Manipulation of baby's head during delivery may damage the VII nerve. This leads to paralysis of facial muscles especially the buccinator, required for sucking the milk.
- *Crocodile tears syndrome:* Lacrimation during eating occurs due to aberrant regeneration after trauma.
- In case of damage to facial nerve proximal to geniculate ganglia, regenerating fibres for submandibular salivary gland grow in endoneural sheaths of preganglionic secretomotor fibres supplying the lacrimal gland. That is why patient lacrimates while eating food. This is called *crocodile tears syndrome.*
- *Ramsay-Hunt syndrome:* Involvement of geniculate ganglia by herpes zoster results in this syndrome. It shows following symptoms:
  a. Hyperacusis.
  b. Loss of lacrimation.
  c. Loss of sensation of taste in anterior two-thirds of tongue.
  d. Bell's palsy and lack of salivation.
  e. Vesicles on the auricle.

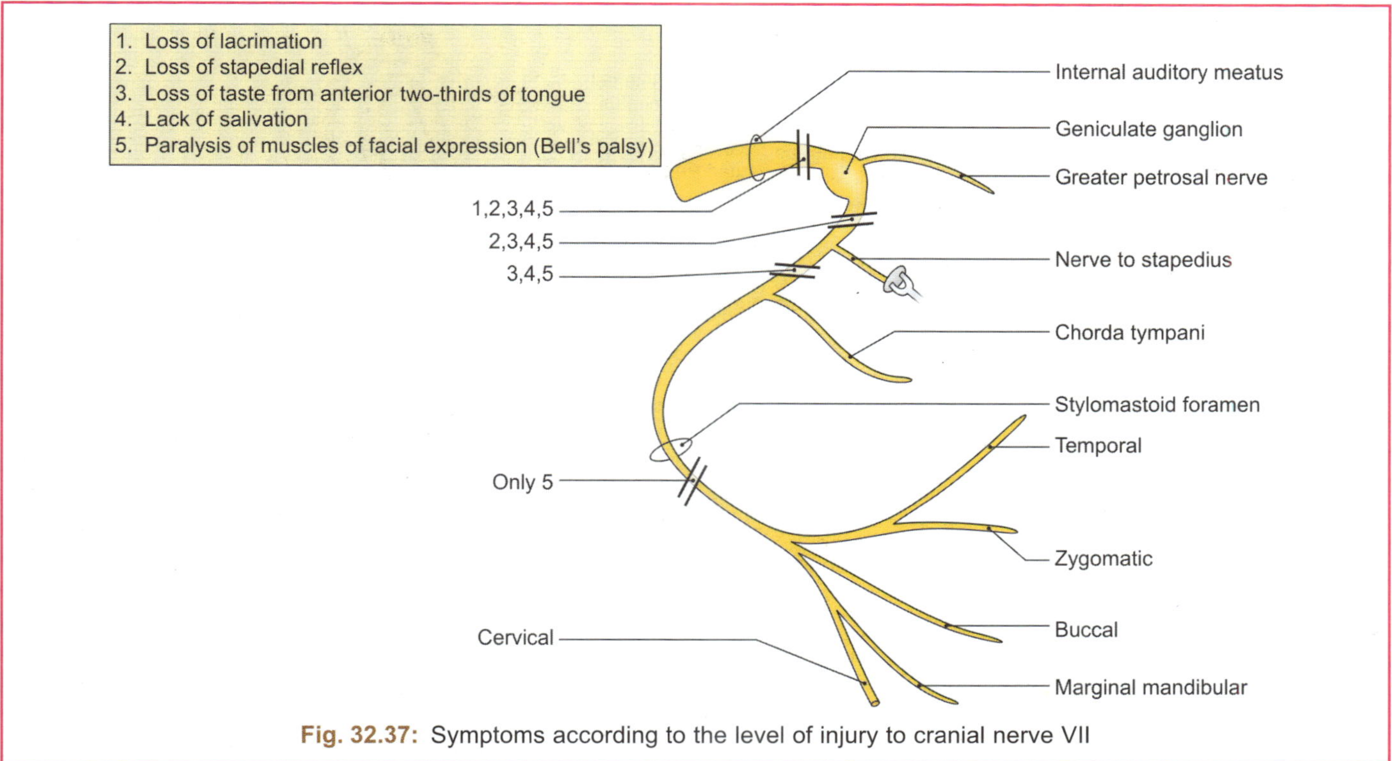

Fig. 32.37: Symptoms according to the level of injury to cranial nerve VII

EIGHTH CRANIAL NERVE

VESTIBULOCOCHLEAR NERVE

This nerve comprises hearing and vestibular parts.

Pathway of Hearing

1 The first neurons of the pathway are located in the spiral ganglion. They are bipolar. Their peripheral processes innervate the spiral organ of Corti (Fig. 32.38), while central processes form the cochlear nerve (Fig. 32.39). This nerve terminates in the dorsal and ventral cochlear nuclei.

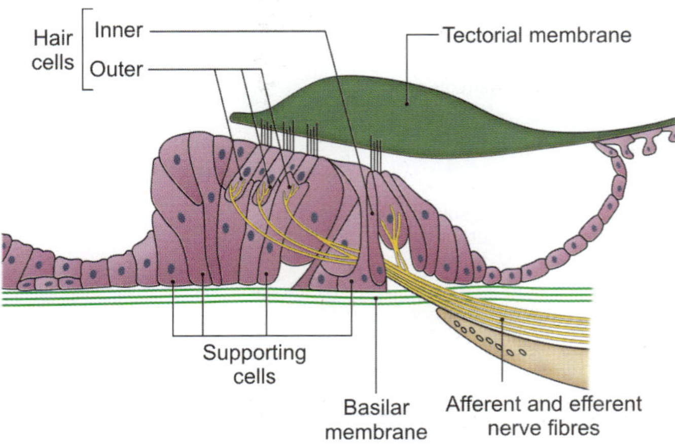

Fig. 32.38: Organ of Corti

2 The second neurons lie in the dorsal and ventral cochlear nuclei. Most of the axons arising in these nuclei cross to the opposite side (in the trapezoid body) and terminate in the superior olivary nucleus. (Many fibres end in the nucleus of trapezoid body or of the lateral lemniscus.) Some fibres are uncrossed (Fig. 32.40).

3 The third neurons lie in the superior olivary nucleus. Their axons form the lateral lemniscus and reach the inferior colliculus.

4 The fourth neurons lie in the inferior colliculus. Their axons pass through the inferior brachium to reach the medial geniculate body. (Some fibres of lateral lemniscus reach the medial geniculate body without relay in the inferior colliculus.)

5 The fifth neurons lie in the medial geniculate body. Their axons form the auditory radiation, which passes through the sublentiform part of the internal capsule to reach the auditory area (Fig. 32.40) in the temporal lobe (Fig. 32.41).

Vestibular Pathway

The vestibular receptors are the maculae of the saccule and utricle (for static balance) (Fig. 32.42) and in the cristae of the ampullae of semicircular ducts (for kinetic balance) (Fig. 32.43). Fibres from cristae of anterior and lateral semicircular canals and some fibres from the two maculae lie in superior vestibular area of internal acoustic meatus.

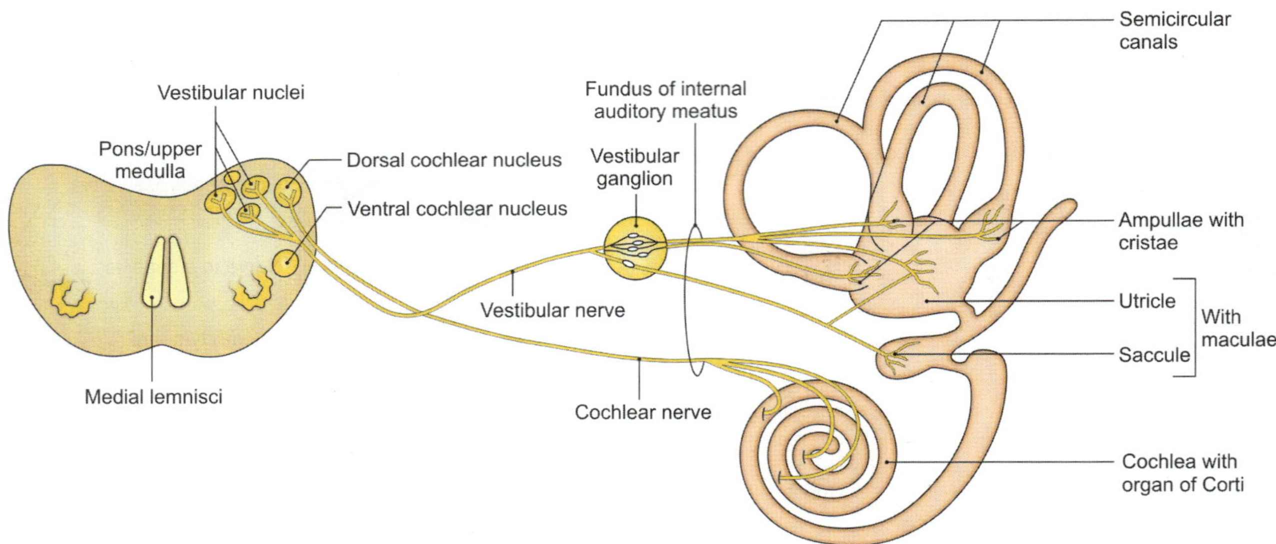

Fig. 32.39: Course of cochlear and vestibular nerves

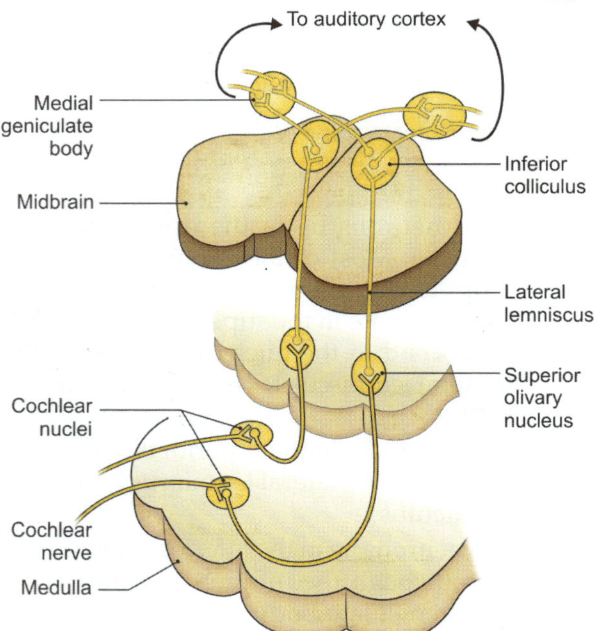

Fig. 32.40: Auditory pathway

Fibres of crista of posterior semicircular canal lie in foramen singulare.

Most of the fibres from maculae of utricle and saccule lie in inferior vestibular area (Fig. 32.34).

These three nerve divisions are peripheral processes of bipolar neurons of the vestibular ganglion. This ganglion is situated in the internal acoustic meatus. The central processes arising from the neurons of the ganglion form the vestibular nerve which ends in the vestibular nuclei.

The second neurons in the pathway of balance lies in the vestibular nuclei (Fig. 32.39). These nuclei send fibres:

a. To the archicerebellum through the inferior cerebellar peduncle (vestibulocerebellar tract).
b. To the motor nuclei of the brainstem (chiefly of the III, IV and VI nerves) through the medial longitudinal bundle (Fig. 32.44).
c. To the anterior horn cells of the spinal cord through the vestibulospinal tract.

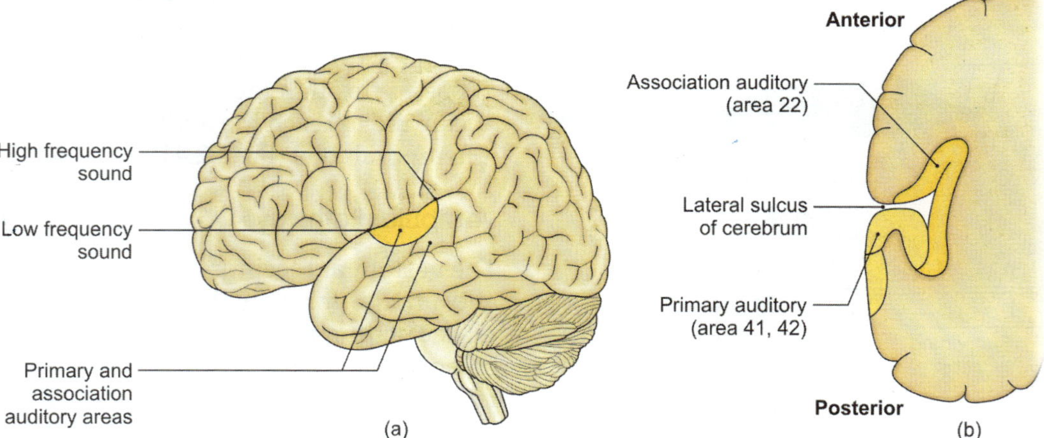

Figs 32.41a and b: Auditory cortex: (a) Posterior ramus of lateral sulcus, and (b) depth of lateral sulcus

Macula
Gelatinous mass
Otoliths
Stereocilia
Hair cell
Supporting columnar cells

Fig. 32.42: Structure of the macula

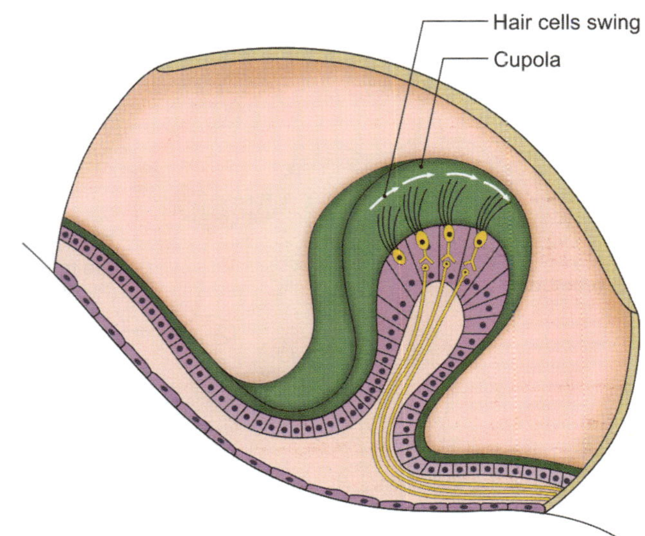

Fig. 32.43: Structure of crista ampullaris

Course of vestibulocochlear nerve

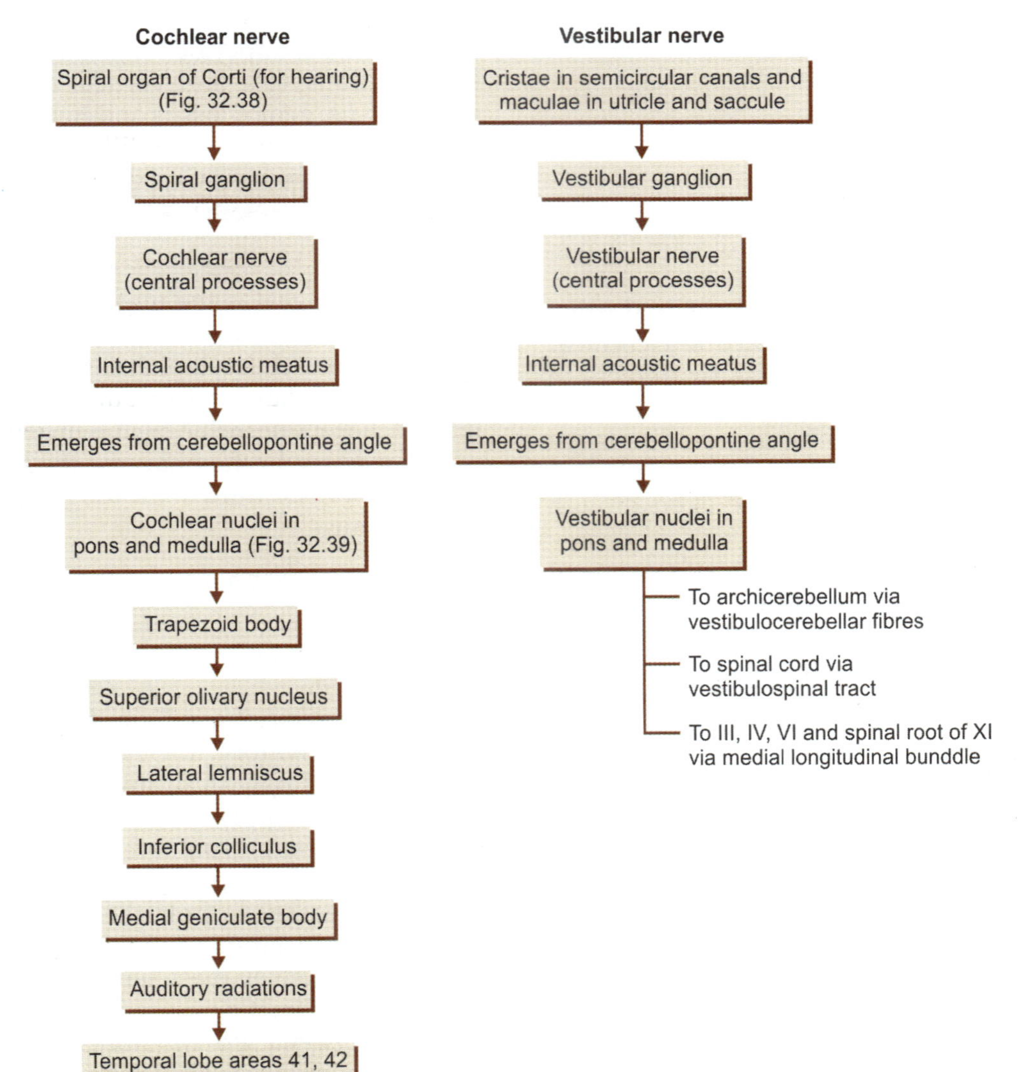

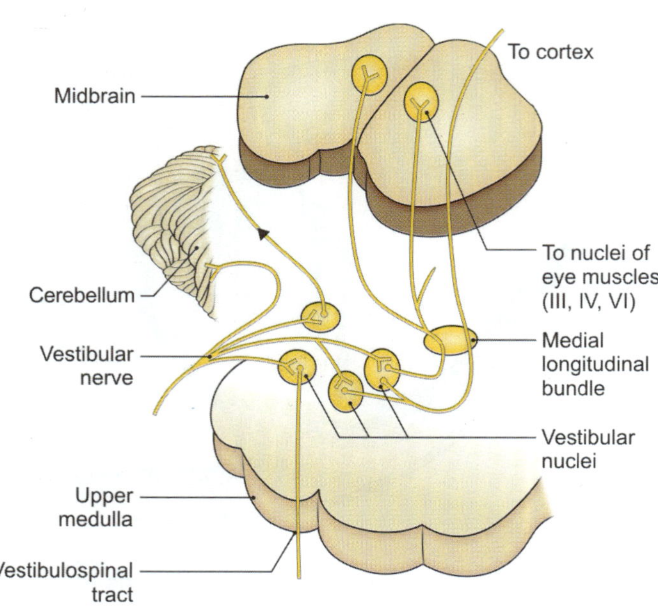

Fig. 32.44: Vestibular pathway

Through the vestibular pathway, the impulses arising in the labyrinth can influence the movements of the eyes, the head, the neck and the trunk.

CLINICAL ANATOMY

Deafness

Three types of hearing loss are seen:

1. Conductive deafness is the failure of sound waves to reach to the cochlea.
2. Sensorineural deafness is the failure of production or transmission of action potential due to cochlear disease, cochlear nerve disease or defects in cochlear nerve central connections.
3. Cortical deafness is a bilateral or dominant posterior temporal lobe lesion. It results in a failure to understand spoken language even though hearing is preserved.

- *Vertigo:* This is an illusion of rotatory movement due to disturbed orientation of the body in space. The patient feels that the environment is moving. It is due to disease of vestibular nerve.
- Tinnitis is a sensation of buzzing, ringing, hissing or singing quality. Tinnitis may be unilateral or bilateral; high or low pitch; continuous or intermittent.
- Meniere's syndrome is characterized by recurrent attacks of tinnitus, vertigo and hearing loss accompanied by a sensitivity to noises. It affects middle aged or older persons. In this condition, there is an increase in volume of endolymph.
- Acoustic neuroma is a slow growing benign tumour of neurolemmal cells. It causes an early loss of hearing.

LAST FOUR CRANIAL NERVES

Ninth nerve is the nerve of third branchial arch and supplies the only muscle of that arch, the stylopharyngeus. It carries sensory fibres from the posterior one-third of tongue, tonsil, pharynx, middle ear, taste fibres from posterior one-third of tongue and circumvallate papillae. Lastly, it provides secretomotor fibres to parotid gland.

Vagus in the neck gives pharyngeal, carotid sinus and laryngeal branches. These are gracefully borrowed from cranial root of accessory nerve. Vagus gives auricular and cardiac branches as its "own". That is why syringing the ear may cause slowing of the heart rate and even its inhibition. Vagus is the parasympathetic nerve of foregut and midgut.

Accessory nerve comprises two roots—cranial root given to vagus and spinal root supplies two muscles of neck, one shrugging muscle, the trapezius, and other, the chin turning muscle, the sternocleidomastoid.

Hypoglossal supplies 7 out of 8 muscles of tongue, except palatoglossus. The muscles supplied are 4 intrinsic, i.e. superior longitudinal, inferior longitudinal, transverse and vertical and 3 extrinsic, i.e. styloglossus, genioglossus and hyoglossus.

NINTH CRANIAL NERVE

GLOSSOPHARYNGEAL NERVE

Glossopharyngeal is the ninth cranial nerve. It is the nerve of the third branchial arch.

It is motor to the stylopharyngeus. It is secretomotor to the parotid gland and gustatory to the posterior one-third of the tongue including the circumvallate papillae.

It is sensory to the pharynx, the tonsil soft palate, the posterior one-third of the tongue, carotid body and carotid sinus.

Functional Components

a. *Special visceral efferent* fibres arise in nucleus ambiguus and supply the stylopharyngeus muscle (Fig. 32.45).
b. *General visceral efferent* fibres (preganglionic) arise in inferior salivatory nucleus and travel to the otic ganglion. Postganglionic fibres arising in the ganglion to supply the parotid gland (Table 32.2).
c. *General visceral afferent* fibres are peripheral processes of cells in inferior ganglion of the nerve. They carry general sensations from the pharynx, carotid body and carotid sinus to the ganglion. The central processes convey these sensations to the nucleus of the solitary tract.
d. *Special visceral afferent* fibres are also peripheral processes of cells in the inferior ganglion. They carry

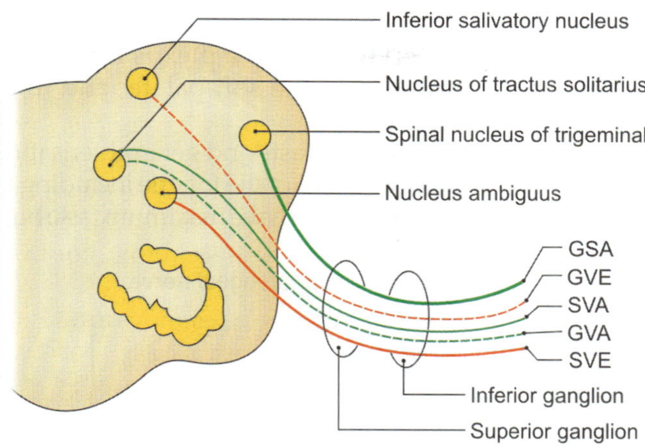

Fig. 32.45: Functional components and nuclei of IX nerve

sensations of taste from the posterior one-third of the tongue including circumvallate papillae to the ganglion. The central processes convey these sensations to the nucleus of the solitary tract.

e. *General somatic afferent* fibres are the peripheral processes of the cells in the inferior ganglion of the nerve. These carry general sensations (pain, touch, temperature) from posterior one-third of tongue and tonsil. The central processes carry these sensations to nucleus of spinal tract of trigeminal nerve.

Nuclei

The three nuclei in the upper part of medulla are named below:

1 Nucleus ambiguus (branchiomotor).
2 Inferior salivary nucleus (parasympathetic).
3 Nucleus of tractus solitarius (gustatory) (Fig. 32.46).

Course and Relations

1 In their *intraneural course,* the fibres of the nerve pass forwards and laterally, between the olivary nucleus and the inferior cerebellar peduncle, through the reticular formation of the medulla.
2 At the base of the brain, the nerve is attached by 3 to 4 filaments to the upper part of the posterolateral

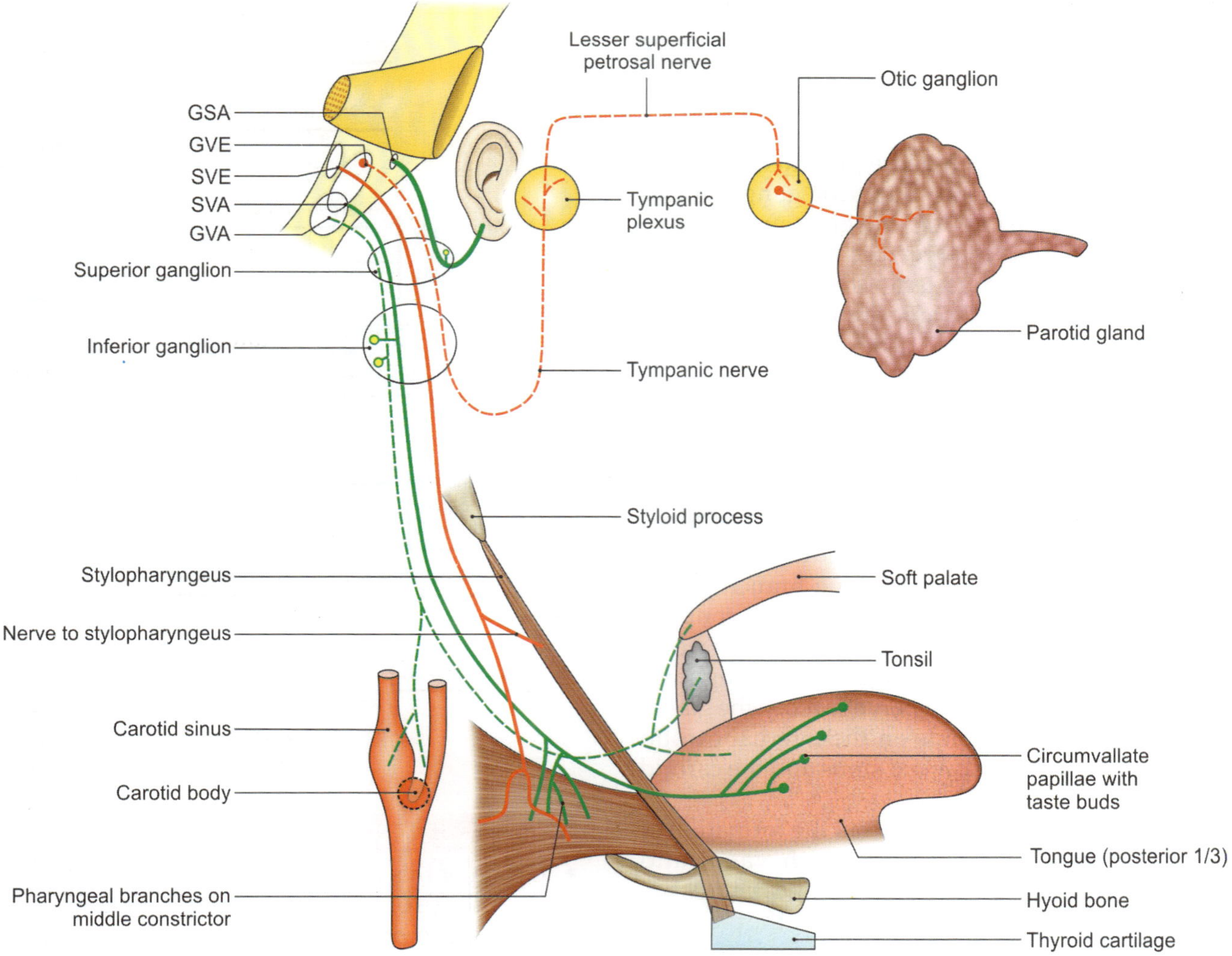

Fig. 32.46: Distribution of functional components of glossopharyngeal nerve

sulcus of the medulla, just above the rootlets of the vagus nerve (*see* Fig. 33.1).

3 In their intracranial course, the filaments unite to form a single trunk which passes forwards and laterally towards the jugular foramen, crossing and grooving the jugular tubercle of the occipital bone.
4 The nerve *leaves the skull* by passing through the middle part of the *jugular foramen,* anterior to the vagus and accessory nerves. It has a separate sheath of dura mater.
5 In the jugular foramen, the nerve is lodged in a deep groove leading to the cochlear canaliculus, and is separated from the vagus and accessory nerves by the inferior petrosal sinus.

   In its *extracranial course,* the nerve descends:
   i. Between the internal jugular vein and the internal carotid artery, deep to the styloid process and the muscles attached to it.
   ii. It then turns forwards winding round the lateral aspect of the stylopharyngeus, passes between the external and internal carotid arteries, and reaches the side of the pharynx (Fig. 32.46). Here it gives pharyngeal branches.
   iii. It enters the submandibular region by passing deep to the hyoglossus (*see* Fig. 15.4), where it breaks up into tonsillar and lingual branches.

6 At the base of skull, ninth nerve presents a superior and an inferior ganglion. Superior ganglion is a detached part of the inferior, and gives no branches. The inferior ganglion is larger, occupies notch on the lower border of petrous temporal, and gives out communicating and tympanic branches (Fig. 32.46).

Branches and Distribution

1 The *tympanic nerve* (Table 32.2) is a branch of the inferior ganglion of the glossopharyngeal nerve. It enters the middle ear through the tympanic canaliculus, takes part in the formation of the tympanic plexus in the middle ear and distributes its fibres to the middle ear, the auditory tube, the mastoid antrum and air cells. One branch of the plexus is called the lesser petrosal nerve. It contains preganglionic secretomotor fibres for the parotid gland and relays in the otic ganglion. Postganglionic fibres join auriculotemporal nerve to reach the gland.
2 The *carotid branch* descends on the internal carotid artery and supplies the carotid sinus and the carotid body.
3 The *pharyngeal branches* take part in the formation of the pharyngeal plexus, along with vagal and sympathetic fibres. The glossopharyngeal fibres are distributed to the mucous membrane of the pharynx.
4 The *muscular branch* supplies the stylopharyngeus (Fig. 32.46).
5 The *tonsillar branches* supply the tonsil and join the lesser palatine nerves to form a plexus from which fibres are distributed to the soft palate and to the palatoglossal arches.
6 The *lingual branches* carry taste and general sensations from the posterior one-third of the tongue including the circumvallate papillae which have maximum taste buds.

Course of glossopharyngeal nerve

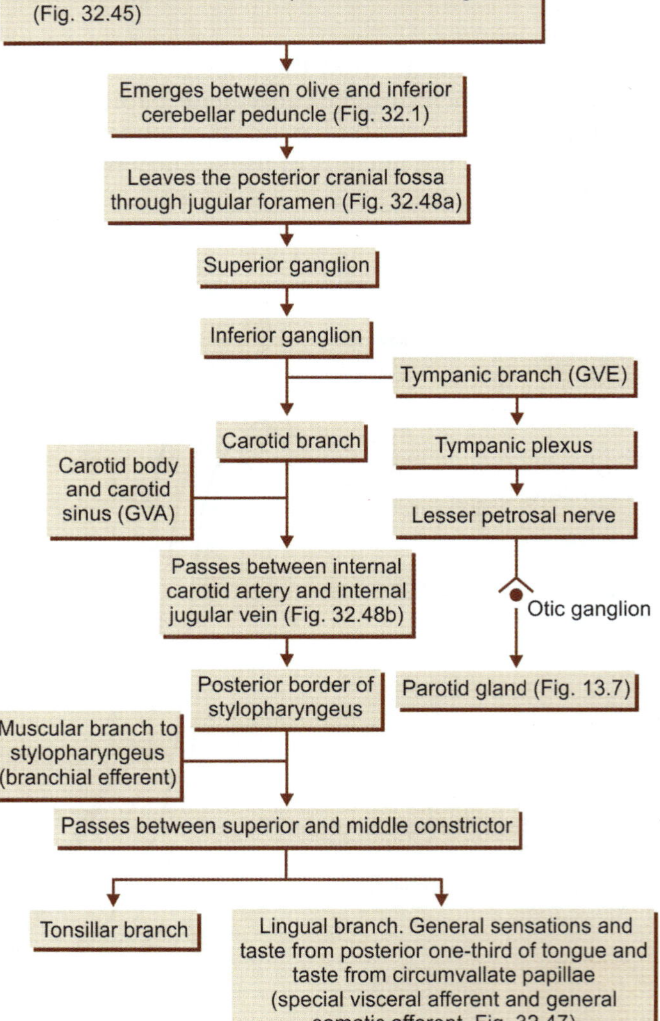

CLINICAL ANATOMY

- Lesion of this nerve causes:
  a. Absence of secretions of parotid gland.
  b. Absence of taste from posterior one-third of tongue and the circumvallate papillae.

c. Loss of pain sensations from tongue tonsil, pharynx and soft palate.
d. Gag reflex is absent.

- *Glossopharyngeal neuralgia:* It is a short sharp severe attacks of pain affecting posterior part of pharynx or tonsillar area.
- Jugular foramen syndrome is due to injury at the jugular foramen resulting in multiple cranial nerve palsies.
- The glossopharyngeal nerve is tested clinically in the following ways:
  a. On tickling the posterior wall of the pharynx, there is reflex contraction of the pharyngeal muscles. No such contraction occurs when the ninth nerve is paralysed.
  b. Taste sensibility on the posterior one-third of the tongue can also be tested. It is lost in ninth nerve lesions.
- Isolated lesions of the ninth nerve are almost unknown. They are usually accompanied by lesions of the vagus nerve.
- Pharyngitis may cause referred pain in the ear as both are supplied by IX nerve. However, in these cases eustachian catarrh should be excluded.

TENTH CRANIAL NERVE

VAGUS NERVE

Vagus nerve is the tenth cranial nerve. It is so called because of its extensive ('vague') course, through the head, the neck, the thorax and the abdomen. The fibres of the cranial root of the accessory nerve are also distributed through it (Figs 32.47 to 32.50).

The vagus nerve bears two ganglia—superior and inferior. The *superior ganglion* is rounded and lies in the jugular foramen. The *inferior* ganglion is cylindrical and lies near the base of the skull (Fig. 32.50).

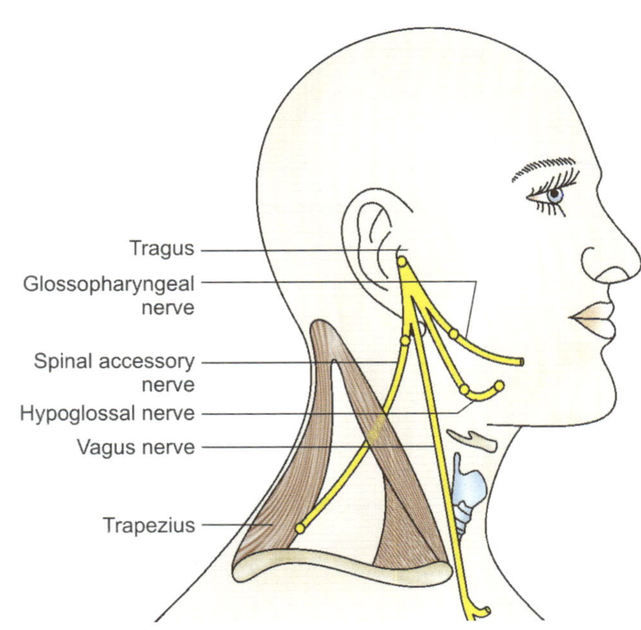

Fig. 32.47: Position of cranial nerves IX, X, XI, XII

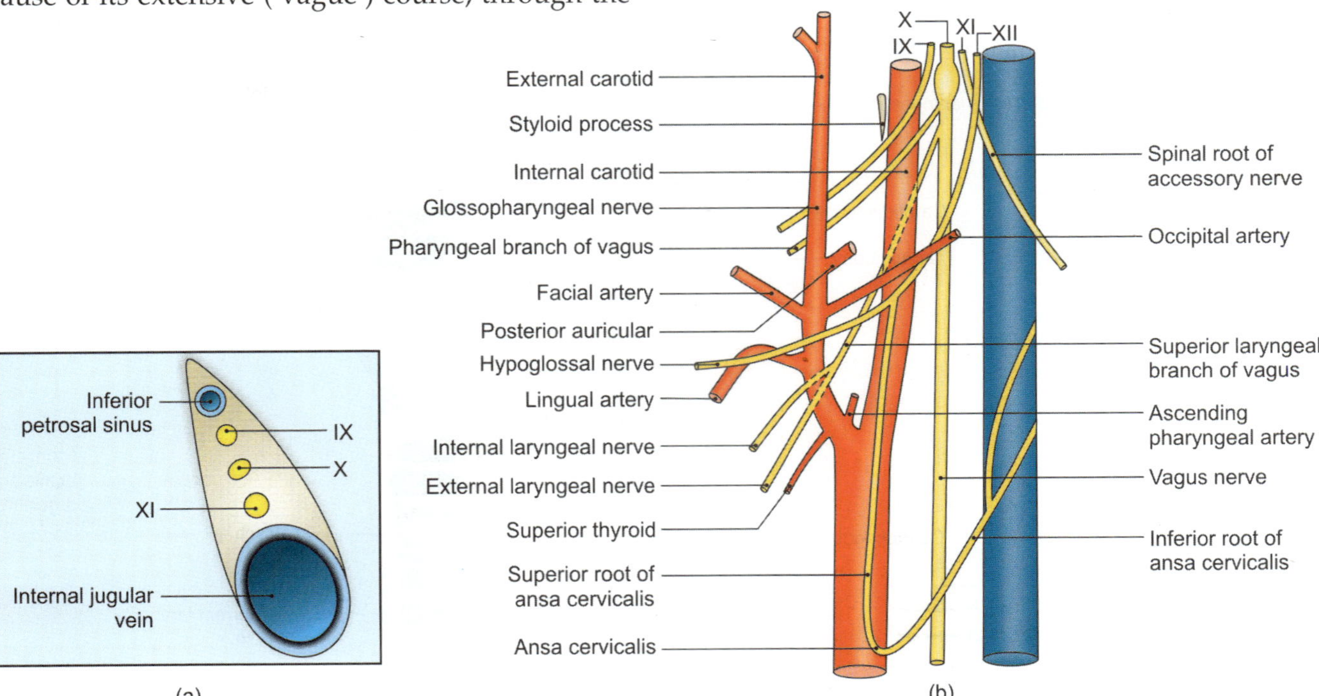

Figs 32.48a and b: (a) Structures passing through jugular foramen, and (b) relation of cranial nerves IX, X, XI, XII to carotid arteries and internal jugular vein

Dorsal nucleus of vagus
Nucleus of tractus solitarius
Spinal nucleus of trigeminal
Nucleus ambiguus
GSA
GVE
SVA
GVA
SVE
Inferior ganglion
Superior ganglion

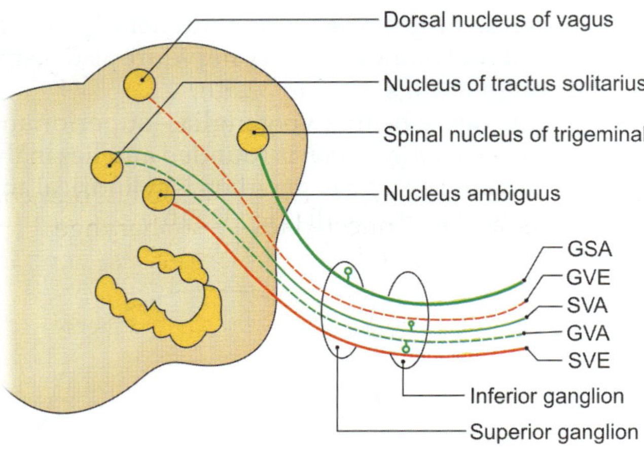

Fig. 32.49: Functional components and nuclei of X nerve

Functional Components

a. *Special visceral efferent* fibres arise in the nucleus ambiguus and supply the muscles of the palate, pharynx and larynx (Fig. 32.50).

b. *General visceral efferent* fibres arise in the dorsal motor nucleus of the vagus. These are preganglionic parasympathetic fibres. They are distributed to thoracic and abdominal viscera. The postganglionic neurons are situated in ganglia lying close to (or within) the viscera to be supplied.

c. *General visceral afferent* fibres are peripheral processes of cells located in the inferior ganglion of the nerve. They bring sensations from the pharynx, larynx, trachea, oesophagus and from the abdominal and

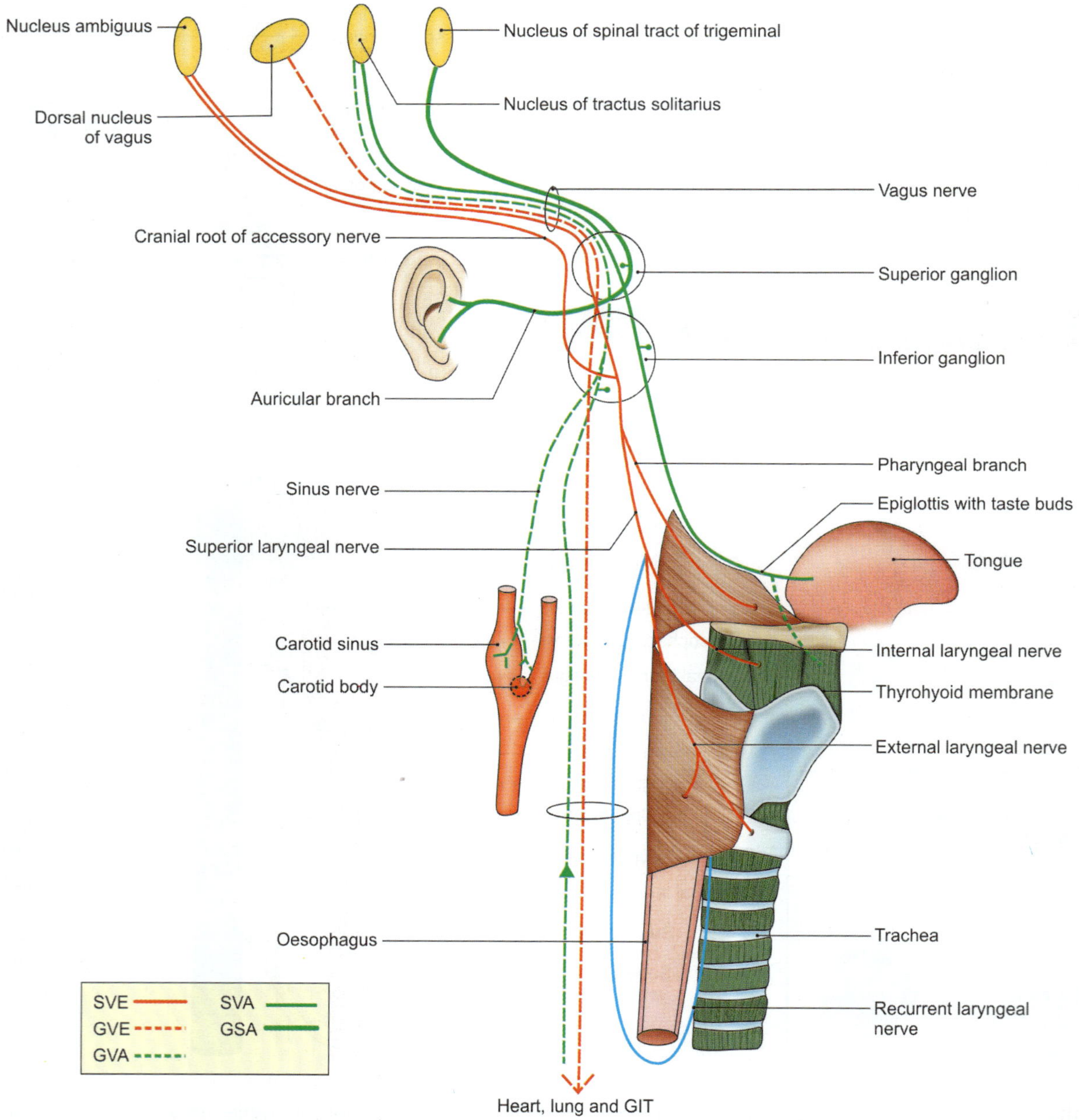

Nucleus ambiguus
Nucleus of spinal tract of trigeminal
Dorsal nucleus of vagus
Nucleus of tractus solitarius
Vagus nerve
Cranial root of accessory nerve
Superior ganglion
Inferior ganglion
Auricular branch
Pharyngeal branch
Sinus nerve
Epiglottis with taste buds
Superior laryngeal nerve
Tongue
Carotid sinus
Internal laryngeal nerve
Carotid body
Thyrohyoid membrane
External laryngeal nerve
Oesophagus
Trachea
Recurrent laryngeal nerve
SVE
GVE
GVA
SVA
GSA
Heart, lung and GIT

Fig. 32.50: Distribution of functional components of vagus nerve

thoracic viscera. These are conveyed by the central processes of the ganglion cells to the nucleus of the tractus solitarius. Some of these fibres terminate in the dorsal nucleus of the vagus.

d. *Special visceral afferent* fibres are also peripheral processes of neurons in the inferior ganglion. They carry sensations of taste from the posteriormost part of the tongue and from the epiglottis. The central processes of the cells concerned terminate in the lower part of the nucleus of the tractus solitarius.
e. *General somatic afferent* fibres are peripheral processes of neurons in the superior ganglion and are distributed to the skin of the external ear. The central processes of the ganglion cells terminate in relation to the spinal nucleus of the trigeminal nerve.

Nuclei

1 *Nucleus ambiguus (branchiomotor):* Mostly a part of the cranial root of accessory nerve; partly of vagus.
2 *Dorsal nucleus of vagus (parasympathetic):* It is a mixed nucleus, being both motor (visceromotor and secretomotor) and sensory (viscerosensory). Its fibres form the main bulk of the nerve.
3 *Nucleus of tractus solitarius (gustatory):* Distributed through internal laryngeal nerve to the taste buds of epiglottis and vallecula.
4 Nucleus of spinal tract of trigeminal.

Course and Relations in Head and Neck

1 In the *intracranial course*, fibres run forwards and laterally through the reticular formation of medulla, between the olivary nucleus and inferior cerebellar peduncle (Fig. 33.5).
2 The nerve is attached, by about ten rootlets, to the posterolateral sulcus of medulla (Fig. 32.1).
3 In the intracranial course, the rootlets unite to from a large trunk which passes laterally across the jugular tubercle along with the glossopharyngeal and cranial root of accessory nerves, and reaches the jugular foramen.
4 The nerve *leaves the cranial cavity* by passing through the middle part of the jugular foramen, between the sigmoid and inferior petrosal sinuses. In the foramen, it is joined by the cranial root of the accessory nerve.
5 Leaving the skull, the nerve descends within the carotid sheath, in between and posterior to the internal jugular vein (laterally), and the internal and common carotid arteries (medially) (Figs 11.8 and 32.50).
6 At the *root of the neck,* the right vagus enters the thorax by crossing the first part of the subclavian artery, and then inclining medially behind the brachiocephalic vessels, to reach the right side of the trachea. The left vagus enters the thorax by passing between the left common carotid and left subclavian arteries, behind the internal jugular and brachiocephalic veins.
7 Vagus bears two ganglia, superior and inferior. The *superior ganglion* is rounded and lies in the jugular foramen. It gives meningeal and auricular branches of vagus, and is connected to glossopharyngeal and accessory nerves and to superior cervical ganglion of sympathetic chain. The *inferior ganglion* is cylindrical (2.5 cm) and lies near the base of skull. It gives pharyngeal, carotid, superior laryngeal branches and is connected to hypoglossal nerve, superior cervical ganglion and the loop between first and second cervical nerves.

Branches in Head and Neck

In the jugular foramen, the superior ganglion gives off:

1 Meningeal, and
2 Auricular branches.

The ganglion also gives off communicating branches to the glossopharyngeal and cranial root of accessory nerves and to the superior cervical sympathetic ganglion.

The branches arising in the neck are:

1 Pharyngeal
2 Carotid
3 Superior laryngeal
4 Right recurrent laryngeal
5 Cardiac.

Meningeal branch supplies dura of the posterior cranial fossa. The fibres are derived from sympathetic and upper cervical nerves.

The *auricular branch* arises from the superior ganglion of the vagus. It passes behind the internal jugular vein, and enters the *mastoid canaliculus* (within the petrous temporal bone). It crosses the facial canal 4 mm above the stylomastoid foramen, emerges through the *tympanomastoid fissure*, and ends by supplying the concha and root of the auricle, the posterior half of the external auditory meatus, and the tympanic membrane (outer surface).

The *pharyngeal branch* arises from the lower part of the inferior ganglion of the vagus, and contains chiefly the fibres of the cranial root of accessory nerve. It passes between the external and internal carotid arteries, and reaches the upper border of the middle constrictor of the pharynx where it takes part in forming the pharyngeal plexus. Its fibres are ultimately distributed to the muscles of the pharynx and soft palate (except the tensor veli palatini which is supplied by the mandibular nerve) (Fig. 32.50).

The *carotid branches* supply the carotid body and carotid sinus.

The *superior laryngeal nerve* arises from the inferior ganglion of the vagus, runs downwards and forwards on the superior constrictor deep to the internal carotid artery, and reaches the middle constrictor where it divides into the external and internal laryngeal nerves.

The *external laryngeal nerve* is thin. It accompanies the superior thyroid artery, pierces the inferior constrictor and ends by supplying the cricothyroid muscle. It also gives branches to the inferior constrictor and to the pharyngeal plexus.

The *internal laryngeal nerve* is thick. It passes downwards and forwards, pierces the thyrohyoid membrane (above the superior laryngeal vessels) and enters the larynx. It supplies the mucous membrane of the larynx up to the level of the vocal folds.

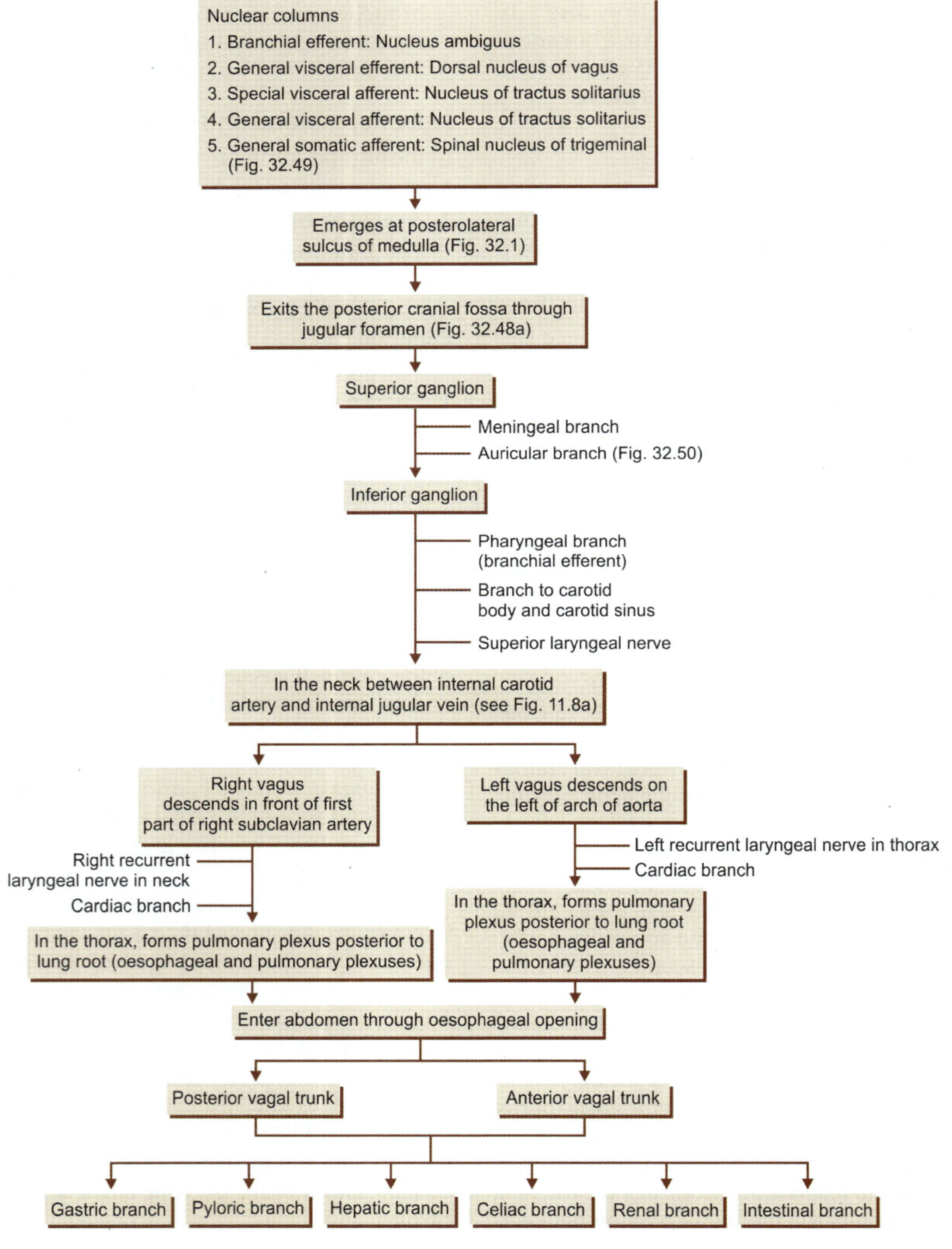

The *right recurrent laryngeal nerve* arises from the vagus in front of the right subclavian artery, winds backwards below the artery, and then runs upwards and medially behind the subclavian and common carotid arteries to reach the tracheoesophageal groove. In the upper part of the groove, it is related to the inferior thyroid artery. It may be superficial or deep to the artery. The nerve then passes deep to the lower border of the inferior constrictor, and enters the larynx behind the cricothyroid joint. It supplies:

a. All intrinsic muscles of the larynx, except the cricothyroid.
b. Sensory nerves to the larynx below the level of the vocal cords.
c. Cardiac branches to the deep cardiac plexus.
d. Branches to the trachea and oesophagus.
e. To the inferior constrictor.

The *left recurrent laryngeal nerve* arises from the vagus in the thorax, as the latter crosses the left side of the arch of the aorta. It loops around the ligamentum arteriosum and reaches the tracheoesophageal groove. Its distribution is similar to that of the right nerve. Usually it is posterior to the inferior thyroid artery.

The *cardiac branches* are superior and inferior. Out of the four cardiac branches of the vagi (two on each side), the left inferior branch goes to the superficial cardiac plexus. The other three cardiac nerves go to the deep cardiac plexus.

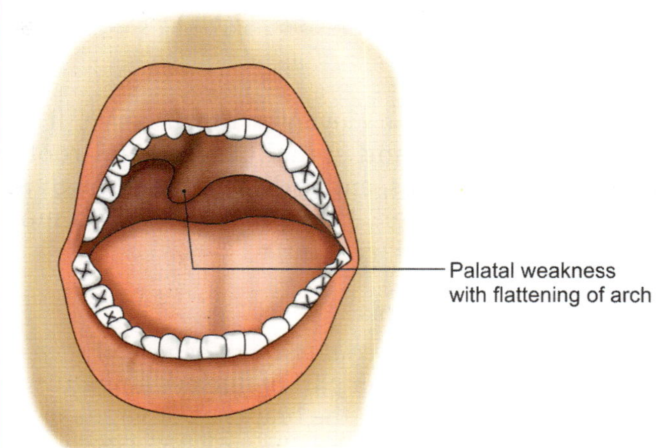

Fig. 32.51: Paralysis of muscles of soft palate on left side

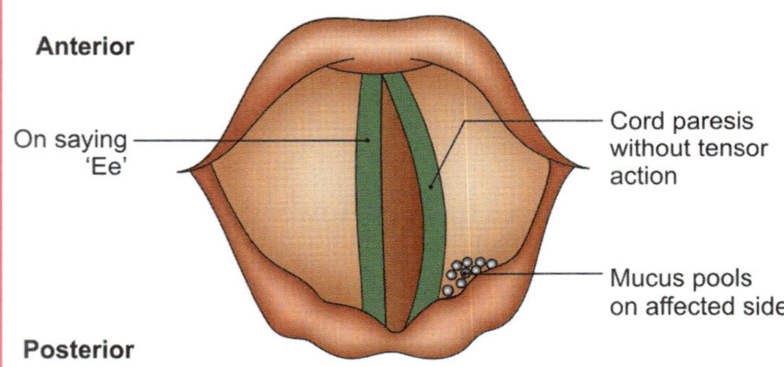

Fig. 32.52: Paralysis of right recurrent laryngeal nerve

CLINICAL ANATOMY

- The vagus nerve is tested clinically by comparing the palatal arches on the two sides. On the paralysed side, there is no arching, and the uvula is pulled to the normal side.
- Paralysis of the vagus nerve produces:
  a. Nasal regurgitation of swallowed liquids,
  b. Nasal twang in voice
  c. Hoarseness of voice
  d. Flattening of the palatal arch (Fig. 32.51).
  e. Cadaveric position of the vocal cord.
  f. Dysphagia.
- Irritation of the auricular branch of the vagus in the external ear (by ear wax, syringing, etc.) may reflexly cause persistent cough (ear cough), vomiting, or even death due to sudden cardiac inhibition.
- Stimulation of the auricular branch may reflexly produce increased appetite.
- Irritation of the recurrent laryngeal nerve by enlarged lymph nodes in children may also produce a persistent cough.
- Some fibres arising in the geniculate ganglion of facial nerve pass into the vagus through communications between the two nerves. They reach the skin of auricle through the auricular branch of vagus. Sometimes a sensory ganglion may have a viral infection (called herpes zoster) and vesicles appear on the area of skin supplied by the ganglion. In herpes zoster of the geniculate ganglion, vesicles appear on the skin of auricle.
- Injury to pharyngeal branch causes dysphagia. Paralysis of muscles of soft palate results in nasal regurgitation of fluids and nasal tone of voice. Lesions of superior laryngeal nerve produces anaesthesia in the upper part of larynx and paralysis of cricothyroid muscle. The voice is weak and gets tired easily.
- Injury to right recurrent laryngeal nerve results in hoarseness and dysphonia due to paralysis of the right vocal cord (Fig. 32.52).
- Paralysis of both vocal cords results in aphonia and inspiratory stridor (high pitched and harsh respiratory sound). It may occur during thyroid surgery.

ELEVENTH CRANIAL NERVE

ACCESSORY NERVE

Accessory nerve is the eleventh cranial nerve. It has two roots—cranial and spinal. The cranial root is accessory to the vagus, and is distributed through the branches of the latter. The spinal root has a more independent course (Fig. 32.53).

Functional Components

1 The cranial root is *special visceral (branchial) efferent*. It arises from the lower part of nucleus ambiguus. It is distributed through the branches of vagus to the muscles of the palate, the pharynx, the larynx, and possibly the heart (Fig. 32.53).
2 The spinal root is also special visceral efferent. It arises from a long spinal nucleus situated in the lateral part of the anterior grey column of the spinal cord extending between segments C1 to C5. Its fibres supply the sternocleidomastoid and the trapezius muscles.

Nuclei

The cranial root arises from the lower part of the *nucleus ambiguus*.

The spinal root arises from a long *spinal nucleus* situated on the lateral part of anterior grey column of spinal cord, extending from C1 to C5 segments. It is in line with nucleus ambiguus.

Course and Distribution of the Cranial Root

1 The cranial root emerges in the form of 4 to 5 rootlets which are attached to the posterolateral sulcus of the medulla. Just below, the rootlets soon join together to form a single trunk.

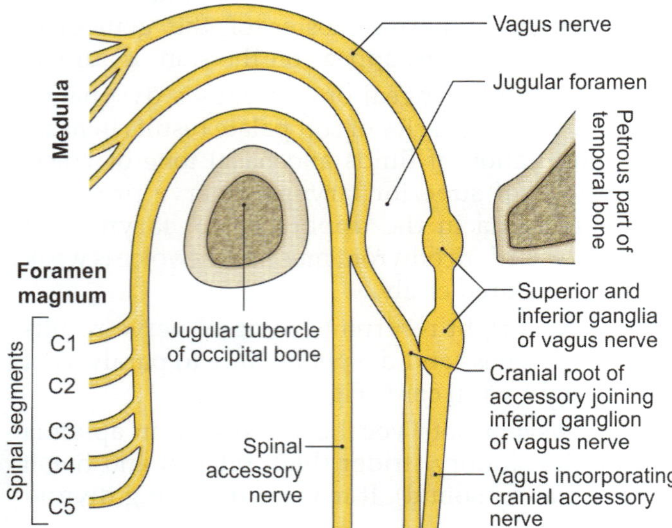

Fig. 32.53: Course of the accessory nerve

2 It runs laterally with the glossopharyngeal vagus and spinal accessory nerves, crosses the jugular tubercle, and reaches jugular foramen.
3 In the jugular foramen, the cranial root unites for a short distance with the spinal root, and again separates from it as it passes out of the foramen.
4 The cranial root finally fuses with the vagus at its inferior ganglion, and is distributed through the branches of the vagus to the muscles of the palate, the pharynx, the larynx and possibly the heart.

Course and Distribution of the Spinal Root

1 It arises from the upper five segments of the spinal cord (Fig. 32.53).
2 It emerges in the form of a row of filaments attached to the cord midway between the ventral and dorsal nerve roots.
3 *In the vertebral canal,* the filaments unite to form a single trunk which ascends in front of the dorsal nerve roots and behind the ligamentum denticulatum.
4 The nerve *enters the cranium* through the foramen magnum lying behind the vertebral artery (Fig. 9.16).
5 Within the cranium, the nerve runs upwards and laterally, crosses the jugular tubercle (with the ninth and tenth cranial nerves) and reaches the jugular foramen.
6 The nerve *leaves the skull* through the middle part of the jugular foramen where it fuses with a short length of the cranial root. It soon separates from the latter and passes out of the foramen.
7 In its *extracranial course*, the nerve descends vertically between the internal jugular vein and the internal carotid artery deep to the parotid and to the styloid process. It reaches a point midway between the angle of mandible and the mastoid process. Then it runs downwards and backwards superficial to the internal jugular vein and deep to the sternocleidomastoid and is surrounded by lymph nodes.
The nerve pierces the anterior border of the sternocleidomastoid at the junction of its upper one-fourth with the lower three-fourths, supplies it and communicates with second and third cervical nerves within the muscle.
The nerve enters the posterior triangle of the neck by emerging through the posterior border of the sternocleidomastoid a little above its middle. In the triangle (Fig. 32.54), it runs downwards and backwards embedded in the fascial roof of the triangle. Here it lies over the levator scapulae. It is related to the superficial lymph nodes. The nerve leaves the posterior triangle by passing deep to the anterior border of the trapezius 5 cm above the clavicle.

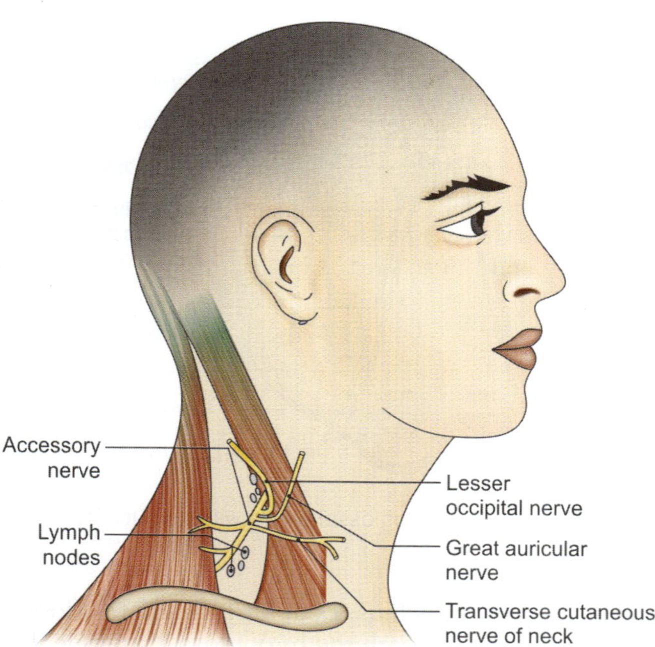

Fig. 32.54: Accessory nerve with some branches of cervical plexus

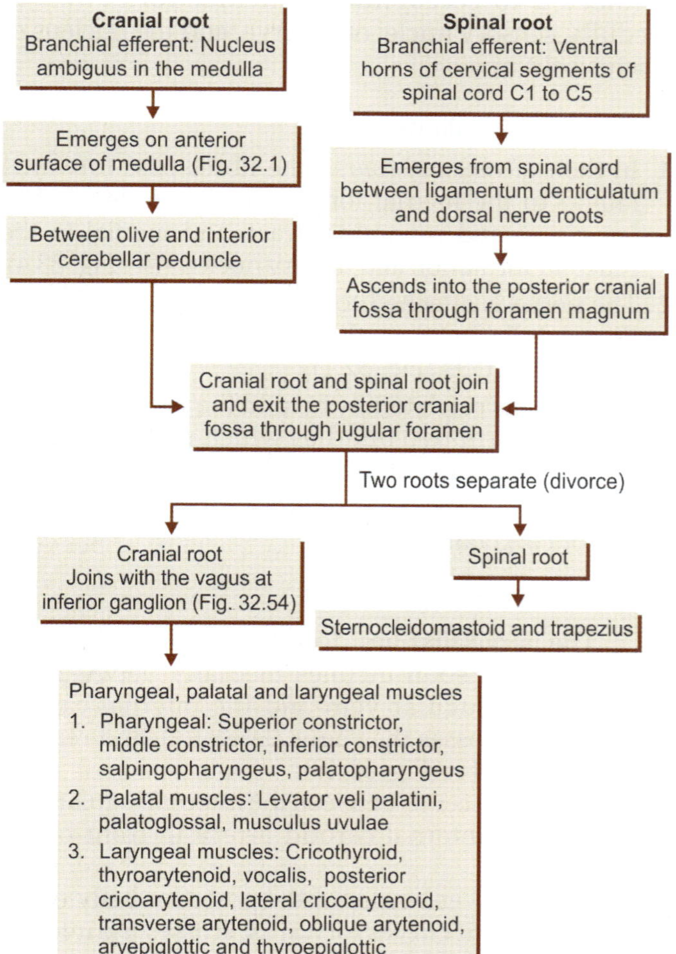

On the deep surface of the trapezius, the nerve communicates with spinal nerves C3 and C4, and ends by supplying the trapezius.

8 *Distribution:* The spinal accessory nerve supplies:
   a. The sternocleidomastoid.
   b. The trapezius.

Cervical nerves provide a proprioceptive supply to these muscles.

CLINICAL ANATOMY

- The accessory nerve is tested clinically:
  a. By asking the patient to shrug his shoulders (trapezius) against resistance and comparing the power on the two sides (Fig. 32.55).
  b. By asking the patient to turn the chin to the opposite side (sternocleidomastoid) against resistance and again comparing the power on the two sides (Fig. 32.56).
- Lesions of spinal root of accessory nerve cause drooping of the shoulder (Fig. 32.57) and inability to turn chin to opposite side.
- Irritation of the nerve during biopsy of enlarged caseous lymph nodes, may produce torticollis or wryneck.
- Supranuclear connections act on the ipsilateral sternocleidomastoid and on the contralateral trapezius. This results in turning of the head away from relevant hemisphere during seizure.
- Unilateral lower motor neuron weakness causes drooping of the shoulder on affected side and weakness in turning the chin to opposite side (Fig. 32.57).

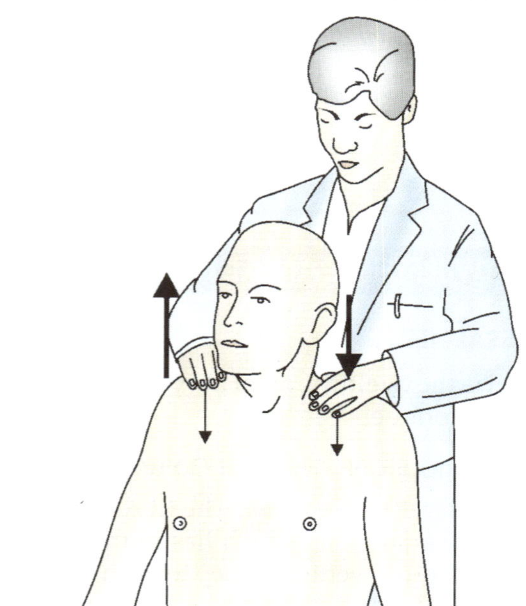

Fig. 32.55: Shrugging shoulders against resistance. Left side is weak

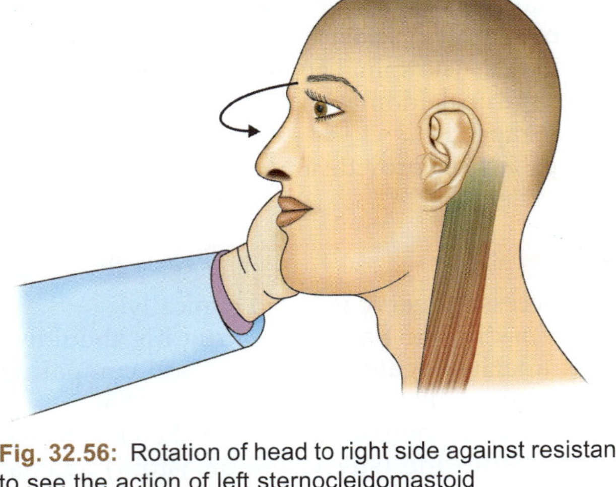

Fig. 32.56: Rotation of head to right side against resistance to see the action of left sternocleidomastoid

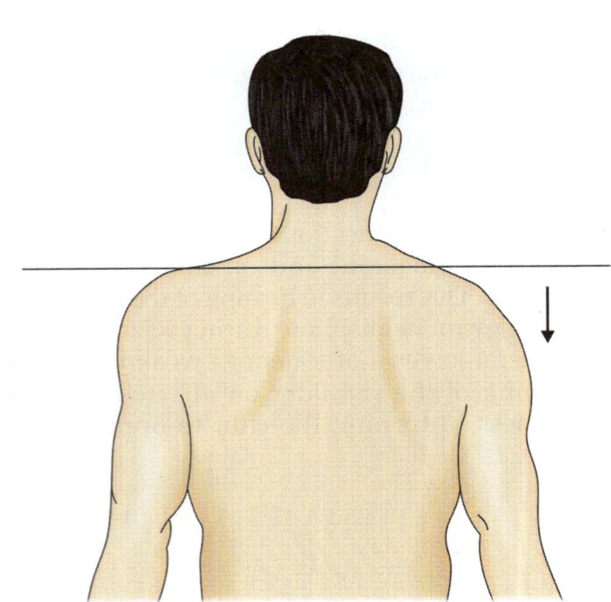

Fig. 32.57: Drooping of the right shoulder due to paralysis of right trapezius

TWELFTH CRANIAL NERVE

HYPOGLOSSAL NERVE

Hypoglossal is the twelfth cranial nerve. It supplies the muscles of the tongue.

Functional Components/Nuclear Columns

1 *General somatic efferent column:* The fibres arise from the hypoglossal nucleus which lies in the medulla, in the floor of fourth ventricle deep to the hypoglossal triangle (Fig. 32.58).
2 *General somatic afferent column:* The nucleus is spinal nucleus of V cranial nerve where proprioceptive fibres from tongue end.

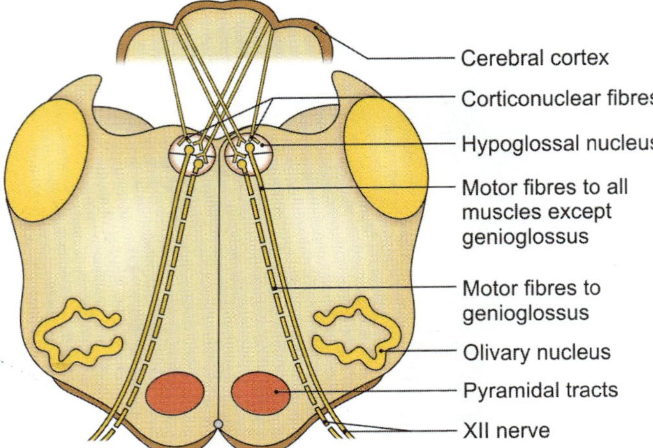

Fig. 32.58: Hypoglossal nerve with its nucleus

Nucleus

The hypoglossal nucleus, 2 cm long, lies in the floor of fourth ventricle beneath the hypoglossal triangle. It is divided into a part for genioglossus and a part for rest of the muscles (Fig. 32.5c).

Connection of the nucleus with opposite pyramidal tract forms supranuclear pathway of the nerve. It is also connected to cerebellum, reticular formation of medulla, sensory nuclei of V nerve, and the nucleus of tractus solitarius.

Course and Relations

1 In their *intraneural course,* the fibres pass forwards lateral to the medial longitudinal bundle, medial lemniscus and pyramidal tract, and medial to the reticular formation and olivary nucleus (*see* Fig. 33.4).
2 The nerve is attached to the anterolateral sulcus of the medulla, between the pyramid and the olive, by 10 to 15 rootlets (Fig. 32.1).

The rootlets run laterally behind the vertebral artery and join to form two bundles which pierce the dura mater separately near the hypoglossal canal.

The nerve leaves the skull through the hypoglossal (anterior condylar) canal.

Extracranial Course

i. The nerve first lies deep to the internal jugular vein, but soon inclines medially between the internal jugular vein and the internal carotid artery, crosses the vagus (laterally), and reaches in front of it (Fig. 32.48).
ii. It then descends between the internal jugular vein and the internal carotid artery in front of the vagus.
iii. At the lower border of the posterior belly of the digastric, it curves forwards, crosses the internal and external carotid arteries and the loop of the

Section III • Brain

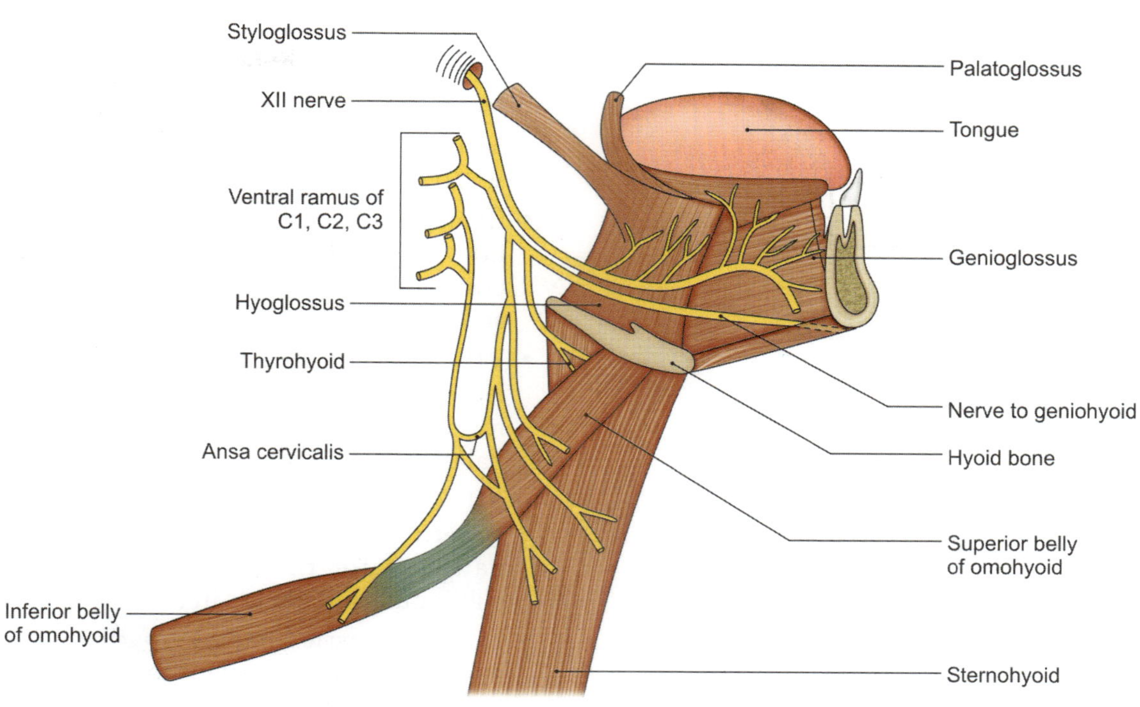

Fig. 32.59: Hypoglossal nerve and ansa cervicalis

lingual artery, and passes deep to the posterior belly of the digastric again to enter the submandibular region (*see* Fig. 15.4).

iv. The nerve then continues forwards on the hyoglossus and genioglossus, deep to the submandibular gland and the mylohyoid, and enters the substance of the tongue to supply all its intrinsic muscles and most of its extrinsic muscles (Fig. 32.59).

Branches and Distribution

In addition to its own fibres, the nerve also carries some fibres that reach it from spinal nerve C1, and are distributed through it.

Branches containing fibres of the hypoglossal nerve proper. They supply the extrinsic and intrinsic muscles of the tongue. Extrinsic muscles are styloglossus, genioglossus, hyoglossus and intrinsic muscles are superior longitudinal, inferior longitudinal, transverse and vertical muscles. Only extrinsic muscle, the palatoglossus is supplied by fibres of the cranial accessory nerve through the vagus and the pharyngeal plexus.

Branches of the hypoglossal nerve containing fibres of nerve C1. These fibres join the nerve at the base of the skull.

1 The *meningeal branch* contains sensory and sympathetic fibres. It enters the skull through the hypoglossal canal, and supplies bone and meninges in the anterior part of the posterior cranial fossa.
2 The *descending branch* continues as the descendens hypoglossi or the upper root of the ansa cervicalis.
3 Branches are also given to the thyrohyoid and geniohyoid muscles (Fig. 32.59).

CLINICAL ANATOMY

- The hypoglossal nerve is tested clinically by asking the patient to protrude his/her tongue. Normally, the tongue is protruded straight forwards. If the nerve is paralysed, the tongue deviates to the paralysed side (Fig. 32.60).
- An infranuclear lesion of the hypoglossal nerve produces paralysis of the tongue on that side. There is gradual atrophy of the paralysed half of the tongue. The tongue looks shrunken.

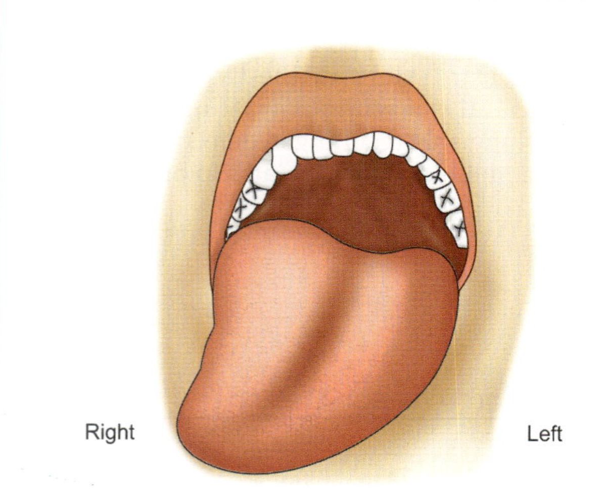

Fig. 32.60: XII nerve paralysis on right side

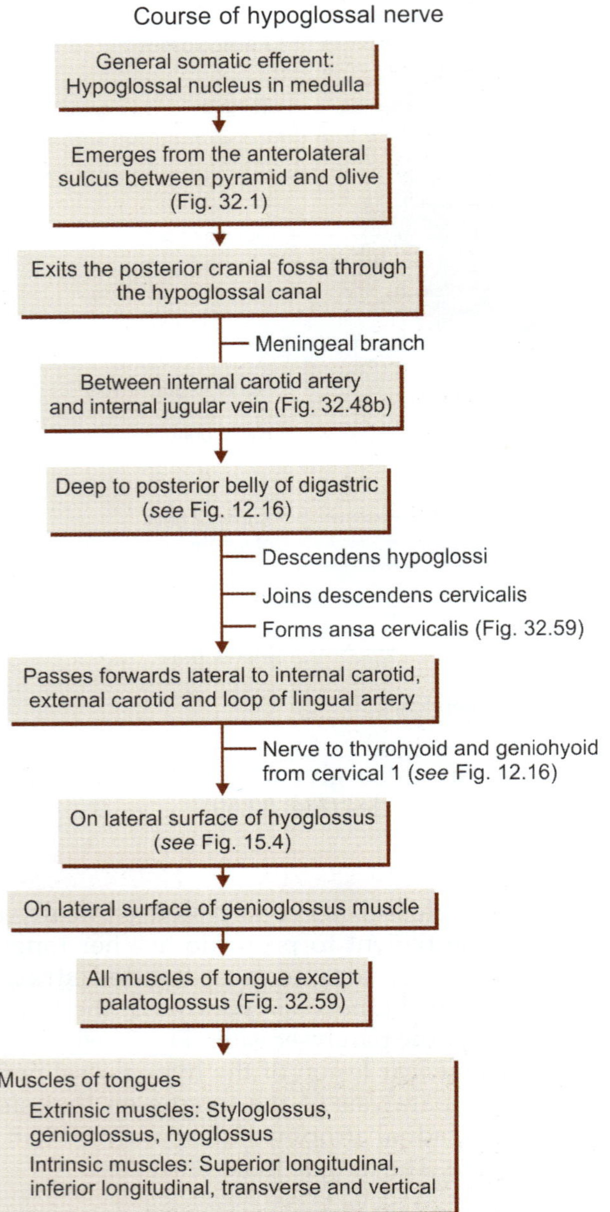

- Supranuclear lesions of the hypoglossal nerve causes paralysis without wasting. The tongue moves sluggishly resulting in defective speech. On protrusion, the tongue deviates to opposite side.

FACTS TO REMEMBER

- Cranial nerves I, II, VIII are almost sensory, cranial nerves III, IV, VI, XI, XII are motor, cranial nerves. V, VII, IX, X are mixed nerves.
- III nerve carries parasympathetic fibres from Edinger-Westphal nucleus of midbrain to the ciliaris and constrictor pupillae muscles for accommodation.
- VII nerve carries parasympathetic fibres from lacrimatory nucleus to pterygopalatine ganglion for the lacrimal gland and glands in nasal cavity, palate and pharynx.
- VII nerve also carries parasympathetic fibres from superior salivatory nucleus to submandibular ganglion for the supply of submandibular, sublingual and glands in the oral cavity.
- IX nerve carries parasympathetic fibres from inferior salivatory nucleus to the otic ganglion for the supply of parotid gland.
- X nerve carries parasympathetic fibres from dorsal nucleus of vagus for the glands in the respiratory tract and glands in the digestive tract till right two-thirds of the transverse colon.
- S2, S3, S4 carry sacral outflow of the parasympathetic system to the distal part of digestive tract and other pelvic viscera.
- V, VII, IX, nerves are the nerves of 1st, 2nd, 3rd arches respectively.
- X, XI, i.e. vagoaccessory complex supplies structures developed from 4th and 6th branchial arches, i.e. muscles of soft palate, pharynx and all the muscles of larynx. The posterior cricoarytenoid is the most important muscle of larynx as it is the only abductor of the vocal cords. XI nerve supplies three out of four extrinsic muscles of the tongue. Most important muscle is the genioglossus. If both the genioglossi get paralysed, the tongue falls backwards and blocks the air passage through the posterior nares.

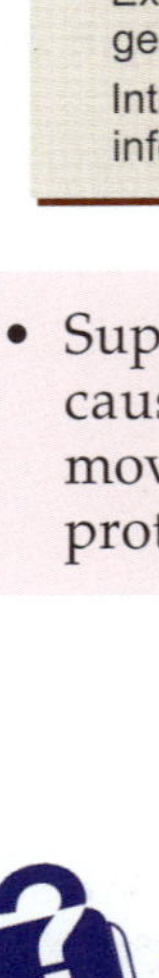

Frequently Asked Questions

1. Describe oculomotor nerve under following headings: Origin, nuclei, course, distribution and clinical anatomy.
2. Describe facial nerve under following headings: Origin, nuclei, course, distribution and clinical anatomy.

3. Write short notes on:
   a. Chorda tympani nerve
   b. Left recurrent laryngeal nerve
   c. Branches of ophthalmic division of V nerve
   d. Branches of mandibular nerve
   e. Roots and branches of pterygopalatine ganglion
   f Ptosis
   g. Branches of hypoglossal nerve and effect of its paralysis

Multiple Choice Questions

1. Cranial nerves which innervate extraocular muscles include:
   a. Oculomotor, abducent and trochlear
   b. Abducent, facial and trigeminal
   c. Trochlear, oculomotor, facial
   d. Oculomotor, facial, trigeminal
2. The three divisions of trigeminal nerve include:
   a. Oculomotor, palatine and lingual
   b. Ophthalmic, maxillary, mandibular
   c. Ophthalmic, palatine, lingual
   d. Frontal, maxillary, mandibular
3. Cranial nerve that does not pass through superior orbital fissure in skull:
   a. Oculomotor b. Trochlear
   c. Facial d. Abducent
4. Cranial nerve that are mainly sensory are:
   a. Optic, vestibulocochlear, vagus
   b. Ophthalmic, optic, facial
   c. Ophthalmic, optic, vestibulocochlear
   d. Optic, olfactory, vestibulocochlear
5. Cranial nerves that carry taste from the tongue are:
   a. Trigeminal, facial, glossopharyngeal
   b. Facial, glossopharyngeal, hypoglossal
   c. Facial, glossopharyngeal, accessory
   d. Facial, glossopharyngeal and vagus
6. The cranial nerve that arise from both brain as well as spinal cord:
   a. Hypoglossal
   b. Accessory
   c. Vagus
   d. Glossopharyngeal
7. Which cranial nerve does not pass through jugular foramen?
   a. Glossopharyngeal
   b. Vagus
   c. Accessory
   d. Hypoglossal
8. Which is not a cranial nerve?
   a. Vagus b. Glossopharyngeal
   c. Phrenic d. Hypoglossal
9. Which structure is not innervated by vagus?
   a. Small intestine b. Heart
   c. Stomach d. Sternocleidomastoid
10. Which cranial nerve innervates muscle that raises the upper eyelid?
    a. Trochlear b. Oculomotor
    c. Abducent d. Facial

Answers

1. a 2. b 3. c 4. d 5. d 6. b 7. d 8. c 9. d 10. b

VIVA VOCE

- Name the cranial nerves in order.
- Name the cranial nerve nuclei of:
  - General somatic efferent column
  - Special somatic afferent column
- Name the ganglia associated with trigeminal nerve.
- Which cranial nerves are sensory?
- Which cranial nerves are motor?
- Which cranial nerves are mixed?
- Right XII nerve is injured, which side will the tongue deviate on protrusion?
- Name the cranial nerve which supplies all muscles of tongue except palatoglossus.
- Name the functional components of III, IX and X cranial nerves.
- Name the largest and thinnest cranial nerves.
- Name the cranial nerve with most extensive distribution.
- Name the nerve having longest intracranial course.
- Name the cranial nerve which is paralysed most frequently.

Chapter

33

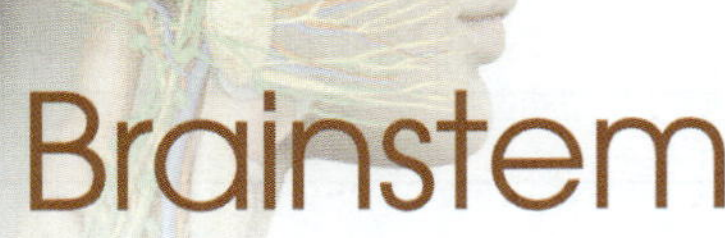

Brainstem

"They think too little, who talk too much."
—Anonymous

INTRODUCTION

The brainstem consists of the medulla oblongata, the pons and the midbrain. It connects the spinal cord to the cerebrum. The various ascending and descending tracts pass through the three components of the brainstem. Medulla contains the respiratory and vasomotor centres. In hanging or capital punishment, the dens of axis breaks and strikes on these centres causing immediate death. Midbrain contains nuclei of oculomotor and trochlear nerves. Pons has the nuclei of trigeminal, abducent, facial and statoacoustic nerves while medulla houses the nuclei of last four cranial nerves, i.e. glossopharyngeal, vagus, accessory and hypoglossal nerves.

MEDULLA OBLONGATA

The medulla is the lowest part of brainstem, extending from the lower border of pons to a plane just above the first cervical nerve where it is continuous with the spinal cord.

External Features

1 The medulla is divided into right and left halves by the anterior and posterior median fissures. Each half is further divided into anterior, lateral and posterior regions by the anterolateral and posterolateral sulci (Fig. 33.1).

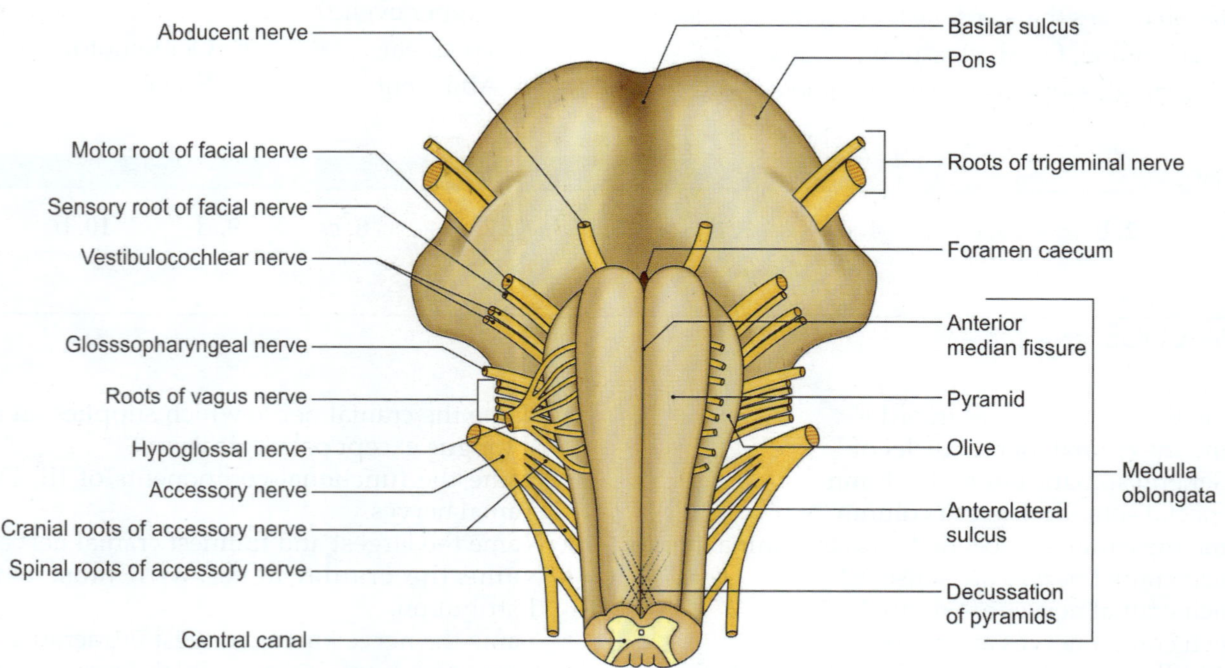

Fig. 33.1: Attachment of cranial nerve to the ventral surface of brainstem

2 The anterior region is in the form of a longitudinal elevation called the *pyramid*. The pyramid is made up of corticospinal fibres. In the lower part of the medulla, many fibres of the right and left pyramids cross in the midline forming the *pyramidal decussation*.
3 The upper part of the lateral region shows an oval elevation, the olive. It is produced by an underlying mass of grey matter called the *inferior olivary nucleus*.
4 The rootlets of the hypoglossal nerve emerge from the anterolateral sulcus between the pyramid and the olive.
5 The rootlets of the cranial nerves IX and X and of the cranial part of the accessory nerve emerge through the posterolateral fissure, behind the olive.
6 The posterolateral region lies between the posterolateral sulcus and the posterior median fissure. The upper part of this region is marked by a V-shaped depression which is the lower part of the floor of the fourth ventricle. Below the floor, we see three longitudinal elevations. From medial to lateral side, these are the fasciculus gracilis, the fasciculus cuneatus and the inferior cerebellar peduncle (Fig. 33.2).

Internal Structure

The internal structure of the medulla can be studied conveniently by examining transverse sections through it at three levels.

Transverse Section through the Lower Part of the Medulla Passing through the Pyramidal Decussation

It resembles a transverse section of the spinal cord in having the same three funiculi and the same tracts (Fig. 33.3).

Grey Matter

1 The decussating pyramidal fibres separate the anterior horn from the central grey matter. The *separated anterior horn* forms the spinal nucleus of the accessory nerve laterally and the supraspinal nucleus for motor fibres of the first cervical nerve medially.
2 The central grey matter (with the central canal) is pushed backwards.
3 The nucleus gracilis and the nucleus cuneatus are continuous with the central grey matter.

White Matter

1 The pyramids, anteriorly.
2 The decussation of the pyramidal tracts forms the most important features of the medulla at this level. The fibres of each pyramid run backwards and laterally to reach the lateral white column of the spinal cord where they form the lateral corticospinal tract.
3 The fasciculus gracilis and the fasciculus cuneatus occupy the broad posterior white column.

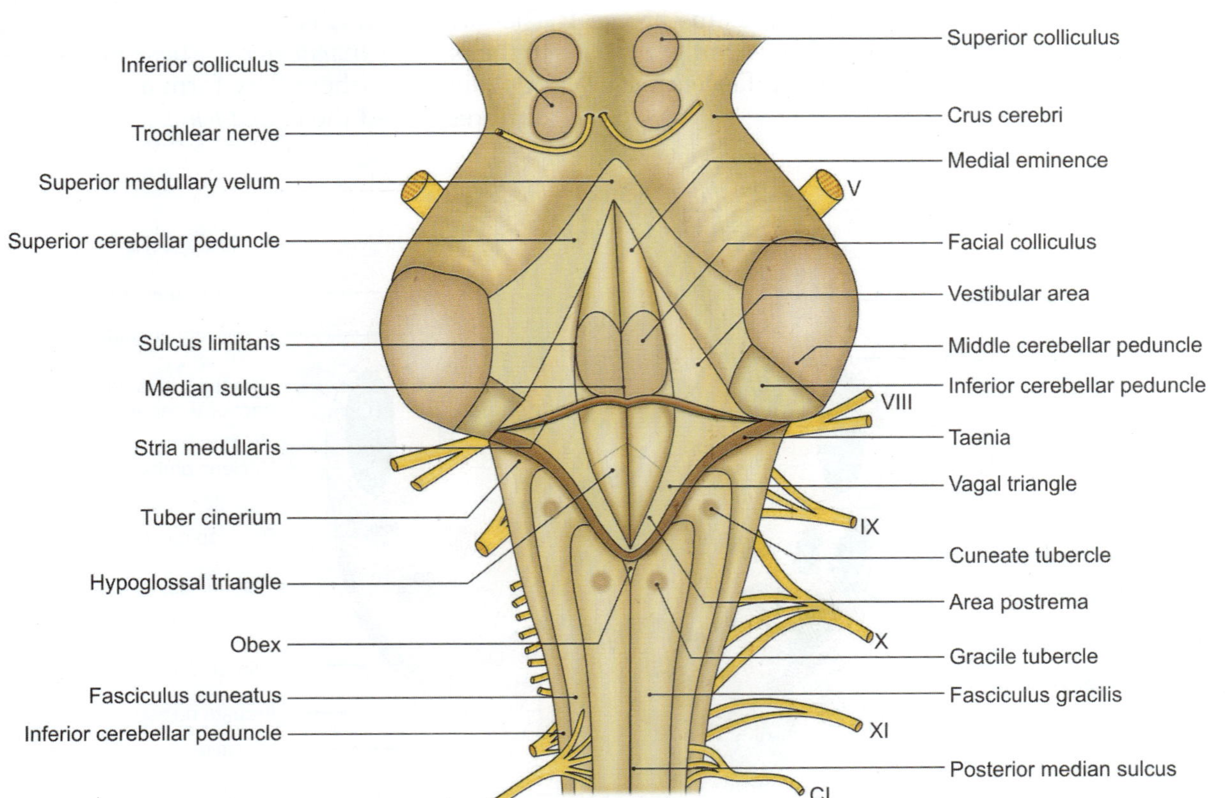

Fig. 33.2: Dorsal aspect of thalamus, brainstem and spinal cord

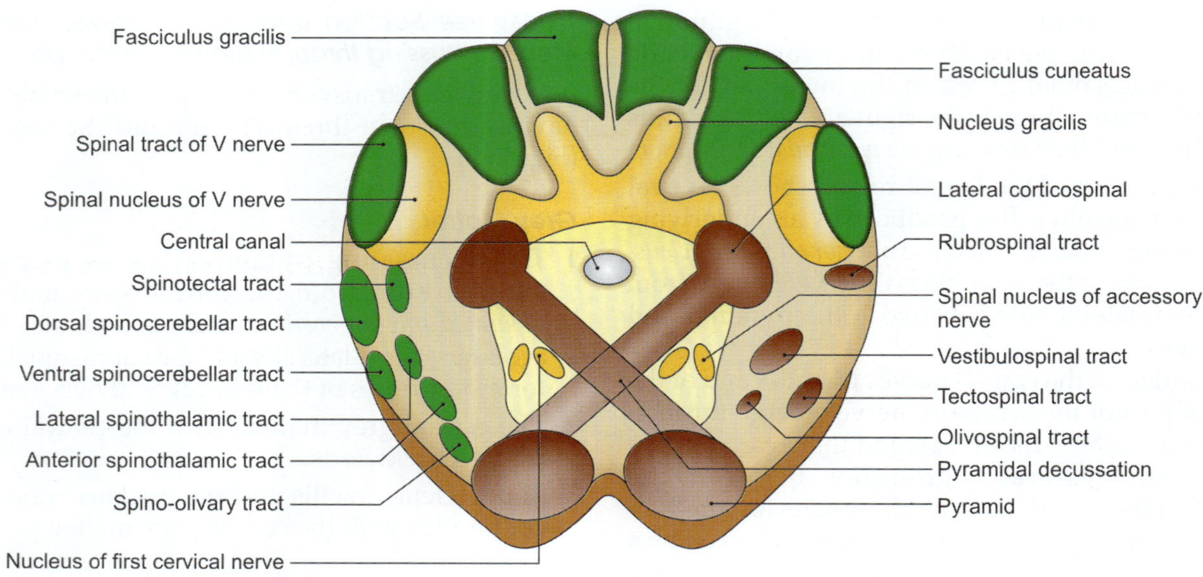

Fig. 33.3: TS of medulla oblongata at the level of pyramidal decussation

4 The other features of the white matter are similar to those of the spinal cord.

Transverse Section through the Middle of Medulla (through the sensory decussation)

Identify the following in Fig. 33.4.

Grey Matter

1 The nucleus gracilis and the nucleus cuneatus are much larger and are separate from the central grey matter. The fasciculus gracilis and the fasciculus cuneatus end in these nuclei.

2 The *nucleus of the spinal tract of the trigeminal nerve* is also separate from the central grey matter.

3 The central grey matter contains the following:
   a. Hypoglossal nucleus
   b. Dorsal nucleus of the vagus.
   c. Nucleus of tractus solitarius.

White Matter

1 The nucleus gracilis and nucleus cuneatus give rise to the *internal arcuate fibres*. These fibres cross to the opposite side where they form a paramedian band of fibres, called the *medial lemniscus*.

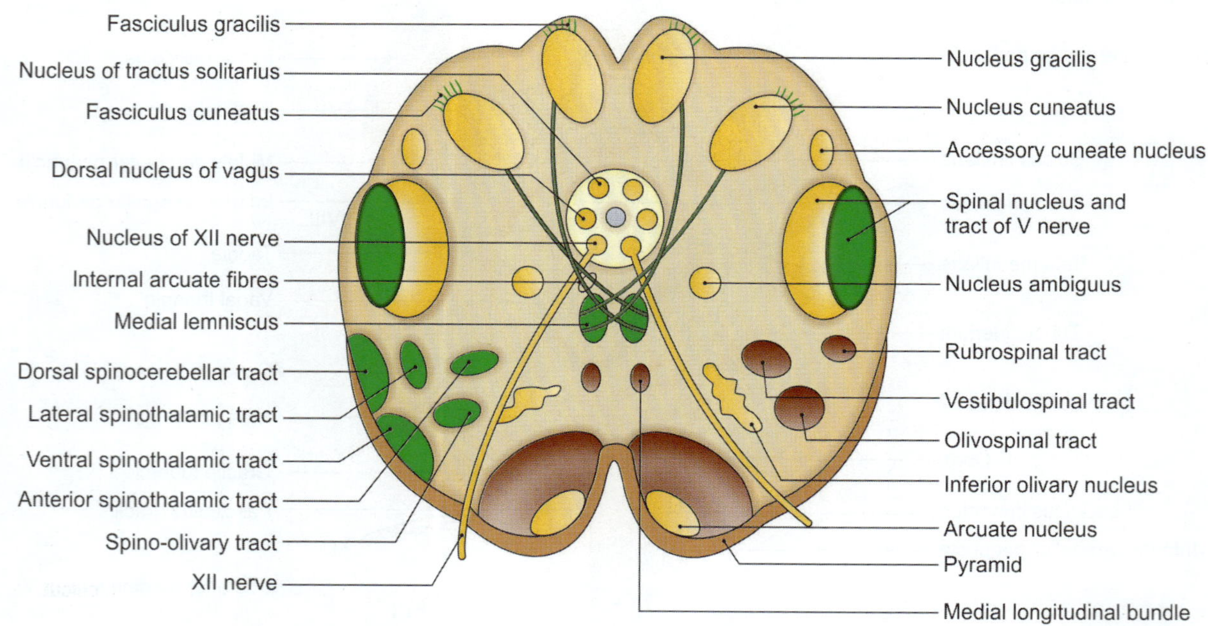

Fig. 33.4: TS of medulla oblongata at the level of sensory decussation

2 The *pyramidal tracts* lie anteriorly.
3 The *medial longitudinal bundle* lies posterior to the medial lemniscus.
4 The *spinocerebellar, lateral spinothalamic* and other tracts lie in the anterolateral area.
5 Emerging fibres of XII nerve.

Transverse Section through the Upper Part of Medulla Passing through the Floor of Fourth Ventricle

Identify the following in Fig. 33.5.

Grey Matter

1 The nuclei of several cranial nerves are seen in the floor of the fourth ventricle:
   a. The *hypoglossal nucleus,* in a paramedian position.
   b. The *dorsal nucleus of the vagus,* lateral to the XII nerve nucleus.
   c. The *nucleus of the tractus solitarius,* ventrolateral to the dorsal nucleus of vagus.
   d. The *inferior and medial vestibular nuclei,* medial to the inferior cerebellar peduncle.
2 The *nucleus ambiguus* lies deep in the reticular formation of the medulla. It gives origin to motor fibres of the cranial nerves IX, X and XI.
3 The dorsal and ventral cochlear nuclei lie on the surface of the inferior cerebellar peduncle.
4 The *nucleus of the spinal tract* of the trigeminal nerve lies in the dorsolateral part.
5 The *inferior olivary nucleus* is the largest mass of grey matter seen at this level.
6 The *arcuate nucleus* lies anteromedial to the pyramidal tract.

Visceral centres are:
   a. Respiratory centre
   b. Cardiac centre for regulation of heart rate
   c. Vasomotor centre for regulation of blood pressure

White Matter

It shows the following important features.
1 The inferior cerebellar peduncle
2 The *olivocerebellar fibres* are seen prominently.
3 Identify the various ascending tracts in the anterolateral part of the medulla.
4 Emerging fibres of IX, X, XI, nerves.

PONS

The pons is the middle part of the brainstem, connecting the midbrain with the medulla. Literally, the word pons, means 'bridge'.

External Features

The pons has *two surfaces,* ventral and dorsal. The *ventral or anterior surface* is convex in both directions and is transversely striated. In the median plane, it shows a vertical *basilar sulcus* which lodges the basilar artery (Fig. 33.1).

Laterally, the surface is continuous with the middle cerebellar peduncle. The trigeminal nerve is attached to this surface at the junction of the pons with the peduncle. The nerve has two roots, a small motor root which lies medial to the much larger sensory root. The abducent, facial and vestibulocochlear nerves are attached at the lower border of the ventral surface.

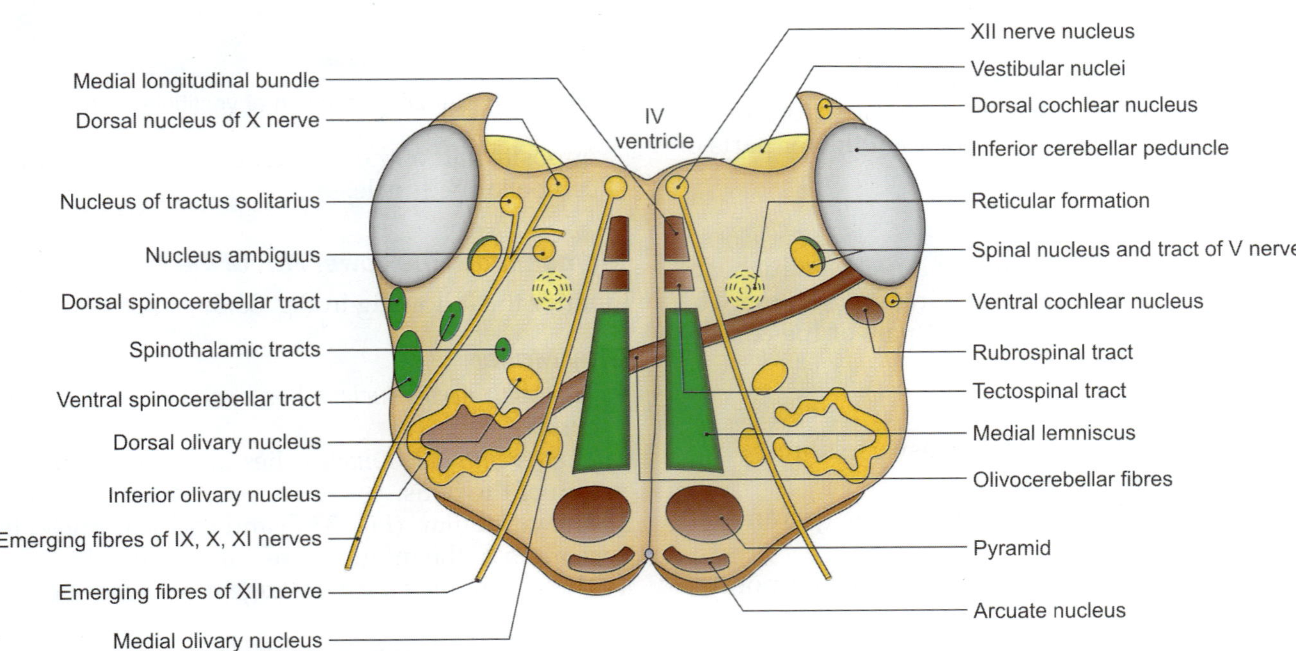

Fig. 33.5: TS of medulla oblongata at the level of olivary nucleus passing through floor of fourth ventricle

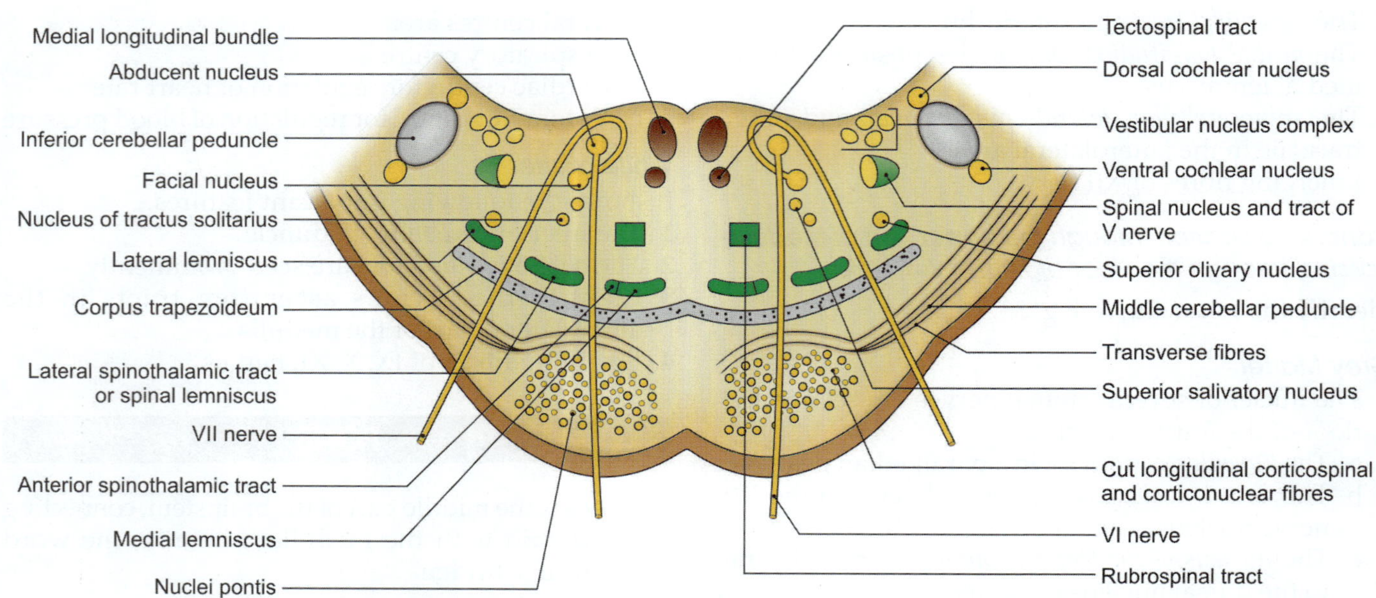

Fig. 33.6: TS of lower part of pons or TS at the level of facial colliculus

The *dorsal or posterior surface* is hidden by the cerebellum, and forms the upper half of the floor of the fourth ventricle (Fig. 33.2).

Internal Structure of Pons

In transverse sections, the pons is seen to be divisible into ventral and dorsal parts. The ventral or *basilar part* is continuous inferiorly with the pyramids of the medulla, and on each side with the cerebellum through the middle cerebellar peduncle. The dorsal or tegmental part is a direct upward continuation of the medulla (excluding the pyramids).

Basilar Part of Pons

The basilar part of the pons has a uniform structure throughout its length. However, the structure of the tegmental part differs in the upper and lower parts of the pons.

Grey Matter

It is represented by the *pontine nuclei* which are scattered among longitudinal and transverse fibres. The pontine nuclei form an important part of the cortico-pontocerebellar pathway.

White Matter

It consists of longitudinal and transverse fibres.

1 The longitudinal fibres include:
   a. The *corticospinal* and *corticonuclear* (pyramidal) tracts.
   b. The *corticopontine* fibres ending in the pontine nuclei.
2 The transverse fibres are *pontocerebellar* fibres beginning from the pontine nuclei and going to the opposite half of the cerebellum, through the middle cerebellar peduncle.

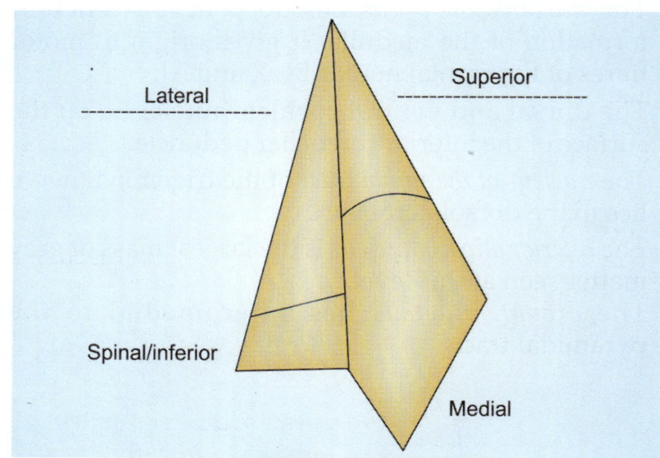

Fig. 33.7: Surface projection of vestibular nerve nuclei

Tegmentum in the Lower Part of the Pons

Identify the following in Fig. 33.6.

Grey Matter

1 The *sixth nerve nucleus* lies beneath the facial colliculus.
2 The *seventh nerve nucleus* lies in the reticular formation of the pons.
3 The vestibular (Fig. 33.7) and cochlear nuclei lie in relation to the inferior cerebellar peduncle.
4 The spinal nucleus of the trigeminal nerve lies in the lateral part.
5 Other nuclei present include the salivatory and lacrimatory nuclei.

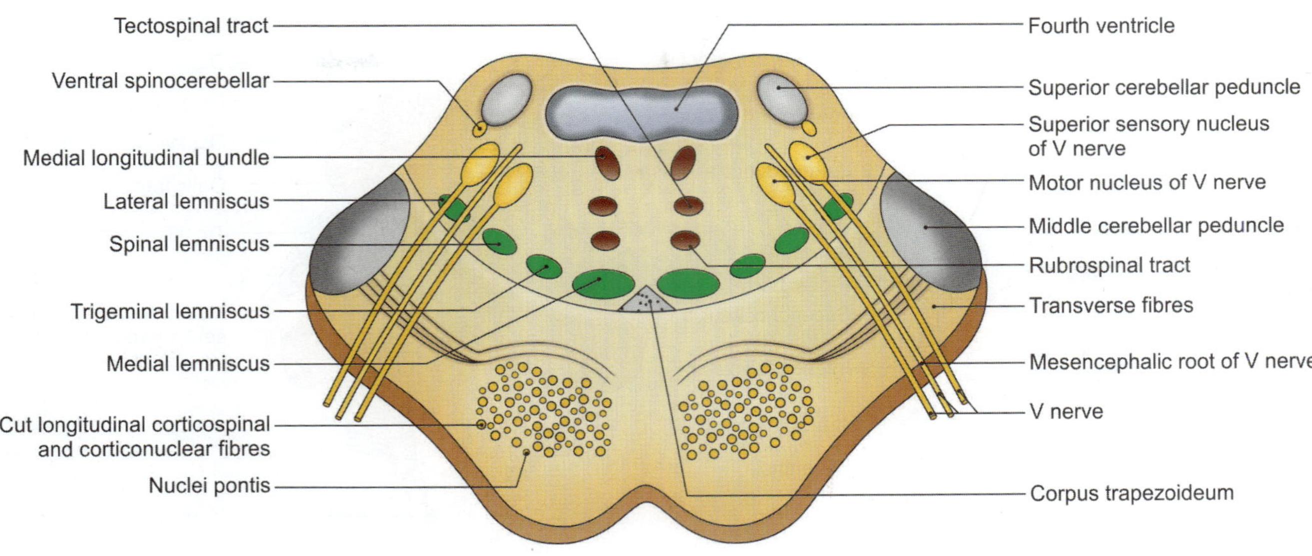

Fig. 33.8: TS of upper pons

White Matter

1 The *trapezoid body* is a transverse band of fibres lying just behind the ventral part of the pons. It consists of fibres that arise in the cochlear nuclei of both sides. It is a part of the auditory pathway.
2 The medial lemniscus forms a transverse band on either side of the midline.
3 The lateral spinothalamic tract (spinal lemniscus).
4 The inferior cerebellar peduncle.
5 The fibres of the facial nerve follow a peculiar course. They first pass backwards and medially to reach the medial side of the abducent nucleus. They then form a loop dorsal and lateral to the abducent nucleus.

Tegmentum in the Upper Part of Pons

Identify the following in Fig. 33.8.

Grey Matter

The special features are the *motor, mesencephalic and superior sensory nuclei of the trigeminal nerve.*

White Matter

1 Immediately behind the ventral part of the pons, we see a transverse band of fibres that is made up (from medial to lateral side) of the medial lemniscus, the trigeminal lemniscus, the spinal lemniscus, and the lateral lemniscus (MTSL).
2 The superior cerebellar peduncles lie dorsolateral to the fourth ventricle.
3 The medial longitudinal bundle is made up of fibres that interconnect the nuclei of the cranial nerves III, IV, VI and VIII and the spinal part of the accessory nerve.

MIDBRAIN

The midbrain is also called the *mesencephalon.* It connects the hindbrain with the forebrain. Its cavity is known as the cerebral aqueduct. It connects the third ventricle with the fourth ventricle (Fig. 33.9).

Subdivisions

When one examines a transverse section through the midbrain following major subdivisions are seen.

A. The *tectum* is the part posterior to aqueduct. It is made up of the right and left superior and inferior colliculi (Fig. 33.9).
B. Each half of the midbrain anterior to the aqueduct is called the *cerebral peduncle.* Each cerebral peduncle is subdivided into:
   a. Crus cerebri, anteriorly.
   b. Substantia nigra, in the middle.
   c. Tegmentum, posteriorly.

Internal Structure of Midbrain

It is studied conveniently by examining sections, at the level of the inferior colliculi and at the level of the superior colliculi.

Transverse Section of Midbrain at the Level of Inferior Colliculi

Grey Matter

1 The central (periaqueductal) grey matter contains:
   a. The *nucleus of the trochlear nerve* in the ventromedial part; and
   b. The *mesencephalic nucleus* of the trigeminal nerve in the lateral part (Fig. 33.10).

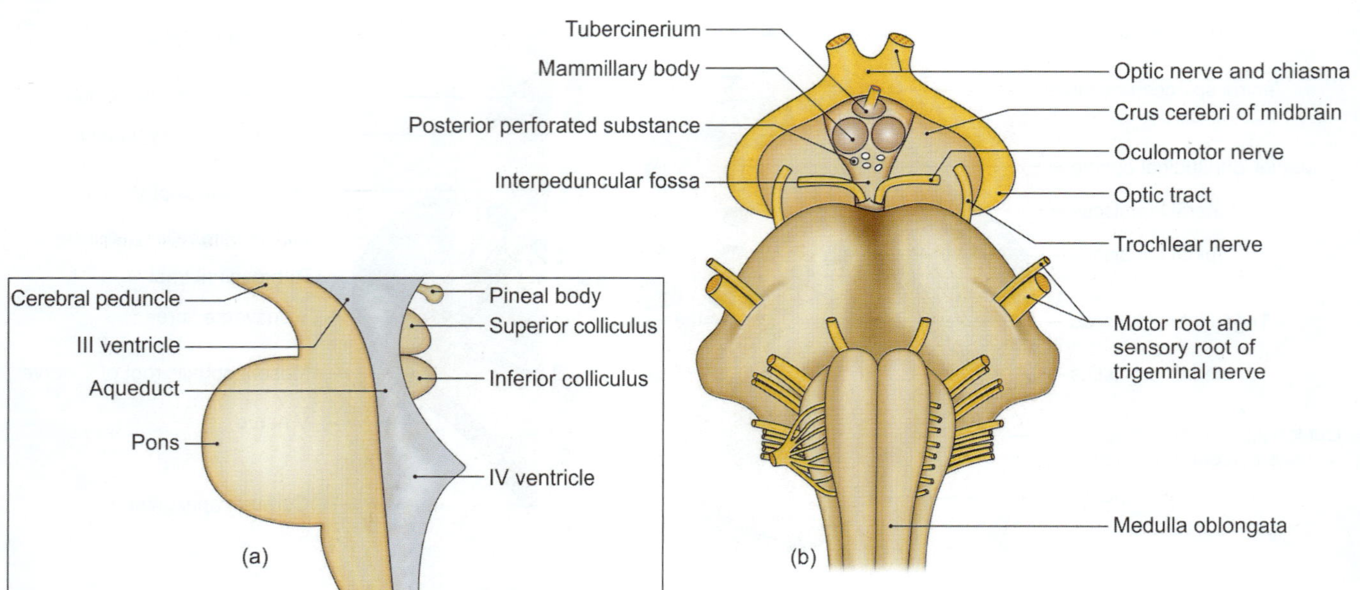

Figs 33.9a and b: (a) Sagittal section of midbrain with pons, and (b) ventral aspect of midbrain

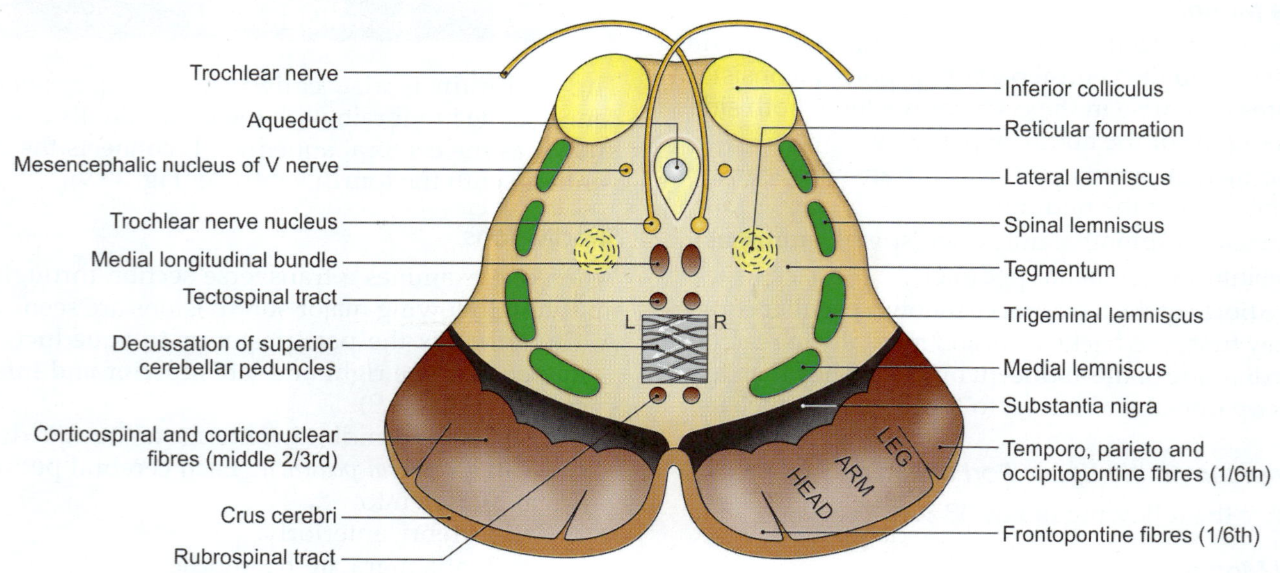

Fig. 33.10: TS of midbrain at the level of inferior colliculus

2 The *inferior colliculus* receives afferents from the lateral lemniscus, and gives efferents to the medial geniculate body.
3 The *substantia nigra* is a lamina of grey matter made up of deeply pigmented nerve cells.

White Matter

1 The *crus cerebri* contains:
   a. The corticospinal tract in the middle (Fig. 33.10).
   b. Frontopontine fibres in the medial one-sixth.
   c. Temporopontine, parietopontine and occipitopontine fibres in the lateral one-sixth.

2 The *tegmentum* contains ascending tracts as follows.
   a. The *lemnisci* (medial, trigeminal, spinal and lateral) are arranged in the form of a band in which they lie in the order mentioned (from medial to lateral side).
   b. The *decussation of the superior cerebellar peduncles* is seen in the median plane.
   c. The *medial longitudinal bundle* lies in close relation to the trochlear nucleus.
   d. The tectospinal and rubrospinal tracts.

3 The trochlear nerve passes laterally and dorsally round the central grey matter. It decussates in the

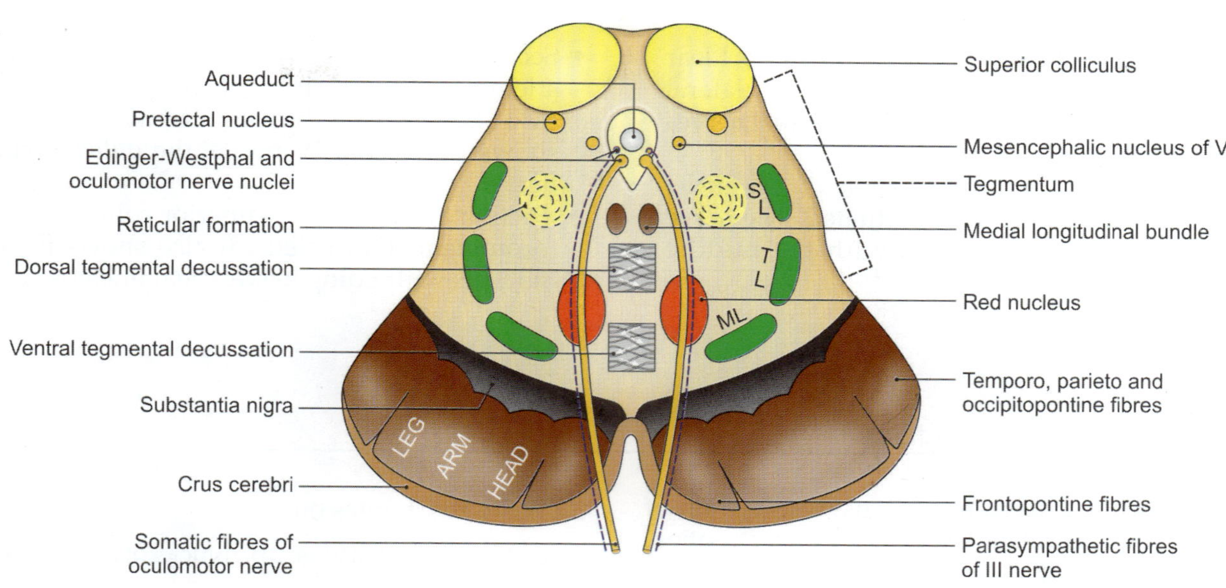

Fig. 33.11: TS of midbrain at the level of superior colliculus

superior medullary velum, and emerges lateral to the frenulum veli.

Transverse Section of Midbrain at the Level of Superior Colliculi

Grey Matter

1 The central grey matter contains:
   a. Nucleus of *oculomotor nerve* with Edinger-Westphal nucleus in the ventromedial part.
   b. *Mesencephalic nucleus* of the trigeminal nerve in the lateral part. The oculomotor nuclei of the two sides are very close to each other (Fig. 33.11).
2 *Superior colliculus* receives afferents from the retina (visual).
3 *Pretectal nucleus* lies deep to the superolateral part of the superior colliculus.
4 *Red nucleus* is about 0.5 cm in diameter. It has an inhibitory influence on muscle tone.
5 *Substantia nigra* has already been described.

White Matter

1 The *crus cerebri* has the same tracts as described above.
2 The *tegmentum* contains the following:
   a. The same lemnisci as seen in the lower part except for the lateral lemniscus which has terminated in the inferior colliculus.
   b. The decussation of the tectospinal tracts forms the dorsal tegmental decussation.
   c. The decussation of the rubrospinal tracts forms the ventral tegmental decussation.
   d. Medial longitudinal bundle.
   e. Emerging fibres of oculomotor nerve.
3 The *tectum* shows the posterior commissure connecting the two superior colliculi.

CLINICAL ANATOMY

- *Pontine haemorrhage:* This entity has following features:
   a. Bilateral paralysis of face and limbs due to involvement of VII nerve nucleus and all corticospinal fibres.
   b. Deep coma due to damage to the reticular formation.
   c. Hyperpyrexia due to cutting off of the temperature regulating fibres from the hypothalamus.
   d. Pinpoint pupil due to damage to sympathetic ocular fibres. Pontine haemorrhage is usually fatal.
- *Tumours of pons:* Astrocytoma is the most common tumour of brainstem, usually in childhood. Signs and symptoms vary according to area of origin of tumour.
- *Argyll-Robertson pupil:* In this condition, light reflex is lost but accommodation reflex is retained due to lesion in the vicinity of pretectal nucleus.

FACTS TO REMEMBER

- Pyramidal decussation cuts off the anterior horn which forms nucleus of 1st cervical nerve and nucleus of spinal accessory nerve.
- Nucleus gracilis and nucleus cuneatus are equivalent of the nuclei in the posterior horn of spinal cord. These are present in the medulla oblongata. Fasciculus gracilis and fasciculus cuneatus relay in their respective nuclei.

- At the lower section of pons, fibres of cochlear nuclei form trapezoid body which forms lateral lemniscus. Nuclei of VI, VII and VIII cranial nerves are present here.
- At the upper section of pons some of the nuclei forming trigeminal nerve are situated. The nerve lies at the junction of pons with the middle cerebellar peduncle.
- Section, at the level of inferior colliculus shows 4 lemnisci: Medial, trigeminal, spinal and lateral (MTSL) from medial to lateral side. It also shows nucleus of IV nerve, the delicate cranial nerve.
- Section at the level of superior colliculus shows prominent red nucleus. It also shows III nerve nucleus with Edinger-Westphal nucleus.

Frequently Asked Questions

1. Draw a labelled diagram of transverse section of medulla oblongata at the level of sensory decussation.
2. Draw a labelled diagram of midbrain at the level of superior colliculus.
3. Write short notes on:
   a. Medial lemniscus
   b. Nuclei of trigeminal nerve
   c. Lateral lemniscus
   d. Pontine nuclei

Multiple Choice Questions

1. The pontine nuclei form an important part of:
   a. Corticorubral pathway
   b. Corticoponto-cerebellar pathway
   c. Vestibulocerebellar pathway
   d. Olivocerebellar pathway
2. Which of these fasciculus lies most medially?
   a. Fasciculus cuneatus
   b. Fasciculus gracilis
   c. Inferior cerebellar peduncle
   d. None of the above
3. Which is not the content of central grey matter in section of lower part of medulla?
   a. Hypoglossal nucleus
   b. Nucleus of spinal tract of trigeminal nerve
   c. Nucleus ambiguus
   d. Spinal nucleus of XI nerve
4. What is true about crus cerebri?
   a. The corticospinal tract is in its middle part
   b. Frontopontine fibres in medial 1/6 part
   c. Temporopontine, parietopontine and occipito-pontine fibres in lateral 1/6 part
   d. All of the above
5. Pons contains which of following set of nuclei?
   a. IX, X, XI, XII
   b. V, VI, VII, VIII
   c. III, IV
   d. IV, V, VI, VII

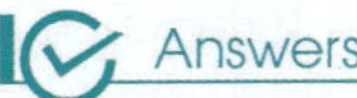

Answers

1. b **2.** b **3.** d **4.** d **5.** b

VIVA VOCE

- Name the components of brainstem.
- Which cranial nerves are attached to medulla oblongata?
- Which nerves arise from nucleus ambiguus?
- Which cranial nerves end in tractus solitarius?
- Name the nuclei which give fibres to X nerve.
- Name the cranial nerves attached to the pons.
- What is law of neurobiotaxis?
- Name the cranial nerves attached to midbrain.
- Which cranial nerve has a dorsal attachment?
- What is the function of Edinger-Westphal nucleus?
- Name the artery involved in lateral medullary syndrome.
- Name two important decussations of the medulla oblongata.
- Which cranial nerve nuclei are connected by medial longitudinal bundle?

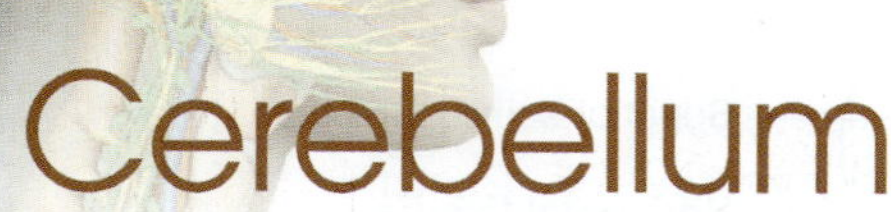

Chapter

34

Cerebellum

"Change yourself and the circumstances will change."
—Anonymous

INTRODUCTION

Cerebellum, though small in size, subserves important functions for maintaining tone, posture equilibrium and movements of the body. Cerebellum controls the same side of the body directly or indirectly. The grey matter is highly folded to accommodate millions of neurons in a small area and the arrangement is called "arbor vitae" (vital tree of life). The structure of cerebellum is uniform throughout, i.e. it is homotypical. Damage to cerebellum gives rise to very typical symptoms.

The cerebellum (little brain) is the largest part of the hindbrain. It is situated in the posterior cranial fossa behind the pons and medulla. It is an infratentorial structure that coordinates voluntary movements of the body (Fig. 34.1).

Relations

- *Anteriorly:* Fourth ventricle, pons and medulla.
- *Posteroinferiorly:* Squamous occipital bone.
- *Superiorly:* Tentorium cerebelli (Fig. 34.2).

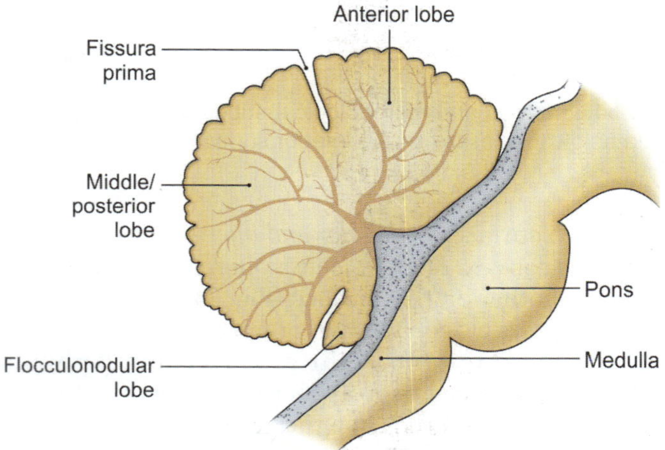

Fig. 34.1: Anatomical lobes of the cerebellum

EXTERNAL FEATURES

The cerebellum consists of two cerebellar hemispheres that are united to each other through a median *vermis.*

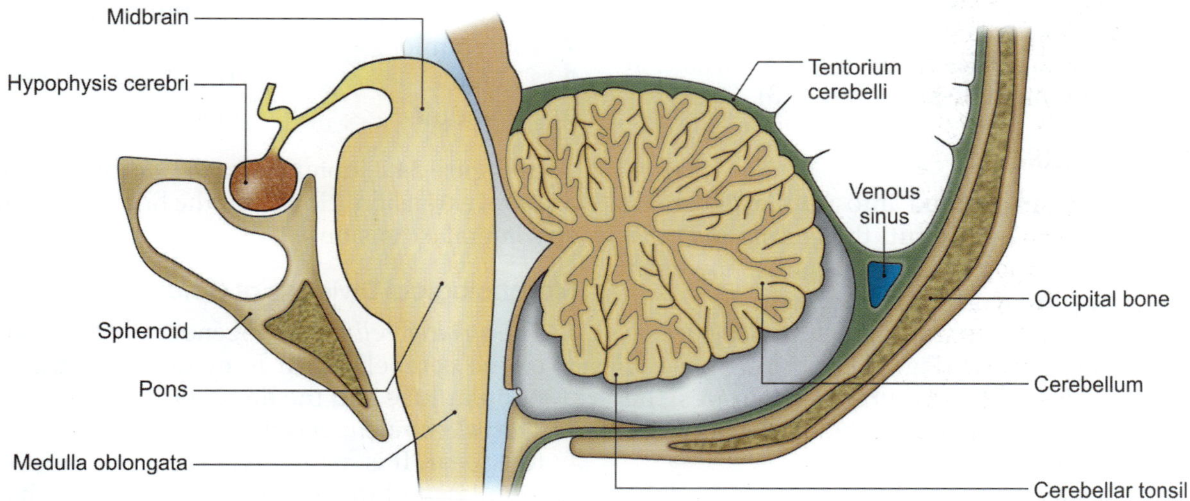

Fig. 34.2: Relations of cerebellum

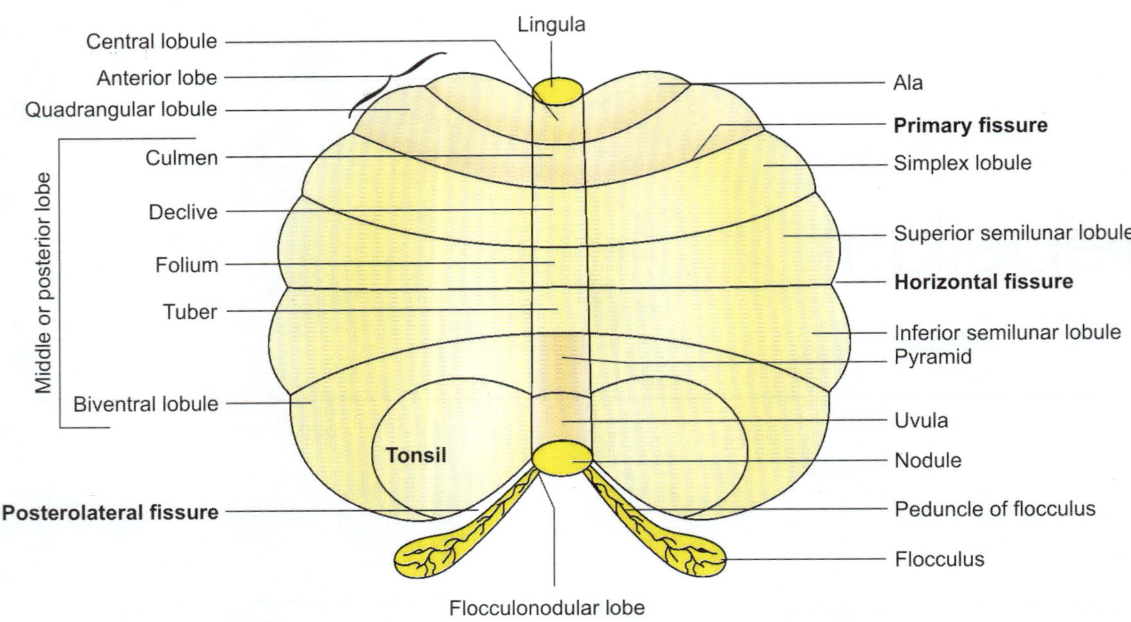

Fig. 34.3: Lobes and morphological subdivisions of cerebellum. Area above horizontal fissure represents superior surface and area below the fissure shows inferior surface

It has two surfaces—*superior and inferior*. The superior surface is convex. The two hemispheres are continuous with each other on this surface (Fig. 34.3). The inferior surface shows a deep median notch called the *vallecula* which separates the right and left hemispheres (Fig. 34.3). The anterior aspect of the cerebellum is marked by a deep notch in which the pons and medulla are lodged. Posteriorly, there is a narrow and deep notch in which the falx cerebelli lies.

Each hemisphere is divided into three *lobes*. The *anterior lobe* lies on the anterior part of the superior surface. It is separated from the middle lobe by the *fissura prima*. The *middle lobe* is the largest of three lobes. It is limited in front by the fissura prima (on the superior surface), and by the posterolateral fissure (on the inferior surface). The *flocculonodular lobe* is the smallest lobe of the cerebellum. It lies on the inferior surface, in front of the posterolateral fissure (Fig. 34.3).

PARTS OF CEREBELLUM

The cerebellum is subdivided into numerous small parts by fissures. Each fissure cuts the vermis and both hemispheres. Out of the numerous fissures, however, only the following are worth remembering.

1 The *horizontal fissure* separates the superior surface from the inferior surface (Fig. 34.3).
2 The *primary fissure (fissure prima)* separates the anterior lobe from the middle lobe on the superior surface of the cerebellum.
3 The *posterolateral fissure* separates the middle lobe from the flocculonodular lobe on the inferior surface.

The various parts of cerebellum (Fig. 34.3) where both the superior and inferior surfaces of the cerebellum are drawn in one plane. The upper part of the diagram, above the horizontal fissure represents the superior surface; and the lower part, below the horizontal fissure represents the inferior surface.

	Parts of vermis	*Subdivisions of the cerebellar hemisphere*
1	Lingula	—
2	Central lobule	Ala
3	Culmen	Quadrangular lobule
4	Declive	Simple lobule
5	Folium	Superior semilunar lobule
6	Tuber	Inferior semilunar lobule
7	Pyramid	Biventral lobule
8	Uvula	Tonsil
9	Nodule	Flocculus

In Figure 34.3, note that each part of the vermis has a lateral extension. However, the lingula does not have any lateral extension.

Morphological Divisions of Cerebellum

1 The *archicerebellum* phylogenetically is the oldest part of the cerebellum. It is made up of the flocculonodular lobe and the lingula (Fig. 34.4).
2 The *paleocerebellum* is the next part of the cerebellum to appear. It is made up of the anterior lobe (minus lingula), and the pyramid and uvula of the inferior vermis (Fig. 34.3).

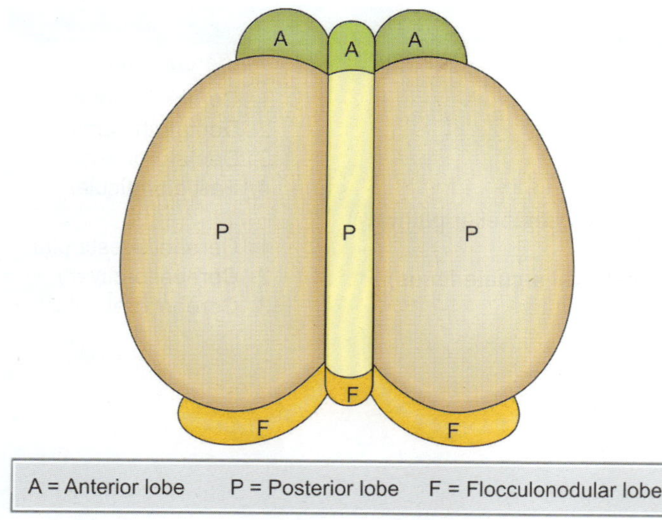

Fig. 34.4: Functional subdivisions of cerebellum

3 The *neocerebellum* is the newest part of the cerebellum to develop. It is made up of the posterior/middle lobe (the largest part of the cerebellum) minus the pyramid and uvula of the inferior vermis.

Functionally, the anterior and posterior lobes are organized into 3 longitudinal zones, lateral, intermediate and vermis (Figs 34.4 and 34.5).

Lateral Zone

Connected with association areas of the brain and is involved in planning and programming muscular activities.

Intermediate Zone

Concerned with control of muscles of hands, fingers, feet and toes.

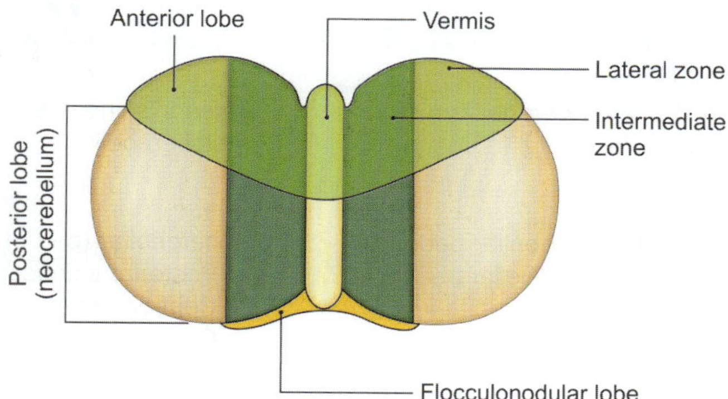

Fig. 34.5: Functions of cerebellum according to the zones

Vermis

Concerned with control of muscles of trunk, neck, shoulders and hips.

Flocculonodular Lobe

This lobe functions with vestibular system in controlling equilibrium.

Connections of Cerebellum

The fibres entering or leaving the cerebellum are grouped to form three peduncles which connect the cerebellum to the midbrain, the pons and the medulla. The constituent fibres in them are given in Table 34.1 and Fig. 34.6.

Grey Matter of Cerebellum

It consists of the cerebellar cortex and the cerebellar nuclei. There are four pairs of nuclei:

1 *Nucleus dentatus* is neocerebellar.
2 *Nucleus globosus.*

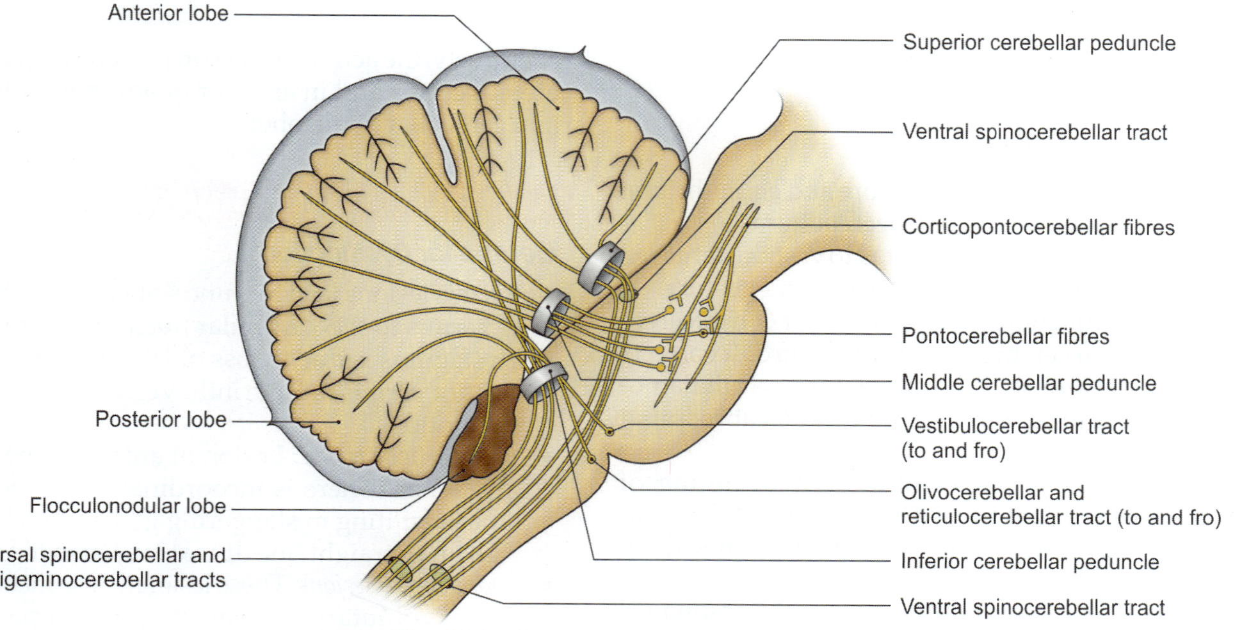

Fig. 34.6: Connections of cerebellum

Table 34.1: Constituents of the cerebellar peduncles

Peduncle	Afferent tracts	Efferent tracts
A. Superior cerebellar peduncle	1. Anterior spinocerebellar 2. Tectocerebellar	1. Cerebellorubral 2. Dentatothalamic 3. Dentato-olivary 4. Fastigioreticular
B. Middle cerebellar peduncle	Pontocerebellar (part of the corticopontocerebellar pathway)	—
C. Inferior cerebellar peduncle	1. Posterior spinocerebellar 2. Cuneocerebellar (posterior external arcuate fibres) 3. Olivocerebellar 4. Parolivocerebellar 5. Reticulocerebellar 6. Vestibulocerebellar 7. Anterior external arcuate fibres 8. Striae medullares 9. Trigeminocerebellar	1. Cerebellovestibular 2. Cerebello-olivary 3. Cerebelloreticular

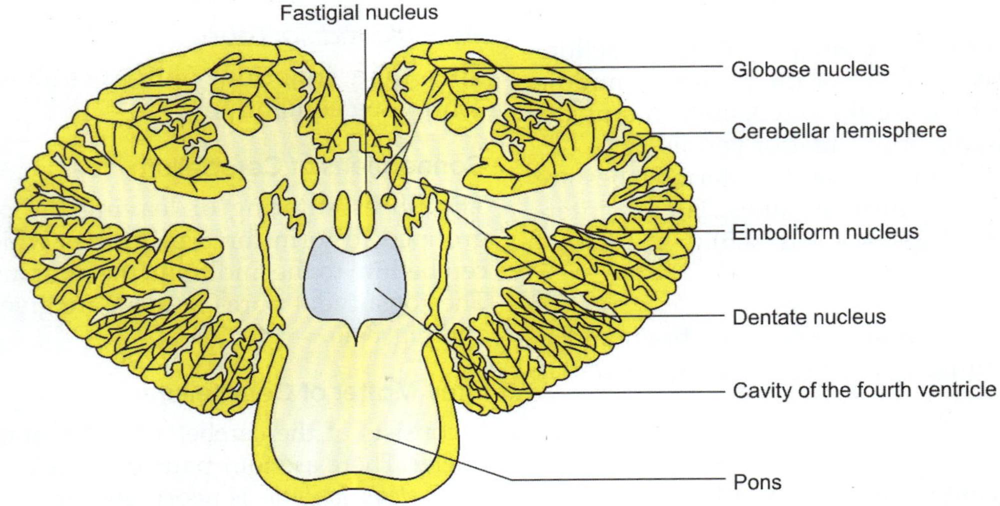

Fig. 34.7: Positions of intracerebellar nuclei

3 *Nucleus emboliformis* are paleocerebellar.
4 *Nucleus fastigii* is archicerebellar (Fig. 34.7).

Functions of Cerebellum

The cerebellum controls tone, posture and equili-brium. This is chiefly done by the paleocerebellum.

Flocculonodular lobe is connected to vestibular nuclei. It is involved in maintenance of balance and posture.

Cerebellum functions as "comparator". It receives information from cerebrum and spinal cord. It corrects and modifies ongoing movements through thalamo-cortical projections, reticulospinal and rubrospinal tracts.

Neocerebellum is responsible for fine tuning of motor performance for precise movements. It helps in planning and production of skilled movements along with cerebrum.

It has been seen by functional magnetic resonance imaging (FMRI) that if fingers of right hand are moved repetitively, the activity is seen in precentral gyrus of left cerebral cortex and in anterior quadrangular lobule of right cerebellar hemisphere.

CLINICAL ANATOMY

Cerebellar Dysfunction

- Vermis lesions lead to truncal ataxia as connection of vermis to the vestibular nuclei are involved.
- Nystagmus is due to loss of labyrinthine connections of vermis to labyrinth. Vermis is also related to emotions.
- *Anterior lobe lesion:* Lesion of anterior lobe causes gait ataxia. There is incoordination of the lower limbs resulting in staggering gait and inability to walk in a straight line. It is also seen in alcoholics.
- *Neocerebellar lesions:* These lesions cause incoordination of voluntary movements of the upper limbs.

It results in intention tremor, action tremor and overshoot movements.

- Speech is also defective. Phonation is defective due to loss of smoothness in expiratory muscles. Articulation is defective as there is less coordination between muscles of lip, tongue and palate.
- If there is thrombosis of one of six arteries nurturing cerebellum, "cerebellum cognitive affective syndrome" develops. These patients show inattention, grammatical errors in speech and patchy memory loss. Involvement of vermis results in dulling of emotional response. It is characterised by:
  - a. Muscular hypotonia
  - b. Intention tremors (tremors only during movements) tested by finger-nose and heel-knee tests.
  - c. Adiadochokinesia which is inability to perform rapid and regular alternating movements, like pronation and supination.
  - d. Nystagmus is to and fro oscillatory movements of the eyeballs while looking to either side.
  - e. Scanning speech is jerky and explosive speech.
  - f. Ataxic or unsteady gait.

FACTS TO REMEMBER

- Cerebellum or little brain acts like younger sibling of the large cerebrum. It controls tone, posture, equilibrium and fine movements of the body. It cannot initiate the movement.
- It is connected to medulla oblongata by inferior cerebellar peduncle.
- It is connected to pons by middle cerebellar peduncle.
- It is connected to midbrain by superior cerebellar peduncle.
- Number of neurons are about half of the cerebrum, though it is much smaller than the cerebrum.
- Its structure is uniform throughout, i.e. homotypical.
- Its control is ipsilateral.

Frequently Asked Questions

1. Name the afferent and efferent fibers of the three cerebellar peduncles.
2. Discuss the functions and clinical anatomy of cerebellum.
3. Write short notes on:
   a. Dental nucleus
   b. Parts of vermis and subdivision of cerebellar hemisphere
   c. Histology of cerebellar cortex

Multiple Choice Questions

1. The ratio of cerebellum to cerebrum in an adult is:
   a. 1:8 b. 1:16
   c. 1:4 d. 1:20
2. Purkinje cells are situated in:
   a. Cerebral cortex
   b. Junction of molecular and granular layers of cerebellum
   c. Granular layer of cerebellum
   d. Nucleus emboliformis
3. Which lobe is smallest in cerebellum?
   a. Flocculonodular b. Middle
   c. Anterior d. Posterior
4. Which of following region of cerebellum is concerned with planning and programming muscular activities?
   a. Intermediate zone b. Vermis
   c. Lateral zone d. Flocculonodular zone

Answers

1. a **2.** b **3.** a **4.** c

VIVA VOCE

- Name the nuclei present in white matter of the cerebellum.
- Name the peduncles which connect cerebellum to 3 parts of the brainstem.
- What are the symptoms of anterior lobe lesion of the cerebellum?
- Name the three functional zones with their respective functions.
- Name the characteristic cell seen in a histological slide of cerebellum.
- What are the symptoms of neocerebellar lesion?
- Name the morphological divisions of cerebellum.

Chapter 35

Cerebrum, Diencephalon, Basal Nuclei and White Matter

"Industry keeps body healthy, the mind clear, the heart whole and the purse full."
—Anonymous

INTRODUCTION

The cerebrum is made of two cerebral hemispheres which are incompletely separated from each other by the median *longitudinal fissure.* The two hemispheres are connected to each other across the median plane by the corpus callosum. Each hemisphere contains a cavity, called the lateral ventricle.

CEREBRAL HEMISPHERE

External Features

Each hemisphere has the following features.

Three Surfaces

1. The *superolateral surface* is convex and is related to the cranial vault (Figs 35.1 and 35.2).
2. The *medial surface* is flat and vertical. It is separated from the corresponding surface of the opposite hemisphere by the falx cerebri and the longitudinal fissure (Fig. 35.3).
3. The *inferior surface* is irregular. It is divided into an anterior part, the *orbital surface*, and a posterior part, the *tentorial surface.* The two parts are separated by a deep cleft called the stem of the lateral sulcus (Fig. 35.4).

Four Borders

1. *Superomedial border* separates the superolateral surface from the medial surface (Fig. 35.1).
2. *Inferolateral border* separates the superolateral surface from the inferior surface. The anterior part of this border is called the *superciliary border.* There is a depression on the inferolateral border situated about 5 cm in front of the occipital pole. It is called the preoccipital notch.
3. *Medial orbital border* separates the medial surface from the orbital surface.
4. *Medial occipital border* separates the medial surface from the tentorial surface.

Three Poles

1. *Frontal pole,* at the anterior end.
2. *Occipital pole,* at the posterior end.
3. *Temporal pole,* at the anterior end of the temporal lobe (Fig. 35.1).

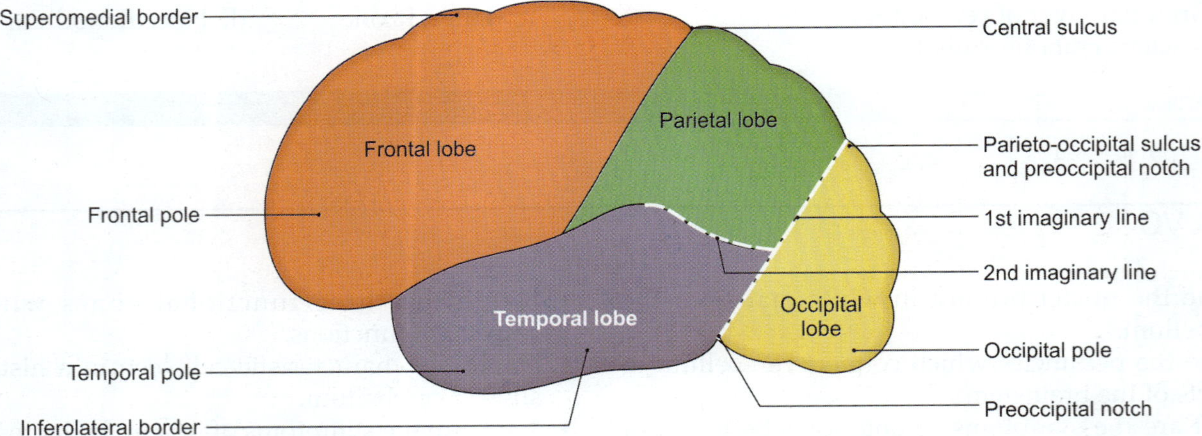

Fig. 35.1: Superolateral surface of cerebral hemisphere

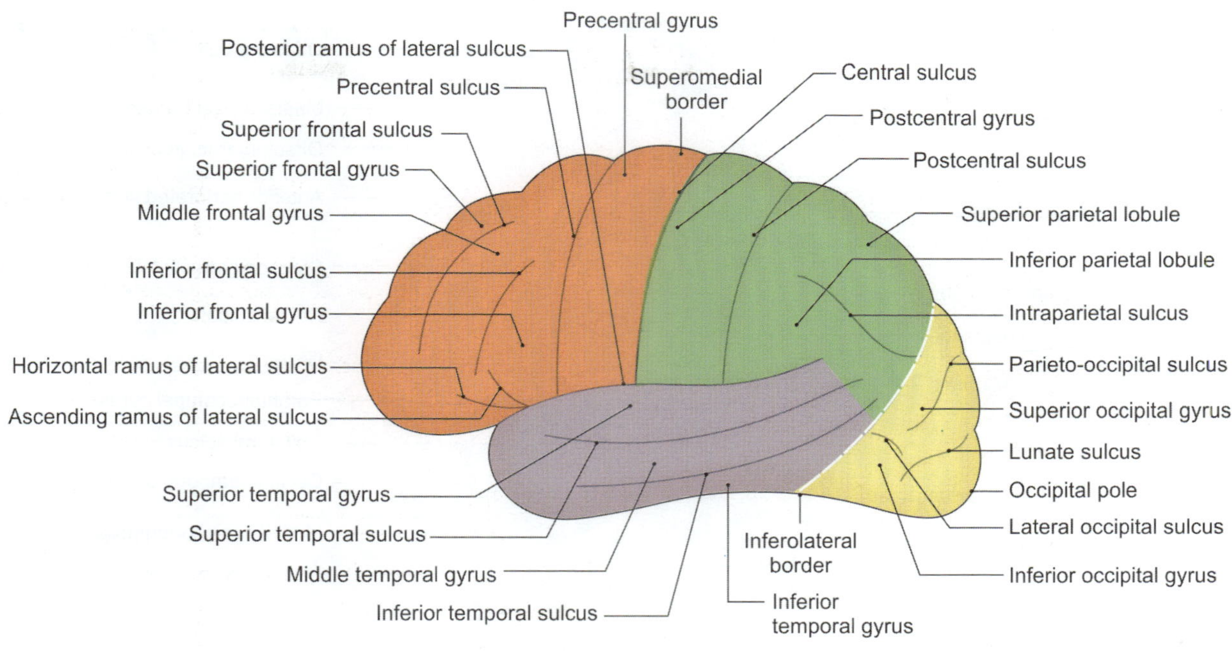

Fig. 35.2: Sulci and gyri on superolateral surface of left cerebral hemisphere

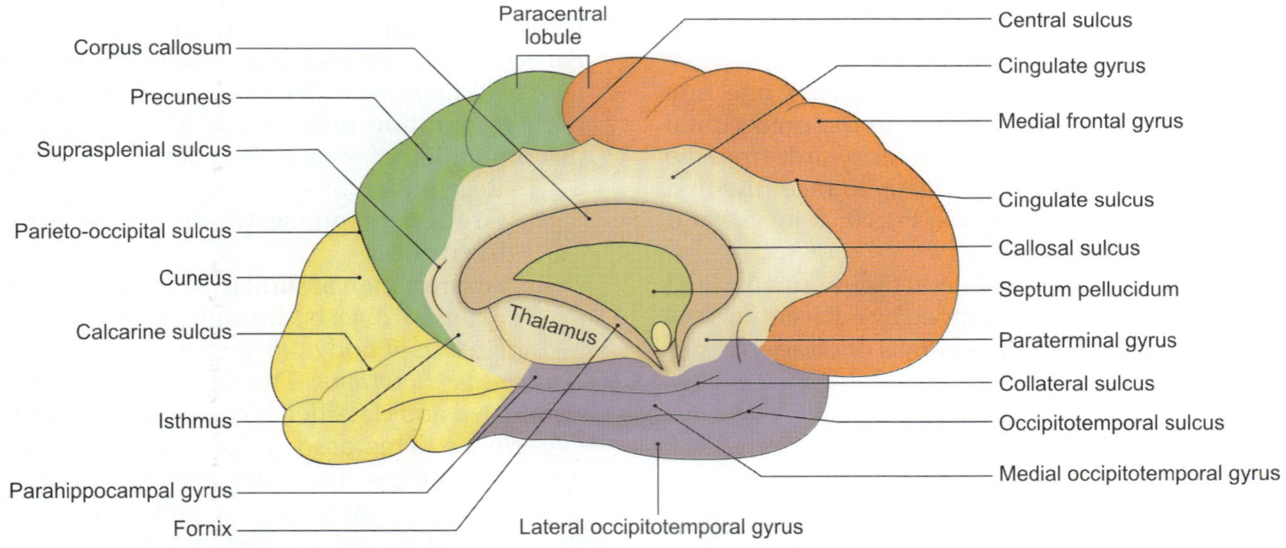

Fig. 35.3: Sulci and gyri on the medial surface of left cerebral hemisphere

Lobes of Cerebral Hemisphere

Each cerebral hemisphere is divided into four lobes—frontal, parietal, occipital and temporal. Their positions correspond, very roughly, to that of the corresponding bones. The lobes are best appreciated on the superolateral surface (Fig. 35.2). The sulci separating the lobes on this surface are as follows:

1. The *central sulcus* begins at the superomedial border of the hemisphere a little behind the midpoint between the frontal and occipital poles. It runs on the superolateral surface obliquely downwards and forwards and ends a little above the posterior ramus of the lateral sulcus (Figs 35.2 and 35.3).
2. It is seen that the *lateral sulcus* separates the orbital and tentorial parts of the inferior surface. Laterally, this sulcus reaches the superolateral surface where it divides into anterior, ascending and posterior branches. The largest of these, the *posterior ramus of the lateral sulcus* passes backwards and slightly upwards over the superolateral surface.
3. The *parieto-occipital* sulcus is a sulcus of the medial surface. Its upper end cuts off the superomedial border about 5 cm in front of the occipital pole.

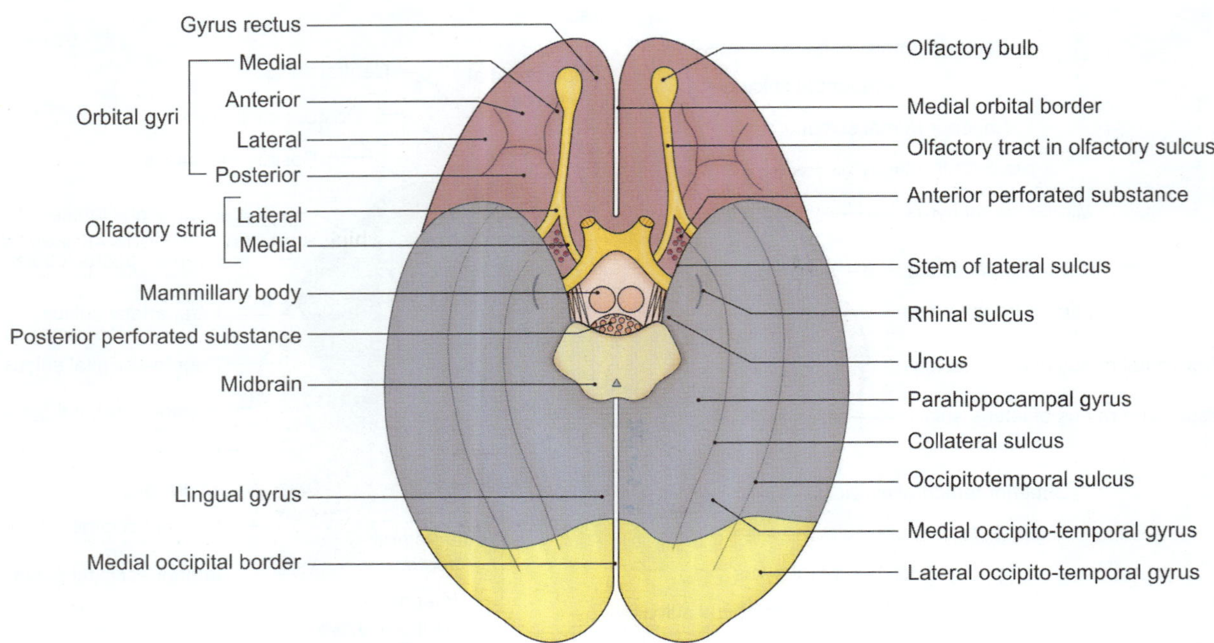

Fig. 35.4: Gyri and sulci on the inferior aspect of cerebral hemisphere

4 The *preoccipital notch* is an indentation on the infero-lateral border, about 5 cm in front of the occipital pole.

The division is completed by drawing one line joining the parieto-occipital sulcus to the preoccipital notch; and another line continuing backwards from the posterior ramus of the lateral sulcus to meet the first line. Sulci and gyri are shown in Figs 35.2 to 35.4 and Table 35.1.

Insula lies deep in floor of lateral fissure surrounded by a circular sulcus and overlapped by adjacent cortical areas, the opercula. Functional areas of cortex are put in Table 35.2.

Functions of Cerebral Cortex

1 *Cerebral dominance:* One cerebral hemisphere dominates the other one in relation to handedness, speech, perception of language and spatial judgement. In 80–95% subjects, the left hemisphere dominates the right one. Since left hemisphere controls the right half of the body, all these subjects are right-handed. The left hemisphere is verbal, mathematical, analytical and has direct link to consciousness.

   The right hemisphere is active in understanding geometrical figures, and important for temporal synthesis and spatial comprehension. It helps in recognition of faces, figures and appreciating music. Localisation of speech on left side in 70% of left handed and 98% of right handed is well known. Association of negative emotions with right prefrontal activity and of positive emotions with left prefrontal activity is also known. Mahatma Gandhi Father of the Nation, Bill Clinton, Bill Gates, Amitabh Bachchan and Abhishek Bachchan are all left handed.

2 *Discriminatory aspects:* Sensory cortex is not concerned with recognition only, but is also involved with discrimination of sensory function as:
   i. Recognition of spatial relationship
   ii. Graded response to stimuli of different intensities
   iii. Appreciation of similarities and differences in external objects, brought into contact with surface of body.

3 *Associative functions:* The information thus discriminated and classified is correlated with previous experience. This association forms the basis of memory patterns. These are transmitted to frontal cortex which synthesizes it and forms basis of thinking and related intellectual activities.

4 The motor area of one cerebral hemisphere controls voluntary movements of opposite side of the body (Table 35.2).

DIENCEPHALON

The diencephalon is a middle structure which is largely embedded in the cerebrum, and therefore hidden from surface view (Fig. 35.7). Its cavity forms the greater part of the third ventricle. The hypothalamic sulcus, extending from the interventricular foramen to the cerebral aqueduct, divides each half of the diencephalon into dorsal and ventral parts. Further subdivisions are:

Table 35.1: Sulci and gyri of the cerebrum

Surface/Lobe	*Sulci*	*Gyri*
I. Superolateral surface		
1. Frontal lobe (Fig. 35.2)	A. Precentral B. Superior frontal C. Inferior frontal	(a) Precentral (b) Superior frontal (c) Middle frontal (d) Inferior frontal which also contains horizontal and anterior ascending rami of the lateral sulcus, and the pars orbitalis, pars triangularis and pars opercularis
2. Parietal lobe	A. Postcentral B. Intraparietal	(a) Postcentral (b) Superior parietal lobule (c) Inferior parietal lobule, which is divided into 3 parts: (i) the anterior, supramarginal, (ii) the middle, angular, and (iii) the posterior, over the upturned end of inferior temporal sulcus
3. Temporal lobe	A. Superior temporal B. Inferior temporal	(a) Superior temporal, with 3 transverse temporal gyri (b) Middle temporal (c) Inferior temporal
4. Occipital lobe	A. Transverse occipital B. Lateral occipital C. Lunate D. Superior and inferior polar	(a) Arcus parieto-occipitalis (b) Superior occipital (c) Inferior occipital (d) Gyrus descendens
II. Medial surface (Fig. 35.3)	A. Anterior parolfactory B. Posterior parolfactory C. Cingulate D. Callosal E. Suprasplenial or subparietal F. Parieto-occipital G. Calcarine	(a) Paraterminal (b) Parolfactory (subcallosal area) (c) Medial frontal (d) Paracentral lobule (e) Cingulate (f) Cuneus (g) Precuneus
III. Inferior surface (Fig. 35.4)	A. Olfactory B. H-shaped orbital sulci C. Collateral D. Rhinal E. Occipitotemporal	(a) Gyrus rectus (b) Anterior orbital (c) Posterior orbital (d) Medial orbital (e) Lateral orbital (f) Lingual (g) Uncus (h) Parahippocampal (i) Medial occipitotemporal (j) Lateral occipitotemporal

Dorsal Part of Diencephalon

1 Thalamus (dorsal thalamus).

2 Metathalamus, including the medial and lateral geniculate bodies (included with thalamus).

3 Epithalamus, including the pineal body and habenula.

Ventral Part of Diencephalon

1 Hypothalamus, and
2 Subthalamus (ventral thalamus).

THALAMUS

The thalamus (inner chamber) is a large mass of grey matter situated in the lateral wall of the third ventricle

Table 35.2: Functional areas of the cerebral cortex

Lobe	*Area*	*Area no.*	*Location*	*Representation of body parts*	*Function*	*Effect of lesion*
Frontal lobe (Fig. 35.5)	Motor area	4	Precentral gyrus and paracentral lobule	Upside down	Controls voluntary activities of the opposite half of body	Contralateral paralysis and Jacksonian fits
	Premotor area	6	Posterior parts of superior, middle and inferior frontal gyri	—	Controls extrapyramidal system	Often mixed with pyramidal effect
	Frontal eye field	6, 8	Posterior part of middle frontal gyrus	—	Controls horizontal conjugate movements of the eyes	Horizontal conjugate movements are lost
	Motor speech area (Broca's area)	44, 45	Pars triangularis and pars opercularis	—	Controls the spoken speech	Aphasia (motor)
	Prefrontal area	—	The remaining large, anterior part of frontal lobe	—	Controls emotion, concentration, attention and judgement	Loss of orientation
Parietal lobe (Fig. 35.6)	Sensory (somesthetic) area	3, 1, 2	Postcentral gyrus and paracentral lobule	Upside down	Perception of exteroceptive (touch, pain and temperature) and proprioceptive impulses	Loss of appreciation of the impulses received
	Parietal area	—	Between sensory and visual areas	—	Stereognosis and sensory speech	Astereognosis and sensory aphasias
Occipital lobe	Visuosensory area or striate area	17	In and around the postcalcarine sulcus	Macular area has largest representation	Reception and perception of the isolated visual impressions of colour, size, form, motion, illumination and transparency	Homonymous hemianopia with macular sparing
	Visuopsychic area, parastriate and peristriate areas	18, 19	Surround the striate area	—	Correlation of visual impulses with past memory and recognition of objects seen, and also the depth	Visual agnosia
Temporal lobe	Auditosensory area	41, 42	Posterior part of superior temporal gyrus and anterior transverse temporal gyrus	—	Reception and perception of isolated auditory impressions of loudness, quality and pitch	Impaired hearing
	Auditopsychic area	22	Rest of the superior temporal gyrus	—	Correlation of auditory impressions with past memory and identification (interpretation) of the sounds heard	Auditory agnosia

Fig. 35.5: Functional areas of superolateral aspect of simian cerebral hemisphere

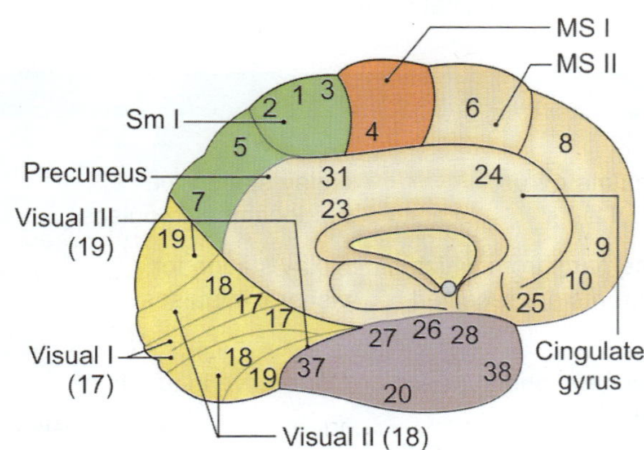

Fig. 35.6: Functional areas on the medial surface of cerebral hemisphere

and in the floor of the central part of the lateral ventricle. It has anterior and posterior ends and superior, inferior, medial and lateral surfaces (Table 35.3).

The *anterior end* with anterior nucleus is narrow and forms the posterior boundary of the interventricular foramen (Fig. 35.8).

The *posterior end* is expanded, and is known as the pulvinar. It overhangs the lateral and medial geniculate bodies, and the superior colliculus with its brachium (Fig. 35.9).

The *superior surface* is divided into a lateral ventricular part which forms the floor of the central part of the lateral ventricle, and a medial extraventricular part which is covered by the tela choroidea of the third ventricle.

The *inferior surface* rests on the subthalamus and the hypothalamus (Fig. 35.8).

The *medial surface* forms the posterosuperior part of the lateral wall of the third ventricle. The medial surfaces of two thalami are interconnected by an interthalamic adhesion (Fig. 35.8).

The *lateral surface* forms the medial boundary of the posterior limb of the internal capsule.

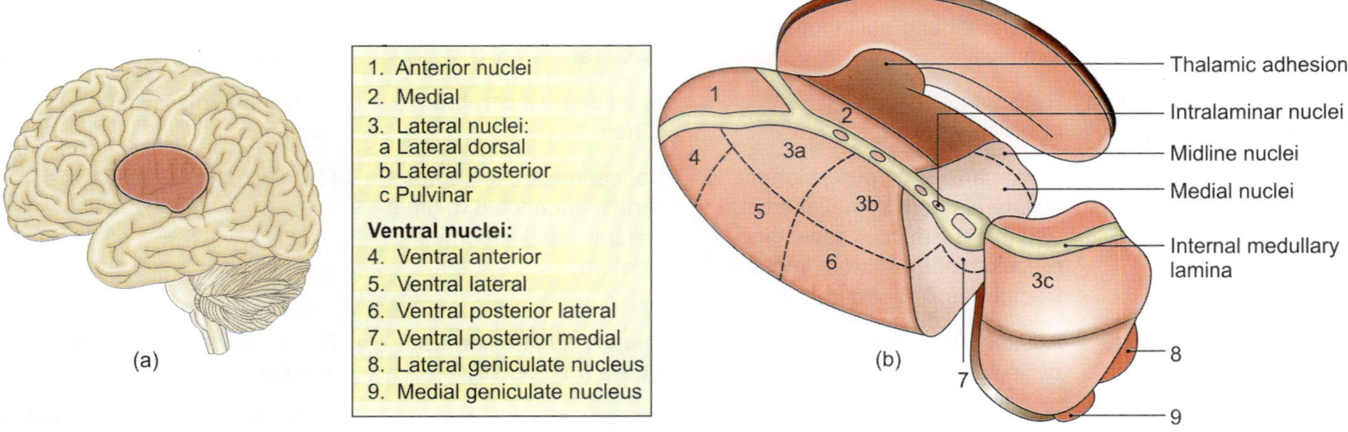

Figs 35.7a and b: Three-dimensional view of thalamus and with its location in the cerebral hemisphere

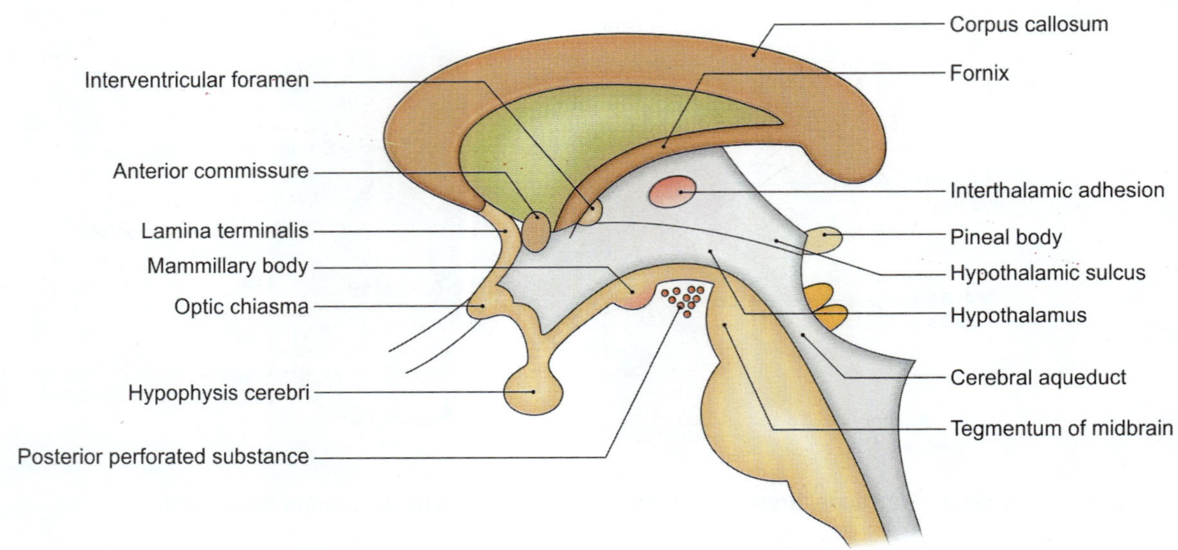

Fig. 35.8: Thalamus and hypothalamus as seen in sagittal section

Table 35.3: Connection of thalamus

Nucleus	*Afferents*	*Efferents*	*Function*
Anterior nucleus (Fig. 35.9)	Mammillothalamic tract	To cingulate gyrus (Fig. 35.11)	Relay station for hippocampal impulses
Medial nucleus	From hypothalamus, frontal lobe in front of area 6, corpus striatum, and other thalamus nuclei	To same parts from which the afferents are received	Relay station for visceral impulses
Lateral nucleus: Lateral dorsal, lateral posterior and pulvinar	From precuneus and superior parietal lobule; also from ventral and medial nuclei Temporal and occipital lobes	To precuneus and superior parietal lobule Temporal and occipital lobes	Correlative in function
Ventral anterior nucleus	From globus pallidus (subthalamic fasciculus)	To areas 6 and 8 of cortex (Fig. 35.10)	Relay station for striatal impulses
Ventral lateral nucleus	From cerebellum (dentatothalamic fibres) and red nucleus	To motor areas 4 and 6	Relay station for cerebellar impulses
Ventral posterolateral nucleus (Fig. 35.9)	Spinal and medial lemnisci	To postcentral gyrus (areas 3, 1, 2)	Relay station for exteroceptive (touch, pain and temperature) and proprioceptive impulses from body, except face and head
Ventral posteromedial nucleus	Trigeminal and solitariothalamic lemnisci	To postcentral gyrus (areas no. 3, 1, 2)	Relay station for impulses from the face, head and taste impulses
Intralaminar,midline, and reticular nuclei	Reticular formation of brainstem	To all parts of cerebral cortex	Participate in arousal reactions
Centromedian nucleus	From parts of corpus striatum; collaterals from spinal, medial, trigeminal lemnisci, ascending reticulothalamic fibres. Impulses from areas 4, 6 of cerebral cortex	Not connected to cerebral cortex, connected to other thalamic nuclei, corpus striatum	Receive pain fibres
Medial geniculate body	Auditory fibres from inferior colliculus	Primary auditory areas 41, 42 (Fig. 35.10)	Relay station for auditory impulses
Lateral geniculate body (Fig. 35.9)	Optic tract	Primary visual cortex (Fig. 35.11)	Relay station for visual impulses (area 17)

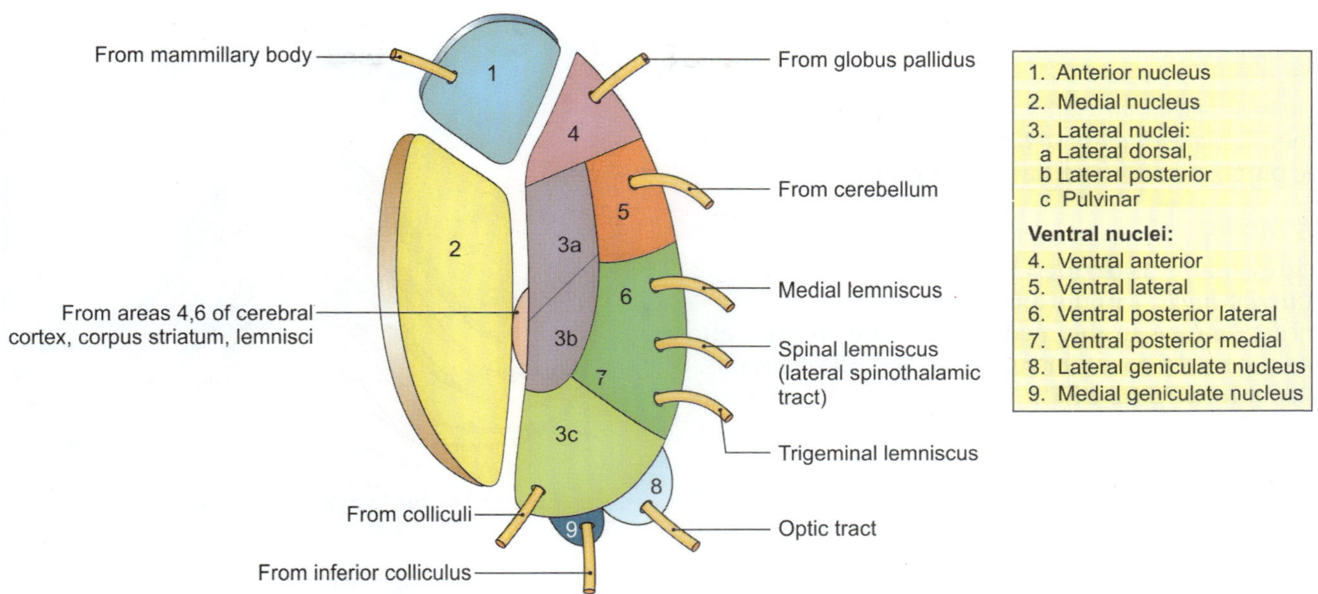

Fig. 35.9: Parts of the thalamus. The afferents to the nuclei of thalamus are also indicated

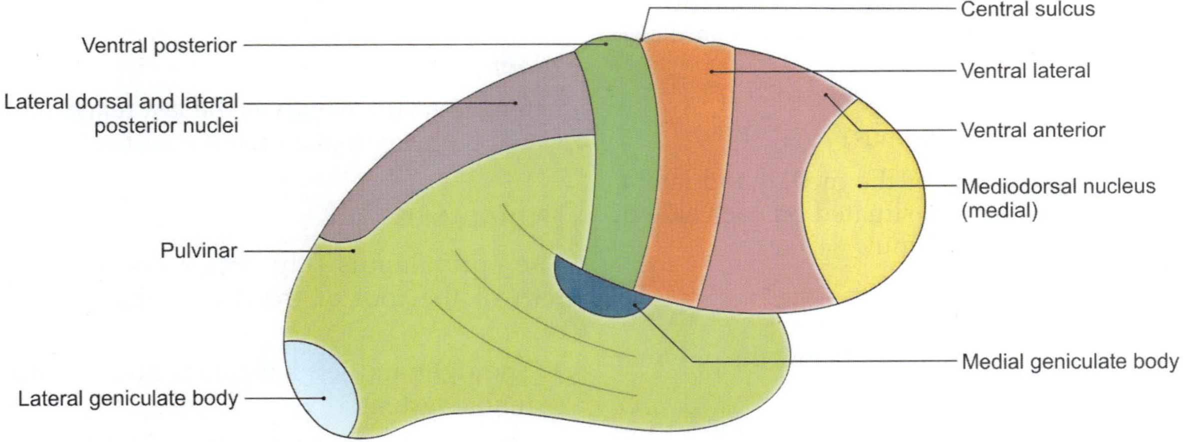

Fig. 35.10: Projection from thalamic nuclei to superolateral surface of cerebral hemisphere

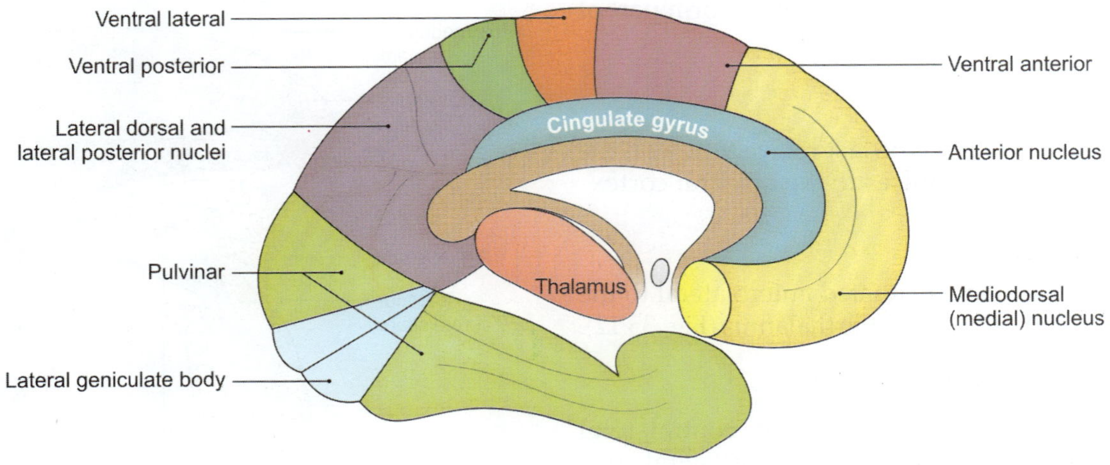

Fig. 35.11: Projection from thalamic nuclei to medial surface of cerebral hemisphere

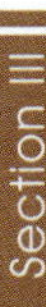

Structure and Nuclei of Thalamus

White Matter

The *external medullary lamina* covers the lateral surface.

The *internal medullary lamina* divides the thalamus into three parts, anterior, medial and lateral.

Grey Matter

The grey matter is divided to form several nuclei.

1 *Anterior nucleus* in the anterior part.
2 *Medial nucleus* in the medial part. The anterior and medial nuclei together represent the *paleothalamus.*
3 The lateral part of the thalamus is largest and represents the *neothalamus.* It is divided into the *lateral nucleus* in the dorsolateral part, and the *ventral nucleus* in the ventromedial part. The ventral nucleus is subdivided into anterior, intermediate and posterior groups. The posterior group is further subdivided into the posterolateral and posteromedial groups.
4 Intralaminar nuclei including centromedian nucleus (located in the internal medullary lamina), midline nuclei (periventricular grey on the medial surface) and reticular nuclei (on the lateral surface) are also present.

METATHALAMUS (Part of Thalamus)

The metathalamus consists of the medial and lateral geniculate bodies, which are situated on each side of the midbrain, below the thalamus.

Medial Geniculate Body

It is an oval elevation situated just below the pulvinar of the thalamus.

- *Afferents:* (1) lateral lemniscus; and (2) fibres from both inferior colliculi.
- *Efferents:* They give rise to the acoustic (auditory) radiation going to the auditory area of the cortex (in the temporal lobe) through the sublentiform part of the internal capsule.

Function

Medial geniculate body is the last relay station on the pathway of auditory impulses to the cerebral cortex.

Lateral Geniculate Body

It is a small oval elevation situated anterolateral to the medial geniculate body, below the thalamus (Fig. 35.12).

Structure

It is six-layered. Layers 1, 4 and 6 receive contralateral optic fibres, and layers 2, 3 and 5 receive ipsilateral optic fibres.

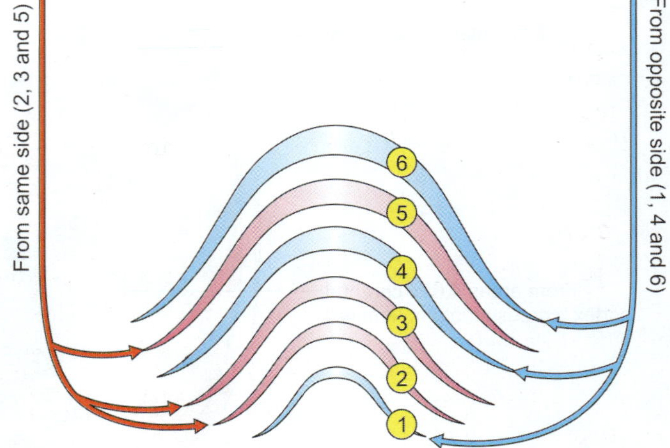

Fig. 35.12: Six layers of lateral geniculate body

Connections

Afferents: Optic tract (lateral root).

Efferents: They give rise to optic radiations going to the visual area of cortex through retrolentiform part of internal capsule.

Function

Lateral geniculate body is the last relay station on the visual pathway to the occipital cortex.

EPITHALAMUS

The epithalamus (Fig. 35.13) occupies the caudal part of the roof of the diencephalon and consists of:

1 The right and left habenular nuclei. Forms part of limbic system.
2 The pineal body or epiphysis cerebri.

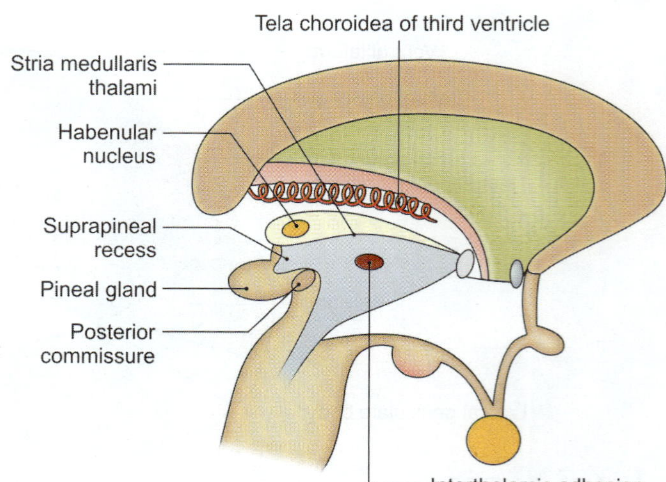

Fig. 35.13: Components of the epithalamus

Pineal Body/Gland

The pineal body is a small, conical organ, projecting backwards and downwards between the two superior colliculi.

It consists of a conical *body* about 8 mm long, and a *stalk* or *peduncle.*

Structure

The pineal gland is composed of two types of cells, pinealocytes and neuroglial cells, with a rich network of blood vessels and sympathetic fibres.

Calcareous concretions are constantly present in the pineal after the 17th year of life and may form aggregations *(brain sand).* Spaces or cysts may also be present.

Functions

It is an endocrine gland of great importance. It produces hormones that may have an important regulatory influence on many other endocrine organs. The best known hormone is melatonin which causes changes in skin colour in some species. The synthesis and discharge of melatonin is remarkably influenced by exposure of the animal to light. It is secreted more during dark periods.

HYPOTHALAMUS

The hypothalamus is a part of the diencephalon (Fig. 35.14). It lies in the floor and lateral wall of the third ventricle. It has been designated as the head ganglion of the autonomic nervous system.

Boundaries

As seen in a sagittal section of the brain, it is bounded *anteriorly* by the lamina terminalis; *inferiorly* by the floor of the third ventricle (from the optic chiasma to the posterior perforated substance); and *posterosuperiorly* by the hypothalamic sulcus (Fig. 35.8).

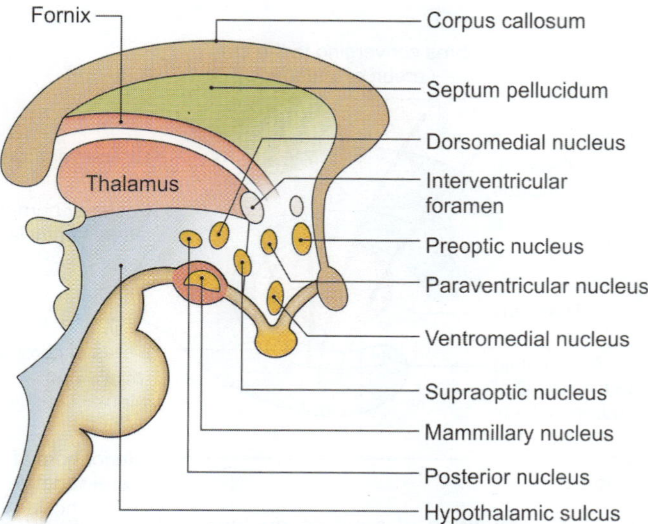

Fig. 35.14: Nuclei of medial zone of hypothalamus

Parts of the Hypothalamus

Optic Part

1 Supraoptic nucleus, above the optic chiasma.
2 Paraventricular nucleus, just above the supraoptic nucleus.

Tuberal Part

3 Ventromedial nucleus.
4 Dorsomedial nucleus.
5 Tuberal nucleus, lateral to the ventromedial nucleus.

Mammillary Part

6 Posterior nucleus, caudal to the ventromedial and dorsomedial nuclei.
7 Lateral nucleus, lateral to the posterior nucleus.

Important Connections

Afferents

The hypothalamus receives visceral sensations through the spinal cord and brainstem (reticular formation). It is also connected to several centres associated with olfactory pathways, including the piriform cortex; with the cerebellum; and with the retina.

Efferents

1 Supraopticohypophyseal tract from the optic nuclei to the pars posterior, the pars tuberalis and the pars intermedia of the hypophysis cerebri.
2 Mammillothalamic tract.
3 Mammillotegmental tract.

Functions of Hypothalamus

Endocrine Control

By forming *releasing hormones* or *release inhibiting hormones,* the hypothalamus regulates secretion of thyrotropin (TSH), corticotropin (ACTH), somatotropin (STH), prolactin, luteinizing hormone (LH), follicle stimulating hormone (FSH) and melanocyte stimulating hormone, by the pars anterior of the hypophysis cerebri.

Neurosecretion

Oxytocin and vasopressin (antidiuretic hormone, ADH) are secreted by the hypothalamus and transported to the infundibulum and the posterior lobe of the hypophysis cerebri.

General Autonomic Effect

The anterior parts of the hypothalamus chiefly mediate parasympathetic activity, and the posterior parts, chiefly mediate sympathetic activity.

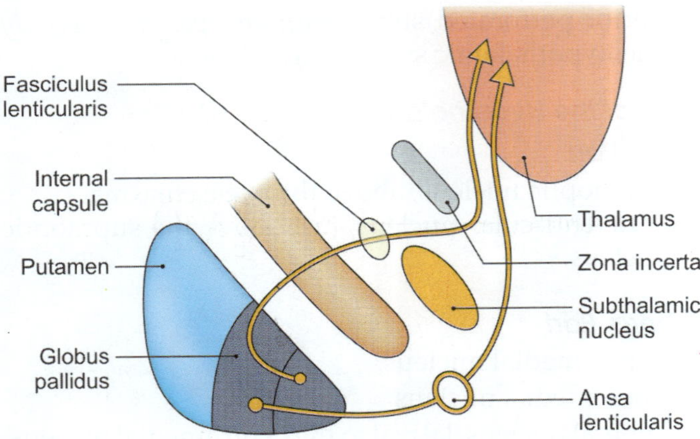

Fig. 35.15: Important fibre bundle running through subthalamic region

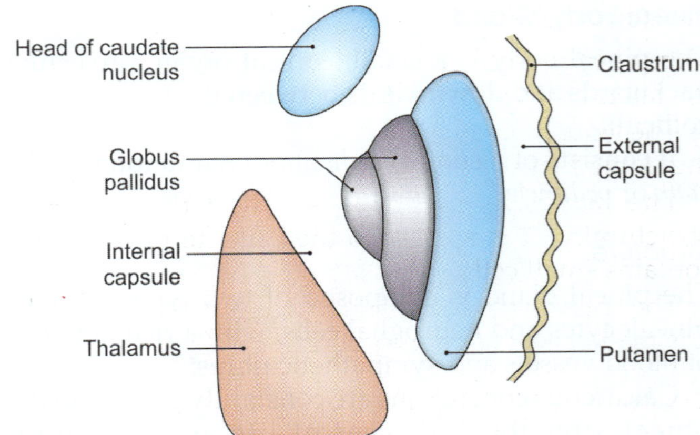

Fig. 35.16: Horizontal section through corpus striatum, thalamus and internal capsule

Temperature Regulation

The hypothalamus maintains a balance between heat production and heat loss of the body.

Regulation of Food and Water Intake

The *hunger* or *feeding centre* is placed laterally, the *satiety centre,* medially.

Sexual Behaviour and Reproduction

Through its control of the anterior pituitary, the hypothalamus controls gametogenesis, various reproductive cycles (uterine, ovarian, etc.) and the maturation and maintenance of secondary sexual characteristics.

Biological Clocks

Many tissues and organ-systems of the body show a cyclic variation in their functional activity during the 24 hours of a day (circadian rhythm). Sleep and wakefulness is an outstanding example of a circadian rhythm.

Emotion, Fear, Rage, Aversion, Pleasure and Reward

These faculties are controlled by the hypothalamus, the limbic system and the prefrontal cortex.

SUBTHALAMUS

The subthalamus lies between the midbrain and thalamus, medial to internal capsule and the globus pallidus (Fig. 35.15). It is a site for integration of number of motor centres.

BASAL NUCLEI

The basal nuclei are subcortical, intracerebral masses of grey matter forming important parts of the extrapyramidal system. They include the following.

1. The *corpus striatum* (Fig. 35.16), which is partially divided by the internal capsule into two nuclei:
   a. The *caudate nucleus.*
   b. The *lentiform nucleus.*
2. The *amygdaloid body* forms a part of the limbic system.
3. *Claustrum.*

The four nuclei (caudate, lentiform, amygdaloid and claustrum) are joined to the cortex at the anterior perforated substance.

CORPUS STRIATUM

Corpus striatum comprises the caudate nucleus and lentiform nucleus.

Caudate Nucleus

It is a C-shaped or comma-shaped nucleus which is surrounded by the lateral ventricle. The concavity of 'C' encloses the thalamus and the internal capsule (Fig. 35.17).

The nucleus has a head, a body, and a tail.

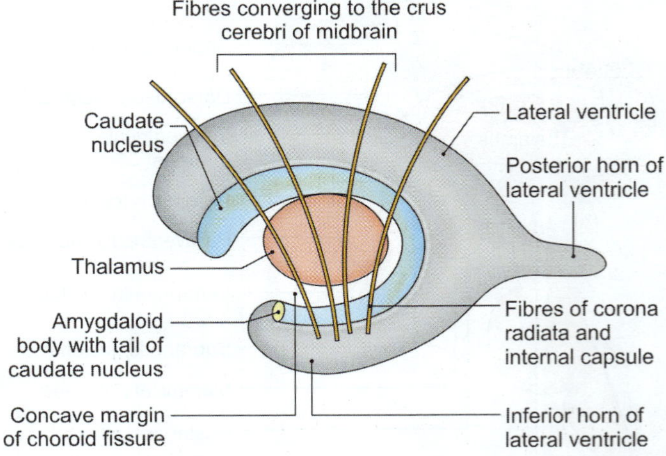

Fig. 35.17 Relations of caudate nucleus to lateral ventricle, thalamus and internal capsule

Lentiform Nucleus

This is a large lens-shaped (biconvex) nucleus, forming the lateral boundary of the internal capsule.

The lentiform nucleus is divided into two parts by a thin lamina of white matter.

The larger lateral part is called the *putamen*. Structurally, it is similar to the caudate nucleus and contains small cells.

The smaller medial part is called the *globus pallidus*. It is made up of large (motor) cells.

Connections of Corpus Striatum

The caudate nucleus and putamen are afferent nuclei, while the globus pallidus is the efferent nucleus, of the corpus striatum. The connections are shown in Table 35.4 and Fig. 35.18.

Functions of Corpus Striatum

1 The corpus striatum regulates muscle tone and thus helps in smoothening voluntary movements.
2 It controls automatic associated movements, like the swinging of arms during walking. Similarly, it controls the coordinated movements of different parts of the body for emotional expression.
3 It influences the precentral motor cortex which is supposed to control the extrapyramidal activities of the body.
4 These do not receive any sensory input from spinal cord unlike the cerebellum. Basal ganglia contribute to congnitive function of the brain.

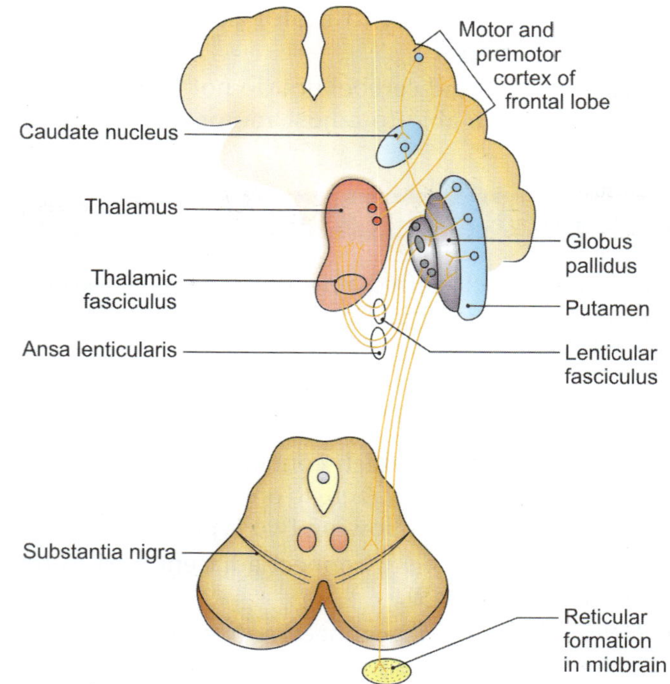

Fig. 35.18: Connections of corpus striatum

5 These help cortex in execution of learned patterns of movements subconsciously.
6 Corpus striatum, cerebellum and motor areas of cerebrum jointly are responsible for planning, execution and control of movements.
7 Corpus striatum and cerebellum without sending fibres to spinal cord modify the effect on spinal cord

Table 35.4: Connections of the corpus striatum (Fig. 35.18)

Nucleus	*Afferents*	*Efferents*
A. Caudate nucleus and putamen.	From: 1. Cerebral cortex (areas 4 and 6) 2. Thalamus (medial, intralaminar and midline nuclei) 3. Substantia nigra	Chiefly to globus pallidus, but also to substantia nigra and thalamus.
B. Globus pallidus	Mainly from: 1. Caudate nucleus 2. Putamen Also from: 1. Thalamus 2. Subthalamic nucleus 3. Substantia nigra	Efferents form three bundles, namely: 1. Ansa lenticularis, ventrally 2. Fasciculus lenticularis, dorsally 3. Subthalamic fasciculus from the middle part of the globus pallidus These bundles terminate in the following. (a) Thalamus (b) Hypothalamus (c) Subthalamic nucleus (d) Red nucleus (e) Olivary nucleus (f) Substantia nigra (g) Reticular nuclei

through projections to motor cortex and extra-pyramidal fibres.

8 Basal ganglia and cerebellum do not initiate movements but are able to adjust motor commands.

WHITE MATTER OF CEREBRUM

The fibres are classified into three groups, association fibres, projection fibres, of white matter and commissural fibres.

ASSOCIATION (ARCUATE) FIBRES

These are the fibres which connect different cortical areas of the same hemisphere to one another. These are subdivided into the following two types.

- *Short association fibres* connect adjacent gyri to one another (Fig. 35.19).
- *Long association fibres* connect more widely separated gyri to one another. Some examples are:
  1. The *uncinate fasciculus,* connecting the temporal pole to the motor speech area and to the orbital cortex.
  2. The *cingulum,* connecting the cingulate gyrus to the parahippocampal gyrus.
  3. The *superior longitudinal fasciculus,* connecting the frontal lobe to occipital and temporal lobes.
  4. The *inferior longitudinal fasciculus,* connecting the occipital and temporal lobes.

PROJECTION FIBRES

These are fibres which connect the cerebral cortex to other parts of the CNS, e.g. the brainstem and spinal cord. The internal capsule is made up of projection fibres.

COMMISSURAL FIBRES

Corpus Callosum

The corpus callosum is the largest commissure of the brain. It connects the two cerebral hemispheres. Since it is the neopallial commissure, it attains enormous size in man (10 cm long).

Parts of Brain Connected

The corpus callosum connects all parts of the cerebral cortex of the two sides, except the lower and anterior parts of the temporal lobes which are connected by the anterior commissure.

Parts of Corpus Callosum

1. The *genu* is the anterior end. It lies 4 cm behind the frontal pole (Fig. 35.20).
2. The *rostrum* is directed downwards and backwards from the genu, and ends by joining the lamina terminalis, in front of the anterior commissure.
3. The *trunk* or body is the middle part, between the genu and the splenium. Its *superior surface* is convex from before backwards and concave from side to side.
4. The *splenium* is the posterior end forming the thickest part of the corpus callosum. It lies 6 cm in front of the occipital pole.

Fibres of Corpus Callosum (Fig. 35.21)

1. The rostrum connects the orbital surfaces of the two frontal lobes.
2. The *forceps minor* is made up of fibres of the genu that connect the two frontal lobes.
3. The *forceps major* is made up of fibres of the splenium connecting the two occipital lobes.
4. The *tapetum* is formed by some fibres from the trunk and splenium of the corpus callosum.

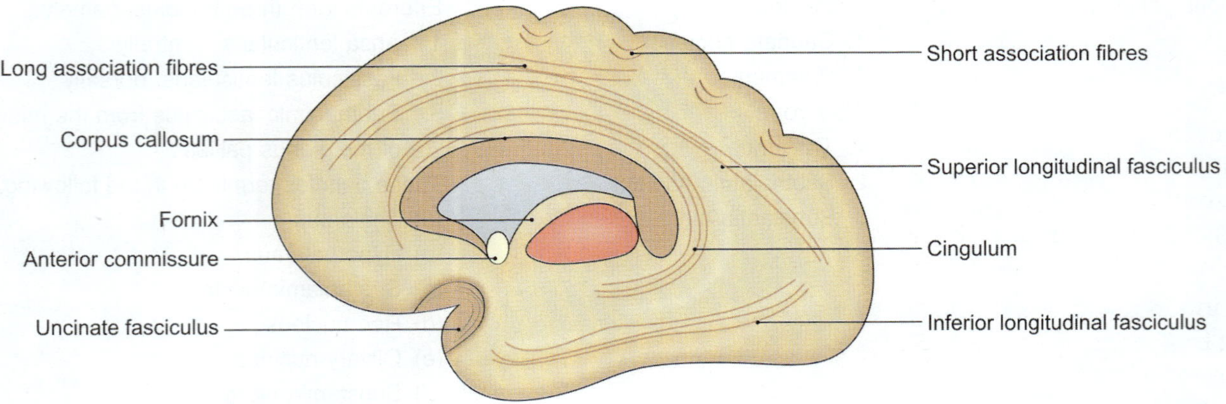

Fig. 35.19: Association fibres

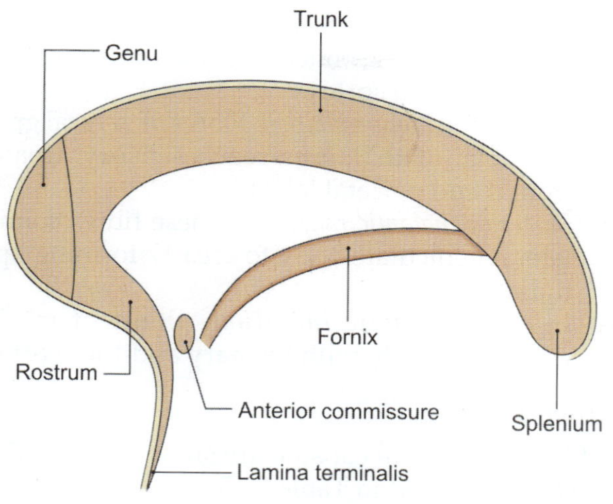

Fig. 35.20: Parts of corpus callosum

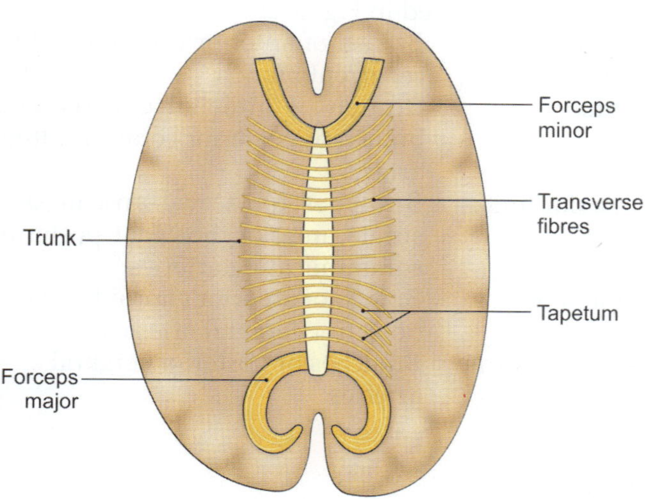

Fig. 35.21: Fibres of corpus callosum

Functional Significance

The corpus callosum helps in coordinating activities of the two hemispheres.

INTERNAL CAPSULE

Gross Anatomy

The internal capsule is a large band of fibres, situated in the inferomedial part of each cerebral hemisphere. In horizontal sections of the brain, it appears V-shaped with its concavity directed laterally. The concavity is occupied by the lentiform nucleus (Fig. 35.22).

The internal capsule contains fibres going to and coming from the cerebral cortex. It can be compared to a narrow gate where the fibres are densely crowded. Small lesions of the capsule can give rise to widespread derangements of the body.

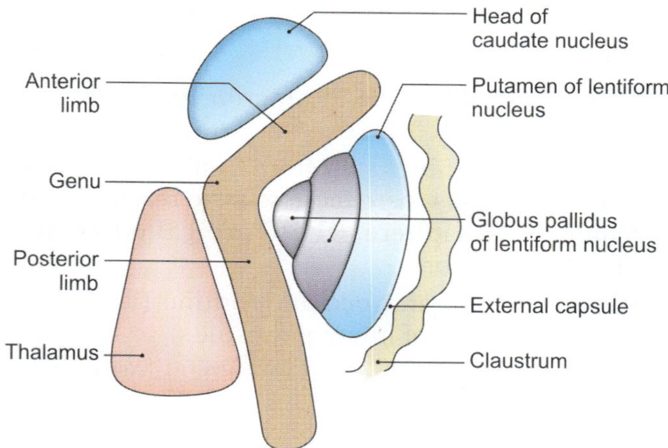

Fig. 35.22: Boundaries and parts of internal capsule

When traced *upwards,* the fibres of the capsule diverge and are continuous with the corona radiata. When traced *downwards*, its fibres converge and many of them are continuous with the crus cerebri of the midbrain.

The internal capsule is divided into the following parts.

1. The *anterior limb* lies between the head of the caudate nucleus and the lentiform nucleus (Fig. 35.23).
2. The *posterior limb* lies between the thalamus and the lentiform nucleus.
3. The *genu* is the bend between the anterior and posterior limbs.
4. The *sublentiform part* lies below the lentiform nucleus. It can be seen in a coronal section, whereas the rest of the parts are seen in a horizontal section.
5. The *retrolentiform part* lies behind the lentiform nucleus.

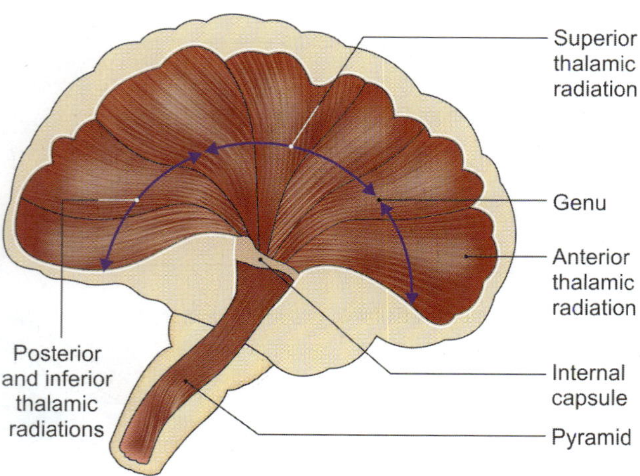

Fig. 35.23: Fibres of various parts of internal capsule

Fibres of Internal Capsule

Motor Fibres

Corticopontine fibres lie in anterior limb, genu and posterior limb (Fig. 35.24).

Frontopontine fibres start from frontal lobe to reach the pontine nuclei where these relay to reach opposite cerebellar hemisphere. These are called cortico-pontocerebellar fibres.

Parietopontine and occipitopontine fibres lie in retrolentiform part of internal capsule.

Temporopontine fibres lie in sublentiform part of internal capsule.

Pyramidal Fibres

Corticonuclear to nuclei of III, IV, V, VI, VII, XII and nucleus ambiguus for IX, X, XI nerves of opposite side.

Corticospinal: Fibres for anterior horn cells of muscles of head and neck lie in genu.

Fibres for upper limb, trunk and lower limb lie in posterior limb of internal capsule in sequential order (Fig. 35.24).

Extrapyramidal Fibres

These fibres start from cerebral cortex as corticostriate and corticorubral fibres and reach corpus striatum and red nucleus.

Sensory Fibres

Thalamocortical fibres form thalamic radiations (3rd order neuron fibres):

i. *Anterior thalamic radiation*: Fibres from anterior and dorsomedial nuclei of thalamus terminate in frontal lobe cortex.
ii. *Superior thalamic radiation*: Fibres of ventral group of nuclei of thalamus reach sensory areas of frontal and parietal lobes.
iii. *Posterior thalamic radiation*: These fibres connect lateral geniculate body to area 17 forming optic radiation.
iv. *Inferior thalamic radiation*: Connect medial geniculate body with primary auditory cortex.

Constituent Fibres

The fibres of internal capsule are shown in Fig. 35.24. These are presented in Table 35.5.

Blood Supply

The arteries supplying different parts of the internal capsule are depicted in Fig. 35.25.

Anterior limb:	Branch of anterior cerebral and its recurrent branch.
Genu:	Branch of internal carotid and branch of posterior communcating artery.
Posterior limb:	Branches of lateral and medial striate, anterior choroidal, posterior communicating arteries
Sublentiform part:	Branch of anterior choroidal and posterior cerebral arteries
Retrolentiform part:	Branches of posterior cerebral arteries

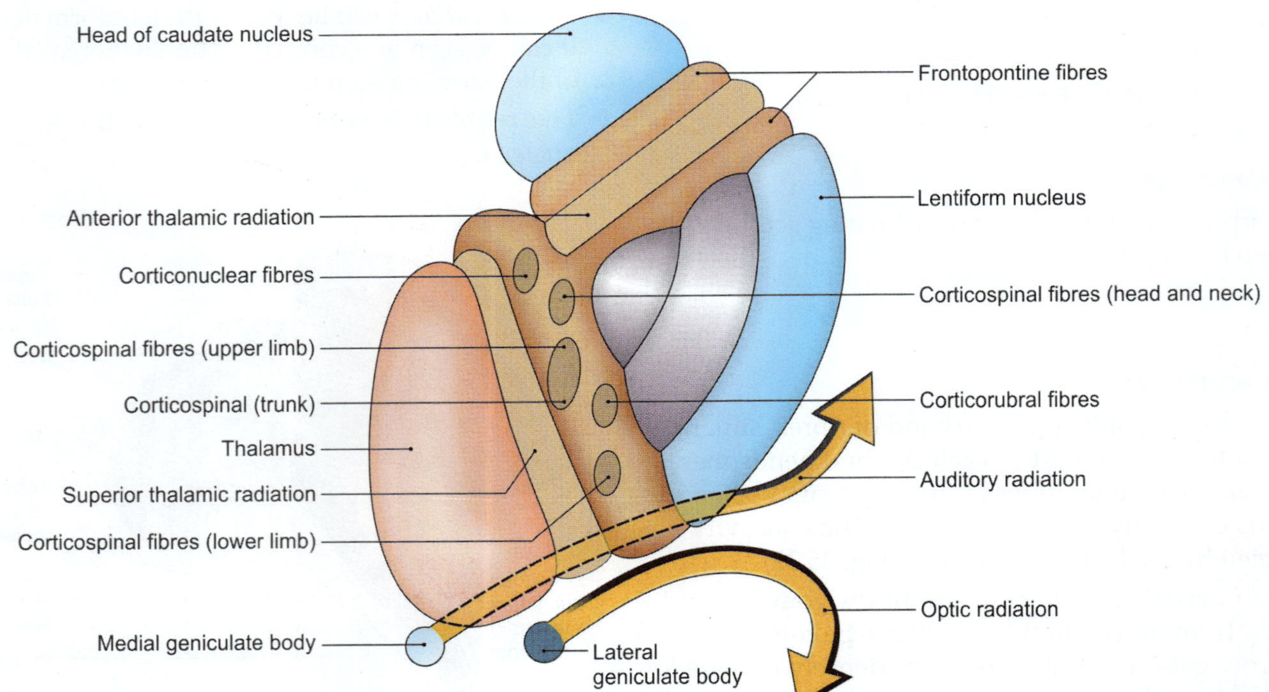

Fig. 35.24: Fibre components of internal capsule

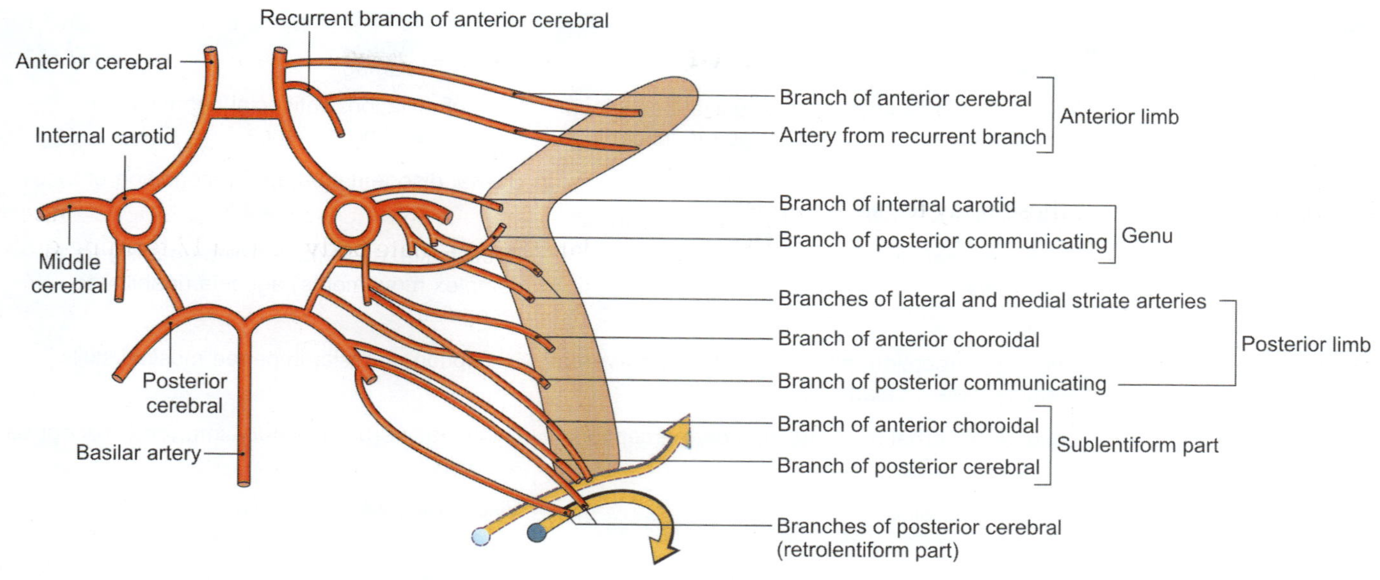

Fig. 35.25: Arteries supplying the internal capsule

Table 35.5: Fibres in the internal capsule (Fig. 35.24)

Part	*Descending tracts*	*Ascending tracts*	*Arterial supply*
Anterior limb	Frontopontine fibres (a part of the corticopontocerebellar pathway)	Anterior thalamic radiation (fibres from anterior and medial nuclei of thalamus)	Recurrent branch of anterior cerebral Direct branches from anterior cerebral
Genu	Corticonuclear fibres (a part of the pyramidal tract going to motor nuclei of cranial nerves and forming their supranuclear pathway	Anterior part of the superior thalamic radiation (fibres from posterior ventral nucleus of thalamus)	Direct branches from internal carotid Posterior communicating
Posterior limb	1. Corticospinal tract (pyramidal tract for the upper limb, trunk and lower limb) 2. Corticopontine fibres 3. Corticorubral fibres	1. Superior thalamic radiation 2. Fibres from globus pallidus to subthalamic nucleus	Lateral striate branches of middle cerebral Medial striate branches of middle cerebral Anterior choroidal
Sublentiform part	1. Parietopontine and temporopontine fibres 2. Fibres between temporal lobe and thalamus	Auditory radiation Fibres connecting thalamus to temporal lobe	Branches of posterior cerebral Anterior choroidal
Retrolentiform part	1. Parietopontine and occipitopontine fibres 2. Fibres from occipital cortex to superior colliculus and pretectal region	Posterior thalamic radiation made up of: 1. Mainly optic radiation 2. Partly fibres connecting thalamus to the parietal and occipital lobes	Branches of posterior cerebral

CLINICAL ANATOMY

- Table 35.6 depicts summary of functions and effects of damage of lobes of brain.
- *Ageing:* Usually after 60–70 years or so there are changes in the brain (Fig. 35.26). These are:
  a. Prominence of sulci due to cortical shrinkage.
  b. The gyri get narrow and sulci get broad.
  c. The subarachnoid space becomes wider. There is enlargement of the ventricles.
- *Dementia:* In this condition, there is slow and progressive loss of memory, intellect and personality. The consciousness of the subject is normal.

Table 35.6: Summary of functions and effects of damage of lobes of brain

Lobar functions	*Functions*	*Effects of damage*
Frontal	Personality, emotional control, social behaviour, contralateral motor control, language, micturition	Lack of initiation, antisocial behaviour, impaired memory and incontinence
Parietal lobe	Spatial orientation, recognition of faces, appreciation of music	Spatial disorientation, non-recognition of faces
Parietal lobe (dominant)	Language, calculation, analytical, logical, geometrical	Dyscalculia, dyslexia, apraxia (inability to do complex movements) agnosia (inability to recognize)
Temporal (non-dominant)	Auditory perception, pitch perception, non-verbal memory, smell, balance	Reception aphasia, impaired musical skills
Temporal (dominant)	Language, verbal memory, auditory perception	Dyslexia, verbal memory impaired, receptive aphasia
Occipital	Visual processing	Visual loss, visual agnosia

Dementia usually occurs due to Alzheimer's disease.

- *Alzheimer's disease:* The changes of normal aging are pronounced in the parietal lobe, temporal lobe, and in the hippocampus (Fig. 35.26).
- *Parkinsonism:* Lesions of corpus striatum leads to parkinsonism with loss of automatic associated movements, mask like face and lead pipe rigidity. L-dopa is used as a therapy in this condition.

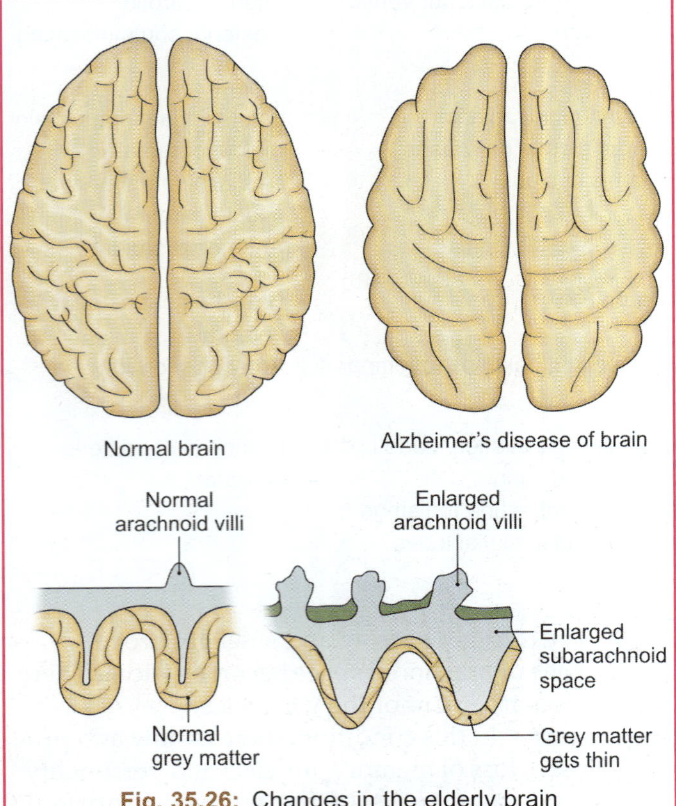

Fig. 35.26: Changes in the elderly brain

FACTS TO REMEMBER

- Human's status as the most highly evolved animal so far is due to larger size of the cerebrum, especially the frontal lobes.
- Cerebrum comprises 3 borders: superomedial, inferolateral and medial; 3 surfaces: superolateral, medial and inferior; 3 poles: frontal, occipital and temporal and 4 lobes: frontal, parietal, temporal and occipital.
- Cerebrum receives sensations from the opposite side of body. It controls the movements of the opposite side of body, a few structures are controlled by both sides.
- Body is represented upside down, only the face and area of vocalization is represented straight.
- Thalamus is the inner chamber receiving and coordinating motor, sensory, visceral, visual, auditory and emotional impulses.
  - Commissural fibre components are anterior commissure, posterior commissure, habenular commissure. The largest is the corpus callosum. These connect identical areas of 2 hemispheres.
  - Association fibres connect different areas of same hemisphere.
  - Projection fibres connect upper areas of brain with lower ones.
- Internal capsule is the most typical example of projection fibres. Internal capsule is supplied by lateral striate branch of middle cerebral artery which is an end artery. Its lockage or rupture leads to upper motor neuron paralysis of the opposite side of the body.

Frequently Asked Questions

1. Describe the superolateral surface of the cerebral hemisphere under the following headings: Sulci, gyri and functional areas.
2. Describe the connections of the various including the nuclei of thalamus. What are their functions?
3. Write short notes on:
   a. Corpus callosum
   b. Motor speech area
   c. Lateral geniculate body
   d. Components of basal ganglia and their functions
   e. Interpenduncular fossa
   f. Association fibers
4. Describe the parts of internal capsule. Name their component fibres. Enumerate its arteries. Add a note on its clinical importance.

Multiple Choice Questions

1. Broca's area is located in which lobe?
   a. Parietal
   b. Frontal
   c. Temporal
   d. Occipital
2. Which of the following structures is related to auditory pathway?
   a. Lateral geniculate body
   b. Trapezoid body
   c. Medial lemniscus
   d. Spinal lemniscus
3. Brodmann's number given to auditosensory area is:
   a. 41, 42   b. 44, 45
   c. 3, 1, 2   d. 18, 19
4. Afferents to lateral geniculate body is:
   a. Optic tract
   b. Globus pallidus
   c. Auditory fibres from inferior colliculus
   d. Reticular formation of brainstem
5. Parkinsonism is due to lesion in:
   a. Corpus luteum   b. Corpus striatum
   c. Corpus callosum   d. Substantia gelatinosa

Answers

1. b **2.** b **3.** a **4.** a **5.** b

VIVA VOCE

- Name the poles and lobes of cerebral hemisphere.
- Name the borders and surfaces of cerebral hemisphere.
- What is insula? Name its functions.
- Where is motor speech area present?
- What is the function of prefrontal tube?
- Name the biggest commissural fibre bundle on medial surface of cerebral hemisphere.
- What is the function of primary motor area?
- What is sylvian point?
- Name the Brodmann's area on the frontal lobe.
- What is the number of visual area?
- Where is the Broca's speech area present? Name its number.
- Where is the hearing area present and its number?
- How is the body represented in the postcentral gyrus?
- Name the nuclei of the thalamus.
- What are the afferents and efferents of ventral posterolateral nucleus?
- Name the afferent and efferent connection of lateral geniculate body.
- Name the functions of pineal gland.
- Name the parts of caudate nucleus.
- Name the features of parkinsonism.
- Name the association and commissural fibres.
- Name the basal ganglia.
- What are the parts of internal capsule?
- What is the blood supply of posterior limb of internal capsule?
- Name dorsal tier nuclei of thalamus.
- Name ventral tier nuclei of thalamus.
- What is neostriatum? What is paleostriatum?
- What are the parts of corpus callosum?

Chapter 36

Blood Supply of Spinal Cord and Brain

"Everything is easy, when you are crazy about it and nothing is easy, when you are lazy about it."
—Anonymous

The nervous tissue is too delicate to bear anoxia beyond three minutes. The blood supply to nervous tissue per unit tissue is maximum in the body. It shows the importance of the grey matter. The blood supply may be erratic due to haemorrhage, thrombosis or embolism of the arteries supplying the nervous tissue. Further the arteries are "end arteries" once these reach the deeper level.

BLOOD SUPPLY OF SPINAL CORD

The spinal cord receives its blood supply from three longitudinal arterial channels that extend along the length of the cord. The *anterior spinal artery* is present in relation to the anterior median sulcus. Two posterior spinal arteries (one on each side) run along the posterolateral sulcus (i.e. along the line of attachment of the dorsal nerve roots). In addition to these channels, the pia mater covering the spinal cord has an arterial plexus (called the *arteria vasocorona)* which also sends branches into the substance of the cord (Fig. 36.1).

Fig. 36.1: Blood supply of spinal cord

The veins draining the spinal cord are arranged in the form of six longitudinal channels. These are anteromedian and posteromedian channels that lie in the midline; and anterolateral and posterolateral channels that are paired.

ARTERIES OF BRAIN

Two vertebral and two carotid arteries carry the total arterial supply to the brain (Fig. 36.2).

Vertebral Arteries

The vertebral artery on each side is a branch of first part of subclavian artery. Its course is divided into four parts:
- 1st part lies from its origin to the foramen transversarium of 6th cervical vertebra.
- 2nd part courses through foramen transversaria of 6th to 1st cervical vertebrae.
- 3rd part lies on the posterior arch of atlas vertebra.
- 4th part of the vertebral artery enters the cranium through foramen magnum. Then it curves round the

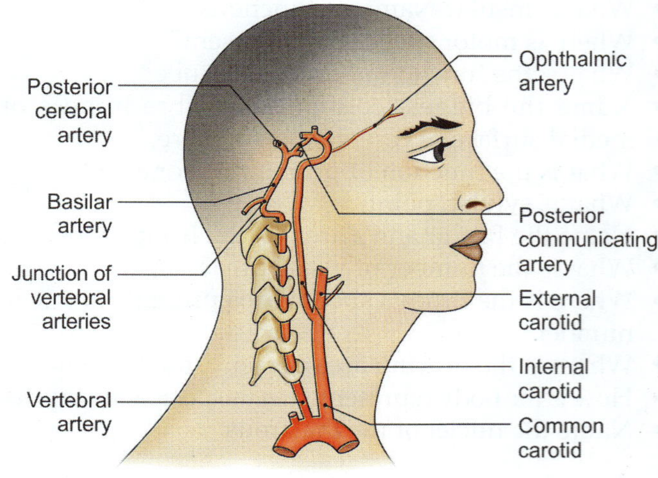

Fig. 36.2: Arteries of brain

ventrolateral aspect of the medulla oblongata to unite with its fellow at the lower border of pons and forms the median basilar artery.

Intracranial Branches

Posterior Spinal Artery

It is the first intracranial branch (Fig. 36.3).

Posterior Inferior Cerebellar Artery

It is the largest branch which arises from vertebral artery after it pierces the meninges.

Anterior Spinal Artery

It is formed by the union of a branch from each vertebral artery on ventral surface of medulla oblongata close to the pons.

Medullary Branches

As vertebral artery ascends along medulla oblongata, it gives number of branches to the medulla oblongata.

Meningeal Branches

A few meningeal branches are given.

Basilar Artery

It is formed by the union of two vertebral arteries at the lower border of pons. It lies in the median groove of pons and at the upper border of pons ends by dividing into two posterior cerebral arteries.

Branches

a. Anterior inferior cerebellar artery
b. Labyrinthine branch
c. Pontine branches
d. Superior cerebellar artery
e. Terminal: Two posterior cerebral arteries.

Branches of Posterior Cerebral Arteries

i. *Posteromedial central branches:* These pierce the posterior perforated substance in the interpeduncular fossa to supply midbrain.
ii. *Posterior choroidal artery:* Supplies choroid plexus of the lateral and the third ventricles.
iii. *Cortical branches* namely temporal branches, parieto-occipital branch and occipital branch to cerebral cortex as shown in Fig. 36.4.

Internal Carotid Artery

Each internal carotid artery enters the cranial cavity after traversing the carotid canal and superior aspect of foramen lacerum. It then courses through the cavernous sinus, pierces the dural roof of sinus and gives following branches: (1) Ophthalmic artery, (2) posterior communicating artery, (3) anterior choroidal artery, (4) anterior cerebral and (5) continues as middle cerebral.

Branches

i. *Anterior cerebral artery:* It is a terminal branch of internal carotid artery and runs above the optic nerve to follow the curve of corpus callosum. Cortical branches supply the medial surface of hemisphere by giving:
   a. Orbital
   b. Frontal
   c. Parietal branches (Fig. 36.5).
ii. *Middle cerebral artery:* It is the larger terminal branch of internal carotid artery that lies in line with the internal carotid artery (Fig. 36.6). It runs laterally in the stem of lateral sulcus. It gives off:

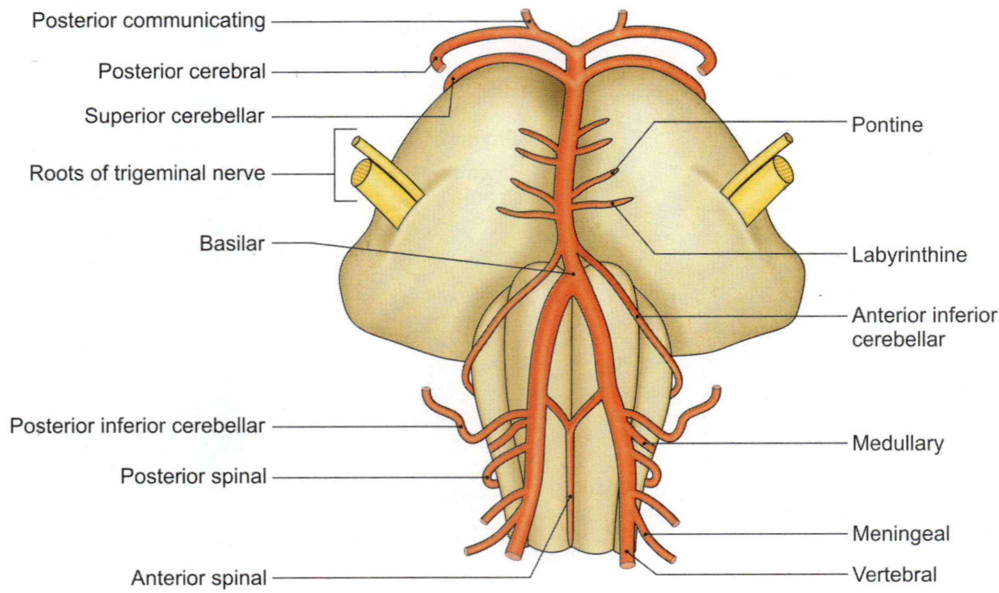

Fig. 36.3: Arteries related to brainstem

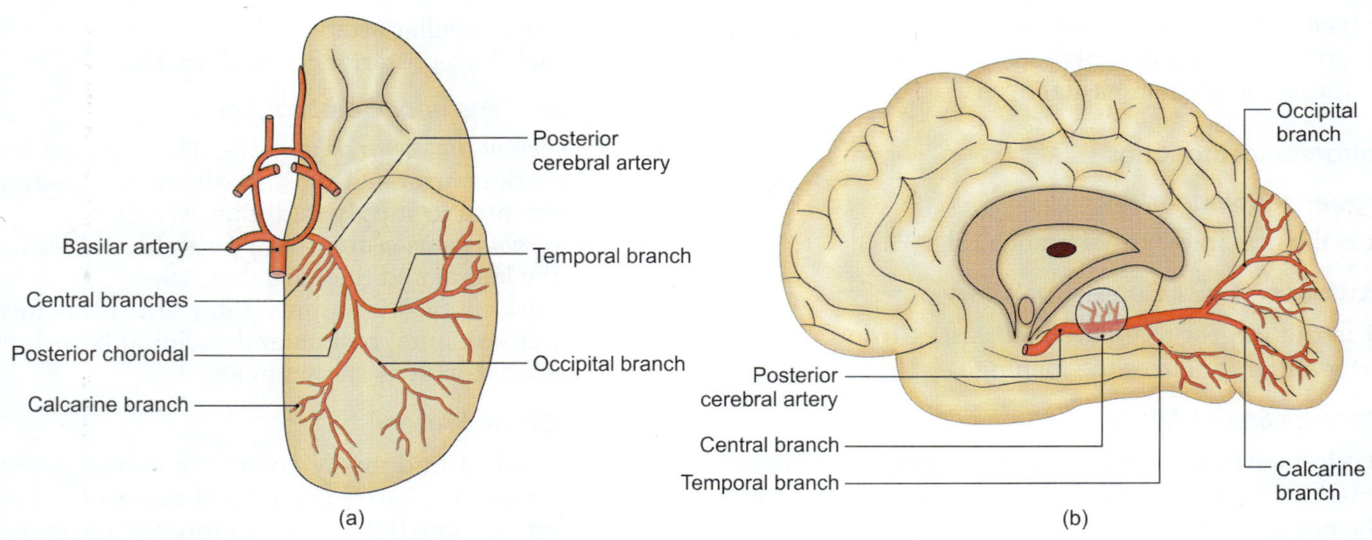

Figs 36.4a and b: Posterior cerebral artery on: (a) Inferior surface of left cerebral hemisphere; (b) medial surface of right cerebral hemisphere

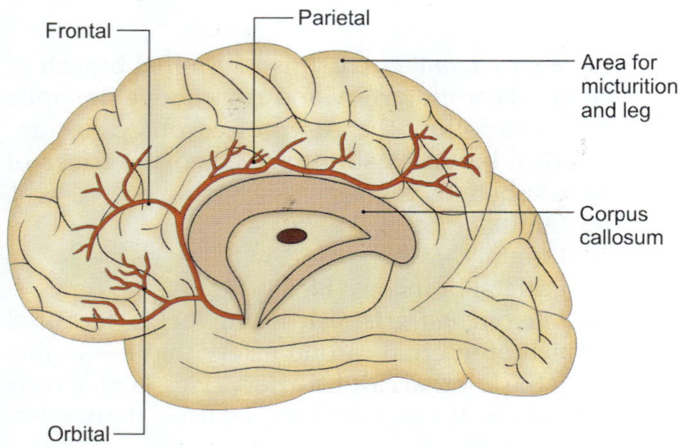

Fig. 36.5: Medial surface of right cerebral hemisphere

a. Deep or perforating branches which supply anterior limb of interal capsule and part of basal nuclei. The artery then passes out to the lateral surface of hemisphere at the insula of the lateral sulcus. It ends by giving cortical branches.
b. Temporal (Fig. 36.7)
c. Frontal and
d. Parietal branches.

CIRCULUS ARTERIOSUS OR CIRCLE OF WILLIS

It is an arterial circle, situated at the base of brain in the interpeduncular fossa. It is formed by the anterior and cerebral branches of internal carotid, terminal parts of internal carotid, posterior communicating and the posterior cerebral branches of basilar arteries (Figs 36.8 and 36.9).

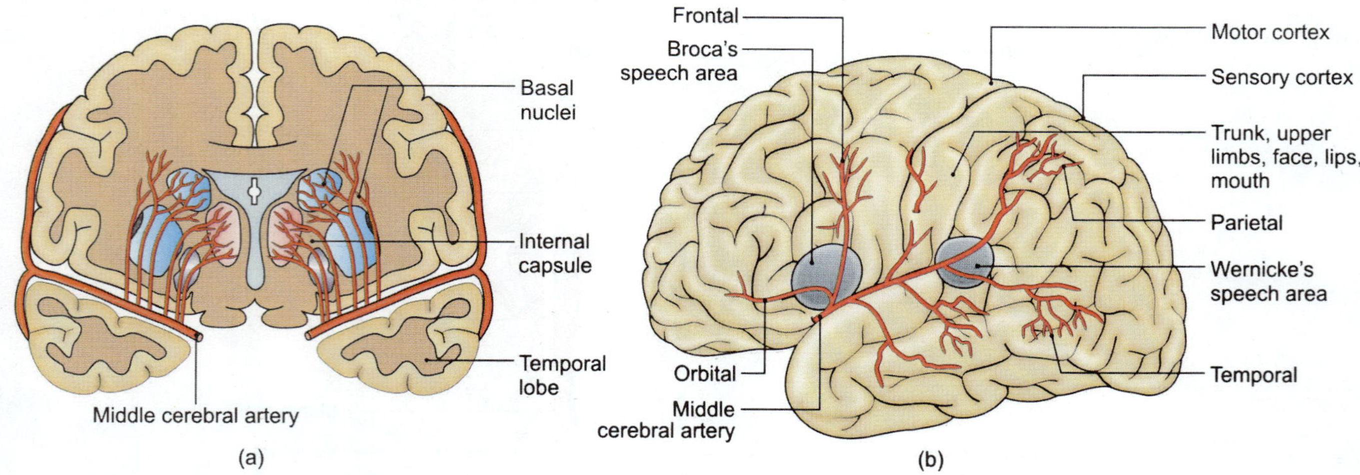

Figs 36.6a and b: (a) Deep branches of middle cerebral artery; (b) cortical branches of middle cerebral artery

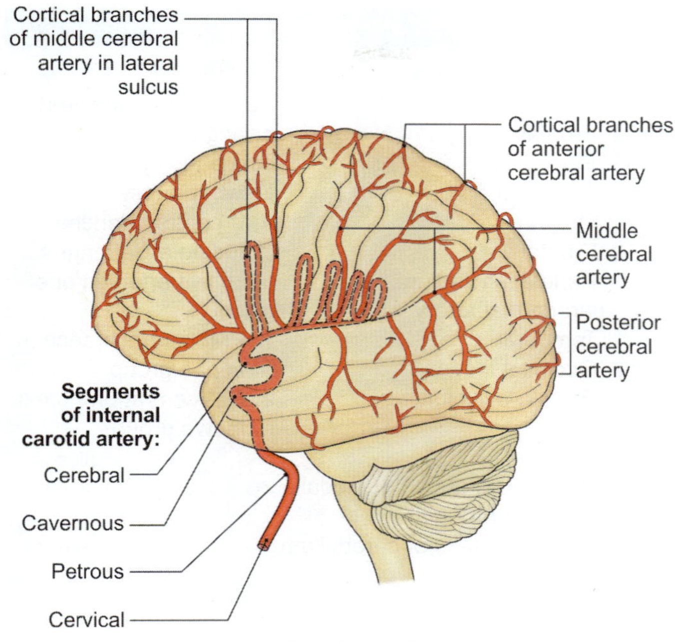

Fig. 36.7: The cortical branches of three cerebral arteries illustrated on the lateral surface of cerebral hemisphere

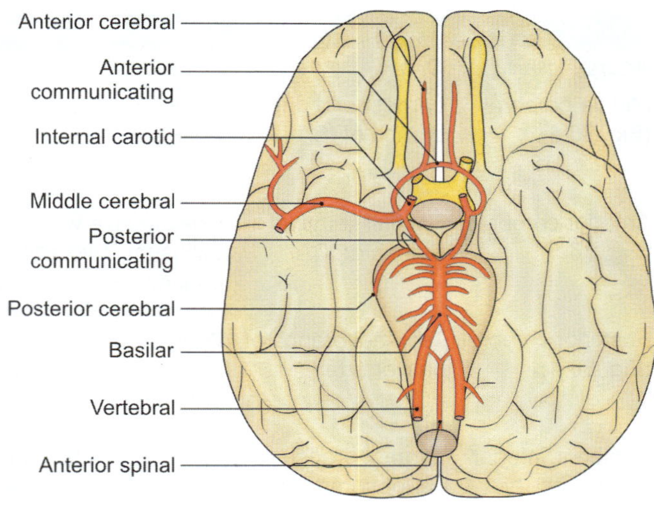

Fig. 36.8: Arteries seen on the inferior surface of brain

The two anterior cerebral arteries are connected by anterior communicating artery. The middle and posterior cerebral arteries of same side are united by the posterior communicating artery.

The circulus arterious attempts to equalize the flow of blood to different parts of brain and provides a collateral circulation in the event of obstruction to one of its components. There is hardly any mixing of bloodstreams on right and left sides of the circulus arteriosus.

Branches

The branches of the circulus arteriosus are cortical and the central. Cortical or external branches run on the surface of the cerebrum, anastomose freely and if these get blocked, they give rise to small infarcts.

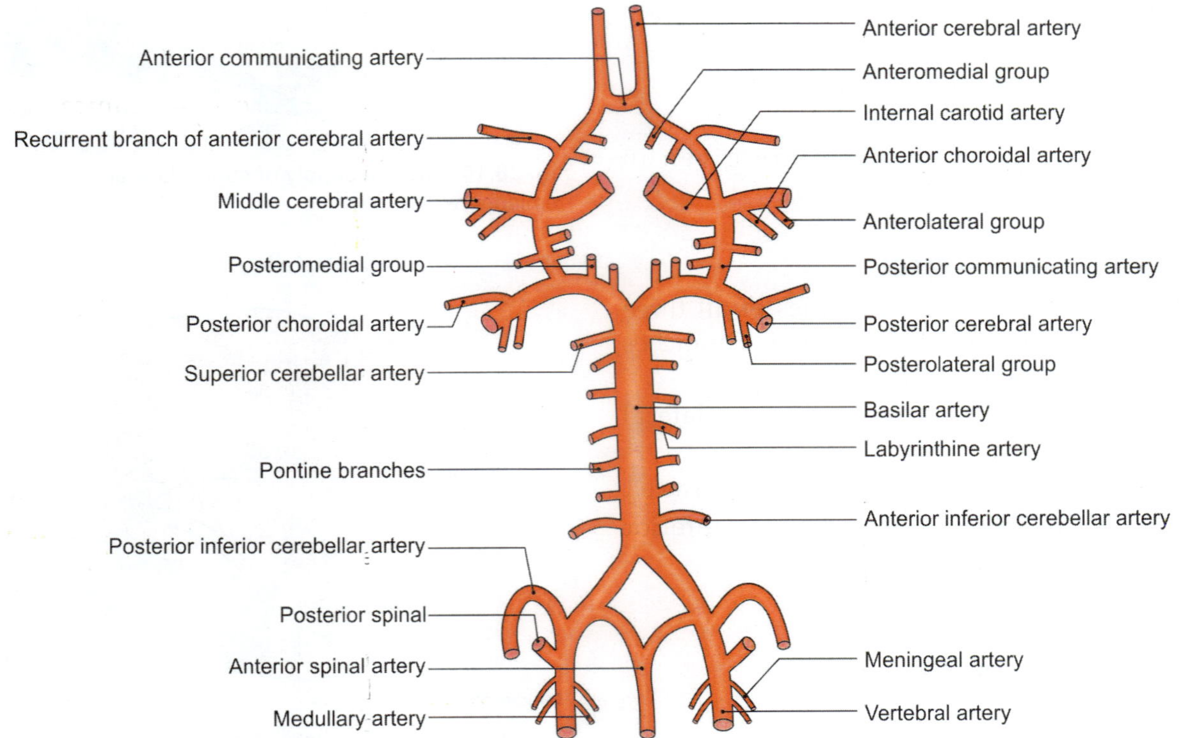

Fig. 36.9: Circle of Willis and the branches of arteries supplying the brain

Table 36.1: Important arteries of brain

Artery	Origin	Course	Cortical branches	Central branches
Middle cerebral (Fig. 36.6)	Largest and direct branch of ICA	In the lateral sulcus and on the insula	1. Orbital 2. Frontal 3. Parietal 4. Temporal	AL* central branches, arranged as lateral striate artery in two groups
Anterior cerebral (Fig. 36.5)	Smaller terminal branch of ICA	Coextensive with corpus callosum. Two arteries are connected by the anterior communicating artery	1. Orbital 2. Frontal 3. Parietal, including paracentral artery	AM* central branches, including a Heubner's recurrent artery in one group
Posterior cerebral (Fig. 36.4)	Terminal branch of basilar artery	Winds round cerebral peduncle to reach the tentorial surface of cerebrum	1. Temporal 2. Occipital 3. Parieto-occipital	1. PM* central branches in one group 2. PL* central branches in two groups
Posterior inferior cerebellar	Largest branch of vertebral artery	Tortuous course in relation of olive, lower border of pons and vallecula of cerebellum	It supplies: 1. Posterolateral part of medulla 2. Lower part of pons 3. Inferior surface of cerebellum	

* AL = anterolateral; AM = anteromedial; PM = posteromedial; PL = posterolateral.

The central branches perforate the white matter to supply the thalamus, the corpus striatum, and the internal capsule. These do not anastomose and if these get blocked, they give rise to large infarcts.

The central branches are arranged in six groups:

1. *Anteromedial:* The largest branch is called the medial striate or recurrent artery of Heubner. It supplies corpus striatum and internal capsule which has motor fibres for face, tongue and shoulder. These are in one group.
2. *Anterolateral:* These are in two groups one on each side.
3. *Posterolateral* in two groups one on each side.
4. *Posteromedial* in one group.

Important arteries of the brain are given in Table 36.1.

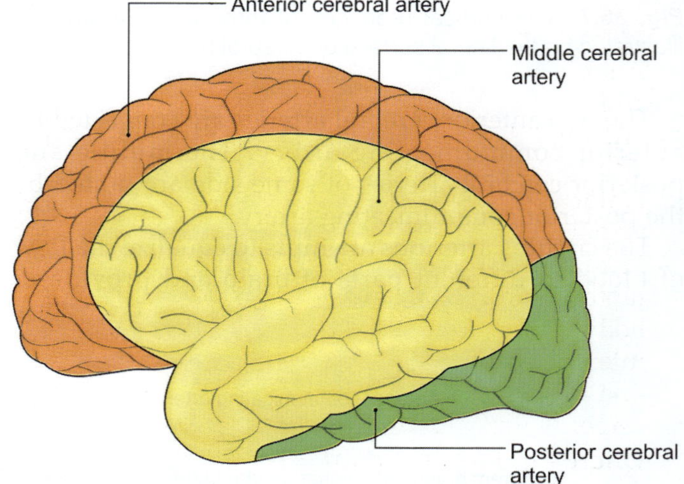

Fig. 36.10: Arterial supply of superolateral surface of cerebral hemisphere

Arterial Supply of Different Areas

Cerebral cortex is supplied by branches of all three cerebral arteries. All the three surface receive branches from all three arteries (Figs 36.10 to 36.12).

- Middle cerebral is main artery on superolateral surface.
- Anterior cerebral is chief artery on medial surface.
- Posterior cerebral is principal artery on inferior surface.

Cerebellum

The little brain is supplied by:

a. Superior cerebellar (Fig. 36.13),
b. Anterior inferior cerebellar and
c. Posterior inferior cerebellar arteries.

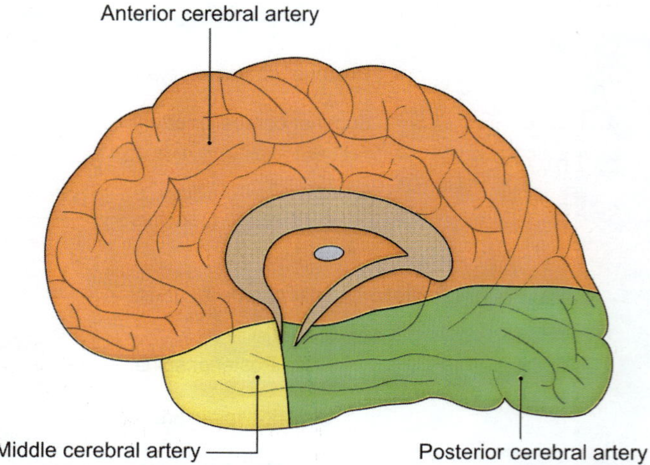

Fig. 36.11: Arterial supply of medial and tentorial surfaces of cerebral hemisphere

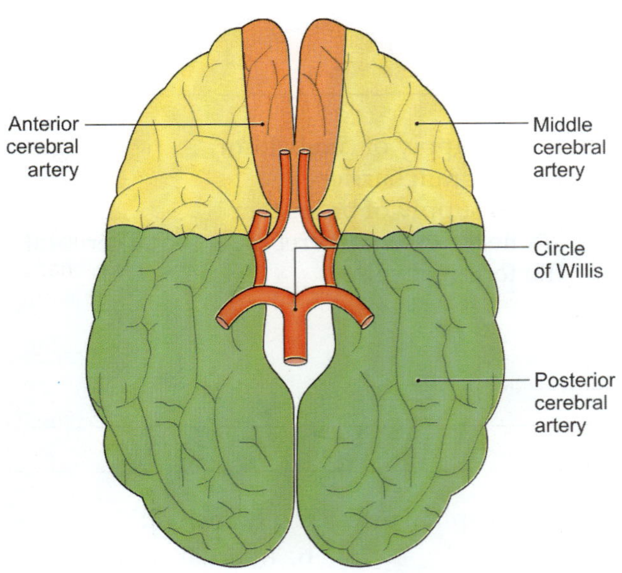

Fig. 36.12: Arterial supply of inferior surface of cerebral hemisphere

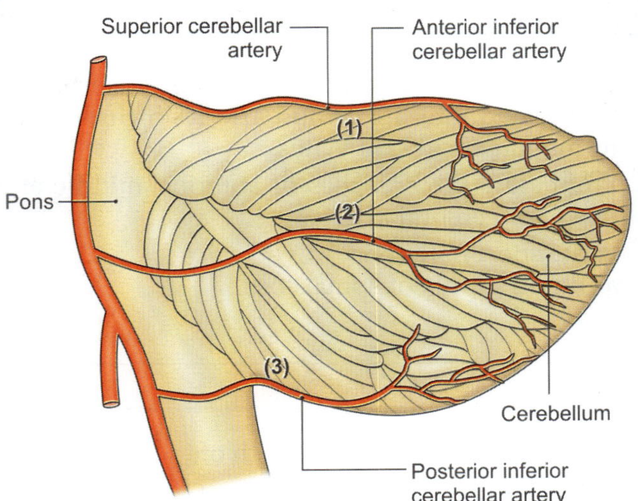

Fig. 36.13: Arterial supply of opened up cerebellum

CLINICAL ANATOMY

- Anterior spinal artery supplies anterior two-thirds while posterior spinal artery supplies posterior one-third of spinal cord. Posterior column gets affected in posterior spinal artery thrombosis. Anterolateral columns get affected in anterior spinal artery thrombosis.
- Hemiplegia is a common condition. It is an upper motor neuron type of paralysis of one-half of the body, including the face. It is usually due to an internal capsule lesion caused by thrombosis of one of the lenticulostriate branches of middle cerebral artery (cerebral thrombosis).

  One of the lenticulostriate branches is most frequently ruptured (cerebral haemorrhage); it is known as Charcot's artery of cerebral haemorrhage. This lesion also produces hemiplegia with deep coma, and is ultimately fatal.
- Cerebral vascular disease is quite common in old age and manifest in different ways.
  a. Haemorrhage—cortical or subcortical
  b. Thrombosis
  c. Embolism.

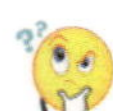

FACTS TO REMEMBER

- Posterior inferior cerebellar artery is the largest branch of vertebral artery. It supplies postero-lateral part of medulla oblongata, lower part of pons, inferior surface of cerebellum including choroidal branches to 4th ventricle.
- Posterior cerebral arteries are the terminal branches of the basilar artery. It chiefly supplies the visual cortex.
- Middle cerebral artery is the larger terminal branch of internal carotid and supplies most of the supero-lateral surface of the cerebral cortex.
- Anterior cerebral is the smaller terminal branch of the internal carotid artery. It runs along the corpus callosum supplying maximum area on the medial surface of the cerebral hemisphere.
- Two lobes of the cerebellum are supplied by 3 pairs of cerebellar arteries. These are superior cerebellar, anterior inferior cerebellar and posterior inferior cerebellar arteries.
- Anterior two-thirds of spinal cord is supplied by larger anterior spinal artery. Only posterior one-third of the cord is supplied by posterior spinal arteries.

Frequently Asked Questions

1. Describe the intracranical course of vertebral, basilar and internal carotid arteries including the formation of circle of Willis.
2. Enumerate the branches of anterior, middle and posterior cerebral arteries.
3. Write short notes on:
   a. Blood supply of spinal cord
   b. Blood supply of cerebellum
   c. Blood–brain barrier
   d. Blood supply of brainstem
   e. Name the external cerebral, internal cerebral and the terminal veins

Multiple Choice Questions

1. Labyrinthine artery is a branch of:
   a. Basilar b. Vertebral
   c. Internal carotid d. Posterior inferior cerebellar
2. Which of the following arteries supply visual fibres?
   a. Anterior and middle cerebral
   b. Middle cerebral
   c. Middle and posterior cerebral
   d. Posterior cerebral
3. Anterior spinal artery is a branch of:
   a. Vertebral b. Internal carotid
   c. Basilar d. Labyrinthine
4. Which is the largest direct branch of internal carotid artery?
   a. Middle cerebral
   b. Anterior cerebral
   c. Posterior cerebral
   d. Posterior inferior cerebellar

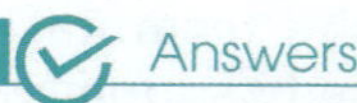

Answers

1. a **2.** c **3.** a **4.** a

VIVA VOCE

- Name the arteries and veins present in relation to the spinal cord.
- How much of spinal cord is supplied by anterior spinal artery?
- Name the branches of vertebral and basilar arteries.
- How is the circle of Willis formed?
- Does middle cerebral artery take part in formation of circle of Willis?
- Which artery is predominant on medial surface?
- Which artery is predominant on superolateral surface?
- Which artery is predominant on the inferior surface?
- Name the artery involved in hemiplegia.
- Name the type of branches from cerebral arteries.
- Name the functional areas of brain supplied by middle cerebral artery.
- What are the functions of 'blood–brain barrier'?
- Name the paired and unpaired venous sinuses.

Chapter 37

Miscellaneous

"If you salute your work, you do not have to salute anybody. If you pollute your work, you have to salute everybody."
—Anonymous

SUMMARY OF THE VENTRICLES OF THE BRAIN

LATERAL VENTRICLE

The lateral ventricle comprises a central body and three horns—anterior, posterior and inferior. The body lies between trunk of corpus collosum and thalamus. Anterior horn lies between corpus callsum and head of caudate nucleus in the frontal lobe.

- Posterior horn extends into occipital lobe.
- Inferior horn is the largest horn and extends into the temporal lobe.

THIRD VENTRICLE

The third ventricle lies between the two thalami. The components of its boundaries and recesses are enumerated:

Anterior wall: Lamina terminalis, anterior commissure, anterior column of fornix (*see* Fig. 35.8).

Posterior wall: Pineal body, cerebral aqueduct.

Floor: Optic chiasma, tubercinerium, infundibulum, mamillary body, posterior perforated substance, tegmentum of midbrain.

Roof: Ependyma, tela choroidea (*see* 35.13).

Lateral wall: Medial surface of thalamus, medial aspect of hypothalamus, epithalamus, interventricular foramen.

Recesses: Infundibular recess, optic recess, pineal recess, suprapineal recess (*see* Fig. 35.13).

FOURTH VENTRICLE

The cavity of fourth ventricle is situated dorsal to pons and upper part of medulla oblongata and ventral to the cerebellum. Its boundaries, recesses, apertures and continuations are mentioned here.

Lateral Boundaries: Gracile tubercle, cuneate tubercle, inferior cerebellar peduncles, superior cerebellar peduncles (*see* Fig. 33.2).

Floor

Upper part: Facial colliculus on the dorsal surface of pons (*see* Fig. 33.2).

Intermediate part: Vestibular nuclei, medullary striae.

Lower part: Upper part of medulla oblongata containing hypoglossal and vagal triangles.

Roof: Superior medullary velum, thin sheet of pia mater and ependyma with median aperture, inferior medullary velum.

Recesses in roof: One median dorsal, two lateral dorsal and two lateral.

Apertures: One median—foramen of Magendie, two lateral—foramina of Lushka (*see* Fig. 30.6).

Continuity: Above with cerebral aqueduct. Below with central canal of spinal cord (*see* Fig. 30.6).

NUCLEAR COMPONENTS OF CRANIAL NERVES

CN I. OLFACTORY

Part of forebrain

CN II. OPTIC

Part of forebrain

CN III. OCULOMOTOR

a. General somatic efferent column for 5 extraocular muscles at level of superior colliculus (*see* Fig. 32.1)
b. General visceral efferent column for 2 sets of intraocular muscles (Flowchart 37.1).
c. General somatic afferent—mesencephalic nucleus of CN V. It receives proprioceptive impulses from extraocular muscles (Fig. 37.1).

CN IV. TROCHLEAR

a. General somatic efferent column for supply of only superior oblique muscle at level of inferior colliculus (*see* Fig. 32.17).

b. General somatic afferent—mesencephalic nucleus of CN V. It receives proprioceptive impulses from the superior oblique muscle.

CN V. TRIGEMINAL

a. Special visceral efferent column for 4 muscles of mastication and 4 other muscles at upper level of pons (*see* Fig. 32.27).
b. General somatic afferent column:
   i. Spinal nucleus of CN V for pain and temperature from face (*see* Fig. 32.24).
   ii. Superior sensory nucleus of CN V for touch and pressure from face.
   iii. Mesencephalic nucleus of CN V for proprioceptive impulses from extraocular muscles, muscles of tongue and mastication.

CN VI. ABDUCENT

a. General somatic efferent column for lateral rectus at lower level of pons (*see* Fig. 32.20).
b. General somatic afferent—mesencephalic nucleus of CNV. It receives proprioceptive impulses from the lateral rectus muscle.

CN VII. FACIAL

a. Special visceral efferent column for muscles of facial expression at lower level of pons (*see* Fig. 32.28).
b. General visceral efferent for lacrimal, nasal, palatal and submandibular, sublingual glands (Flowchart 37.1).
c. Special visceral and general visceral afferents (nucleus of tractus solitarius) for carrying taste from most of anterior two-thirds of tongue and afferents from glands supplied by it.
d. General somatic afferent from part of skin of auricle.

CN VIII. VESTIBULOCOCHLEAR

Special somatic afferent column:

Two parts:

- *Vestibular nuclei:* Medial, superior, spinal, lateral.
- *Cochlear nuclei:* Dorsal and ventral.

All at pontomedullary junction.

CN IX. GLOSSOPHARYNGEAL

a. Special visceral efferent for one muscle of larynx—the stylopharyngeus and medulla oblongata (Fig. 32.45).
b. General visceral efferent for parotid gland (Chart 37.1).
c. Special and general visceral afferent (nucleus of tractus solitarius) for sensations of taste from posterior one-third of tongue and circumvallate

Flowchart 37.1: General visceral efferents for intraocular muscles

Edinger-Westphal nucleus

↓
III nerve
↓
Nerve to inferior oblique
↓
Branch to ciliary ganglion
↓
Relay
↓
Short ciliary nerves supply ciliaris and constrictor pupillae muscles

Superior salivatory nucleus

↓
VII nerve
↓
Chorda tympani branch via lingual nerve
↓
Submandibular ganglion
↓
Relays to supply submandibular gland directly and sublingual salivary gland via lingual nerve

Lacrimatory nucleus

↓
VII nerve
↓
Greater petrosal nerve + deep petrosal nerve (sympathetic)
↓
Nerve of pterygoid canal
↓
Pterygopalatine ganglion
↓
Relays to supply glands of nose, palate, pharynx and lacrimal fibres pass along zygomatic nerve
↓
Zygomaticotemporal nerve, communicating branch, lacrimal nerve to supply lacrimal gland

Inferior salivatory nucleus of IX nerve

↓
Tympanic branch
↓
Tympanic plexus
↓
Lesser petrosal nerve
↓
Relays in otic ganglion
↓
Fibres join auriculotemporal nerve
↓
Parotid gland

Vagus carries preganglionic fibres for the glands in respiratory system and foregut and midgut derivatives of GIT.

S2, S3, S4 preganglionic fibres relay in the ganglia in the walls of the organs developing from hindgut and cloaca.

papillae. Also carries general sensations from posterior one-third of tongue, carotid body and carotid sinus.

d. General somatic afferent for proprioceptive fibres from the muscle.

CN X. + CN XI. VAGUS AND CRANIAL PART OF CN XI

a. Special visceral efferent for muscles of larynx, pharynx, soft palate in medulla oblongata.
b. General visceral efferent for glands of respiratory system and gastrointestinal tract till right two-thirds of transverse colon (*see* Fig. 32.49).
c. Special and general visceral afferents carry (nucleus of tractus solitarius) taste from posterior most part of tongue, epiglottis and afferents from foregut and midgut derivatives.
d. General somatic afferent from skin of external auditory meatus.

CN XI. SPINAL PART OF ACCESSORY NERVE

a. Special visceral efferent column in C1–C4 ventral horn cells of spinal cord for sternocleidomastoid and trapezius.
b. General somatic afferent—dorsal horns of C2–C4 segments of spinal cord. These receive proprioceptive impulses from the above two muscles.

CN XII. HYPOGLOSSAL

a. General somatic efferent column for all 4 intrinsic muscles of tongue and three extrinsic muscles—styloglossus, genioglossus and hyoglossus in medulla oblongata (*see* Fig. 32.58).
b. General somatic afferent—spinal nucleus of CN V. It receives proprioceptive impulses from the muscles of tongue.

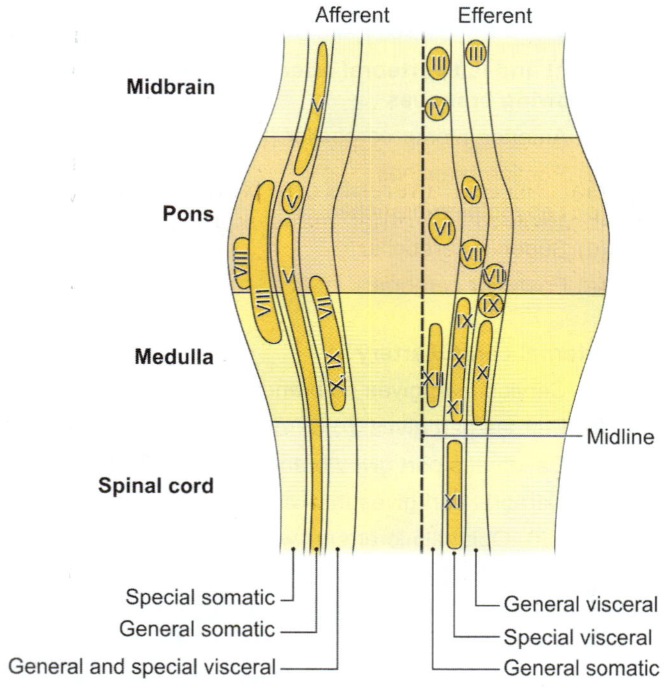

Fig. 37.1: Position of cranial nerve nuclear columns in brainstem

EFFERENT PATHWAYS OF CRANIAL PART OF PARASYMPATHETIC NERVOUS SYSTEM

Preganglionic parasympathetic fibres are present in 4 cranial nerves, e.g. cranial nerves III, VII, IX, X and along spinal nerves S2, S3, S4 . Four ganglia namely ciliary, pterygopalatine, submandibular and otic are concerned with efferent parasympathetic fibres. Their pathways are shown in Flowchart 37.1.

Arteries of the Brain

The arteries of the brain have been tabulated in Table 37.1.

Table 37.1: Arteries of brain

1. **Vertebral artery, a branch of 1st part of subclavian artery, is divided into four parts**
   (a) ***First part:*** Lies deep in the neck in the vertebral triangle; gives no branches.
   (b) ***Second part:*** Passes in the foramen transversaria of C6–C1 vertebrae; gives spinal branches for supply of meninges and spinal cord (*see* Fig. 17.2).
   (c) ***Third part:*** Lies in the suboccipital triangle, on the posterior arch of atlas vertebra and gives branches to muscles of suboccipital triangle (*see* Fig. 18.5).
   (d) ***Fourth part:*** Enters the cranial cavity through foramen magnum. Joins with the same artery of opposite side to form basilar artery at the lower border of pons. The fourth part gives:
      (i) Meningeal branches (*see* Fig. 36.3)
      (ii) Posterior spinal artery
      (iii) Anterior spinal artery
      (iv) Posterior inferior cerebellar artery
      (v) Medullary branches.

Contd...

Table 37.1: Arteries of brain *(Contd...)*

2. **Right and left vertebral arteries unite at the lower border of the pons to form a median basilar artery, which gives following branches**
   (a) Anterior inferior cerebellar (Fig. 36.9)
   (b) Pontine branches
   (c) Labyrinthine branches
   (d) Superior cerebellar
   (e) Posterior cerebral

3. **Internal carotid artery**
   (a) Cervical part gives no branches.
   (b) Petrous part gives: (i) Caroticotympanic for the middle ear, and (ii) pterygoid branch.
   (c) Cavernous part gives branches to: (i) Trigeminal ganglion and (ii) superior and inferior hypophyseal branches.
   (d) Cerebral part gives following branches:
      (i) Ophthalmic artery which supplies outer layers of eyeball and through central artery of retina (end artery), the retina (*see* Fig. 21.9).
      (ii) Anterior cerebral
      (iii) Middle cerebral
      (iv) Posterior communicating
      (v) Anterior choroidal

4. **Circle of Willis**
   Circle of Willis is formed by union of posterior cerebral of vertebral artery and posterior communicating branch and anterior cerebral branch of internal carotid arteries on each side (*see* Fig. 36.9). It gives
   (a) ***Central branches:*** These are long thin, numerus end arteries with supply deeper structures like internal capsule and basal ganglia.
   (b) ***Choroidal branches*** of internal carotid and posterior cerebral arteries supply choroid plexuses of the ventricles.
   (c) ***Cortical branches:*** These are:
      (i) *Anterior cerebral:* Chief artery on the medial surface of cerebral hemisphere till parieto-occipital sulcus. It also supplies 1 cm. wide area on the superolateral surface, along the superomedial border. The area includes motor and sensory areas of lower limb and perineum.
      (ii) *Middle cerebral:* Main artery of the superolateral surface supplying major parts of motor and sensory areas. It also supplies motor speech area, auditory and vestibular areas.
      (iii) *Posterior cerebral:* Chief artery of the tentorial surface and occipital lobe. This is the artery of visual cortex.

Section

IV

Other Regions of Human Body

Ichchak dana, beechak dana, dane upar dana
Hands naache, feet naache, brain hai khushnama
Ichchak dana.
Closed cage mai baitha ek naajuk bechara
lub dub, lub dub hi karta hai ye aawara
Lekin iska bahut sensitive hai mijajana
agar tute to mushkil hai samjhana
is liye kisi ka "ye" na dukhana
Ichchak dana
Bolo kya—heart, bolo kya—heart
—Krishna Garg

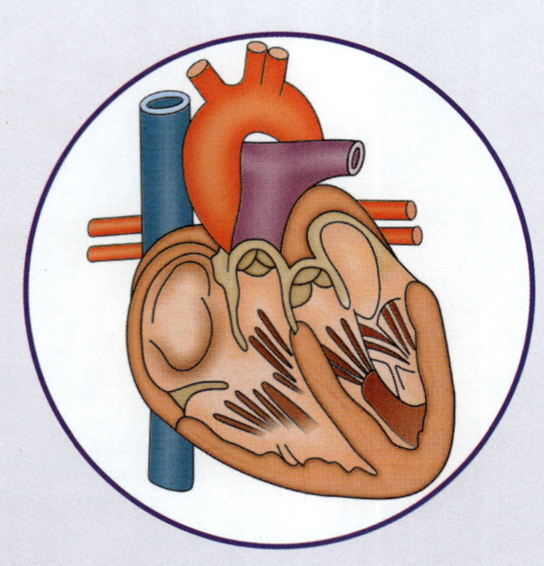

Chapter 38

Upper Limb

"One pronates while giving and supinates while getting."
—Anonymous

Parts of the Upper Limb

The upper limb is made up of four parts: (A) Shoulder region; (B) arm or brachium; (C) forearm or antebrachium; and (D) hand or manus. Further subdivisions of these parts are given in Table 38.1 and Fig. 38.1.

BONES OF UPPER LIMB

Out of 206 total bones in man, the upper limbs contain as many as 64 bones. Each side consists of 32 bones, the distribution of which is shown in Table 38.1.

CLAVICLE

The clavicle is a long bone (Fig. 38.2). It supports the shoulder so that the arm can swing clearly away from the trunk. The clavicle transmits the weight of the limb to the sternum. The bone has a cylindrical part called the shaft, and two ends—lateral and medial.

Shaft

The shaft is divisible into the lateral one-third and the medial two-thirds.

The *lateral one-third of the shaft* is flattened. The anterior border is concave forwards. The posterior border is convex backwards.

Table 38.1: Parts of the upper limb

Parts	*Subdivision*	*Bones*	*Joints*
A. Shoulder region	1. Pectoral region on the front of the chest 2. Axilla or armpit 3. Scapular region on the back	Bones of the shoulder girdle (a) Clavicle (b) Scapula	• Sternoclavicular joint • Acromioclavicular joint
B. Upper arm (arm or brachium) from shoulder to the elbow	—	Humerus (glenohumeral joint)	Shoulder joint
C. Forearm (antebrachium) from elbow to the wrist	—	(a) Radius (b) Ulna	• Elbow joint • Radioulnar joints
D. Hand	1. Wrist	(a) Carpus, made up of 8 carpal bones	• Wrist joint (radiocarpal joint) • Intercarpal joints
	2. Hand proper	(b) Metacarpus, made up of 5 metacarpal bones	• Carpometacarpal joints
	3. Five digits, numbered from lateral to medial side First = Thumb or pollex Second = Index or forefinger Third = Middle finger Fourth = Ring finger Fifth = Little finger	(c) 14 phalanges—two for the thumb, and three for each of the four fingers	• Intermetacarpal joints • Metacarpophalangeal joints • Proximal and distal interphalangeal joints

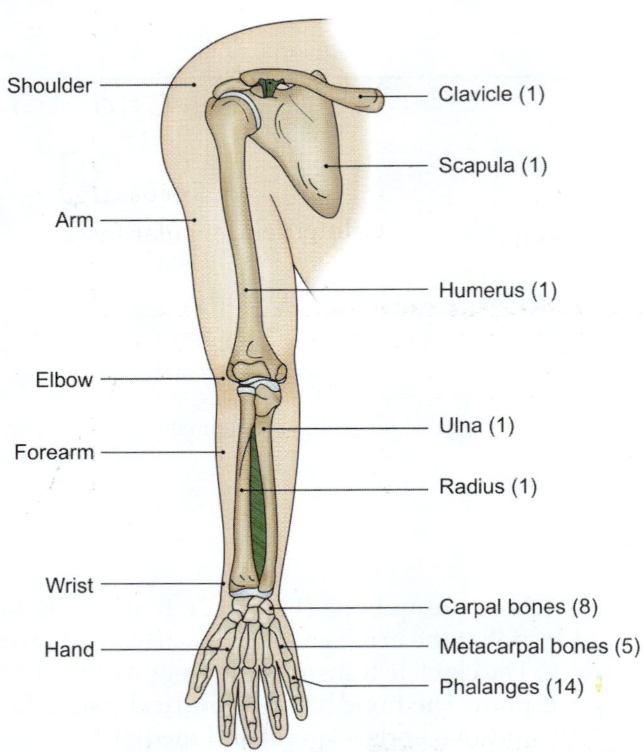

Fig. 38.1: Parts and 32 bones of the upper limb

The *medial two-thirds of the shaft* is rounded. The anterior surface is convex forwards. The lateral half of this surface has a longitudinal subclavian groove.

Side Determination

1 The lateral end is flat, and the medial end is large and quadrilateral.
2 The shaft is slightly curved, so that it is convex forwards in its medial two-thirds, and concave forwards in its lateral one-third.
3 The inferior surface is grooved longitudinally in its middle one-third.

Features

1 Clavicle articulates with the acromion to form the acromioclavicular joint.
2 It also articulates with the manubrium to form the sternoclavicular joint.

3 *Lateral one-third of shaft*
   a. The anterior border and adjacent surfaces give origin to the *deltoid* (Fig. 38.5).
   b. The posterior border and adjacent surfaces provide insertion to the *trapezius*.

4 *Medial two-thirds of the shaft*
   a. The anterior surface gives origin to the *pectoralis major* (Fig. 38.2).
   b. The rough superior surface gives origin to the clavicular head of the *sternocleidomastoid*.

SCAPULA

The scapula is a thin bone placed on the posterolateral aspect of the thoracic cage. The scapula has two surfaces, three borders, three angles, and three processes (Fig. 38.3).

Surfaces

1 The *costal surface* or subscapular fossa is concave and is directed medially and forwards.
2 The *dorsal surface* gives attachment to the spine of the scapula which divides the surface into a smaller *supraspinous fossa* and a larger *infraspinous fossa*.

Borders

1 The *superior border* is thin and shorter.
2 The *lateral border* is thick.
3 The *medial border* is thin.

Angles

1 The *superior angle*
2 The *inferior angle*
3 The *lateral* or *glenoid angle* is broad and bears the glenoid cavity.

Processes

1 The *spine* or *spinous process* (Fig. 38.3)
2 The *acromion*, lateral continuation of the spine
3 The *coracoid* process

Side Determination

1 The lateral or glenoid angle is large and bears the glenoid cavity.

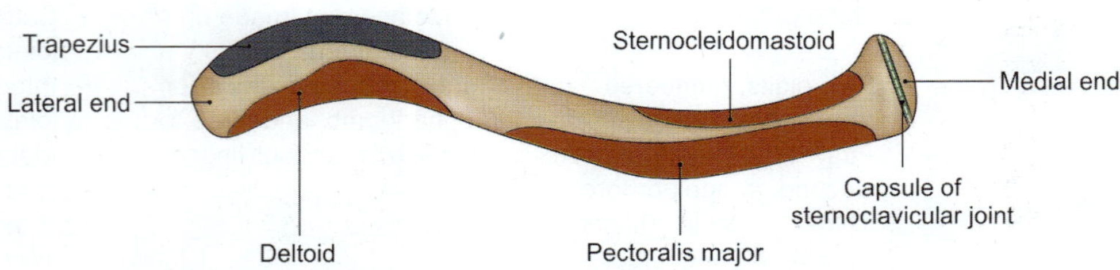

Fig. 38.2: Attachments of right clavicle: Superior aspect

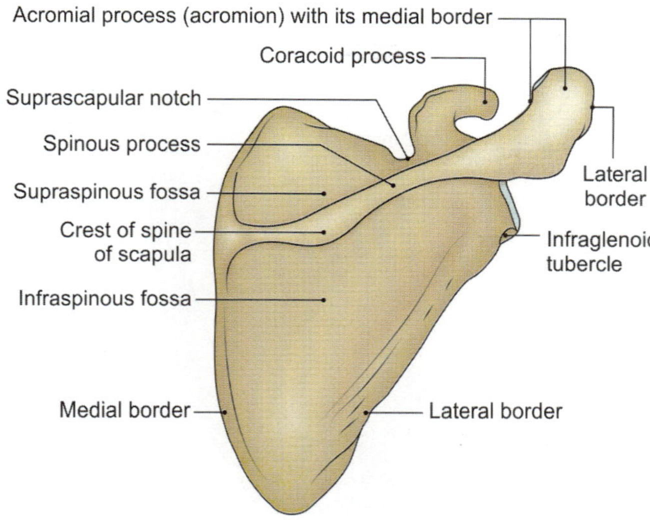

Fig. 38.3: General features of right scapula: Dorsal surface

2 The dorsal surface is convex and is divided by the triangular spine into the supraspinous and infraspinous fossae. The costal surface is concave to fit on the convex chest wall.
3 The thickest lateral border runs from the glenoid cavity above to the inferior angle below.

Relevant Muscles

1 The *deltoid* arises from the lower border of the spine and from the lateral border of the acromion (Fig. 38.5). The acromial fibres are multipennate.
2 The *trapezius* is inserted into the upper border of the crest of the spine and into the medial border of the acromion.
3 The *serratus anterior* is inserted along the medial border of the costal surface.

HUMERUS

The humerus is the bone of the arm. It is the longest bone of the upper limb. It has an upper end, a shaft and a lower end (Fig. 38.4).

Upper End

1 The *head* is directed medially, backwards and upwards. It articulates with the glenoid cavity of the scapula to form the shoulder joint.
2 The line separating the head from the rest of the upper end is called the *anatomical neck.*
3 The *lesser tubercle* is an elevation on the anterior aspect of the upper end.
4 The *greater tubercle* is an elevation that forms the lateral part of the upper end.
5 The *intertubercular sulcus* or bicipital groove separates the lesser tubercle medially from the anterior part of the greater tubercle.

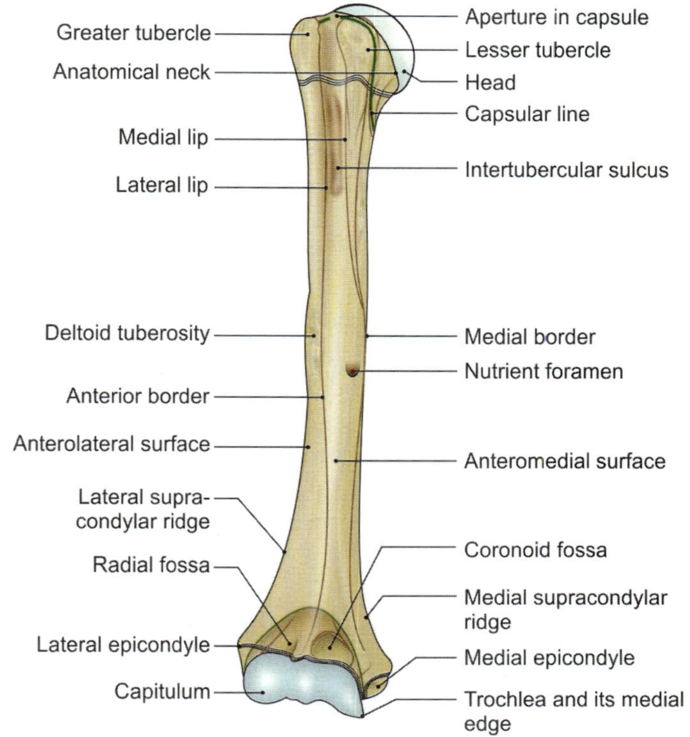

Fig. 38.4: General features of right humerus seen from front

6 The narrow line separating the upper end of the humerus from the shaft is called the *surgical neck*.

Shaft

The shaft is rounded in the upper half and triangular in the lower half. It has three borders and three surfaces.

Borders

1 The upper one-third of the *anterior border* forms the lateral lip of the intertubercular sulcus. In its middle part, it forms the anterior margin of the *deltoid tuberosity*.
2 The *lateral border* is prominent only at the lower half.
3 The upper part of the *medial border* forms the medial lip of the intertubercular sulcus. It is prominent in the lower half of humerus.

Surfaces

1 The *anterolateral surface* lies between the anterior and lateral borders. A little above the middle, it is marked by a V-shaped *deltoid tuberosity*.
2 The *anteromedial surface* lies between the anterior and medial borders.
3 The *posterior surface* lies between the medial and lateral borders. It shows an obliquely placed radial groove in its middle part.

Lower End

The lower end of the humerus forms the condyle which is expanded from side to side, and has articular and non-articular parts. The *articular part* includes the following.

1 The *capitulum* articulates with the head of the radius (Fig. 38.4).
2 The *trochlea* is a pulley-shaped surface. It articulates with the trochlear notch of the ulna.

The *non-articular part* includes the following.

1 The *medial epicondyle.*
2 The *lateral epicondyle* (Fig. 38.4).
3 The *coronoid fossa* is a depression just above the anterior aspect of the trochlea (Fig. 38.4).
4 The *radial fossa* is a depression present just above the anterior aspect of the capitulum.
5 The *olecranon fossa* lies just above the posterior aspect of the trochlea.

Side Determination

1 The upper end is rounded to form the head which is directed medially and backwards.
2 The lesser tubercle projects from the front of the upper end and is limited laterally by the intertubercular sulcus or bicipital groove.
3 Medial epincondyle is prominent at the lower medial end of the bone.

Relevant Muscles

1 The *pectoralis major* is inserted into the lateral lip of the intertubercular sulcus. The insertion is bilaminar.
2 The *deltoid* is inserted into the deltoid tuberosity (Fig. 38.5).
3 The *superficial flexor muscles* of the forearm arise by a common origin from the anterior aspect of the medial epicondyle.
4 The *superficial extensor muscles* of the forearm have a common origin from the lateral epicondyle.
5 Three nerves are directly related to the humerus and are, therefore, liable to injury: The axillary at the surgical neck, the radial at the radial groove, and the ulnar behind the medial epicondyle (Fig. 38.6).

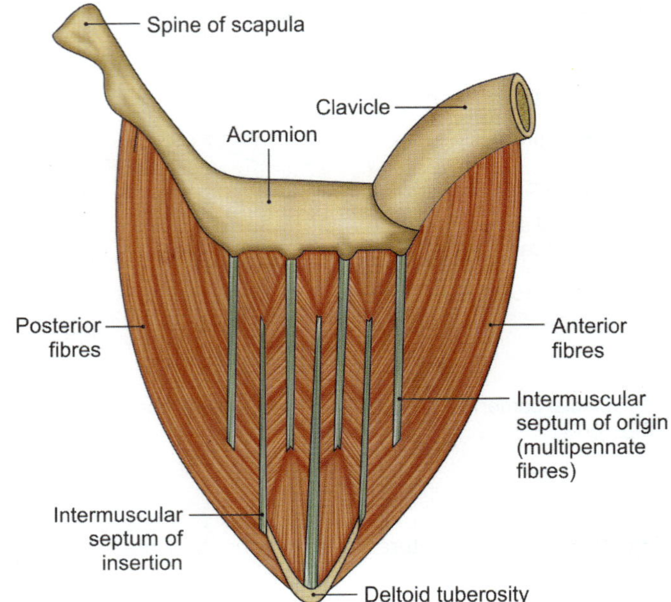

Fig. 38.5: The origin and insertion of the deltoid muscle

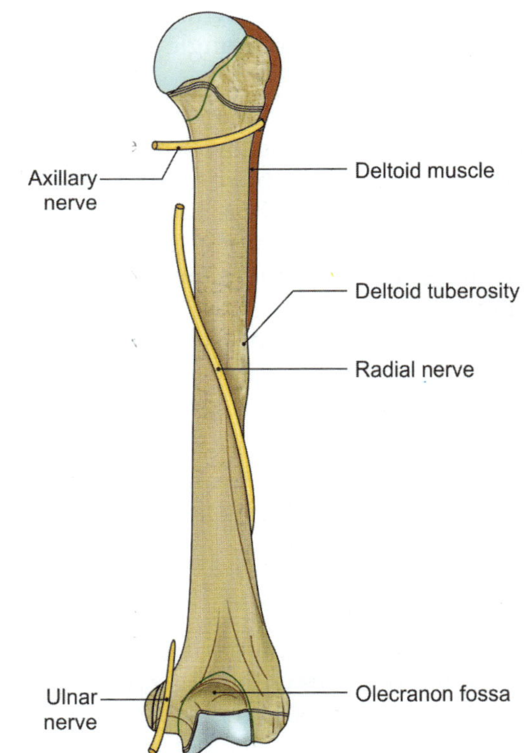

Fig. 38.6: Relation of axillary, radial and ulnar nerves to the back of humerus

RADIUS

The radius is the lateral bone of the forearm. It has an upper end, a shaft and a lower end.

Upper End

1 The *head* is disc-shaped which articulates with the capitulum of the humerus at the elbow joint.
2 The *neck* is below the head.
3 The *tuberosity* lies just below the medial part of the neck (Fig. 38.7).

Shaft

It has three borders anterior, posterior and medial or interosseous borders and three surfaces, anterior, lateral and posterior surfaces.

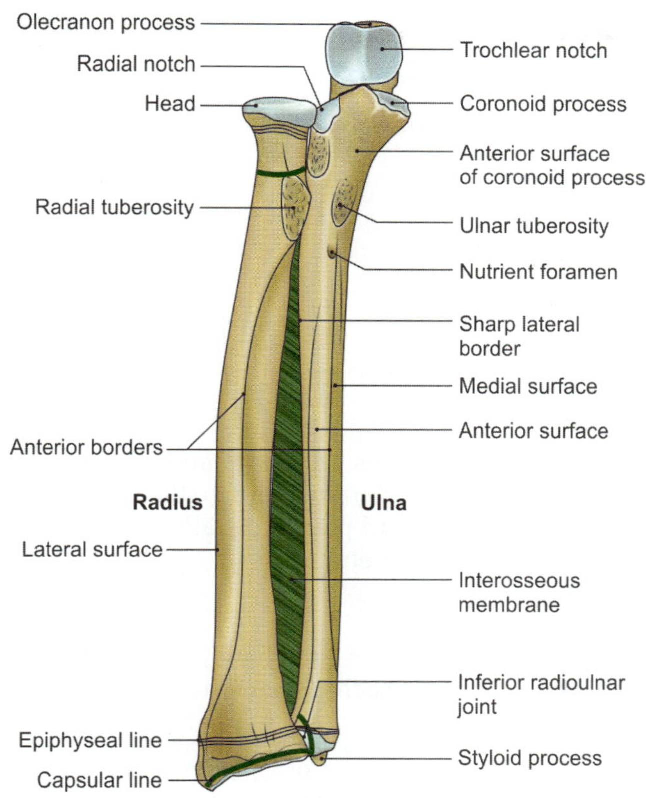

Fig. 38.7: Anterior surfaces of radius and ulna

Lower End

The lower end is the widest part of the bone. It has 5 surfaces.

1. The *anterior surface*
2. The *posterior surface*
3. The *medial surface*
4. The *lateral surface*
5. The *inferior surface*

Side Determination

The smaller circular upper end is concave followed by a constricted neck.

The wider lower end is thick with a pointed styloid process on its lateral aspect and a prominent dorsal tubercle on its posterior surface. Medial or interosseous border is thin and sharp.

Relevant Muscles

1. The *biceps brachii* is inserted into the rough posterior part of the radial tuberosity (Fig. 38.8).
2. The *brachioradialis* is inserted into the lowest part of the lateral surface just above the styloid process.

ULNA

The ulna is the medial bone of the forearm. It has upper end, an shaft and a lower end.

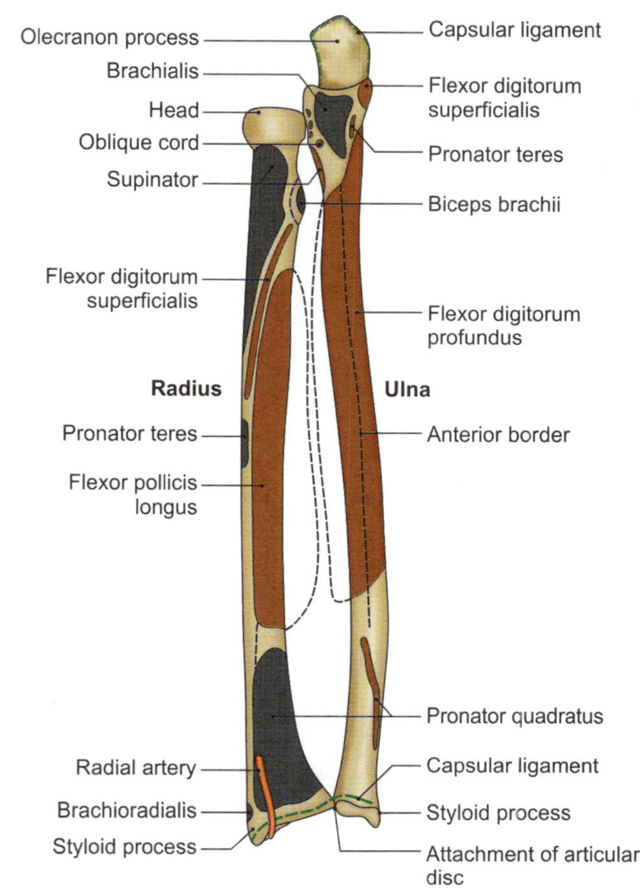

Fig. 38.8: Attachments of right radius and ulna: Anterior aspect

Upper End

The upper end presents the olecranon and coronoid processes, and the trochlear and radial notches.

1. The *olecranon process* projects upwards from the shaft (Fig. 38.7).
2. The *coronoid process* projects forwards from the shaft just below the olecranon.
3. The *trochlear notch* forms an articular surface that articulates with the trochlea of the humerus to form the elbow joint.
4. The *radial notch* articulates with the head of the radius to form the superior radioulnar joint.

Shaft

The shaft has three borders: sharp interosseous or lateral border, anterior border, posterior border and three surfaces, medial, anterior and posterior surfaces.

Lower End

The lower end is made up of the head and the styloid process. The head articulates with the ulnar notch of the radius to form the inferior radioulnar joint.

Side Determination

1 The upper end is hook-like with its concavity directed forwards.
2 The lateral border of the shaft is sharp and crest-like.
3 Pointed styloid process lies medial to the rounded head of ulna.

Relevant Muscles

1 The *triceps brachii* is inserted into the posterior part of the superior surface of the olecranon.
2 Brachialis is inserted into the coronoid process.
3 Flexor digitorum profundus arises from most of the shaft (Fig. 38.8).

CARPAL BONES

The carpus is made up of 8 carpal bones, which are arranged in two rows.

1 The proximal row contains (from lateral to medial side):

   i. The scaphoid, ii. the lunate, iii. the triquetral, and iv. the pisiform bones (Fig. 38.1).

2 The distal row contains in the same order:

   i. the trapezium, ii. the trapezoid, iii. the capitate, and iv. the hamate bones.

Mnemonics

She Looks Too Pretty, Try To Catch Her

She	*Scaphoid*
Look	*Lunate*
Too	*Triquetral*
Pretty	*Pisiform*
Try	*Trapezium*
To	*Trapezoid*
Catch	*Capitate*
Her	*Hamate*

METACARPAL BONES

1 The metacarpal bones are 5 miniature long bones, which are numbered from lateral to the medial side.
2 Each bone has a head placed distally, a shaft and a base at the proximal end.

PHALANGES

There are 14 phalanges in each hand, 3 for each finger and 2 for the thumb. Each phalanx has a base, a shaft and a head.

MUSCLES OF THE PECTORAL REGION

Muscles of the pectoral region are described in Tables 38.2 and 38.3. Mammary gland is briefly described at the end of this chapter.

Table 38.2: Muscles of the pectoral region

Muscle	*Origin from*	*Insertion into*
Pectoralis major (Figs 38.2 and 38.9)	• Anterior surface of medial half of clavicle • Half the breadth of anterior surface of manubrium and sternum up to 6th costal cartilages • Second to sixth costal cartilages • Aponeurosis of the external oblique muscle of abdomen	It is inserted by a bilaminar tendon on the lateral lip of the bicipital groove The two laminae are continuous with each other inferiorly
Serratus anterior (Fig. 38.9)	Serratus anterior muscle arises by eight digitations from the upper eight ribs	The muscle is inserted into the costal surface of the scapula along its medial border and inferior angle

Table 38.3: Muscles of the pectoral region

Muscle	*Nerve supply*	*Actions*
Pectoralis major	Medial and lateral pectoral nerves	• Acting as a whole the muscle causes: Adduction and medial rotation of the shoulder (arm) • Clavicular part produces: Flexion of the arm • Sternocostal part is used in: – Extension of flexed arm against resistance – Climbing
Serratus anterior	The nerve to the serratus anterior is a branch of the brachial plexus. It arises from roots C5, C6 and C7	a. The fibres inserted into the inferior angle of the scapula pull it forwards and rotate the scapula so that the glenoid cavity is turned upwards b. The muscle steadies the scapula during weight carrying

AXILLA

The axilla or armpit is a pyramidal space situated between the upper part of the arm and the chest wall. It resembles a four-sided pyramid, and comprises of an apex, a base and four walls.

Apex

It is directed upwards and medially towards the root of the neck.

It is truncated (not pointed), and corresponds to a triangular interval bounded anteriorly by the clavicle, posteriorly by the superior border of the scapula, and medially by the outer border of the first rib.

Base or Floor

It is directed downwards, and is formed by skin, superficial and axillary fasciae.

Four Walls

These are anterior, posterior, medial and lateral (Fig. 38.9).

CONTENTS OF AXILLA

1 Axillary artery and its branches (Table 38.14)
2 Axillary vein and its tributaries.
3 Infraclavicular part of the brachial plexus.
4 Five groups of axillary lymph nodes and the associated lymphatics. These are lateral, anterior, posterior, central and apical groups.
5 Axillary fat and areolar tissue in which the other contents are embedded.

BRACHIAL PLEXUS

The plexus consists of roots, trunks, divisions, cords and branches (Fig. 38.10).

Roots

These are constituted by the anterior primary rami of spinal nerves C5, C6, C7, C8 and T1.

Trunks

Roots C5 and C6 join to form the *upper* trunk. Root C7 forms the *middle* trunk. Roots C8 and T1 join to form the *lower* trunk.

Divisions of the Trunks

Each trunk divides into ventral and dorsal divisions (which ultimately supply the anterior and posterior aspects of the limb). These divisions join to form cords.

Cords

i. The lateral cord is formed by the union of ventral divisions of the upper and middle trunks.
ii. The medial cord is formed by the ventral division of the lower trunk.
iii. The posterior cord is formed by union of the dorsal divisions of all the three trunks.

Branches

The roots value of each branch is given in brackets.

A. *Branches of the Roots*

1 Nerve to serratus anterior (long thoracic nerve) (C5, C6, C7)
2 Nerve to rhomboids (dorsal scapular nerve) (C5)

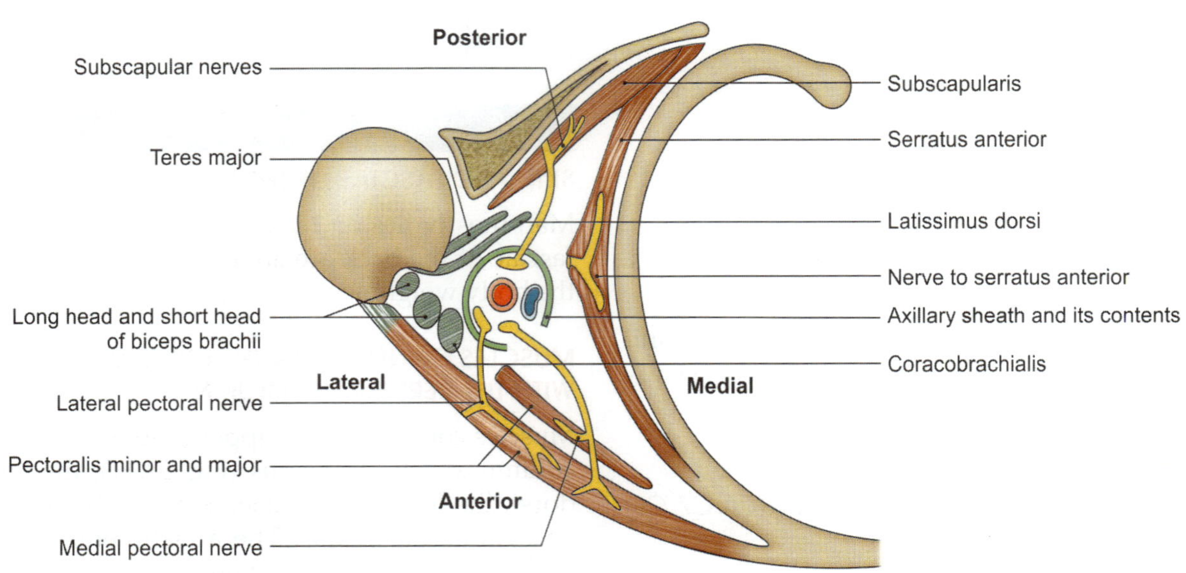

Fig. 38.9: Walls and contents of axilla

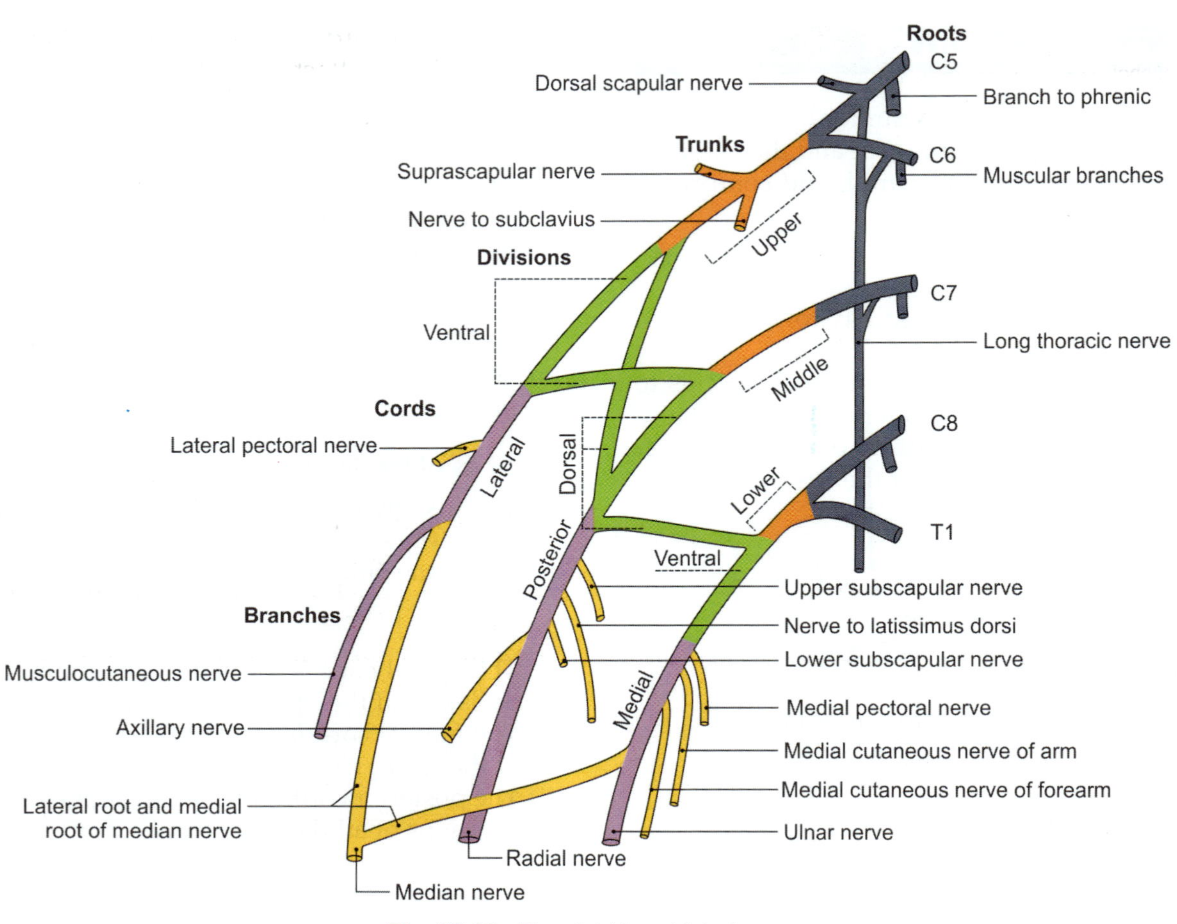

Fig. 38.10: The right brachial plexus

B. *Branches of the Trunks*

These arise only from the upper trunk which gives two branches.

1 Suprascapular nerve (C5, C6)
2 Nerve to subclavius (C5, C6)

C. *Branches of the Cords*

(A) Branches of lateral cord

1 Lateral pectoral (C5–C7)
2 Musculocutaneous (C5–C7)
3 Lateral root of median (C5–C7) (Fig. 38.10)

(B) Branches of medial cord

1 Medial pectoral (C8, T1)
2 Medial cutaneous nerve of arm (C8, T1)
3 Medial cutaneous nerve of forearm (C8, T1)
4 Ulnar (C7, C8, T1). C7 fibres reach by a communicating branch from lateral root of median nerve.
5 Medial root of median (C8, T1)

(C) Branches of posterior cord

1 Upper subscapular (C5, C6)
2 Nerve to latissimus dorsi (thoracodorsal) (C6, C7, C8)
3 Lower subscapular (C5, C6)
4 Axillary (circumflex) (C5, C6)
5 Radial (C5–C8, T1).

AXILLARY VEIN

The axillary vein is the continuation of the basilic vein. The axillary vein is joined by the venae comitantes of the brachial artery a little above the lower border of the teres major. It lies on the medial side of the axillary artery. At the outer border of the first rib, it becomes the subclavian vein.

BACK

SKIN AND FASCIAE OF THE BACK

Man mostly lies on his back. Therefore, the skin and fasciae of the back are adapted to sustain pressure of the body weight.

MUSCLES CONNECTING THE UPPER LIMB WITH THE VERTEBRAL COLUMN

Muscles connecting the upper limb with the vertebral column are the trapezius (Fig. 38.11), the latissimus dorsi, the levator scapulae, and the rhomboid minor and rhomboid major. The attachments of first two important muscles are given in Table 38.4, and their nerve supply with actions in Table 38.5.

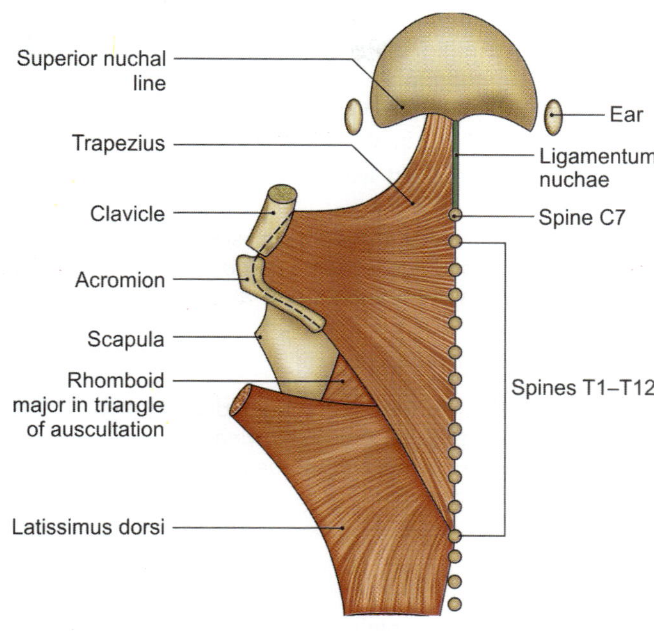

Fig. 38.11: The trapezius and latissimus dorsi muscles

SCAPULAR REGION

MUSCLES OF THE SCAPULAR REGION

These are the deltoid, the supraspinatus, the infraspinatus, the teres minor, the subscapularis, and the teres major. The deltoid is described below.

Deltoid

Origin

1 The anterior border of the lateral one-third of the clavicle (Fig. 38.5).

2 The lateral border of the acromion where four septa of origin are attached.

3 Lower lip of the crest of the spine of the scapula.

Insertion

The deltoid tuberosity of the humerus where three septa of insertion are attached.

Nerve Supply

Axillary nerve (C5, C6). It runs along the surgical neck of humerus to supply deltoid (Fig. 38.12).

Structure

The acromial part of deltoid is an example of a multipennate muscle. Many fibres arise from four septa of origin that are attached above to the acromion. The fibres converge on to three septa of insertion which are attached to the deltoid tuberosity (Fig. 38.5). A multipennate arrangement allows a large number of muscle fibres to be packed into a relatively small volume. As the strength of contraction of a muscle is proportional to the number of muscle fibres present in it (and not on their length), a multipennate muscle is much stronger than other muscles having the same volume.

Actions

1 The acromial fibres are powerful abductors of the arm at the shoulder joint from beginning to 90°.

2 The anterior fibres are flexors and medial rotators of the arm.

3 The posterior fibres are extensors and lateral rotators of the arm.

Table 38.4: Attachments of muscles connecting the upper limb to the vertebral column (Fig. 38.11)

Muscle	*Origin from*	*Insertion into*
1. Trapezius The right and left muscles together form a trapezium that covers the upper half of the back	• Medial one-third of superior nuchal line • External occipital protuberance • Ligamentum nuchae, C7 spine, • T1–T12 spines	• Upper fibres into the posterior border of lateral one-third of clavicle (Fig. 38.2) • Middle fibres into the medial margin of the acromion and upper lip of the crest of spine of the scapula • Lower fibres on the apex of triangular area at the medial end of the spine, with a bursa intervening
2. Latissimus dorsi It covers a large area of the lower back, and is overlapped by the trapezius (Fig. 38.11)	• Posterior one-third of the outer lip of iliac crest • Posterior layer of lumbar fascia; • Spines of T7–T12, Lower four ribs, Inferior angle of the scapula	The muscle winds round the lower border of the teres major, and forms the posterior fold of the axilla The tendon is twisted upside down, and is inserted into floor of the intertubercular sulcus

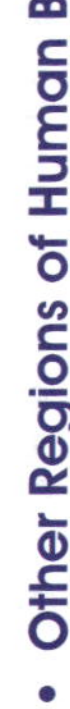

Table 38.5: Nerve supply and actions of muscles connecting the upper limb to the vertebral column

Muscle	*Nerve supply*	*Actions*
Trapezius	• Spinal part of accessory nerve is motor • Branches from C3, C4 are proprioceptive	• Upper fibres act with levator scapulae, and elevate the scapula as in shrugging • Middle fibres act with rhomboids, and retract the scapula • Upper and lower fibres act with serratus anterior, and rotate the scapula forwards round the chest wall, thus playing an important role in abduction of the arm beyond 90° • Steadies the scapula
Latissimus dorsi	Thoracodorsal nerve (C6, C7, C8) (nerve to latissimus dorsi)	• Adduction, extension, and medial rotation of the shoulder as in swimming, rowing, climbing, pulling, folding the arm behind the back, and scratching the opposite scapula • Helps in violent expiratory effort like coughing, sneezing, etc. • Essentially a climbing muscle • Holds inferior angle of the scapula in place

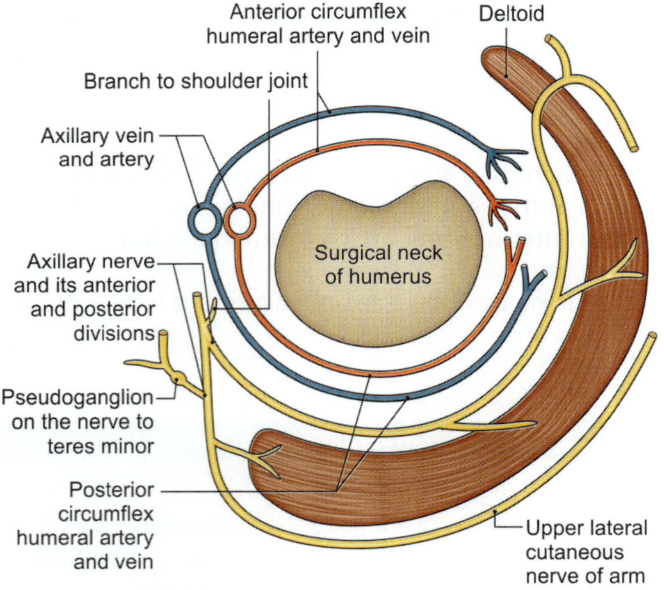

Fig. 38.12: Horizontal section of the deltoid region showing the nerves and vessels around the surgical neck of humerus

Structures under Cover of the Deltoid

i. The upper end of the humerus, muscles attached to greater and lesser tubercles and bicipital groove.
ii. The coracoid process, and its attached muscles and ligments (Fig. 38.13).
iii. Axillary nerve and accompanying blood vessels (Fig. 38.12).

All bursae around the shoulder joint, including the subacromial or subdeltoid bursa.

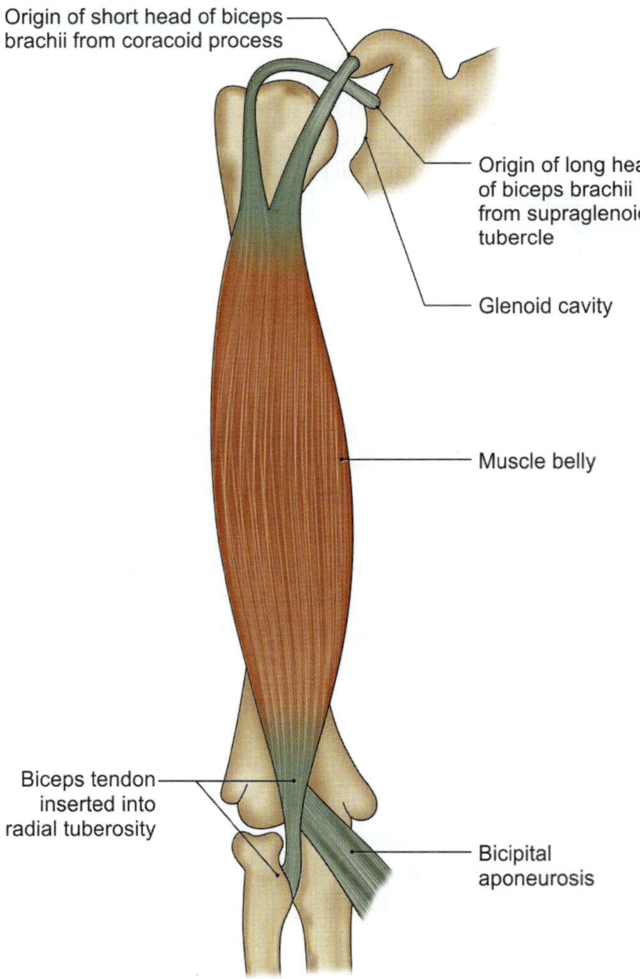

Fig. 38.13: The biceps brachii muscle in extended elbow

CLINICAL ANATOMY

Deltoid muscle is used for giving intramuscular injections. Injection is given 5–6 cm below acromion to protect the axillary nerve.

ARM

The arm extends from the shoulder joint till the elbow joint. The skeleton of the arm is a 'solo' bone, the humerus.

COMPARTMENTS OF THE ARM

The arm is divided into anterior and posterior compartments by extension of deep fascia which are called the *medial* and *lateral intermuscular septa*.

ANTERIOR COMPARTMENT

Muscles

Muscles of the anterior compartment of the arm are the coracobrachialis, the biceps brachii and the brachialis. These are described in Tables 38.6 and 38.7.

CUBITAL FOSSA

Cubital fossa is a triangular hollow situated on the front of the elbow.

Boundaries

Laterally – Medial border of the brachioradialis (Fig. 38.14).
Medially – Lateral border of the pronator teres.
Base – It is directed upwards, and is represented by an imaginary line joining the front of two epicondyles of the humerus.
Apex – It is directed downwards, and is formed by the meeting point of the lateral and medial boundaries.

Roof

The roof of the cubital fossa is formed by:
a. Skin.
b. Superficial fascia containing the median cubital vein and few nerves.
c. Deep fascia.
d. Bicipital aponeurosis.

Table 38.6: Attachments of muscles

Muscle	*Origin from*	*Insertion into*
1. Coracobrachialis	• The tip of the coracoid process with the short head of the biceps brachii	The middle 5 cm of the medial border of the humerus
2. Biceps brachii (Fig. 38.13)	It has two heads of origin : • The short head arises with coracobrachialis from the tip of the coracoid process • The long head arises from the supraglenoid tubercle of the scapula and from the glenoidal labrum. The tendon is intracapsular	• Posterior rough part of the radial tuberosity. The tendon is separated from the anterior part of the tuberosity by a bursa • The tendon gives off an extension called the bicipital aponeurosis which separates median cubital vein from brachial artery
3. Brachialis	• Lower half of the front of the humerus, including both the anteromedial and anterolateral surfaces and the anterior border Superiorly the origin embraces the insertion of the deltoid • Medial and lateral intermuscular septa	• Coronoid process and ulnar tuberosity • Rough anterior surface of the coronoid process of the ulna (Fig. 38.8)

Table 38.7: Nerve supply and actions

Muscle	*Nerve supply*	*Actions*
1. Coracobrachialis	Musculocutaneous nerve (C5–C7)	Flexes the arm at the shoulder joint
2. Biceps brachii	Musculocutaneous nerve (C5, C6)	• It is strong supinator when the forearm is flexed All screwing movements are done with it • It is a flexor of the elbow • The short head is a flexor of the arm • The long head prevents upwards displacement of the head of the humerus
3. Brachialis	• Musculocutaneous nerve is motor • Radial nerve is proprioceptive	Flexes forearm at the elbow joint

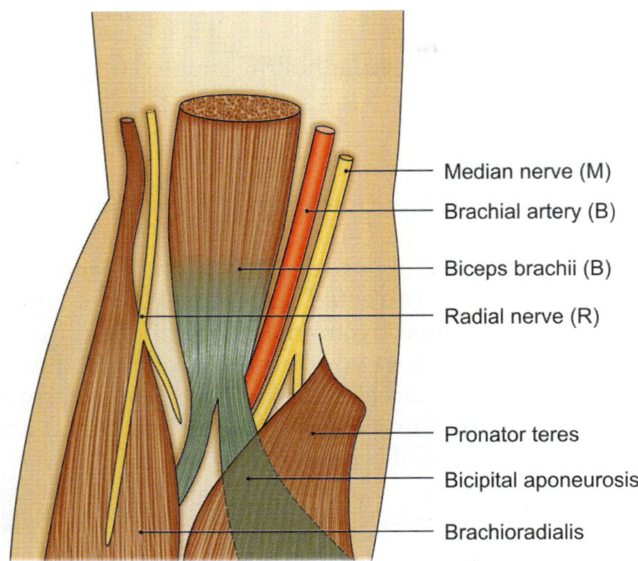

Fig. 38.14: Contents of the right cubital fossa

Floor

It is formed by:

a. Brachialis.

b. Supinator muscles.

Contents

The fossa is actually very narrow. The contents described are seen after retracting the boundaries. From medial to the lateral side, the contents are as follows.

1. *The median nerve* (Fig. 38.14).
2. The termination of the *brachial artery*, and the beginning of the radial and ulnar arteries lie in the fossa.
3. The tendon of the *biceps brachii*, with the bicipital aponeurosis.
4. The *radial nerve*

POSTERIOR COMPARTMENT

The region contains the triceps muscle, the radial nerve and the profunda brachii artery.

TRICEPS BRACHII MUSCLE

Origin

Triceps brachii muscle arises by the following three heads (Fig. 38.15).

1. The *long head* arises from the infraglenoid tubercle of the scapula. It is the longest of the three heads.
2. The *lateral head* arises from an oblique ridge on the upper part of the posterior surface of the humerus.
3. The *medial head* arises from a large triangular area on the posterior surface of the humerus below the radial groove.

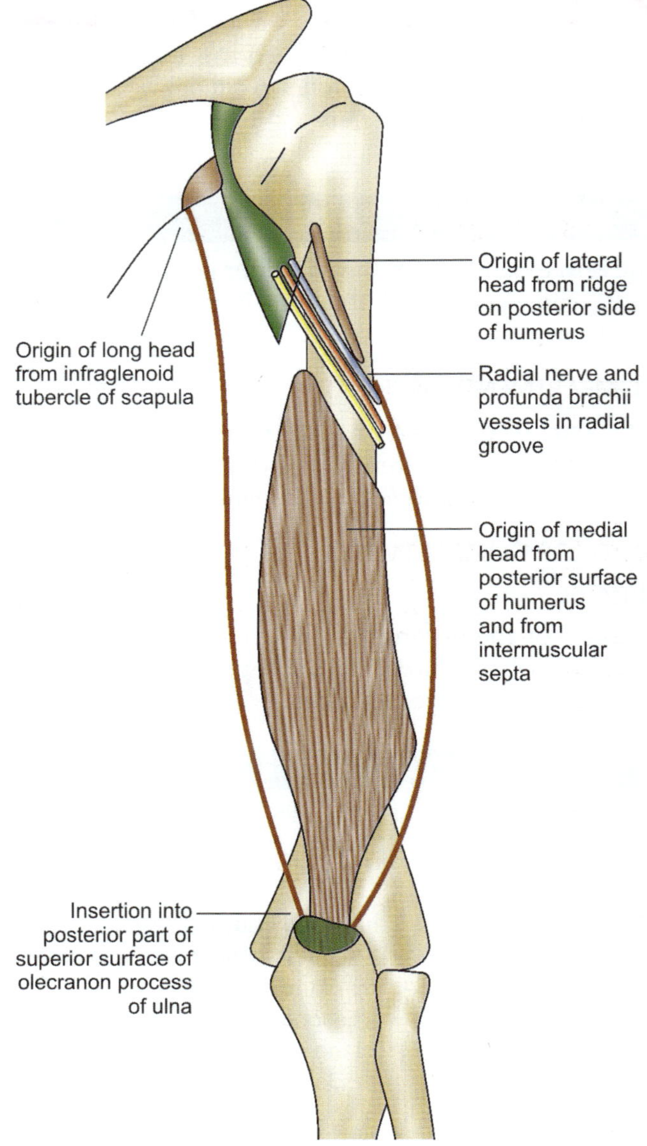

Fig. 38.15: The triceps brachii muscle

Insertion

The long and lateral heads converge and fuse to form a superficial flattened tendon which covers the medial head and all heads are inserted into the posterior part of the superior surface of the olecranon process.

Nerve Supply

Each head receives a separate branch from the radial nerve (C7, C8). The branches arise in the axilla and in the radial groove.

Actions

The triceps is a powerful active extensor of the elbow. The long head supports the head of the humerus in the abducted position of the arm. Gravity extends the elbow passively.

CLINICAL ANATOMY

- Brachial pulsations are felt or auscultated in front of the elbow just medial to the tendon of biceps while recording the blood pressure (Fig. 38.16). The figure shows other palpable arteries as well.
- The cubital region is important for the following reasons.
  a. The median cubital vein is often the vein of choice for intravenous injections and for obtaining blood samples.
  b. The blood pressure is universally recorded by auscultating the brachial artery in front of the elbow (Fig. 38.17).

The palpable arteries in head and neck are common carotid, internal carotid, facial and superficial temporal. The abdominal aorta is palpable near the umbilicus. The brachial and radial arteries are palpable in upper limb. Femoral, posterior tibial and dosalis pedis are palpable in lower limb.

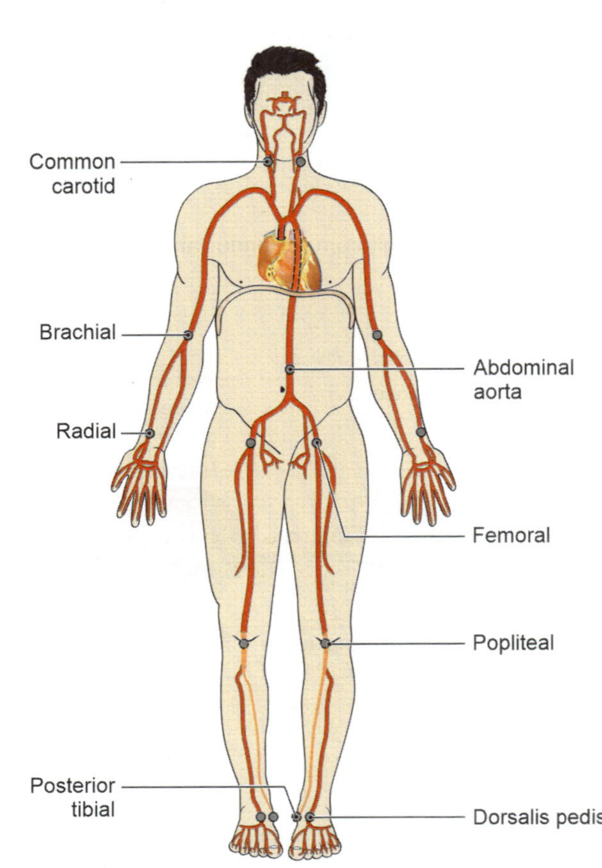

Fig. 38.16: Palpable arteries in the body

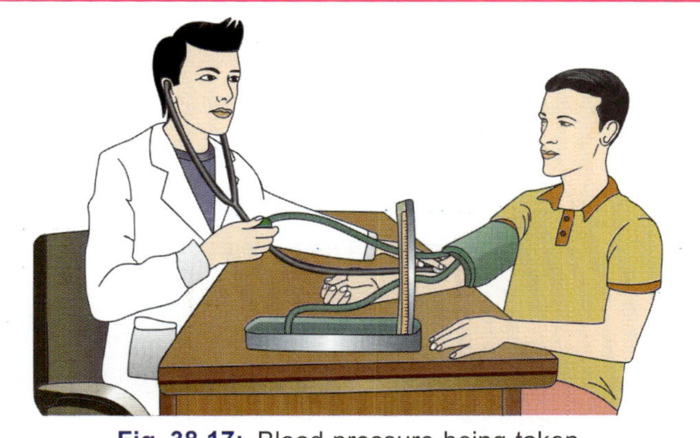

Fig. 38.17: Blood pressure being taken

FOREARM AND HAND

FRONT OF FOREARM

The front of the forearm presents the following components for study.

Components

1 Eight muscles—five superficial and three deep.
2 Two arteries—radial and ulnar.
3 Three nerves—median, ulnar and radial.

SUPERFICIAL MUSCLES

These are pronator teres, flexor carpi radialis, palmaris longus, flexor digitorum superificalis and flexor carpi ulnaris (Fig. 38.18).

DEEP MUSCLES

Deep muscles of the front of the forearm are the flexor digitorum profundus, the flexor pollicis longus and the pronator quadratus (Fig. 38.19).

PALMAR ASPECT OF WRIST AND HAND

Flexor Retinaculum

Flexor retinaculum is a strong fibrous band which bridges the anterior concavity of the carpus and converts it into a tunnel—the *carpal tunnel.*

Attachments

Medially, to:
1 The pisiform bone.
2 The hook of the hamate (Fig. 38.20)

Laterally, to:
1 The tubercle of the scaphoid, and
2 The crest of the trapezium.

INTRINSIC MUSCLES OF THE HAND

The intrinsic muscles of the hand serve the function of adjusting the hand during gripping and also for

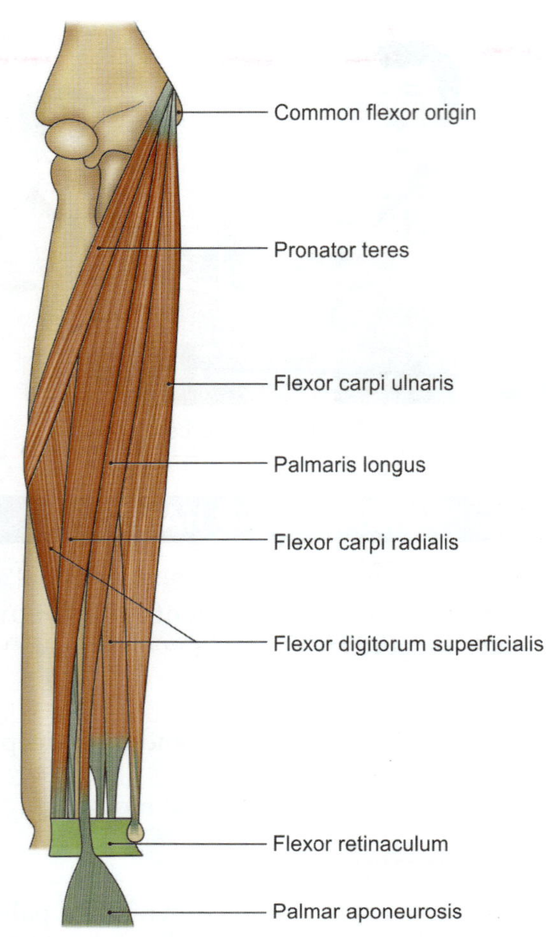

Fig. 38.18: The superficial muscles of the front of the right forearm

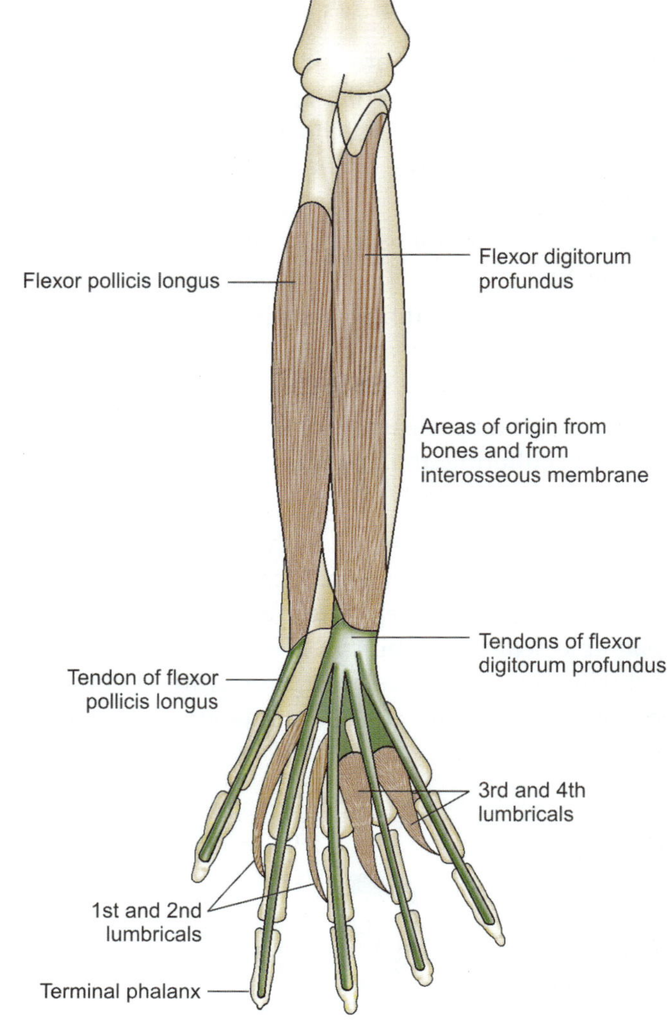

Fig. 38.19: The flexor digitorum profundus and the flexor pollicis longus

carrying out fine skilled movements. The origin and insertion of these muscles is within the territory of the hand.

There are 20 muscles in the hand, as follows.

1 a. *Three muscles of thenar eminence*
   i. Abductor pollicis brevis.
   ii. Flexor pollicis brevis.
   iii. Opponens pollicis.
  b. *One adductor of thumb:* Adductor pollicis.
2 *Four hypothenar muscles*
   i. Palmaris brevis.
   ii. Abductor digiti minimi.
   iii. Flexor digiti minimi.
   iv. Opponens digiti minimi.

Muscles (ii)–(iv) are muscles of hypothenar eminence.

3 *Four lumbricals.*
4 *Four palmar interossei* (Fig. 38.21).
5 *Four dorsal interossei.*

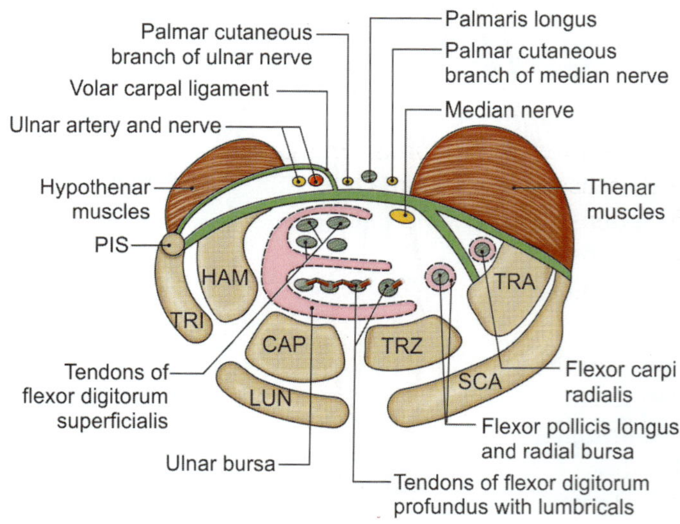

Fig. 38.20: Flexor retinaculum of wrist

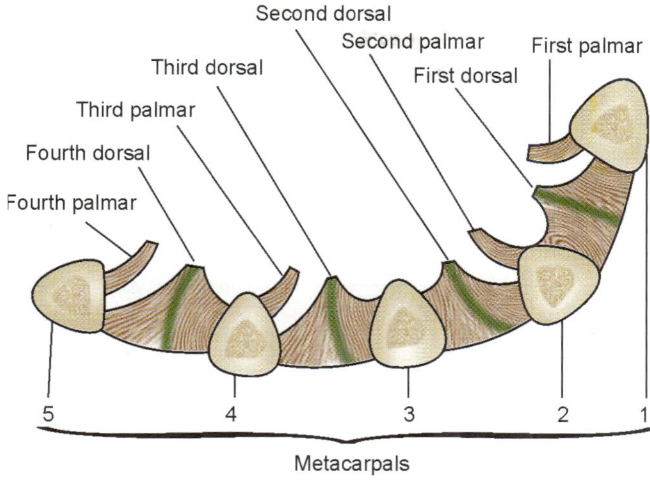

Fig. 38.21: The origin of the interossei muscles

DORSAL ASPECT OF WRIST

Extensor Retinaculum

The deep fascia on the back of the wrist is thickened to form the extensor retinaculum which holds the extensor tendons in place. It is an oblique band, directed downwards and medially. It is about 2 cm broad vertically.

Attachments

Laterally, to the lower part of the *anterior* border of the radius. Medially, to:

i. Triquetral.
ii. Pisiform and to the ridges on dorsal aspect of distal end of radius.

Superficial Muscles

There are seven superficial muscles and five deep muscles on the back of the forearm:

1 Anconeus
2 Brachioradialis
3 Extensor carpi radialis longus
4 Extensor carpi radialis brevis
5 Extensor digitorum
6 Extensor digiti minimi
7 Extensor carpi ulnaris.

Deep Muscles

These are as follows.

1 Supinator
2 Abductor pollicis longus
3 Extensor pollicis brevis
4 Extensor pollicis longus
5 Extensor indicis

CLINICAL ANATOMY

The radial artery is used for feeling the arterial pulse at the wrist. The pulsation can be felt well on the anterolateral side of forearm above the wrist joint because of the presence of the flat radius behind the artery (Fig. 38.16).

SUPERFICIAL VEINS

Superficial veins of the upper limb assume importance in medical practice because these are most commonly used for intravenous injections and transfusion; also used for withdrawing blood for testing.

General Remarks

1 Most of the superficial veins of the limb join together to form two large veins—cephalic (preaxial) and basilic (postaxial).
2 The superficial veins are accompanied by cutaneous nerves and superficial lymphatics, and not by arteries. The superficial lymph vessels lie along the veins, and the deep lymph vessels along the arteries.
3 The superficial veins are best utilised for intravenous injections.

Individual Veins

Dorsal Venous Arch

Dorsal venous arch lies on the dorsum of the hand (Fig. 38.22a). Its afferents (tributaries) include:

i. Three dorsal metacarpal veins.
ii. A dorsal digital vein from the medial side of the little finger.
iii. A dorsal digital vein from the radial side of the index finger.
iv. Two dorsal digital veins from the thumb.
v. Most of the blood from the palm courses through veins passing around the margins of the hand and also by perforating veins passing through the interosseous spaces. Its efferents are the cephalic and basilic veins.

Cephalic Vein

It begins from the lateral end of the dorsal venous arch. It runs upwards:

i. Through the roof of the anatomical snuff box,
ii. winds round the lateral border of the distal part of the forearm.
iii. continues upwards in front of the elbow and along the lateral border of the biceps brachii.
iv. pierces the deep fascia at the lower border of the pectoralis major (Fig. 38.22b).
v. runs in the deltopectoral groove up to the infraclavicular fossa where it pierces the clavipectoral fascia and joins the axillary vein.

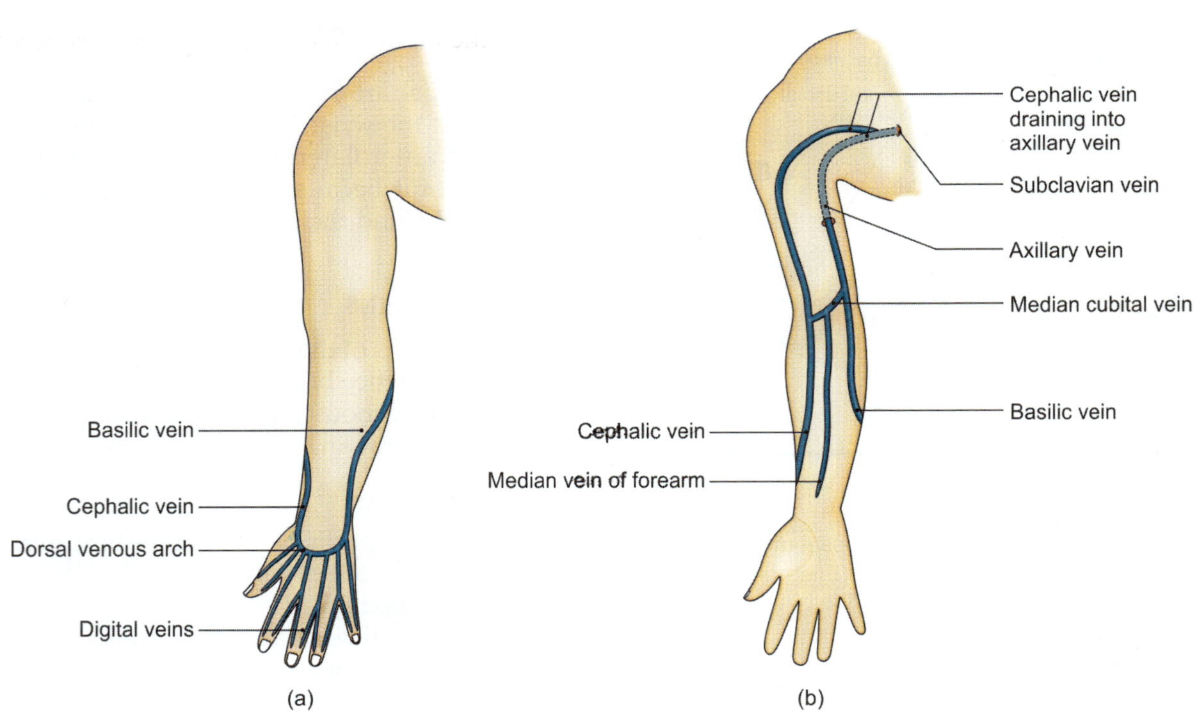

Figs 38.22a and b: The superficial veins of the upper limb: (a) On the back, and (b) on the front of the limb

At the elbow, the greater part of its blood is drained into the basilic vein through the median cubital vein, and partly also into the deep veins through the perforator vein.

Basilic Vein

It begins from the medial end of the dorsal venous arch.

It runs upwards:

i. Along the back of the medial border of the forearm,
ii. Winds round this border near the elbow.
iii. Continues upwards in front of the elbow (medial epicondyle) and along the medial margin of the biceps brachii up to the middle of the arm where it pierces the deep fascia, and
iv. Runs along the medial side of the brachial artery up to the lower border of teres major where it becomes the axillary vein.

About 2.5 cm above the medial epicondyle of the humerus, it is joined by the median cubital vein.

Median Cubital Vein

Median cubital vein is a large communicating vein which shunts blood from the cephalic to the basilic vein.

It begins from the cephalic vein 2.5 cm below the bend of the elbow, runs obliquely upward and medially, and ends in the basilic vein 2.5 cm above the medial epicondyle. It is separated from the brachial artery by the bicipital aponeurosis.

CLINICAL ANATOMY

The median cubital vein is the vein of choice for intravenous injections, for withdrawing blood from donors, and for cardiac catheterisation, because it is fixed by the perforator and does not slip away during piercing (Fig. 38.23). When the median cubital vein is absent, the basilic is preferred over the cephalic because the former is a more efficient channel.

It may receive tributaries from the front of the forearm and is connected to the deep veins through a perforator vein which pierces the bicipital aponeurosis. The perforator vein fixes the median cubital vein and thus makes it ideal for intravenous injections (Fig. 38.22).

Median Vein of the Forearm

Median vein of the forearm begins from the palmar venous network, and ends in any one of the veins in front of the elbow mostly in median cubital vein.

JOINTS OF UPPER LIMB

Joints are sites where two or more bones or cartilages articulate. Free movements occur at the synovial joints. Shoulder joint is the most freely mobile joint. Shoulder joint get excessive mobility at the cost of its own

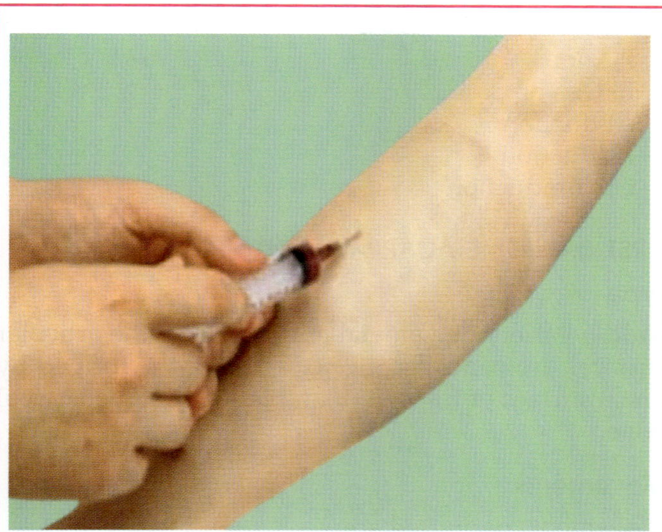

Fig. 38.23: Intravenous injection being given in the median cubital vein

stability, since both are not feasible to the same degree. The carrying angle in relation to elbow joint is to facilitate carrying objects like buckets without hitting the pelvis.

Supination and pronation are basic movements for the survival of human being. During pronation, the food is picked and by supination it is put at the right place—the mouth. While 'giving', one pronates, while 'getting' one supinates.

The first carpometacarpal joint allows movements of opposition of thumb with the fingers for picking up or holding things. Thumb is the most important digit. Remember *Muni* Dronacharya asked Eklavya to give his right thumb as *Guru-Dakshina*, so that he is not able to outsmart Arjuna in archery.

SHOULDER GIRDLE

Sternoclavicular Joint

The sternoclavicular joint is a synovial joint of saddle variety.

Acromioclavicular Joint

The acromioclavicular joint is a plane synovial joint.

SHOULDER JOINT

Type

The shoulder joint is a synovial joint of the ball and socket variety. Glenoid cavity of scapula and head of humerus form the shoulder joint.

Movements at Shoulder Joint

Movements of shoulder joint are depicted in Table 38.8.

Table 38.8: Muscles bringing about movements at the shoulder joint

Movements	*Main muscles*	*Accessory muscles*
1. Flexion	• Clavicular head of the pectoralis major • Anterior fibres of deltoid	• Coracobrachialis • Short head of biceps brachii
2. Extension	• Posterior fibres of deltoid • Latissimus dorsi	• Teres major • Long head of triceps brachii • Sternocostal head of the pectoralis major
3. Adduction	• Pectoralis major • Latissimus dorsi • Short head of biceps brachii • Long head of triceps brachii	• Teres major • Coracobrachialis
4. Abduction	• Supraspinatus 0°–90° • Deltoid 0°–90° • Serratus anterior 90°–180° • Upper and lower fibres of trapezius 90°–180°	—
5. Medial rotation	• Pectoralis major • Anterior fibres of deltoid • Latissimus dorsi • Teres major	• Subscapularis
6. Lateral rotation	• Posterior fibres of deltoid • Infraspinatus • Teres minor	—

ELBOW JOINT

The elbow joint is a hinge variety of synovial joint between the the capitulum and trochlea of the lower end of humerus and the upper ends of radius and ulna bones.

i. Upper surface of the head of the radius articulates with the capitulum.
ii. Trochlear notch of the ulna articulates with the trochlea of the humerus.

RADIOULNAR JOINTS

The radius and the ulna are joined to each other at the superior and inferior radioulnar joints. The radius and ulna are also connected by the interosseous membrane which constitutes middle radioulnar joint. Movements at these joints are supination and pronation (Table 38.9).

Interosseous Membrane

The interosseous membrane connects the shafts of the radius and ulna. It is attached to the interosseous borders of these bones. The fibres of the membrane run downwards and medially from the radius to ulna. It transmits weight from radius to ulna.

WRIST (RADIOCARPAL) JOINT

Type

Wrist joint is a synovial joint of the ellipsoid variety between lower end of radius and three lateral bones of proximal row of carpus.

Movements

1 Flexion
2 Extension
3 Abduction
4 Adduction
5 Circumduction

FIRST CARPOMETACARPAL JOINT

Type

Saddle variety of synovial joint (because the articular surfaces are concavoconvex). This joint is formed by distal surface of trapezium and base of 1st metacarpal bone.

Movements

Movements permitted are:

1 Flexion with medial rotation
2 Extension with lateral rotation
3 Abduction
4 Adduction
5 Opposition

NERVES OF UPPER LIMB

MUSCULOCUTANEOUS NERVE

Musculocutaneous nerve is so named as it supplies muscles of front of arm and skin of lateral side of forearm.

Root Value

Ventral rami of C5, C6 and C7 segments of spinal cord.

Table 38.9: Radioulnar joints

Features	*Superior radioulnar joint*	*Inferior radioulnar joint*
Type	Pivot type of synovial joint	Pivot type of synovial joint
Articular surfaces	• Circumference of head of radius • Osseofibrous ring, formed by the radial notch of the ulna and the annular ligament	• Head of ulna • Ulnar notch of radius
Ligaments	• The annular ligament. It forms four-fifths of the ring within which the head of the radius rotates. It is attached to the margins of the radial notch of the ulna, and is continuous with the capsule of the elbow joint above	• The capsule surrounds the joint • The apex of articular disc is attached to the base of the styloid process of the ulna, and the base to the lower margin of the ulnar notch of the radius
Blood supply	Anastomoses around the lateral side of the elbow joint	Anterior and posterior interosseous arteries
Nerve supply	Musculocutaneous, median, and radial nerves	Anterior and posterior interosseous nerves
Movements	Supination and pronation	Supination and pronation

Course

Musculocutaneous nerve is a branch of the lateral cord of brachial plexus, lies lateral to axillary and upper part of brachial artery. At the crease of elbow, it becomes cutaneous by piercing the deep fascia. There the nerve is called the lateral cutaneous nerve of forearm (Fig. 38.24).

Branches

Muscular	Coracobrachialis, long head of biceps brachii, short head of biceps brachii, and brachialis.
Cutaneous	Lateral side of forearm (both on the front and the back).
Articular	Elbow joint.

AXILLARY OR CIRCUMFLEX NERVE

Axillary nerve is called axillary as it runs through the upper part of axilla though it does not supply any structure there. It is called circumflex as it courses around the surgical neck of humerus (Fig. 38.12) to supply the prominent deltoid muscle.

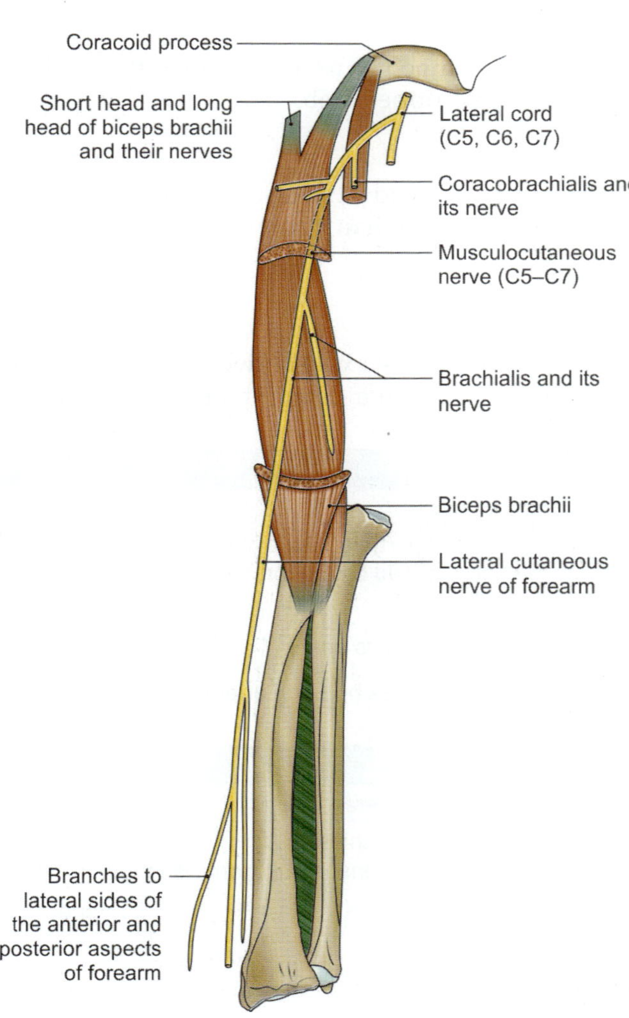

Fig. 38.24: The course of the musculocutaneous nerve

Root Value

Ventral rami of C5, C6 segments of spinal cord.

Course

Axillary or circumflex nerve is the smaller terminal branch of posterior cord. It passes backwards and divides into anterior and posterior divisions.

Branches

The branches of axillary nerve are presented in Table 38.10.

RADIAL NERVE

Radial nerve is the thickest branch of brachial plexus.

Axilla

Radial nerve lies against the muscles forming the posterior wall of axilla (Fig. 38.25).

Radial Sulcus/Groove

Radial nerve then enters the radial sulcus, where it lies between the long and medial heads of triceps brachii along with profunda brachii vessels.

Front of Arm

Radial nerve enters the lower anterolateral part of arm to reach the cubital fossa, where it ends by dividing into its two terminal branches—the superficial and deep (posterior interosseous) branches (Fig. 38.14).

Posterior Interosseous (Deep Branch)

It lies in the lateral part of cubital fossa. Then it enters into the back of forearm. There the nerve supplies many muscles. It ends in a pseudoganglion, branches of which supply the wrist joint (Fig. 38.25).

Superficial Branch

Superficial branch is given off in the cubital fossa and runs on the lateral side of forearm accompanied by radial artery in the upper two-thirds of forearm. Then it curves posteriorly to descend till the anatomical snuff box. It gives branches to supply the skin of lateral half of dorsum of hand (Fig. 38.25).

Branches of Radial Nerve

The branches of radial nerve are presented in Table 38.11.

MEDIAN NERVE

Median nerve is called median as it runs in the median plane of the forearm.

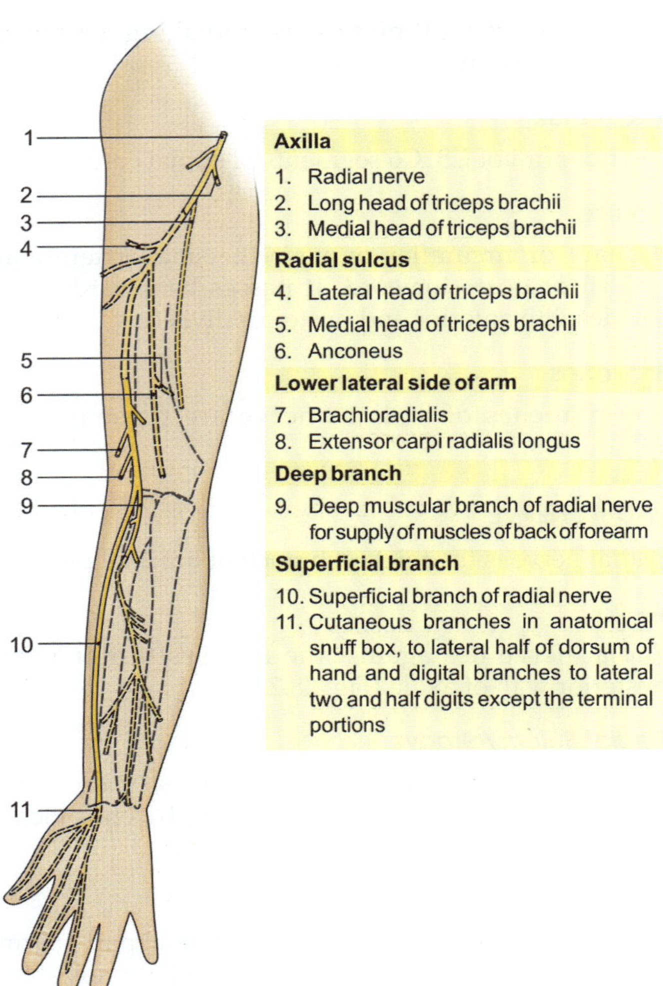

Fig. 38.25: Distribution of right radial nerve

Root Value

Ventral rami of C5–C8, T1 segments of spinal cord.

Median nerve is formed by two roots—lateral root from lateral cord and medial root from medial cord of brachial plexus. Medial root crosses the axillary artery to join the lateral root. The median nerve runs on the lateral side of axillary artery till the middle of arm, where it crosses in front of the artery to lie medial to the artery. Then it passes anterior to elbow joint, and courses through the forearm (Fig. 38.26).

It gives a number of branches in cubital fossa and forearm. It enters palm under the flexor retinaculum.

In the palm, median nerve lies medial to the muscles of thenar eminence, which it supplies. It also gives cutaneous branches to lateral three and a half-digits and their nail beds including skin of distal phalanges on their dorsal aspect.

Branches of Median Nerve

The branches of median nerve are presented in Table 38.12.

ULNAR NERVE

Ulnar nerve is named so as it runs along the medial or ulnar side of the upper limb.

Root Value

Ventral rami of C8 and T1. It also gets fibres of C7 from the lateral root of median nerve.

Course

Axilla

Ulnar nerve lies in the axilla between the axillary vein and axillary artery on a deeper plane and lies medial

Table 38.10: Branches of axillary nerve

	Trunk	*Anterior division*	*Posterior division*
Muscular	—	Deltoid (most part)	Deltoid (posterior part) and teres minor. The nerve to teres minor is characterised by the presence of a pseudoganglion
Cutaneous	—	—	Upper lateral cutaneous nerve of arm
Articular and vascular	Shoulder joint	—	To posterior circumflex humeral artery

Table 38.11: Branches of radial nerve

	Axilla	*Radial sulcus*	*Lateral side of arm*
Muscular	Long head of triceps brachii Medial head of triceps brachii	Lateral head of triceps brachii Medial head of triceps brachii Anconeus	Brachioradialis Extensor carpi radialis longus
Cutaneous	Posterior cutaneous nerve of arm	Posterior cutaneous nerve of forearm Lower lateral cutaneous nerve of arm	— —
Vascular	—	To profunda brachii artery	

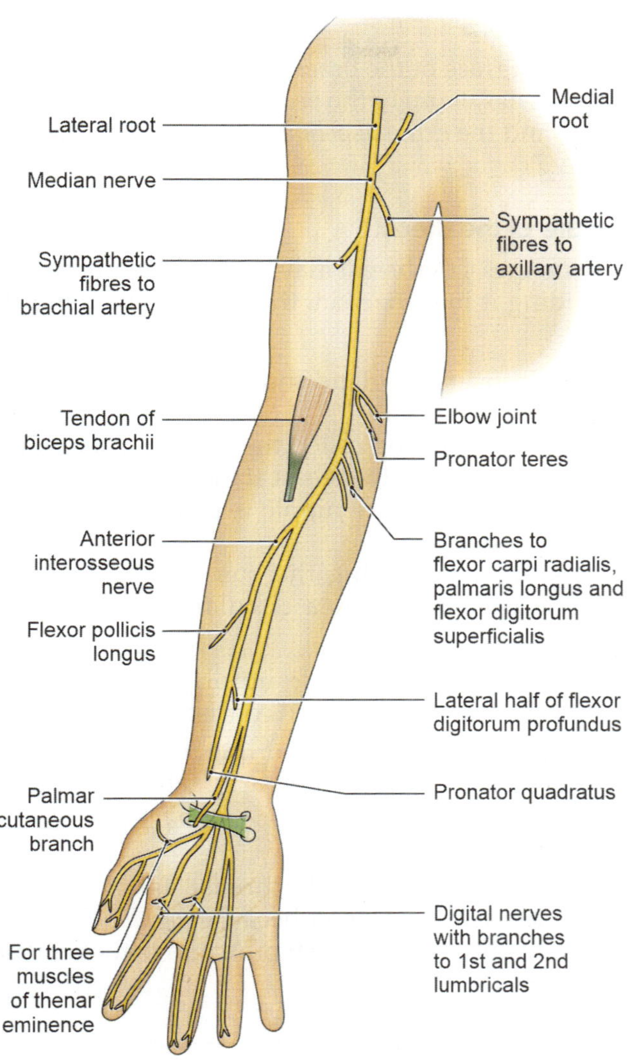

Fig. 38.26: Distribution of median nerve

to brachial artery. It pierces the medial intermuscular septum to lie on its back and descends on the back of medial epicondyle of humerus where it can be palpated. Palpation causes tingling sensations. That is why humerus is called "funny bone".

Forearm

Ulnar nerve enters the forearm. It is accompanied by the ulnar artery in lower two-thirds of forearm (Fig. 38.27). Finally, it lies on the medial part of flexor retinaculum to enter palm (Fig. 38.20). At the distal border of retinaculum the nerve divides into its superficial and deep branches.

Branches

The branches of ulnar nerve are presented in Table 38.13.

ARTERIES OF UPPER LIMB

Arteries of upper limb, their origin, course, termiantion and area of distribution are given in Table 38.14.

THE BREAST/MAMMARY GLAND

The breast is found in both sexes, but is rudimentary in the male. It is well developed in the female after puberty. The breast is a *modified sweat gland.* The breast lies in the superficial fascia of the pectoral region.

Extent

- Vertically, it extends from the second to the sixth rib.
- Horizontally, it extends from the lateral border of the sternum to the mid-axillary line.

Table 38.12: Branches of median nerve

	Axilla and arm	*Cubital fossa*	*Forearm*	*Palm*
Muscular	Pronator teres in lower part of arm	Flexor carpi radialis, flexor digitorum superficialis, palmaris longus	Anterior interosseous which supplies: lateral half of flexor digitorum profundus, pronator quadratus, and flexor pollicis longus	Recurrent branch for abductor pollicis brevis, flexor pollicis brevis, opponens pollicis, 1st lumbrical and 2nd lumbrical from the digital nerves
Cutaneous	—	—	Palmar cutaneous branch for lateral two-thirds of palm	• Two digital branches to lateral and medial sides of thumb • One to lateral side of index finger • Two to adjacent sides of index and middle fingers • Two to adjacent sides of middle and ring fingers. These branches also supply dorsal aspects of distal phalanges of lateral three and a half digits

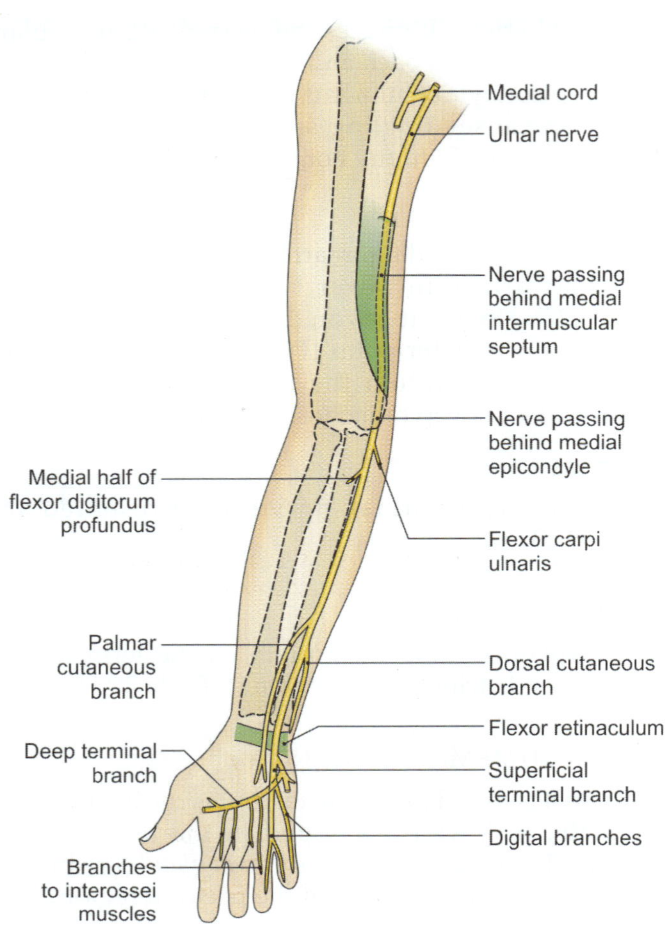

Fig. 38.27: Course and branches of ulnar nerve

Deep Relations

The deep surface of the breast is related to the parts of three muscles, namely the *pectoralis major*, the *serratus anterior*, and the *external oblique muscle* of the abdomen (Fig. 5A.71).

Structure of the Breast

The structure of the breast may be conveniently studied by dividing it into the skin, the parenchyma, and the stroma.

The skin: It covers the gland and presents the following features.

1. A conical projection called the *nipple* is present just below the centre of the breast at the level of the fourth intercostal space. The nipple is pierced by 15 to 20 *lactiferous ducts.*
2. The skin surrounding the base of the nipple is pigmented and forms a circular area called the *areola*.

The parenchyma: It is made up of glandular tissue which secretes milk. The gland consists of 15 to 20 *lobes*.

The stroma: It forms the supporting framework of the gland. It is partly fibrous and partly fatty.

Lymphatic Drainage

Lymphatic drainage of the breast assumes great importance to the surgeon because *carcinoma* of the breast spreads mostly along lymphatics to the regional

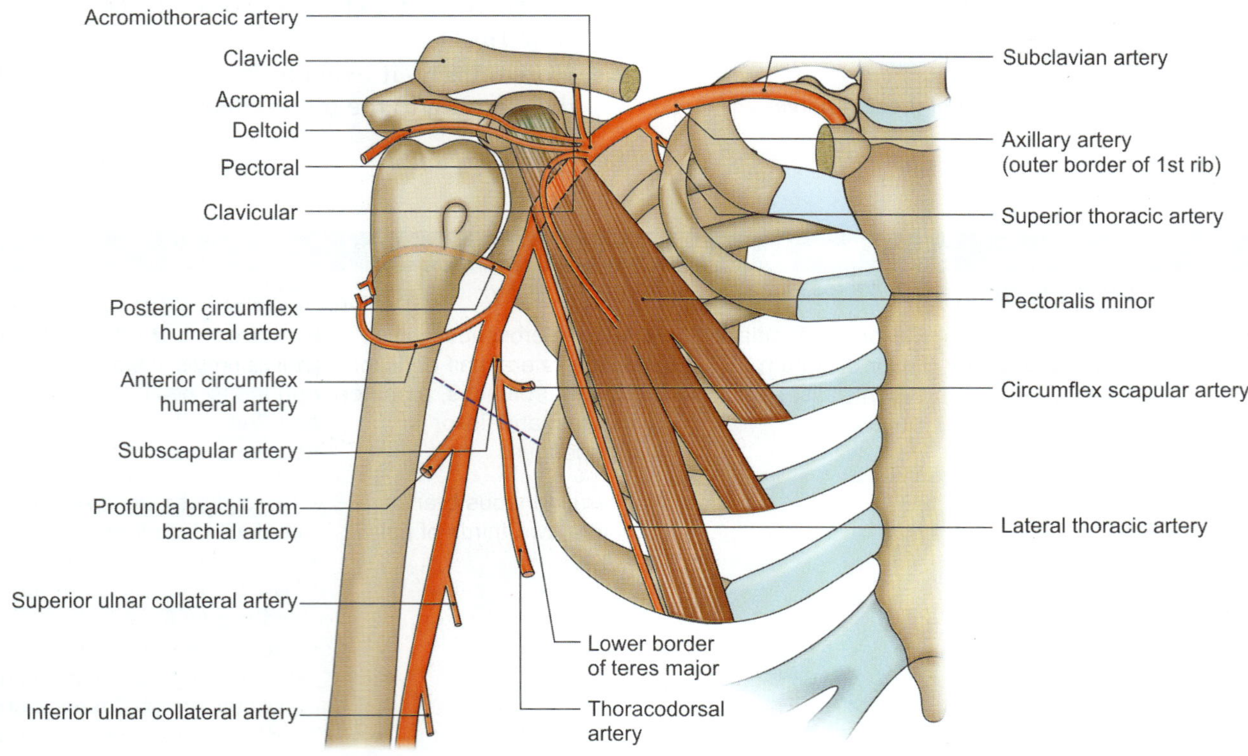

Fig. 38.28: The branches of the axillary and brachial arteries

Table 38.13: Branches of ulnar nerve		
	Forearm	Hand
Muscular	Medial half of flexor digitorum profundus, flexor carpi ulnaris	Superficial branch—palmaris brevis. Deep branch—hypothenar eminence muscles, medial two lumbricals, 4–1 dorsal and palmar interossei and adductor pollicis
Cutaneous/digital	Dorsal cutaneous branch for medial half of dorsum of hand. Palmar cutaneous branch for medial one-third of palm. Digital branches to medial one and a half fingers, nail beds and dorsal distal phalanges	
Vascular/Articular	Also supplies digital vessels and joints of medial side of hand	

Table 38.14: Arteries of upper limb		
Artery	*Origin, course and termination*	*Area of distribution*
AXILLARY (Fig. 38.28)	Starts at the outer border of first rib as continuation of subclavian artery, runs through axilla and continues as brachial artery at the lower border of teres major muscle	Supplies all walls of axilla, pectoral region including mammary gland
Superior thoracic	From 1st part of axillary artery	Supplies upper part of thoracic wall; the pectoral muscles
Thoracoacromial	From 2nd part of axillary artery, pierces clavipectoral fascia and divides into branches	Supplies pectoral and deltoid muscles; acromion and clavicle
Lateral thoracic	From 2nd part of axillary artery runs along inferolateral border of pectoralis minor	Supplies the muscles of thoracic wall including the mammary gland
Anterior circumflex humeral	From 3rd part of axillary artery, runs on the anterior aspect of intertubercular sulcus and anastomoses with large posterior humerus circumflex humeral artery	Supplies the neighbouring shoulder joint and the muscles
Posterior circumflex humeral	From third part of axillary artery, lies along the surgical neck of humerus with axillary nerve	Supplies huge deltoid muscle, overlying skin and the shoulder joint
Subscapular	Largest branch of axillary artery runs along the muscles of posterior wall of axilla	Supplies muscles of posterior wall of axilla, i.e. teres major, latissimus dorsi, subscapularis. Takes part in anastomoses around scapula
BRACHIAL ARTERY (Fig. 38.28)	Starts at the lower border of teres major as continuation of axillary artery. Runs on anterior aspect of arm and ends by dividing into radial and ulnar arteries at neck of radius in the cubital fossa	Supplies muscles of the arm, humerus bone and skin of whole of arm. Takes part in anastomoses around elbow joint
Profunda brachii artery	Largest branch of brachial artery. Runs with radial nerve in the radial sulcus of humerus. Reaching the lateral side of arm ends by dividing into anterior and posterior branches	Supplies muscles of back of arm and its branches anastomose with branches of radial artery and ulnar artery on lateral epicondyle of humerus
RADIAL ARTERY (Fig. 38.29)	Starts as smaller branch of brachial artery, lies on the lateral side of forearm, then in the anatomical snuff box to reach the palm, where it continues as deep palmar arch, which gives digital branches via superficial palmar arch.	Muscles of lateral side of forearm, including the overlying skin. Gives a branch for completion of superficial palmar arch. Digital branches to thumb and lateral side of index finger
ULNAR ARTERY (Fig. 38.29)	Originates as the larger terminal branch of brachial artery at neck of radius. Courses first obliquely in upper one-third and then vertically in lower two-thirds of forearm. Lies superficial to flexor retinaculum and ends by dividing into superficial and deep branches The former forms superficial palmar arch	Gives branches to take part in the anastomoses around elbow joint. Branches supply muscles of front of forearm, back of forearm and nutrient arteries to forearm bones

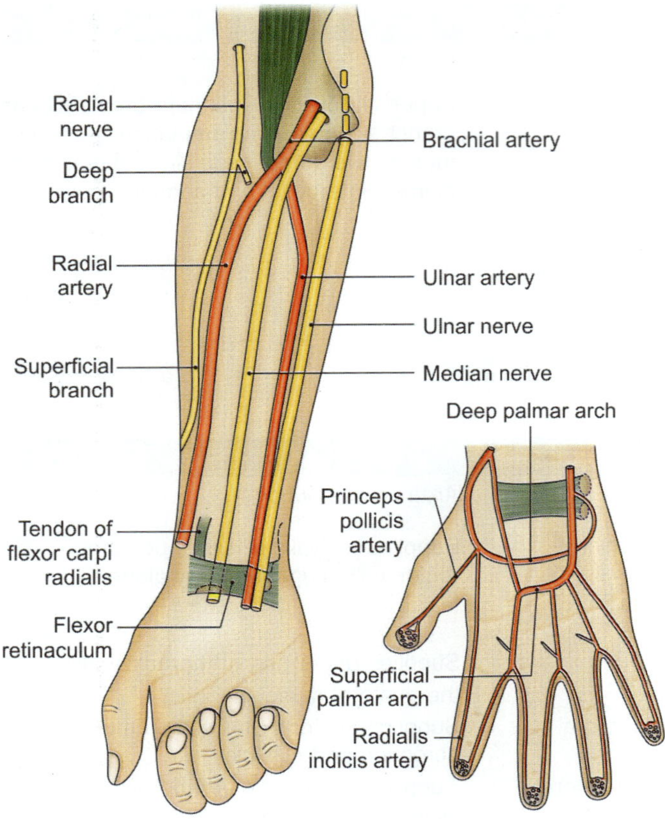

Fig. 38.29: The radial and ulnar nerves and vessels in the forearm and palm

lymph nodes. The subject can be described under two heads, the lymph nodes, and the lymphatics.

Lymph Nodes

Lymph from the breast drains into the following lymph nodes.

1 The axillary lymph nodes, chiefly the *anterior* (or pectoral) group. The *posterior, lateral, central* and *apical* groups of nodes also receive lymph from the breast either directly or indirectly (Fig. 38.30).

2 The *internal mammary* (parasternal) nodes which lie along the internal thoracic vessels.

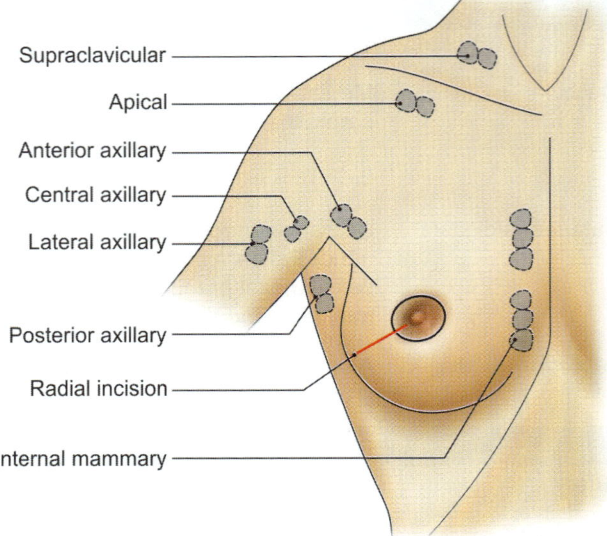

Fig. 38.30: Lymph nodes draining the breast

3 Some lymph from the breast also reaches the *supraclavicular nodes,* the *cephalic* (deltopectoral) node, *the posterior intercostal* nodes (lying in front of the heads of the ribs), the *subdiaphragmatic* and *subperitoneal* lymph plexuses.

Lymphatic Vessels

The *superficial lymphatics* drain the skin over the breast except for the nipple and areola. The lymphatics pass radially to the surrounding lymph nodes (axillary, internal mammary, supraclavicular and cephalic).

The *deep lymphatics* drain the parenchyma of the breast. They also drain the nipple and areola.

Some further points of interest about the lymphatic drainage are as follows.

1 About 75% of the lymph from the breast drains into the *axillary nodes;* 20% into the *internal mammary nodes;* and 5% into the *posterior intercostal nodes.*

2 Lymphatics from the lower and inner quadrants of the breast may communicate with the subdiaphragmatic and subperitoneal lymph plexuses and then piercing the anterior abdominal wall. So cancer may spread into the abdominal lymph nodes.

Chapter 39

Thorax

"One thousand Americans and same number of Indians stop smoking everyday—by dying."
—Anonymous

INTRODUCTION

Thorax forms the upper part of the trunk of the body. It not only permits boarding and lodging of the thoracic viscera, but also provides necessary shelter to some of the abdominal viscera.

BONES OF THORAX

The bones of thorax are:

1. Sternum
2. Twelve pairs of ribs
3. Twelve thoracic vertebra described with the vertebral column

STERNUM

The sternum forms anterior boundary of the thoracic cage. It consists of three parts:

a. Manubrium sterni is the upper part (Fig. 39.1).
b. Body of sternum is the middle part
c. *Xiphoid process* is the lower smallest part
   a. Manubrium sterni shows a suprasternal notch along the upper border and two clavicular facets on the sides. Manubrium sterni articulates with each clavicle above and laterally, and body of sternum inferiorly. The site of articulation with body of sternum is marked by a prominent ridge called sternal angle or angle of Louis. The 2nd costal cartilage articulates partly with manubrium and partly with body of sternum. The intercostal space below 2nd costal cartilage is the 2nd intercostal space. It is used for counting the intercostal spaces. On the posterior aspect of manubrium is the arch of aorta and its three branches, e.g. brachiocephalic, left common carotid and left subclavian arteries.
   b. *Body of sternum* It comprises anterior and posterior surfaces and two lateral borders, which have facets for articulation with 3rd to 6th costal cartilages. The anterior surface including that of manubrium sterni gives origin to pectoralis major muscle. The posterior surface is related to pleura on the right side and pericardium on the left side due to lateral deviation of left pleura (Fig. 39.2).
   c. *Xiphoid process* It is a narrow process which gives attachment to linea alba and two slips of thoraco-abdominal diaphragm. It articulates above with the lower part of body of sternum. Its tip is free and lies in epigastric fossa.

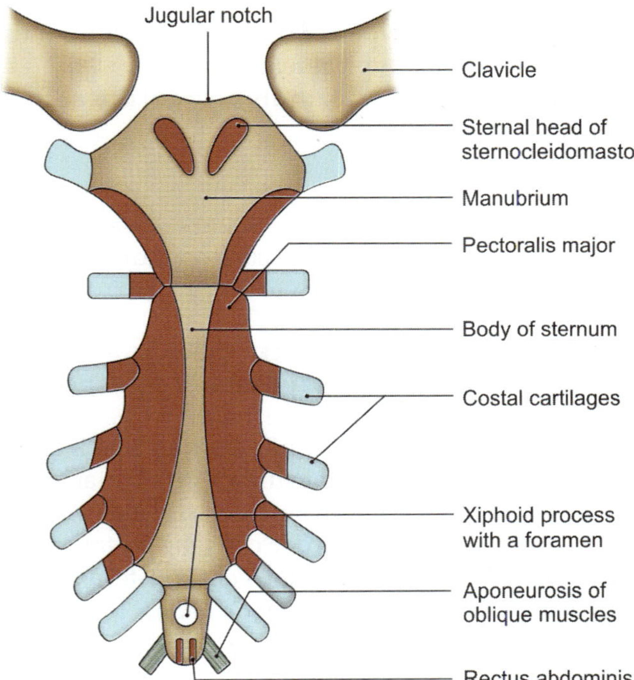

Fig. 39.1: The sternum—anterior aspect

CLINICAL ANATOMY

Manubrium is punctured to take out bone marrow in cases of severe anaemia or leukaemia, etc. The procedure is called *sternal puncture*.

RIBS

There are twelve pairs of ribs which form the thoracic cage. This cage encloses heart, lungs and some abdominal viscera like liver, stomach, spleen. The ribs are classified as:

1 *True or vertebrosternal ribs:* These are upper 7 ribs. These articulate with vertebrae posteriorly and via costal cartilages to sternum anteriorly.
2 *False or vertebrochondral ribs:* These are 8th 9th and 10th ribs. These articulate with vertebrae posteriorly. Their costal cartilages articulate with next higher cartilage anteriorly and not to sternum directly.
3 *Floating or vertebral ribs*: These are 11th and 12th ribs. These only articulate posteriorly with the vertebrae. Their anterior ends are free and tipped with costal cartilages.

The ribs can also be classified as—Typical ribs. The 3rd to 9th ribs are typical ribs. Typical ribs are those which show same typical features.

1st, 2nd, 10th, 11th and 12th are atypical ribs as these depict atypical features.

Typical Rib

Typical rib comprises a head, neck, tubercle and a shaft

Head articulates with sides of corresponding thoracic vertebra and one higher vertebra also, to form costovertebral joints (Fig. 39.3).

Neck is the intervening part. Tubercle articulates with facet on tip of transverse process of corresponding vertebra to form cutotransverse joint.

Shaft consists of thick upper border and a sharp lower border. Its rough outer surface gives attachment to muscles. Its inner smooth surface is related to costal pleura. Along the lower border runs the costal groove containing posterior intercostal vein, posterior intercostal artery and intercostal nerve (VAN).

Atypical Ribs

The 1st rib is short and wide with anteriorly placed groove on its upper surface for subclavian vein. The posterior groove is for lower trunk of brachial plexus and subclavian artery. The two grooves are separated by scalene tubercle. The rib has no costal groove and articulates with 1st thocacic vertebra only (Fig. 39.4).

The 10th rib only articulates with side of 10th thoracic vertebra only.

The 11th and 12th ribs have no angles and no tubercles. They articulate only with their respective thoracic vertebrae. These do not reach anterior aspect of thorax.

The costovertebral, costotransverse, manubriosternal and chondrosternal joints permit movements of the thoracic cage during breathing.

SUPERIOR APERTURE/INLET OF THORAX

The narrow upper end of the thorax, which is continuous with the neck, is called the inlet of the thorax (Fig. 39.5). It is kidney-shaped. Its transverse diameter is 10–12.5 cm. The anteroposterior diameter is about 5 cm.

Structures Passing through the Inlet of Thorax

Viscera

Trachea, oesophagus, apices of the lungs with pleura, remains of the thymus. Figure 39.6 depicts the structures passing through the inlet of the thorax.

Large Vessels

Brachiocephalic artery on right side.

Left common carotid artery and the left subclavian artery on the left side. Right and left brachiocephalic veins.

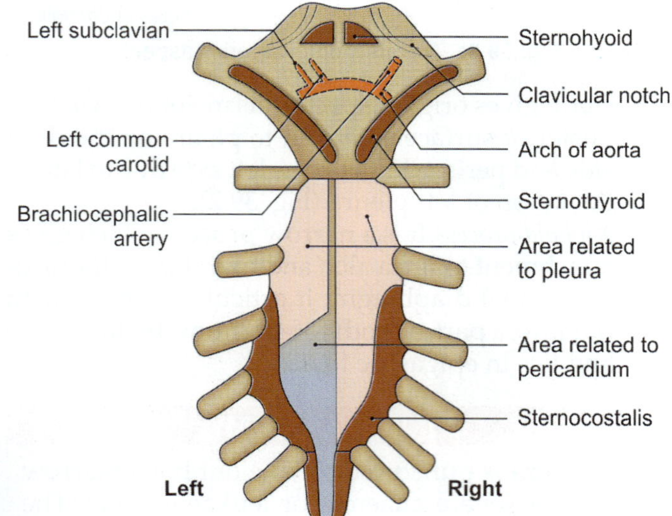

Fig. 39.2: Attachments on the posterior surface of the sternum

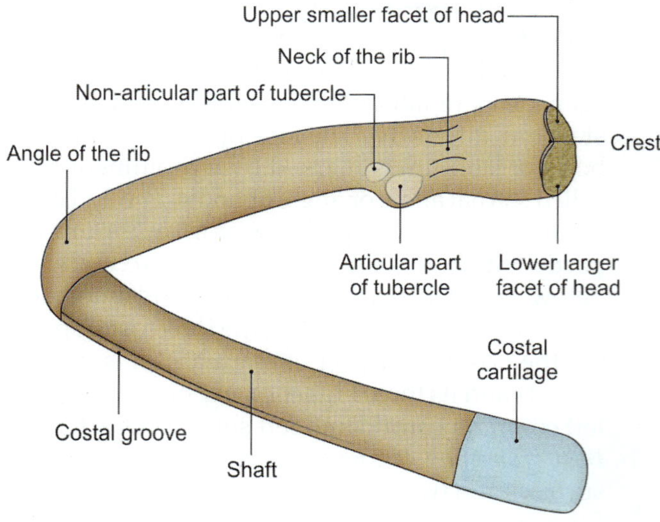

Fig. 39.3: A typical rib of the left side

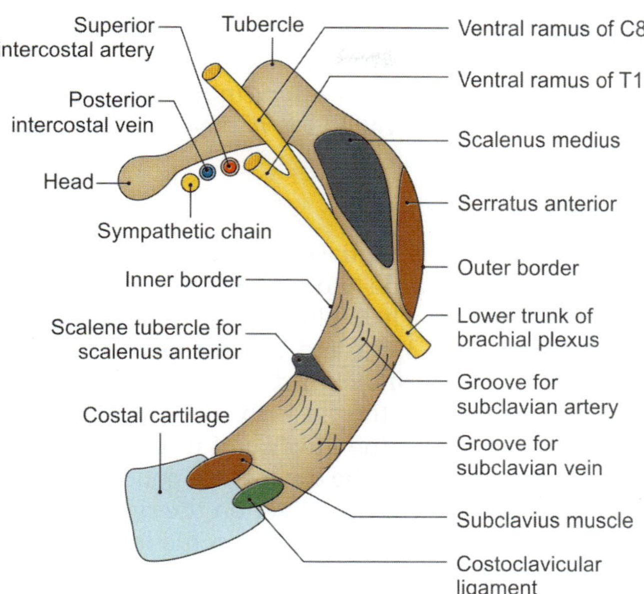

Fig. 39.4: Superior view of the first rib (left side)

Nerves

- Right and left phrenic nerves (Fig. 39.6).
- Right and left vagus nerves.
- Right and left sympathetic trunks.
- Right and left first thoracic nerves as they ascend across the first rib to join the brachial plexus.

Muscles

Sternohyoid, sternothyroid and longus colli.

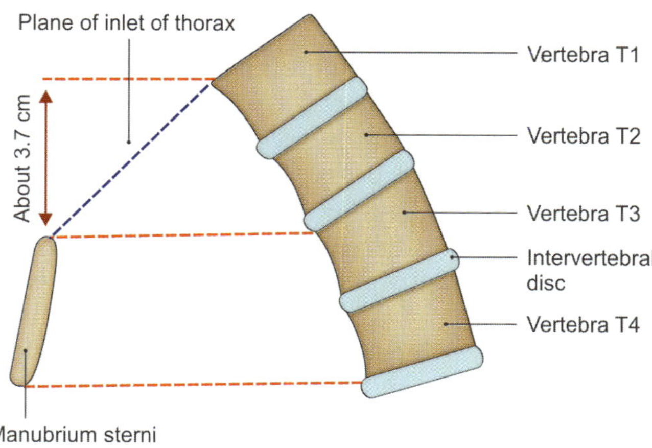

Fig. 39.5: The plane of the inlet of the thorax

INFERIOR APERTURE OF THORAX

Boundaries

- *Anteriorly:* Infrasternal angle between the two costal margins.
- *Posteriorly:* Inferior surface of the body of the twelfth thoracic vertebra.
- *On each side:* Costal margin formed by the cartilages of seventh to twelfth ribs.

Diaphragm at the Outlet/Inferior Aperture of Thorax

The diaphragm is a dome-shaped muscle forming the partition between the thoracic and abdominal cavities. It is the chief muscle of respiration.

Muscle fibres, form the periphery of the partition. They arise from circumference of the thoracic outlet and are inserted into a central tendon (Fig. 39.7).

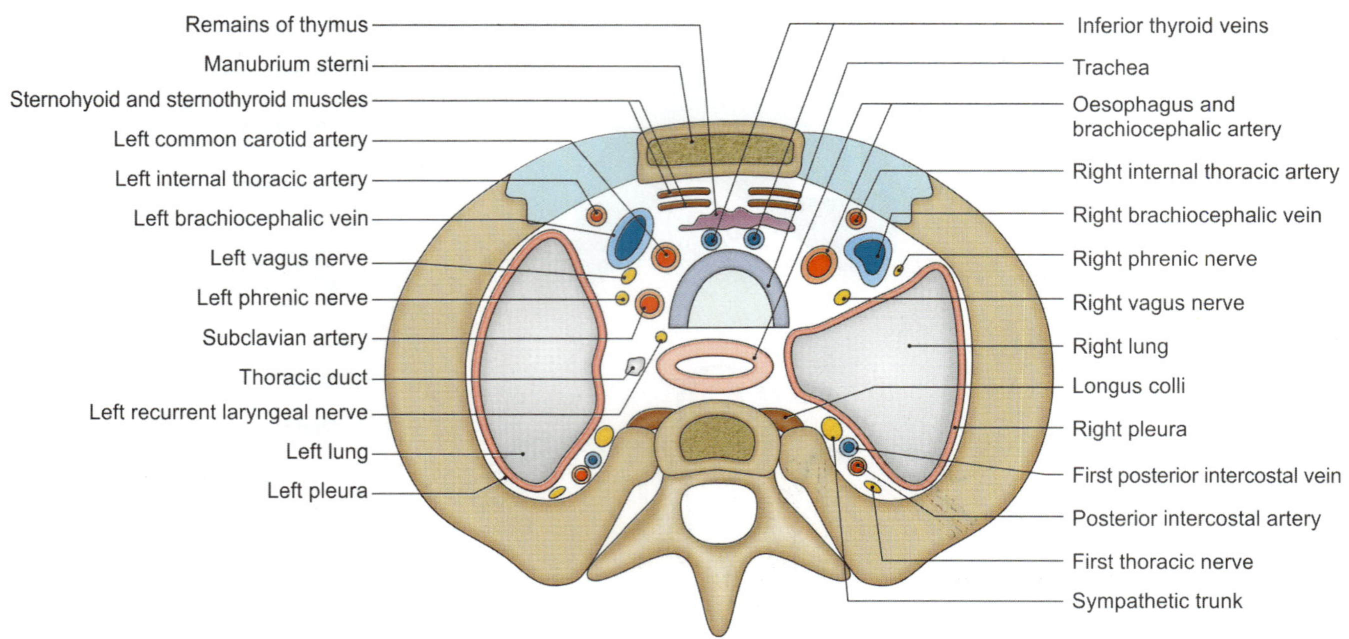

Fig. 39.6: Structures passing through the inlet of the thorax

Origin

The muscle fibres may be grouped into three parts—sternal, costal and lumbar.

The *sternal part* arises by two fleshy slips from the back of the xiphoid process.

The *costal part* arises from the inner surfaces of the cartilages and the adjacent parts of the lower six ribs on each side, interdigitating with the transversus abdominis.

The *lumbar part* arises from the medial and lateral lumbocostal arches and from the lumbar vertebrae by right and left *crura*.

a. The *medial lumbocostal arch* or medial arcuate ligament is a tendinous arch in the fascia covering the upper part of the psoas major. Laterally, it is attached to the front of the transverse process of vertebra L1.
b. The *lateral lumbocostal arch* or lateral arcuate ligament is a tendinous arch in the fascia covering the upper part of the quadratus lumborum. It is attached medially to the front of the transverse process of vertebra L1, and laterally to the lower border of the 12th rib.
c. The *right crus* is larger and stronger than the left crus, because it has to pull down the liver during each inspiration. It arises from the anterolateral surfaces of the bodies of the upper three lumbar vertebrae and the intervening intervertebral discs (Fig. 39.8).
d. The *left crus* arises from the corresponding parts of the upper two lumbar vertebrae. The medial margins of the two crura form a tendinous arc across the front of the aorta, called the *median arcuate ligament* (Fig. 39.7).

Muscle Fibres

1 From the circumferential origin described above, the fibres arch upwards and inwards to form the right and left domes. The right dome is higher than the left dome (Figs 39.9a and b). In full expiration, it reaches the level of the fourth intercostal space. The left dome reaches the fifth rib. The central tendon lies at the level of the lower end of the sternum at 6th costal cartilage. The downward concavity of the dome is occupied by the liver on the right side and by the fundus of the stomach on the left side.
2 The medial fibres of the right crus run upwards and to the left, and encircle the oesophagus.
3 In general, all fibres converge towards the central tendon for their insertion (Fig. 39.9a).

Insertion

The *central tendon* of the diaphragm lies below the pericardium and is fused to the latter. The tendon is *trilobar* in shape, made up of three leaflets. The middle leaflet is triangular in shape with its apex directed towards the xiphoid process. The right and left leaflets are tongue-shaped and curve laterally and backwards, the left being a little narrower than the right.

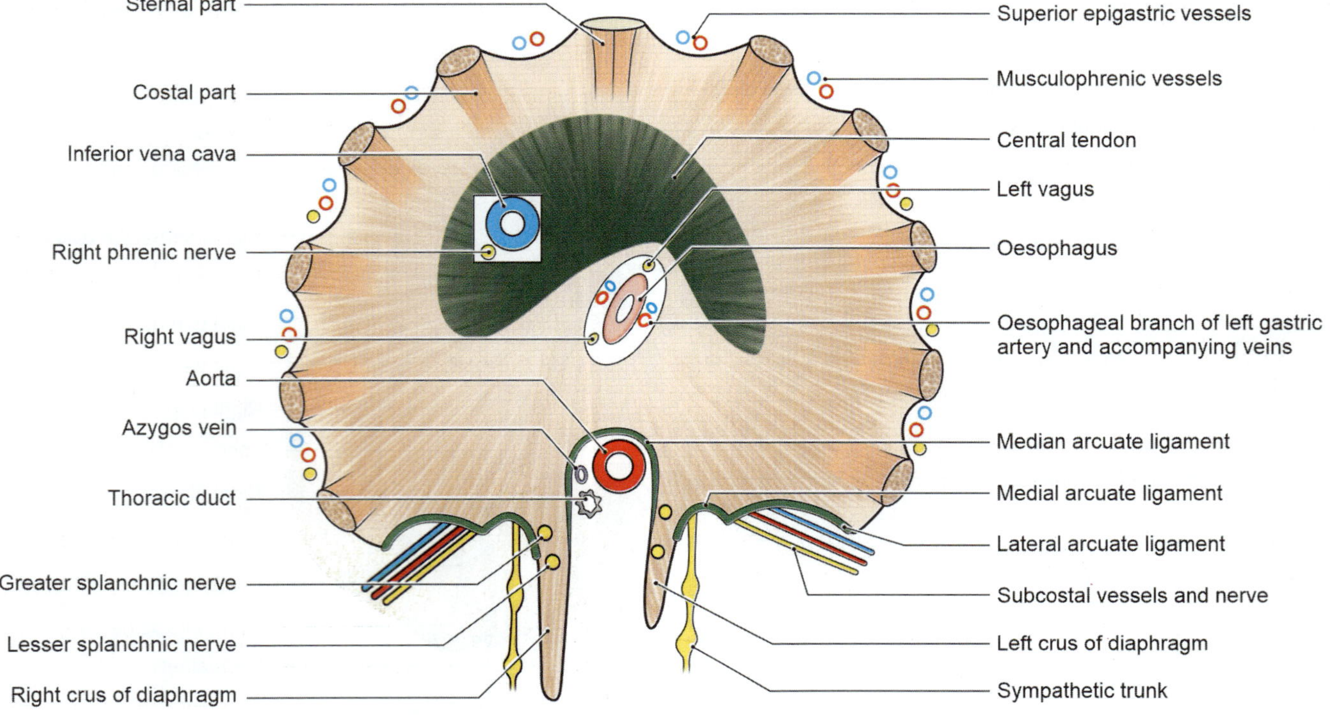

Fig. 39.7: The diaphragm as seen from below

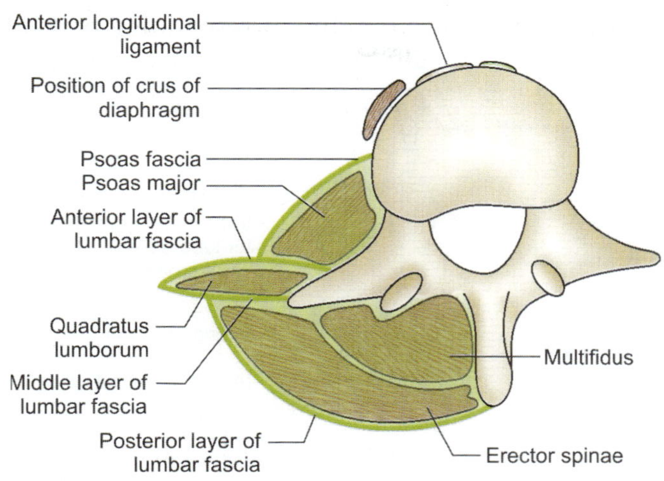

Fig. 39.8: Position of right crus of diaphragm on the third lumbar vertebra

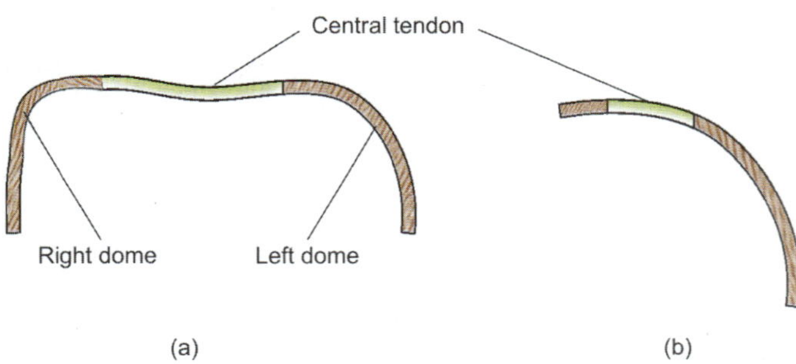

Fig. 39.9: Shape of the diaphragm: (a) Anteroposterior view shows the right and left domes, (b) in left lateral view, it resembles an inverted J

Structures Passing through the Diaphragm

There are three large, and several small, openings in the diaphragm which allow passage to structures from thorax to abdomen or *vice versa* (Fig. 39.10).

Large Openings in the Diaphragm

A. The *aortic opening* is osseoaponeurotic. It lies at the lower border of the twelfth thoracic vertebra. It transmits:
   i. Aorta
   ii. Thoracic duct
   iii. Azygos vein
B. The *oesophageal opening* lies in the muscular part of the diaphragm, at the level of the tenth thoracic vertebra. It transmits:
   i. Oesophagus
   ii. Gastric (vagus) nerves
   iii. Oesophageal branches of the left gastric artery, with some oesophageal veins that accompany the arteries.
C. The *vena caval opening* lies in the central tendon of the diaphragm at the level of the eighth thoracic vertebra. It transmits:

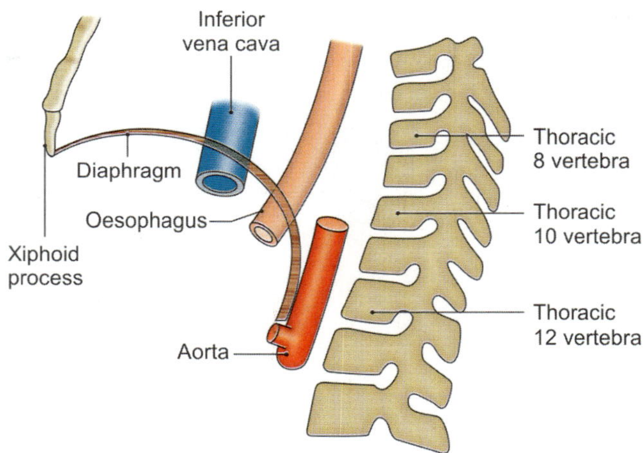

Fig. 39.10: Structures passing through the diaphragm

   i. The inferior vena cava.
   ii. Branches of the right phrenic nerve.

VERTEBRAL COLUMN

Vertebral Column as a Whole

The vertebral column is also called the spine, the spinal column, or back bone. It is the central axis of the body. It supports the body weight and transmits it to the ground through the lower limbs.

The vertebral column is made up of 33 vertebrae; seven cervical, twelve thoracic, five lumbar, five sacral and four coccygeal. In the thoracic, lumbar and sacral regions, the number of vertebrae corresponds to the number of spinal nerves, each nerve lying below the corresponding vertebra. In the cervical region, there are eight nerves, the upper seven lying above the corresponding vertebrae and the eighth below the seventh vertebra. In the coccygeal region, there is only one coccygeal nerve.

The length of the spine is about 70 cm in males and about 60 cm in females. The intervertebral discs contribute one-fifth of the length of the vertebral column.

Parts of a Typical Vertebra

A typical vertebra is made up of the following parts.

1. The *body* lies anteriorly. It is shaped like a short cylinder, being rounded from side to side and having flat upper and lower surfaces that are attached to those of adjoining vertebrae by intervertebral discs (Fig. 39.11).
2. The *pedicles:* Right and left pedicles are short rounded bars that project backwards, and somewhat laterally, from the posterior aspect of the body.
3. Each pedicle is continuous, posteromedially, with a vertical plate of bone called the *lamina*.

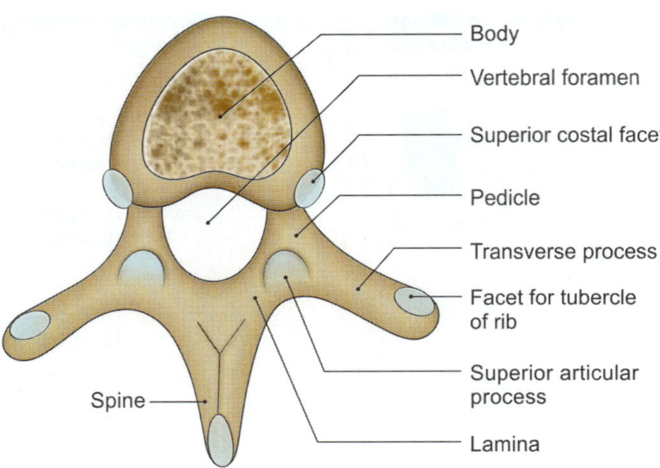

Fig. 39.11: Typical thoracic vertebra—superior aspect

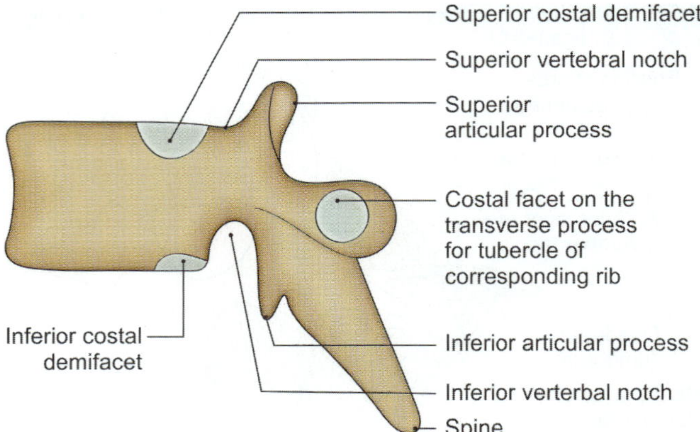

Fig. 39.12: Typical thoracic vertebra—lateral view

4 Bounded anteriorly by the posterior aspect of the body, on the sides by the pedicles, and behind by the lamina, there is a large *vertebral foramen.*

5 Passing backwards and usually downwards from the junction of the two laminae there is the spine or spinous process.

6 Passing laterally and usually somewhat downwards from the junction of each pedicle and the corresponding lamina, there is a *transverse process.* The spinous and transverse processes serve as levers for muscles acting on the vertebral column.

7 Projecting upwards from the junction of the pedicle and the lamina there is on either side, a *superior articular process;* and projecting downwards there is an *inferior articular process.*

8 The pedicle is much narrower in vertical diameter than the body and is attached nearer its upper border. As a result, there is a large *inferior vertebral notch* below the pedicle. Above the pedicle, there is a much shallower *superior vertebral notch.*

Thoracic Vertebrae

Identification

The thoracic vertebrae are identified by the presence of costal facets on the sides of the vertebral bodies. The costal facets may be two or only one on each side.

There are 12 thoracic vertebrae, out of which the second to eighth are typical, and the remaining five (first, ninth, tenth, eleventh and twelfth) are atypical.

Typical Thoracic Vertebra

A. The body is heart-shaped with roughly the same measurements from side to side and anteroposteriorly. On each side, it bears two costal demifacets. The *superior costal demifacet* is larger and placed on the upper border of the body near the pedicle. It articulates with the head of the numerically corresponding rib. The *inferior costal demifacet* is smaller and placed on the lower border in front of the inferior vertebral notch. It articulates with the next lower rib (Fig. 39.12).

B. *The vertebral foramen* is comparatively small and circular.

C. *The vertebral arch:*

1 The *pedicles* are directed straight backwards.

2 The *laminae* overlap each other from above.

3 The *superior articular processes* project upwards from the junction of the pedicles and laminae.

4 The *inferior articular processes* are fused to the laminae.

5 The *transverse processes*: The anterior surface of each process bears a facet near its tip, for articulation with the tubercle of the corresponding rib.

6 The *spine* is long, directed downwards and backwards. The fifth to ninth spines are the longest, more vertical and overlap each other. The upper and lower spines are less oblique in direction.

THORACIC WALL

The thoracic cage forms the skeletal framework of the wall of the thorax. The gaps between the ribs are called intercostal spaces. They are filled by the intercostal muscles and contain the intercostal nerves, vessels and lymphatics.

Intercostal Muscles

These are:

i. The external intercostal muscle.

ii. The internal intercostal muscle.

iii. The transversus thoracis muscle which is divisible into three parts, namely the subcostalis, the intercostalis intimi and the sternocostalis. The attachments of these muscles are given in Table 39.1.

Table 39.1: The attachments of the intercostal muscles (Fig. 39.10)

Muscle	*Origin*	*Insertion*
1. External intercostal	Lower border of the rib above the space	Outer lip of the upper border of the rib below
2. Internal intercostal	Floor of the costal groove of the rib above	Inner lip of the upper border of the rib below
3. Transversus thoracis		
(a) Subcostalis	Inner surface of the rib near the angle	Inner surface of two or three ribs below
(b) Intercostalis intimi	Middle two-fourths of the ridge above the costal groove	Inner lip of the upper border of the rib below
(c) Sternocostalis	• Lower one-third of the posterior surface of the body of the sternum • Posterior surface of the xiphoid	Costal cartilages of the 2nd to 6th ribs

Direction of Fibres

In the anterior part of the intercostal space:

1 The fibres of the external intercostal muscle run downwards, forwards and medially.
2 The fibres of the internal intercostal run downwards, backwards and laterally, i.e. at right angle to those of the external intercostal.
3 The fibres of the transversus thoracis run in the same direction as those of the internal intercostal (Fig. 39.13).

Nerve Supply

All intercostal muscles are supplied by the intercostal nerves of the spaces in which they lie.

Actions of the Intercostal Muscles

1 The main action of the intercostal muscles is to prevent intercostal spaces being drawn in during inspiration and from bulging outwards during expiration.
2 The external intercostals, interchondral portions of the internal intercostals elevate the ribs during inspiration.

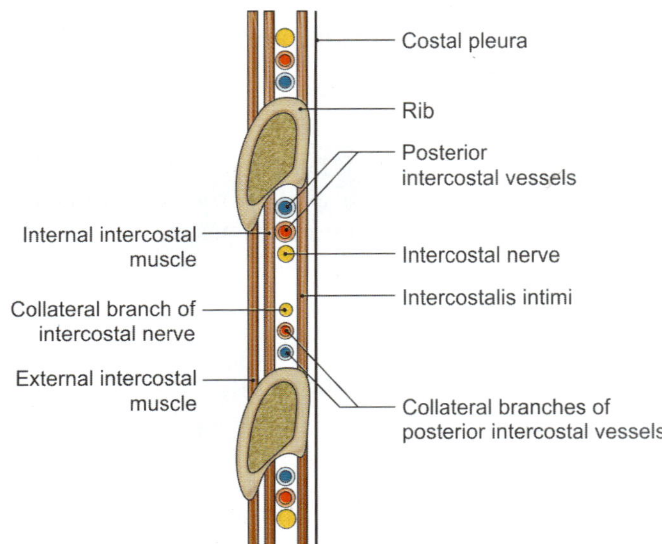

Fig. 39.13: Vertical section through an intercostal space

THE PLEURA

The spongy lungs occupying a major portion of thoracic cavity are enveloped in a serous cavity—the pleural cavity. There is always slight negative pressure in this cavity. During inspiration the pressure becomes more negative, and air is drawn into the lungs covered with its visceral and parietal layers. Visceral layer is inseparable from the lung and is supplied by the same arteries, veins and nerves as the lungs. In a similar manner, the parietal pleura follows the walls of the thoracic cavity with cervical, costal, diaphragmatic and mediastinal parts. Pleural cavity limits the expansion of the lungs (Fig. 39.14). There are two pleural sacs, one on either side of the mediastinum. Each pleural sac is invaginated from its medial side by the lung, so that it has an outer layer, the *parietal pleura,* and an inner layer, the *visceral* or *pulmonary pleura.*

Pulmonary Pleura

The serous layer of pulmonary pleura covers the surfaces and fissures of the lung.

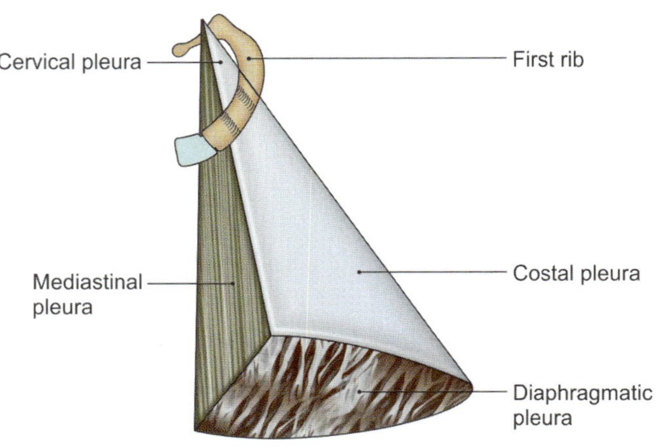

Fig. 39.14: The parietal pleura as a half cone

Parietal Pleura

The parietal pleura is thicker than the pulmonary pleura, and is subdivided into the following four parts.

i. Costal—lines thoracic wall
ii. Diaphragmatic—lines susperior aspect of diaphragm.
iii. Mediastinal—lines mediastinum and covers root of lung.
iv. Cervical—surrounds the apex of the lung (Fig. 39.14).

Recesses of Pleura

The *costomediastinal recess* lies anteriorly, behind the sternum and costal cartilages, between the costal and mediastinal pleurae, particularly in relation to the cardiac notch of the left lung (Fig. 39.15).

The *costodiaphragmatic recess* lies inferiorly between the costal and diaphragmatic pleura. Vertically, it measures about 5 cm, and extends from the eighth to tenth ribs along the midaxillary line.

The parietal pleura is pain sensitive. The costal and peripheral parts of the diaphragmatic pleurae are supplied by the intercostal nerves, and the mediastinal pleura and central part of the diaphragmatic pleurae by the phrenic nerves.

The pulmonary pleura is supplied by autonomic nerves. The sympathetic nerves are derived from second to fifth spinal segments while parasympathetic nerves are drawn from the vagus nerve. The nerves accompany the bronchial vessels. This part of the pleura is not sensitive to pain.

LUNGS

Introduction

The lungs are a pair of respiratory organs situated in the thoracic cavity. Each lung invaginates the corresponding pleural cavity. The right and left lungs are separated by the mediastinum.

The lungs are spongy in texture. In the young, the lungs are brown or grey in colour. Gradually, they become mottled black because of the deposition of inhaled carbon particles. The right lung weighs about 700 g; it is about 50 to 100 g heavier than the left lung.

Features

Each lung is conical in shape (Fig. 39.16). It has:

1 An apex at the upper end.
2 A base resting on the diaphragm.
3 Three borders, i.e. anterior, posterior and inferior.
4 Two surfaces, i.e. costal and medial. The medial surface is divided into vertebral and mediastinal parts.

The *anterior border* is very thin. It is shorter than the posterior border. On the right side, it is vertical and corresponds to the anterior or costomediastinal line of pleural reflection. The anterior border of the left lung shows a wide cardiac notch below the level of the fourth costal cartilage. The heart and pericardium are not covered by the lung in the region of this notch.

The *posterior border* is thick and ill defined. It corresponds to the medial margins of the heads of the ribs. It extends from the level of the seventh cervical spine to the tenth thoracic spine.

The *inferior border* separates the base from the costal and medial surfaces.

The *costal surface* is large and convex. It is in contact with the costal pleura and the overlying thoracic wall.

The *medial surface* is divided into a posterior or vertebral part, and an anterior or mediastinal part. The vertebral part is related to the vertebral bodies, intervertebral discs, the posterior intercostal vessels and the splanchnic nerves. The mediastinal part is related to the mediastinal septum, and shows a cardiac

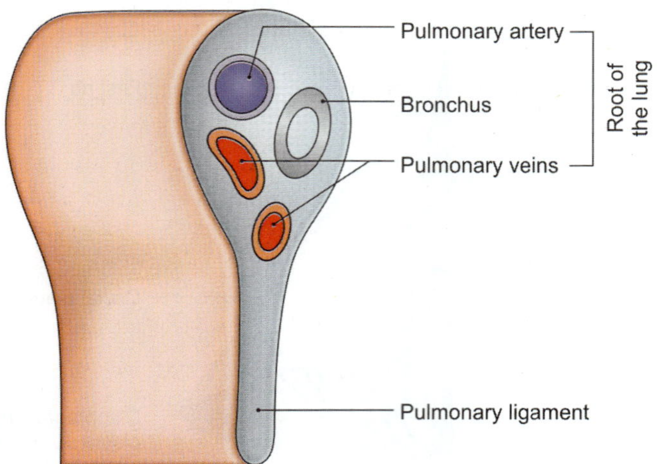

Fig. 39.15: Pleura at the root of the left lung

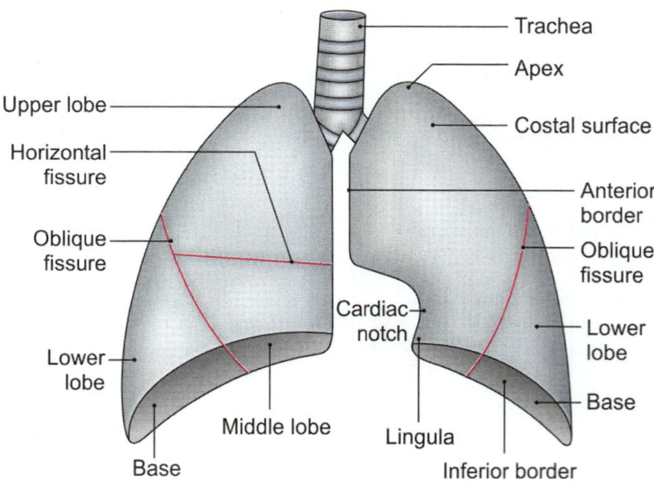

Fig. 39.16: The trachea and lungs as seen from the front

impression, the hilum and a number of other impressions of vessels and nerves.

Fissures and Lobes of the Lungs

The right lung is divided into 3 lobes (upper, middle and lower) by two fissures, oblique and horizontal. The left lung is divided into two lobes (upper and lower) by the oblique fissure (Fig. 39.16).

Root of the Lung

Root of the lung is a short, broad pedicle which connects the medial surface of the lung to the mediastinum. It is formed by structures which either enter or come out of the lung at the hilum. The roots of the lungs lie opposite the bodies of the fifth, sixth and seventh thoracic vertebrae.

Arrangement of Structures in the Root (Fig. 39.17)

A. From before backwards, tt is similar on the two sides.

1. Superior pulmonary vein
2. Pulmonary artery
3. Bronchus

B. From above downwards, it is different on the two sides.

	Right side	*Left side*
1	Eparterial bronchus	—
2	Pulmonary artery	Pulmonary artery
3	Hyparterial bronchus	Bronchus
4	Inferior pulmonary vein	Inferior pulmonary vein

Differences between the Right and Left Lungs

These are given in Table 39.2.

Table 39.2: Differences between the right and left lungs

Right lung	*Left lung*
1. It has 2 fissures and 3 lobes	1. It has only one fissure and 2 lobes
2. Anterior border is straight	2. Anterior border is interrupted by the cardiac notch
3. Larger and heavier, weighs about 700 g	3. Smaller and lighter, weighs about 600 g
4. Shorter and broader	4. Longer and narrower

Nerve Supply

1. Parasympathetic nerves are derived from the vagus. These fibres are:
   i. Motor to the bronchial muscles, and on stimulation cause bronchospasm.
   ii. Secretomotor to the mucous glands of the bronchial tree.
   iii. Sensory fibres are responsible for the stretch reflex of the lungs, and for the cough reflex.
2. Sympathetic nerves are derived from second to fifth spinal segments. These are inhibitory to the smooth muscle and glands of the bronchial tree. That is how sympathomimetic drugs, like adrenaline, cause bronchodilatation and relieve symptoms of bronchial asthma.

Both parasympathetic and sympathetic nerves first form anterior and posterior pulmonary plexuses situated in front of and behind the lung roots. From the plexuses nerves are distributed to the lungs along the blood vessels and bronchi.

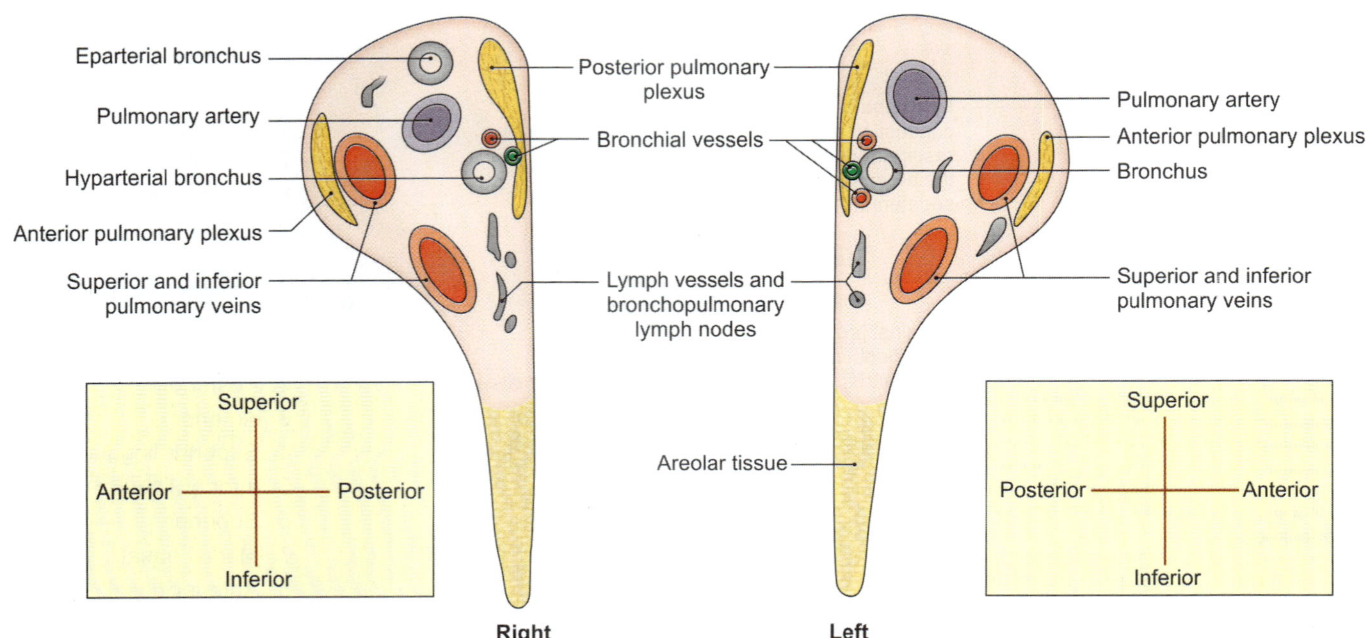

Fig. 39.17: Roots of the right and left lungs seen in section

Bronchial Tree

The *trachea* divides at the level of the lower border of the fourth or fifth thoracic vertebra into two primary principal bronchi, one for each lung. The *right principal bronchus* is 2.5 cm long. It is shorter, wider and more in line with the trachea than the left principal bronchus. Inhaled particles, therefore, tend to pass more frequently to the right lung, with the result that infections are more common on the right side than on the left.

The *left principal bronchus* is 5 cm. It is longer, narrower and more oblique than the right bronchus. Right bronchus makes an angle of 25° with tracheal bifurcation, while left bronchus makes an angle of 45° with the trachea.

Each principal bronchus enters the lung through the hilum, and divides into *secondary lobar bronchi,* one for each lobe of the lungs. Thus there are three lobar bronchi on the right side, and only two on the left side. Each lobar bronchus divides into *tertiary or segmental bronchi,* one for each bronchopulmonary segment; which are 10 on the right side and 10 on the left side. The segmental bronchi divide repeatedly to form very small branches called *terminal bronchioles.* Still smaller branches are called *respiratory bronchioles* (Fig. 39.18).

Each respiratory bronchiole aerates a small part of the lung known as a *pulmonary unit.* The respiratory bronchiole ends in microscopic passages which are termed:

i. Alveolar ducts.
ii. Atria.
iii. Air saccules.
iv. Pulmonary alveoli. Gaseous exchanges mainly take place in the alveoli.

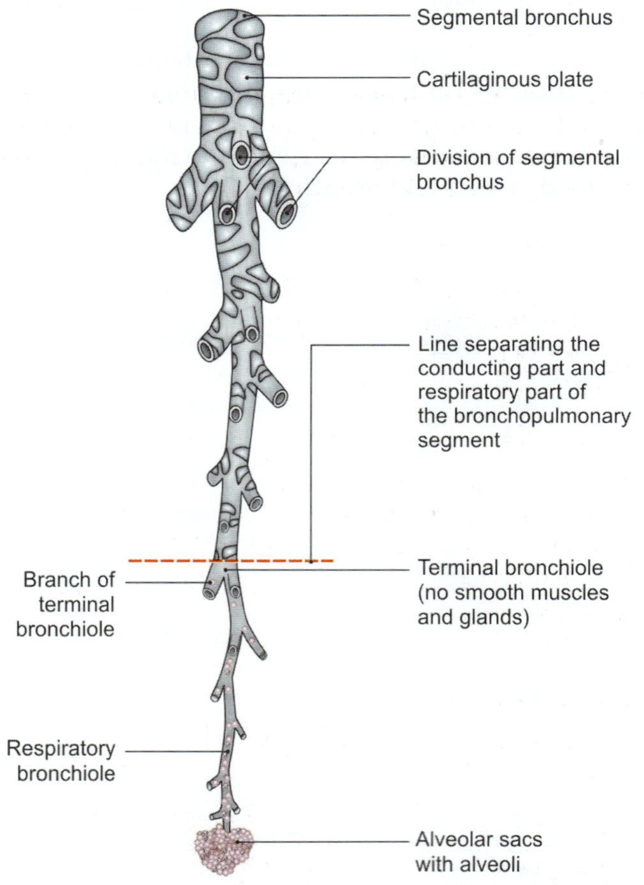

Fig. 39.18: A bronchopulmonary segment

Bronchopulmonary Segments

The most widely accepted classification of segments is given in Table 39.3. There are 10 segments on the right side and 10 on the left side (Fig. 39.19).

Definition

- These are well-defined anatomic, functional and surgical sectors of the lung.
- Each one is aerated by a tertiary or segmental bronchus.
- Each segment is pyramidal in shape with its apex directed towards the root of the lung (Fig. 39.18).

MEDIASTINUM

Introduction

Mediastinum is the middle space left in the thoracic cavity in between the lungs. Its most important content is the heart enclosed in the pericardium in the middle

Table 39.3: The bronchopulmonary segments

Lobes	*Segments*
Right lung	
A. Upper	1. Apical
	2. Posterior
	3. Anterior
B. Middle	4. Lateral
	5. Medial
C. Lower	6. Superior
	7. Medial basal
	8. Anterior basal
	9. Lateral basal
	10. Posterior basal
Left lung	
A. Upper	1. Apical
• Upper division	2. Posterior
	3. Anterior
• Lower division	4. Superior lingular
	5. Inferior lingular
B. Lower	6. Superior
	7. Medial basal
	8. Anterior basal
	9. Lateral basal
	10. Posterior basal

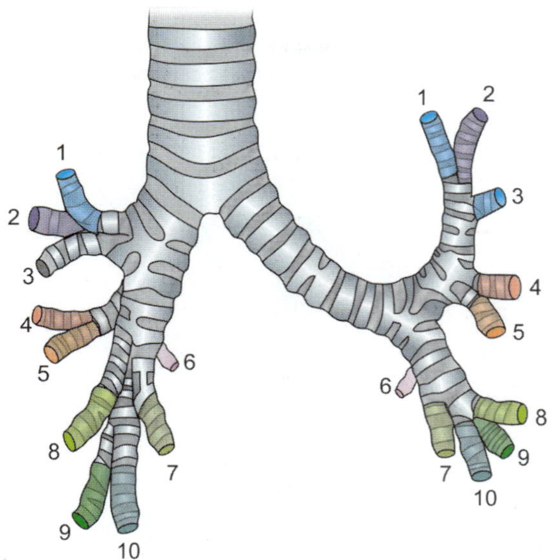

Fig. 39.19: Bronchopulmonary segments of the lungs (Table 39.3)

part of the inferior mediastinum or the middle mediastinum. Above it, lies superior mediastinum. Anterior and posterior to the heart are anterior mediastinum and posterior mediastinum respectively (Fig. 39.20).

Superior Mediastinum

Boundaries

- *Anteriorly*: Manubrium sterni
- *Posteriorly*: Upper four thoracic vertebrae
- *Superiorly*: Plane of the thoracic inlet
- *Inferiorly*: An imaginary plane passing through the sternal angle in front, and the lower border of the body of the fourth thoracic vertebra behind.
- *On each side*: Mediastinal pleura.

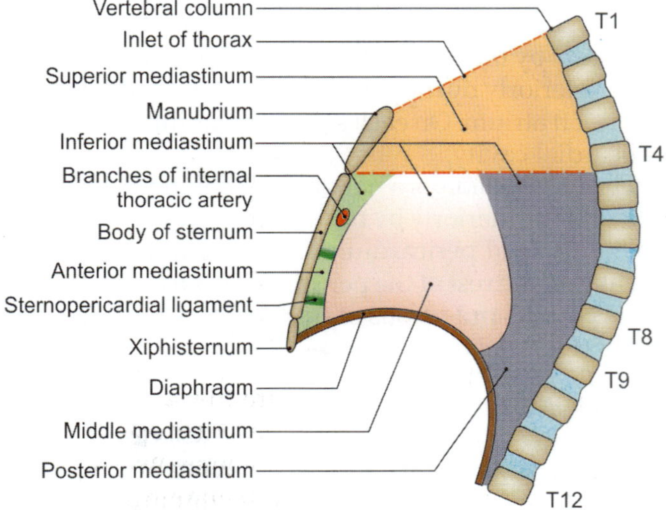

Fig. 39.20: Subdivisions of the mediastinum

Contents

1 Trachea and oesophagus.
2 *Muscles:* Origins of (i) sternohyoid, (ii) sternothyroid, (iii) lower ends of longus colli.
3 *Arteries:* (i) Arch of aorta, (ii) brachiocephalic artery, (iii) left common carotid artery, (iv) left subclavian artery (Fig. 39.21).
4 *Veins:* (i) Right and left brachiocephalic veins, (ii) upper half of the superior vena cava, (iii) left superior intercostal vein.
5 *Nerves:* (i) Vagus, (ii) phrenic, (iii) cardiac nerves of both sides, (iv) left recurrent laryngeal nerve.
6 Thymus.
7 Thoracic duct.
8 *Lymph nodes:* Paratracheal, brachiocephalic, and tracheobronchial.

Inferior Mediastinum

The inferior mediastinum is divided into anterior, middle and posterior mediastina. These are as follows.

Anterior Mediastinum

Anterior mediastinum is a very narrow space in front of the pericardium, overlapped by the thin anterior borders of both lungs. It is continuous through the superior mediastinum with the pretracheal space of the neck.

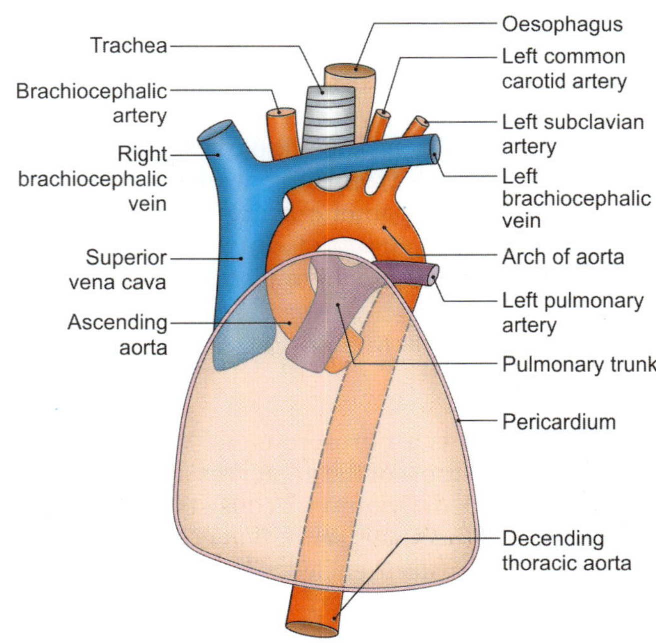

Fig. 39.21: Arrangement of the large structures in the superior mediastinum. Note the relationship of superior vena cava, ascending aorta and pulmonary trunk to each other in the middle mediastinum, i.e. within the pericardium. The bronchi are not shown

Middle Mediastinum

Middle mediastinum is occupied by the pericardium and its contents, along with the phrenic nerves and the pericardiaco-phrenic vessels.

Boundaries

- *Anteriorly*: Sternopericardial ligaments.
- *Posteriorly*: Oesophagus, descending thoracic aorta, azygos vein.
- *On each side*: Mediastinal pleura.

Contents

1 *Heart* enclosed in pericardium.
2 *Arteries:* (i) Ascending aorta, (ii) pulmonary trunk, (iii) two pulmonary arteries.
3 *Veins:* (i) Lower half of the superior vena cava, (ii) terminal part of the azygos vein, (iii) right and left pulmonary veins.
4 *Nerves:* (i) Phrenic, (ii) deep cardiac plexus.
5 *Lymph nodes:* Tracheobronchial nodes.
6 *Tubes:* (i) Bifurcation of trachea, (ii) the right and left principal bronchi.

Posterior Mediastinum

Boundaries

- *Anteriorly:* Pericardium
- *Posteriorly*: Lower eight thoracic vertebrae and intervening discs.
- *On each side*: Mediastinal pleura.

Contents

1 Oesophagus.
2 *Arteries:* Descending thoracic aorta and its branches.
3 *Veins:* (i) Azygos vein, (ii) hemiazygos vein, (iii) accessory hemiazygos vein.
4 *Nerves:* (i) Vagi, (ii) splanchnic nerves, greater, lesser and least, arising from the lower eight thoracic ganglia of the sympathetic chain.
5 *Lymph nodes and lymphatics:*
   i. Posterior mediastinal lymph nodes lying alongside the aorta.
   ii. The thoracic duct.

PERICARDIUM

The pericardium is a fibroserous sac which encloses the heart and the roots of the great vessels. It is situated in the middle mediastinum. It consists of the *fibrous pericardium* and the *serous pericardium* (Fig. 39.22).

Fibrous pericardium encloses the heart and fuses with the vessels which enter/leave the heart. Heart is situated within the fibrous and serous pericardial sacs. As heart develops, it invaginates itself into the serous sac, without causing any breach in its continuity, the last part to enter is the region of atria, from where the visceral pericardium is reflected as the parietal pericardium. Thus parietal layer of serous pericardium

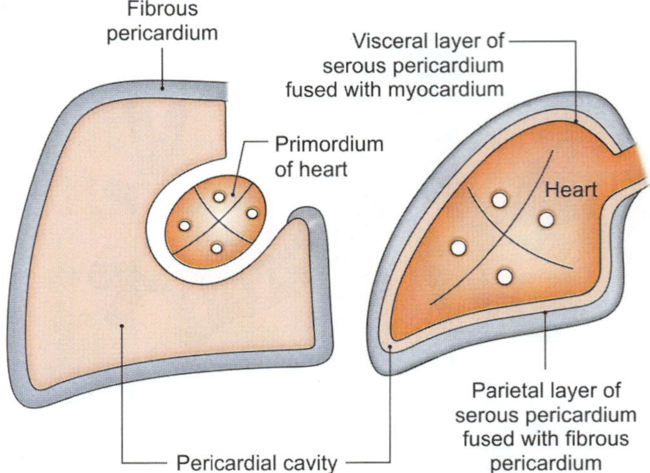

Fig. 39.22: Development of the layers of serous pericardium

gets adherent to the inner surface of fibrous pericardium, while the visceral layer of serous pericardium gets adherent to the outer layer of heart and forms its epicardium.

The *pericardial cavity* is a potential space between the parietal pericardium and the visceral pericardium. It contains only a thin film of serous fluid which lubricates the apposed surfaces and allows the heart to beat smoothly.

Contents of the Pericardium

i. Heart with cardiac vessels and nerves.
ii. Ascending aorta.
iii. Pulmonary trunk.
iv. Lower half of the superior vena cava.
v. Terminal part of the inferior vena cava.
vi. The terminal parts of the pulmonary veins.

Sinuses of Pericardium

The *transverse sinus* is a horizontal gap between the arterial and venous ends of the heart tube. It is bounded anteriorly by the ascending aorta and pulmonary trunk, and posteriorly by the superior vena cava and inferiorly by the left atrium. On each side, it opens into the general pericardial cavity.

The *oblique sinus* is a narrow gap behind the heart. It is bounded anteriorly by the left atrium, and posteriorly by the parietal pericardium. Below, and to the left, it opens into the rest of the pericardial cavity. The oblique sinus permits pulsations of the left atrium to take place freely (Fig. 39.23).

Nerve Supply

The fibrous and parietal pericardia are supplied by the phrenic nerve. They are sensitive to pain. The epicardium is supplied by autonomic nerves of the heart, and is not sensitive to pain. Pain of pericarditis

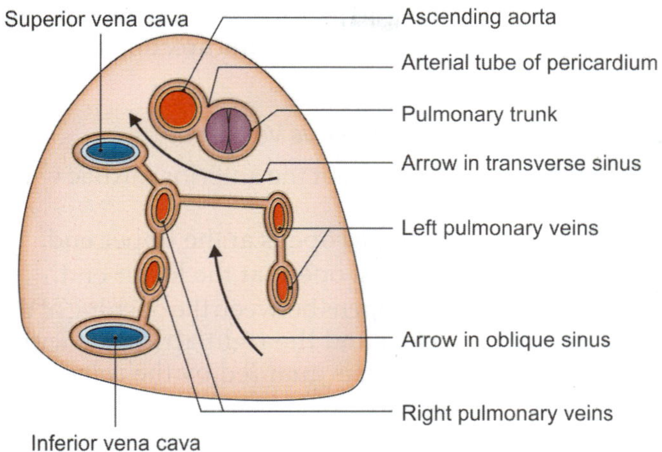

Fig. 39.23: The pericardial cavity seen after removal of the heart. Note the reflections of pericardium and the mode of formation of the transverse and oblique sinuses

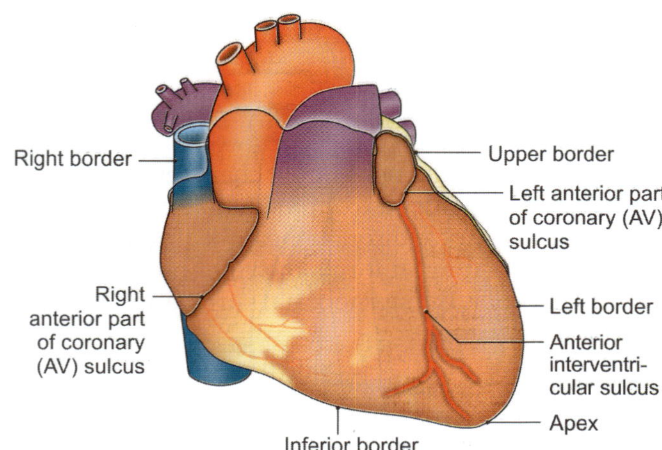

Fig. 39.24: Gross features: Sternocostal surface of heart

originates in the parietal pericardium alone. On the other hand, cardiac pain or angina originates in the cardiac muscle or in the vessels of the heart.

HEART

Introduction

The heart is a conical hollow muscular organ situated in the middle mediastinum. It is enclosed within the pericardium. It pumps blood to various parts of the body to meet their nutritive requirements. The Greek name for the heart is *cardia* from which we have the adjective *cardiac*. The Latin name for the heart is *cor* from which we have the adjective *coronary*.

The heart is placed obliquely behind the body of the sternum and adjoining parts of the costal cartilages, so that one-third of it lies to the right and two-thirds to the left of the median plane. The direction of blood flow, from atria to the ventricles, is downwards, forwards and to the left. The heart measures about 12 × 9 cm and weighs about 300 g in males and 250 g in females.

External Features

The human heart has four chambers. These are the right and left atria and the right and left ventricles.

The heart has an apex directed downwards, forwards and to the left, a base (or posterior surface) directed backwards; and anterior, inferior and left surfaces (Fig. 39.24).

Grooves or Sulci

The atria are separated from the ventricles by a circular *atrioventricular* or *coronary sulcus*. The *interatrial groove* is faintly visible posteriorly, while anteriorly it is hidden by the aorta and pulmonary trunk. The *anterior interventricular groove* is nearer to the left margin of the heart. It runs downwards and to the left. The *posterior interventricular groove* is situated on the diaphragmatic or inferior surface of the heart. It is nearer to the right margin of this surface. The two interventricular grooves meet at the inferior border near the apex.

Apex of the Heart

Apex of the heart is formed entirely by the left ventricle. It is directed downwards, forwards and to the left and is overlapped by the anterior border of the left lung. It is situated in the left fifth intercostal space 9 cm lateral to the midsternal line just medial to the midclavicular line. In the living subject, pulsations may be seen and felt over this region.

Base of the Heart

The base of the heart is also called its posterior surface. It is formed mainly by the left atrium and by a small part of the right atrium.

Borders of the Heart

The *upper border* is slightly oblique, and is formed by the two atria, chiefly the left atrium. The *right border* is more or less vertical and is formed by the right atrium. The *inferior border* is nearly horizontal and is formed mainly by the right ventricle. A small part of it near the apex is formed by left ventricle. The *left border* is oblique and curved. It is formed mainly by the left ventricle, and partly by the left auricle.

Surfaces of the Heart

The *anterior* or *sternocostal surface* is formed mainly by the right atrium and right ventricle, and partly by the left ventricle and left auricle.

The *inferior* or *diaphragmatic surface* rests on the central tendon of the diaphragm. It is formed in its left two-thirds by the left ventricle, and in its right one-third by the right ventricle. The *left surface* is formed mostly by the left ventricle, and at the upper end by the left auricle.

Right Atrium

The right atrium is the right upper chamber of the heart. It receives venous blood from the whole body, pumps it to the right ventricle through the right atrioventricular or tricuspid opening. It forms the right border, part of the upper border, the sternocostal surface and the base of the heart.

External Features

1 The chamber is elongated vertically, receiving the superior vena cava at the upper end and the inferior vena cava at the lower end.
2 The upper end is prolonged to the left to form the right *auricle.*
3 Along the right border of the atrium, there is a shallow vertical groove called the *sulcus terminalis.* It is produced by an internal muscular ridge called the *crista terminalis* (Fig. 39.25). The upper part of the sulcus contains the *sinuatrial* or *SA node* which acts as the pacemaker of the heart.

Tributaries or Inlets of the Right Atrium

i. Superior vena cava.
ii. Inferior vena cava.
iii. Coronary sinus.
iv. Anterior cardiac veins.
v. Venae cordis minimi (Thebesian veins).

Right Atrioventricular Orifice

Blood passes out of the right atrium through the right atrioventricular or tricuspid orifice and goes to the right ventricle. The tricuspid orifice is guarded by the tricuspid valve which maintains unidirectional flow of blood (Fig. 39.26).

Smooth Posterior Part or Sinus Venarum

Most of the tributaries except the anterior cardiac veins open into it.

i. The *superior vena cava* opens at the upper end.
ii. The *inferior vena cava* opens at the lower end.
iii. The *coronary sinus* opens between the opening of the inferior vena cava and the right atrioventricular orifice. The opening is guarded by the *valve of the coronary sinus.*
iv. The venae cordis minimi are numerous small veins present in the walls of all the four chambers. They open into the right atrium through small foramina.

Rough Anterior Part or Pectinate Part, Including the Auricle

It presents a series of transverse muscular ridges called *musculi pectinati.*

Interatrial Septum

1 It presents the *fossa ovalis,* a shallow saucer- shaped depression, in the lower part.
2 The *annulus ovalis* or *limbus fossa ovalis* is the prominent margin of the fossa ovalis.

RIGHT VENTRICLE

The right ventricle is a triangular chamber which receives blood from the right atrium and pumps it to the lungs through the pulmonary trunk and pulmonary arteries. It forms the inferior border and a large part of the sternocostal surface of the heart (Fig. 39.24).

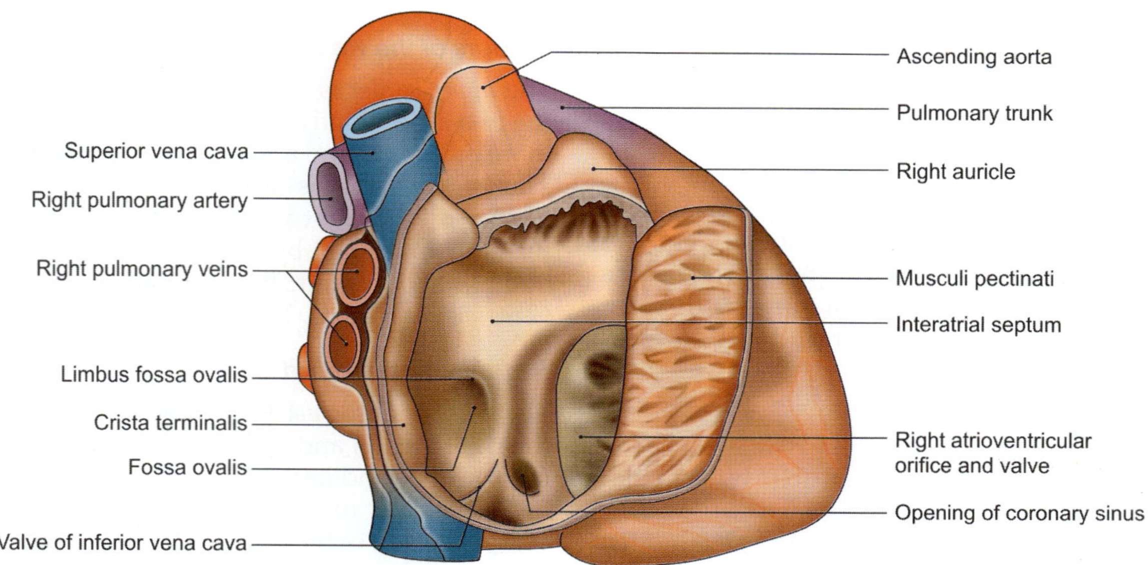

Fig. 39.25: Interior of the right atrium

Features

1 Externally, the right ventricle has two surfaces—anterior or sternocostal and inferior diaphragmatic.

2 The interior has two parts.

   i. The *inflowing part* is rough due to the presence of muscular ridges called *trabeculae carneae*.

   ii. The *outflowing part* or *infundibulum* is smooth and forms the upper conical part of the right ventricle which gives rise to the pulmonary trunk.

   The two parts are separated by a muscular ridge called the *supraventricular crest* or infundibuloventricular crest situated between the tricuspid and pulmonary orifices.

3 The interior shows two orifices:

   i. The right atrioventricular or tricuspid orifice, guarded by the tricuspid valve.

   ii. The pulmonary orifice guarded by the pulmonary valve (Fig. 39.26).

4 The interior of the inflowing part shows *trabeculae carneae* or muscular ridges of three types:

   i. *Ridges* or fixed elevations

   ii. *Bridges*

   iii. *Pillars* or papillary muscles with one end attached to the ventricular wall, and the other end connected to the cusps of the tricuspid valve by chordae tendinae. There are three papillary muscles in the right ventricle, anterior, posterior and septal. Each papillary muscle is attached by chordae to the contiguous sides of two cusps (Fig. 39.27).

5 The cavity of the right ventricle is crescentic in section because of the forward bulge of the interventricular septum (Fig. 39.26).

6 The wall of the right ventricle is thinner than that of the left ventricle in a ratio of 1:3.

LEFT ATRIUM

The left atrium is a quadrangular chamber situated posteriorly. Its appendage, the left auricle projects anteriorly to overlap the infundibulum of the right ventricle. The left atrium forms the left two-thirds of the base of the heart, the greater part of the upper border, parts of the sternocostal and left surfaces and of the left border. It receives oxygenated blood from the lungs through four pulmonary veins, and pumps it to the left ventricle through the left atrioventricular or bicuspid or mitral orifice which is guarded by the valve of the same name.

Features

1 The posterior surface of the atrium forms the anterior wall of the oblique sinus of pericardium.

2 The anterior wall of the atrium is formed by the interatrial septum.

3 Two pulmonary veins open into the atrium on each side of the posterior wall (4 veins).

4 The greater part of the interior of the atrium is smooth walled.

Left Ventricle

The left ventricle receives oxygenated blood from the left atrium and pumps it into the aorta. It forms the

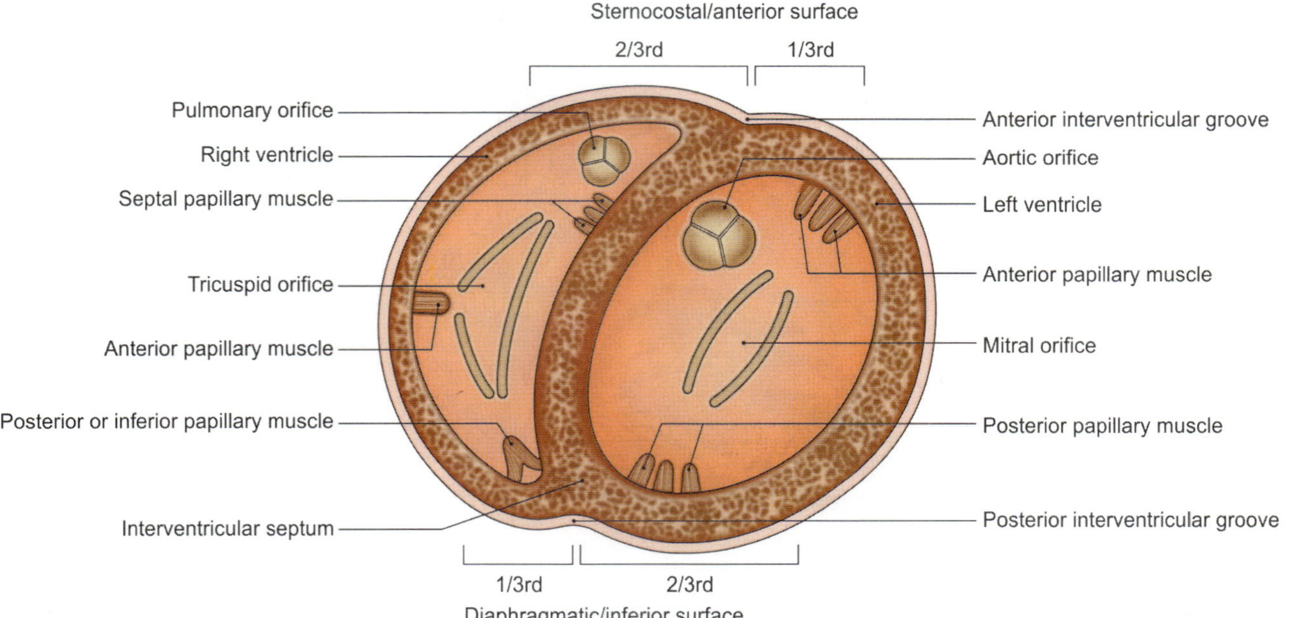

Fig. 39.26: Schematic transverse section through the ventricles of the heart showing the atrioventricular orifices, papillary muscles, and the pulmonary and aortic orifices

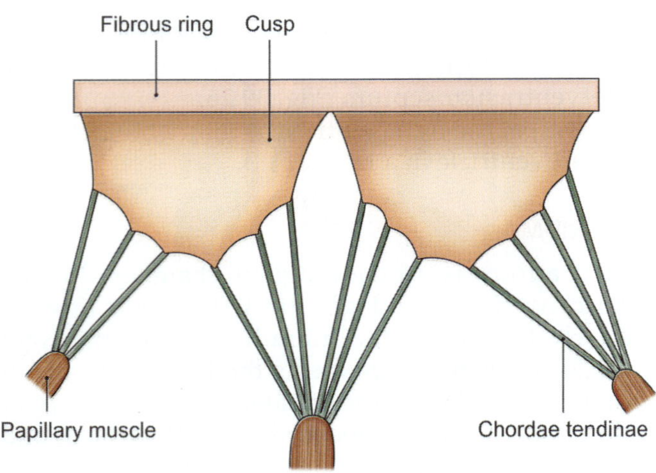

Fig. 39.27: Structure of an atrioventricular valve

apex of the heart, a part of the sternocostal surface, most of the left border left surface, and the left two-thirds of the diaphragmatic surface (Figs 39.24 and 39.28).

Features

1 Externally, the left ventricle has three surfaces—anterior or sternocostal, inferior or diaphragmatic, and left.
2 The interior is divisible into two parts:
   i. The lower rough part with trabeculae carneae develops from the primitive ventricle of the heart tube.
   ii. The upper smooth part or aortic vestibule gives origin to the ascending aorta.
3 The interior of the ventricle shows two orifices:
   i. The left atrioventricular or bicuspid or mitral orifice, guarded by the bicuspid or mitral valve.
   ii. The aortic orifice, guarded by the aortic valve (Fig. 39.28).
4 There are two well-developed papillary muscles—anterior and posterior. Chordae tendinae from both muscles are attached to both the cusps of the mitral valve.
5 The cavity of the left ventricle is circular in cross-section (Fig. 39.26).
6 The walls of the left ventricle are three times thicker than those of the right ventricle.

Valves of Heart

The valves of the heart maintain unidirectional flow of the blood and prevent its regurgitation in the opposite direction. There are two pairs of valves in the heart, a pair of atrioventricular valves and a pair of semilunar valves. The right atrioventricular valve is known as the tricuspid valve because it has three cusps. The left atrioventricular valve is known as the bicuspid valve because it has two cusps. It is also called the mitral valve.

The semilunar valves include the aortic and pulmonary valves, each having three semilunar cusps. The cusps are folds of endocardium, strengthened by an intervening layer of fibrous tissue.

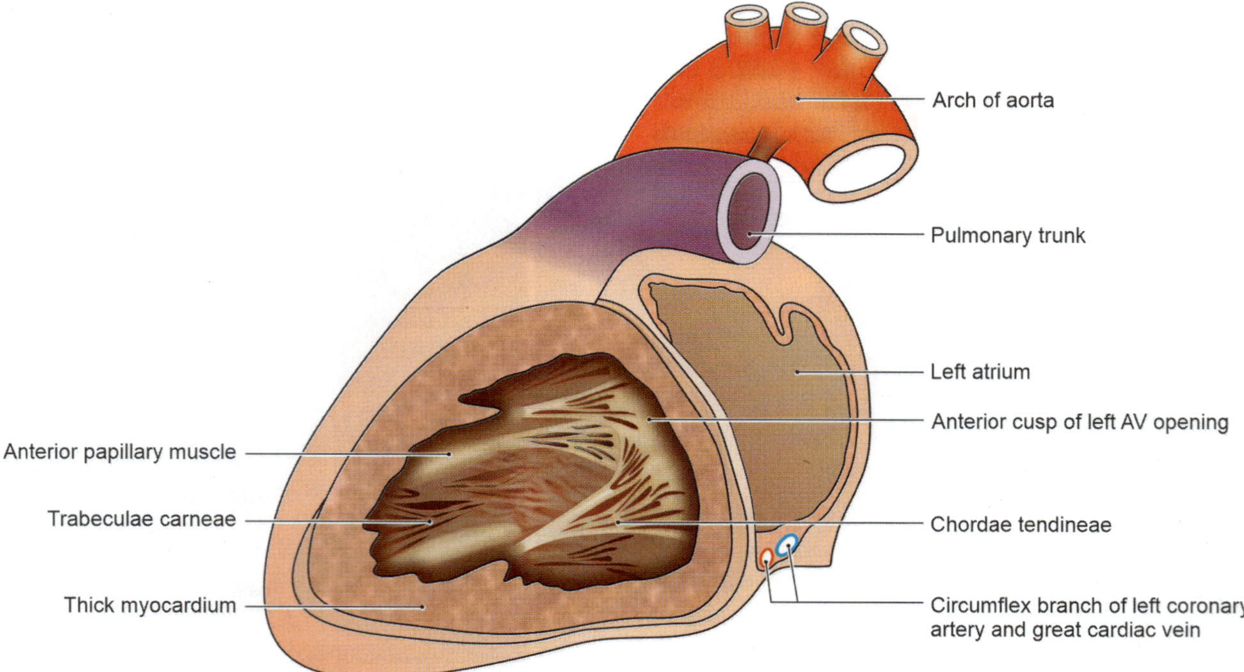

Fig. 39.28: Sagittal section of the heart. Note that the left atrium lies posterosuperior to the left ventricle, and that the mitral valve is placed almost vertically

Conducting System

The conducting system is made up of myocardium that is specialised for initiation and conduction of the cardiac impulse. Its fibres are finer than other myocardial fibres, and are completely cross-striated. The conducting system has the following parts.

1 *Sinuatrial node or SA node:* It is known as the 'pacemaker' of the heart. It generates an impulse at the rate of about 70/min and initiates the heartbeat.
2 *Atrioventricular node or AV node:* It is smaller than the SA node and is situated in the lower and dorsal part of the atrial septum just above the opening of the coronary sinus.
3 *Atrioventricular bundle or AV bundle or bundle of His:* It is the only muscular connection between the atrial and ventricular musculatures. It begins as the atrioventricular (AV) node, crosses AV ring and descends along the posteroinferior border of the membranous part of the ventricular septum. At the upper border of the muscular part of the septum, it divides into right and left branches.
4 *The right branch* of the AV bundle passes down the right side of the interventricular septum.
5 *The left branch* of the AV bundle descends on the left side of the interventricular septum and is distributed to the left ventricle after dividing into Purkinje fibres.
6 *The Purkinje fibres* form a subendocardial plexus. They are large pale fibres striated only at their margins. They usually possess double nuclei.

Arteries of the Heart

See Table 39.4.

Veins of the Heart

These are the great cardiac vein, the middle cardiac vein, the right marginal vein, the posterior vein of the left ventricle, the oblique vein of the left atrium, the right marginal vein, the anterior cardiac veins, and the venae cordis minimi (Fig. 39.30). All veins, except the

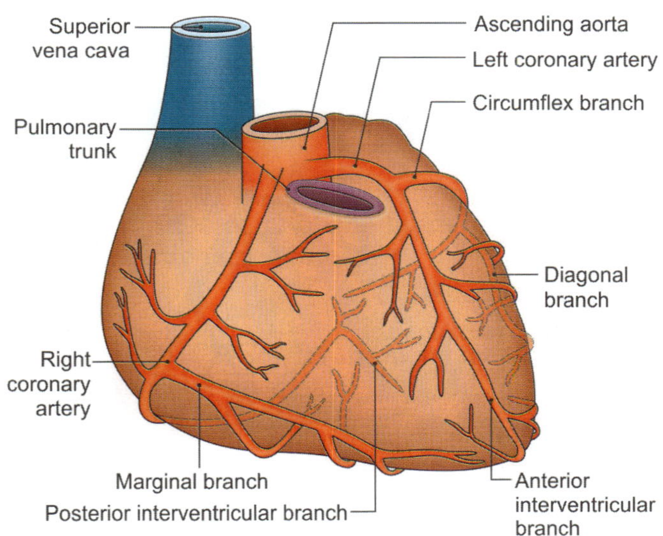

Fig. 39.29: Arterial supply of heart

last two, drain into the coronary sinus which opens into the right atrium. The anterior cardiac veins and the venae cordis minimi open directly into the right atrium.

Nerve Supply of Heart

Parasympathetic nerves reach the heart via the vagus. These are cardioinhibitory; on stimulation they slow down the heart rate. Sympathetic nerves are derived from the upper four to five thoracic segments of the spinal cord. These are cardio-acceleratory, and on stimulation they increase the heart rate, and also dilate the coronary arteries. Both parasympathetic and sympathetic nerves form the superficial and deep cardiac plexuses, the branches of which run along the coronary arteries to reach the myocardium (Fig. 39.30).

The *superficial cardiac plexus* is situated below the arch of the aorta in front of the right pulmonary artery. It is formed by:

i. The superior cervical cardiac branch of the left sympathetic chain.

Table 39.4: Comparison of right and left coronary arteries (Fig. 39.29)

Right coronary artery	*Left coronary artery*
1. Origin: Anterior aortic sinus of ascending aorta	1. Left posterior aortic sinus of ascending aorta
2. Course: Between pulmonary trunk and right auricle	2. Between pulmonary trunk and left auricle
3. Descends in atrioventricular groove on the right side	3. Descends in atrioventricular groove on the left side
4. Turns at the inferior border to run in posterior part of atrioventricular groove	4. Turns at left border to run in posterior part of atrioventricular groove. It is now called as circumflex branch
5. Termination: Ends by anastomosing with the circumflex branch of left coronary artery	5. Its circumflex branch ends by anastomosing with right coronary artery
6. Branches: To right atrium, right ventricle (marginal artery) and posterior interventricular branch for both ventricles and interventricular septum	6. Left atrium, left ventricle and anterior interventricular branch for both ventricles and interventricular septum Anterior interventricular branch ends by anastomosing with posterior interventricular branch

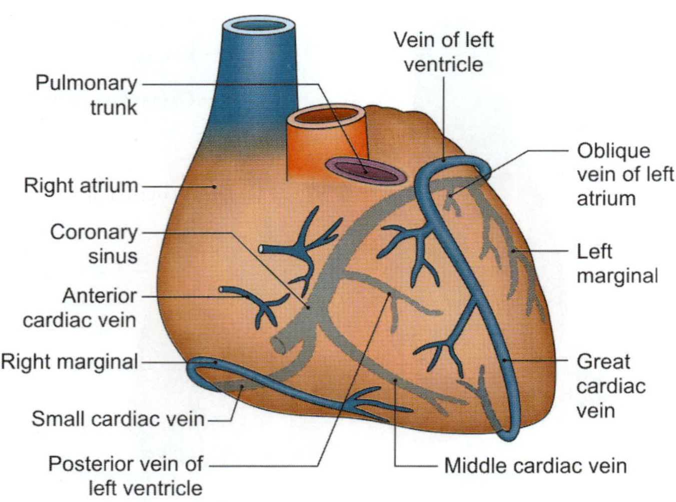

Fig. 39.30: Veins of the heart

ii. The inferior cervical cardiac branch of the left vagus nerve. It gives branches to the deep cardiac plexus, the right coronary artery, and to the left anterior pulmonary plexus.

The *deep cardiac plexus* is situated in front of the bifurcation of the trachea, and behind the arch of the aorta. It is formed by all the cardiac branches derived from all the cervical and upper thoracic ganglia of the sympathetic chain, and the cardiac branches of the vagus and recurrent laryngeal nerves, except those which form the superficial plexus. The right and left halves of the plexus distribute branches to the corresponding coronary and pulmonary plexuses. Separate branches are given to the atria.

TRACHEA

The trachea is a wide tube lying more or less in the midline, in the lower part of the neck and in the superior mediastinum. Its upper end is continuous with the lower end of the larynx. At its lower end the trachea ends by dividing into the right and left principal bronchi (Fig. 39.31).

The trachea is 10 to 15 cm in length. Its external diameter measures about 2 cm in males and about 1.5 cm in females.

The upper end of the trachea lies at the lower border of the cricoid cartilage, opposite the sixth cervical vertebra.

SUPERIOR VENA CAVA

Superior vena cava is a large venous channel which collects blood from the upper half of the body and drains it into the right atrium. It is formed by the union of the right and left brachiocephalic or innominate veins behind the lower border of the first right costal cartilage close to the sternum. Each brachiocephalic vein is formed behind the corresponding sternoclavicular joint by the union of the internal jugular and subclavian veins.

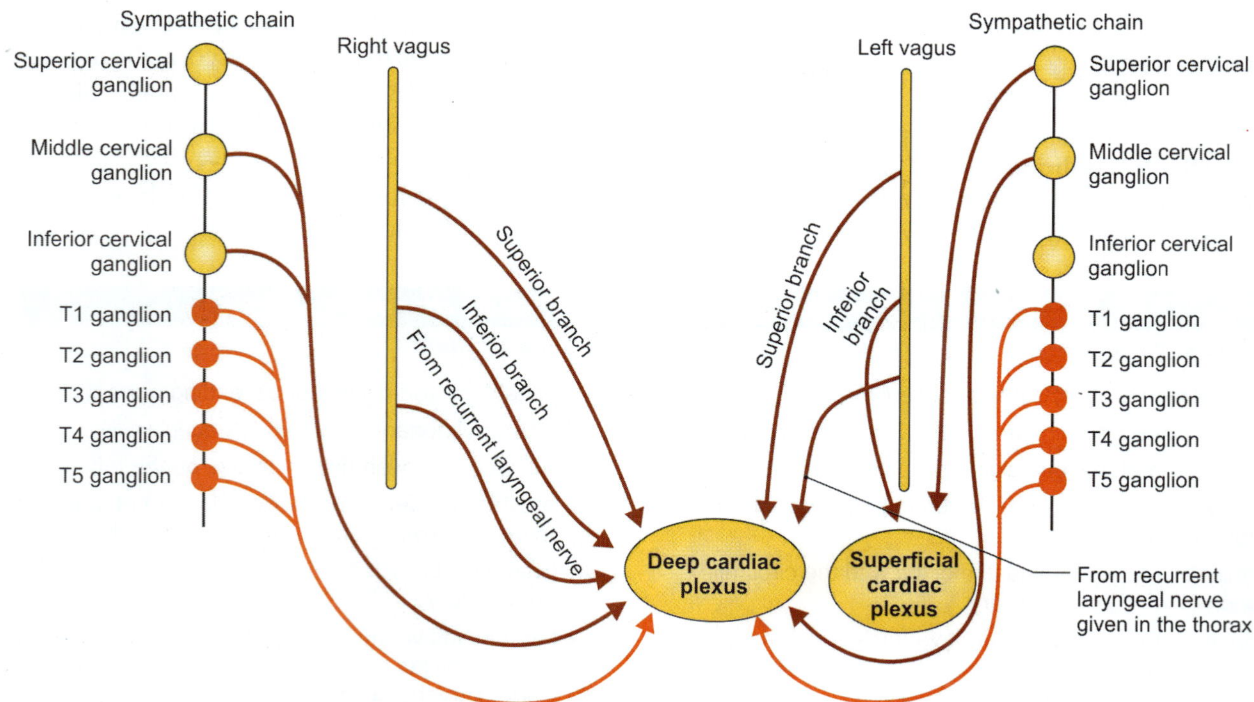

Fig. 39.31: Formation of superficial and deep cardiac plexuses

Course

The superior vena cava is about 7 cm long. It begins behind the lower border of the sternal end of the first right costal cartilage, pierces the pericardium opposite the second right costal cartilage, and terminates by opening into the upper part of the right atrium behind the third right costal cartilage (Fig. 39.32). It has no valves.

OESOPHAGUS

The oesophagus is a narrow muscular tube, forming the food passage between the pharynx and stomach. It extends from the lower part of the neck to the upper part of the abdomen (Fig. 39.33). The oesophagus is about 25 cm long.

The oesophagus begins in the neck at the lower border of the cricoid cartilage where it is continuous with the lower end of the pharynx.

It descends in front of the vertebral column through the superior and posterior parts of the mediastinum, and pierces the diaphragm at the level of tenth thoracic vertebra. It ends by opening into the stomach at its cardiac end at the level of eleventh thoracic vertebra.

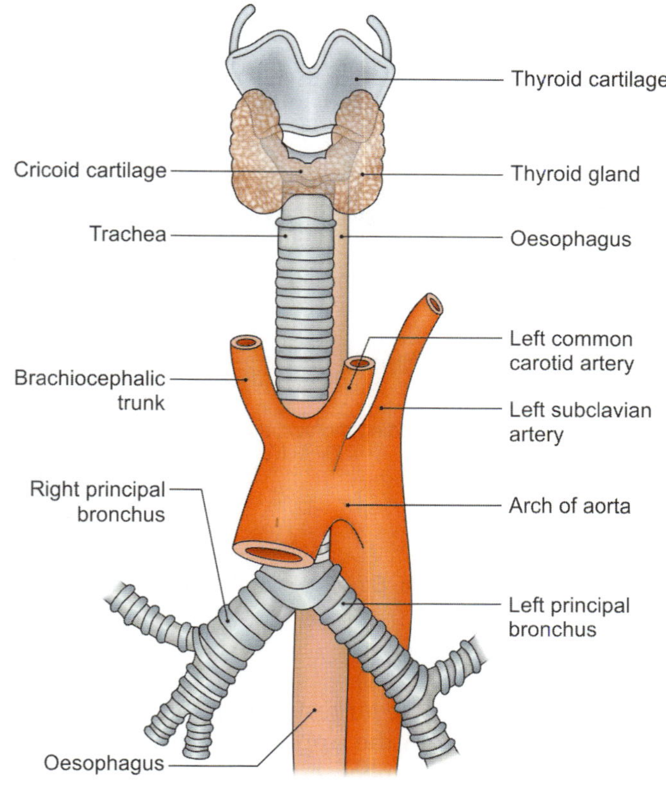

Fig. 39.32: Trachea and its relations

Curvatures

In general, the oesophagus is vertical, but shows slight curvatures in the following directions. There are two side to side curvatures, both towards the left (Fig. 39.34). One is at the root of the neck and the other near the lower end. It also has anteroposterior curvatures that correspond to the curvatures of the cervicothoracic spine.

Constrictions

1. At its beginning, 15 cm from the incisor teeth.
2. Where it is crossed by the aortic arch, 22.5 cm from the incisor teeth.
3. Where it is crossed by the left bronchus, 27.5 cm from the incisor teeth.
4. Where it pierces the diaphragm, 37.5 cm from the incisor teeth.

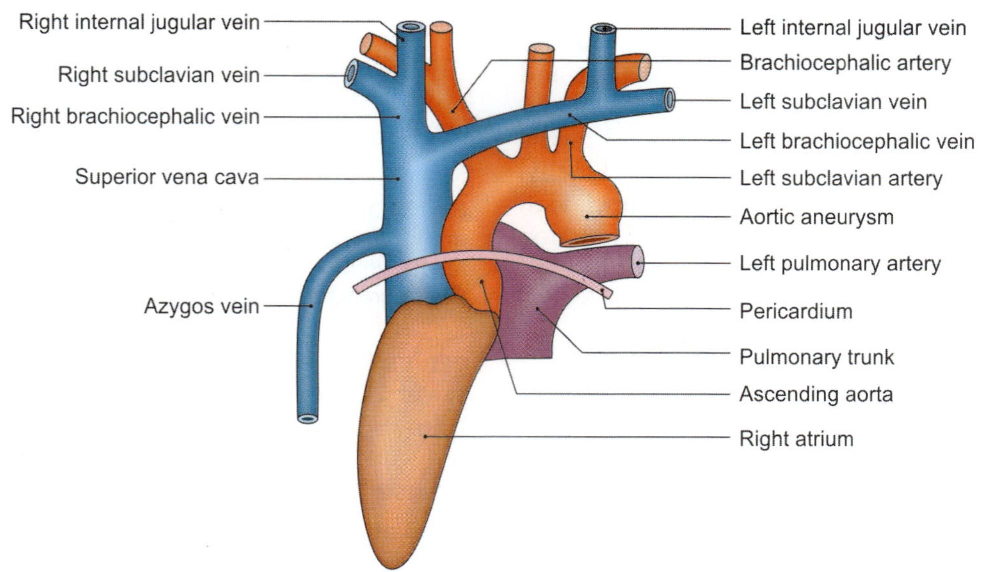

Fig. 39.33: The superior vena cava and its relations

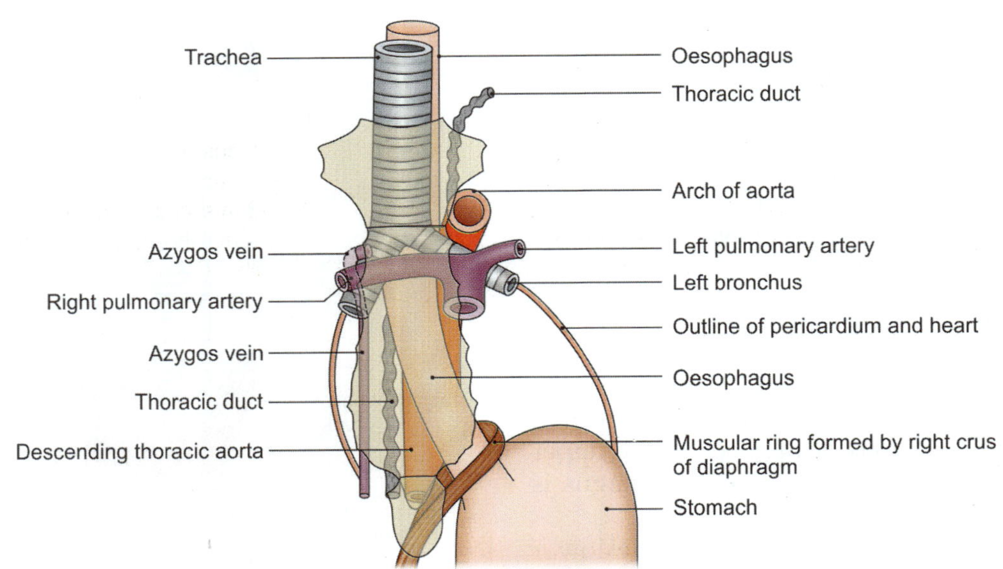

Fig. 39.34: Structures in the posterior mediastinum seen after removal of the heart and pericardium

THORACIC DUCT

The thoracic duct is the largest lymphatic vessel in the body. It extends from the upper part of the abdomen to the lower part of the neck, crossing the posterior and superior parts of the mediastinum. It is about 45 cm long. It has a beaded appearance because of the presence of many valves in its lumen (Figs 39.34 and 39.35).

Course

The thoracic duct begins as a continuation of the upper end of the cisterna chyli near the lower border of the twelfth thoracic vertebra and enters the thorax through the aortic opening of the diaphragm.

It then ascends through the posterior mediastinum crossing from the right side to the left at the level of the fifth thoracic vertebra. It then runs through the superior mediastinum along the edge of the oesophagus and reaches the neck.

In the neck, it arches laterally at the level of the transverse process of seventh cervical vertebra. Finally, it descends in front of the first part of the left subclavian artery and ends by opening into the angle of junction between the left subclavian and left internal jugular veins. **Arteries of thorax** are described in Table 39.5.

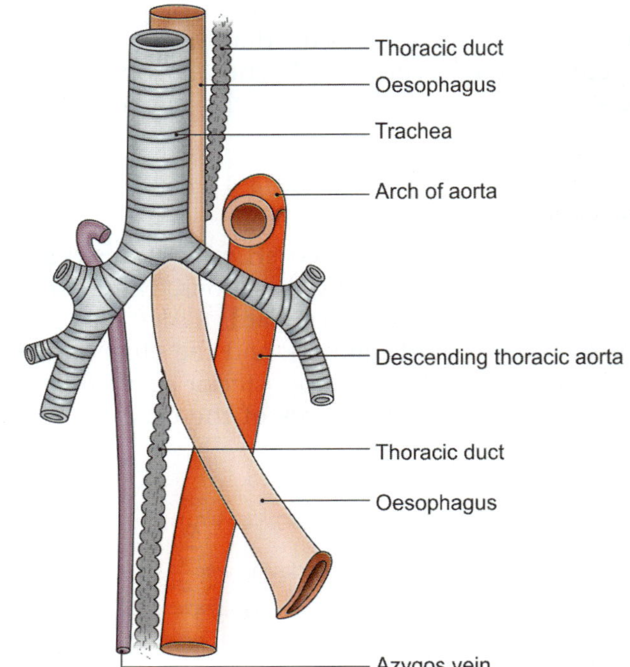

Fig. 39.35: Structures in the posterior part of the superior mediastinum, and their continuation into the posterior mediastinum. Note the relationship of the arch of the aorta to the left bronchus, and that of the azygos vein to the right bronchus

TYPICAL INTERCOSTAL NERVE

Typical intercostal nerves are any of the nerves belonging to 3rd to 6th intercostal spaces.

Beginning

Typical thoracic spinal nerve after it has given off dorsal primary ramus or dorsal ramus is called the intercostal nerve. It runs in the intercostal space, i.e. between the lower border of rib above and upper border of rib below.

Course

Typical intercostal nerve enters the posterior part of intercostal space by passing behind the posterior intercostal vessels. So the intercostal nerve lies lowest in

Table 39.5: Arteries of thorax

Artery	*Origin, course and termination*	*Area of distribution*
INTERNAL THORACIC (Fig. 39.37)	Arises from inferior aspect of 1st part of subclavian artery. Its origin lies 2 cm above the sternal end of the clavicle. It runs downwards, forwards and medially behind the clavicle and behind the 1–6 costal cartilages and 1–5 intercostal spaces to terminate in the 6th intercostal space by dividing into superior epigastric and musculophrenic arteries	It supplies pericardium, thymus, upper six intercostal spaces in their anterior parts, mammary gland, rectus sheath and also 7–9 intercostal spaces. Thus it supplies anterior thoracic and anterior abdominal walls from the clavicle to the umbilicus
ASCENDING AORTA (FIg. 39.21)	Arises from the upper end of left ventricle. It is about 5 cm long and is enclosed in the pericardium. It runs upwards, forwards and to the right and continues as the arch of aorta at the sternal end of upper border of 2nd right costal cartilage. At the root of aorta, there are three dilatations of the vessel wall called the aortic sinuses. These are anterior, left posterior and right posterior	Supplies the heart musculature with the help of right coronary and left coronary arteries, described in Table 39.4.
ARCH OF AORTA (Fig. 39.21)	It begins behind the upper border of 2nd right sternochondral joint. Runs upwards, backwards and to left across the left side of bifurcation of trachea. Then it passes behind the left bronchus and on the left side of of body of T4 vertebra by becoming continuous with the descending thoracic aorta	Through its three branches namely brachiocephalic, left common carotid and left subclavian arteries, arch of aorta supplies part of brain, head, neck and upper limb
Brachiocephalic artery	1st branch of arch of aorta. Runs upwards and soon divides into right common carotid and right subclavian arteries	Through these two branches part of the right half of brain, head, neck are supplied. The distribution of 2 branches on right side is same as on the left side
Left common carotid artery	It runs upwards on the left side of trachea till the upper border of thyroid cartilage. The artery ends by dividing into internal carotid and external carotid arteries	The two branches supply brain, structures in the head and neck
Left subclavian artery	It is the last branch of arch of aorta. Runs to left in the root of neck behind scalenus anterior muscle, then on the upper surface of 1st rib. At the outer border of 1st rib, it continues as the axillary artery	Gives branches which supply part of brain, part of thyroid gland, muscles around scapula, 1st and 2nd posterior intercostal spaces
Descending thoracic aorta (Figs 39.21 to 39.35)	Begins on the left side of the lower border of body of T4 vertebra. Descends with inclination to right and ends at the lower border of T12 vertebra by continuing as abdominal aorta	3–11 posterior intercostal spaces, subcostal area, lung tissue, oesophagus, pericardium, mediastinum and diaphragm

the neurovascular bundle. The order from above downwards is vein, artery and nerve (VAN) (Fig. 39.13). At first the bundle runs between posterior intercostal membrane and subcostalis, then between inner intercostal and innermost intercostal and lastly between inner intercostal and sternocostalis muscles.

At the anterior end of intercostal space, the intercostal nerve passes in front of internal thoracic vessels, pierces internal intercostal muscle and anterior intercostal membrane to continue as anterior cutaneous branch which ends by dividing into medial and lateral cutaneous branches.

Branches

1 Communicating branches to the sympathetic ganglion close to the beginning of ventral ramus. The anterior ramus containing sympathetic fibres from lateral horn of spinal cord gives off a white ramus communicans to the sympathetic ganglion. These fibres get relayed in the ganglion. Some of these relayed fibres pass via grey ramus communicans to ventral ramus. Few pass backwards in the dorsal ramus and rest pass through the ventral ramus. These sympathetic fibres are sudomotor, pilomotor and vasomotor to the skin and vasodilator to the skeletal vessels.
2 Before the angle, nerve gives a collateral branch that runs along the upper border of lower rib. This branch supplies intercostal muscles, costal pleura and periosteum of the rib (Fig. 39.13).
3 Lateral cutaneous branch arises along the midaxillary line. It divides into anterior and posterior branches.

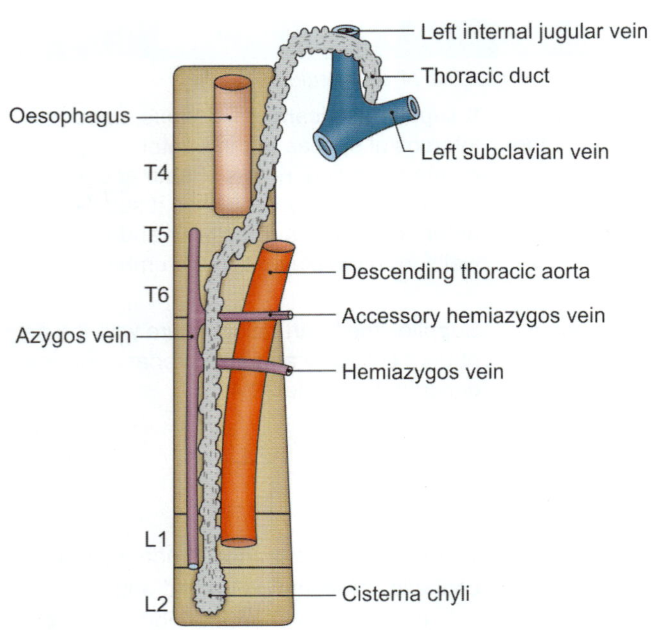

Fig. 39.36: The course of the thoracic duct

4 The nerve keeps giving muscular, periosteal and branches to the costal pleura during its course.
5 Anterior cutaneous branch is the terminal branch of the nerve.

ATYPICAL INTERCOSTAL NERVES

The thoracic spinal nerves which do not follow absolutely thoracic course are designated as atypical intercostal nerves. Thus intercostal one, two, are atypical as these two nerves partly supply the upper limb.

The first thoracic nerve entirely joins the brachial plexus as its last rami or root. It gives no contribution to the first intercostal space. That is why the nerve supply of skin of first intercostal space is from the supraclavicular nerves (C3, C4).

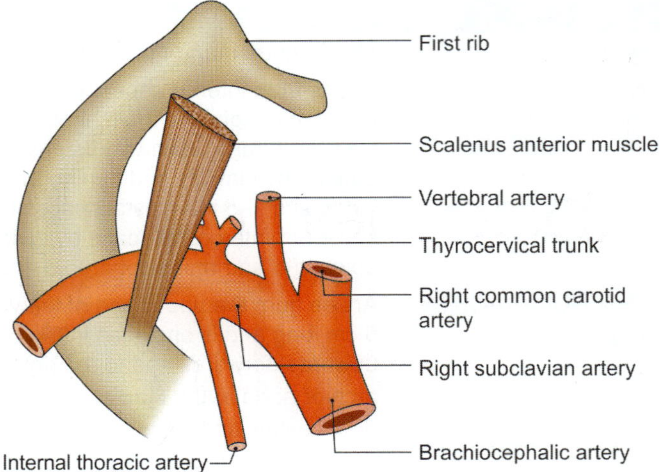

Fig. 39.37: The origin of the internal thoracic artery from the first part of the subclavian artery

The second thoracic or second intercostal nerve runs in the second intercostal space. But its lateral cutaneous branch as intercostobrachial nerve is rather big and it supplies skin of the axilla as well. Third to sixth intercostal nerves are typical.

Also seventh, eight, ninth, tenth, eleventh intercostal nerves are atypical, as these course partly through thoracic wall and partly through anterolateral abdominal wall. Lastly the twelfth thoracic is known as subcostal nerve. It also passes through the anterolateral abdominal muscles. These nerves supply, parietal peritoneum, muscles and overlying skin.

Chapter 40

Abdomen and Pelvis

"Man may be the captain of his fate, but is also the victim of his blood sugar."
—Anonymous

Abdominal cavity including the pelvic cavity is the largest cavity of the human body. It only has five lumbar vertebrae and the bony pelvis as its own bones.

Viscera of abdomen also lie in the lower part of the thoracic cavity, separate from heart and lungs by the thoracoabdominal diaphragm.

Abdominal cavity is supported by layered muscles of the anterolateral abdominal wall (Table 40.1) and muscles of posterior abdominal walls (Table 40.2). The muscles have been put in Figs 40.1 to 40.5.

RECTUS SHEATH

Definition

This is an aponeurotic sheath covering the rectus abdominis. It has two walls—anterior and posterior.

Formation

Details about the formation of the walls are as follows

Above the costal margin (Fig. 40.6a):

Anterior wall: External oblique aponeurosis.

Posterior wall: It is deficient; the rectus muscle rests directly on the 5th, 6th and 7th costal cartilages.

Between the costal margin and the arcuate line (midway between umbilicus and pubic symphysis):

Anterior wall:

1 External oblique aponeurosis.
2 Anterior lamina of the aponeurosis of the internal oblique.

Posterior wall:

1 Posterior lamina of the aponeurosis of the internal oblique.

Table 40.1: Muscles of anterolateral abdominal wall

Name	*Origin*	*Insertion*	*Nerve supply*	*Action*
External oblique (Fig. 40.1)	Middle of outer surfaces of 5th–12th i.e., lower eight ribs	Xiphoid process, linea alba, pubic tubercle, iliac crest	Th 7th–Th 12th nerves iliohypo-gastric and ilioinguinal nerves	Supports abdominal contents; in flexion and rotation of trunk. Assists in micturition, defaecation,parturition and vomiting. Active during expiration.
Internal oblique (Fig. 40.2)	Lumbar fascia, iliac crest, lateral two-thirds of inguinal ligament	7–12 ribs and costal cartilages, xiphoid process, linea alba, symphysis pubis	Same as above	Same as above
Transversus abdominis (Fig. 40.3)	Inner aspects of 7th–12th costal cartillages, lumbar fascia, iliac crest, lateral one-third of inguinal ligament	Xiphoid process, linea alba, symphysis pubis	Same as above	Compresses abdominal contents
Rectus abdominis (Fig. 40.4)	Symphysis pubis and pubic crest	Fifth, sixth, and seventh costal cartilages	Th7–Th12 nerves	Flexes vertebral column

Table 40.2: Muscles of posterior abdominal wall

Name	*Origin*	*Insertion*	*Nerve supply*	*Action*
Psoas major (Fig. 40.5)	Transverse processes, bodies, and intervertebral discs of T12, L1–L5 vertebrae	With iliacus into lesser trochanter of femur	Lumbar plexus. Ventral rami of L1–L4 nerves	Flexes thigh on trunk. If thigh is fixed, it flexes trunk on thigh
Quadratus lumborum	Iliac crest, tips of transverse processes of lumbar vertebrae	Anterior aspect of twelfth rib	Same as above	Fixes twelfth rib during inspiration: laterally rotate lumbar vertebrae; flexes vertebral column to same side
Iliacus	Iliac fossa	With psoas major into lesser trochanter of femur	Femoral nerve	Flexes thigh on trunk. If thigh is fixed, it flexes the trunk on the thigh

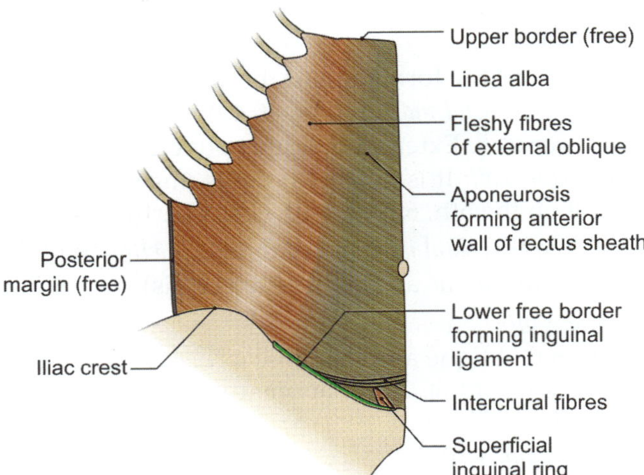

Fig. 40.1: External oblique muscle of the abdomen

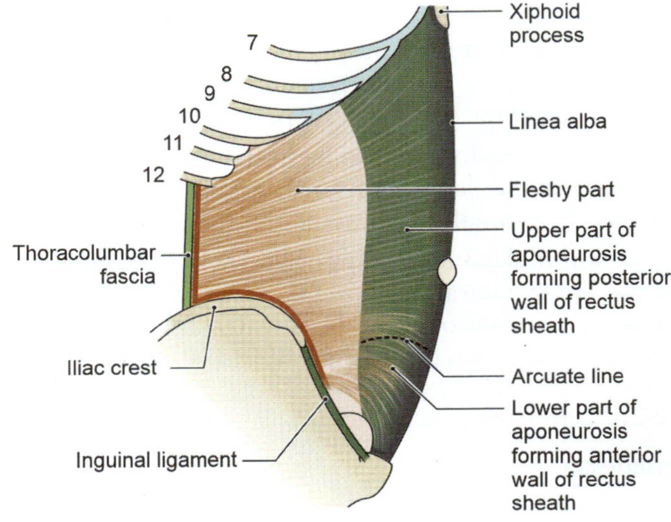

Fig. 40.3: Transversus abdominis muscle

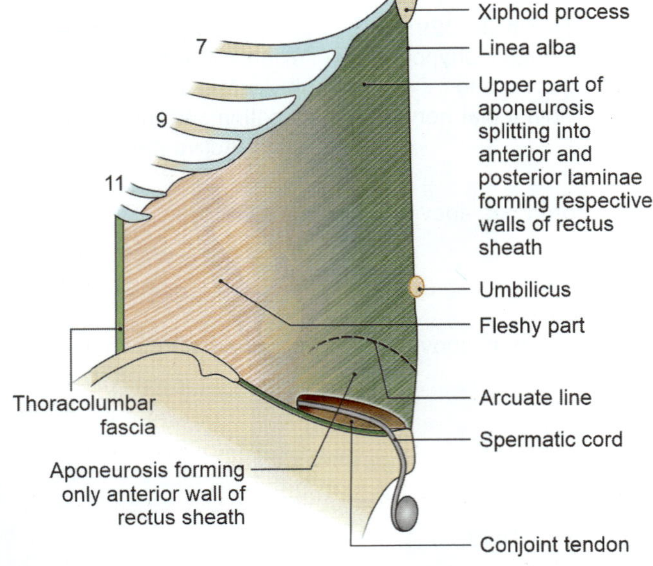

Fig. 40.2: Internal oblique muscle of the abdomen

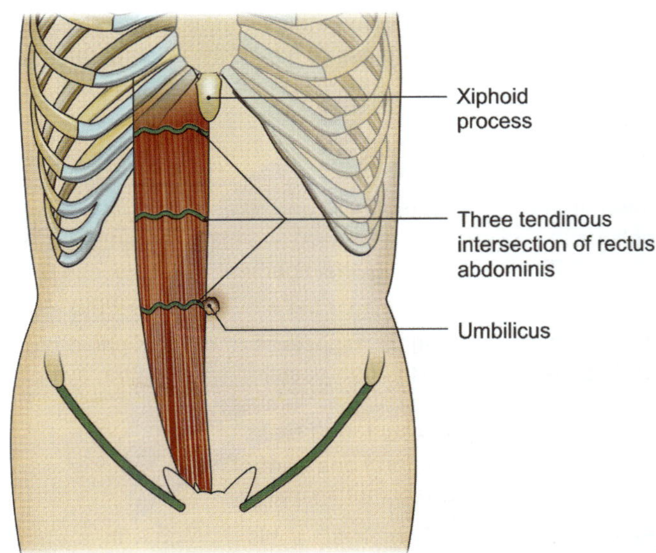

Fig. 40.4: Rectus abdominis muscle

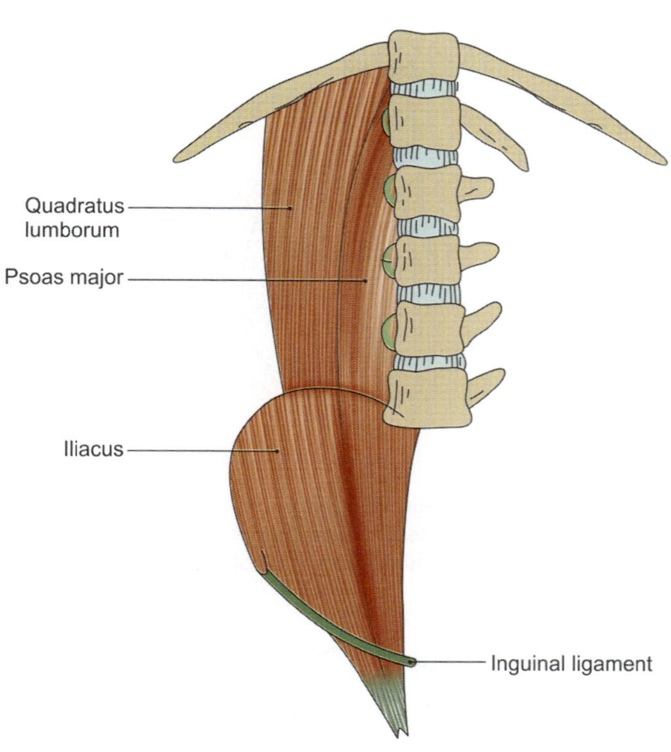

Fig. 40.5: Muscles of the posterior abdominal wall

The aponeurosis of internal oblique muscle only splits into an anterior and a posterior laminae, one lies anterior to rectus abdominis and other lying posterior to the muscle.

2 Aponeurosis of the transversus muscle (Fig. 40.6b).

Midway between the umbilicus and the pubic symphysis, the posterior wall of the rectus sheath ends in the arcuate line. The line is concave downwards.

Below the arcuate line.

Anterior wall: Aponeuroses of all the three flat muscles of the abdomen (Fig. 40.6c).

Posterior wall: It is deficient. The rectus muscle rests on the fascia transversalis.

Contents

Muscles

1 *Rectus abdominis* is the chief and largest content.
2 *Pyramidalis*

Arteries and Veins

1 The *superior epigastric artery and vein*
2 The *inferior epigastric artery and vein*

Nerves

These are the terminal parts of the lower six thoracic nerves, that is the *lower five intercostal nerves* and the *subcostal nerves*.

Functions

1 It checks bowing of rectus muscle during its contraction and thus increases the efficiency of the muscle.
2 It maintains the strength of the anterior abdominal wall.

ABDOMINAL CAVITY

Nine Regions of the Abdomen

For the purpose of describing the location of viscera, the abdomen is divided into nine regions by four imaginary planes, two horizontal and two vertical. The horizontal planes are the transpyloric and

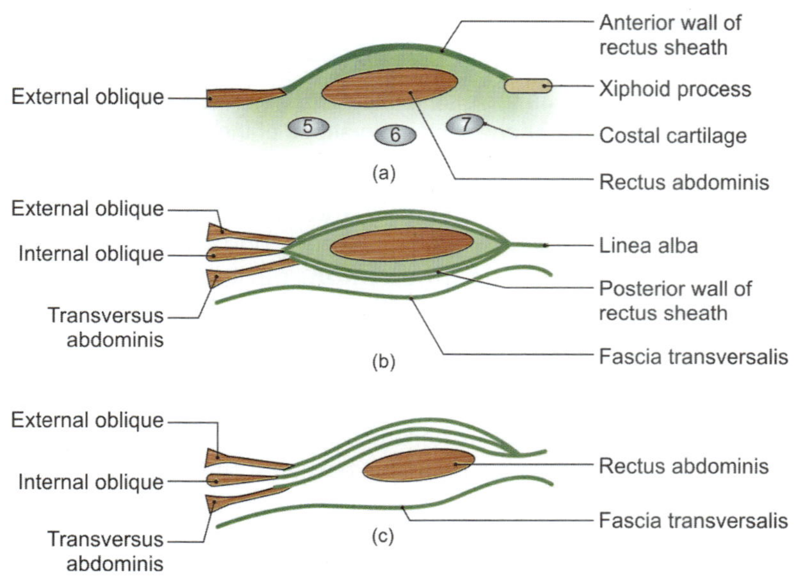

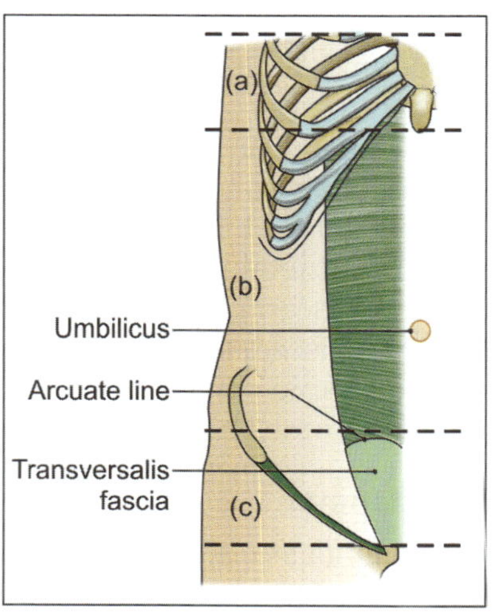

Fig. 40.6: Transverse sections through the rectus abdominis, and its sheath: (a) Above the costal margin, (b) between costal margin and arcuate line, (c) below arcuate line

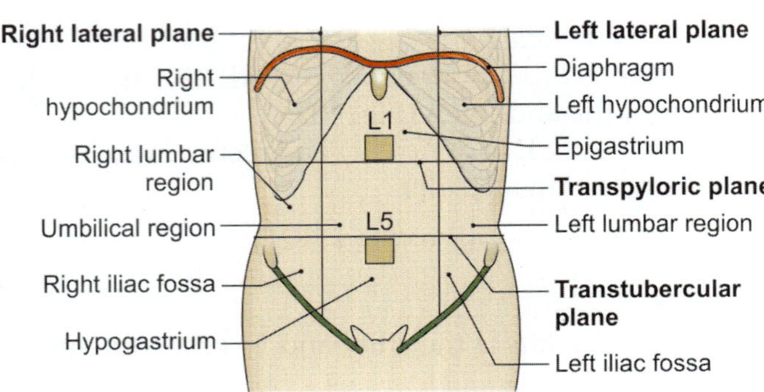

Fig. 40.7: Regions of the abdomen

transtubercular planes. The vertical planes are the right lateral and the left lateral planes (Fig. 40.7).

The *transpyloric plane* of Addison passes midway between the suprasternal notch and the pubic symphysis. It lies roughly a hand's breadth below the xiphisternal joint. Anteriorly, it passes through the tips of the ninth costal cartilage; and posteriorly through the body of vertebra L1 near its lower border.

The *transtubercular plane* passes through the tubercles of the iliac crest and the body of vertebra L5 near its upper border.

The *right and left lateral planes* correspond to the midclavicular or mammary lines. Each of these vertical planes passes through the midinguinal point and crosses the tip of the ninth costal cartilage.

The nine regions marked out in this way are arranged in three vertical zones—median, right and left. From above downwards, the median regions are *epigastric, umbilical* and *hypogastric.* The right and left regions, in the same order, are *hypochondriac, lumbar* and *iliac.*

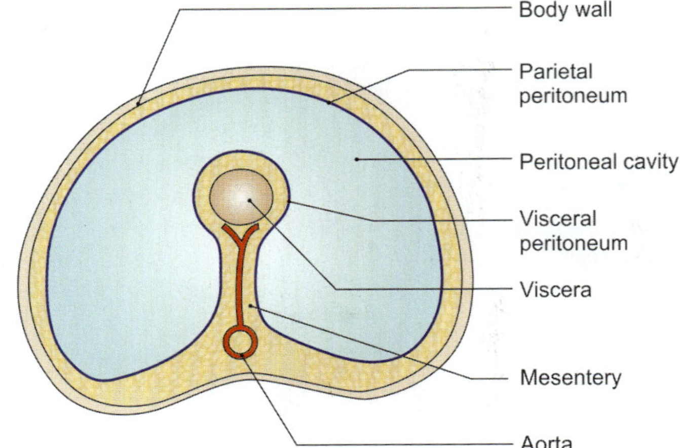

Fig. 40.8: Diagrammatic transverse section of the abdomen showing the arrangement of the peritoneum. The peritoneal cavity is actually a potential space and not so spacious as shown

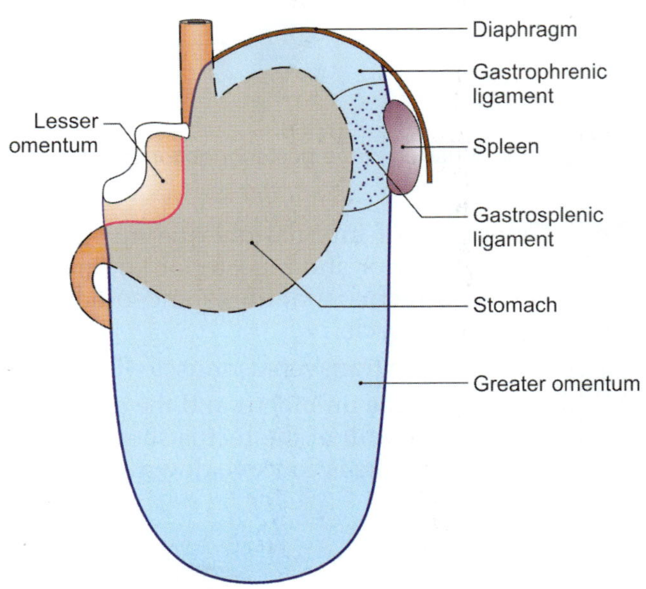

Fig. 40.9: Anterior view of the peritoneal folds attached to the greater and lesser curvatures of the stomach

THE PERITONEUM

Introduction

The peritoneum is a large serous membrane lining the abdominal cavity.

The peritoneum is in the form of a closed sac which is invaginated by a number of viscera. As a result, the peritoneum is divided into:

1 An outer or parietal layer (Fig. 40.8).
2 An inner or visceral layer; and folds of peritoneum by which the viscera are suspended. The peritoneum which is a simple cavity, before being invaginated by viscera becomes highly complicated (Fig. 40.9).

Parietal Peritoneum

1 It lines the inner surface of the abdominal and pelvic walls and the lower surface of the diaphragm. It is loosely attached to the walls by extraperitoneal connective tissue and can, therefore, be easily stripped.
2 Its blood supply and nerve supply are the same as those of the overlying body wall. Because of the somatic innervation, parietal peritoneum is *pain sensitive* (Fig. 40.8).

Visceral Peritoneum

1 It lines the outer surface of the viscera, to which it is firmly adherent and cannot be stripped. In fact it forms a part and parcel of the viscera.
2 Its blood supply and nerve supply are the same as those of the underlying viscera. Because of the autonomic innervation, visceral peritoneum evokes pain when viscera is stretched, ischaemic or distended.

Folds of Peritoneum

1 Many organs within the abdomen are suspended by folds of peritoneum (Fig. 40.9). Such organs are mobile. Other organs are fixed and immobile. They rest directly on the posterior abdominal wall, and may be covered by peritoneum on one side. Such organs are said to be *retroperitoneal.*
2 Apart from allowing mobility, the peritoneal folds provide pathways for passage of vessels, nerves and lymphatics.

Peritoneal Cavity

The peritoneal cavity is divided broadly into two parts. The main, larger part is known as the *greater sac,* and the smaller part, situated behind the stomach, the lesser omentum and the liver, is known as the *lesser sac.* The two sacs communicate with each other through the *epiploic foramen* or *foramen of Winslow* or *opening into the lesser sac.*

Functions of Peritoneum

1 *Movements of viscera:* The chief function of the peritoneum is to provide a slippery surface for free movements of abdominal viscera.
2 *Protection of viscera:* The peritoneum contains various phagocytic cells which guard against infection. Lymphocytes present in normal peritoneal fluid provide both cellular and humoral immunological defence mechanisms.
3 *Absorption and dialysis:* The mesothelium acts as a semipermeable membrane across which fluids and small molecules of various solutes can pass.
4 *Healing power and adhesions:* The mesothelial cells of the peritoneum can transform into fibroblasts which promote healing of wounds.
5 *Storage of fat:* Peritoneal folds are capable of storing large amounts of fat, particularly in obese persons.

Greater Omentum

This is a large fold of peritoneum which hangs down from the greater curvature of the stomach like an apron and covers the loops of intestines to a varying extent. It is made up of four layers of peritoneum all of which are fused together to form a thin fenestrated membrane containing variable quantities of fat (Fig. 40.10).

Functions

1 It is a storehouse of fat.
2 It protects the peritoneal cavity against infection because of the presence of macrophages in it. Collections of macrophages form small, dense patches, known as *milky* spots, which are visible to the naked eye.
3 It also limits the spread of infection by moving to the site of infection and sealing it off from the surrounding areas. On this account, the greater omentum is also known as the *policeman of the abdomen.*

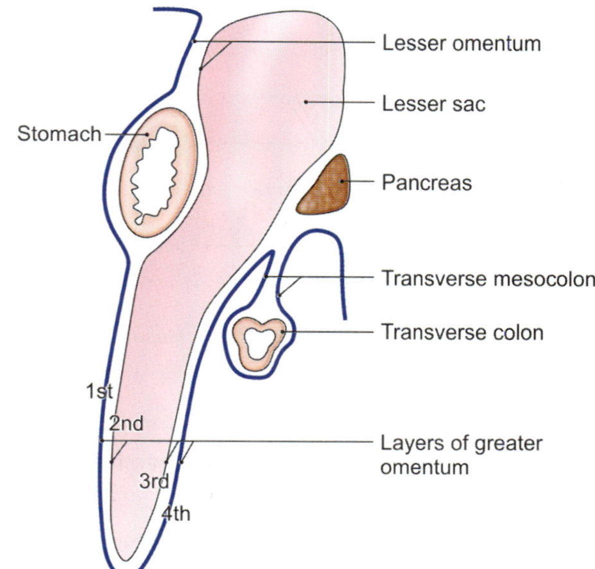

Fig. 40.10: Position of greater omentum, lesser omentum and lesser sac

Lesser Omentum

This is a fold of peritoneum which extends from the lesser curvature of the stomach and the first 2 cm of the duodenum to the liver. Behind the lesser omentum, there lies a part of the lesser sac. The lesser omentum has a free right margin behind which there is the epiploic foramen. The greater and lesser sacs communicate through this foramen (Fig. 40.10).

The right free margin of the lesser omentum contains: (a) The hepatic artery proper, (b) the portal vein, (c) the bile duct.

Mesentery

The mesentery of the small intestine or mesentery proper is a broad, fan-shaped fold of peritoneum which suspends the coils of jejunum and ileum from the posterior abdominal wall (Figs 40.11 and 40.12).

Mesoappendix

It is a small, triangular fold of peritoneum which suspends the vermiform appendix from the posterior surface of the lower end of the mesentery close to the ileocaecal junction. It contains vessels, nerves, lymph nodes and lymphatics of the appendix.

Transverse Mesocolon

This is a broad fold of peritoneum which suspends the transverse colon from the upper part of the posterior abdominal wall.

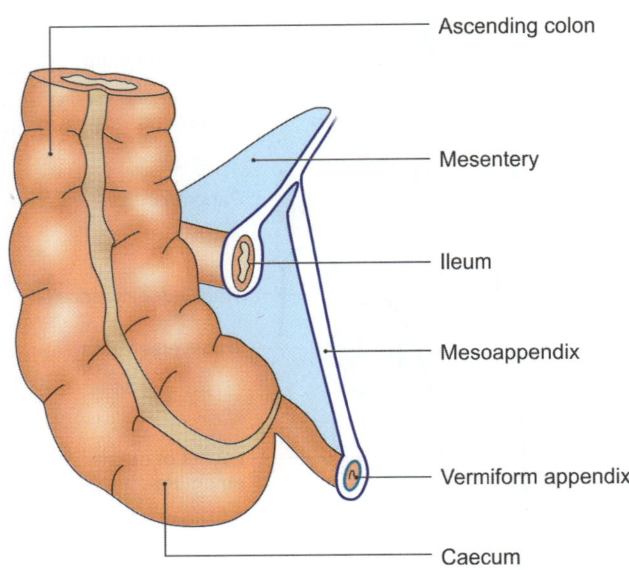

Fig. 40.11: The attachment of the mesoappendix to the posterior (left) surface of the lower end of the mesentery

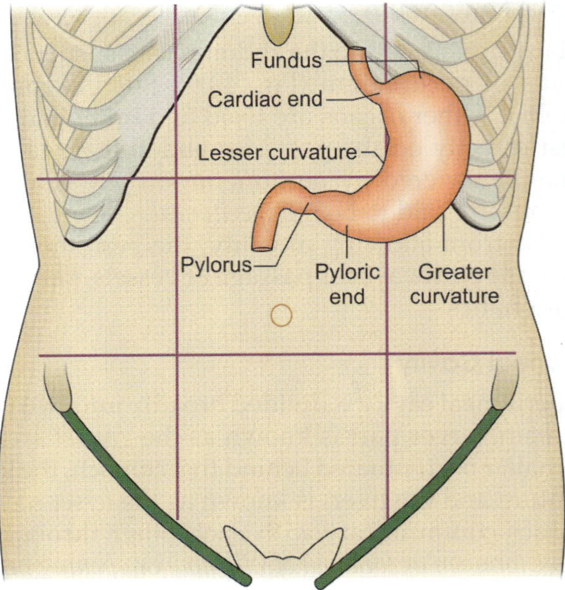

Fig. 40.13: External features of the stomach

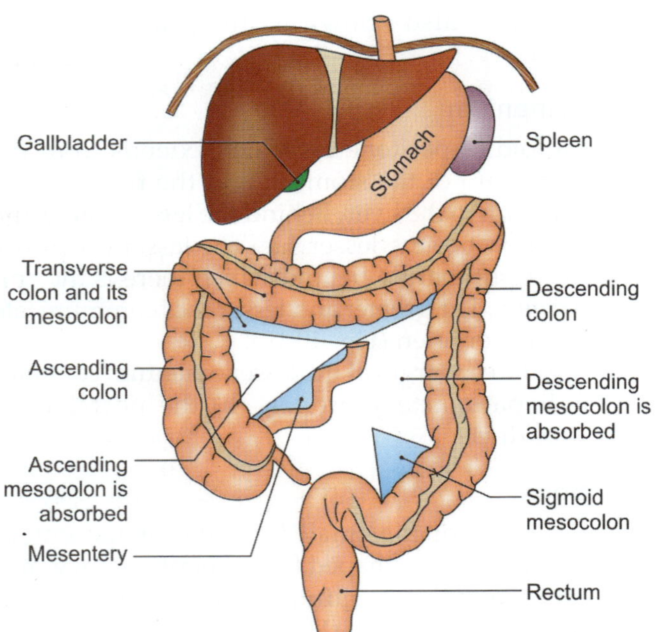

Fig. 40.12: Anterior view of the small and large intestines showing the parts of the dorsal mesentery that persist and other parts which are absorbed

Sigmoid Mesocolon

This is a triangular fold of peritoneum which suspends the sigmoid colon from the pelvic wall.

DIGESTIVE SYSTEM

Figure 40.12 shows some of the abdominal organs.

OESOPHAGUS

The oesophagus (Fig. 40.13) is a tubular, muscular structure about 10 inches (25 cm) long, which is continuous above with the laryngeal part of the pharynx opposite the sixth cervical veterbra. In the thorax, it passes downwards and to the left. It passes through the diaphragm at the level of the tenth thoracic vertebra and ends by opening into the stomach (cardiac end) at the level of T 11 vertebra.

Relations of the thoracic part of the oesophagus.

1 *Anteriorly*
The trachea in the superior mediastinum.
2 *Posteriorly*
The bodies of the thoracic vertebrae, in the superior mediastinum.
3 *To the right side* Right lung and pleura
4 *To the left side*
i. Arch of aorta, descending thoracic aorta
ii. Left lung and pleura.

Blood supply: The abdominal part is supplied by oesophageal branches of left gastric artery, a branch of the coeliac trunk of the abdominal aorta.

Veins from abdominal part drain into vena azygos, i.e. systemic veins and partly into portal vein. So the abdominal part of the oesophagus is a site of portosystemic anastomoses.

STOMACH

The stomach acts as mechanical mixer, chemical digester and temporary storehouse of food. It is the most dilated part of digestive tube. Its capacity in adults is 1 to 1.5 litres.

1 *Position:* Left hypochondriac and epigastric regions.

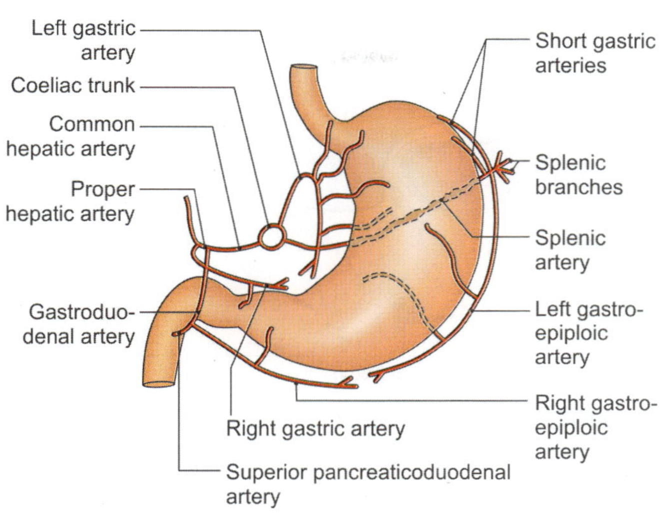

Fig. 40.14: Arteries supplying the stomach

2 *Parts:* The junction of oesophagus and stomach is the cardio-oesophageal junction. The stomach consists of:
 - 2 ends—the proximal **cardiac** and distal **pyloric end.**
 - 2 borders—the lesser curvature and the greater curvature.
 - 2 surfaces—anterosuperior and postero- inferior surface. The latter rests on a number of organs, i.e. pancreas, spleen, left kidney forming the stomach bed.

 Part of the stomach above the gastro-oesophageal junction is called the fundus of the stomach. The main part is the body and the distal part is the **pyloric part.** This part possesses a sphincter, the **pyloric sphincter** at its distal part.

3 *Blood supply:* Stomach gets its arterial supply from the three branches of **coeliac trunk,** a branch of abdominal aorta (Fig. 40.14). Veins drain into the **portal vein.**

Sympathetic nerves supply the blood vessels and also carry pain impulses. Vagus is secretory to the glands and causes peristalsis and inhibits the pyloric sphincter as well.

INTESTINES

Intestines follow the stomach. There are two parts of intestines, small and large. Small intestine has villi which are absent in large intestine.

Small Intestine

It is the intestine between pylorus of stomach and ileocaecal valve. It is 5 meters long. The mucosal folds run circularly across the wall and are permanent. It is subdivided into 3 parts—proximal 25 cm is **duodenum,** middle 2/5th is **jejunum** and distal 3/5th is **ileum.**

Duodenum

Duodenum is 'C' shaped with **head of pancreas** lying in its concavity. The **bile duct** and the **pancreatic duct** open by a **common opening** into the duodenum, 10 cm from the pylorus at major duodenal papilla (Fig. 40.15).

Jejunum and Ileum

These two parts form most of the small intestine. These are suspended from the posterior abdominal wall by a fold of peritoneum called the **mesentery.**

Arterial blood supply is from the superior mesenteric artery which gives 12 to 15 branches for small intestine and 3 branches—middle colic, right colic and ileocolic for large intestine as well. **Veins** drain into superior mesenteric vein which with splenic vein forms the portal vein.

The lymph vessels drain into para-aortic lymph nodes and from there into the upper part of cisterna chyli, at the beginning of the thoracic duct.

Nerve supply is from vagus and sympathetic nerves. These nerves, form plexuses within the wall of intestine. These are submucosal or **Meissner's plexus** and myenteric or **Auerbach's plexus** in between two coats of muscularis externa. These plexuses cause peristaltic movements of propelling the contents of small intestine towards large intestine.

Large Intestine

It is the last part of the digestive tube and follows the small intestine. It starts at ileocaecal junction. Its parts are caecum, vermiform appendix, colon, rectum and anal canal.

Caecum

Lies in the right iliac fossa. The ileocaecal valve guards the opening of ileum into the caecum. Present 2 cm below this opening is the opening of the vermiform appendix. Caecum is continuous with the ascending colon.

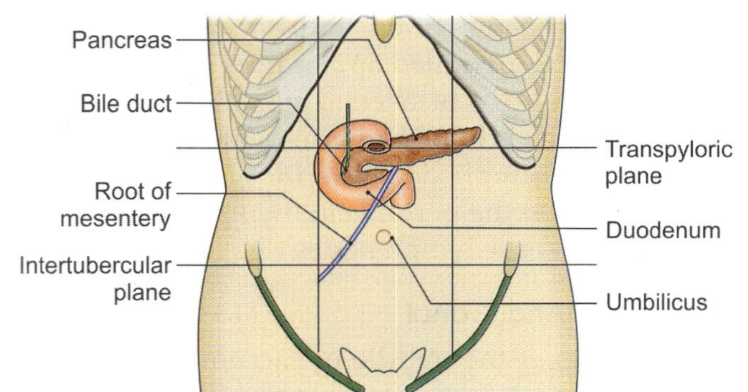

Fig. 40.15: Position of duodenum, pancreas, root of mesentery and opneing of the bile duct

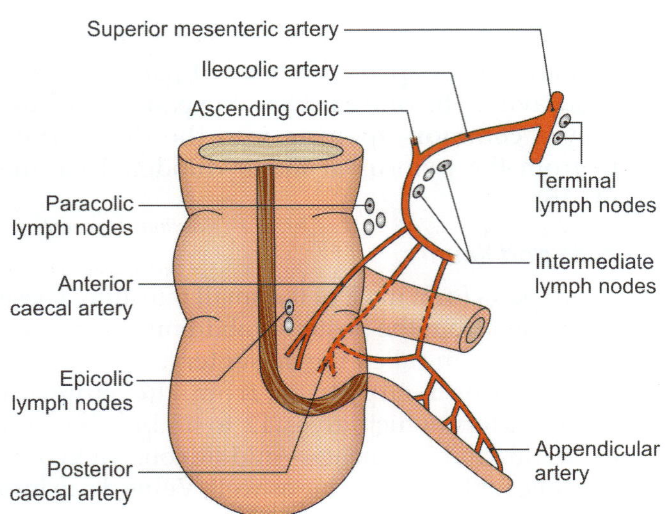

Fig. 40.16: Arterial supply of caecum and appendix. Various groups of lymph nodes are also seen

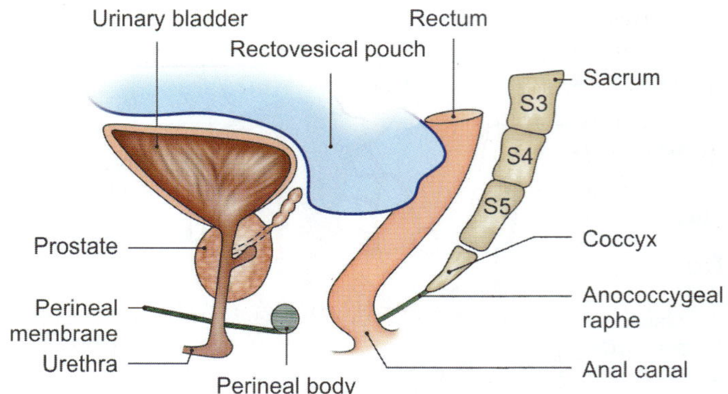

Fig. 40.17: Sagittal section through the male pelvis showing the location of the rectum and some of its anterior and posterior relations

Vermiform Appendix

It is the narrowest part of the digestive tube. It is usually 8 cm long and 0.5 cm wide. It has a base and a tip. The tip may occupy different positions.

Arterial supply is from appendicular artery, one of the caecal branches of superior mesenteric artery (Fig. 40.16).

Colon

It forms the greatest length of large intestine, and is subdivided into **ascending colon** on right side of abdominal cavity, **transverse colon** across the abdomen, **descending colon** on the left side and **pelvic colon** in the pelvis.

In **colon**, the longitudinal muscle fibres are arranged in three thick bands called **taeniae coli** situated at regular intervals around it. They stop at the junction of the sigmoid colon and rectum. These bands of muscle are slightly shorter than the total length of colon. They give a sacculated or puckered appearance forming a series of pouches called **haustra.** Small pouches of visceral peritoneum filled with fat are attached to taeniae coli and are called **appendices epiploicae.**

Arterial supply of ascending and most of the transverse colon is by superior mesenteric artery. Rest of the colon is supplied by inferior mesenteric artery. **Veins** drain into the portal vein. Lymph vessels drain into the para-aortic lymph nodes (Fig. 40.16).

Rectum and Anal Canal

Rectum starts at the middle of sacrum and is 15 cm long. It follows forward curvature of sacrum and coccyx and ends 2.5 cm below and in front of coccyx where it continues as anal canal (Fig. 40.17).

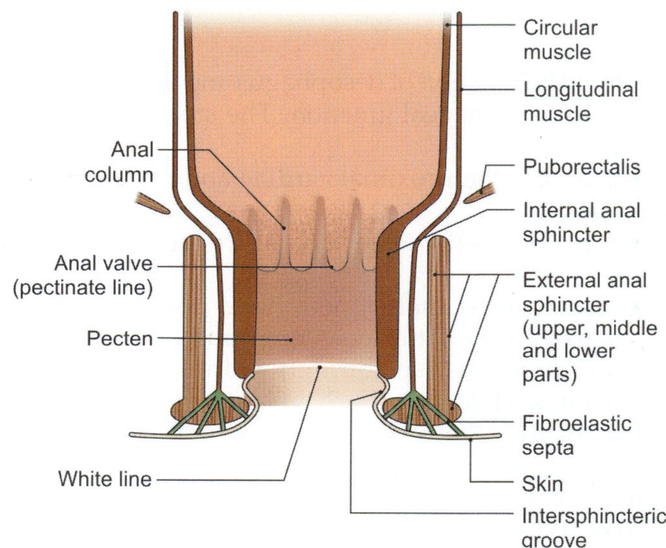

Fig. 40.18: Coronal section through the wall of the anal canal

Anal canal is the last 4 cm of digestive tube. From the anorectal junction it passes downwards and backwards to the anus. In the wall of anal canal, the inner circular layer of smooth muscle becomes thickened to form **internal anal sphincter** while outside this is **external anal sphincter** of skeletal muscle. Internal sphincter is supplied by autonomic nerves while external anal sphincter by inferior rectal nerve (Fig. 40.18).

The mucous membrane of anal canal shows in upper part three folds at positions 3, 7 and 11 which keep anal canal mostly closed. These are due to plexus of veins. If enlarged these form **haemorrhoids or piles** which may cause pain or bleeding or both.

Rectum and anal canal are supplied by **superior rectal artery** (continuation of inferior mesenteric artery), **middle and inferior rectal arteries,** branches of internal pudendal artery.

Veins draining along superior rectal artery end in portal vein, while those running along middle and inferior rectal arteries end in pudendal and systemic veins. Thus anal canal is a site of **portosystemic anastomoses.**

THE LIVER

Definition

The liver is a large, solid, gland situated in the right upper quadrant of the abdominal cavity. In the living subject, the liver is reddish brown in colour, soft in consistency, and very friable. It weighs about 1600 g in males and about 1300 g in females.

Location

The liver occupies the whole of the right hypochondrium, the greater part of the epigastrium, and extends into the left hypochondrium reaching up to the left lateral line (Fig. 40.19).

The liver is the largest gland in the body. It secretes bile and performs various other metabolic functions.

The liver is also called the 'Hepar' from which we have the adjective 'hepatic' applied to many structures connected with the organ.

External Features

The liver is wedge-shaped. It resembles a four-sided pyramid laid on one side.

Five Surfaces

It has five surfaces. These are: (1) Anterior, (2) posterior, (3) superior, (4) inferior, and (5) right.

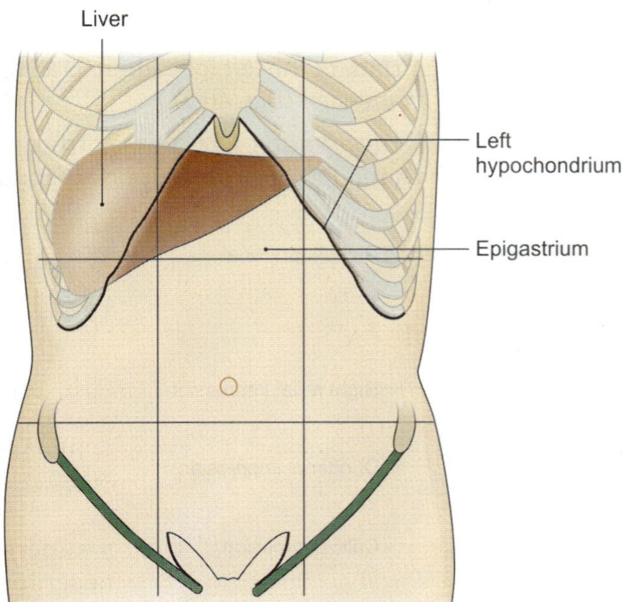

Fig. 40.19: Location of the liver

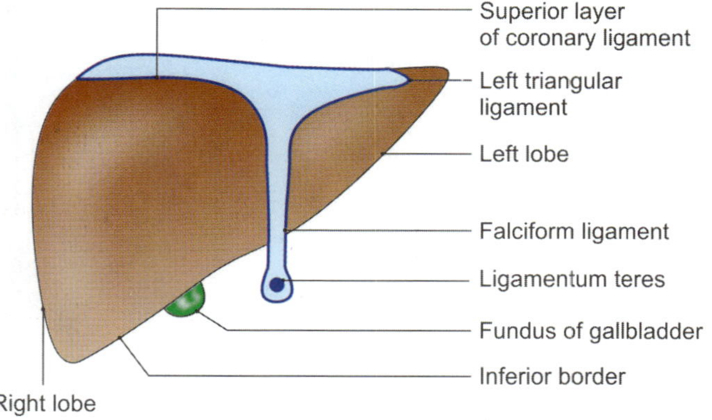

Fig. 40.20: Liver seen from the front

Out of these, the inferior surface is well-defined because it is demarcated, anteriorly, by a sharp inferior border. The other surfaces are more or less continuous with each other and are imperfectly separated from one another by ill-defined, rounded borders (Fig. 40.20).

One Prominent Border

The *inferior border* is sharp anteriorly where it separates the anterior surface from the inferior surface. It is somewhat rounded laterally where it separates the right surface from the inferior surface.

Two Lobes

The liver is divided into right and left lobes by the attachment of the falciform ligament anteriorly and superiorly; by the fissure for the ligamentum teres inferiorly; and by the fissure for the ligamentum venosum posteriorly.

The *right lobe* is much larger than the left lobe, and forms five-sixth of the liver. It contributes to all the five surfaces of the liver, and presents the caudate and quadrate lobes.

The *quadrate lobe* is situated on the inferior surface, and is rectangular in shape. It is bounded anteriorly by the inferior border, posteriorly by the porta hepatis, on the right by the fossa for the gallbladder, and on the left by the fissure for the ligamentum teres (Fig. 40.21).

The *caudate lobe* lies between inferior vena cava and attachment of lesser omentum to the liver.

The *porta hepatis* is a deep, transverse fissure about 5 cm long, situated on the inferior surface of the right lobe of the liver. It lies between the caudate lobe above and the quadrate lobe below and in front. The portal vein, the hepatic artery and the hepatic plexus of nerves enter the liver through the porta hepatis, while the right and left hepatic ducts and a few lymphatics leave it. The relations within the porta hepatis are from behind forwards the portal vein, the hepatic artery and the hepatic ducts. The lips of the porta hepatis provide attachment to the lesser omentum (Fig. 40.21).

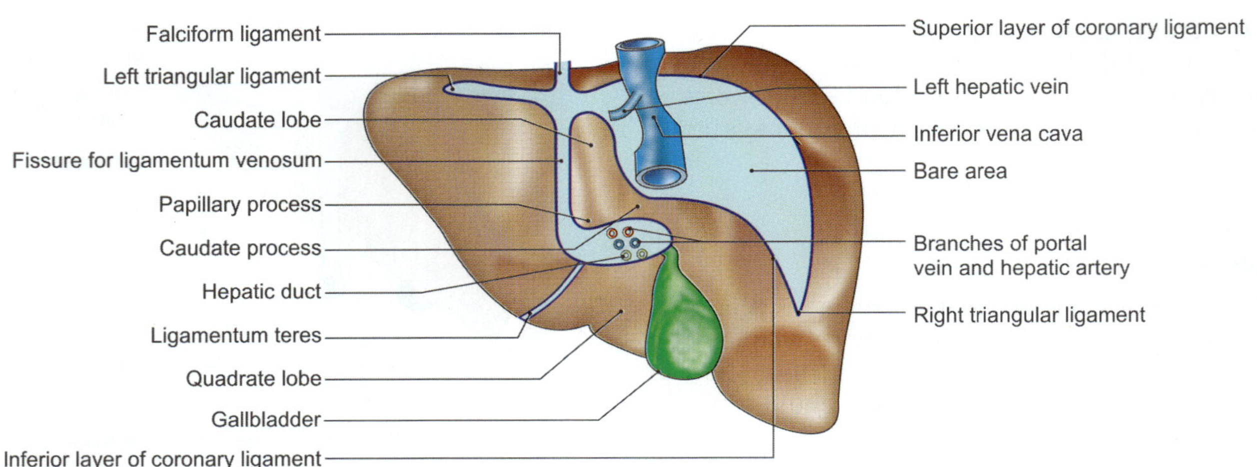

Fig. 40.21: Liver seen from below

The *left lobe* of the liver is much smaller than the right lobe and forms only one-sixth of the liver. It is flattened from above downwards.

Relations

Peritoneal Relations

Most of the liver is covered by peritoneum. The important area not covered by peritoneum is the triangular *bare area* on the posterior surface of the right lobe.

Visceral Relations

Anterior Surface

The anterior surface is triangular and slightly convex. It is related to the xiphoid process and to the anterior abdominal wall in the median plane, and to diaphragm on each side.

Posterior Surface

The posterior surface is triangular. Its middle part shows a deep concavity for the vertebral column. Other relations are as follows.

1. The *bare area* is related to the diaphragm, and to the right suprarenal gland near the lower end of the groove for the inferior vena cava (Fig. 40.22).
2. The *groove for the inferior vena cava* lodges the upper part of the vessel, and its floor is pierced by the hepatic veins.
3. The *posterior surface of the left lobe* is marked by the oesophageal impression.

Superior Surface

The superior surface is quadrilateral and shows a concavity in the middle. This is the cardiac impression. On each side of the impression, the surface is convex to fit the dome of the diaphragm. The diaphragm separates this surface from the pericardium and the heart in the middle, and from pleura and lung on each side.

Inferior Surface

The inferior surface is quadrilateral and is directed downwards, backwards and to the left. It is marked by impressions for neighbouring viscera as follows.

1. On the inferior surface of the left lobe, there is a large concave *gastric impression* (Fig. 40.22).
2. The *fissure for the ligamentum teres* passes from the inferior border to the left end of the porta hepatis.

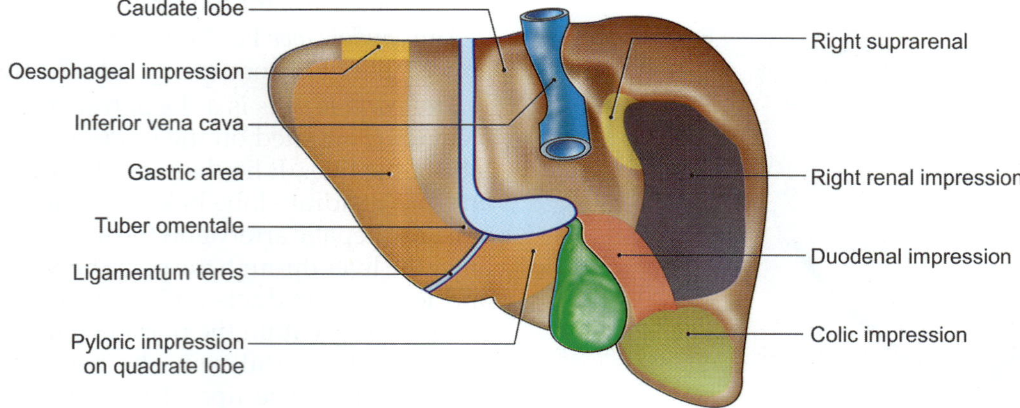

Fig. 40.22: Relations of the inferior surface of the liver

The ligamentum teres represents the obliterated left umbilical vein.

3 The *quadrate lobe* is related to the lesser omentum, the pylorus, and the first part of the duodenum.
4 The *fossa for the gallbladder* lies to the right of the quadrate lobe.
5 To the right of this fossa, the inferior surface of the right lobe bears the *colic impression* for the hepatic flexure of the colon, the renal impression for the right kidney, and the duodenal impression for the second part of the duodenum.

Right Surface

The right surface is quadrilateral and convex. It is related to diaphragm along its entire extent.

Blood Supply

The liver receives 20% of its blood supply through the hepatic artery, and 80% through the portal vein. Before entering the liver, both the hepatic artery and the portal vein divide into right and left branches.

Venous Drainage

Hepatic sinusoids drain into interlobular veins, which join to form sublobular veins. These in turn unite to form the hepatic veins which drain directly into the inferior vena cava.

Hepatic Segments

From surgical point of view, the segments of liver are important as each segment contains its own branch of hepatic artery and hepatic duct. The smaller left lobe of liver contains only two segments. These are left superior and left inferior segments.

Anatomical right lobe is divided by two imaginary lines into three parts—medial (close to falciform ligament), anterior and posterior. Each of them is subdivided into superior and inferior parts by horizontal line. Thus, there are medial superior segment, medial inferior segment, anterior superior segment, anterior inferior segment, posterior superior segment and posterior inferior segment.

In total, there are six segments in the anatomical right lobe and two segments in the left lobe of liver.

Liver Biopsy

Liver biopsy is done through right 8th intercostal space to see the abnormality in the liver.

EXTRAHEPATIC BILIARY APPARATUS

The extrahepatic biliary apparatus comprises all the structures which conduct the bile from the liver to the duodenum. These are:

1 Right and left hepatic ducts (Fig. 40.23).

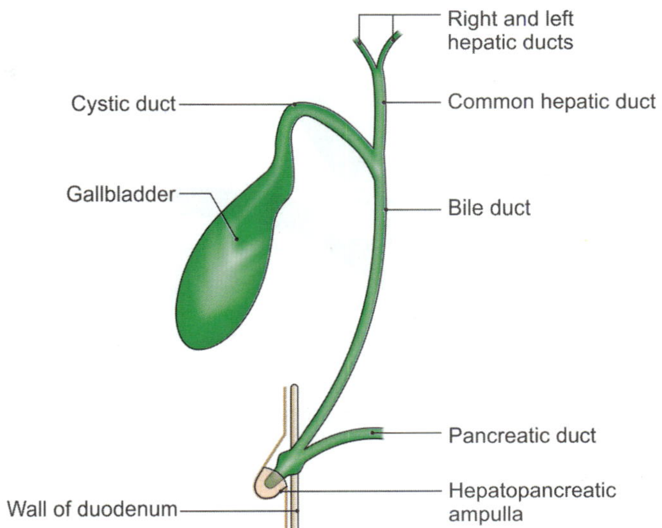

Fig. 40.23: Parts of the biliary apparatus

2 Common hepatic duct.
3 Gallbladder and cytic duct.
4 Bile duct.

Hepatic ducts: Bile ductules of the two functional lobes of liver join to form right and left hepatic ducts. These join to form common hepatic duct—3 cm long which passes downwards. It is soon joined by the cystic duct and then renamed as bile duct.

Gallbladder: It is fibromuscular sac lying on the inferior surface of liver. It stores the bile temporarily and even concentrates it. It is made up of three parts—fundus, body and neck. Fundus is covered by peritoneum all around and lies against tip of right 9th costal cartilage. Body and neck lie in the fossa for gallbladder. The neck continues as the cystic duct. Cystic duct joins the common hepatic duct at the upper end of lesser omentum (Fig. 40.24).

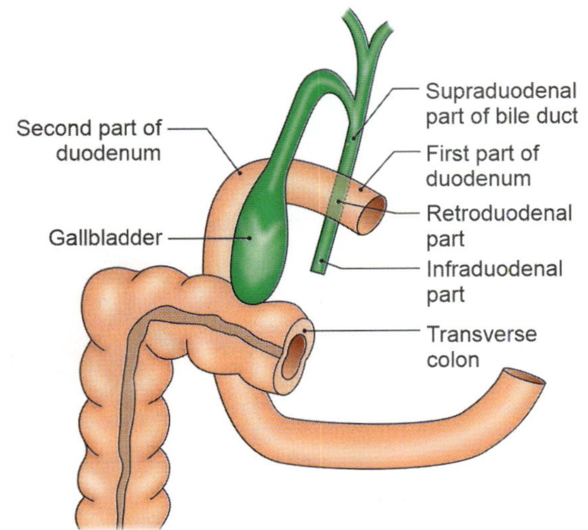

Fig. 40.24: Relations of the gallbladder—Anterior view after removal of the liver

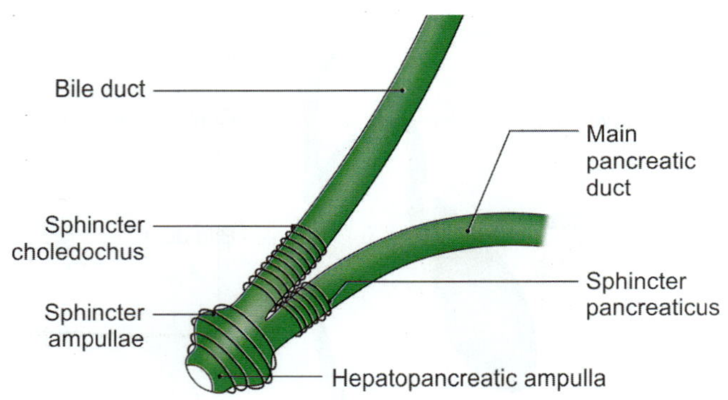

Fig. 40.25: Sphincters in the region of the junction of the bile duct and the main pancreatic duct with the duodenum

Bile duct: It is formed by the union of common hepatic duct and cystic ducts. Its parts are:

a. Supraduodenal
b. Retroduodenal
c. Infraduodenal (Fig. 40.24)
d. Intraduodenal

Arterial supply: Cystic artery a branch of right hepatic artery supplies gallbladder, cystic duct, hepatic ducts and bile duct.

Veins drain into branch of portal vein.

CLINICAL ANATOMY

Cholecystitis is an inflammation of gallbladder and cholelithiasis is calculi in the gallbladder.

SPLEEN

Spleen is the largest mass of lymphoid tissue situated in the left hypochondrium. Its long axis lies along 10th rib (Fig. 40.26). Spleen is supported and connected to neighboring viscera by gastrosplenic and lienorenal ligaments.

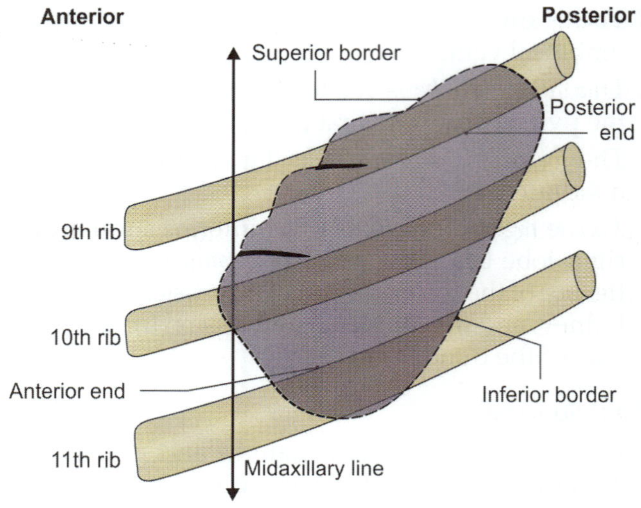

Fig. 40.26: Position of spleen in relation to left 9th–11th ribs—diaphragmatic surface. Recent view: Spleen lies along 10th–12th ribs.

The spleen possesses two surfaces—the diaphragmatic and visceral surface.

The diaphragmatic surface is related to diaphragm.

Relations of Visceral Surface

1 Gastric impression lies in the upper part of spleen including the notched upper border. The hilum is also included in the gastric area.
2 Renal impression lies in the lower part of spleen and is related to upper lateral part of anterior surface of kidney (Fig. 40.27).
3 Colic impression is situated near the lateral end of spleen. Left colic flexure is related here.
4 Pancreatic impression is present near the lateral end of the hilum of spleen.

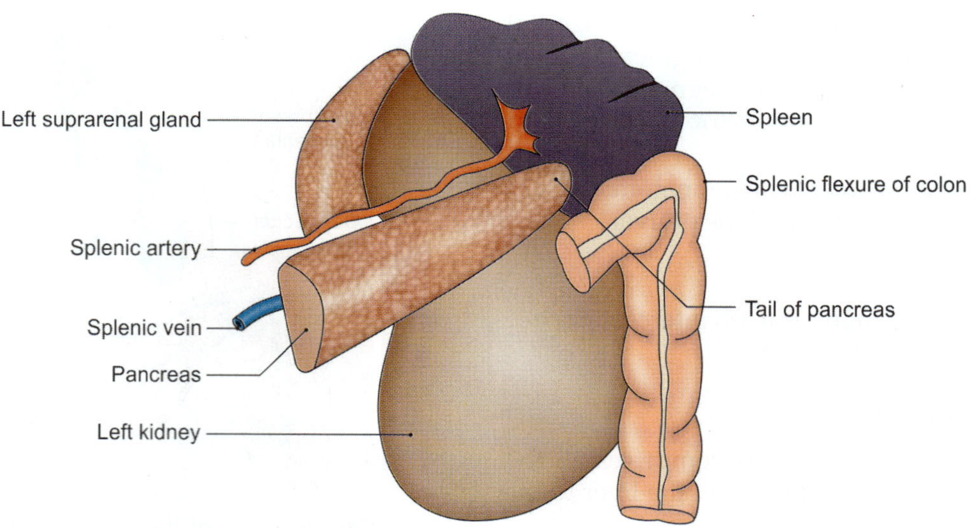

Fig. 40.27: Visceral relations of the spleen

Blood Supply

Spleen is supplied by branches of tortuous splenic artery. Veins drain into splenic vein.

PANCREAS

Pancreas is both an endocrine (ductless) and an exocrine gland. It lies on the posterior abdominal wall. Its parts are head, neck, body and tail. Most of it lies behind the peritoneum. Head lies in the concavity of 1st, 2nd and 3rd parts of duodenum (Fig. 40.28).

Neck lies anterior to the region of formation of portal vein by the union of superior mesenteric and splenic veins.

Body extends across the posterior abdominal wall, tail in the lienorenal ligament and extends till the hilum of spleen.

Relations

Head: It is closely fitting into the C-shaped concavity of three parts of duodenum. Head is related anteriorly to transverse colon.

Posterior relations: Bile duct, abdominal aorta and inferior vena cava.

Neck: Behind neck is formation of portal vein.

Body: It is prismoid in shape and has three borders, anterior, inferior and superior; and three surfaces, anterior, inferior and posterior.

Tail of pancreas: It is lodged in the lienorenal ligament with splenic vessels. Tail contains **maximum amount of islets of Langerhans.** It should be carefully separated during splenectomy.

Ducts of pancreas: The main duct is joined by bile duct to form hepatopancreatic ampulla which opens into 2nd part of duodenum on top of major duodenal papilla (Fig. 40.29).

Arterial supply: Splenic artery gives number of branches to the pancreas, as it runs along its superior border. One artery is large and is called arteria pancreatica magna.

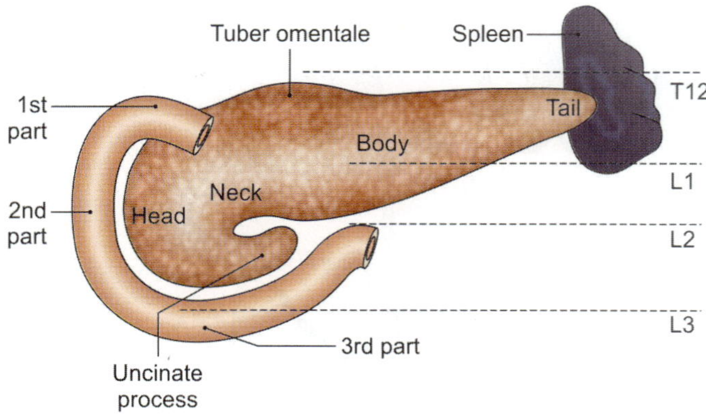

Fig. 40.28: Location of the pancreas

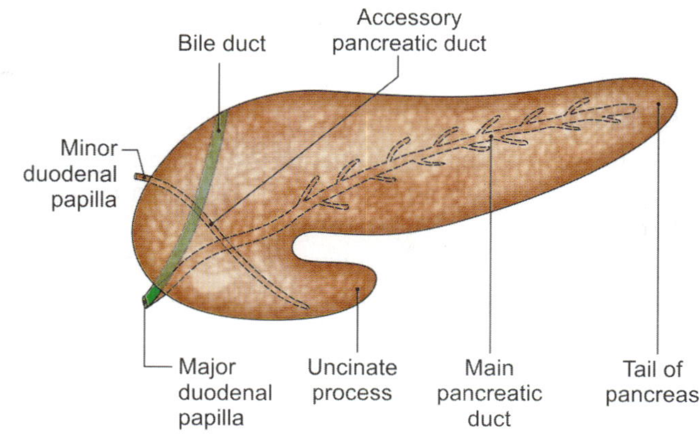

Fig. 40.29: The pancreatic ducts

Venous drainage: Into splenic and superior mesenteric veins. Both these join to form the portal vein.

PORTAL VEIN

Portal vein is a large vein which collects blood from:

a. The abdominal part of the alimentary tract
b. The gallbladder
c. The pancreas
d. The spleen, and conveys it to the liver. In the liver, the portal vein breaks up into sinusoids which are drained by the hepatic veins to the inferior vena cava.

Formation

The portal vein is about 8 cm long. It is formed by the union of the superior mesenteric and splenic veins behind the neck of the pancreas at the level of second lumbar vertebra. Inferior mesenteric vein drains into splenic vein (Fig. 40.30).

Course

It runs upwards and a little to the right, first behind the neck of the pancreas, next behind the first part of

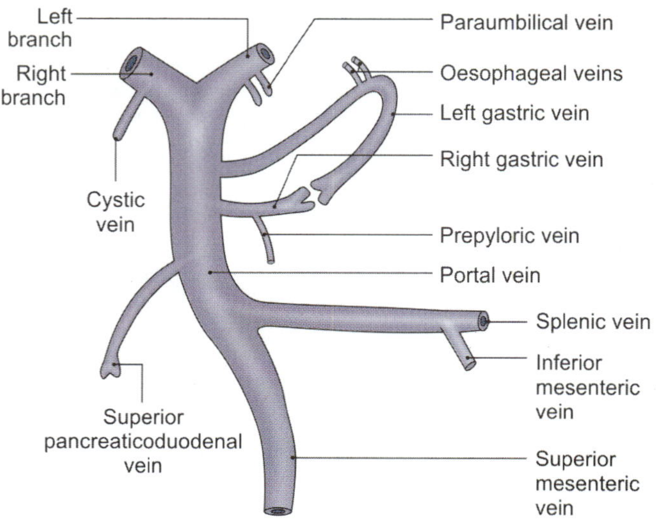

Fig. 40.30: Tributaries of the portal vein

the duodenum, and lastly in the right free margin of the lesser omentum.

Termination

The vein ends at the right end of the porta hepatis by dividing into right and left branches which enter the liver.

Branches of Portal Vein

1 The *right branch* is shorter and wider than the left branch. After receiving the cystic vein, it enters the right lobe of the liver (Fig. 40.30).
2 The left branch is longer and narrower than the right branch and furnishes branches to the caudate and quadrate lobes.

Tributaries

Portal vein receives the following veins.

i. Left gastric
ii. Right gastric
iii. Superior pancreaticoduodenal
iv. Cystic in right
vi. Paraumbilical veins in left branch (Fig. 40.30).

PORTOSYSTEMIC COMMUNICATIONS (PORTOCAVAL ANASTOMOSES)

These communications form important routes of collateral circulation in portal obstruction. The following are the important sites of portosystemic communications.

1 *Umbilicus:* The left branch of the portal vein anastomoses with the veins of the anterior abdominal wall (systemic) through the paraumbilical veins. In portal obstruction, the veins around the umbilicus enlarge forming the *caput medusae* (Fig. 40.31).

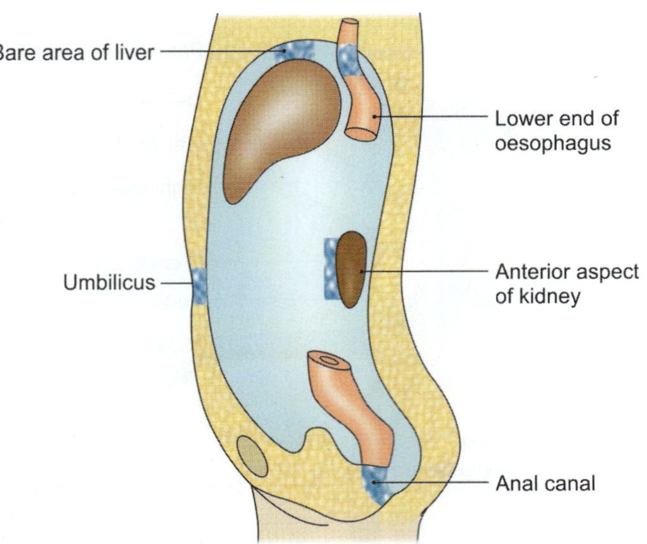

Fig. 40.31: Sites of portosystemic anastomosis

2 *Lower end of oesophagus:* Oesophageal tributaries of the left gastric vein (portal) anastomose with the oesophageal tributaries of the accessory hemiazygos vein (systemic).
3 *Anal canal:* The superior rectal vein (portal) anastomoses with the middle and inferior rectal veins (systemic) (Fig. 40.31).
4 *Bare area of the liver:* Hepatic venules (portal) anastomose with the phrenic and intercostal veins (systemic).
5 *Posterior abdominal wall:* Veins of retro-peritoneal organs, like the duodenum, the ascending colon and the descending colon (portal) anastomose with the retroperitoneal veins of the abdominal wall and of the renal capsule (systemic).
6 *Liver:* Rarely, the ductus venosus remains patent and connects the left branch of the portal vein directly to the inferior vena cava.

URINARY SYSTEM

THE KIDNEYS

The kidneys are also called *renes* from which one has the derivative *renal,* and *nephros.* From nephros the terms *nephron, nephritis,* etc. are derived.

External Features

Each kidney is bean-shaped. It has upper and lower poles, concave medial and convex lateral borders. It has anterior and posterior surfaces (Fig. 40.32).

Hilum

The following structures are seen in the hilum from anterior to posterior side:

1 The renal vein.
2 The renal artery.
3 The renal pelvis, which is the expanded upper end of the ureter.

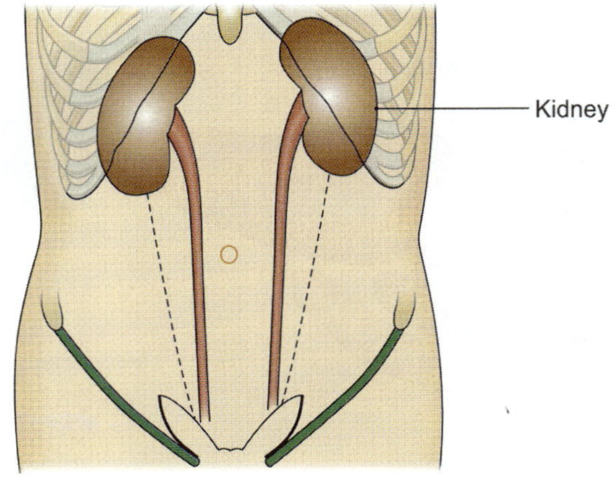

Fig. 40.32: Position of kidneys from anterior aspect

So it is possible to determine the side to which a kidney belongs by examining the structures in the hilum.

Location and Gross Features

The kidneys occupy the epigastric, hypochondriac, lumbar and umbilical regions. Vertically, they extend from the upper border of twelfth thoracic vertebra to the centre of the body of third lumbar vertebra. The right kidney is slightly lower than the left, and the left kidney is a little nearer to the median plane than the right.

Each kidney is about 11 cm long, 6 cm broad, and 3 cm thick. On an average, the kidney weighs 150 g in males and 135 g in females. The kidneys are reddish brown in colour (Fig. 40.32).

The long axis of the kidney is directed downwards and laterally, so that the upper poles are nearer to the median plane than the lower poles.

Relations of the Kidneys

The kidneys are retroperitoneal organs and are only partly covered by peritoneum anteriorly.

Relations common to the two kidneys

1. The upper pole of each kidney is related to the corresponding suprarenal gland.
2. The medial border of each kidney is related to: (i) The suprarenal gland, above the hilus, and (ii) To the ureter below the hilus.
3. *Posterior relations:* These are shown in Fig. 40.33. The structures related to the hilum are renal vein, renal artery and the renal pelvis from anterior to posterior side.

Anterior relations of right kidney and left kidney are shown in Fig. 40.34.

Capsules or Coverings of Kidney

1. *Perirenal or perinephric fat*
2. *Renal fascia*
3. *Pararenal* or *paranephric body (fat)*

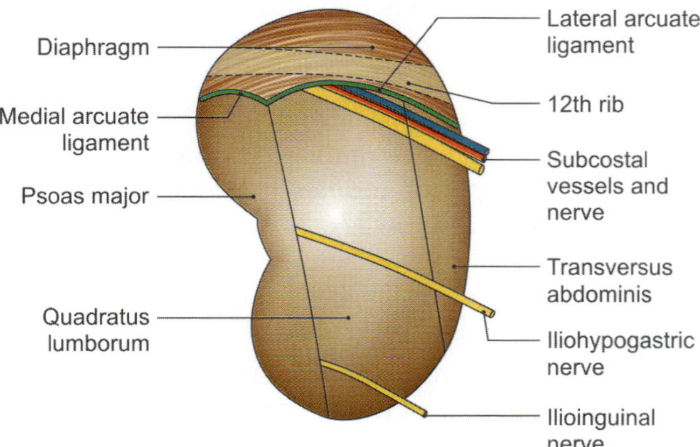

Fig. 40.33: Posterior relations of the right kidney

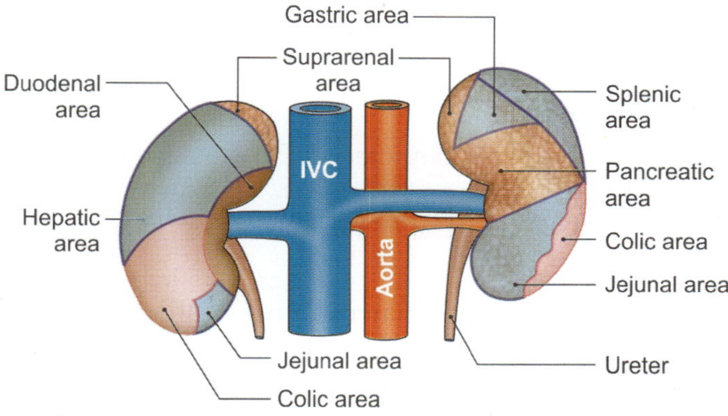

Fig. 40.34: Anterior relations of the kidneys. Areas covered by peritoneum are shaded

Structure

Naked eye examination of a coronal section of the kidney shows:

a. An outer, reddish brown cortex,
b. An inner, pale medulla, and
c. A space, the renal sinus (Fig. 40.35)

The *renal medulla* is made up of about 10 conical masses, called the *renal pyramids.* Their apices form the *renal papillae which* indent the minor calices.

The *renal cortex* is divisible into two parts: (a) *cortical arches,* which form caps over the bases of the pyramids; and (b) *renal columns,* which dip in between the pyramids.

Each pyramid along with the overlying cortical arch forms a lobe of the kidney.

The *renal sinus* is a space that extends into the kidney from the hilus. It contains: (a) Branches of the renal artery, (b) tributaries of the renal vein, and (c) the renal pelvis. The pelvis divides into 2 major calyces, and these in their turn divide into 7 to 13 minor calyces. Each minor calyx (*kalyx* = cup of a flower) ends in an

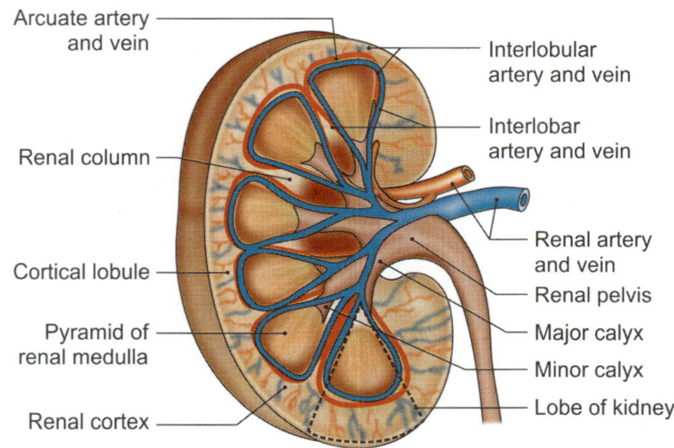

Fig. 40.35: A coronal section through the kidney showing the naked eye structure

expansion which is indented by one to three renal papillae.

Blood Supply

The blood supply is depicted in Flowchart 40.1.

THE URETERS

Definition

The ureters are a pair of narrow, thick-walled muscular tubes which convey urine from the kidneys to the urinary bladder (Fig. 40.36).

These lie deep to the peritoneum, closely applied to the posterior abdominal wall in the upper part, and to the lateral pelvic wall in the lower part.

Dimensions

Each ureter is about 25 cm (10 in) long, of which the upper half (5 in) lies in the abdomen, and the lower half (5 in) in the pelvis. It measures about 3 mm in diameter, but it is slightly constricted at five places.

Course

The ureter begins within the renal sinus as a funnel-shaped dilatation, called the *renal pelvis.* The pelvis issues from the hilus of the kidney, descends along its medial margin, and at the lower end of the kidney it becomes the ureter proper (Fig. 40.36).

Normal Constrictions

The ureter is slightly constricted at five places:

1 At the pelviureteric junction,

Flowchart 40.1: Blood supply of kidney

Abdominal aorta L2	Inferior vena cava
↓	↑
Renal artery	Renal vein
↓	↑
5 segmental arteries each segmental art	5 segmental vein segmental vein
↓	↑
Lobar art	Lobar vein
↓	↑
Interlobar art	Interlobar vein
↓	↑
Arcuate art	Arcuate vein
↓	↓
Interlobular art	Interlobular vein
↓	↑
Afferent arteriole	Peritubular plexus
↓	↑
Glomerulus	
↓	
Efferent arteriole	

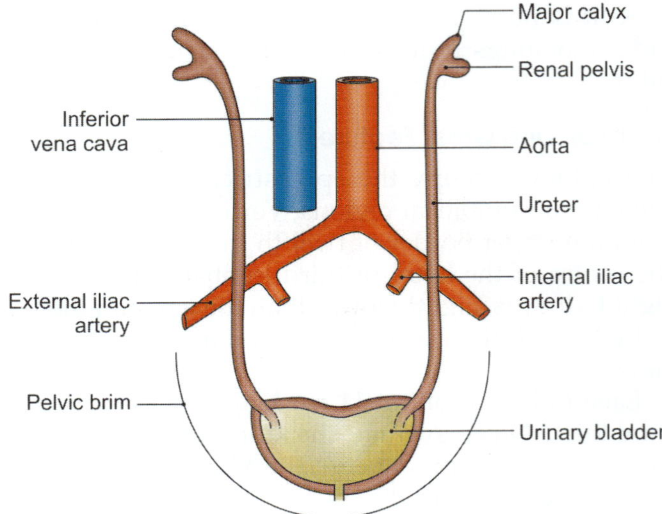

Fig. 40.36: The location of the ureters on the posterior abdominal and lateral pelvic walls

2 At the brim of the lesser pelvis, and

3 Where it is crossed by ductus deferens or uterine artery

4 At its passage through the bladder wall

5 At its opening in the trigone.

URINARY BLADDER

Introduction

Urinary bladder is the temporary storehouse of urine which gets emptied through the urethra.

The urinary bladder is a muscular reservior of urine, which lies in the anterior part of the pelvic cavity. The detrusor muscle of urinary bladder is arranged in whorls and spirals and is adapted for mass contraction rather than peristalsis.

Position

The bladder is situated immediately behind the pubic bones in the pelvic cavity. It is a receptacle for the storage of urine and has maximum capacity of about 500 ml in an adult.

Parts

An empty bladder is pyramidal in shape, having an apex, a base, a superior and two inferolateral surfaces. It also has a neck (Fig. 40.37).

Relations

1 *Base or posterior surface*

It is triangular in shape. Its superolateral angles have the openings of ureters and one inferior angle.

2 *Superior surface*

3 *Inferolateral surface*

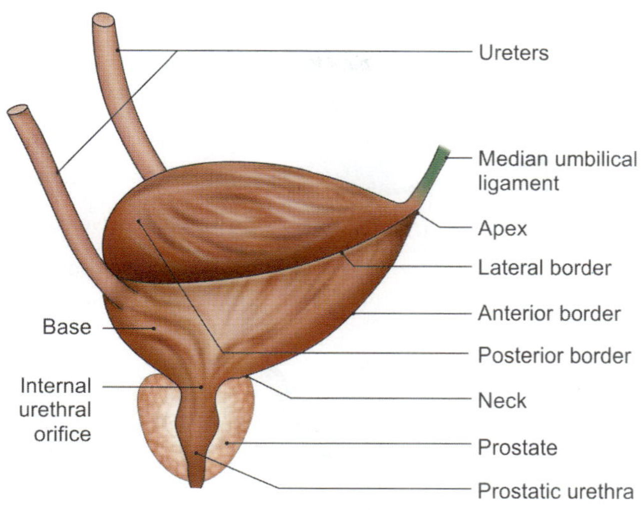

Fig. 40.37: The shape of the urinary bladder

Neck of Bladder

Rests on the upper surface of prostate.

Arterial Supply

Superior and inferior vesical arteries—branches of internal iliac artery in male. Superior vesical and vaginal arteries—branches of internal iliac artery in female.

Venous Drainage

Vesical venous plexus which communicates with prostatic plexus and drains into internal iliac vein.

Ligaments of the Bladder

These are condensations of pelvic fascia around the neck and base of the bladder. They are continuous with the fascia on the superior surface of the levator ani.

1 The *lateral true ligament*.
2 The *posterior ligament*

Interior of the Bladder

It can be examined by cystoscopy, at operation or at autopsy.

In an empty bladder, the greater part of the mucosa shows irregular folds due to its loose attachment to the muscular coat (Fig. 40.38).

In a small triangular area over the lower part of the base of the bladder, the mucosa is smooth due to its firm attachment to the muscular coat. This area is known as the *trigone* of the bladder. The apex of the trigone is directed downwards and forwards. The internal urethral orifice, opening into the urethra is located here. The ureters open at the posterolateral angles of the trigone. Their openings are 2.5 cm apart in the empty bladder, and 5 cm apart in a distended bladder.

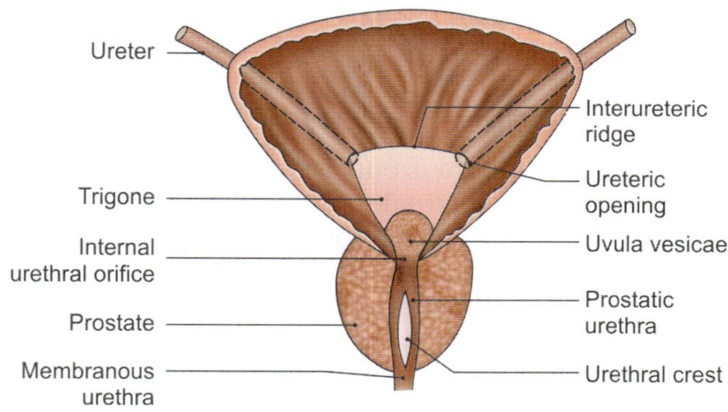

Fig. 40.38: Coronal section through the bladder and prostate to show the interior of the bladder.

THE MALE URETHRA

Male urethra is a membranous canal, 18–20 cm long, for the external discharge of urine and seminal fluid.

Extent and Location

Parts of urethra are short posterior and long anterior parts.

Posterior Part Comprises

1 Preprostatic part
2 The prostatic part passes thrugh the prostate
3 The membranous part traverses the perineal membrane (Fig. 40.39).

Anterior Part Comprises

1 Bulbar urethra in perineum
2 Penile urethra in the penis.

Sphincters of the Urethra

1 The *internal urethral sphincter* or *sphincter vesicae* is involuntary in nature.

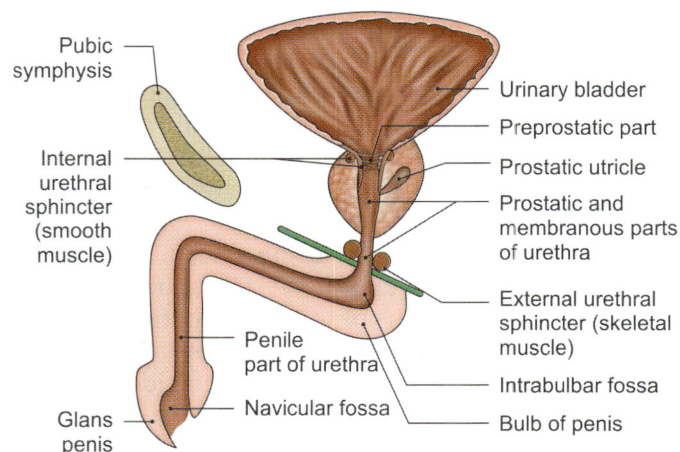

Fig. 40.39: Left view of a sagittal section through the male urethra showing its subdivisions

2 The *external urethral sphincter* or *sphincter urethrae* is voluntary in nature.

THE FEMALE URETHRA

1 The female urethra is only 4 cm long.
2 It begins at the internal urethral orifice, at the neck of the urinary bladder roughly 5 cm behind the middle of the pubic symphysis. It runs downwards and forwards embedded in the anterior wall of the vagina, traverses the perineal membrane, and ends at the external orifice in the vestibule.
3 The female urethra is easily dilatable, and catheters or cystoscopes can be easily passed through it.

FEMALE REPRODUCTIVE SYSTEM

Introduction

Female reproductive organs include external and internal genital organs. The internal genital organs comprise a pair of ovaries, a pair of uterine/fallopian tubes, single uterus and vagina.

INTERNAL GENITAL ORGANS

THE OVARIES

Ovaries are the female sex glands, situated in the true pelvis. During reproductive life of the female, these produce secondary oocytes, oestrogens and progesterone hormones.

Location

These are situated in the lateral pelvic wall in ovarian fossa.

Gross Features

Ovary is half the size of the testis. It is 3 cm × 1.5 cm × 1.0 cm in dimensions. It is smooth and greyish pink before ovulation, but later on its surface gets puckered (Fig. 40.40).

Ovary has two surfaces—the medial and lateral.
Two ends—the tubal and uterine ends.
Two borders—the free and attached borders.

Blood Supply

Ovary is supplied by the ovarian artery, a branch of abdominal aorta at level of L2 vertebra. In addition it also supplies lateral part of the fallopian tube.

The ovarian vein drains into inferior vena cava on right side and into left renal vein on left side.

UTERINE TUBES

Fallopian tube/oviduct/uterine tube/salphinx are two muscular tubes situated between ovaries and the lateral ends of the uterus. Each tube is 10 cm in length. Its course is tortuous. It has four parts. These are infundibulum, ampulla, isthmus and intramural parts (Fig. 40.41) from lateral to medial side.

Secondary oocyte is propelled by the contraction of smooth muscle of the uterine tube to its ampulla where fertilisation takes place. Cilia lining the tube move the fluid so that the oocyte receives proper nutrients during its journey from ovary to the uterus. The uterine tube opens into the superior angle of the cavity of body of uterus.

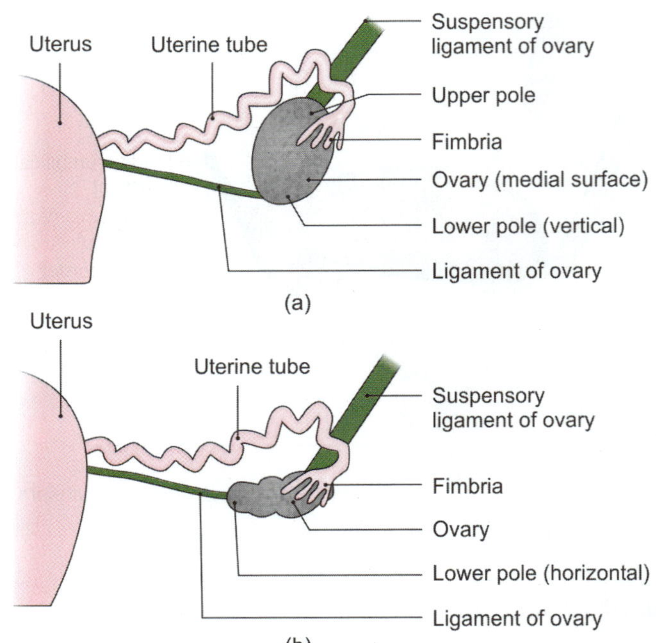

Figs 40.40a and b: Positions of the ovary. (a) It is vertical in nullipara; and (b) horizontal in multipara (after one or more deliveries) due to the pull by the pregnant uterus. The surface of the ovary is smooth before puberty, but puckered after puberty due to the scars of ovulation

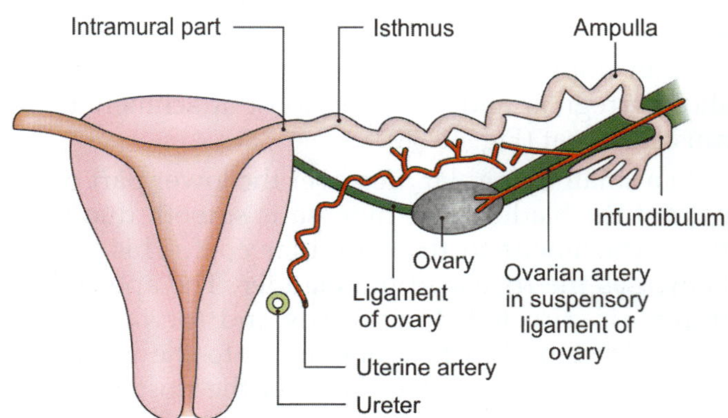

Fig. 40.41: The subdivisions, relations and blood supply of the uterine tube

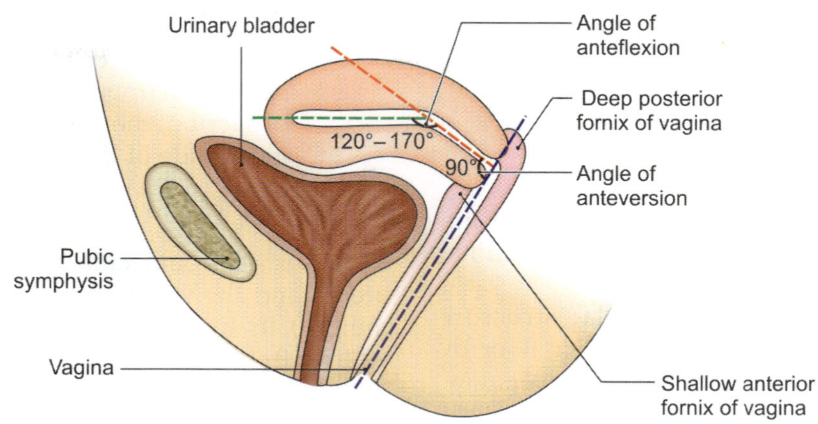

Fig. 40.42: Angulations of the uterus and vagina, and their axes

Blood Supply and Lymph Drainage

Fallopian tube in its medial two-thirds is supplied by uterine artery and in its lateral one-third by ovarian artery. Veins follow the arteries and drain into uterine venous plexus and pampiniform plexus.

THE UTERUS

The uterus or hystera is the organ which protects and provides nutrition to the fertilised ovum enabling it to grow into a fully formed foetus. It is narrow, pear-shaped organ with thick, muscular walls. In young nulliparous adult woman, it measures 8 cm × 5 cm × 2.5 cm.

Positions

Normally, in majority of women, long axis of the uterus is bent forward on the long axis of the vagina forming an angle of 90°. This position is referred to as anteversion of the uterus (Fig. 40.42).

The long axis of the uterus is bent forwards at the level of internal os with the long axis of the cervix forming an angle of about 170°. This position is called anteflexion of the uterus.

Parts

The uterus is divided into: (i) the fundus, (ii) the body, and (iii) cervix.

The fundus is the part of the uterus that lies above the entrance of the uterine tubes.

The body lies below the entrance of the uterine tubes and becomes narrow to become continuous with the cervix.

Blood Supply of Uterus

Each uterine artery is a branch of the internal iliac artery.

It runs medially in the base of the broad ligament and **crosses above the ureter,** bends at right angles to reach the cervix at the level of internal os. It then ascends along the lateral margin of the uterus within the broad ligament and ends by anastomosing with the ovarian artery (Fig. 40.43).

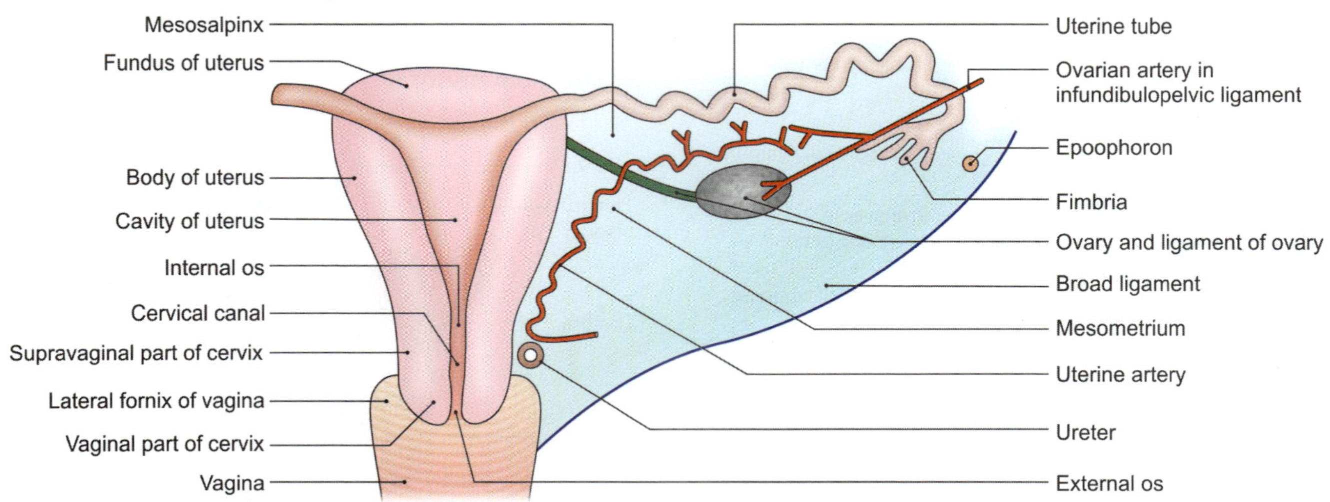

Fig. 40.43: Posterosuperior view of the uterus and the right broad ligament

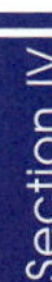

Uterine vein follows the artery and drains into the internal iliac vein.

Supports

The supports of the uterus are:

1 *Muscular (Active)*
   i. *Pelvic diaphragm:* Formed by two levator ani muscles resists the rise in the intra-abdominal pressure (Fig. 40.44).
   ii. *Perineal body:* This fibromuscular structure maintains the integrity of the pelvic floor by acting as an anchor for the pelvic diaphragm.

2 *Fibromuscular*
   i. *Pubocervical ligaments:* These are derived from pelvic fascia and connect the cervix to the posterior surface of the pubis.
   ii. *Transverse cervical (cardinal) ligaments of Mackenrodt:* Fibromuscular condensations of pelvic fascia that pass from the cervix and the upper end of vagina to the lateral pelvic walls (Fig. 40.45).
   iii. *Uterosacral ligaments (sacrocervical):* Fibromuscular bands of pelvic fascia passing to cervix and upper end of vagina from lower end of sacrum, thereby forming two ridges one on either side of the rectouterine pouch.

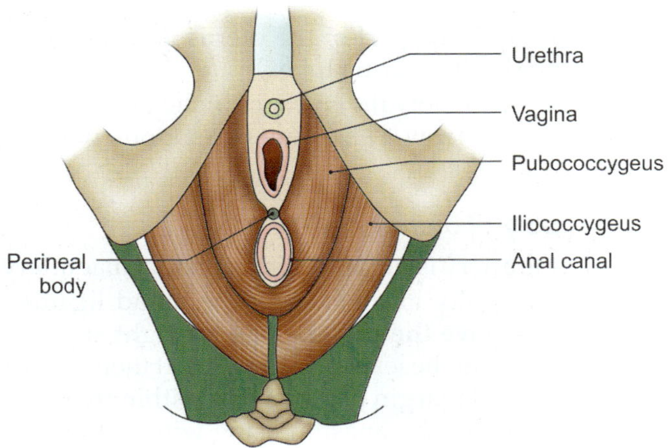

Fig. 40.44: Superior view of the pelvic diaphragm (the levator ani and coccygeus)

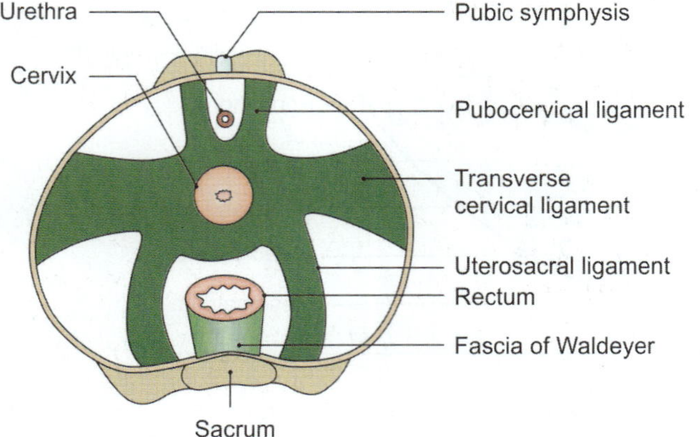

Fig. 40.45: Condensation of pelvic fascia forming the supports of the pelvic organs. Superior view of the ligamentous supports of the uterus and rectum

THE VAGINA

Vagina is a fibromuscular canal between the cervix of uterus and the vestibule (cleft between the two labia minora). Its anterior wall is 7.5 cm long while posterior wall is 10 cm long. The upper two-thirds of vagina lies in the pelvic cavity while lower one-third is situated in the perineum (Fig. 40.46).

Fornices of Vagina

The interior of the upper end of the vagina or vaginal vault is in the form of a circular groove that surrounds the protruding cervix. The groove becomes progressively deeper from before backwards and is arbitrarily divided into four parts called the vaginal fornices. The *anterior fornix lies* in front of the cervix and is shallowest. The *posterior fornix* lies behind the cervix and is deepest. The *lateral fornices* lie one on each side of the cervix.

Arterial Supply

The vagina is a very vascular organ, and is chiefly supplied by the vaginal branch of the internal iliac artery.

Venous Drainage

The rich vaginal venous plexus drains into the internal iliac veins through the vaginal veins which accompany the vaginal arteries.

EXTERNAL GENITAL ORGANS/ PUDENDUM or VULVA

Pudendum includes:

1 The mons pubis,
2 The labia majora,
3 The labia minora,

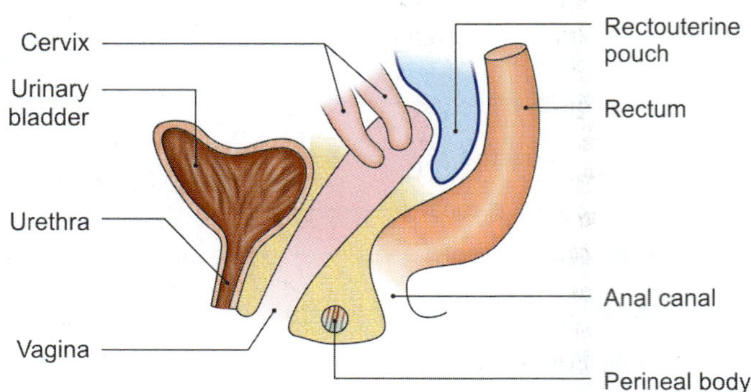

Fig. 40.46: Vagina and some related structures as seen in sagittal section

4 The clitoris,
5 The vestibule of the vagina,
6 The bulbs of the vestibule, and
7 The greater vestibular glands.

MALE REPRODUCTIVE SYSTEM

Organs

(1) The penis, (2) the scrotum, (3) the testes, (4) the epididymes, (5) the spermatic cords, (6) the ductus deferens, (7) the seminal vesicles, and (8) prostate. The urethra has been described in the Urinary System.

PENIS

The penis is the male organ of copulation. It is made up of: (a) A root or attached portion, and (b) a body or free portion (Fig. 40.47).

Root of Penis

The root of the penis is composed of three masses of erectile tissue, namely the two crura and one bulb. Each cryra is covered by the ischiocavernosus. The *bulb* is covered by the *bulbospongiosus.*

Body of Penis

The penis has a ventral surface that faces backwards and downwards, and a dorsal surface that faces forwards and upwards.

The free portion of the penis is completely enveloped by skin. It is composed of three elongated masses of erectile tissue. These masses are the right and left corpora cavernosa, and a median corpus spongiosum.

The two *corpora cavernosa* are the forward continuations of the crura. They are in close apposition with each other throughout their length. The corpora cavernosa do not reach the end of the penis. Each of them terminates under cover of the *glans penis* in a blunt conical extremity. They are surrounded by a strong fibrous envelope called the *tunica albuginea.*

The *corpus spongiosum* is the forward continuation of the bulb of the penis. Its terminal part is expanded to form a conical enlargement, called the glans penis. Throughout its whole length, it is traversed by the urethra.

The base of the *glans penis* has a projecting margin, the *corona glandis,* which overhangs an obliquely grooved constriction, known as the *neck of the penis.* Within the glans, the urethra shows a dilatation (in its roof) called the *navicular fossa.*

The *skin* covering the penis is very thin and dark in colour. It is loosely connected with the fascial sheath of the organ. At the neck, it is folded to form the *prepuce* or *foreskin,* which covers the glans to a varying extent and can be retracted backwards to expose the glans. On the undersurface of the glans there is a median fold of skin called the *frenulum.*

Figure 40.48 shows the structures seen in transverse section through the body of the penis.

Arteries of the Penis

The internal pudendal artery gives off three branches which supply the penis.

1 The *deep artery of the penis* runs in the corpus cavernosum.
2 The *dorsal artery of the penis* runs on the dorsum, deep to the deep fascia, and supplies the glans penis and

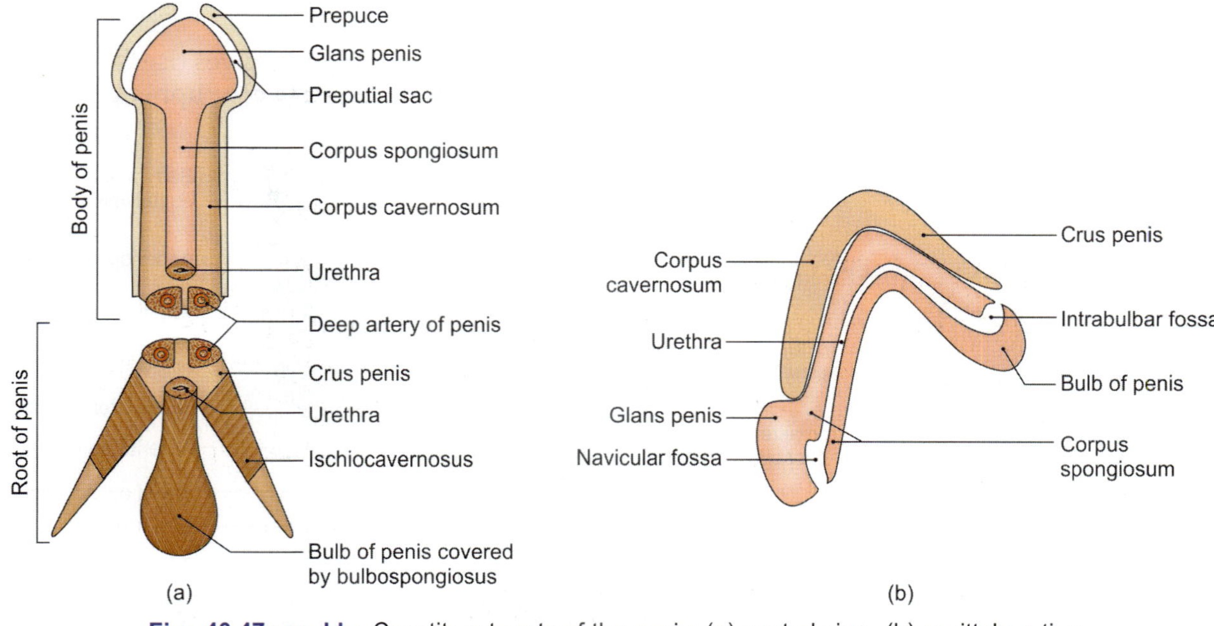

Figs 40.47a and b: Constituent parts of the penis: (a) ventral view, (b) sagittal section

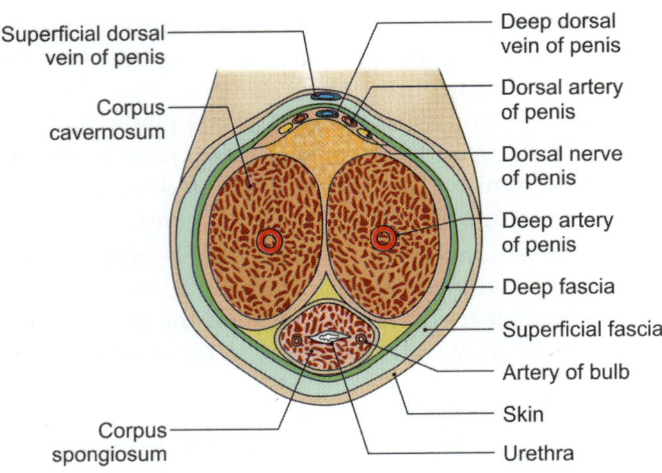

Fig. 40.48: Transverse section through the body of the penis

the distal part of the corpus spongiosum, the prepuce and the frenulum.

3 The artery of the bulb of the penis supplies the bulb and the proximal half of the corpus spongiosum.

SCROTUM

The scrotum is a cutaneous bag containing the right and left testes, the epididymes and the lower parts of the spermatic cords.

1 Externally, the scrotum is divided into right and left parts by a ridge or raphe (Fig. 40.49).

2 Under the influence of cold, and in young and robust persons, the scrotum is short, corrugated and closely applied to the testis. This is due to contraction of the subcutaneous muscle of the scrotum, called the *dartos*, which helps in regulation of the temperature within the scrotum.

Layers of Scrotum

The scrotum is made up of the following layers from without inwards (Fig. 40.49).

1 Skin.

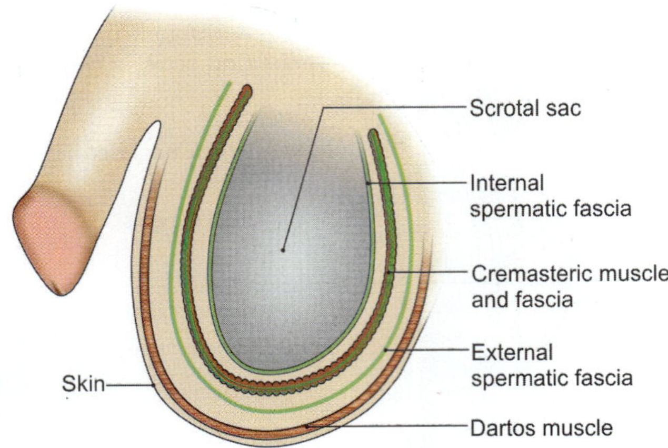

Fig. 40.49: Layers of the scrotum

2 Dartos muscle

3 The external spermatic fascia.

4 The cremasteric fascia.

5 The internal spermatic fascia.

Blood Supply

The scrotum is supplied by the arteries—superficial external pudendal, deep external pudendal and scrotal branches of internal pudendal.

TESTIS

The testis is the male gonad. It is homologous with the ovary of the female. It is suspended in the scrotum by the spermatic cord.

The testis is oval in shape, and is compressed from side to side. It is 3.75 cm long, 2.5 cm broad from before backwards, and 1.8 cm thick from side to side. An adult testis weighs about 10 to 15 g.

External Features

The testis has:

1 Two poles or ends—upper and lower,

2 Two borders, anterior and posterior,

3 Two surfaces—medial and lateral (Fig. 40.50)

Structure of the Testis

The glandular part of the testis consists of 200 to 300 lobules. Each lobule contains two to three seminiferous tubules. Each tubule is highly coiled on itself. The tubules are lined by cells which represent stages in the formation of spermatozoa.

The *seminiferous tubules join* together at the apices of the lobules to form 20 to 30 *straight tubules which* enter the mediastinum (Fig. 40.51). Here they anastomose with each other to form a network of tubules, called the *rete testis*.

In its turn, the rete testis gives rise to 12 to 30 *efferent ductules* which emerge near the upper pole of the testis

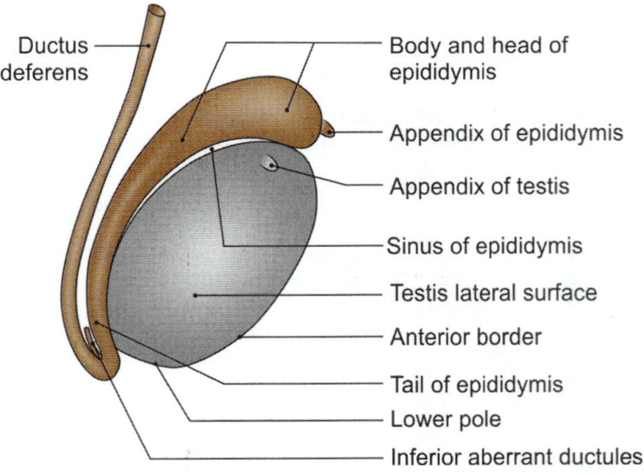

Fig. 40.50: Side view of the testis and epididymis, with the embryonic remnants present in the region

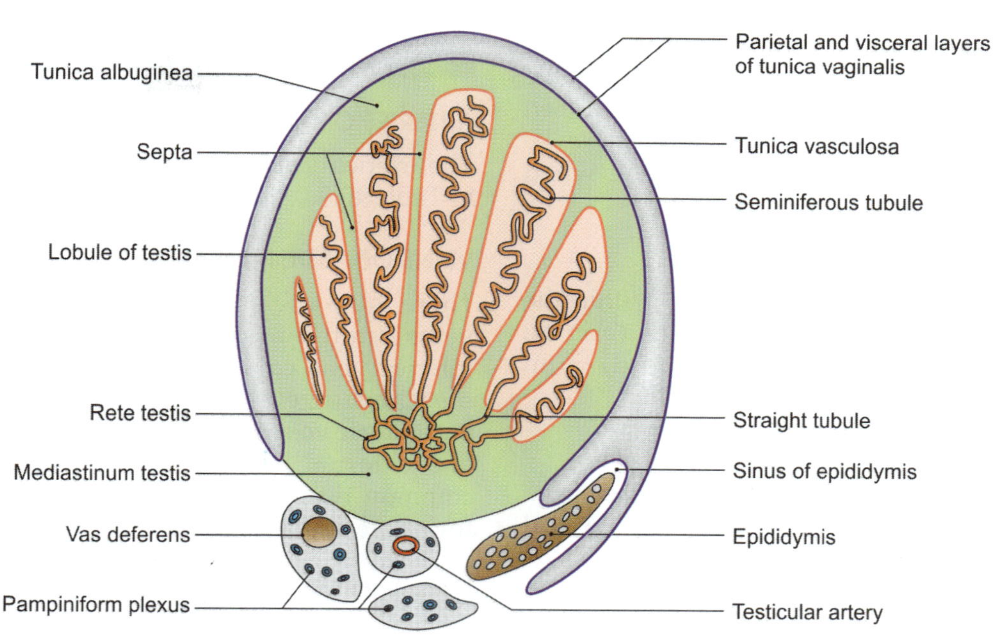

Fig. 40.51: Transverse section through the right testis and surrounding structures

and enter the epididymis. The tubules end in a single duct which is coiled on itself to form the head, body and tail of the epididymis. It is continuous with the ductus deferens.

Arterial Supply

The *testicular artery* is a branch of the abdominal aorta given off at the level of vertebra L2.

Venous Drainage

The veins emerging from the testis form the *pampiniform plexus* (pampiniform = like a vine). The plexus condenses into four veins at the superficial inguinal ring, and into two veins at the deep inguinal ring. These veins accompany the testicular artery. Ultimately, one vein is formed which drains into the *inferior vena cava* on the *right side*, and into the *left renal vein* on the *left side*.

EPIDIDYMIS

The epididymis is an organ made up of highly coiled tube that act as reservoir of spermatozoa.

Parts: Its upper end is called the *head.* The head is enlarged and is connected to the upper pole of the testis by *efferent ductules.* The middle part is *called* the *body.* The lower part is called the *tail.*

SPERMATIC CORD

Constituents of the Spermatic Cord

These are as follows:

1 The ductus deferens (Fig. 40.52).
2 The testicular and cremasteric arteries, and the artery of the ductus deferens.

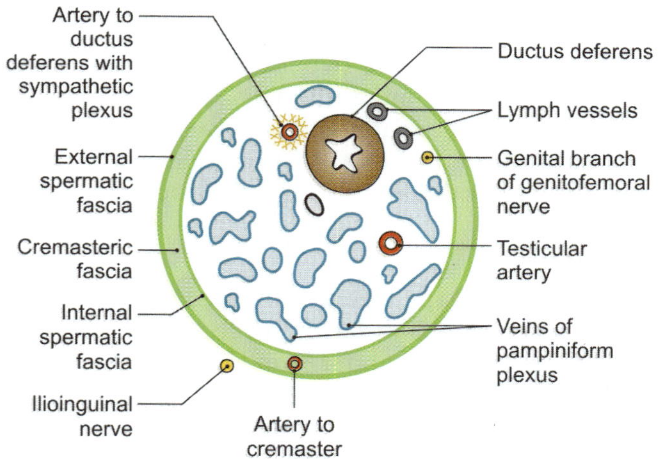

Fig. 40.52: Transverse section through the spermatic cord

3 The pampiniform plexus of veins.
4 Lymph vessels from the testis.
5 The genital branch of the genitofemoral nerve, and the plexus of sympathetic nerves around the artery to the ductus deferens.
6 Remains of the processus vaginalis.

Coverings of Spermatic Cord

From within outwards, these are as follows:

1 The *internal spermatic fascia*
2 The *cremasteric fascia*
3 The *external spermatic fascia*

THE DUCTUS DEFERENS

The *ductus deferens* is also called the *vas deferens* or the *deferent duct.*

The ductus deferens is a thick-walled, muscular tube which transmits spermatozoa from the epididymis to the ejaculatory duct. It feels cord-like and has a narrow lumen except at the terminal dilated part called the *ampulla.*

The ductus deferens is about 45 cm long when straightened.

Location

In its course, the vas lies successively: (1) within the scrotum along the posterior border of the testis, (2) in the inguinal canal as part of the spermatic cord, (3) in the greater pelvis, and (4) in the lesser pelvis.

Arterial Supply

The artery to the ductus deferens usually arises from one of the terminal branches of the superior vesical artery.

Venous Drainage

Veins from the ductus join the vesical venous plexus which opens into the internal iliac vein.

SEMINAL VESICLES

The seminal vesicles are two lobulated sacs, situated between the bladder and rectum. Each vesicle is about 5 cm long, and is directed upwards and laterally. The lower narrow end forms the duct of the seminal vesicle which joints the ductus deferens to form the ejaculatory duct.

THE PROSTATE

The prostate is shaped like an inverted pyramid—it is a fibromuscular glandular organ that surrounds the prostatic urethra. It is about 3 cm long and 4 cm wide. It surrounds the neck of the bladder (Fig. 40.37).

The prostate is covered by fibrous capsule; outside the capsule is a fibrous sheath—a part of the visceral layer of the pelvic fascia.

Structure

The prostate consists of numerous glands embedded in a mixture of smooth muscle and connective tissue. The ducts of the glands open into the prostatic urethra.

The anterior part of prostate gland is mainly fibromuscular, being overlapped from above by the detrusor muscle of urinary bladder.

Blood Supply

The prostate is supplied by branches from the inferior vesical, middle rectal and internal pudendal arteries.

Lymphatic Drainage

Lymphatics from the prostate drain chiefly into the internal iliac and sacral nodes, and partly into the external iliac nodes.

ARTERIES AND NERVES

ARTERIES OF ABDOMEN AND PELVIS

The arteries of abdomen and pelvis have been tabulated in Table 40.3.

VEINS OF ABDOMEN AND PELVIS

There is no coeliac axis vein. Left and right gastric veins drain into portal vein. Hepatic veins end in inferior vena cava. Splenic vein joins with superior mesenteric vein to form the portal vein. Inferior mesenteric vein drains into splenic vein. Internal iliac and external iliac veins of each side join to form common iliac vein. Two common iliac veins join to form inferior vena cava.

LOWER INTERCOSTAL NERVES

Course

The ventral rami of T7–T11 pass forwards in the intercostal spaces below respective intercostal vessels. As they reach the anterior ends of their respective spaces, these neves enter the rectus sheath. After supplying rectus abdominis, they pierce the anterior wall of the rectus sheath to reach the skin. 7th nerve supplies skin of the epigastrium and 8th below it.

The 10th nerve supplies the band of skin which includes the umbilicus.

Muscular Branches

The intercostal and subcostal nerves and their collateral branches supply intercostal muscles and muscles of anterolateral abdominal wall. T12 supplies pyramidalis also, if present.

SACRAL PLEXUS

It is formed by ventral rami of part of L4, L5, S1, S2, S3. Few muscular branches are given off from the rami. Then these divide into ventral and dorsal divisions.

Important branches arising from ventral divisions are:

- Pudendal nerve (S2, S3, S4), is described below.
- Tibial part of sciatic nerve (L4, L5, S1, S2, S3): Supplies hamstrings, muscles of calf and sole.

Branches from dorsal divisions are:

- Superior gluteal nerve (L4, L5, S1): Supplies gluteus medius, gluteus minimus and tensor fascia latae.
- Inferior gluteal nerve (L5, S1, S2): Supplies only gluteus maximus.
- Common peroneal part of sciatic nerve (L4, L5, S1, S2): Supplies evertors of foot and dorsiflexors of ankle joint and extensor digitorum brevis.

Table 40.3: Arteries of abdomen and pelvis

Artery	*Origin, course, termination*	*Distribution*
VENTRAL BRANCHES OF ABDOMINAL AORTA		
Coeliac trunk (Fig. 40.53)	It is the artery of foregut and the first ventral visceral branch of abdominal aorta arising at upper border of L1 vertebra. It has a course of 1.25 cm and ends by dividing into left gastric, common hepatic and splenic arteries	Coeliac trunk supplies the derivatives of foregut, namely oesophagus, stomach, proximal part of duodenum, spleen, greater part of pancreas, liver and gall bladder
Left gastric artery	Smallest branch of coeliac trunk. First it courses upward till the cardiac end of stomach, then it enters lesser omentum to run along lesser curvature of stomach. Ends by anastomosing with right gastric artery	Oesophageal branches to lower part of oesophagus. This part is also supplied by oesophageal branches of thoracic aorta. Gives gastric branches to both surfaces of stomach
Common hepatic artery	Branch of coeliac trunk. First descends till the upper border of duodenum, where it gives gastroduodenal artery, and continues as proper hepatic artery	Gastroduodenal supplies the stomach and 1st part of duodenum
Proper hepatic artery	It runs upwards in lesser omentum and ends at porta hepatis by dividing into right and left hepatic branches	Right gastric supplies stomach. Cystic artery for gall bladder arises from right hepatic artery. Two hepatic arteries to supply oxygen to the hepatic cells
Splenic artery	It is the largest branch of coeliac trunk. Runs sinuously along upper border of pancreas to reach hilum of spleen, where it ends by dividing 5–7 splenic branches	• Gives numerous pancreatic branches • 5–7 short gastric branches for fundus of stomach • Left gastroepiploic to supply stomach along greater curvature and greater omentum also
Superior mesenteric artery (Fig. 40.54)	It is the artery of midgut, arising from aorta at lower border of L1 vertebra. Courses downwards and to right to terminate in the right iliac fossa by anastomosing with a branch of ileocolic artery	• Distal part of duodenum below the opening of bile duct • Jejunum and ileum • Vermiform appendix • Caecum and ascending colon • Right two-thirds of transverse colon
Inferior pancreatico-duodenal artery	First branch of superior mesenteric artery from its right side	Supplies both duodenum and pancreas
Middle colic	Branch of superior mesenteric from its right side, it passes in the transverse mesocolon and divides into right and left branches	Supplies the transverse colon
Right colic	Branch of superior mesenteric from right side passes to right to reach ascending colon and divides into ascending and descending branches	Supplies the hepatic flexure and ascending colon
Ileocolic artery	Arises from right side of superior mesenteric artery. Runs downwards and to right till the caecum and ends by dividing into superior and inferior branches. Inferior branch ends by anastomosing with superior mesenteric artery	Supplies ascending colon, caecum, vermiform appendix and terminal ileum
12–15 jejunal and ileal branches	Arise from left side of superior mesenteric artery course between layers of mesentery to reach the jejunum and ileum	Supply both surfaces of jejunum and ileum
Inferior mesenteric artery (Fig. 40.55)	This is the artery of the hindgut. It is also a ventral branch of abdominal aorta arising at the left, crosses to left at the level of L3 vertebra. It courses downwards crosses common iliac artery and continues in sigmoid mesocolon, by changing its name to superior rectal artery	It supplies the • Left one-third of transverse colon • The descending colon, the sigmoid colon • The rectum • Upper part of anal canal
Left colic artery	First branch of inferior mesenteric artery. Runs upwards and to the left and ends by dividing into ascending and descending branches	• Left one-third of transverse colon • Descending colon
Sigmoid arteries	2–4 sigmoid arteries pass downwards and to left and anastomose with each other, lowest branch anastomoses with superior rectal artery	• Descending colon • Sigmoid colon

Contd...

Table 40.3: Arteries of abdomen and pelvis (Contd.)

Artery	*Origin, course, termination*	*Distribution*
Superior rectal artery	Continuation of inferior mesenteric artery at the pelvic brim. Divides into right and left branches	Muscles and mucous membrane of rectum Rectum and upper part of anal canal
OTHER BRANCHES OF ABDOMINAL AORTA		
Inferior phrenic arteries	Right and left inferior phrenic arteries give branches to the respective suprarenal glands and end in the thoracoabdominal diaphragm	Suprarenal glands and muscle of the diaphragm
Middle suprarenal arteries	Right and left arteries run upwards on the muscle of diaphragm to end in the suprarenal glands	Suprarenal glands
Renal arteries (Fig. 40.56)	These two large arteries arise at the level of L2 vertebra. Reach the hila of respective kidney to supply kidney	Suprarenals, ureters and kidneys
Gonadal	Arise at level of L2 vertebra. Each artery runs downwards and laterally	Runs as ovarian artery in female and as testicular artery in male
Ovarian arteries	Ovarian artery crosses the pelvic brim to enter the suspensory ligament of ovary. It then enters the hila of respective ovary	Supplies ovary and lateral part of oviduct
Testicular arteries	Each testicular artery joins the spermatic cord at the deep inguinal ring, courses through the inguinal canal. At the upper pole of testis, it divides into branches which supply testis and epididymis	Testis and epididymis
Lumbar arteries	Four pairs of lumbar arteries arise from the dorsal aspect of abdominal aorta. These pass laterally and dorsally to supply muscles of posterior abdominal wall. Gives branch to the vertebral canal also	Muscles of anterolateral and posterior abdominal wall. Spinal cord, muscles and skin of the back are also supplied
Median sacral artery	Single artery from back of aorta above its bifurcation. Ends in front of coccyx	Rectum and muscles of the pelvis
Common iliac artery	The two terminal branches of abdominal aorta. Each runs downwards and laterally and ends by dividing into larger external iliac and smaller internal iliac in front of sacroiliac joint at the level of L5 and S1 vertebrae	No branches are given off
EXTERNAL ILIAC ARTERY		
External Iliac artery	Larger terminal branch of common iliac artery Courses downwards and laterally till the midinguinal point from where it continues as the femoral artery	• Deep circumflex iliac for the muscles attached to the iliac crest • Inferior epigastric which enters the rectus sheath to supply the muscle and overlying skin
INTERNAL ILIAC ARTERY		
Internal iliac artery	Smaller terminal branch of common iliac artery Begins in front of sacroiliac joint, crosses the pelvic brim and ends by dividing into anterior and posterior divisions	The artery supplies most of the pelvic organs, perineum and the gluteal region
ANTERIOR DIVISION		
Superior vesical	Branch of internal iliac artery. Ends by giving branches to urinary bladder and ductus deferens	Superior surface of urinary bladder and the muscular wall of ductus deferens
Obturator artery	Branch of internal iliac artery. Runs on the lateral wall of pelvis, passes through obturator foramen to enter the thigh	Gives branches to obturator internus and iliacus muscles. In thigh it supplies the adductor muscles
Middle rectal artery	Branch of internal iliac artery. Ends by supplying muscle coats of rectum	Supplies muscle coats of rectum, prostate and seminal vesicles
Inferior vesical artery	Branch of internal iliac artery. Only in male ends by supplying trigone of urinary bladder	Supplies urinary bladder, prostate, seminal vesicle and lower part of ureter

Contd...

Table 40.3: Arteries of abdomen and pelvis (Contd.)		
Artery	*Origin, course, termination*	*Distribution*
Inferior gluteal artery	Largest and one of the terminal branches of internal iliac artery. It leaves the pelvis through greater sciatic notch to enter the gluteal region	Branches to muscles of gluteal region It is the axial artery of lower limb
Internal pudendal artery	Smaller terminal branch of internal iliac artery. Runs out of pelvis through greater sciatic notch and leaves the gluteal region by passing through lesser sciatic foramen to enter the pudendal canal. Then it runs in pudendal canal in the lateral wall of ischioanal fossa. Lastly it enters the deep perineal space where it ends by dividing into deep and dorsal arteries	In ischiorenal fossa, inferior rectal artery is given off which supplies mucous membrane, musculature of anal canal including skin overlying it. In perineum, it gives perineal artery for muscles, scrotal or labial branches, deep and dorsal arteries of penis or clitoris
Vaginal artery	Branches of internal iliac artery only in female It ends by supplying the vagina	Supplies vagina, base of urinary bladder
Uterine artery	It is branch of internal iliac artery only in female. It runs downwards and medially till the lateral fornix of vagina and then upwards along vagina, cervix and uterus with a tortuous course and ends by anastomosing with the ovarian artery	Supplies vagina, uterus, medial two-thirds of oviduct The artery crosses in front of ureter
POSTERIOR DIVISION		
Iliolumbar artery	Runs upwards in front of sacroiliac joint and ends by dividing into iliac branch and lumbar branch	Iliac branch supplies iliacus and lumbar branch supplies muscles of back and through its spinal branch, cauda equina is also supplied
Lateral sacral arteries	Two lateral sacral arteries which divide to enter four ventral sacral foramina to supply sacral canal and muscles of back of sacrum	Supply cauda equina and muscles of back of sacrum
Superior gluteal artery	Passes out through greater sciatic notch to reach gluteal region	It supplies muscles of gluteal region especially gluteus medius and minimus

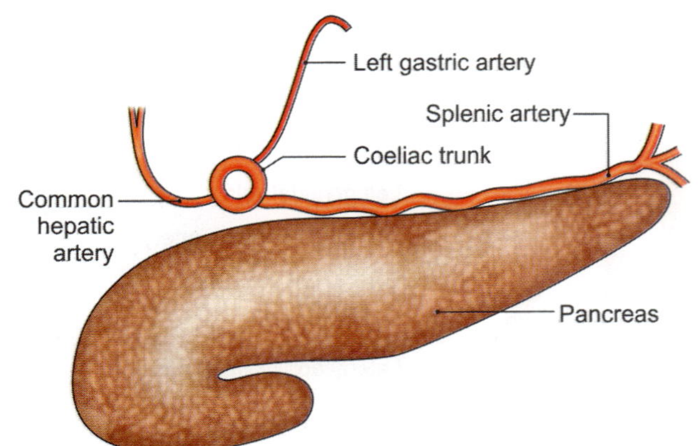

Fig. 40.53: Three branches of the coeliac trunk

PUDENDAL NERVE

Pudendal nerve supplies the skin, external genital organs and muscles of perineum. It is concerned with micturition, defaecation, erection, ejaculation and in females, with parturition. It is accompanied by internal pudendal vessels.

Root value: It arises from the sacral plexus in the pelvis. Its root value is ventral rami of S2, S3, S4 nerves.

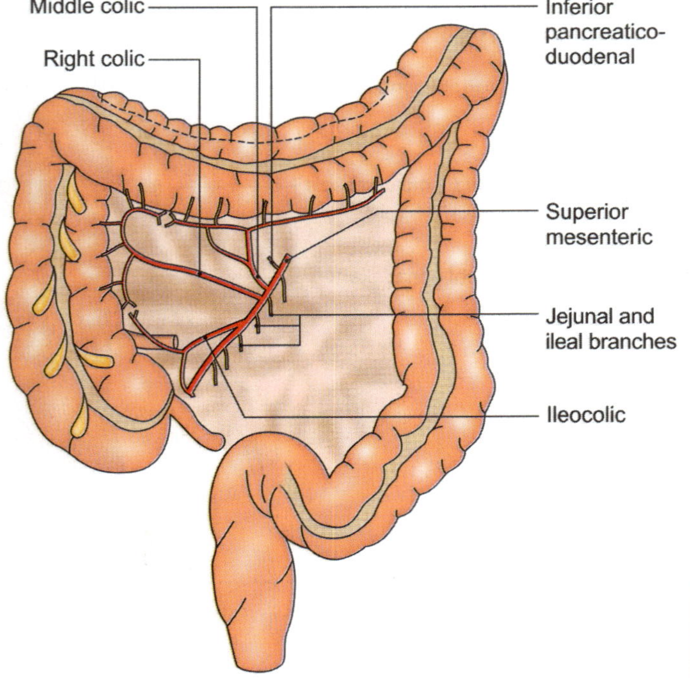

Fig. 40.54: Branches of the superior mesenteric artery

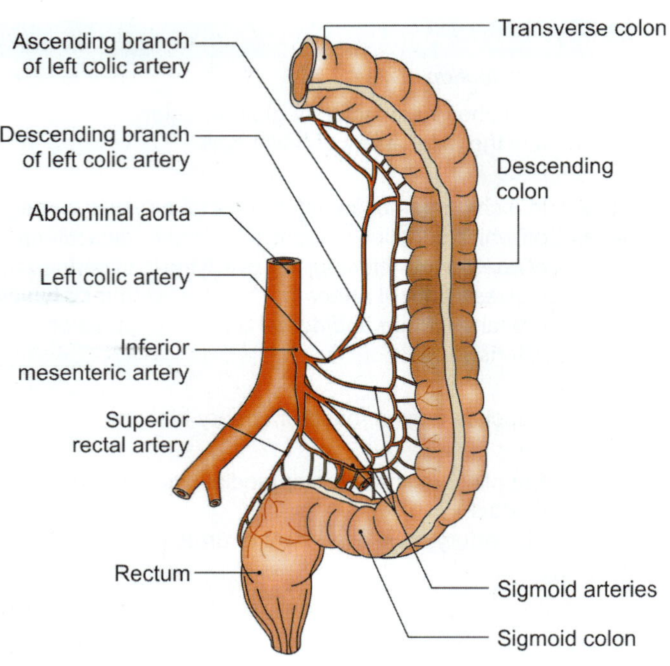

Fig. 40.55: Branches of the inferior mesenteric artery

Clinical Anatomy

Pudendal nerve block is given in some vaginal operations.

ABDOMINAL PART OF SYMPATHETIC TRUNK

Sympathetic trunk runs along the medial border of psoas major muscle. It is continuous with the pelvic part by passing behind the common iliac vessels. There are 4 ganglia in the lumbar or abdominal part. Only upper two ganglia receive white ramus communicans from the ventral primary rami of first and second lumbar nerves.

Branches

1 Grey rami communicans to the lumbar spinal nerves. These pass along the spinal nerves to be distributed to the sweat glands, cutaneous blood vessels and arrector pili muscles (sudomotor, vasomotor and pilomotor).
2 Postganglionic fibres pass medially to the aortic plexus.

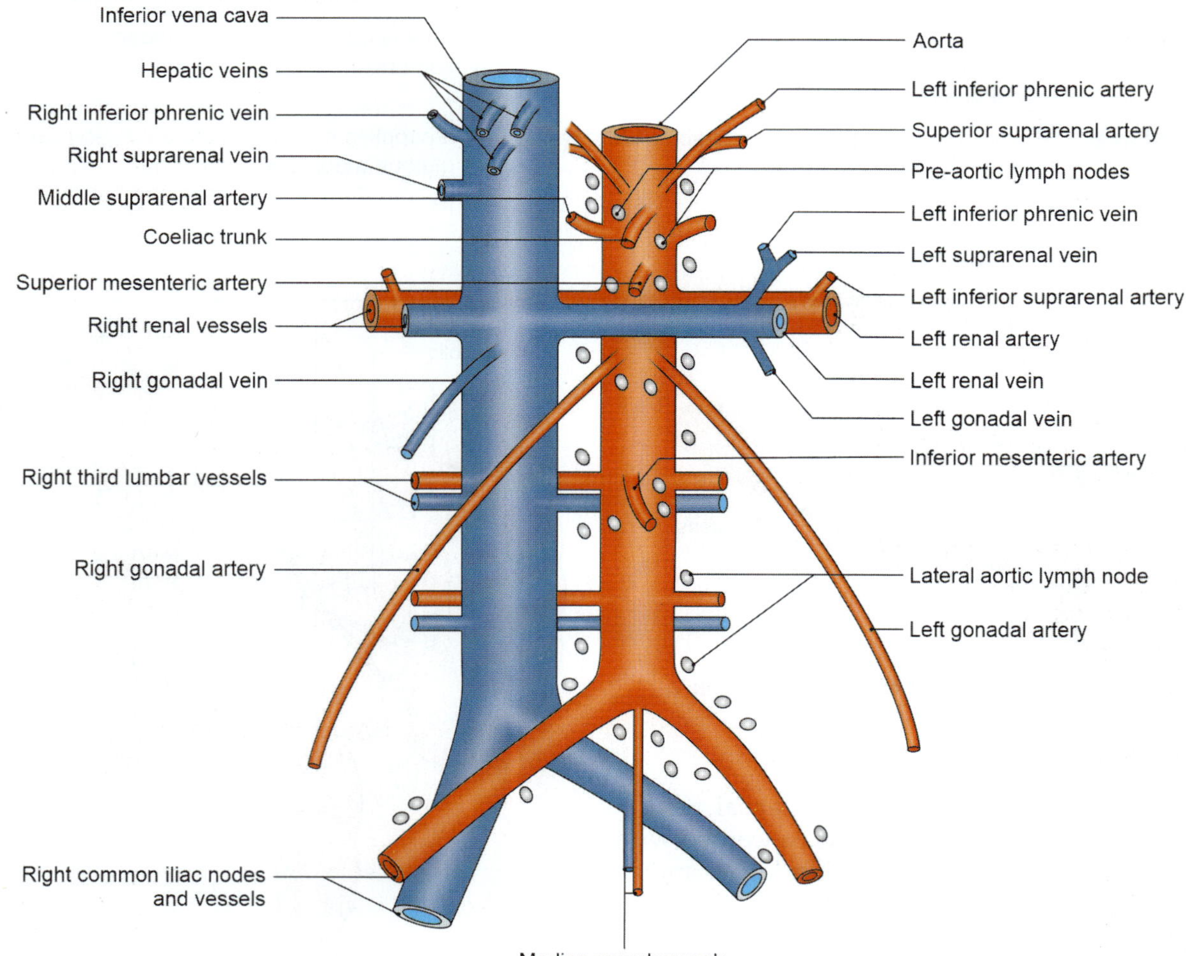

Fig. 40.56: The abdominal aorta, inferior vena cava and associated lymph nodes

3 Postganglionic fibres pass in front of common iliac vessels to form hypogastric plexus, which is also supplemented by branches of aortic plexus.

Aortic Plexus

This plexus is formed by preganglionic sympathetic, postganglionic sympathetic, preganglionic parasympathetic and visceral afferent fibres around the abdominal aorta. The plexus is concentrated around the origin of ventral and lateral branches of abdominal aorta. These are known as coeliac plexus, superior mesenteric plexus, inferior mesenteric plexus, and renal plexus.

Pelvic Part of Sympathetic Trunk

It runs in front of sacrum, medial to ventral sacral foramina. Caudally the two trunks unite and fuse into a single ganglion impar in front of coccyx. There are 4 ganglia in this part of sympathetic trunk. Their branches are:

1 Grey rami communicans to the sacral and coccygeal nerves.
2 Branches to the pelvic plexuses.

Collateral or Prevertebral Ganglia and Plexuses

Coeliac Plexus

It is the largest of the three autonomic plexuses, e.g. coeliac, superior mesenteric and inferior mesenteric plexuses. It is a dense network of nerve fibres which unite the two coeliac ganglia. The ganglia receive the greater splanchnic nerves, lesser splanchnic nerves of both sides including some filaments of vagi and phrenic nerves.

Coeliac ganglia are two irregularly shaped ganglia. Each ganglion receives greater splanchnic nerve. The lower part of the ganglion receives lesser splanchnic nerve and is also called as aorticorenal ganglion. The aorticorenal ganglion gives off the renal plexus which accompanies the renal vessels.

Secondary plexuses arising from coeliac and aorticorenal plexus are distributed along the branches of the aorta, namely phrenic, splenic, left gastric, hepatic, intermesenteric, suprarenal, renal, gonadal, superior and inferior mesenteric plexuses, and abdominal aortic plexus.

Superior hypogastric plexus: This plexus lies between the two common iliac arteries and is formed by:

1 Aortic plexus.
2 Branches from third and fourth lumbar sympathetic ganglia.

It divides into right and left inferior hypogastric plexus (pelvic plexus); which runs on the medial side of internal iliac artery and is supplemented by pelvic splanchnic nerves (parasympathetic nerves). Thus inferior hypogastric plexus contains both sympathetic and parasympathetic nerves. These are for the supply of the pelvic viscera along the branches of the arteries. The plexuses supply gastrointestinal tract and genitourinary tract.

The autonomic nerves supply of various organs and their effects are described.

Gastrointestinal Tract

Oesophagus

It receives its nerve supply from vagus and sympathetic.

Cervical part of oesophagus receives branches from recurrent laryngeal nerve of vagus and middle cervical ganglion of sympathetic trunk.

Thoracic part gets branches from vagal trunks and oesophageal plexus as well as from sympathetic trunks and greater splanchnic nerves.

Abdominal part receives fibres from vagal trunk (i.e. anterior and posterior gastric nerves), thoracic part of sympathetic trunks, greater splanchnic nerves and plexus around left gastric artery. The nerves form a plexus called myenteric plexus between two layers of the muscularis externa and another one in the submucous layer.

Stomach

Sympathetic supply reaches from coeliac plexus along gastric and gastroepiploic arteries. A few branches also reach from thoracic and lumbar sympathetic trunks.

Parasympathetic supply is derived from vagus nerves. The left vagus forms anterior gastric, while right vagus comprises posterior gastric nerve. The anterior gastric nerve supplies cardiac orifice, anterior surface of body as well as fundus of stomach, pylorus and liver.

Posterior gastric nerve supplies posterior surface of body and fundus till pyloric antrum. It gives a number of coeliac branches, which form part of the coeliac plexus.

Vagus is secretomotor to stomach. Its stimulation causes secretion which is rich in pepsin. Sympathetic inhibits peristalsis and is motor to the pyloric sphincter. It also carries pain fibres from stomach. Spasm, ischaemia and distension causes pain.

Small Intestine

The nerves of this part of the gut are derived from coeliac ganglia formed by posterior gastric nerve (parasympathetic) and the plexus around superior mesenteric artery. These nerves form myenteric plexus and submucous plexus. Parasympathetic fibres relay in the ganglion cells present in these plexuses. Sympathetic inhibits the peristaltic movements of intestine but stimulates the sphincters.

Large Intestine

Large intestine except the lower half of anal canal is supplied by both components of autonomic nervous system. The derivatives of midgut, i.e. caecum, vermiform appendix, ascending colon and right two-thirds of transverse colon receive their sympathetic nerve supply from coeliac and superior mesenteric ganglia and parasympathetic from vagus nerve.

Left one-third of transverse colon, descending colon, sigmoid colon, rectum and upper half of anal canal (developed from hindgut and anorectal canal) receive their sympathetic nerve supply from lumbar part of sympathetic trunk and superior hypogastric plexus through the plexuses on the branches of inferior mesenteric artery. Its effect is chiefly vasomotor. Parasympathetic supply of colon is received from pelvic splanchnic nerves.

Pelvic splanchnic nerves give fibres to inferior hypogastric plexuses to supply rectum and upper half of anal canal. Some fibres of inferior hypogastric plexus pass up through superior hypogastric plexus and get distributed along the branches of inferior mesenteric artery to the left one-third of transverse colon, descending and sigmoid colon.

Rectum and Anal Canal

Sympathetic fibres pass along inferior mesenteric and superior rectal arteries also via superior and inferior hypogastric plexuses.

Parasympathetic supply is from pelvic splanchnic nerve, which joins inferior hypogastric plexus. This supply is motor to muscles of rectum and inhibitory to internal sphincter.

The external anal sphincter is supplied by inferior rectal branch of pudendal nerve. Afferent impulses of physiological distension of rectum and sigmoid colon are carried by parasympathetic, whereas pain impulses are conveyed both by sympathetic and parasympathetic nerves.

Pancreas

Branches of coeliac plexus pass along the arteries. Sympathetic is vasomotor. The nerve fibres make synaptic contact with acinar cells before innervating the islets. The parasympathetic ganglia lies in sparse connective tissue of the gland and the islet cells.

Liver

Nerves of the liver are derived from hepatic plexus which contain both sympathetic and parasympathetic fibres. These accompany the blood vessels and bile ducts. Both types of nerve fibres also reach the liver through various peritoneal folds.

Gallbladder

Parasympathetic and sympathetic nerves of gallbladder are derived from coeliac plexus, along the hepatic artery (hepatic plexus) and its branches. Fibres from the right phrenic nerve (C4) through the communication of coeliac and phrenic plexus also reach gallbladder in the hepatic plexus. The reason of pain in the right shoulder (from where impulses are carried by lateral supraclavicular nerve C4) in cholecystitis is the stimulation of phrenic nerve fibres (C4) due to the communication of phrenic plexus and hepatic plexus via coeliac plexus.

Genitourinary Tract

Kidneys

The kidneys are supplied by renal plexus formed from coeliac ganglion, coeliac plexus, lowest thoracic splanchnic nerve, and first lumbar splanchnic nerve. The plexus runs along the branches of renal artery to supply the vessels, renal glomeruli and tubules. These are chiefly vasomotor in function.

Ureter is supplied in its upper part from renal and aortic plexus, middle part from superior hypogastric plexus and lower part from hypogastric nerve and inferior hypogastric plexus.

Vesical Plexus

Sympathetic fibres arise from T11, T12 segments and L1, L2 segments of spinal cord. Parasympathetic fibres arise from sacral S2, S3, S4 segments of spinal cord, which relay in the neurons present in and near the wall of urinary bladder. Parasympathetic is motor to the muscular coat and inhibitory to the sphincter; sympathetic is chiefly vasomotor. Emptying and filling of bladder is normally controlled by parasympathetic only.

Male Reproductive Organs

Testicular plexus accompanies the testicular artery to reach the testis. It is formed by renal and aortic plexus, and also from superior and inferior hypogastric plexuses. This plexus supplies the epididymis and ductus deferens.

Prostatic plexus is formed from inferior hypogastric plexus and branches are distributed to prostate, seminal vesicle, prostatic urethra, ejaculatory ducts, erectile tissue of penis, penile part of urethra and bulbourethral glands. Sympathetic nerves cause vasoconstriction, parasympathetic nerves cause vasodilatation.

Female Reproductive Organs

Ovary and uterine tube receive their nerve supply from plexus around the ovarian vessels. This plexus is derived from renal, aortic plexuses and also superior and inferior hypogastric plexuses. Sympathetic fibres derived from T10 and T11 segments of spinal cord are vasomotor in nature whereas parasympathetic fibres are probably vasodilator in function.

Uterus

It is supplied by uterovaginal plexus, formed from the inferior hypogastric plexus. The sympathetic fibres are derived from T12 and L1 segments of spinal cord. Parasympathetic fibres arise from S2, S3, S4 segments of spinal cord. Sympathetic causes uterine contraction and vasoconstriction, while parasympathetic nerves produce vasodilatation and uterine inhibition. Vagina is supplied by nerves arising from inferior hypogastric plexus and uterovaginal plexus. These supply wall of vagina including vestibular glands and clitoris. Parasympathetic fibres contain vasodilator effect on the erectile tissue.

Chapter

41

Lower Limb

"Do instead of dream, move instead of meditate, work instead of wish."
—Anonymous

BONES OF LOWER LIMB

The lower limbs are chiefly for locomotion. These provide stability to the whole body. Various regions of lower limb are as follows:

Regions	*Subdivision*
1. Gluteal region on the side and back of pelvis	The bone in the region is the hip bone and joints are the hip joint and sacroiliac joint.
2. Thigh from hip joint to knee joint	Bones are femur and patella and joint is the knee joint
3. Leg from knee to the ankle joint	Bones included are tibia, fibula and patella. The joints are superior and inferior tibio-fibular joints.
4. Foot from heel to the toes.	Tarsus made up of 7 tarsal bones, metatarsus made up of 5 metatarsals and 5 toes containing 14 phalangs, 2 in big or first toe and 3 each in 2nd to 5th toes. Joints included are ankle, subtalar, tarso-metatarsal, intermetatarsal, metatarsophalangeal and interphalangeal joints.

HIP BONE

Hip bone is a large bone comprised of three bones fused together, viz ilium situated above and laterally; ischium on the posterior aspect with a tuberosity on which one sits and pubis which lies anteroinferiorly. The two pubic bones articulate with each other to form pubic symphysis, a joint present in the midline in the lowest part of abdomen.

Ilium forms large flat bone below the waist. Its posterior part articulates with the lateral surface of sacrum to form the strong sacroiliac joint, which transmits the weight of the body to the ground via the lower limbs.

On the lateral aspect of hip bone is a deep fossa named the acetabulum, which articulates with the head of femur to form the hip joint.

Side Determination

1 The flat expanded ilium forms upper part of the bone and lies above the acetabulum.
2 Acetabulum is directed laterally.
3 The pubis lies anteriorly.

Ilium

Ilium forms upper expanded part of the hip bone. It has following parts.

1 Iliac crest forming the upper border.
2 Lower end which forms part of the acetabulum.
3 Three borders—anterior, medial and posterior.
4 Three surfaces—gluteal, sacropelvic and iliac.

Iliac Crest

Iliac crest forms the broad convex ridge (Fig. 41.1). It presents anterior superior iliac spine (ASIS) anteriorly. A little behind ASIS is the tubercle of iliac crest.

Gluteal Surface

Gluteal surface shows small posterior gluteal line, longest anterior gluteal line and an ill-defined inferior gluteal line, dividing this surface into four areas.

Iliac Fossa

Iliac fossa is concave smooth area between anterior and medial border. It forms lateral wall of false pelvis.

Sacropelvic Surface

It articulates with lateral mass of sacrum to form strong sacroiliac joint.

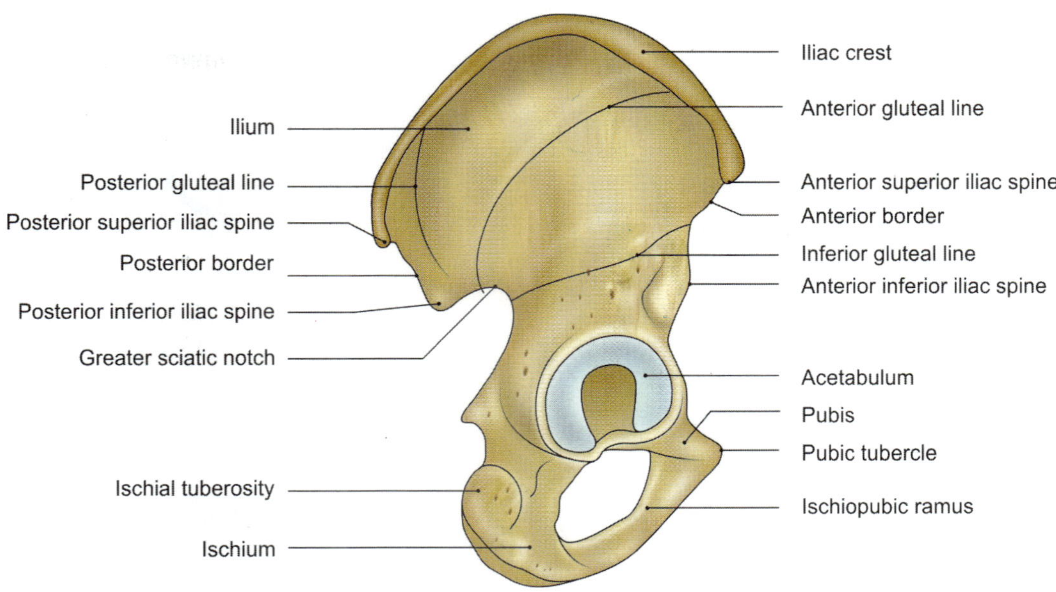

Fig. 41.1: General features of outer surface of hip bone

Attachments

1 Inguinal ligament and sartorius are attached to ASIS.
2 The ventral segment in its anterior two-thirds provides attachment to external oblique, internal oblique and transversus abdominis muscles of abdomen.
3 The gluteal surface gives origin to gluteus maximus, gluteus medius, gluteus minimus and rectus femoris (Fig. 41.1).
4 Iliac fossa gives origin to iliacus muscle.

Pubis

The pubis comprises a body, superior ramus and inferior ramus. Body has superior border or pubic crest, with pubic tubercle placed laterally.

Relevant Attachments

Pubic tubercle gives attachment to medial end of inguinal ligament.

ISCHIUM

Ischium forms posteroinferior part of the hip bone and part of acetabulum. It has a body, one ramus and ischial tuberosity on which one sits.

Muscles attached to ischial tuberosity are semitendinosus with long head of biceps femoris, semimembranosus and ischial part of adductor magnus.

FEMUR

Femur is the longest and strongest bone of the body. It comprises an upper end, a shaft and a lower end.

Upper End

The upper end includes:
1 Rounded head, which takes part in formation of hip joint (Fig. 41.2)
2 The neck, which makes an angle of 125° with the shaft in adults.
3 Greater trochanter giving distal attachment to gluteus medius and gluteus minimus and also to piriformis, obturator internus, two gemelli and obturator externus.
4 Lesser trochanter which provides insertion to iliopsoas the muscle of posterior abdominal wall.
5 Intertrochanteric line anteriorly between neck and shaft.
6 Intertrochanteric crest posteriorly between neck and shaft.

Shaft

The shaft is cylindrical and is convex forwards directed downwards and medially.

The posterior surface in lower one-third is called the popliteal surface.

Lower End

The lower end comprises large lateral and medial condyles, each having a patellar and a tibial surface. Between the two condyles is the intercondylar notch.

Side Identification

i. Head is above and large lower end is below.
ii. Greater trochanter is placed laterally in the upper part of the bone.
iii. Popliteal surface lies in the lower and posterior part of femur.

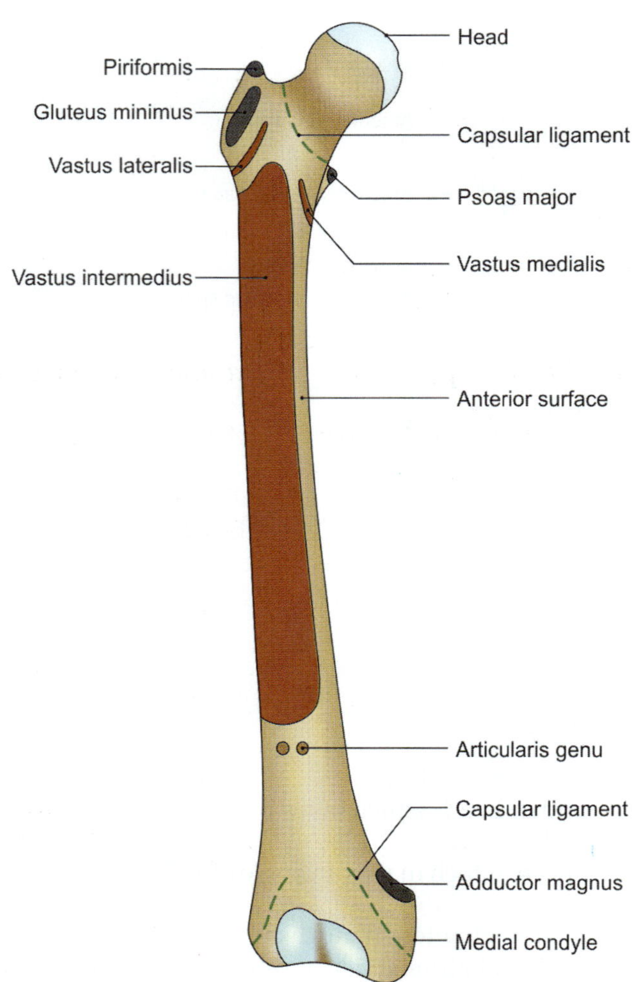

Fig. 41.2: Attachments on the anterior aspect of the right femur

Relevant Attachments

The three heads of quadriceps femoris, i.e. vastus medialis, vastus intermedius and vastus lateralis take origin from the borders and surfaces of shaft of femur (Fig. 41.2).

PATELLA

Patella is the largest sesamoid bone in the tendon of quadriceps femoris muscle. Patella is triangular in shape with base above and apex below. Anterior surface is rough while the posterior surface articulates with the patellar surface of femur.

Vastus lateralis is inserted into upper one-third of lateral border (Fig. 41.3).

Vastus medialis is inserted into upper two-third of medial border. Along the upper border are the insertions of vastus intermedius behind and rectus femoris in front. The ligamentum patellae is attached to the apex of patella.

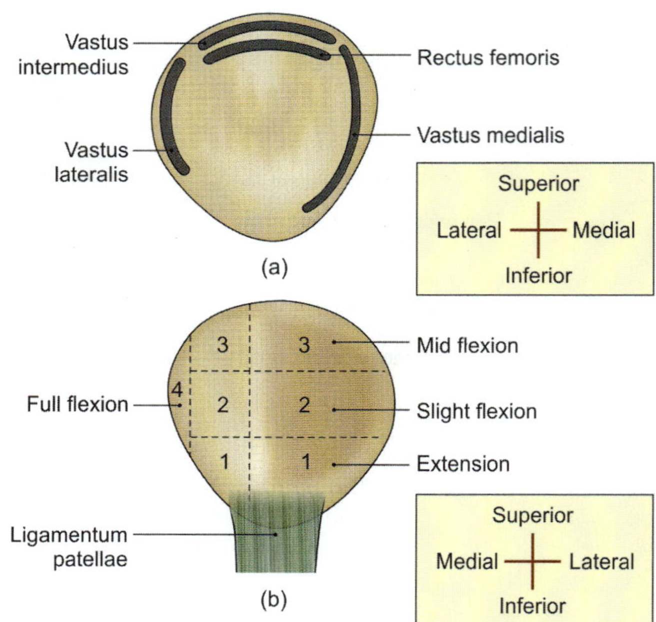

Figs 41.3a and b: Features of the right patella: (a) Anterior view, and (b) posterior view. Areas of patella in contact with patellar surface of femur during movement

TIBIA

Tibia is the larger and medial bone of the leg. It presents an upper end, a shaft and a lower end with medial malleolus.

Upper End

The upper end comprises large medial and lateral condyles with an intercondylar area in between and a tibial tuberosity (Fig. 41.4).

a. Medial condyle articulates with medial condyle of femur.
b. The lateral condyle articulates with lateral condyle of femur. Its lateral aspect articulates with upper end of fibula to form superior tibiofibular joint.
c. The ligamentum patellae, continuation of quadriceps femoris muscle, is attached to the upper smooth part of tibial tuberosity.
d. Structures attached to upper end of tibia are shown in Fig. 41.5.

Shaft

The shaft of tibia is nearly triangular in shape comprising three borders and three surfaces. The three borders are—anterior palpable border or shin, medial border extending down till medial malleolus and lateral border.

The three surfaces are—lateral, medial, and posterior. The posterior surface is marked by an oblique soleal line and a vertical ridge.

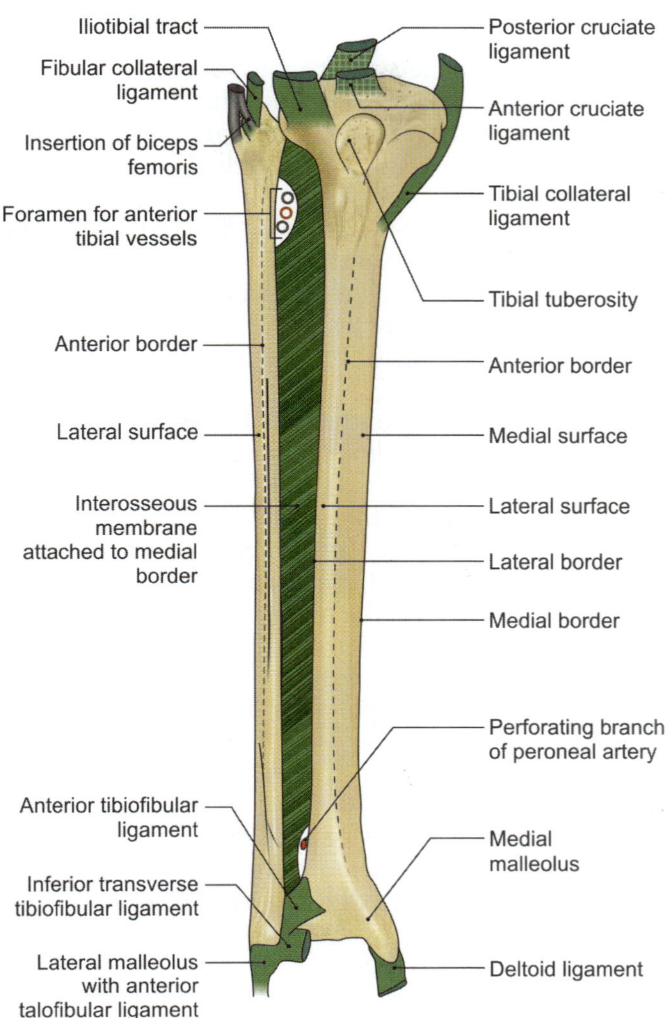

Fig. 41.4: Anterior view of right tibia and fibula including the ligaments

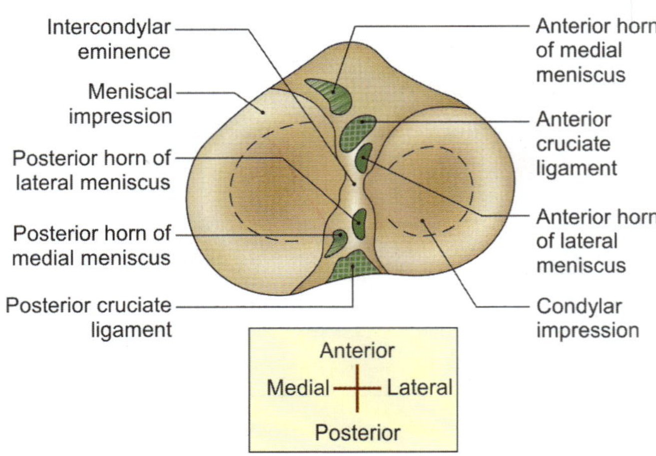

Fig. 41.5: Superior view of the upper end of the right tibia

Broad Lower End

It is prolonged downwards and medially as the medial malleolus. The lateral aspect of lower end is marked by a fibular notch to articulate with lower end of fibula to form inferior tibiofibular joint.

FIBULA

The fibula is the thinner and lateral bone of the leg. It does not participate in the formation of knee joint, whereas it takes part in building up of the ankle joint. Fibula has an upper end, a shaft and a lower end (Fig. 41.4).

1. *Upper end or head:* Its superior surface articulates with lateral condyle of tibia.
2. *Shaft:* The shaft shows three ill-defined anterior, posterior and interosseous borders and three surfaces—medial, lateral, and posterior. The posterior surfaces is divided into two parts by the medial crest.
3. *Lower end:* The lower end is prolonged to form the lateral malleolus. The medial surface of lateral malleolus bears a triangular facet for articulation with talus to form part of the ankle joint.

BONES OF THE FOOT

TARSUS

The tarsus is made up of seven tarsal bones arranged in two rows. The proximal row comprises, talus sitting on the lower calcaneum. The distal row contains medial, intermediate, lateral cuneiforms and cuboid. In between talus and cuneiforms, i.e. between proximal and distal rows is the navicular (Fig. 41.6).

The 7 tarsal bones are larger and stronger than the 8 carpal bones.

METATARSUS

The metatarsus comprises five metatarsal bones. Each bone is a short long bone with base, shaft and a distal end or head.

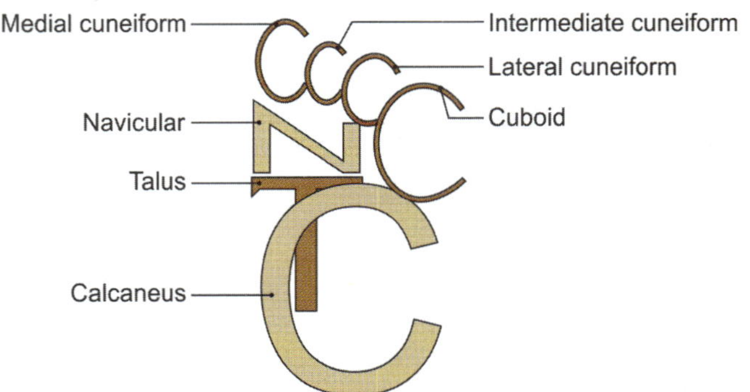

Fig. 41.6: Tarsus

PHALANGES

There are 14 phalanges. Two are present in big toe and are relatively bigger than three each present in second–fifth toes.

FRONT OF THIGH

Front of thigh includes muscles, femoral triangle and adductor canal.

FEMORAL TRIANGLE

It is a triangular depression on the front of the upper one-third of the thigh immediately below the inguinal ligament.

Boundaries

The femoral triangle is bounded *laterally* by the medial border of sartorius; and *medially* by the medial border of the adductor longus (Fig. 41.7). Its base is formed by the inguinal ligament. The *apex,* which is directed downwards, is formed by the point where the medial and lateral boundaries meet. The **roof** is formed by:

i. Skin.
ii. Superficial fascia containing the superficial inguinal lymph nodes, cutaneous veins, cutaneous nerves, superficial branches of the femoral artery with accompanying veins, and the upper part of the great saphenous vein.
iii. *Deep fascia,* with the saphenous opening and the cribriform fascia.

The *floor* of the triangle is formed medially by the adductor longus and pectineus, and laterally by the iliopsoas (Fig. 41.7).

Contents

The contents of the femoral triangle are as follows.

1 *Femoral artery and its branches.* The femoral artery traverses the triangle from its base at the midinguinal point to the apex. In the triangle, it gives off six branches.
2 *Femoral vein and its tributaries.* The femoral vein accompanies the femoral artery.
The femoral vein receives the great saphenous vein.
3 The *femoral sheath* encloses the upper 4 cm of the femoral vessels (Fig. 41.7).
4 *Nerves:*
   a. The *femoral nerve* lies lateral to the femoral artery, *outside the femoral sheath* described at end of lower limb.
   b. The *nerve to the pectineus.*
   c. The *femoral branch of the genitofemoral nerve* occupies the lateral compartment of the femoral sheath along with the femoral artery.
   d. The *lateral cutaneous nerve of the thigh* crosses the lateral angle of the triangle.
5 The *deep inguinal lymph nodes* lie deep to the deep fascia.

Femoral Sheath

This is a funnel-shaped sleeve of fascia enclosing the upper 3 to 4 cm of the femoral vessels. The sheath is formed by downward extension of two layers of the fascia of the abdomen.

The sheath is divided into the following three compartments by septa.

1 The *lateral or arterial compartment* contains the femoral artery and the femoral branch of the genitofemoral nerve.

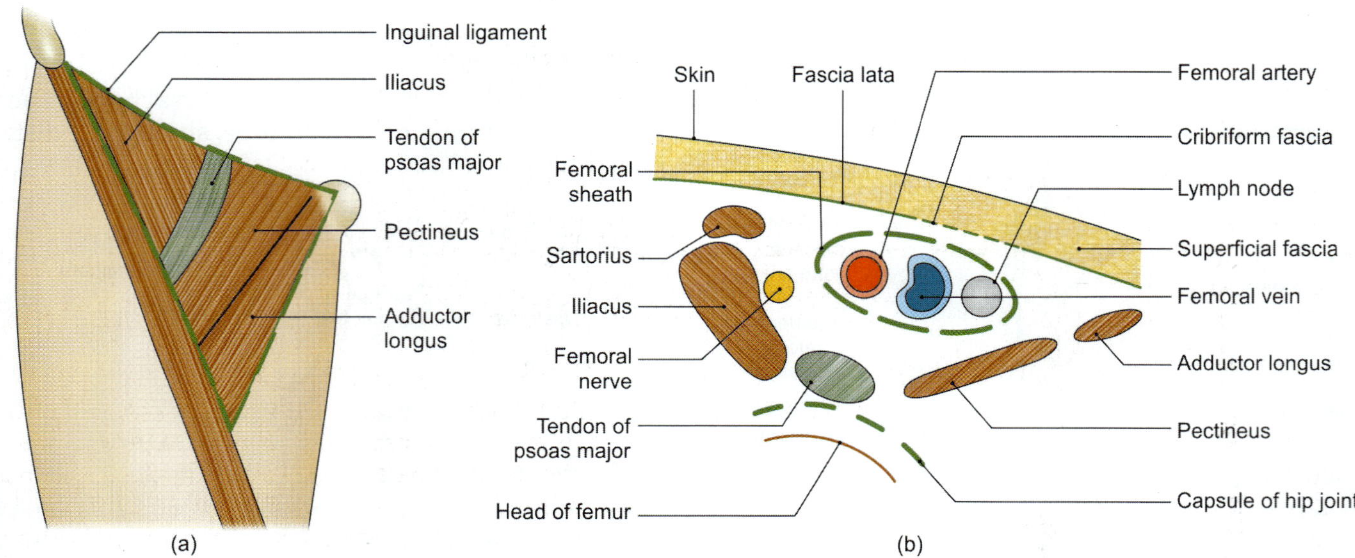

Figs 41.7a and b: Floor of the femoral triangle; surface view

Table 41.1: Muscles of the anterior or extensor compartment of thigh

Muscle	*Origin from*	*Insertion into*
1. **Sartorius** (Fig. 41.9)	• Anterior superior iliac spine and • Upper half of the notch below the spine	Upper part of the medial surface of the shaft of the tibia in front of the insertions of the gracilis and the semitendinosus
2. **Quadriceps femoris**		
A. Rectus femoris (Fig. 41.9) fusiform, superficial fibres bipennate, deep fibres straight	• Straight head—from the upper half of the anterior inferior iliac spine • Reflected head—from the groove above the margin of the acetabulum and the capsule of the hip joint	Base of patella
B. Vastus lateralis forms large part of quadriceps femoris	The origin is linear The line runs along: • Upper part of intertrochanteric line • Anterior and inferior borders of greater trochanter • Lateral lip of gluteal tuberosity • Upper half of lateral lip of linea aspera	• Lateral part of the base of patella. • Upper one-third of the lateral border of patella. • Expansion to the capsule of knee joint, tibia and iliotibial tract
C. Vastus medialis (Fig. 41.9)	The origin is linear. The line runs along: • Lower part of intertrochanteric line • Spiral line • Medial lip of linea aspera • Upper one-fourth of medial supracondylar line	Medial one-third of the base and upper two-thirds of the medial border of the patella
D. Vastus intermedius	• Upper three-fourths of the anterior and lateral surfaces of the shaft of femur	Base of patella *Note.* The patella is a sesamoid bone in the tendon of the quadriceps femoris. The ligamentum patellae is the actual tendon of the quadriceps femoris, which is inserted into the upper part of tibial tuberosity

2 The *intermediate or venous compartment* contains the femoral vein.
3 The *medial or lymphatic compartment* is known as the *femoral canal* and is described below (Fig. 41.8).

Femoral Canal

This is the medial compartment of the femoral sheath. It is conical in shape, being wide above or at base and narrow below. It is about 1.5 cm long, and about 1.5 cm wide at the base.

- Femoral hernia may occur through the femoral canal.

MUSCLES OF FRONT OF THE THIGH

The muscles of the anterior compartment of the thigh are the sartorius, the quadriceps femoris, and the articularis genu described in Table 41.1 and Fig. 41.9.

Nerve supply—Femoral nerve.

Action: Quadriceps femoris is the extensor of knee joint. Rectus femoris is also called "kicking muscle". Sartorius is flexor of hip and knee joints.

ADDUCTOR/HUNTER'S/SUBSARTORIAL CANAL

This is also called the subsartorial canal or Hunter's canal (Fig. 41.10).

Extent

The canal extends from the apex of the femoral triangle, above, to the tendinous opening in the adductor magnus, below.

Shape

The canal is triangular on cross-section.

Boundaries

It has anterior, posterior and medial walls. The anterior wall is formed by the vastus medialis. The posterior wall or floor is formed by the adductor longus, above, and the adductor magnus, below. The medial wall or roof is formed by a strong fibrous membrane joining the anterior and posterior walls. The roof is overlapped by the sartorius.

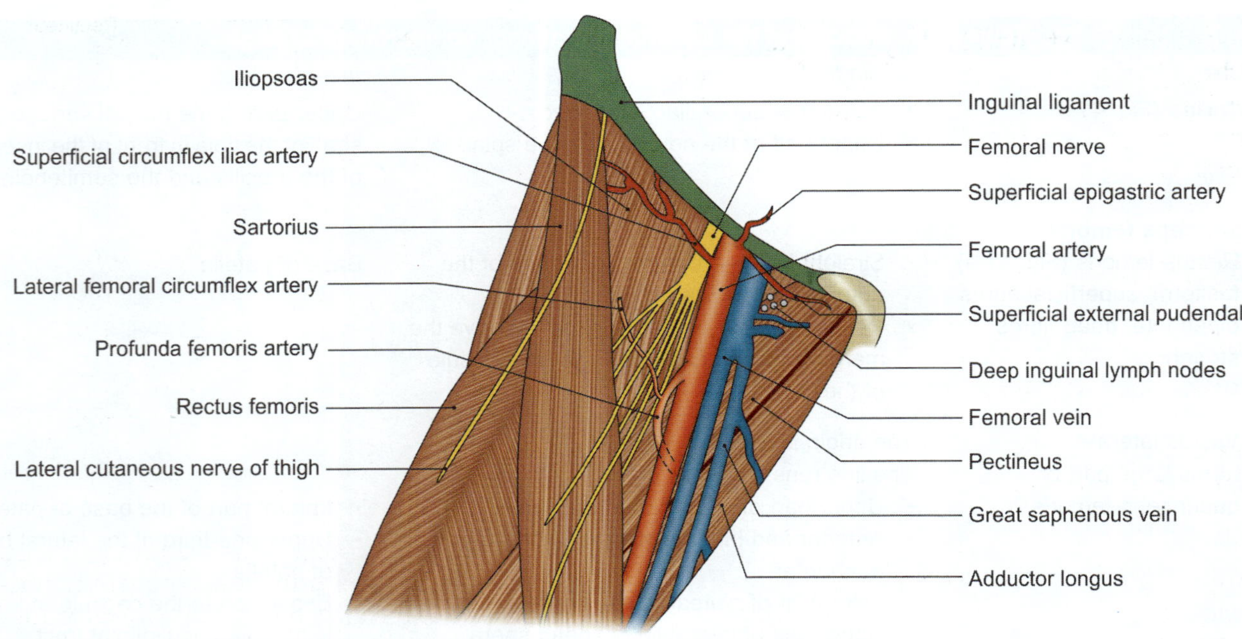

Fig. 41.8: Contents of the femoral triangle

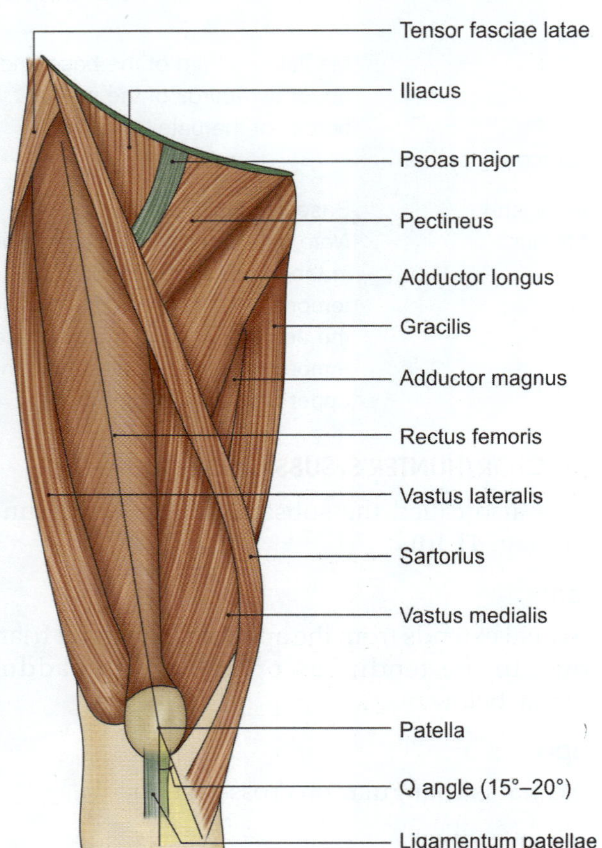

Fig. 41.9: Muscles seen on the front of the thigh

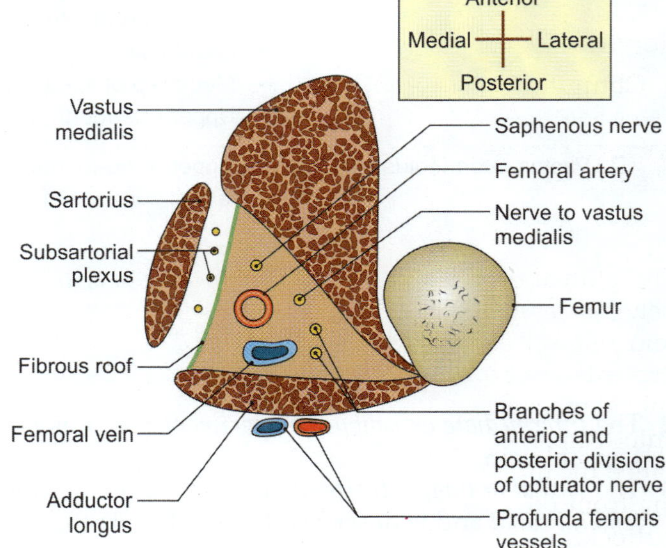

Fig. 41.10: Transverse section through the middle of the adductor canal, seen from above. Note the boundaries and contents of the canal

Contents

These are as follows.

1. The *femoral artery* enters the canal at the apex of the femoral triangle. Described at end of lower limb.
2. The femoral vein (Fig. 41.10)

CLINICAL ANATOMY

- *Femoral hernia:* The femoral canal is an area of potential weakness in the abdominal wall through which abdominal contents may bulge out forming a femoral hernia. A femoral hernia is more common in females because the femoral canal is wider in them than in males. This is associated with the wider pelvis, and the smaller size of the femoral vessels, in the female.

- Pulsations of the femoral artery can be felt at the midinguinal point, against the head of the femur and the tendon of the psoas major.
- Intramuscular injections can be given in vastus lateralis muscle.

MEDIAL SIDE OF THIGH

Boundaries

The adductor or medial compartment of the thigh is bounded anteriorly by the medial intermuscular septum and posteriorly by an ill-defined posterior intermuscular septum (Fig. 41.11).

Contents

i. Adductor longus (Fig. 41.12)
ii. Adductor brevis
iii. Adductor magnus
iv. Gracilis
v. Pectineus.

Nerves

1 Obturator nerve described at end of lower limb.

GLUTEAL REGION

INTRODUCTION

The gluteal region overlies the side and back of the pelvis, extending from the iliac crest above to the gluteal fold below. The lower part of the gluteal region which presents a rounded bulge due to excessive amount of subcutaneous fat is known as the buttock or natis. The anterosuperior part of the region seen in a side view is called the hip. The muscles, nerves and vessels emerging from pelvis are covered by gluteus maximus and buttock.

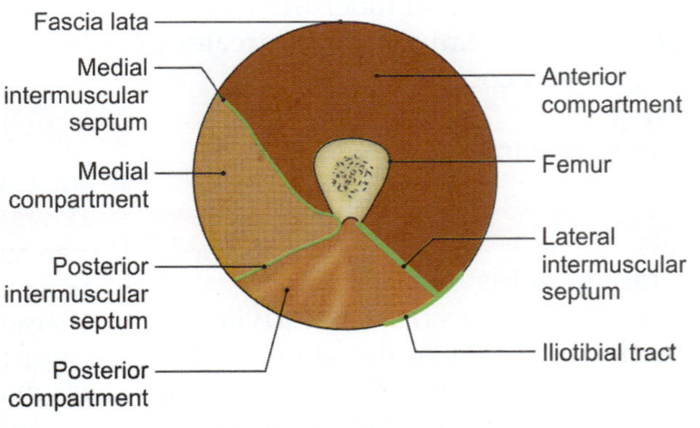

Fig. 41.11: Intermuscular septa and compartments of thigh

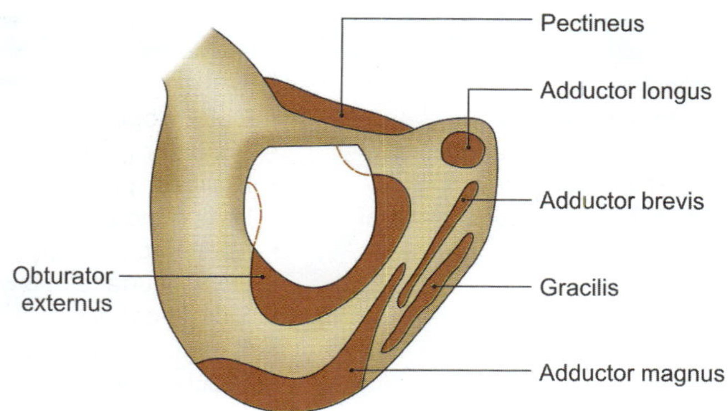

Fig. 41.12: Origin of muscles of medial compartment of the thigh

MUSCLES OF GLUTEAL REGION

These muscles are the gluteus maximus, the gluteus medius, the gluteus minimus, the piriformis, the superior and inferior gemelli, the obturator internus, obturator externus, and quadratus femoris. The tensor fasciae latae which lies on the lateral side of thigh, just in front of gluteal region, is also considered here. The attachments and nerve supply of first three muscles are given in Tables 41.2 and 41.3. Their actions and some other features are considered below.

STRUCTURES UNDER COVER OF GLUTEUS MAXIMUS

These are as follows:

Muscles

1 Gluteus medius (Fig. 41.13).
2 Gluteus minimus.

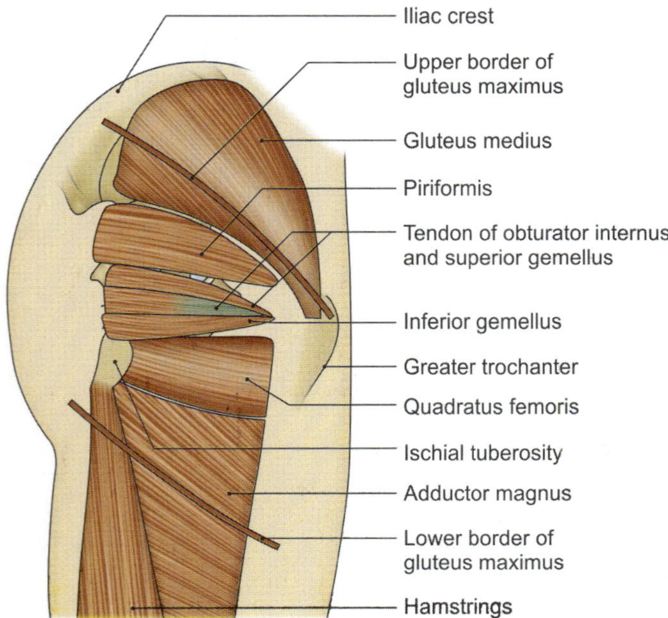

Fig. 41.13: Muscles under cover of the gluteus maximus. The upper and lower borders of this muscle are indicated in thick lines

Table 41.2: Important muscles of the gluteal region—origin and insertion

Muscles	*Origin*	*Insertion*
Gluteus maximus This is a large, quadrilateral powerful muscle covering mainly the posterior surface of pelvis	• Outer slope of the dorsal segment of iliac crest • Posterior gluteal line • Posterior part of gluteal surface of ilium behind the posterior gluteal line • Aponeurosis of erector spinae • Dorsal surface of lower part of sacrum • Side of coccyx • Sacrotuberous ligament • Fascia covering gluteus medius	• The deep fibres of the lower part of the muscle are inserted into the gluteal tuberosity • The greater part of the muscle is inserted into the iliotibial tract
Gluteus medius It is fan-shaped, and covers the lateral surface of the pelvis and hip	Gluteal surface of ilium between the anterior and posterior gluteal lines	Into the greater trochanter of femur, on oblique ridge on the lateral surface. The ridge runs downwards and forwards
Gluteus minimus It is fan-shaped, and is covered by the gluteus medius	Gluteal surface of ilium between the anterior and inferior gluteal lines	Into greater trochanter of femur, on a ridge on the lateral part of the anterior surface

Table 41.3: Important muscles of the gluteal region—nerve supply and actions

Muscles	*Nerve supply*	*Actions*
Gluteus maximus	Inferior gluteal nerve (L5, S1, S2)	Chief extensor of the thigh at the hip joint. This action is very important in rising from a sitting position. It is essential for maintaining the erect posture. Other actions are: a. Lateral rotation of the thigh b. Abduction of the thigh (by upper fibres) c. Along with the tensor fasciae latae, the muscle stabilises the knee through the iliotibial tract It supports both the hip and the knee when these joints are slightly flexed. It is an antigravity muscle as well.
Gluteus medius **Gluteus minimus**	Superior gluteal nerve (L4, L5, S1) Superior gluteal nerve (L4, L5, S1)	The *gluteus medius* and *gluteus minimus* are powerful abductors of the thigh. Their anterior fibres are also medial rotators. However, their most important action is to maintain the balance of the body when the opposite foot is off the ground, as in walking and running. They do this by preventing the opposite side of the pelvis from tilting downwards under the influence of gravity.

Vessels

1 Superior gluteal vessels (Fig. 41.14).
2 Inferior gluteal vessels.
3 Internal pudendal vessels.

Nerves

1 Superior gluteal (L4, L5, S1).
2 Inferior gluteal (L5, S1, S2).
3 Sciatic (L4, S5, S1, S2, S3).
4 Pudendal nerve (S2, S3, S4).

Bones and Joints

1 Ilium.
2 Ischium with ischial tuberosity.
3 Upper end of femur with the greater trochanter.
4 Sacrum and coccyx.
5 Hip joint.
6 Sacroiliac joint.

CLINICAL ANATOMY

Gluteal Muscles

Intramuscular injections are given in the antero-superior quadrant of the gluteal region, i.e. in the glutei medius, to avoid injury to large vessels and nerves which pass through the lower part of this

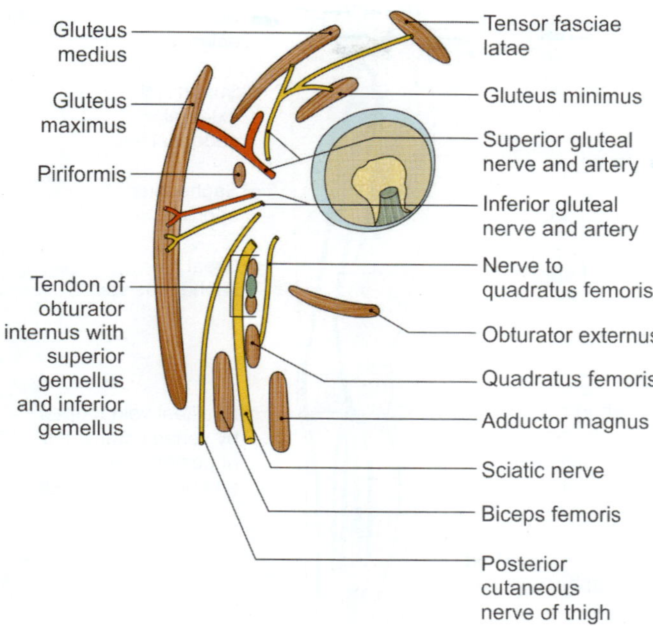

Fig. 41.14: Structures under cover of the gluteus maximus

region (*see* Fig. 42.2). Gluteal region is not the prominence of the buttock only. It is a very big area over the iliac bone.

POPLITEAL FOSSA

The popliteal fossa is a diamond-shaped depression lying behind the knee joint, the lower part of the femur, and the upper part of the tibia.

The *boundaries* of the fossa are as follows:

- *Superolaterally:* The biceps femoris (Fig. 41.15).
- *Superomedially:* The semitendinosus and the semimembranosus, supplemented by the gracilis, the sartorius and the adductor magnus.

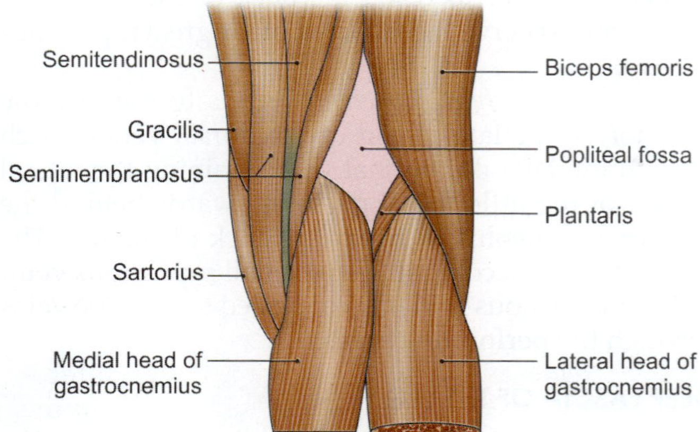

Fig. 41.15: Boundaries of the right popliteal fossa. Part of popliteal artery shown

- *Inferolaterally:* Lateral head of the gastrocnemius supplemented by the plantaris.
- *Inferomedially:* Medial head of the gastro-cnemius.

The **roof** of the fossa is formed by deep fascia or popliteal fascia. The superficial fascia over the roof contains:

1. The small saphenous vein.
2. Cutaneous nerves

The **floor** of the popliteal fossa is formed from above downwards by:

1. The popliteal surface of the femur.
2. The capsule of the knee joint and the oblique popliteal ligament.
3. The strong popliteal fascia covering the popliteus muscle.

The main **contents** of the fossa are:

1. The popliteal artery and its branches.
2. The popliteal vein and its tributaries.
3. The tibial nerve and its branches.
4. The common peroneal nerve and its branches (Fig. 41.16).

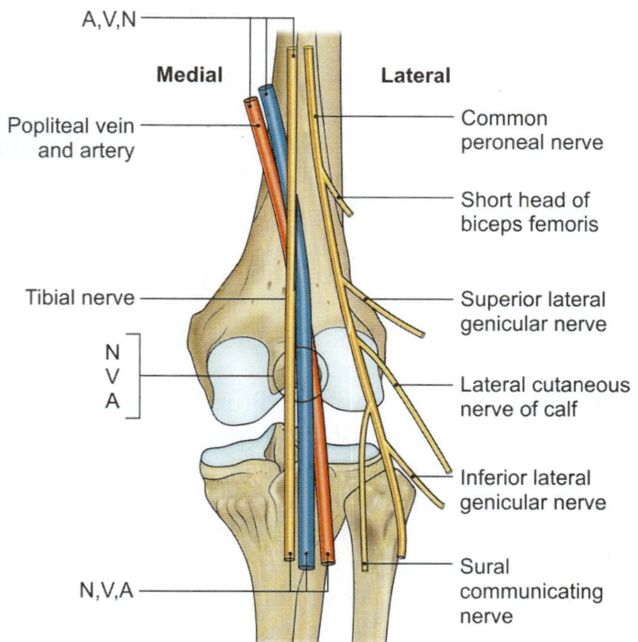

Fig. 41.16: The arrangement of the main nerves and vessels in the popliteal fossa

CLINICAL ANATOMY

Blood pressure in the lower limb is recorded from the popliteal artery. In coarctation of the aorta, the popliteal pressure is lower than the brachial pressure (Fig. 41.17).

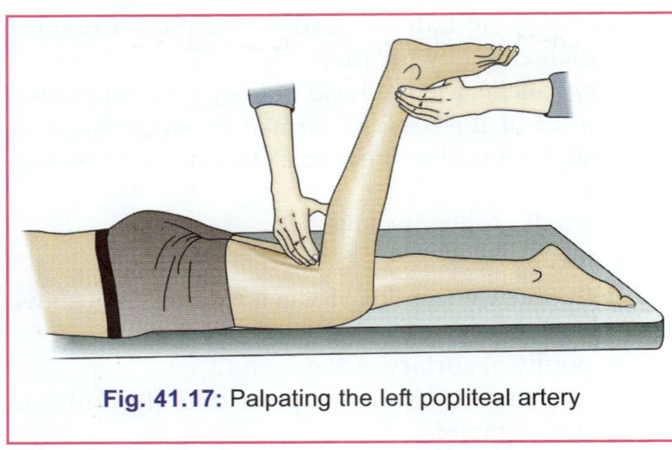
Fig. 41.17: Palpating the left popliteal artery

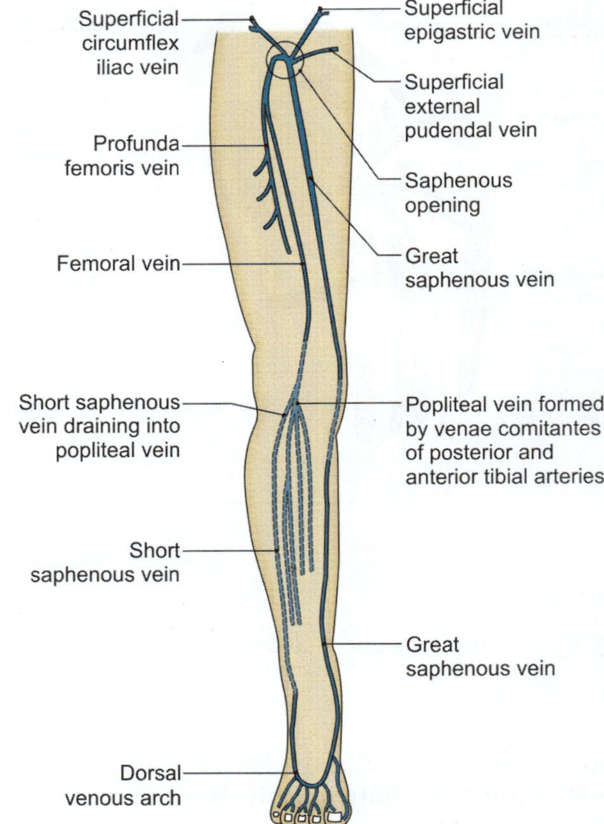

Fig. 41.18: Scheme to show the arrangement of the veins of lower limb. Popliteal, short saphenous and venae comitantes of posterior tibial artery are on posterior aspect

BACK OF THIGH

MUSCLES OF BACK OF THE THIGH

The muscles of the back of the thigh are called the *hamstring muscles*. They are the semitendinosus, the semimembranosus, the long head of the biceps femoris, and the ischial head of the adductor magnus.

The hamstrings share the following characters.

i. Origin from the ischial tuberosity.
ii. Insertion into one of the bones of the leg. The adductor magnus reaches only up to the adductor tubercle of the femur, but is included amongst the hamstrings because the tibial collateral ligament of the knee joint is, morphologically, the degenerated tendon of this muscle.
iii. Nerve supply from the tibial part of the sciatic nerve.
iv. The muscles act as flexors of the knee and extensors of the hip.

- The sciatic nerve may be injured by penetrating wounds, dislocation of the hip, or fracture of the pelvis. This results in loss of all movements below the knee with foot drop; sensory loss on the back of the thigh, the whole of the leg, and the foot except the area innervated by the saphenous nerve.
- Motor loss includes loss of hamstring muscles, loss of dorsiflexors, plantarflexors, evertors and muscles of sole.

FRONT, LATERAL AND MEDIAL SIDES OF LEG AND DORSUM OF FOOT

FRONT OF LEG AND DORSUM OF FOOT

Superficial Veins

1 The *dorsal venous arch* lies on the dorsum of the foot over the proximal parts of the metatarsal bones. It receives four dorsal metatarsal veins each of which is formed by the union of two dorsal digital veins (Fig. 41.18).

2 The *great or long saphenous vein* is formed by the union of the medial end of the dorsal venous arch with the medial marginal vein which drains the medial side of the great toe. It passes upwards in front of the medial malleolus, crosses the lower one-third of the medial surface of tibia obliquely, and runs along its medial border to reach the back of the knee. The saphenous nerve runs in front of the great saphenous vein.

3 The *small or short saphenous vein* is formed by the union of the lateral end of the dorsal venous arch with the lateral marginal vein, draining the lateral side of the little toe. It passes upwards behind the lateral malleolus to reach the back of the leg. The sural nerve accompanies the small saphenous vein.

Both saphenous veins are connected to the deep veins through the perforating veins.

DEEP FASCIA OF THE LEG

The following points about the fascia are noteworthy.

1 Extensions of deep fascia form intermuscular septa that divide the leg into compartments (Fig. 41.21).

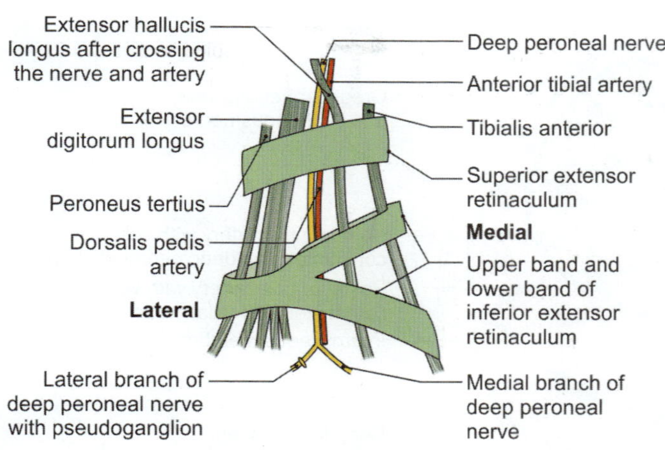

Fig. 41.19: Tendons, vessels and nerves related to the extensor retinacula

The *anterior and posterior* intermuscular septa are attached to the anterior and posterior borders of the fibula. They divide the leg into three compartments, *anterior, lateral, and posterior.* The posterior compartment is subdivided into superficial, intermediate and deep parts by *superficial and deep transverse fascial septa.*

2 Around the ankle, the deep fascia is thickened to form bands called *retinacula.* These are so called because they retain tendons in place. On the front of the ankle, there are the *superior and inferior extensor retinacula.* Laterally, there are the *superior and inferior peroneal retinacula.* Posteromedially, there is the *flexor retinaculum.*

The structures passing under cover of the extensor retinacula are as follows (Fig. 41.19).

1 Tibialis anterior.
2 Extensor hallucis longus.
3 Anterior tibial vessels. } Described at end
4 Deep peroneal nerve } of lower limb
5 Extensor digitorum longus.
6 The peroneus tertius.

MUSCLES OF ANTERIOR COMPARTMENT OF THE LEG

The muscles of the anterior compartment of the leg are the tibialis anterior, the extensor hallucis longus, the extensor digitorum longus and the peroneus tertius (Fig. 41.20).

LATERAL SIDE OF THE LEG

The lateral or peroneal compartment of the leg is bounded *anteriorly* by the anterior intermuscular septum, *posteriorly* by the posterior intermuscular sputum, *medially* by the lateral surface of the fibula, and *laterally* by the deep fascia.

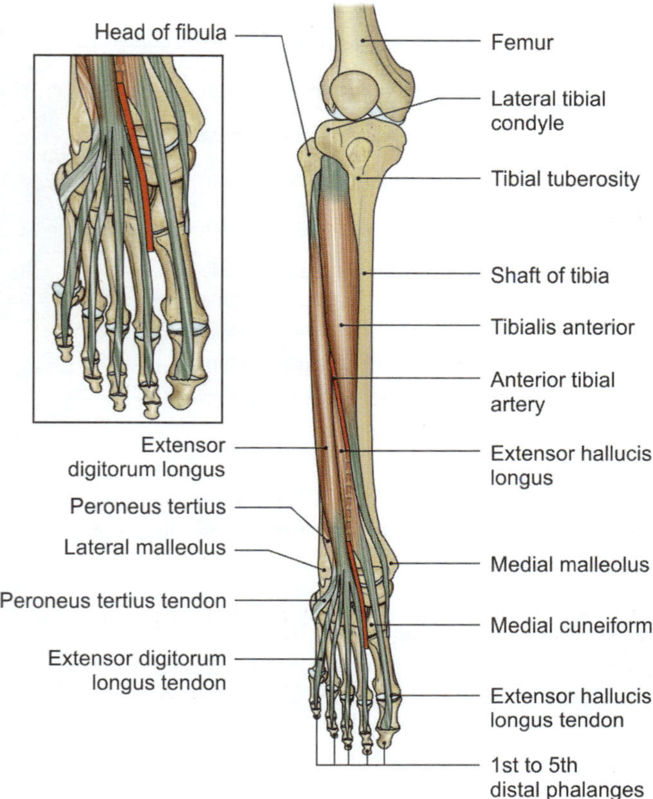

Fig. 41.20: Origin and insertion of the muscles of the anterior compartment of the leg

Contents

- *Muscles:* Peroneus longus and peroneus brevis.
- *Nerve:* Superficial peroneal nerve.
- *Vessels:* The arterial supply is derived from the branches of the peroneal artery.

MEDIAL SIDE OF LEG

Medial side of the leg is formed by the medial surface of the shaft of tibia. The greater part of this surface is subcutaneous and is covered only by the skin and superficial fascia. In the upper part, however, the surface provides attachment to tibial collateral ligament near the medial border, and provides insertion to sartorius, gracilis and semitendinosus in front of the ligament, all of which are covered by a thin layer of deep fascia. The great saphenous vein and the saphenous nerve lie in the superficial fascia as they cross the lower one-third of this surface.

BACK OF LEG

INTRODUCTION

The back or posterior compartment of the leg, also called the calf is the bulkiest of the three compartments

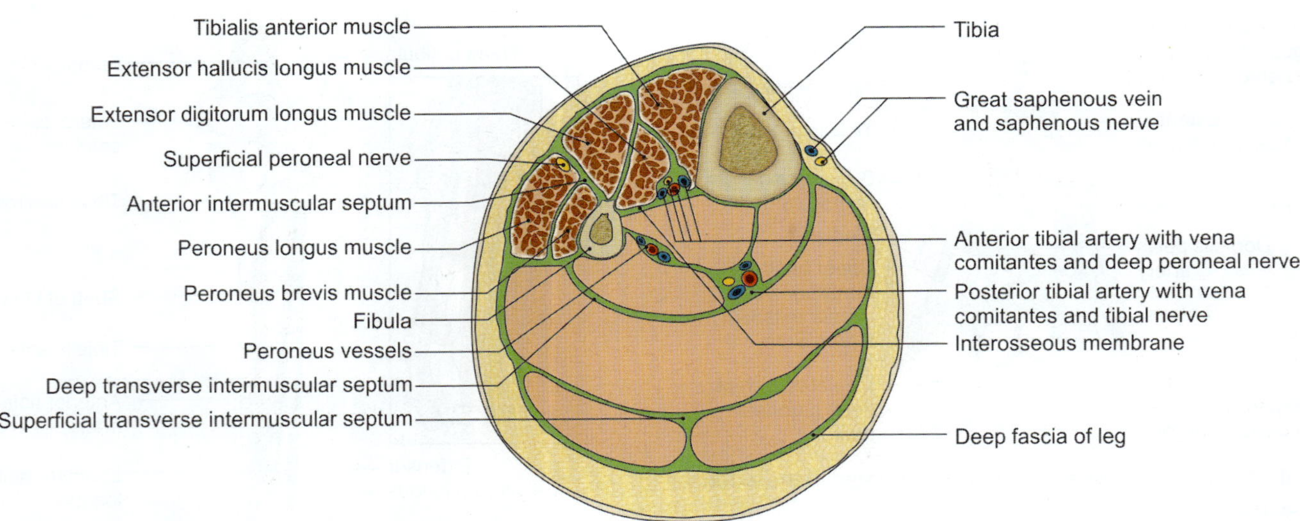

Fig. 41.21: Transverse section through the middle of the leg, showing the three compartments and the contents of the anterior and lateral compartments

of leg, because of the powerful antigravity superficial muscles, e.g. gastrocnemius plantaris, and soleus, which are quite large in size. They raise the heel during walking. These muscles are inserted into the heel. The deeper muscles cross the ankle medially to enter the sole.

Flexor Retinaculum

Some important facts about the retinaculum are as follows.

1 *Attachments:* The flexor retinaculum is attached *anteriorly* to the posterior border and tip of the medial malleolus and *posteriorly* and *laterally* to the medial tubercle of the calcaneum.

2 *Structures passing deep to the retinaculum:* These are from medial to lateral side.
   a.. The tendon of the tibialis posterior.
   b. The tendon of the flexor digitorum longus.
   c. The posterior tibial artery and its terminal branches, along with the accompanying veins.
   d. The tibial nerve and its terminal branches.
   e. The tendon of the flexor hallucis longus (Fig. 41.22).

SUPERFICIAL MUSCLES

The muscles of the back of leg are classified into two groups—superficial and deep. The superficial muscles are the gastrocnemius, the soleus, and the plantaris (Fig. 41.23).

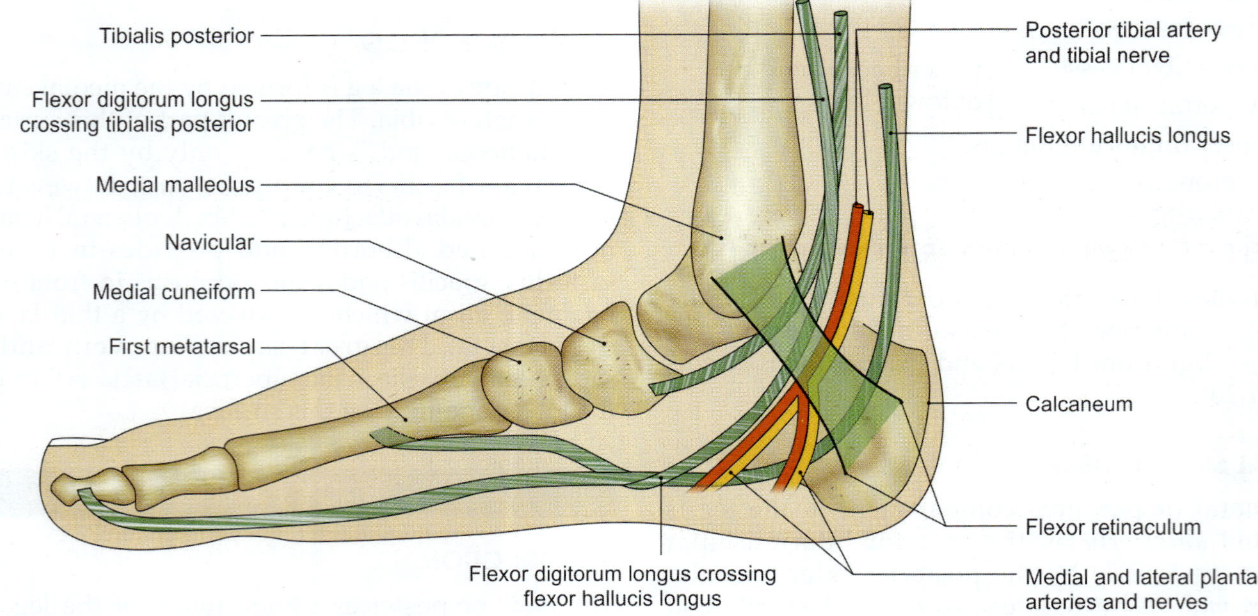

Fig. 41.22: Flexor retinaculum of the ankle, and the structures passing deep to it

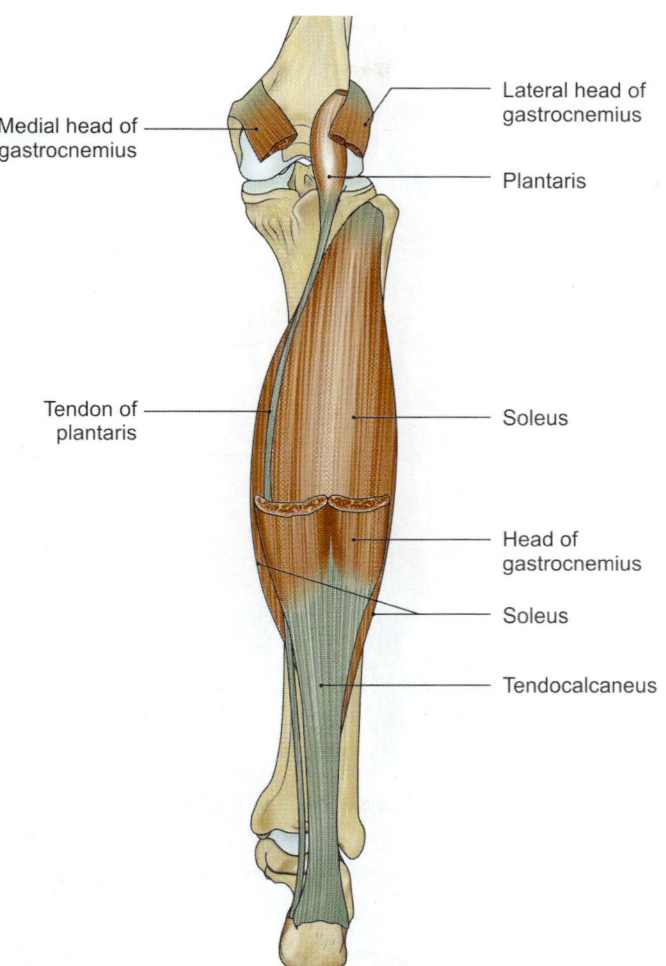

Fig. 41.23: Superficial muscles of the back of the leg

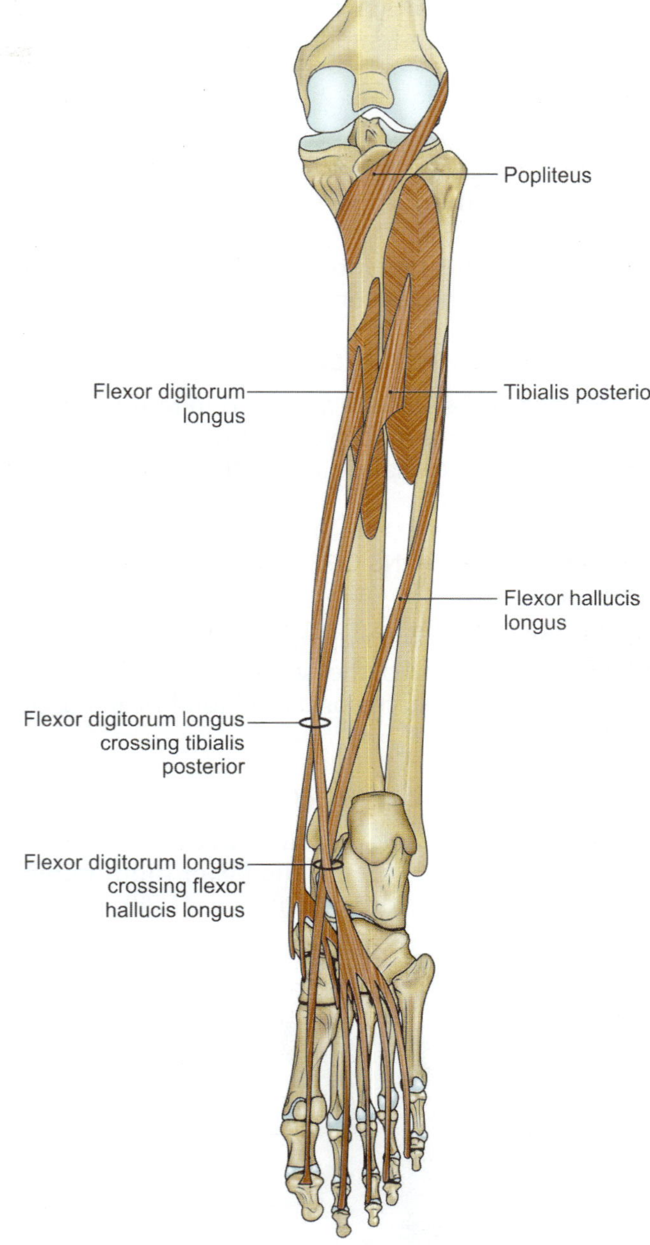

Fig. 41.24: Some attachments of the muscles of the back of the leg. The tibialis posterior also arises from the fibula, but this area cannot be seen in this view

DEEP MUSCLES

The deep muscles of the back of the leg are the popliteus, the flexor digitorum longus, the flexor hallucis longus, and the tibialis posterior (Fig. 41.24).

The posterior tibial pulse can be felt against the calcaneum about 2 cm below and behind the medial malleolus (Fig. 41.25).

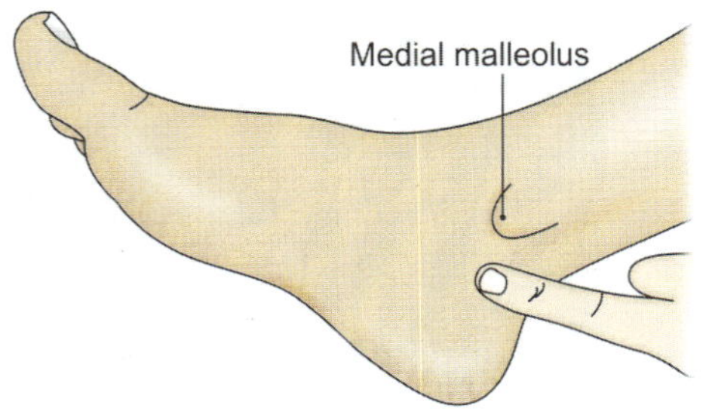

Fig. 41.25: Shows where to palpate the posterior tibial artery

SOLE OF FOOT

INTRODUCTION

The structure of the sole is similar to that of the palm. The skin, superficial fascia, deep fascia, muscles, vessels and nerves, are all comparable in these two homologous parts. However, unlike the hand, the foot is an organ of support and locomotion. Accordingly, the structures of the foot get modified. The great toe has lost its mobility and its power of prehension; the lesser four toes are markedly reduced in size; and the tarsal bones and the first metatarsal are enlarged to form a broad base for better support. The arches of the foot serve as elastic springs for efficient walking, running, jumping and supporting of body weight.

SKIN

The skin of the sole is:

i. Thick for protection;
ii. Firmly adherent to the underlying plantar aponeurosis; and
iii. Creased. These features increase the efficiency of the grip of the sole on the ground.

MUSCLES OF THE FIRST LAYER OF THE SOLE

The muscles of the sole are arranged in four layers.

The muscles of the first layer are the flexor digitorum brevis, the abductor hallucis, and the abductor digiti minimi (Fig. 41.26).

MUSCLES AND TENDONS OF THE SECOND LAYER OF THE SOLE

The contents of this layer are the tendons of the flexor digitorum longus, and of the flexor hallucis longus; and the flexor digitorum accessorius and lumbrical muscles (Fig. 41.27).

MUSCLES OF THE THIRD LAYER OF THE SOLE

The third layer of the sole contains three muscles. These are the flexor hallucis brevis, the flexor digiti minimi brevis, and the adductor hallucis (Fig. 41.28).

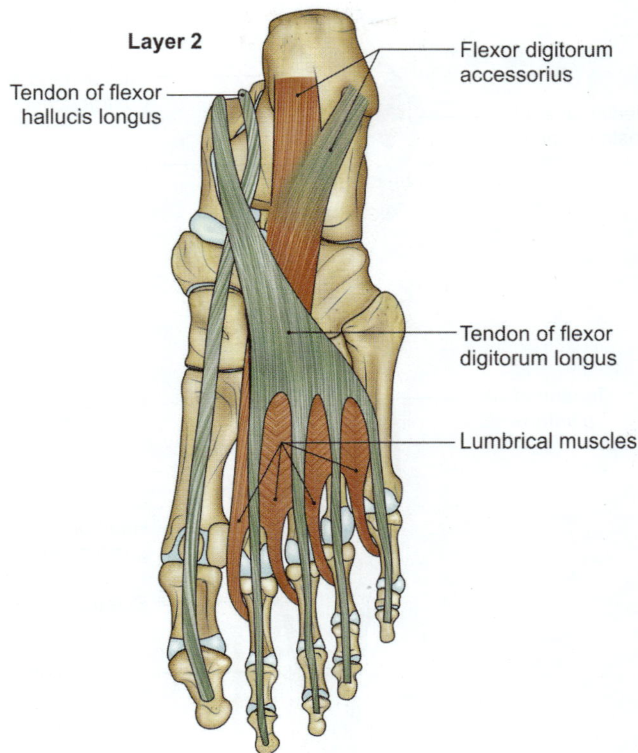

Fig. 41.27: The second layer of the sole

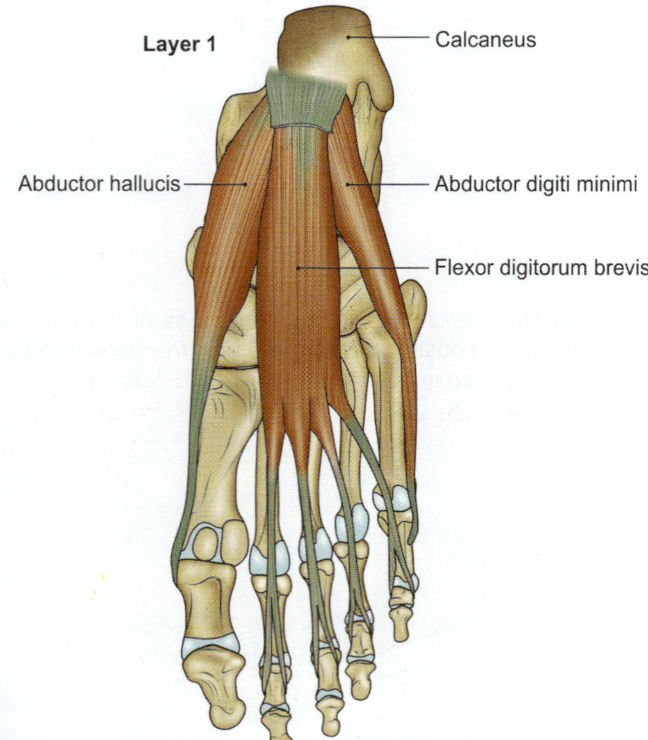

Fig. 41.26: Muscles of the first layer of the sole

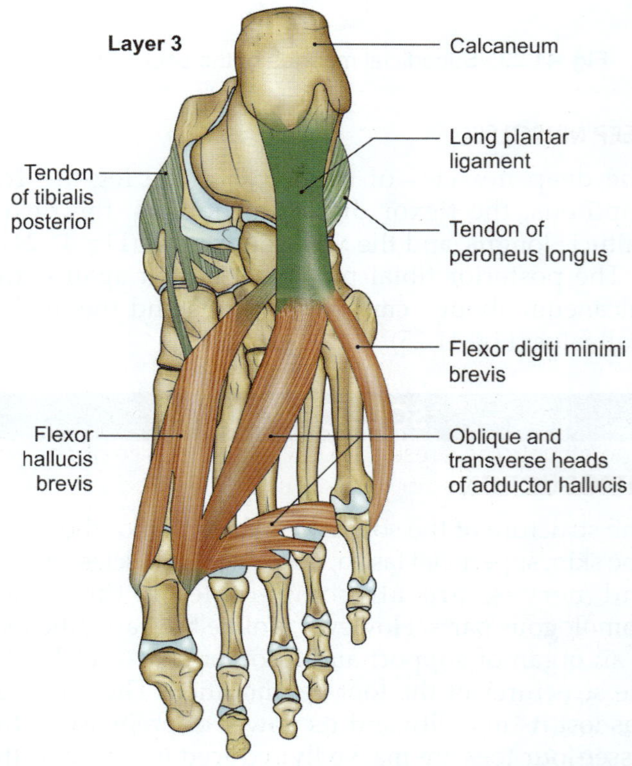

Fig. 41.28: Muscles of third layer of the sole. The tendons of tibialis posterior and peroneus longus belong to the fourth layer

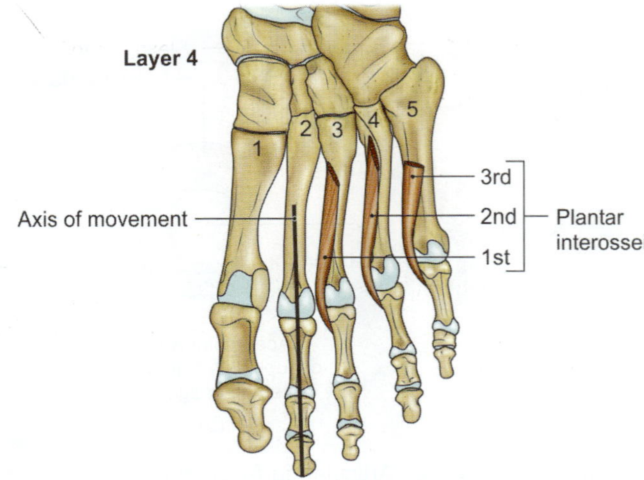

Fig. 41.29: The plantar interossei

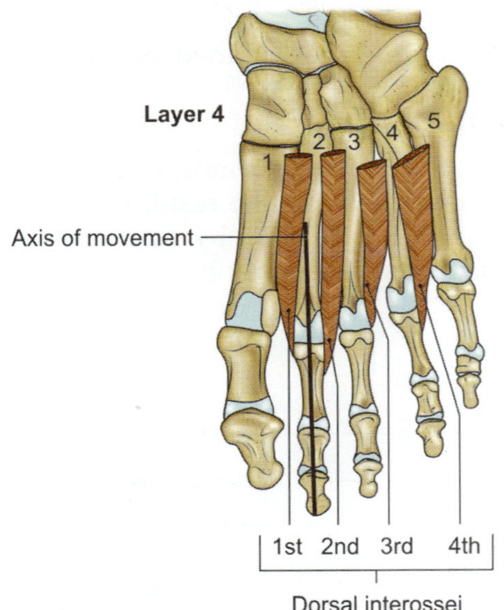

Fig. 41.30: The dorsal interossei

MUSCLES OF THE FOURTH LAYER OF THE SOLE

The structures present in the fourth layer of the sole are the intraosseous muscles, and the tendons of the tibialis posterior and of the peroneus longus (Figs 41.29 and 41.30).

VENOUS DRAINAGE

The saphenous veins can be "easily seen" in the leg. The varicose veins, if occur, look quite ugly under the skin. Effort should be made not to develop the varicose veins. Venous drainage acquires importance as blood has to flow up against the gravity.

Table 41.4: Comparison of the saphenous veins

	Long saphenous vein	*Short saphenous vein*
Beginning	Medial end of dorsal venous plexus	Lateral end of dorsal venous plexus
Position	Anterior to medial malleolus	Posterior to lateral malleolus
Number of valves	15–20 valves	8–10 valves
Relation of a sensory nerve	Saphenous nerve	Sural nerve
Termination	Femoral vein	Popliteal vein

Superficial Veins

They include the great and small saphenous veins, and their tributaries. They lie in the superficial fascia. Their comparison is given in Table 41.4.

Deep Veins

These are the medial plantar, lateral plantar, dorsalis pedis, anterior and posterior tibial, peroneal, popliteal, and femoral veins, and their tributaries.

Perforating Veins

They connect the superficial with the deep veins. Their valves permit only one way flow of blood.

CLINICAL ANATOMY

- *Calf pump* and *peripheral heart*. In the upright position of the body, the venous return from the lower limb depends largely on the contraction of calf muscles. These muscles are, therefore, known as the "calf pump".
  For the same reason, the soleus is called the *peripheral heart*.
- "Cut open procedure" is done on the great saphenous vein as it lies in front of medial malleolus.
- *Varicose veins and ulcers.* If the valves in perforating veins or at the termination of superficial veins become incompetent, the defective veins become "high pressure leaks" through which the high pressure of the deep veins produced by muscular contraction is transmitted to the superficial veins. This results in dilatation of the superficial veins and to gradual degeneration of their walls producing varicose veins and varicose ulcers.

JOINTS OF LOWER LIMB

HIP JOINT

Type

Ball and socket variety of synovial joint.

Articular Surfaces

The head of the femur articulates with the acetabulum of the hip bone to form the hip joint (Fig. 41.31).

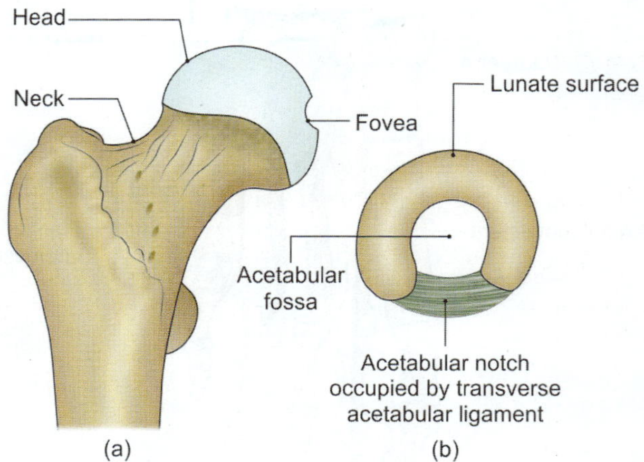

Figs 41.31a and b: Articular surfaces of the hip joint

Ligaments

The ligaments include:
1 The fibrous capsule,
2 The iliofemoral ligament,
3 The pubofemoral ligament,
4 The ischiofemoral ligament,
5 The ligament of the head of the femur,
6 The acetabular labrum, and
7 The transverse acetabular ligament.

The *fibrous capsule* is attached *on the hip bone* to the acetabular labrum including the transverse acetabular ligament, and to bone above and behind the acetabulum; and *on the femur* to the intertrochanteric line in front, and 1 cm medial to the intertrochanteric crest behind.

Relations of the Hip Joint (Fig. 41.32)

Blood Supply

The hip joint is supplied by one obturator artery, two circumflex femoral and two gluteal arteries.

Nerve Supply

The hip joint is supplied by the femoral nerve, through the nerve to the rectus femoris; the anterior division of the obturator nerve; the nerve to the quadratus femoris; and the superior gluteal nerve.

Movements

Movements of the hip joint are depicted in Table 41.5.

KNEE JOINT

The knee is the largest and most complex joint of the body. The complexity is the result of fusion of three joints in one. It is formed by fusion of the lateral femorotibial, medial femorotibial, and femoropatellar joints.

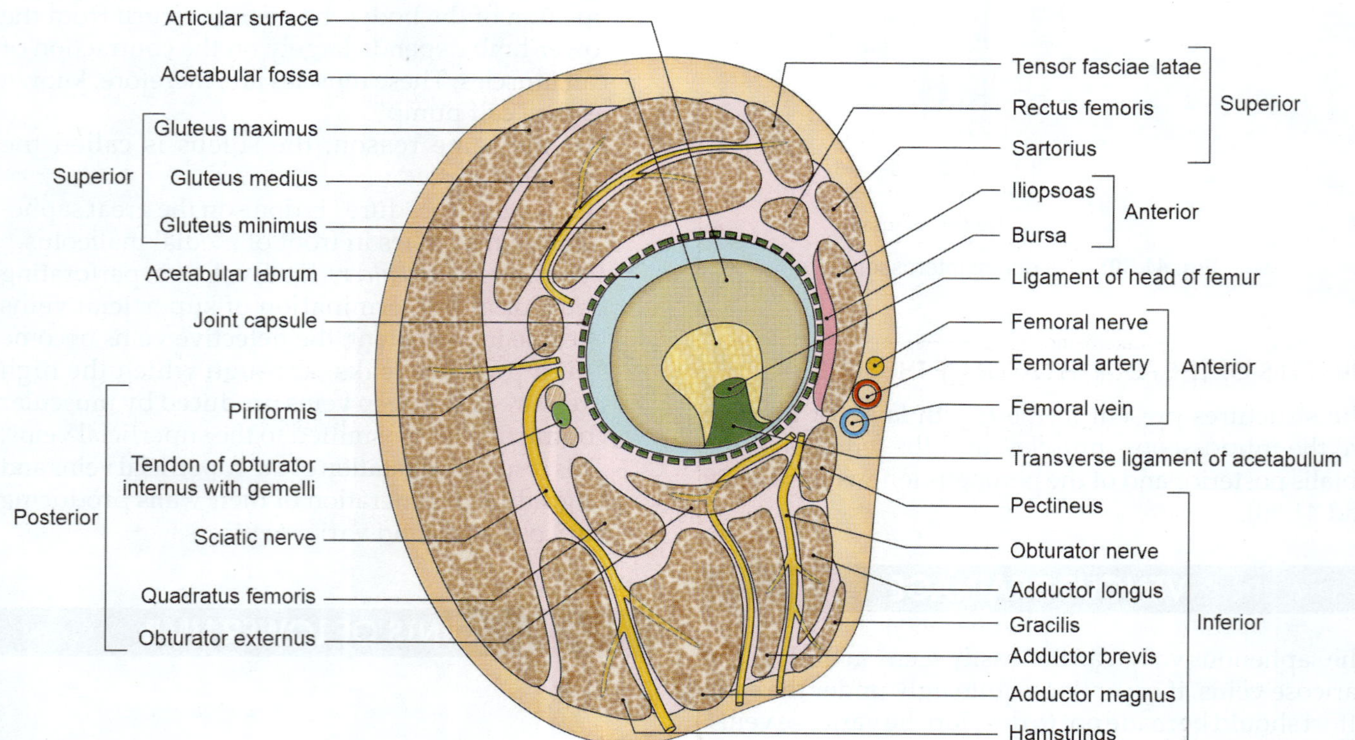

Fig. 41.32: Relations of the hip joint

Table 41.5: Muscles producing movements at the hip joint		
Movement	*Chief muscles*	*Accessory muscles*
1. Flexion	Psoas major and iliacus	Pectineus, rectus femoris, and sartorius; adductors (mainly adductor longus) participate in early stages
2. Extension	Gluteus maximus and hamstrings	—
3. Adduction	Adductors longus, brevis and magnus	Pectineus and gracilis
4. Abduction	Glutei, medius and minimus	Tensor fasciae latae and sartorius
5. Medial rotation	Tensor fasciae latae and the anterior fibres of the glutei medius and minimus	—
6. Lateral rotation	Two obturators, two gemelli and the quadratus femoris	Piriformis, gluteus maximus and sartorius

Type

It is compound synovial joint, incorporating two condylar joints between the condyles of the femur and tibia, and one saddle joint between the femur and the patella.

Articular Surfaces

The knee joint is formed by:

1. The condyles of the femur.
2. The patella
3. The condyles of the tibia. The femoral condyles articulate with the tibial condyles below and behind, and with the patella in front.

Ligaments

The knee joint is supported by the following ligaments.

1. Fibrous capsule.
2. Ligamentum patellae.
3. Tibial collateral or medial ligament.
4. Fibular collateral or lateral ligament.
5. Oblique popliteal ligament.
6. Arcuate popliteal ligament.
7. Anterior cruciate ligament.
8. Posterior cruciate ligament.
9. Medial meniscus.
10. Lateral meniscus.
11. Transverse ligament.

Relations of Knee Joint

Relations of the knee joint are shown in Fig. 41.33.

Blood Supply

The knee joint is supplied by the anastomoses around it. The chief sources of blood supply are:

1. Five genicular branches of the popliteal artery.
2. The descending genicular branch of the femoral artery. The descending branch of the lateral circumflex femoral artery.
3. Two recurrent branches of the anterior tibial artery. The circumflex fibular branch of the posterior tibial artery.

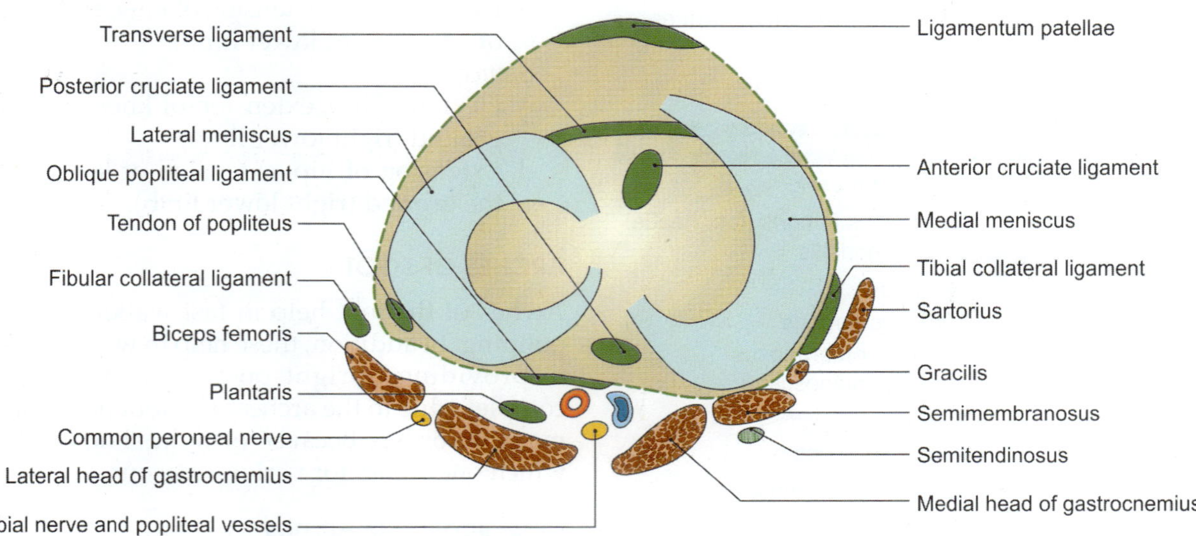

Fig. 41.33: Transverse section through the left knee joint showing its relations

Nerve Supply

1 Femoral nerve—through its branches to the vasti, especially the vastus medialis.
2 Sciatic nerve—through the genicular branches of the tibial and common peroneal nerves.
3 Obturator nerve—through its posterior division.

Movements at the Knee Joint

Active movements at the knee are flexion, extension, medial rotation and lateral rotation (Table 41.6).

Table 41.6: Muscles producing movements at the knee joint

Movement	Principal muscles
A. Extension	Quadriceps femoris (four heads)
B. Locking	Vastus medialis
C. Unlocking	Popliteus
D. Flexion	1. Biceps femoris 2. Semimembranosus 3. Semitendinosus
E. Medial rotation of flexed leg	1. Popliteus 2. Semitendinosus 3. Semimembranosus
F. Lateral rotation of flexed leg	Biceps femoris

ANKLE JOINT

This is a synovial joint of the hinge variety.

Articular Surfaces

The upper articular surface is formed by:

i. The lower end of the tibia including the medial malleolus.
ii. The lateral malleolus of the fibula, and
iii. The inferior transverse tibiofibular ligament. These structures form a deep socket.

The inferior articular surface is formed by articular areas on the upper, medial and lateral aspects of the talus.

Ligaments

The joint is supported by:

i. Fibrous capsule.
ii. The deltoid or medial ligament.
iii. A lateral ligament.

Movements

1 *Active movements* are dorsiflexion and plantar flexion (Table 41.7).
   a. In *dorsiflexion* the forefoot is raised, and the angle between the front of the leg and the dorsum of the foot is diminished. There are no chances of dislocation in dorsiflexion.

Table 41.7: Muscles producing movements

Movement	Principal muscles
A. Dorsiflexion	Tibialis anterior
B. Plantar flexion	1. Gastrocnemius 2. Soleus

   b. In *plantar flexion,* the forefoot is depressed, and the angle between the leg and the foot is increased. High heels cause plantar flexion of ankle joint and chances its dislocations.

Blood Supply

From anterior tibial, posterior tibial, and peroneal arteries.

Nerve Supply

From deep peroneal and tibial nerves.

TIBIOFIBULAR JOINTS

The tibia and fibula articulate at three joints, the superior, middle and inferior tibiofibular joints.

JOINTS OF THE FOOT

a. Intertarsal,
b. Tarsometatarsal,
c. Intermetatarsal,
d. Metatarsophalangeal, and
e. Interphalangeal.

GAIT

- Gait is a motion which carries the body forwards. There are two phases—swing and stance (Fig. 41.34).
  Swing phase:
  a. Flexion of hip, flexion of knee and plantar flexion of ankle (right lower limb).
  b. Flexion of hip, extension of knee and dorsi-flexion of ankle (right lower limb).
  Stance:
  c. Flexion of hip, extension of knee and foot on the ground (right lower limb).
  d. Extension of hip, extension of knee and foot on the ground (right lower limb).

ARCHES OF FOOT

Arches of the foot help in fast walking, running and jumping. In addition, these help in weight-bearing and in providing upright posture. Foot prints are not complete due to the arches. The foot has to suffer from many disorders because of tight shoes or high heels which one wears for various reasons.

Classification of Arches

A. Longitudinal (Table 41.8)

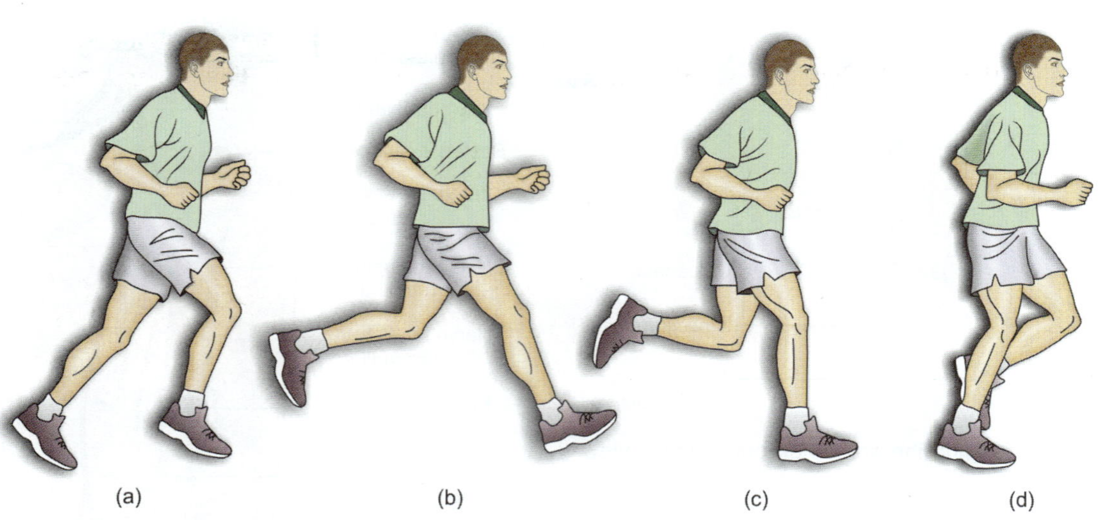

Fig. 41.34: Phases of gait: (a) and (b) Swing phase; (c) and (d) Stance phase

Table 41.8: Comparison of medial longitudinal arch and lateral longitudinal arch

	Medial longitudinal arch (Fig. 41.35)	*Lateral longitudinal arch (Fig. 41.36)*
Features	Higher, more mobile, resilient and shock absorber	Lower, limited mobility transmits weight
Anterior end	Heads of 1st, 2nd, 3rd metatarsal bones	Heads of 4th, 5th metatarsals
Posterior end	Medial tubercle of calcaneum	Lateral tubercle of calcaneum
Summit	Superior articular surface of talus	Articular facet on superior surface of calcaneum at level of subtalar joint
Anterior pillar	Talus, navicular, 3 cuneiforms and 1–3 metatarsals	Cuboid and 4th, 5th metatarsals
Posterior pillar	Medial half of calcaneum	Lateral half of calcaneum
Main joint	Talocalcaneonavicular joint	Calcaneocuboid joint
Bony factor	Wedge-shaped	Wedge-shaped
Intersegmental ties	Spring ligament	Long plantar ligament
		Short plantar ligament
Tie beams	Plantar aponeuroriss (medial part)	Plantar aponeurosis (lateral part)
	Abductor hallucis	Abductor digiti minimi
	Medial part of flexor digitorum brevis	Lateral part of flexor digitorum brevis
Slings	Tibialis posterior	Peroneus longus
	Flexor hallucis longus	Peroneus brevis
	Flexor digitorum longus	
	Sling formed by tibialis anterior and peroneus longus	Sling formed by tibialis anterior and peroneus longus

1 Medial
2 Lateral

B. Transverse
1 Anterior
2 Posterior

NERVES AND ARTERIES OF LOWER LIMB

FEMORAL NERVE

Femoral nerve is the nerve of anterior compartment of thigh. Its cutaneous branch, the saphenous nerve

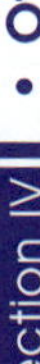

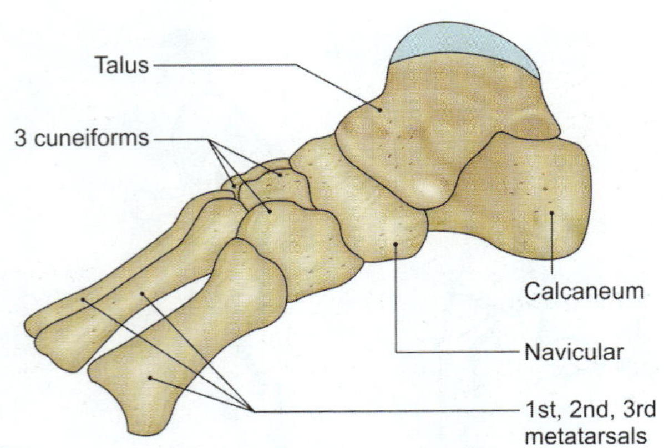

Fig. 41.35: Bones forming the arches of foot—medial view

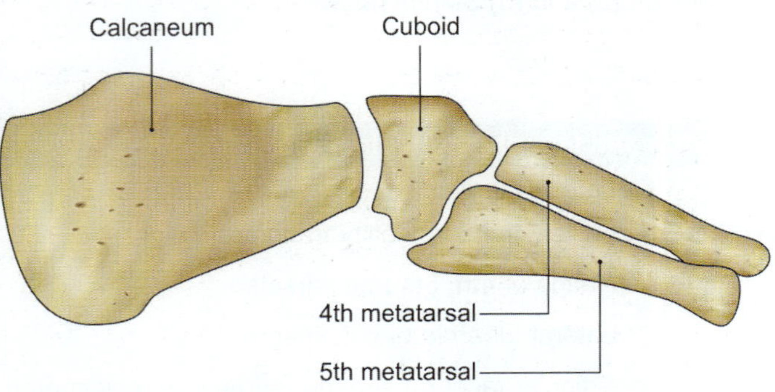

Fig. 41.36: Bones forming the arches of foot—lateral view

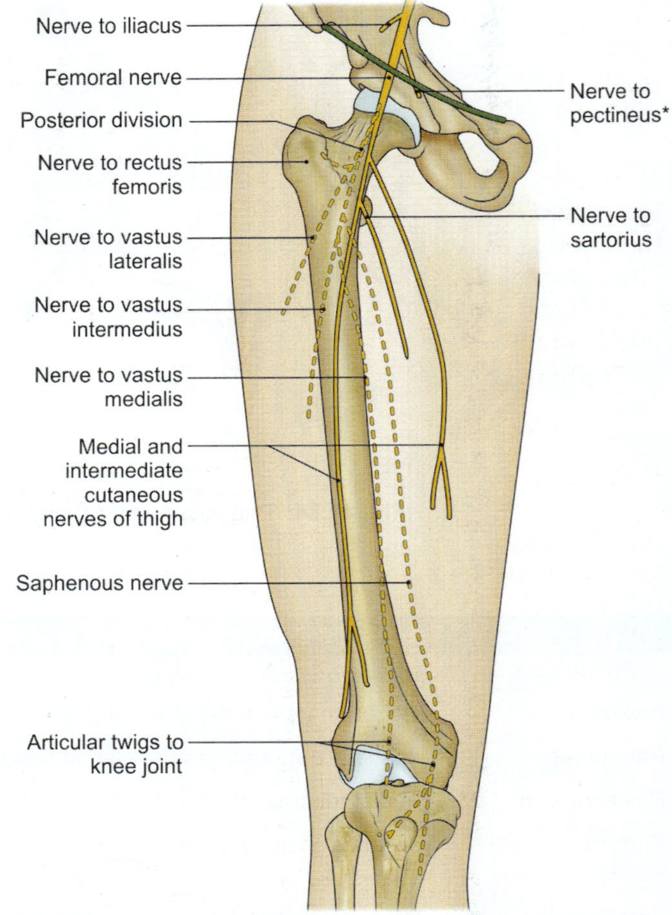

Fig. 41.37: The branches and distribution of femoral nerve

extends to the medial side of leg and medial border of foot till the ball of the big toe.

Root value: Dorsal division of ventral rami of L2, L3, L4 segments of spinal cord.

Beginning and course: It emerges at the lateral border of psoas major muscle in abdomen. It passes downwards between psoas major and iliacus muscles. The nerve enters the thigh behind the inguinal ligament, lateral to femoral sheath. It is not a content of femoral sheath (Fig. 41.37).

Termination: It ends by dividing into two divisions 4 cm below the inguinal ligament. Both these divisions end in number of branches.

Branches: In *abdomen*, femoral nerve supplies iliacus muscle. Just above the inguinal ligament, it gives a branch to pectineus muscle, which passes behind the femoral sheath to reach the muscle. Its branches in the thigh are presented in Table 41.9.

Table 41.9: Branches of femoral nerve in thigh

	Superficial division	*Deep division*
Muscular	Sartorius	Vastus medialis Vastus intermedius Vastus lateralis Rectus femoris
Cutaneous	Medial cutaneous nerve of thigh Intermediate cutaneous nerve of thigh	Saphenous for medial side of leg and medial border of foot till ball of big toe
Articular and vascular	Sympathetic fibres to femoral artery	Knee joint from branches to vasti Hip joint from branch to rectus femoris

OBTURATOR NERVE

Root value: Obturator nerve is a branch of lumbar plexus. It arises from ventral division of ventral rami of L2, L3, L4 segments of spinal cord (Fig. 41.38).

Beginning and course: It emerges on the medial border of psoas major muscle within the abdomen. It crosses the pelvic brim to run downwards and forwards on the lateral wall of pelvis to reach the upper part of obturator foramen.

Termination: It ends by dividing into anterior and posterior divisions.

The branches are presented in Table 41.10.

SUPERIOR GLUTEAL NERVE

Root value: L4, L5, S1.

Course: Enters the gluteal region through greater sciatic notch above piriformis muscle. Runs between gluteus medius and gluteus minimus to end in tensor fascia latae.

Branches: It supplies gluteus medius, gluteus minimus and tensor fascia latae.

INFERIOR GLUTEAL NERVE

Root value: L5, S1, S2.

Course: Enters the gluteal region through greater sciatic notch below piriformis muscle.

Branches: It gives number of branches to the gluteus maximus muscle only. It is the sole supply to the large antigravity, postural muscle with red fibres, responsible for extending the hip joint.

SCIATIC NERVE

Sciatic nerve is the thickest nerve of the body. It is the terminal branch of the lumbosacral plexus.

Root value: Ventral rami of L4, L5, S1, S2, S3. It consists of two parts:

Tibial part: Its root value is ventral division of ventral rami of L4, L5, S1, S2, S3, segments of spinal cord.

Common peroneal part: Its root value is dorsal division of ventral rami of L4, L5, S1, S2 segments of spinal cord.

Course: Sciatic nerve arises in the pelvis. Leaves the pelvis by passing through greater sciatic foramen below the piriformis to enter the gluteal region (Fig. 41.14).

In the gluteal region, it lies deep to the gluteus maximus muscle, and crosses superior gemellus, obturator internus, inferior gemellus, quadratus femoris to enter the back of thigh. During its short course, it lies between ischial tuberosity and greater trochanter with a convexity to the lateral side. It gives no branches in the gluteal region.

In the back of thigh, it lies deep to biceps femoris and superficial to adductor magnus.

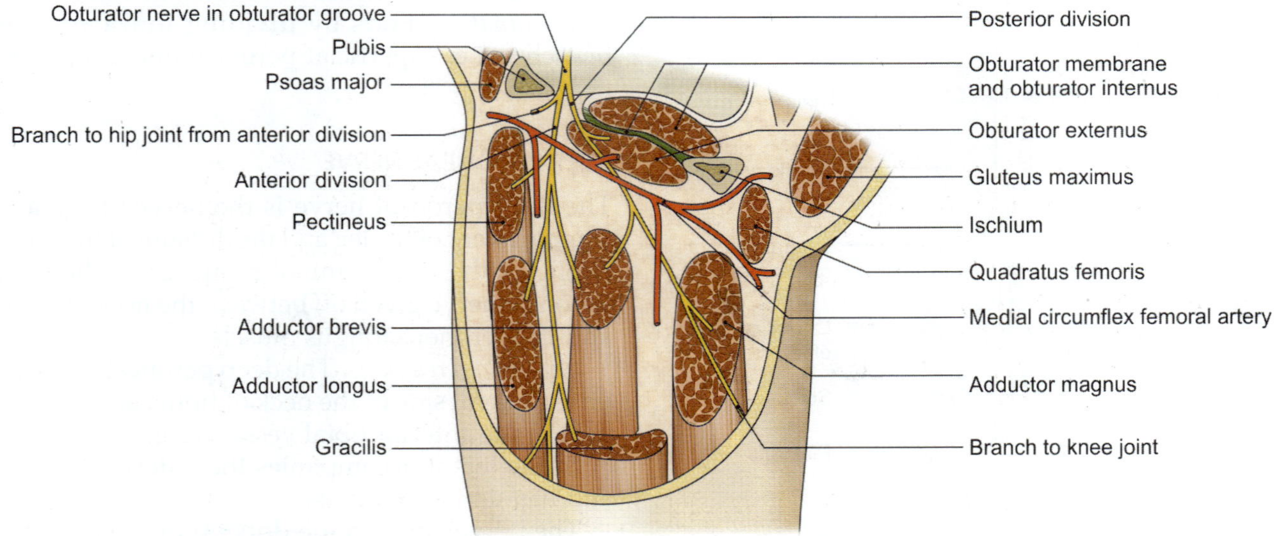

Fig. 41.38: The course and distribution of the obturator nerve

Table 41.10: Branches of obturator nerve

	Anterior division	*Posterior division*
Muscular	Pectineus, adductor longus, adductor brevis, gracilis	Obturator externus, adductor magnus (adductor part)
Articular	Hip joint	Knee joint
Vascular and cutaneous	Femoral artery. Medial side of thigh	Popliteal artery

Table 41.11: Branches of sciatic nerve

	Gluteal region	*Back of thigh; from tibial part*	*From common peroneal part*
Muscular	Nil	Long head of biceps femoris, semitendinosus, semimembranosus, ischial part of adductor magnus	Short head of biceps femoris
Articular	Nil	Hip joint	—
Terminal	Nil	Tibial and common peroneal nerves	—

Termination: It ends by dividing into its two terminal branches in the back of thigh.

Branches: The branches of sciatic nerve are shown in Table 41.11.

TIBIAL NERVE

Root value: Ventral division of ventral rami of L4, L5, S1, S2, S3, segments of spinal cord.

Beginning: It begins as the larger subdivision of sciatic nerve in the back of thigh.

Course: It has a long course first in the popliteal fossa and then in the back of leg.

Popliteal fossa: The nerve descends vertically in the popliteal fossa from its upper angle to the lower angle. It lies superficial to the popliteal vessels. It continues in the back of leg beyond the distal border of popliteus muscle (Fig. 41.39).

In back *of leg:* The nerve descends as the neurovascular bundle with posterior tibial vessels. It lies superficial to tibialis posterior and deep to flexor digitorum longus. Lastly, it passes deep to the flexor retinaculum of ankle.

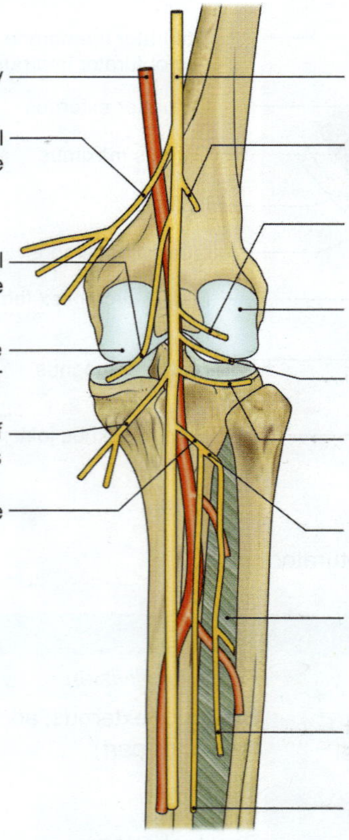

Branches: Its branches are shown in Table 41.12.

Termination: The tibial nerve terminates by dividing into medial plantar and lateral plantar nerves as it lies deep to the flexor retinaculum.

Fig. 41.39: Distribution of tibial nerve

COMMON PERONEAL NERVE

This is the smaller terminal branch of sciatic nerve. Its root value is dorsal division of ventral rami of L4, L5, S1, S2 segments of spinal cord.

Beginning: It begins in the back of thigh as a smaller subdivision of the sciatic nerve.

Course: It lies in the upper lateral part of popliteal fossa, along the medial border of biceps femoris muscle. It turns around the lateral surface of fibula. Then it lies in the substance of peroneus longus muscle (Fig. 41.40).

Branches: Its branches are shown in Table 41.13.

Termination: Ends by dividing into two terminal branches, i.e. superficial peroneal and deep peroneal nerves.

DEEP PERONEAL NERVE

The deep peroneal nerve is the nerve of the anterior compartment of the leg and the dorsum of the foot. This is one of the two terminal branches of the common peroneal nerve given off between the neck of the fibula and the peroneus longus muscle.

Course and relations: The deep peroneal nerve begins on the lateral side of the neck of fibula and comes to lie next to the anterior tibial vessels (Fig. 41.41).

In the leg, it accompanies the anterior tibial artery and has similar relations.

The nerve ends on the dorsum of the foot, close to the ankle joint, by dividing into the lateral and medial terminal branches.

The lateral terminal branch turns laterally and ends in a pseudoganglion deep to the extensor digitorum brevis. Branches arise from the pseudoganglion and supply the extensor digitorum brevis and the tarsal joints.

The medial terminal branch ends by supplying the skin adjoining the first interdigital cleft and the proximal joints of the big toe.

Table 41.12: Branches of tibial nerve

	Popliteal fossa	*Back of leg*
Muscular	Medial head of gastrocnemius Lateral head of gastrocnemius Plantaris Soleus Popliteus. These are given in lower part of fossa	Soleus Flexor digitorum longus Flexor hallucis longus Tibialis posterior
Cutaneous and vascular	Sural nerve. This is given in middle of fossa	Medial calcanean branches and branch to posterior tibial artery
Articular	Superior medial genicular Middle genicular Inferior medial genicular. These are given in upper part of fossa	Ankle joint
Terminal	—	Medial plantar and lateral plantar nerves

Branches and Distribution

Muscular branches: The muscular branches supply the following muscles.

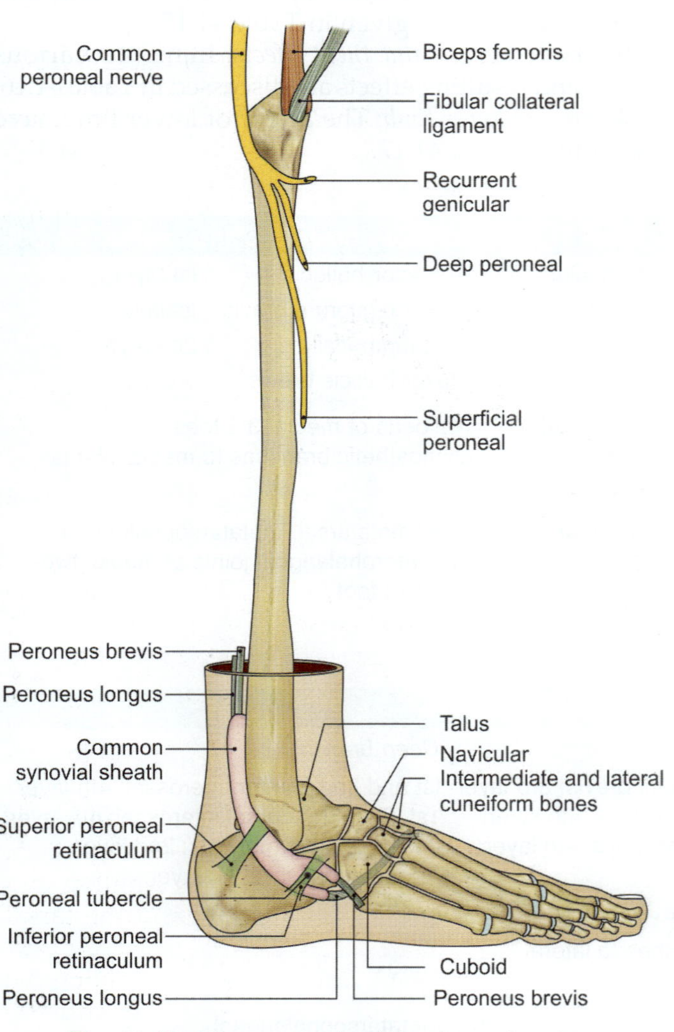

Fig. 41.40: The peroneal or lateral crural region

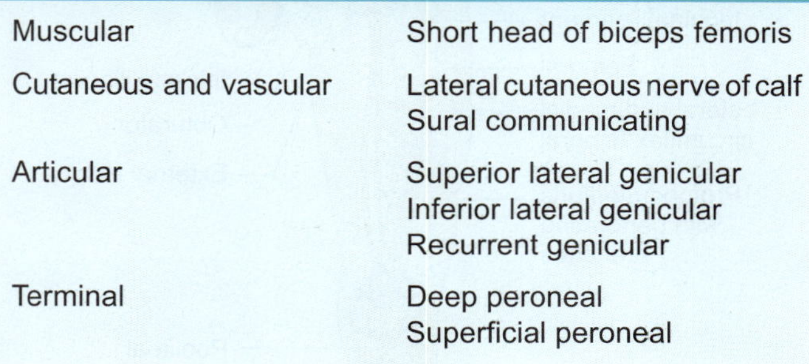

Table 41.13: Branches of common peroneal nerve in popliteal fossa

Muscular	Short head of biceps femoris
Cutaneous and vascular	Lateral cutaneous nerve of calf Sural communicating
Articular	Superior lateral genicular Inferior lateral genicular Recurrent genicular
Terminal	Deep peroneal Superficial peroneal

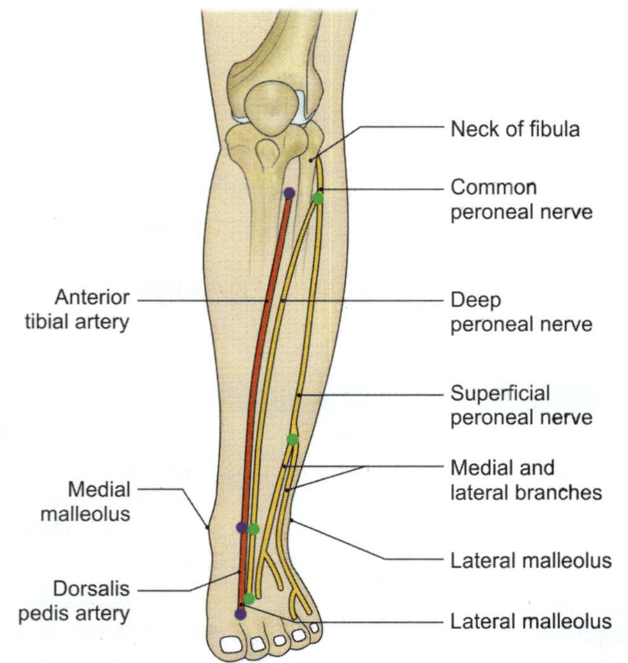

Fig. 41.41: Course of anterior tibial, dorsalis pedis arteries, deep and superficial peroneal nerves

1 Muscles of the anterior compartment of the leg. These include:
   i. Tibialis anterior
   ii. Extensor hallucis longus
   iii. Extensor digitorum longus
   iv. Peroneus tertius.
2 The extensor digitorum brevis (on the dorsum of foot) is supplied by the lateral terminal branch of the deep peroneal nerve.

SUPERFICIAL PERONEAL NERVE

It is the smaller terminal branch of the common peroneal nerve.

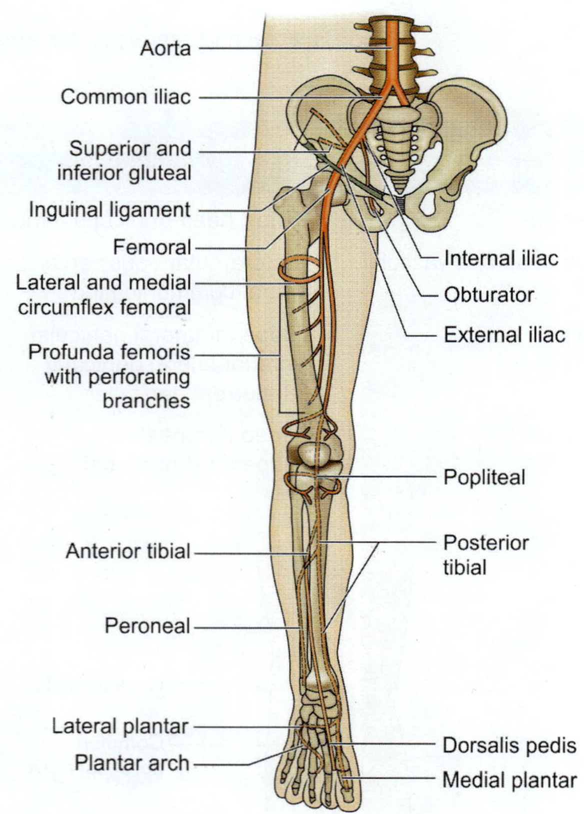

Fig. 41.42: Arteries of lower limb

Origin: It arises in the substance of peroneus longus muscle, lateral to the neck of fibula.

Course: It descends in the lateral compartment of leg deep to peroneus longus. Then it lies between peroneus longus and peroneus brevis muscles and lastly between the peronei and extensor digitorum longus.

It pierces the deep fascia in distal one-third of leg and descends to the dorsum of foot.

Branches: It supplies both peroneus longus and peroneus brevis muscles.

PLANTAR NERVES

The medial and lateral plantar nerves are the terminal branches of the tibial nerve. These nerves begin deep to the flexor retinaculum.

Medial plantar nerve: It is the larger terminal branch of tibial nerve.

Branches: The branches of medial plantar nerve are shown in Table 41.14

Lateral plantar nerve: It is the smaller terminal branch of tibial nerve,

Branches: The structures supplied by the trunk, and its two branches are given in Table 41.15.

Injury to nerves and their effects: Injury to various nerves and resulting effects are discussed in Table 41.16.

Arteries of lower limb: The artery of lower limb have been put in Table 41.17.

Table 41.14: Branches of medial plantar nerve (S2, S3)

Muscular	Abductor hallucis	: Ist layer
	Flexor digitorum brevis	: Ist layer
	First lumbrical	: 2nd layer
	Flexor hallicis brevis	: 3rd layer
Cutaneous and vascular	Nailbeds of medial 3½ toes Sympathetic branches to medial plantar artery	
Articular	Tarsometatarsal, metatarsophalangeal and interphalangeal joints of medial two-thirds of foot	

Table 41.15: Branches of lateral plantar nerve

	Trunk (S2, S3)	*Superficial branch*	*Deep branch*
Muscular	• Abductor digiti minimi: Ist layer • Flexor digitorum accessorius: 2nd layer	• Flexor digiti minimi brevis: 3rd layer • 3rd plantar interosseus: 4th layer • 4th dorsal interosseous: 4th layer	Ist and 2nd plantar interossei: 4th layer 1st, 2nd, 3rd, dorsal interossei: 4th layer 2nd, 3rd, 4th lumbricals: 2nd layer Adductor hallucis: 3rd layer
Cutaneous and vascular	—	Nailbeds of lateral 1½ toes Sympathetic branches to lateral plantar artery	—
Articular	Tarsometatarsal	Interphalangeal	Metatarsophalangeal

Deep Veins of Lower Limb

Veins accompanying the medial and lateral plantar arteries join to form posterior tibial vein. This vein joins with anterior tibial vein joins to form popliteal vein, which courses through adductor canal and femoral triangle as the femoral vein. Femoral vein continues as external iliac vein. Superficial veins have been described earlier in this chapter.

Table 41.16: Injury to nerves and their effects

	Motor loss	*Sensory loss*
Femoral nerve	Quadriceps femoris	Anterior side of thigh, medial side of leg till ball of big toe
Sciatic nerve	Hamstring muscles; dorsiflexors and plantar flexors of ankle joint and evertors of foot Foot drop occurs	Back of leg, lateral side of leg, most of dorsum of foot, sole of foot
Common peroneal	Dorsiflexors of ankle, evertors of foot and foot drop occurs	Lateral and anterior sides of leg, most of dorsum of foot, most of digits
Tibial	Plantar flexors of ankle, intrinsic muscles of sole	Skin of sole. Later trophic ulcers develop
Obturator	Adductors of thigh except hamstring part of adductor magnus	Small area on the medial side of thigh
Superior gluteal	Gluteal medius, gluteus minimus and tensor fascia latae	Nil
Inferior gluteal	Gluteus maximus	Nil
Pudendal nerve	Muscles of perineum	Skin of perineum
Deep peroneal	Muscles of anterior compartment of leg	1st interdigital cleft
Superficial peroneal	Peroneus longus and peroneus brevis	Lateral aspect of leg, most of dorsum of foot
Medial plantar	Four intrinsic muscles of sole	Medial two-thirdss of sole and digital nerves to medial 3½ toes, including nail beds
Lateral plantar	Most of intrinsic muscles of sole	Lateral one-third of sole and digital nerves to lateral 1½ toes, including nailbeds

Table 41.17: Arteries of lower limb

Artery	*Beginning, course, termination*	*Area of distribution*
Femoral artery (Fig. 41.8)	It is the continuation of external iliac artery, begins behind the inguinal ligament at the midinguinal point. Femoral artery courses through femoral triangle and adductor canal. Then it passes through opening in adductor magnus to continue as the popliteal artery	In femoral triangle, femoral artery gives three superficial branches, e.g. superficial external pudendal, superficial epigastric and superficial circumflex iliac, and three deep branches, e.g. profunda femoris, deep external pudendal and muscular branches. In adductor canal, femoral artery gives muscular and descending genicular artery
Popliteal artery (Fig. 41.16)	It is the continuation of femoral artery and lies in the popliteal fossa. Popliteal artery ends by dividing into anterior tibial artery and posterior tibial artery at the distal border of popliteus muscle	Gives five genicular, e.g. • Superior medial genicular • Superior lateral genicular • Middle genicular • Inferior medial genicular • Inferior lateral genicular • Cutaneous branches for skin of popliteal fossa • Muscular branches for the muscles of the fossa
Anterior tibial artery (Fig. 41.21)	Smaller terminal branch of popliteal artery reaches the front of leg through an opening in the interosseous membrane. Runs amongst muscles of front of leg till midway between medial and lateral malleoli, where it ends by changing its name to dorsalis pedis artery	Muscular to the muscles of anterior compartment of leg. Cutaneous to the skin of leg. Articular to the knee joint through anterior and posterior tibial recurrent branches. Also to the ankle joint through anterior medial and anterior lateral malleolar branches

Contd...

Table 41.17: Arteries of lower limb *(Contd...)*

Artery	*Beginning, course, termination*	*Area of distribution*
Dorsalis pedis artery (Fig. 41.19)	Continuation of anterior tibial artery. Runs along medial side of dorsum of foot to reach proximal end of 1st intermetatarsal space where it enters the sole. In the sole it completes the plantar arch	Two tarsal branches for the intertarsal joints. Arcuate artery runs over the bases of metatarsal bones and gives off 2nd, 3rd and 4th dorsal metatarsal arteries.1st dorsal metatarsal artery gives digital branches to big toe and medial side of 2nd toe
Posterior tibial artery (Fig. 41.22)	It begins as the larger terminal branch of popliteal artery at the distal border of popliteus muscle. It descends down medially between the long flexor muscles to reach midway between medial malleolus and medial tubercle of calcaneus where it ends by dividing into medial plantar and lateral plantar arteries	Peroneal artery is the largest branch. Nutrient artery to tibia. Articular branches to the knee joint and ankle joint. Muscular branches to the neighbouring muscles
Peroneal artery	Largest branch of popliteal artery given off 2.5 cm below lower border of popliteus	Muscular branches to muscles of posterior and lateral compartments. Cutaneous to skin of leg. Articular to ankle joint. Perforating branch enters the front of leg through a hole in the interosseous membrane to assist the dorsalis pedis artery
Medial plantar artery (Fig. 41.22)	The smaller terminal branch of posterior tibial artery given off under flexor retinaculum. Runs along the medial border of foot and ends by giving digital arteries	Muscular branches to muscles of medial side of foot. Cutaneous branches to medial side of sole and digital branches to medial 3½ digits. Also gives branches to the joints of foot
Lateral plantar artery	The large terminal branch of posterior tibial artery given off under the flexor retinaculum. It runs laterally between muscles of 1st and 2nd layers of sole till the base of 5th metatarsal bone by becoming continuous with the plantar arch	Muscular branches to muscles of sole, cutaneous branches to skin and fasciae of lateral side of sole
Plantar arch	It is the direct continuation of lateral plantar artery and is completed medially by dorsalis pedis artery The arch lies between 3rd and 4th layers of muscles of sole. The deep branch of lateral plantar nerve lies in its concavity	Four plantar metatarsal arteries, each of them gives two digital branches for adjacent sides of two digits, including medial side of big toe and lateral side of little toe

Section

V

Topics of Importance in Human Anatomy

Tissue structure is histology
Dysfunctional histology is pathology
Pathology forms the basis of medicine
So histology always shines

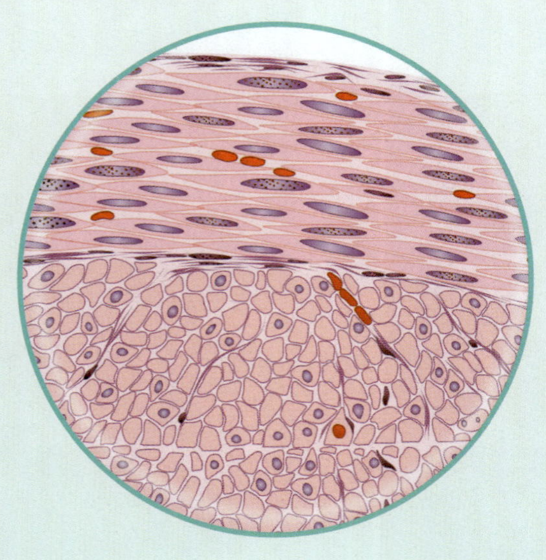

Chapter 42

Clinical Procedures

"Always do your best and the Lord will take care of the rest."
—Anonymous

Following are the clinical procedures which BDS student should practice.

INTRAMUSCULAR INJECTIONS

When a drug cannot be given orally due to nausea/ vomiting/diarrhea, it has to be given by intramuscular route for its action.

Procedure

The part of the muscle where the injection has to be given is cleaned with spirit and allowed to dry. The drug is sucked in a sterile disposable syringe and air is expelled. With the non-dominant hand, the particular muscle is supported. The needle is introduced into the muscle. The piston is withdrawn to see that there is no blood in the syringe. Then the drug is injected at the site. The needle is quickly withdrawn and the part is rubbed with a cotton swab and left to dry.

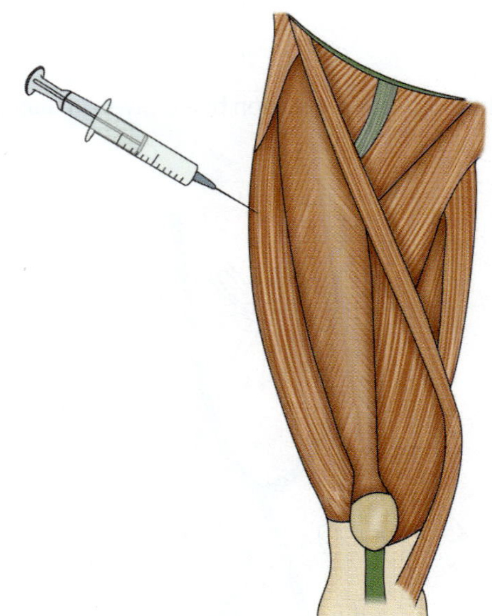

Fig. 42.1: Anterolateral region of thigh

Sites for Injection

1. *Anterolateral aspect of middle third of thigh:* The injection is given in the vastus lateralis muscle. It is done in infants, children and when self-injections are given (Fig. 42.1).
2. *Gluteal region:* The injection is given in the upper and outer quadrant of the gluteal region 5 cm below the tubercle of iliac crest into the gluteus medius muscle. If the injection is given medially it may damage the important sciatic nerve (Fig. 42.2).
3. *Deltoid muscle:* This site is usually preferred as the muscle is well developed and is easily accessible. Injection is given in the middle of the muscle 5–6 cm below the acromion (highest point on the shoulder) to protect the axillary nerve (Fig. 42.3).

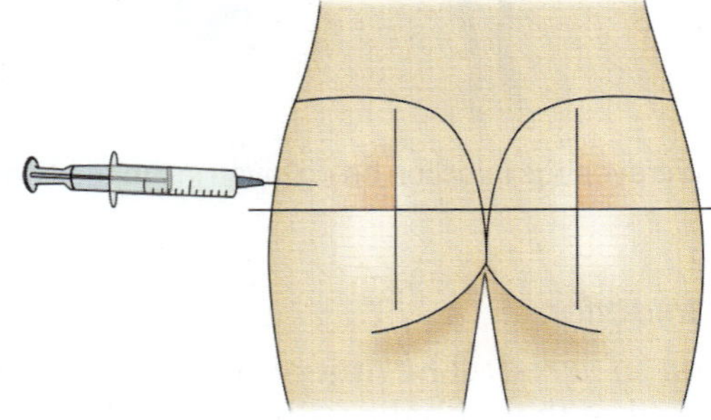

Fig. 42.2: Site of intramuscular injection in the gluteal region

INTRAVENOUS INJECTION

The intravenous injection is given to get immediate effect. Veins carry blood from periphery to the heart. As the drug is delivered into the blood directly, its effect is very quick. The procedure is done under all asceptic precautions. The vein has to be made prominent before the injection. This is done by exercising the part and by tying a tourniquet around the limb a little proximal to the site of injection. This procedure distends the vein.

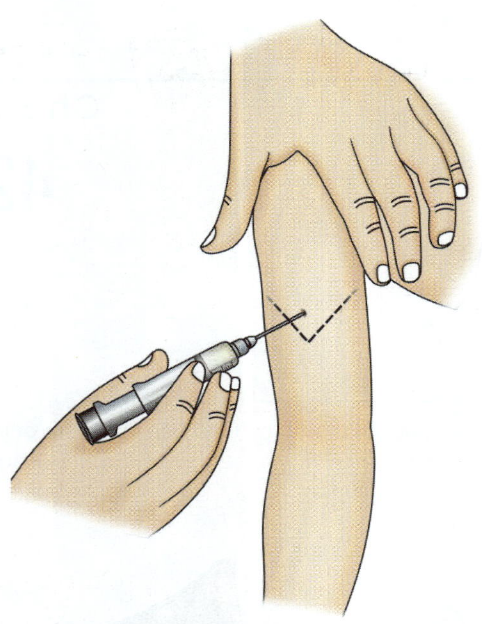

Fig. 42.3: Intramuscular injection being given in deltoid muscle

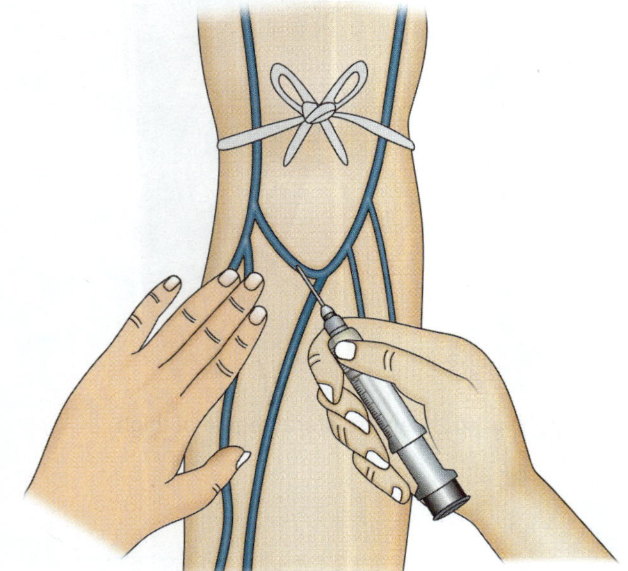

Fig. 42.4: Intravenous injection being given in the median cubital vein

Sites for Injection

1 *Dorsum of wrist:* The injection is given at the beginning of the cephalic vein.
2 *Cubital fossa:* The vein of choice is the median cubital vein. The vein runs across the anterior aspect of elbow joint (Fig. 42.4).
3 *Saphenous vein:* The great saphenous vein or the long saphenous vein lying just anterior to the medial malleolus is the vein of choice in the lower limb. Saphenous nerve lying just anteriorly to the vein should be protected.

SAPHENOUS CUT-OPEN OR CUT-DOWN

A small vertical incision is given in the skin in front of medial malleolus and the flaps are reflected. Under direct vision, a cannula is inserted into the vein. It is connected to intravenous fluid bottle.

PALPATING THE PULSE

At some places in the body, the arteries are superficially placed where these can be palpated. The various arteries are shown in Fig. 42.5.

Radial artery or radial pulse just above and on the lateral side of wrist is most often used for counting the rate, volume and regularity of the pulse.

Brachial artery is auscultated while measuring blood pressure. Superficial temporal, common carotid and facial arteries are mostly used by the anaesthetists, so they are called anaesthetist's arteries.

Femoral artery is felt at the midinguinal point and is used to put catheters into the vessel for some clinical procedures and also for arterial blood sampling.

The femoral vein lies just medial to the artery. Popliteal artery behind the knee joint is used for measuring the blood pressure in the lower limb.

Posterior tibial and dorsalis pedis arteries are used to find out about state of circulation of the blood in the lower limb.

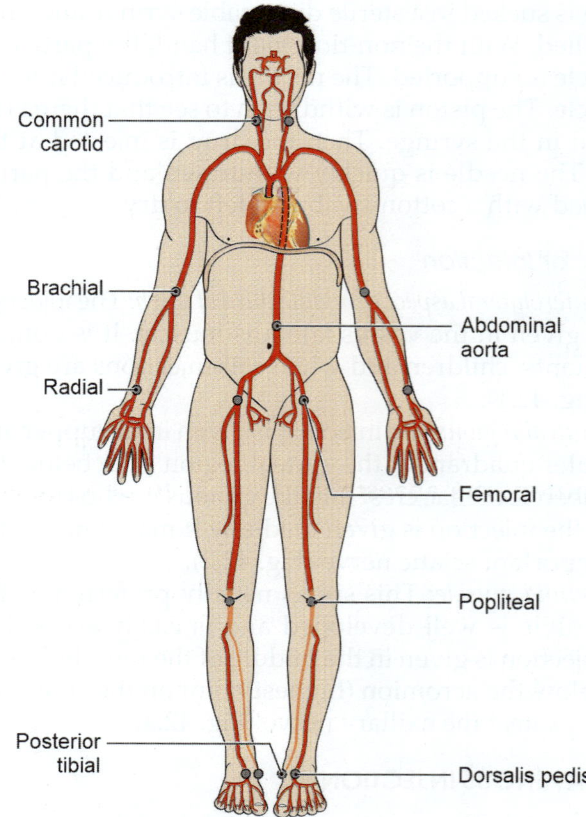

Fig. 42.5: Palpable arteries in the body

MEASUREMENT OF BLOOD PRESSURE

The blood pressure measurement is done by two methods, viz. palpatory method using the radial artery and the auscultatory method using the brachial artery. The cuff of the sphygmomanometer is tied on the middle of the arm. The pressure in the cuff is raised to 180 mm Hg. The cuff is gradually deflated and the reading where the brachial pulse becomes audible is noted as the systolic blood pressure. One continues to hear the sound and the reading where the sound disappear is noted as the diastolic blood pressure (Fig. 42.6).

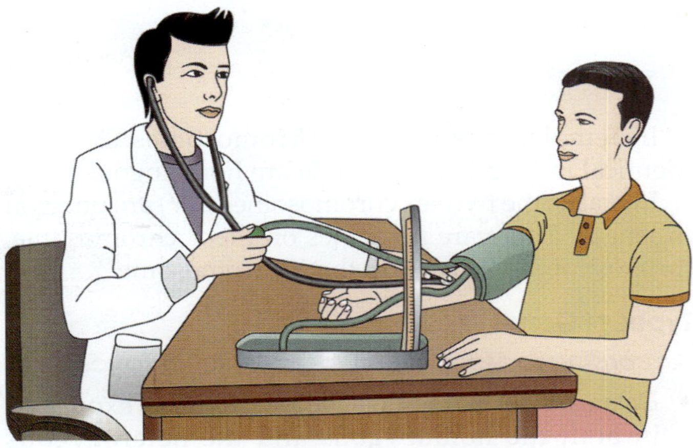

Fig. 42.6: Blood pressure being taken

LUMBAR PUNCTURE

Lumbar puncture in adult: Patient is lying on side with maximally flexed spine. A line is taken between highest points of iliac spine at L4 level.

Skin locally anaesthetized, and lumbar puncture needle with trocar inserted carefully between L3 and L4 spines. Needle courses through skin fat, supra-spinous and interspinous ligaments, ligamentum flava, epidural space, dura, arachnoid, subarachnoid space to enter CSF (Fig. 42.7).

DENTAL PROCEDURES

If any surgical treatment for 3rd upper molar tooth is required, the anaesthetic fluid is to be injected in posterior superior alveolar nerve in the infratemporal fossa (Fig. 42.8).

If any surgical treatment for lower 3rd molar tooth is required, the anaesthetic fluid is to be injected in the inferior alveolar nerve in the submandibular fossa (Fig. 42.9).

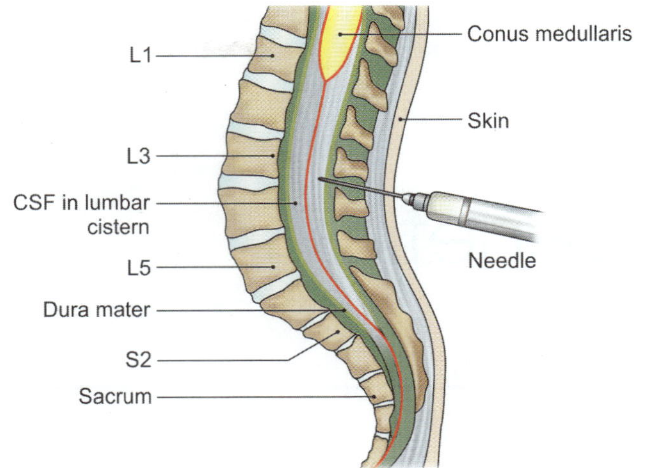

Fig. 42.7: Lumbar puncture in an adult

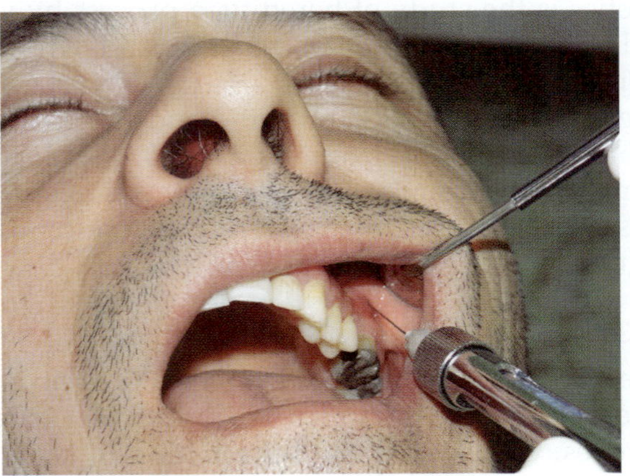

Fig. 42.8: Anaesthesia being given for treatment of 3rd upper molar tooth

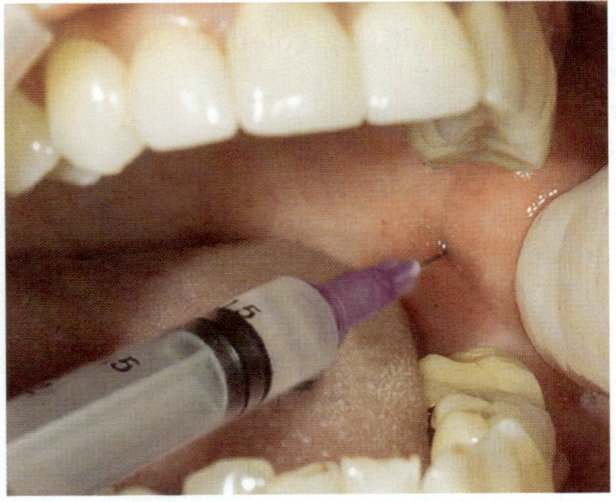

Fig. 42.9: Anaesthesia being given for treatment of 3rd lower molar tooth

Chapter 43

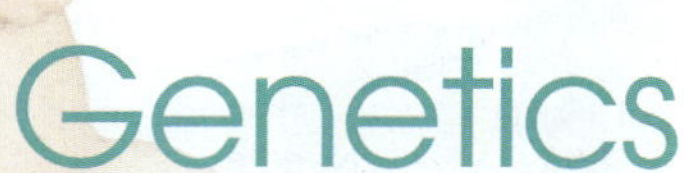

Genetics

"Life can be happier and stressless, if we remember one simple thought; 'we can't have all that we desire, but God will give us all that we deserve'."
—Anonymous

Genetics is the study of heredity, a process by which children inherit certain characteristics (traits) from their parents.

Heredity is controlled by genes and environmental factors. Various environmental factors may cause anomalies in chromosomes, e.g. mother's age over 40 years, viral diseases or exposure to radiation during pregnancy.

THE GENES

Gene, the functional unit of DNA, is the basic unit of heredity in a living organism. All living things depend on genes. Genes hold the information to build and maintain an organism's cells and pass genetic traits to offspring.

Properties of Genes

- To determine traits, e.g. colour of skin, intelligence, height, etc.
- Undergo replication
- May undergo mutation.

Homeobox genes are groups of regulatory genes that control the expression of other genes involved in the normal development, growth and differentiation. Teratogens like retinoic acid can activate these genes to cause abnormal gene expression.

Functions of Genes

- Maintain the genetic specificity of an individual
- Play key role in transmission of traits from the parents to the offspring.
- Synthesise various proteins and enzymes of the cell.

Sites of Genes

Each gene occupies a specific locus on the chromosome. Both chromosomes of a given pair contain similar genes. The genes occupying the same locus on the homologous chromosomes are called alleles.

In females, the two sex chromosomes (XX) are identical in length, hence these are homologous.

In males, the two sex chromosomes (XY) are unequal in length. There are no alleles on the Y chromosome, for most of the loci are on the X chromosome.

Types of Genes

According to Mendelian Pattern of Inheritance

- *Dominant gene:* An allele which is always expressed in both the homozygous and the heterozygous combination.
- *Recessive gene:* When an allele is expressed only in the homozygous state, it is known as recessive gene.
- *Carrier gene:* In the heterozygous state, the recessive gene acts as a carrier gene which is not expressed in the individual but may be expressed in the subsequent generations.
- *Co-dominant gene:* When both the allelic genes are dominant but of two different types, both traits may have concurrent expression, e.g. blood group AB.
- *Sex-linked genes:* The genes located on X or Y chromosomes are sex-linked genes.
- *Sex-limited genes:* These genes are borne by the autosomes, but the trait borne is preferentially in one sex only, e.g. baldness seen predominantly in males.
- *Structural genes:* These are segments of DNA which code for specific sequence of amino acids in the protein.
- *Regulatory genes:* These are segments of DNA which control functions of structural genes.

SOME IMPORTANT TERMS

Inheritance: It is process of transmission of characters/ traits from generation to generation.

Reproduction: It is essential requisite for inheritance to take place. The inheritance of traits from parents to offspring takes place through genes which carry all information about all types of traits.

Locus: The position of a gene in the chromosome is called locus.

Alleles: Genes occupying identical loci in a pair of homologous chromosomes.

Homozygous alleles: When both allelic genes regulating a particular character are similar.

Heterozygous alleles: When both allelic genes regulating a particular character are dissimilar.

Multiple alleles: When in a population, more than two different alleles exist at a given locus on a chromosome.

Mutation: It is a phenomenon which results in alteration in base pair in DNA. Under abnormal conditions, adenine may pair with cytosine or guanine, instead of thymine. This forms the basis of mutation. Some mutations involve changes in whole set of chromosomes like aneuploidy, polyploidy.

Modes of Inheritance

(Mendel's Laws of Inheritance)

1. *Law of uniformity*: The crossing over between two homozygotes of different types results in offspring that are identical and heterozygotic. The inherited characters do not blend.
2. *Law of segregation:* Segregation of alleles occurs during the process of gamete formation (meiosis) and randomly united at fertilization.
3. *Law of independent assortment*: This law states that the traits are transmitted to the offspring independently of one another.

THE CHROMOSOMES

Structure of Chromosomes

1. All chromosomes consist of two parallel identical filaments called chromatids joined together at a narrowed constriction called centromere (Fig. 43.1).
2. As per the position of centromere, chromosomes are grouped in 3 types in humans (Table 43.1).

Groups of Chromosomes

The chromosomes are arranged in descending order of length. The first pair is the longest and the 22nd pair is the shortest. Sex chromosomes are grouped separately.

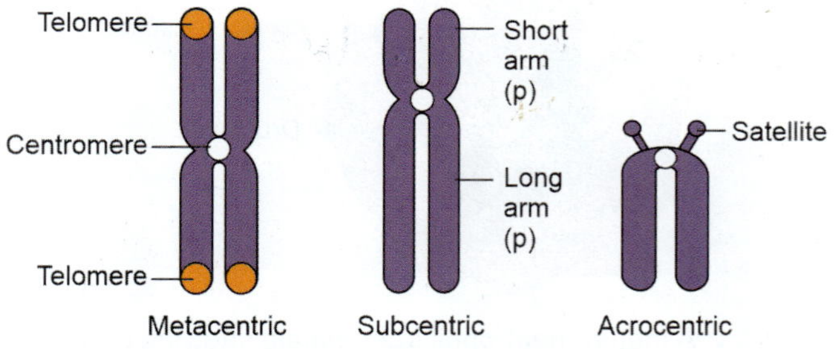

Fig. 43.1: Types of chromosomes

Table 43.1: Types of chromosomes

Type	*Position of centromere in chromosome*
Metacentric	Middle
Subcentric	Near one end
Acrocentric	Between midpoint and end of the chromosome

The chromosomes are divided into 7 groups. They are denoted as A to G (Fig. 43.2 and Table 43.2).

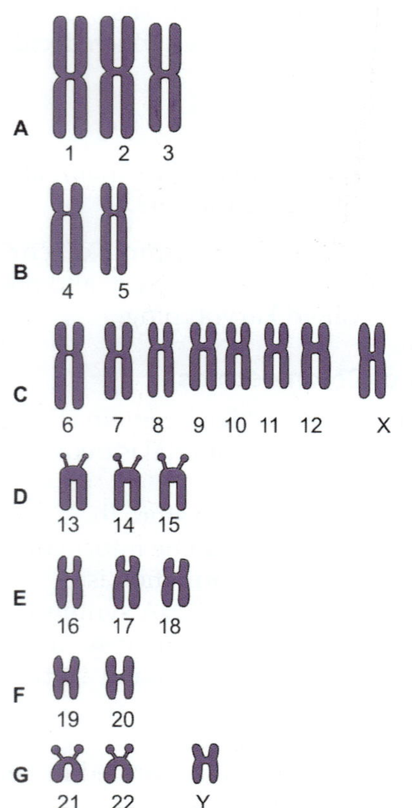

Fig. 43.2: Groups of chromosomes

Table 43.2: Groups of chromosomes

Group	*Chromosome number*	*Feature*
A	1 to 3	Large, metacentric
B	4 and 5	Large, submetacentric
C	6 to 12 and X	Medium sized, submetacentric and X chromosome
D	13 to 15	Medium sized, acrocentric with satellite
E	16 to 18	Short subcentric
F	19 and 20	Short metacentric
G	21, 22 and Y	Very short, acrocentric, and Y chromosome

Function of tRNA is to match a specific amino acid to specific codon of mRNA.

Each cell contains fixed number of chromosomes which is characteristic of that species or organism. In somatic cell (body cell) of human, the number is 46, which is diploid number. In gametes, i.e. ovum and sperm it is 23, called haploid number. During fertilization, union of two haploid cells restores diploid number of chromosomes.

Classification of Chromosomes

According to functions:

a. Autosomes: 22 pairs in humans.
b. A pair of sex chromosomes which decides the sex of the individual:
   i. In male—XY
   ii. In female—XX

According to the position of the centromere (Denver's classification): Shown in Table 43.3.

Clinical significance: Mapping of chromosomes according to the length of their arm and position of the centromere is called karyotyping.

Chemistry of Chromosomes

Human chromosome chiefly contains DNA and only a little RNA. The genetic material is deoxyribose nucleic acid (DNA).

Functions of DNA are to store the genetic information and to transfer the genetic information.

Transfer of genetic information is:

1 From DNA to DNA for DNA synthesis
2 From DNA to RNA for protein synthesis

RNA is present in nucleus and in the cytoplasm. There are three types of RNA:

i. messenger RNA: m-RNA
ii. transfer RNA: t-RNA—formed in nucleus.
iii. ribosomal RNA: r-RNA

Messenger RNA acts as an intermediate agent between DNA of the nucleus and amino acids of the cytoplasm. It plays an important role in synthesis of proteins from the pools of amino acids present in the cytoplasm.

3 mRNA is produced in nucleus from DNA and is rich incystosine and guanine. Plays important role in formation of protein at ribosome.

Table 43.3: Position of the centromere

No.	Particulars	Metacentric	Submetacentric	Acrocentric
1	Centromere	Centrally	Subcentrally	Near one end (Fig. 43.1)
2	Arms	Equal	p arm (short) q arm (long)	p arm shortest q arm longest

Barr Body (Sex Chromatin)

Barr body is an inactivated X chromosome attached to nuclear membrane. It was discovered by Barr and Bertram in 1949 in the neuron of female cats. It is attached to nuclear membrane and is planoconvex in shape and darkly stained. It is also known as sex chromatin (Fig. 43.3).

In female (XX): There are two X chromosomes. One of them is inactivated within 2 weeks of conception. The inactivated X chromosome becomes the Barr body. Normally, a single Barr body is present and only one X is functional. This is called Lyon's hypothesis.

In male (XY): Since there is only one X chromosome, there is no Barr body. Y chromosome is smaller and is for determination of male sex.

Table 43.4: Number of Barr bodies in different syndromes

Name of chromosome	Number of Barr bodies	Syndrome/normal
XX	One	Normal female
XXX	Two	Triple XXX
XO	—	Turner's syndrome
XY	No Barr body	Normal male
XXY	One	Klinefelter's syndrome

Sex chromatin can be stained by scraping from cheek mucosa.

Mature polymorphonuclear leucocytes in females have a drumstick like body. It is present in 6% females (Fig. 43.4).

Clinical significance: It is helpful in determination of sex in case of ambiguity and also in diagnosis of various syndromes like Turner's, Klinefelter's.

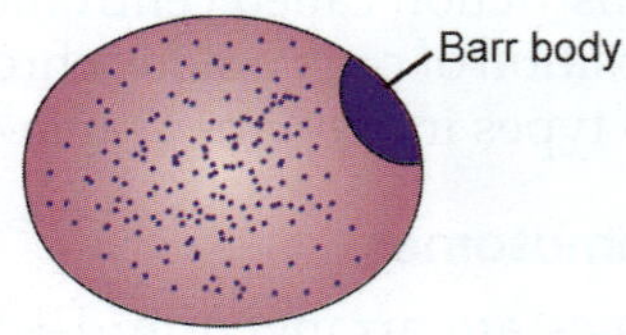

Fig. 43.3: Nucleus of a female cell showing Barr body

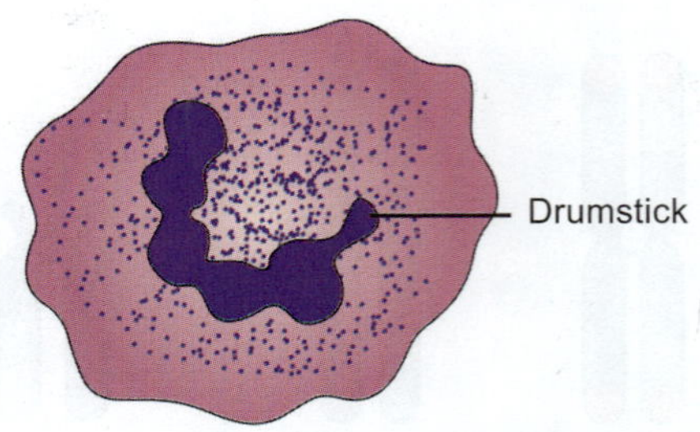

Fig. 43.4: A mature neutrophil from female showing drumstick-like body

Karyotyping

Introduction: Identification of chromosomes according to the length of arms including position of centromere is called karyotyping.

Procedure: It is done by the culture of lymphocytes. The cells are grown in culture media containing phytohaemagglutinin (PHA). The cell division is arrested in metaphase by adding colchicine. The spreads of the chromosomes are counted and photographed under the microscope. The images of each chromosome are cut out and arranged in pairs according to the classification. This procedure is called karyotyping. One needs to note:

i. Total length of chromosomes.
ii. Position of centromere.
iii. Relative length of two arms.
iv. Banding pattern.

The chromosomes are arranged according to their length in a descending order. Identical chromosomes are paired in karyotyping. The chromosomes paired are numbered 1 to 22 in descending order of length, i.e. pair number 1 is long, pair number 22 is short. They are grouped into 7 groups. They are noted as A to G. The chromosomes are placed separately.

Karyotyping helps to

i. Identify pattern of abnormal chromosome.
ii. Determine the sex.

Individual chromosomes can be recognized with quinacrine banding (Q-banding) and Giemsa banding (G-banding). These methods have helped in mapping specific genes on the chromosomes (Fig. 43.5).

MITOCHONDRIAL DNA

A human cell has genetic material contained in the cell nucleus (the nuclear genome) and in the mitochondria (the mitochondrial genome). In human beings, the nuclear genome is divided into 23 pairs of linear DNA molecules called chromosomes. The mitochondrial genome is circular DNA molecule distinct from the nuclear DNA. Although the mitochondrial DNA is very small compared to nuclear chromosomes, it codes for 13 proteins involved in mitochondrial energy production as well as specific tRNAs.

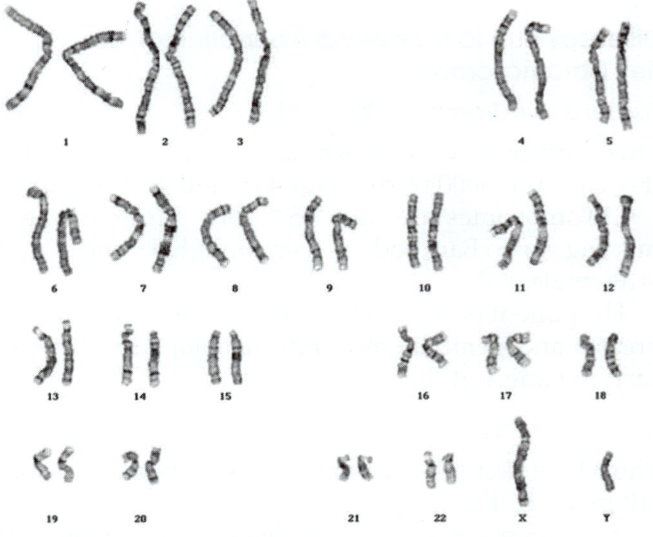

Fig. 43.5: Giemsa banding of the chromosomes

Mitochondrial Inheritance

- The body receives its entire mitochondrial DNA only from the mother, because during fertilization mitochondria of sperm do not pass into the ovum.
- The diseases which occur due to mutation in the mitochondrial DNA are inherited entirely through mother.

The diseases are

- *Leber's hereditary optic neuropathy (LHON):* A condition characterized by sudden onset of blindness in adults.
- *Pearson marrow-pancreas syndrome (PMPS):* It is a condition characterized by a loss of bone marrow cells during childhood. It is fatal.

CHROMOSOMAL ABERRATIONS

It is the change in the structural components of the chromosome. The deletion or an addition of a segment from other chromosome results in structural aberration. The change in number results in numerical aberration. The number may be 45 or 47. Aberrations are seen in elderly primigravida or mother suffering from viral infections during pregnancy or those exposed to radiation during pregnancy.

Various chromosomal aberrations are classified:

Disease due to Autosomal Numerical Chromosomal Aberration

Down's syndrome/Trisomy 21

- It is the most common congenital anomaly due to numerical aberration of chromosomes. This syndrome was described by Dr Down in 1866. There is aneuploidy. In aneuploidy the chromosomes may be 2n+1, 2n–1, i.e. 47 or 45. Fertilisation with disomic gamete will result in 47 chromosomes (Fig. 43.6).
- In Down syndrome there is trisomy of chromosome 21. The number of chromosomes is 47, i.e. 47XX or 47 XY. Sex may be male or female. It is seen to occur as one in 700 newborns (Fig. 43.7).

This condition is commonly seen in elderly primigravida or mother suffering from viral infection during pregnancy. In elderly primigravida the reason is the ageing of the ovum. The sperms are formed fresh every time, so ageing factor does not apply for the sperms.

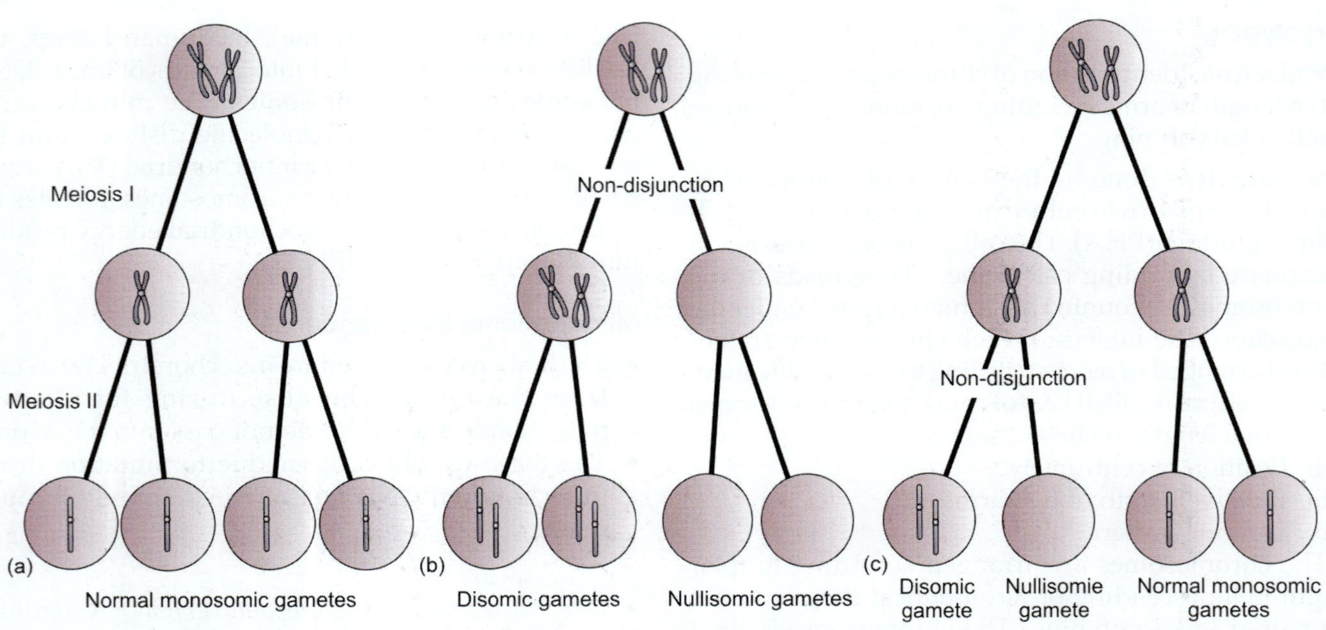

Figs 43.6a to c: (a) Normal meiosis showing segregation of a single pair of chromosomes, (b) gametes at non-disjunction in meiosis I, (c) gametes at non-disjunction in meiosis II

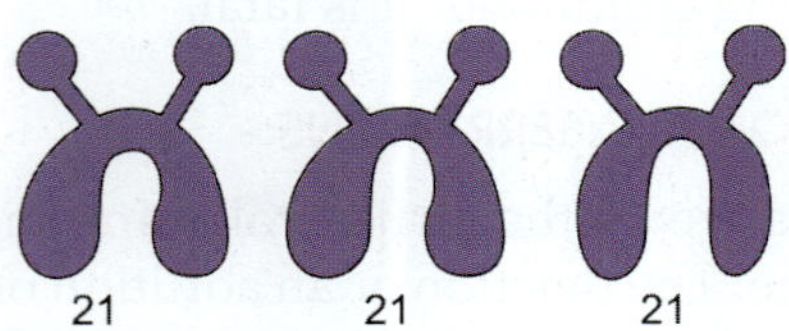
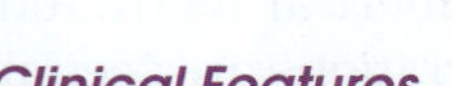

Fig. 43.7: Down syndrome

Clinical Features

- Mental retardation
- Palpebral fissure is slanting upwards at lateral end
- Tongue protrudes out of the mouth
- Palate is narrow so the oral cavity cannot accommodate the tongue
- Nasal bridge is flat
- Epicanthic fold is present on the eyes
- Short broad hands have simian crease.

Disease due to Autosomal Structural Chromosomal Aberration

The autosomal structural chromosomal aberration may be translocations, deletions, duplications, ring chromosomes. Most of these result from unequal exchange between homologons repeated sequences on the same or different chromosomes. One syndrome due to deletion of part of an arm is described below.

Edward syndrome, Trisomy 18

Patau syndrome, Trisomy 13

Both these syndrome infants die within 1st month.

Cri du Chat Syndrome

This is due to deletion of a part of 'p' arm of chromosome 5 (Fig. 43.8). The following symptoms are seen:

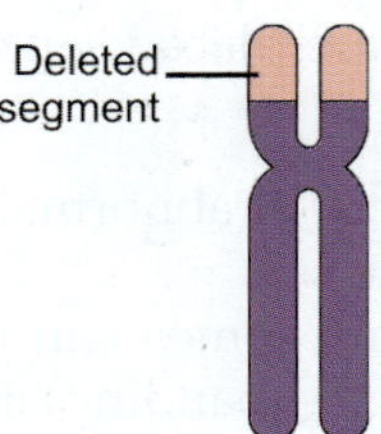

Fig. 43.8: Cri du chat syndrome

- Septal defects in heart
- "Cat like cry" due to underdevelopment of larynx.
- Severe mental retardation.

There may be microdeletions, translocations, isochromosomes or inversions.

Diseases due to Numerical Aberration of Sex Chromosomes

Turner's Syndrome (45X)

This syndrome was discovered by Mr. Turner in 1938. It occurs 1 in 5000 births (Figs 43.9 and 43.10).

Chromosomes are only 45X. One chromosome is missing, so no Barr body is seen though the individual is a female.

The patient is of short height with webbed neck. The breasts and genitalia are underdeveloped with wide carrying angle at the elbow.

Klinefelter's Syndrome (47XXY)

The Klinefelter's syndrome was described in cases of tall males in 1942.

Its incidence is 1 in 1000 male newborns (Figs 43.11 and 43.12).

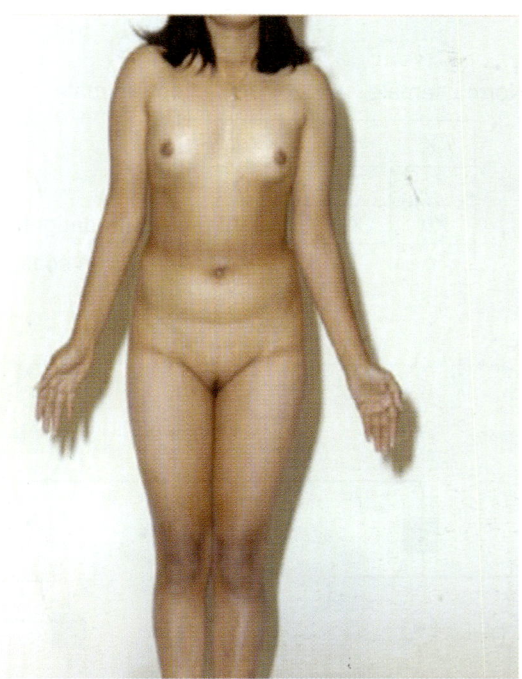

Fig. 43.9: Turner's syndrome showing webbing of the neck

Fig. 43.10: Turner's syndrome, only one X chromosome

The genotype is 47 XXY.

The individual is male with an extra X chromosome. Since there are two X chromosomes, Barr body is present.

External genitalia including testes are underdeveloped. In contrast, breasts are well developed.

Single Gene Inherited Diseases

Autosomal Dominant Inheritance

Characters: Commonest mating normal with heterozygote.

1. Parents show the trait.
2. There is horizontal and vertical transmission (50% affected at every conception).
3. Trait appears in each generation.
4. Normal (unaffected) individual does not carry the gene and does not transmit the trait.
5. No sex predilection.
6. Both the chromosomes carry the trait. Mating is heterozygous.

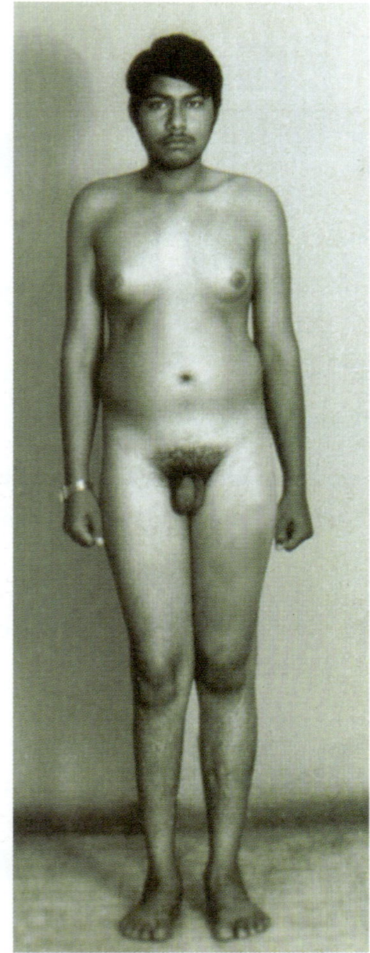

Fig. 43.11: Klinefelter's syndrome

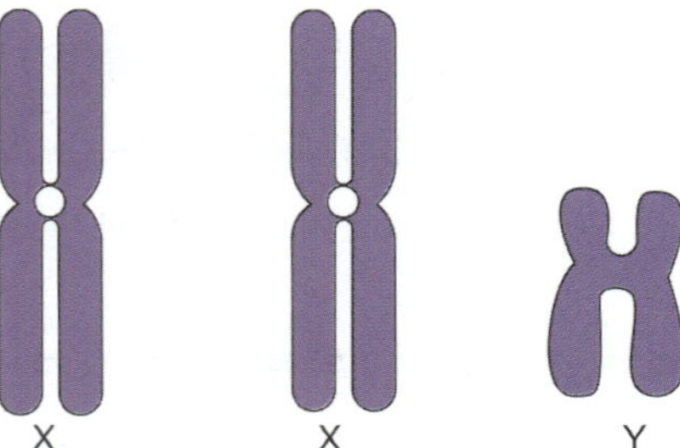

Fig. 43.12: Klinefelter's syndrome

The disease is inherited both male and female in each generation. Examples are seen in brachydactyly, syndactyly, achondroplasia, Huntington's chorea. Pedigree chart is shown in Fig. 43.13.

Autosomal Recessive Inheritance

This condition is common in homozygous mating 25% are affected in every conception.

Carriers are present and look normal. Parents are from consanguineous marriage. Examples are cystic

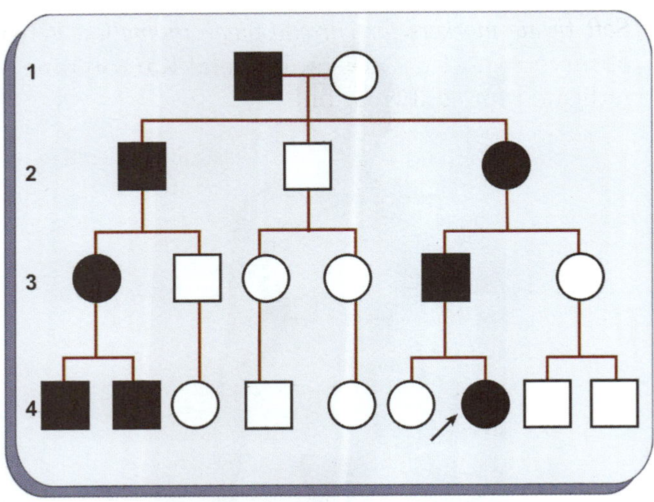

Fig. 43.13: Pedigree chart of autosomal dominant trait

fibrosis, phenylketoneuria in the siblings and not parents. Examples are albinism and deaf mutism. Pedigree chart is shown in Fig. 43.16.

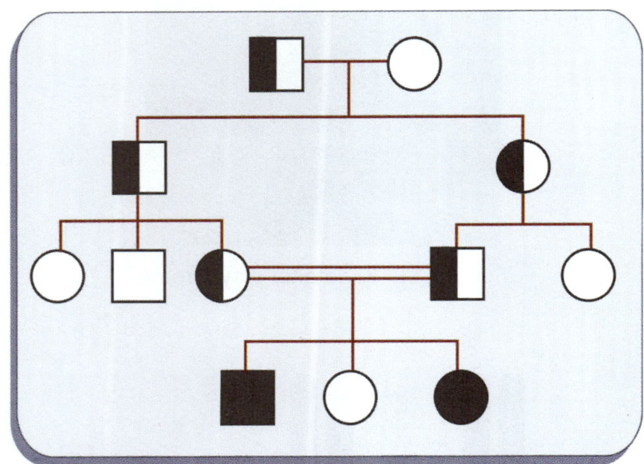

Fig. 43.14: Pedigree chart of autosomal recessive trait

X-linked Dominant Condition

The X-linked dominant trait is seen in homozygous and heterozygous females. It is also seen in male having a gene under question on his single X chromosome. Common in females, ratio of female: male is 2:1.

Example is seen in vitamin D resistant rickets.

X-linked Recessive Traits

The females are always the carriers and do not show the symptoms.

The females are rarely affected (Punnet chart 43.1).

Disease is not transferred from father to son. Pedigree chart is shown in Fig. 43.15.

Examples are hemophilia, colour blindness and Duchenne muscular dystrophy.

Punnet chart 43.1

Normal female — Haemophilic male

XX		X h Y	
	X	X	
Xh	X h X	X h X	Both daughters carrier
Y	XY	XY	Both sons normal

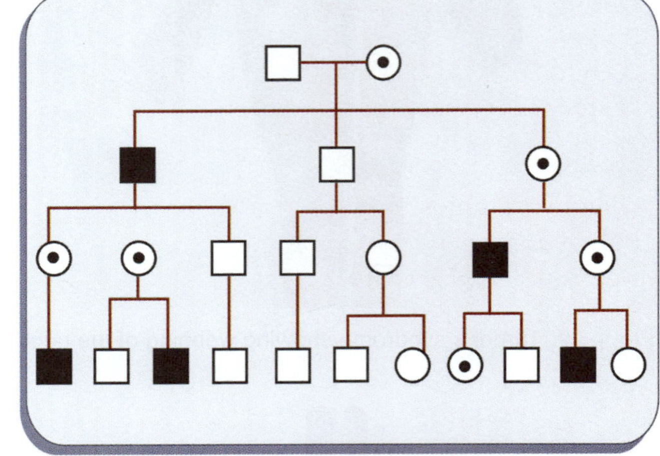

Fig. 43.15: Pedigree chart of X-linked recessive trait; when affected mother reproduce

Y-linked Conditions

Male only has single Y chromosome. The gene is unpaired. If present it should be expressed. The gene is passed from affected male to his sons but none to his daughters as she does not get Y chromosome.

Example is hypertrichosis, i.e. growth of hair on the outer rim of the pinna of the auricle.

PRENATAL DIAGNOSIS

Genetic abnormalities in a conceptus can result in the following:

1 Spontaneous miscarriages: First trimester losses, mostly associated with chromosomal abnormalities.
2 Gross congenital abnormalities in newborn are 2–3%. This leads to perinatal morbidity and mortality.
3 Abnormalities in childhood and adult life, e.g. blindness, deafness, malignancies.

Prenatal diagnosis helps the doctors in early detection and appropriate management in high-risk cases.

PRENATAL DIAGNOSIS THERAPY

Indications of Prenatal Diagnosis

In addition to routine assessment of normal growth of conceptus and to screen for the various congenital malformations, prenatal diagnosis with special tests is indicated in *high risk pregnancies* which include:

Maternal Risk Factors

- Advanced maternal age (>35 years)
- Family history or previous child with neural tube defects.
- Previous gestation with chromosomal abnormalities.
- One or both parents carrier of X-linked or autosomal traits.
- A child born with an unbalanced translocation.
- History of recurrent miscarriages.

Prenatal Risk Factors

- Oligohydramnios,
- Polyhydramnios,
- Decreased fetal activity,
- Severe intrauterine growth retardation,
- Presence of soft tissue markers of chromosomal anomaly on routine ultrasonography.

METHODS OF DIAGNOSIS

I. Pre-implantation Genetic Diagnosis (PGD)

Following techniques are used whenever indicated:

- Polar body biopsy,
- Blastomere biopsy (from 6 to 8 cell stage) and
- Trophectoderm biopsy.

II. Prenatal Diagnostic Techniques

1 *Ultrasonography:* It is a non-invasive technique used for routine antenatal check up to assess fetal growth as well as to detect structural abnormalities whenever indicated.

Assessment of fetal growth is done by serial ultrasonography for following parameters:

- Fetal age and growth is assessed by crown rump length (CRL) during 5th to 10th week of gestation.
- Other parameters which help in assessment of fetal growth are biparietal diameter (BPD) of the skull, femur length and abdominal circumference.

Congenital malformations that can be determined by ultrasonography include the:

- Neural tube defects (anencephaly and spina bifida)
- Abdominal wall defects such as omphalocele and gastroschisis.
- Heart defects, and
- Facial defects including cleft lip and cleft palate.

Soft tissue markers for chromosomal anomalies: When observed on ultrasonography, fetal Karyotyping is indicated for confirmation.

Blood flow velocity: Blood flow velocity is measured in the Doppler ultrasonography to detect the vascular resistance secondary to fetal hypoplasia and IUGR.

2 *Maternal serum screening tests* recommended to search for *biochemical markers* of fetal status are:

i. *Serum a-fetoprotein levels*
   - *Elevated* in twinning, neural tube defects, intestinal atresia, and fetal demise.
   - *Lowered* in trisomies and aneuploidy

ii. *Human chorionic gonadotropins (HCG)* levels are also lowered in trisomies and aneuploidy.

iii. *Circulating fetal cells in maternal blood* for molecular DNA genetic analysis.

3 *Amniocentesis:* In this technique about 20–30 ml of amniotic fluid is withdrawn with the help of a needle inserted into the amniotic cavity transabdominally under ultrasound guidance. It is indicated to perform following tests:

- *Biochemical analysis* for a-fetoprotein and acetyl choline esterase.
- *Karyotyping* (cytogenetics) from the fetal cells present in the fluid.
- *Molecular genetic* DNA diagnosis genome detection etc. by using various tests including polymerase chain reaction (PCR).
- *Fetal maturity assessment* from the levels of creatinine and lecithin.

4 *Cordocentesis*, i.e. percutaneous umbilical cord blood sampling is used for:

- *Fetal blood disorders* such as anaemia, hemoglobinopathies, thrombocytopenia, polycyathemia.
- *Response to infection* by IgM antibody levels in fetal blood.
- *Rapid karyotyping* and *molecular* DNA genetic diagnosis.

5 *Fetal tissue biopsies* indicated in certain specific conditions are as below:

- *Chorionic villus sampling* (CVS) involves transabdominally needle aspiration of about 5 to 30 mg of villus tissue from the placenta. The material obtained is used for karyotyping, molecular DNA genetic analysis and enzyme analysis.
- *Fetal skin biopsy* is indicated with history of hereditary skin disorders.
- *Fetal liver biopsy* may sometimes be required for enzyme essay.

6 *Fetal urine analysis* is needed to comment on prognosis in obstructive uropathy.
7 *Antepartum biophysical monitoring (ABM)* required for fetal distress and hypoxia include:
   - Nonstress test,
   - Contraction stress test, and
   - Biophysical profile (BPP).

III. Postnatal Tests to Detect Congenital Malformations

1 *Clinical evaluation at birth.* Gross anomaly can be seen on routine clinical examination of newborn. Look specifically for:
   - Imperforate anus, and
   - Tracheoesophageal fistulae.
2 *Imaging techniques* like ultrasonography, MRI, radiography, etc can be employed in a newborn if indicated to detect:
   - Anomalies of gastrointestinal tract like oesophageal or duodenal atresia, extent of imperforate anus,
   - Cardiac abnormalities,
   - Intracranial abnormalities and
   - Gross skeletal abnormalities.

GENETIC COUNSELLING

Cytogenetic analysis of cells from amniotic fluid should be done in females over 35 years who had viral infection especially German measles or those who were exposed to radiation during pregnancy. If diagnosed as any syndrome, parents need to be counselled in favour of termination of the pregnancy. Future pregnancy should be discussed and parents be counselled accordingly.

Chapter

44

Embryology

"Laugh like you have never cried; play like you have never lost; love like you have never been hurt; live like there is no tomorrow."

—Anonymous

SCOPE OF EMBRYOLOGY

1. Embryology throws light on the genesis of structure and functions of human organism.
2. Knowledge of normal development is necessary to understand the mechanism of abnormal development. This would help in prevention and treatment of such abnormalities.
3. Many of the adult anatomical relationships of organs, their nerve supply, blood supply and variations can be easily understood from the knowledge of embryology.
4. Embryology forms the basis of concept of growth, repair, regeneration of tissues and the understanding of development of various embryonic tumours.

GAMETOGENESIS

The development of human being begins with fertilization, a process by which two highly specialised cells, the spermatozoon from the male and the mature oocyte from the female, fuse to give rise to a new organism, the zygote.

The spermatozoa are produced in the primary sex organs, namely, the testis in the male and the process is called Spermatogenesis. The mature oocytes are formed in the ovaries in the female and the process of their formation is called Oogenesis. These two processes collectively are known as Gametogenesis.

Before fertilization, the male and female germ cells (gamete) undergo a number of changes which pertain to the chromosomes of the nucleus as well as to the cytoplasm. These changes are an integral part of germ cell maturation.

Chromosomal Changes during Maturation of Germ Cells

The human somatic cell contains 46 chromosomes (44 autosomes and 2 sex chromosomes). The sex chromosomes in the female are represented by two X-chromosomes and in the male by one X and a much shorter Y chromosome. The human somatic cell thus contains 23 pairs of chromosomes, one chromosome of each pair being derived from the mother and the other from the father.

The aim of maturation in germ cells is to reduce the number of chromosomes to half of that in somatic cell (from 46 to 23). This is accomplished by two specialised divisions known as meiotic divisions.

First Meiotic Division

Just before the first meiotic division the gamete (primary oocyte/primary spermatocyte) show pairing of homologous chromosomes and this involves duplication of DNA. Thus at the beginning of this stage, the cells contain double the normal amount of DNA (4n) and each of the 46 chromosomes is a double structure (Fig. 44.1).

The **Prophase** of the first meiotic division is prolonged and divided into following stages:

i. *Leptotene:* Chromosomes which were thin and thread-like, become shorter, thicker and prominent in this stage.
ii. *Zygotene:* The homologous chromosomes approach each other. They pair point for point and lie side by side.
iii. *Pachytene:* The chromosomes get shorter, thicker and each is formed of two chromatids joined at the centromere. The bivalents thus have four chromatids and this is called a tetrad. The two central chromatids from each bivalent chromosome become partially coiled so that they cross over at a number of points. During this process, exchange of DNA takes place. At the site of crossing, the chromatids adhere together and this point is called **chiasmata**.
iv. *Diplotene:* In this, the bivalent chromosomes move apart. At the chiasmata, there is a break in the

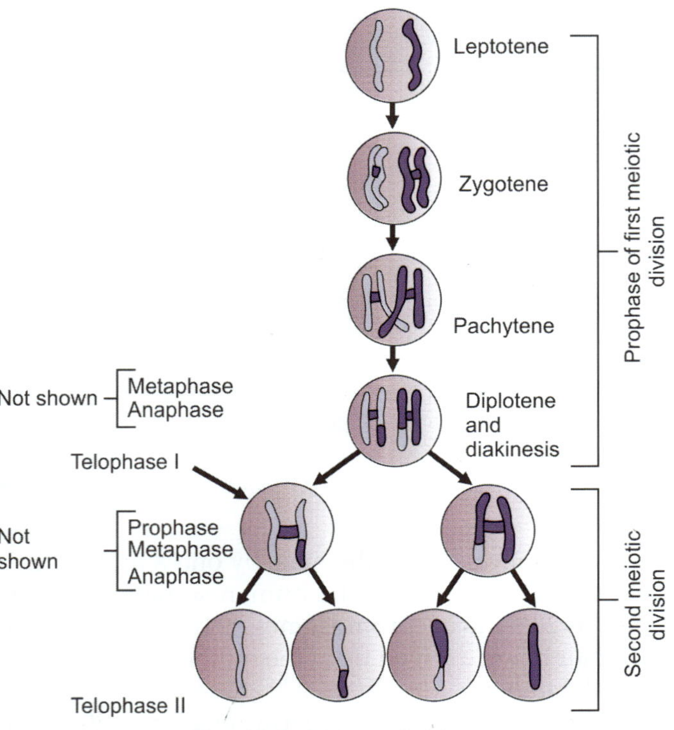

Fig. 44.1: Meiotic division

chromatids and broken pieces get attached to the opposite chromatids thereby bringing about an exchange in gene blocks between homologous chromosomes.

v. *Diakinesis:* In this last stage of prophase, the chromosomes are distinct and the bivalent pairs move away from the each other.

Metaphase: The nuclear membrane disappears and spindle is formed. The two chromatids, attached at the centromere, are oriented on the spindle.

Anaphase: Paired chromosomes migrate to opposite poles. The centromere does **not** divide.

Telophase: Chromosomes are reduced to haploid number in each nucleus.

At the end of the first meiotic division, each daughter cell contains 23 double structured chromosomes, still attached at the centromere. The DNA content in each daughter cell is same as that in a normal somatic cell (2n).

Second Meiotic Division

This follows the first meiotic division and in this, **no DNA synthesis occurs.** This division resembles mitosis with following modifications:

i. The chromatids split along the centromere in anaphase. Centromere divides.
ii. The separating chromatids are genetically dissimilar.
iii. Each germ cell has haploid number of chromosomes (23) and half the amount of DNA of a normal somatic cell.

At the time of fertilization, when one male and one female gamete fuse, the diploid number of chromosomes (46) and 2n DNA are restored.

I. MALE REPRODUCTIVE SYSTEM

Parts of reproductive organs

Two gonads	– Testes (Fig. 44.2)
Duct system	– Epididymis
	– Head, body, tail
(one on each side)	– Ductus deferens
	– Ejaculatory duct
	associated glands
–	Prostate (single)
	– Pair of seminal vesicles
	common passage
	for urine and ejaculate
	– Urethra

Spermatogenesis

Spermatogenesis is the process by which spermatozoa are produced in the testis. These get differentiated from primordial germ cells (Flowchart 44.1 and Fig. 44.4).

Spermiogenesis

The process by which the spermatids are transformed into motile spermatozoa is known as spermiogenesis.

Flowchart 44.1: Spermatogenesis

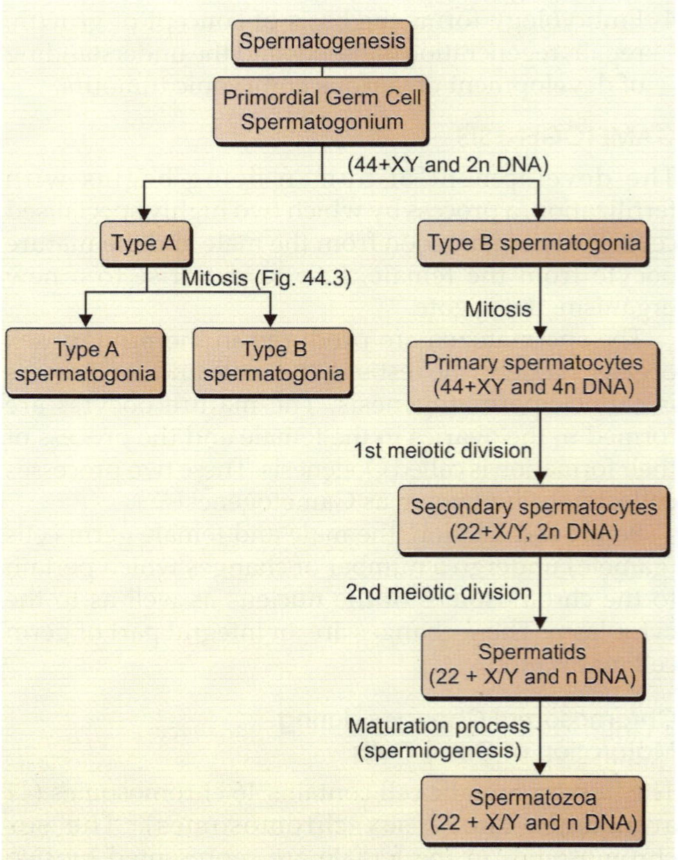

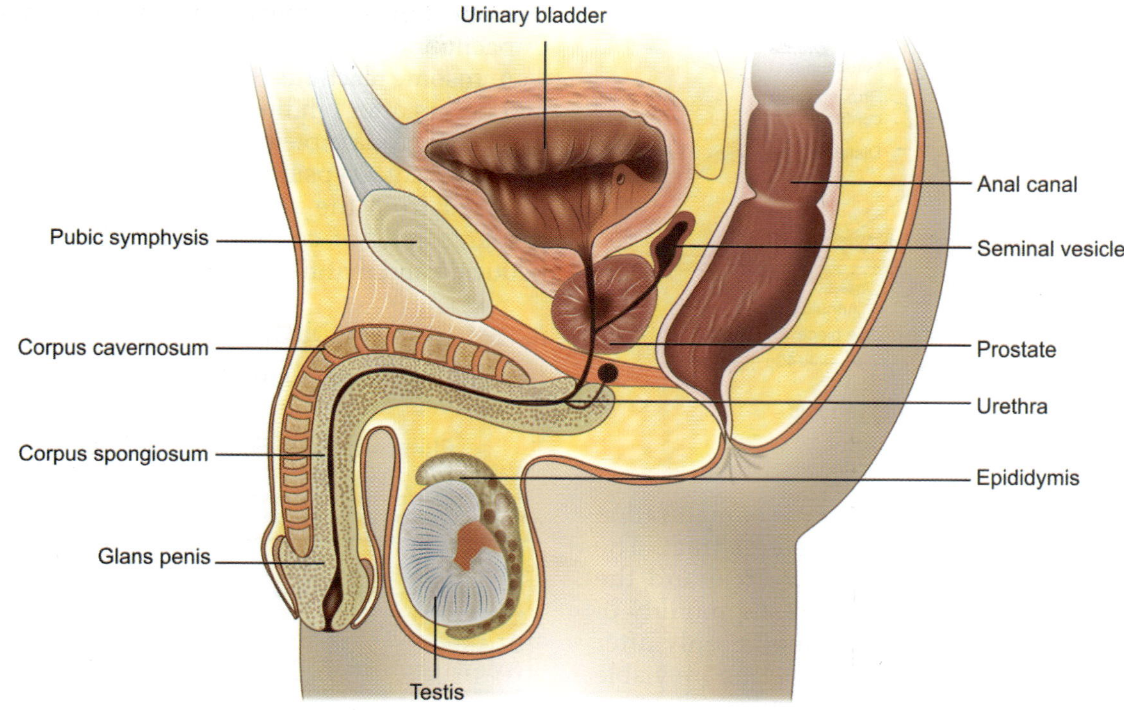

Fig. 44.2: Male reproductive system

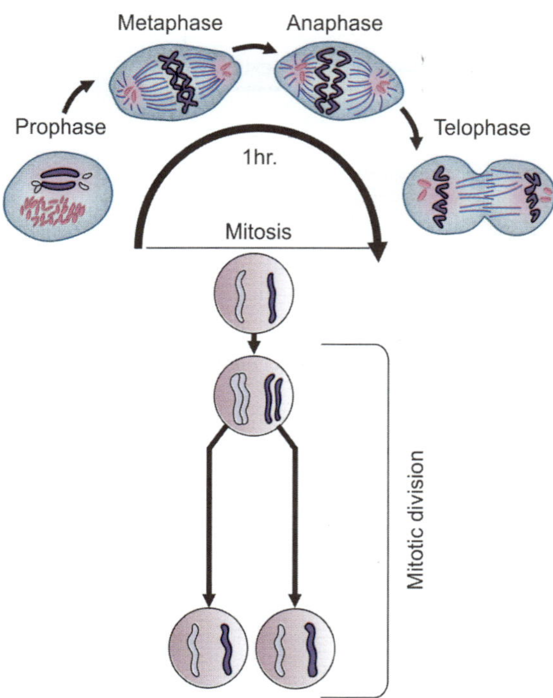

Fig. 44.3: Cell division

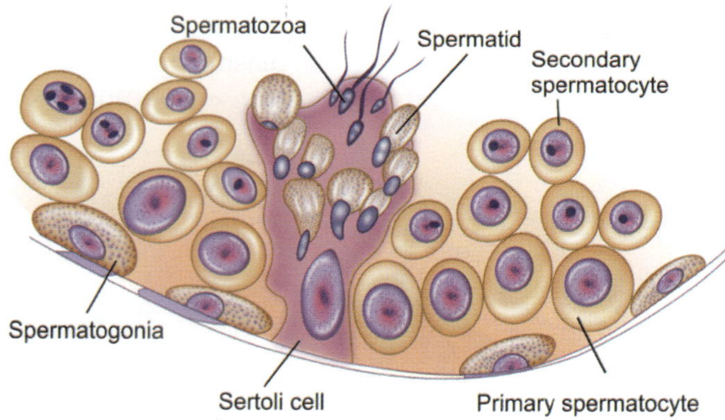

Fig. 44.4: Spermatogenesis

The spermatid is a small cell with a spherical nucleus, a Golgi complex, mitochondria and a centriole. The changes that take place in these during spermiogenesis are:

1 Appearance of deeply staining body, the acrosomic cap in the Golgi complex (Fig. 44.5).
2 Nucleus becomes denser, more ovoid and forms the head. This is capped by the acrosomic cap.
3 The centriole divides into two parts:
   a. One of the centrioles moves to the neck and gives rise to the axial filament.
   b. The other centriole moves distally and gets surrounded by a small ring, the annulus.
4 The axial filament between the head and the annulus is surrounded by mitochondria. This part of the spermatozoon is known as the middle piece.
5 The axial filament elongates and forms the principle piece or the tail.
6 The cytoplasm of the cell disintegrates and only the cell membrane remains as a covering of the spermatozoon.

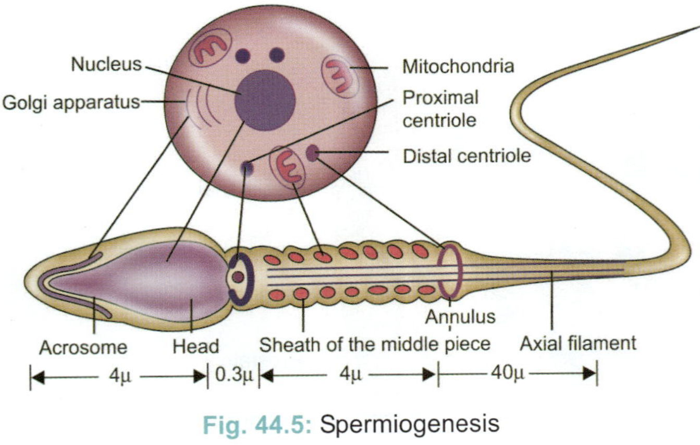

Fig. 44.5: Spermiogenesis

Maturation of Spermatozoon

The spermatozoon undergoes a process of maturation when it passes though the male genital tract. The secretions of epididymis, seminal vesicle and the prostate have an effect on maturation and motility of spermatozoa and it becomes fully motile only after ejaculation into female genital tract. Sperms are viable for 48–72 hours but their capacity to fertilize is limited to 24 hours.

Capacitation: In the female genital tract, the sperms undergo an activation process called capacitation. It consists of enzymatic changes that result in the removal of a glycoprotein coat and seminal plasma proteins from the plasma membrane over the acrosome. No morphological changes are seen in this process. Capacitation makes a sperm species specific.

Acrosome reaction: This reaction follows capacitation and occurs after binding to the zona pellucida. This is induced by zona proteins. During acrosome reaction, the enzymes, e.g. trypsin-like substances and acrosin are released from the acrosome. These are required to disperse cells of corona radiata, to penetrate zona pellucida and mature oocyte cell membrane.

II. FEMALE REPRODUCTIVE SYSTEM

Parts are shown in Flowchart 44.2 and Fig. 44.6.

Flowchart 44.2: Female reproductive organs

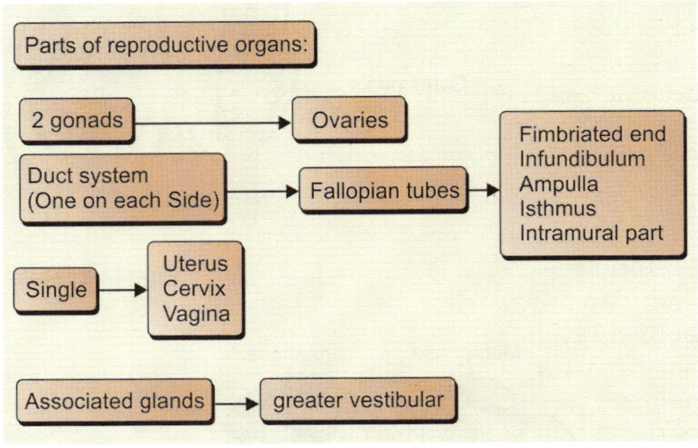

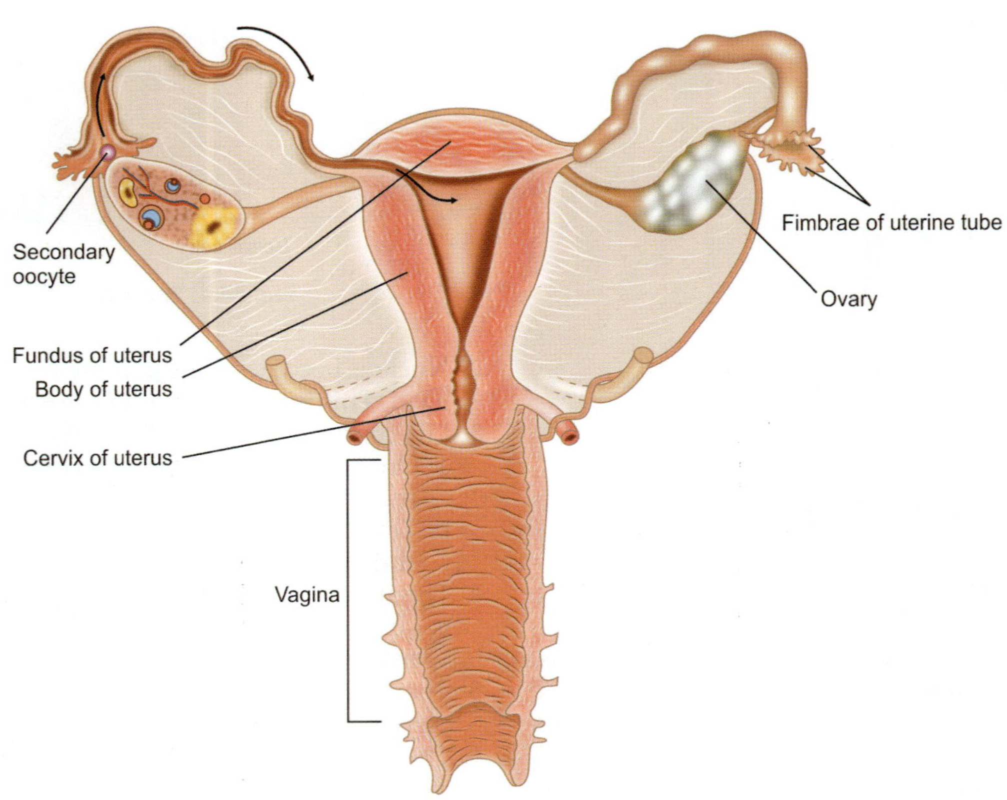

Fig. 44.6: Female reproductive system

Oogenesis

Oogenesis is the process by which the oocytes are produced in the ovaries. It involves pre- and postnatal development (Flowchart 44.3).

Primordial germ cells (endodermal) reach the gonad at the end of 4th week of intrauterine life and are known as **oogonia**. By the end of 3rd month of intrauterine life, after a number of mitotic divisions, these cells become arranged in clusters which are surrounded by a layer of flat epithelial cells derived from surface epithelium covering the ovary. These are called Primordial follicles (Fig. 44.7). The **oogonia** cells are now called **primary oocytes**. When primary oocyte gets bigger, the follicle is called primary follicle. Primary oocyte undergoes first meiotic division and becomes secondary oocyte. The follicle is now secondary follicle. One of the secondary follicles matures further to become Graafian follicle (Fig. 44.8).

Structure of Oocyte at Ovulation

When the **oocyte** is shed from the Graafian follicle of ovary after 12–30 years it is a **secondary oocyte** still undergoing division. It is surrounded by a thick acellular mucopolysaccharide layer known as **zona pellucida**. The follicular cells adherent to the liberated oocyte are called **corona radiata**. Between the cell membrane of the oocyte and the zona pellucida is the perivitelline space. The size of the oocyte is about 120 um in diameter. It is viable for a period of approximately 24 hours.

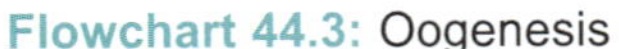

Flowchart 44.3: Oogenesis

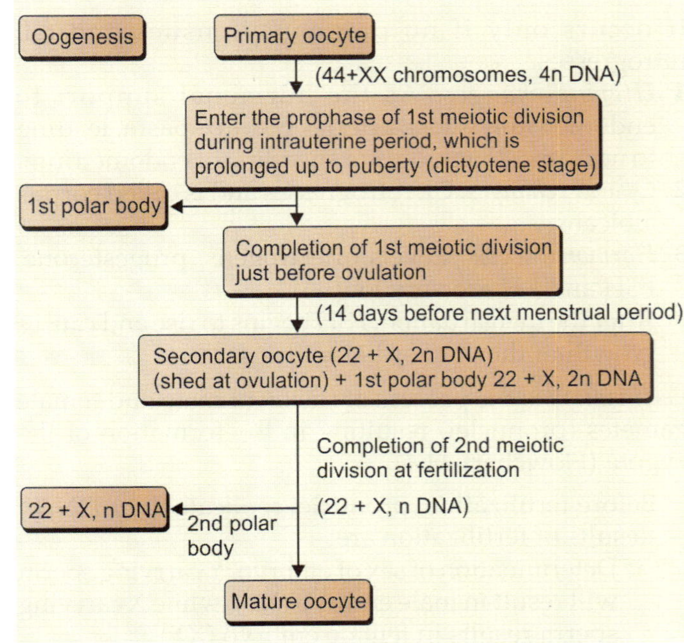

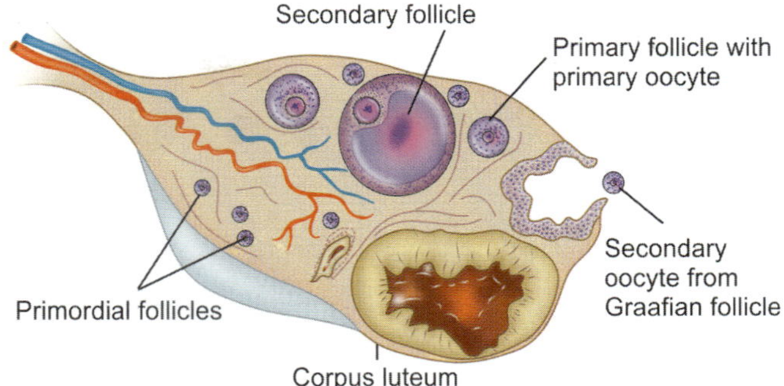

Fig. 44.7: Oocytes and follicles in the ovary

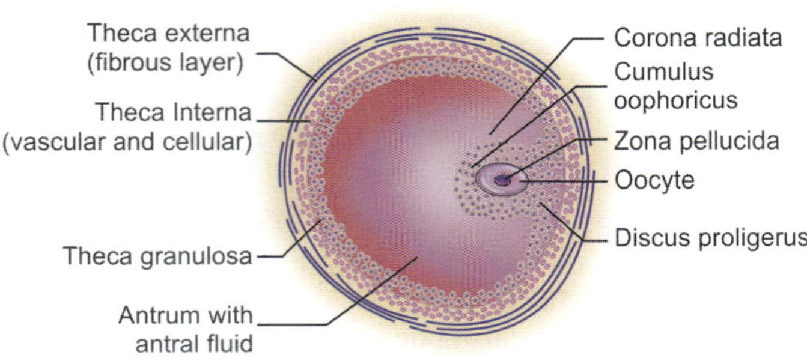

Fig. 44.8: Graafian follicle

Fertilization of mature oocyte by the spermatozoon results in the formation of the zygote.

CYCLICAL CHANGES IN FEMALE GENITAL TRACT

Cyclical changes occur in uterus and ovary, resulting in the menstrual cycles. On an average each cycle lasts for 28 days. It is divided into three phases:

1. Proliferative phase
2. Secretory phase
3. Menstrual phase

I. Proliferative Phase

It follows the menstrual phase during which part of the endometrium is shed off. This phase lasts from 5th to 14th day of the cycle.

1. *Uterine changes*
   Repair of endometrium and glands. (*i*) proliferation of epithelial cells, (*ii*) increase in stroma, (*iii*) increase in length of the glands.
   This is also called estrogenic/preovulatory/follicular phase (Fig. 44.9).
2. *Ovarian changes*
   Many secondary follicles grow in the beginning of the cycle. Approximately on day 6, one follicle grows faster and matures into a Graafian follicle. The cells of the follicle secrete estrogens.

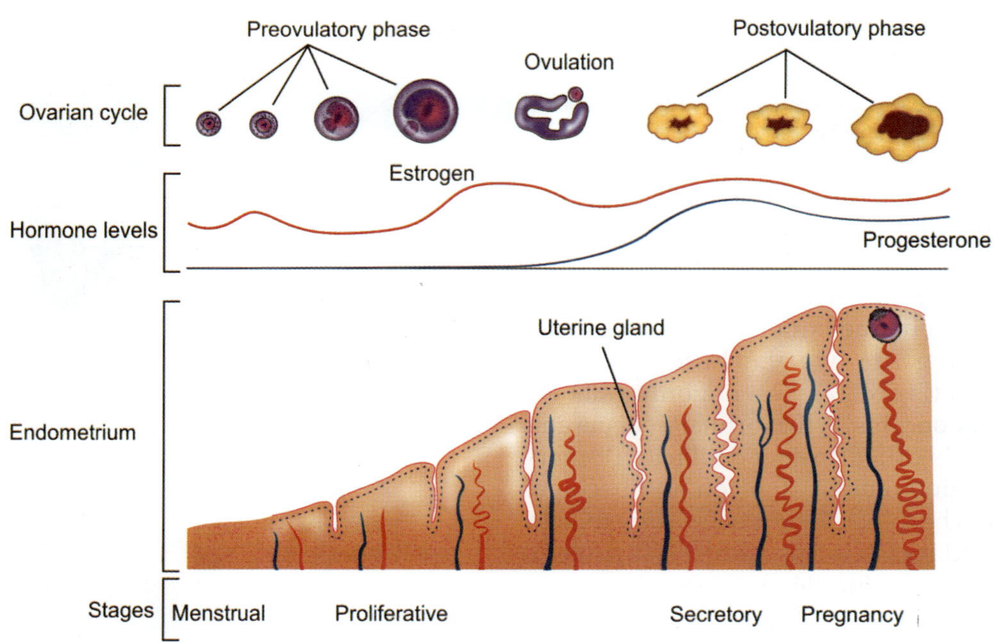

Fig. 44.9: Cyclical changes in ovary and uterus with the hormone levels

3 *Hormonal control*

i. Follicle-stimulating hormone (FSH) from anterior pituitary is responsible for the growth of the ovarian follicles and transformation of one of the follicles into Graafian follicle.
ii. Amount of estrogens secreted by the follicle rises and is responsible for the proliferative changes in the uterine endometrium.
iii. Estrogens reach a peak level amount on 14th day of the cycle and this level is maintained for some time.
iv. Peak level of estrogens affect the secretion of Luteinizing hormone (LH) positively. LH is secreted in large amounts: this is called LH surge. This surge is responsible for ovulation with discharge of secondary oocyte from the ovary and converting the Graafian follicle into corpus luteum (CL).
v. Corpus luteum secretes large amounts of progesterone and small amounts of estrogens. The secretary phase of the endometrium develops under the effect of progesterone.

II. Secretory Phase

1 *Uterine changes:* The endometrium starts secreting a fluid, so this phase receives the name of secretory phase. Lasts from 15th to 28th day:

i. Endometrial glands get dilated and tortuous.
ii. Endometrial arteries get coiled and are called spiral arteries.
iii. Epithelial cells acquire lot of glycogen.

2 *Ovarian changes:*

i. Corpus luteum (CL) grows and secretes progesterone and estrogens.
ii. Corpus luteum continues as CL of pregnancy if it ensues. If no pregnancy occurs, CL retrogresses after 20th day and is known as CL of menstruation.

3 Hormonal changes:

i. Progesterone and estrogens rise and then decline if no pregnancy occurs but remain high in case of pregnancy.
ii. FSH and LH hormones decline in amount.

III. Menstrual Phase

It occurs only if no pregnancy ensues and CL retrogresses.

1 *Uterine changes:* As the hormonal support to endometrium is lost, arteries go into spasm, leading to necrosis, sloughing and shedding of endometrium.

2 *Ovarian changes:* CL retrogresses and is called corpus albicans.

3 *Hormonal levels:* Levels of estrogens, progesterone, FSH and LH are very low.
After the menstruation, FSH begins to rise and causes growth of the primordial follicles.

Fertilization is the process of fusion of male and female gametes (pronuclei) resulting in the formation of the zygote (Flowchart 44.4).

Before fertilization, pronuclei replicate their DNA. Results of fertilization are:

i. Determination of sex of embryo. Y carrying sperm will result in male embryo (XY), while X carrying sperm results in female embryo (XX).

Flowchart 44.4: Fertilization

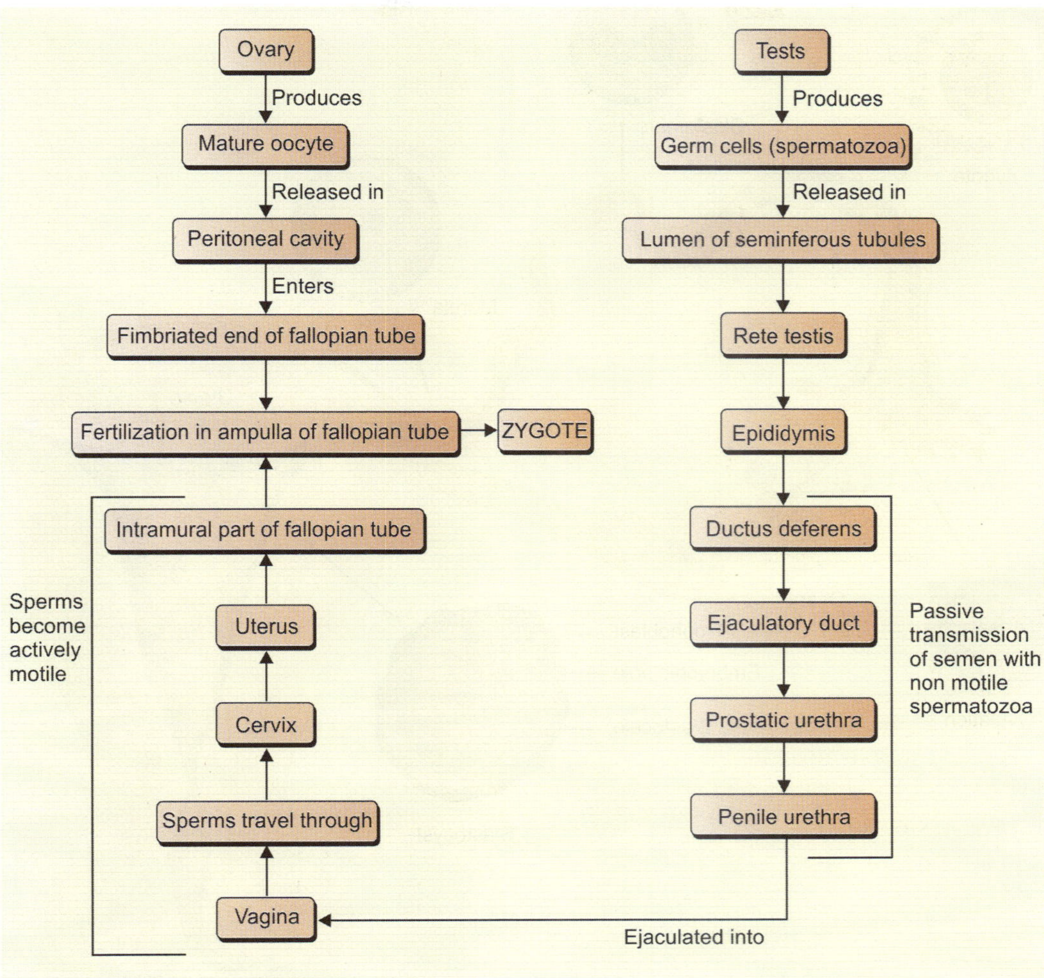

ii. Restoration of diploid number of chromosomes, half from mother and half from father with a new combination (Fig. 44.10).
iii. Beginning of cleavage: Immediately after fertilization the zygote starts the mitotic division. Just prior to mitotic division each gamete duplicates its DNA content.

Just after fertilization the process of cleavage starts. Zygote divides into two cells, which go on multiplying till stage of 16 cells is reached. This is known as **morula.** Zona pellucida is intact so that the cell size does not increase and ectopic pregnancy in fallopian tube does not occur. It slowly reaches the uterine cavity on 3rd or 4th day of fertilization. Some of the central cells of morula degenerate to form a cavity called the blastocele. This stage is known as **Blastocyst.** At this stage zona pellucida fully dissolves allowing the blastocyst to implant into the uterine endometrium (Fig. 44.10).

Blastocyst: It is the stage due to formation of blastocele. Number of cells collect at one pole of the blastocyst. This is called as **Inner cell mass.** The remaining cells around the inner cell mass and blastocyst are called the **outer cell mass**. The inner cell mass forms the embryo and the outer cell mass forms the trophoblast. The pole of the blastocyst with inner cell mass is known as **Embryonic Pole,** and the opposite pole is called as **Abembryonic Pole.**

By 7th day the blastocyst is partially embedded in the endometrium.

Bilaminar disc: The cells of inner cell mass differentiate themselves into (a) columnar cell forming epiblast and (b) cuboidal cells forming hypoblast. These two layers form the flattened circular bilaminar embryonic disc. The epiblast cells partially surround the amniotic cavity. Similarly hypoblast cells partially surround the primitive yolk sac (Fig. 44.11a).

Extraembryonic mesoderm: Appears between outer trophoblast and inner amniotic cavity and yolk sac. Clefts appear in this mesoderm to form two layers – outer somatopleuric mesoderm and inner splanchnopleuric mesoderm and extraembryonic coelom in between the two by the second week (Fig. 44.11b).

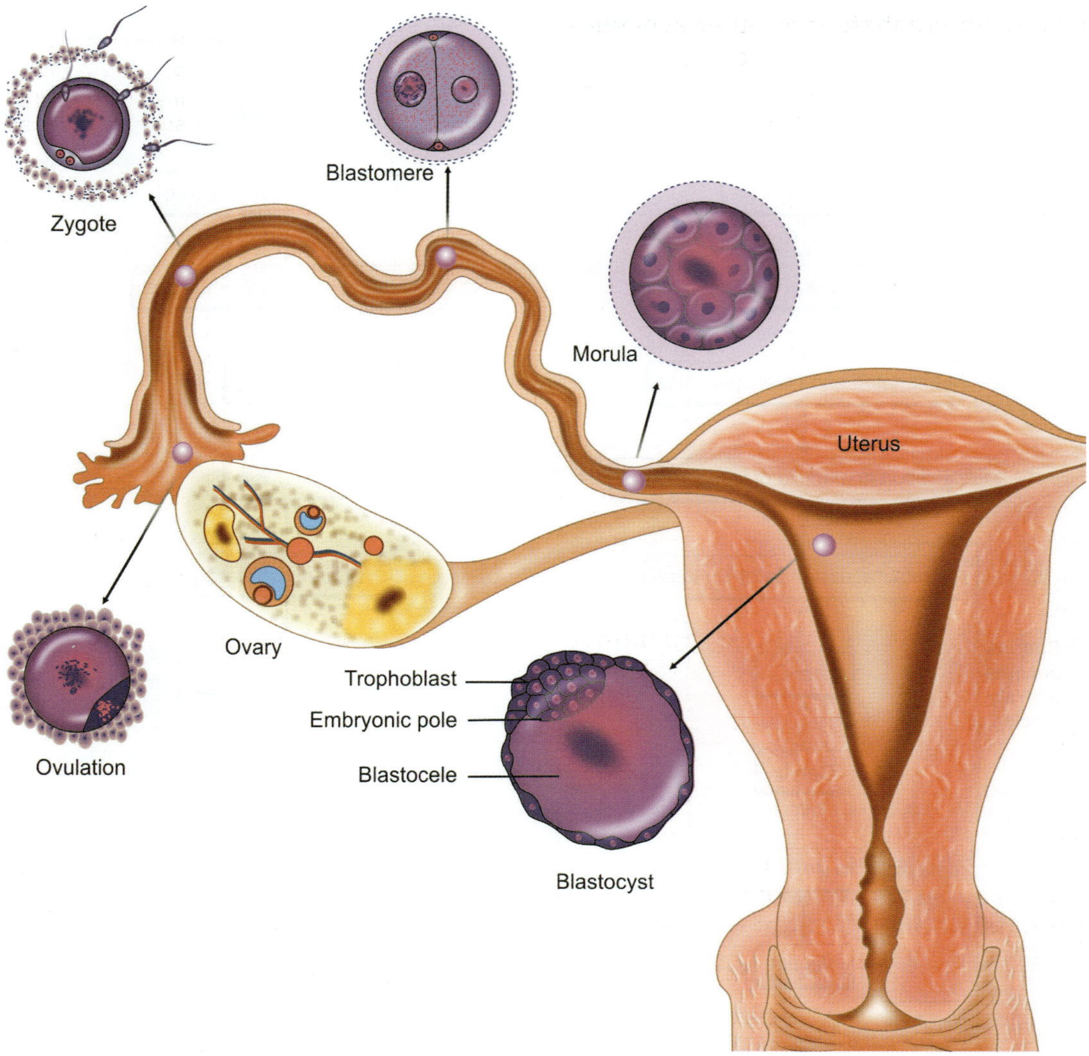

Fig. 44.10: Fertilization to blastocyst formation

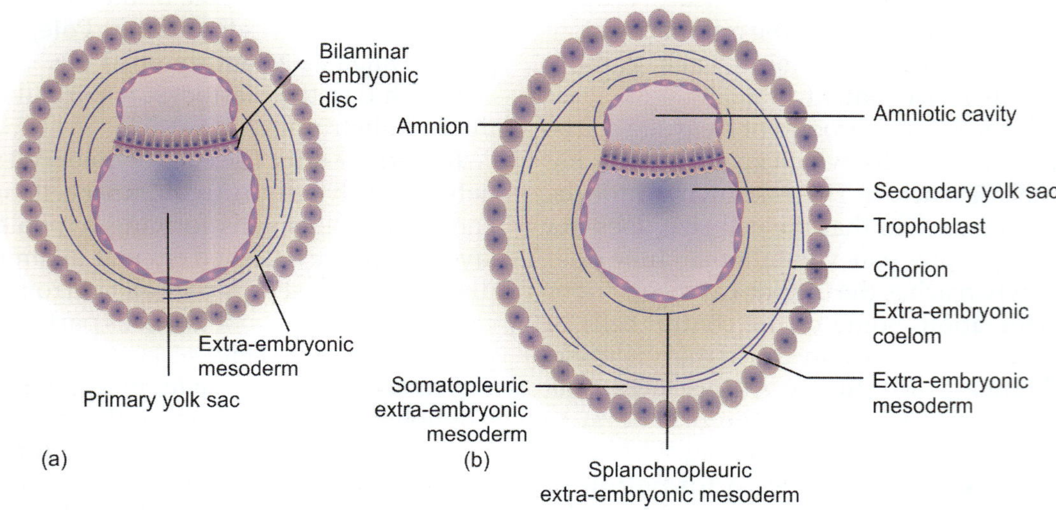

Figs 44.11a and b: (a) Formation of bilaminar disc, (b) formation of extra-embryonic mesoderm

The trophoblast differentiate into outer syncytiotrophoblast and an inner cytotrophoblast. The outer layer erodes into the endometrium while the inner layer is the multiplying layer. This results in implantation of blastocyst in the uterus. During this week lacunae develop in syncytiotrophoblast. These lacunae get continuous with maternal sinusoids eroded by this layer. These two layers form villi around the blastocyst. These are the **Primary Chorionic Villi.**

Trilaminar Disc: The third week of development is characterized by the appearance of a proliferative zone, the **primitive streak**, at the caudal end of the now slipper-shaped embryonic disc. It is capped by the **primitive node** with a pit. From the primitive node, epiblast cells invaginate to form **notochord** (Fig. 44.12). The intraembryonic mesoderm is formed by cells from primitive streak migrating laterally between ectoderm and endoderm. These cells spread all over except at two areas—prochordal plate (buccopharyngeal membrane) and cloacal membrane. By this process trilaminar embryonic disc is formed which is pear shaped (Figs 44.12b and c).

Prenotochordal cells invaginate through the primitive pit and move forwards till the bucco-pharyngeal membrane. Though this notochordal process initially fuses with the endoderm, it soon detaches itself to form the notochord. It forms the central axis of the embryonic disc and gives it a bilateral symmetry. Notochord inducts the overlying ectoderm to form neural plate which is modified to form neural tube and neural crest.

Mesoderm divides into 3 parts:

1 *Paraxial* forming somites from occipital to sacral regions–Each somite shows two parts: dermomyotome and sclerotome (Figs 44.13a and b).
2 *Intermediate cell mass* forms most of the genitourinary system

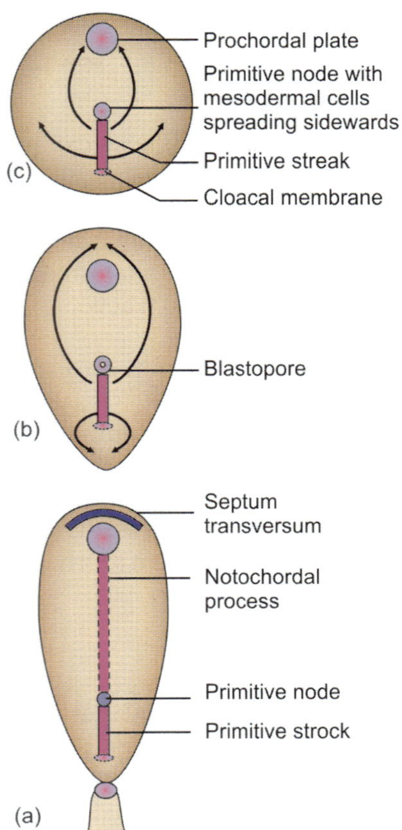

Figs 44.12a to c: Stages in formation of intra-embryonic mesoderm

3 *Lateral plate forms:*
- Body wall
- Body cavities.

Derivatives of Neural Crest

Adrenal medulla, sympathetic ganglia, dorsal root ganglia, sensory ganglia of V, VII, VIII, IX, X cranial nerves; 4 parasympathetic ganglia; pia and arachnoid

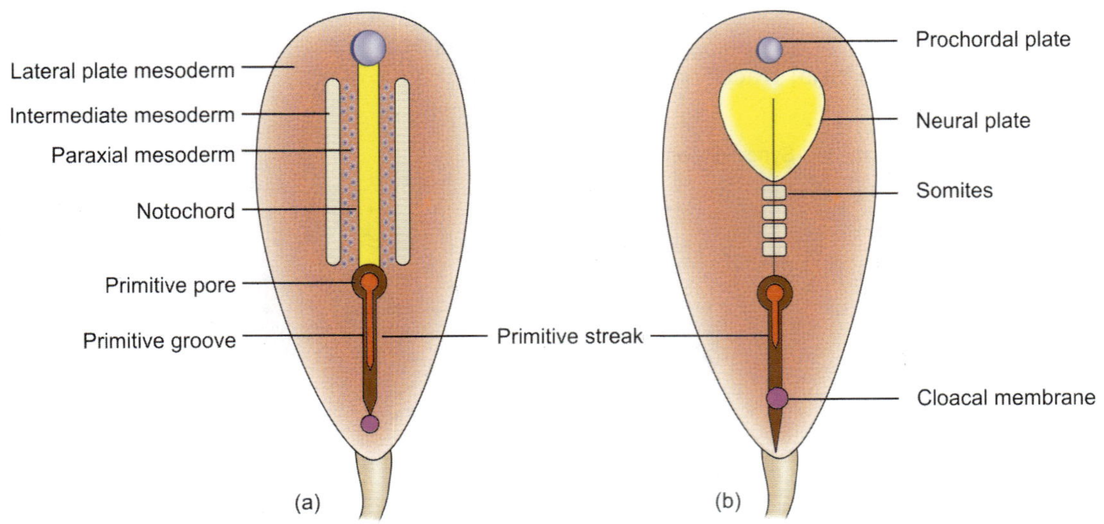

Figs 44.13a and b: (a) Subdivisions of intra-embryonic mesoderm (b) formation of neural plate and somites

maters, mesenchyme of head region, part of face and heart development, etc.

Derivatives of Ectoderm

1 Epidermis of skin, hair, nails, sweat and sebaceous glands and mammary gland.
2 Epithelium of lips, cheeks, gums, floor of mouth and palate, nasal cavities and paranasal sinuses.
3 Epithelium of lower part of anal canal and terminal parts of urinary and genital tracts.
4 Enamel of teeth.
5 Rathke's pouch which gives rise to anterior part of pituitary.
6 The lens of the eye, anterior epithelium of cornea, outer layer of tympanic membrane.
7 The central nervous system including the retina, the optic nerve, epithelium over the ciliary body and iris.
8 The peripheral nervous system (derivatives of neural crest).
9 The musculature of the iris.

Derivatives of Mesoderm

1 The connective tissues, cartilages and bones.
2 Dentine of teeth.
3 Visceral musculature including cardiac muscle and musculature of blood vessels.
4 The lymph nodes, lymph vessels and spleen.
5 Blood cells.
6 Connective tissue sheaths of muscles, tendons and nerve endings, synovial membranes of joints and bursae.
7 Dermis of skin.
8 Somatic musculature.
9 Pachymeninx or duramater.
10 Urinary system except part of the urinary bladder.
11 Cortex of suprarenal gland.
12 Pericardium, pleura and peritoneum.
13 Parts of genital system.

Derivatives of Endoderm

1 Epithelium of the gastrointestinal tract (except the lower end of anal canal).
2 Parenchyma of liver, pancreas, thyroid, parathyroid and thymus.
3 Epithelium of pharyngotympanic tube, middle ear cavity, inner layer of tympanic membrane and lining of mastoid air cells.
4 The lining epithelium of pharynx, tongue, larynx, trachea, bronchi and alveoli of lungs.
5 Epithelium of urinary bladder.
6 Epithelium of most of the female urethra, part of male urethra, prostate and vagina.
7 Primordial germ cells.

FETAL MEMBRANES AND PLACENTA

All structures not forming any part of the embryo and yet derived from the zygote constitute fetal membranes. These are:
1 Chorion
2 Placenta (Flowchart 44.5)
3 Yolk sac
4 Allantois
5 Amnion
6 Umbilical cord

Chorion: This is formed by fusion of extraembryonic somatopleuric mesoderm and trophoblasts. This shows villi like projections on the surface of blastula. The villi are of three types: *(a) primary villi* consisting of syncytio and cytotrophoblast, *(b) secondary villi* with the mesoderm core (Fig. 44.14), *(c)* the mesodermal core gets invaded by fetal capillaries and thereby the secondary villi become tertiary. In early weeks of development, the villi cover the entire surface of the chorion but later, the villi on the embryonic pole continue to grow and form chorion frondosum whereas those on the abembryonic pole degenerate and form chorion laeve or smooth chorion (Flowchart 44.5).

Morphology of Placenta

Placenta at term:
Gross appearance:

Shape	:	Discoid (flat and circular disc)
Diameter	:	Approx. 20 cm

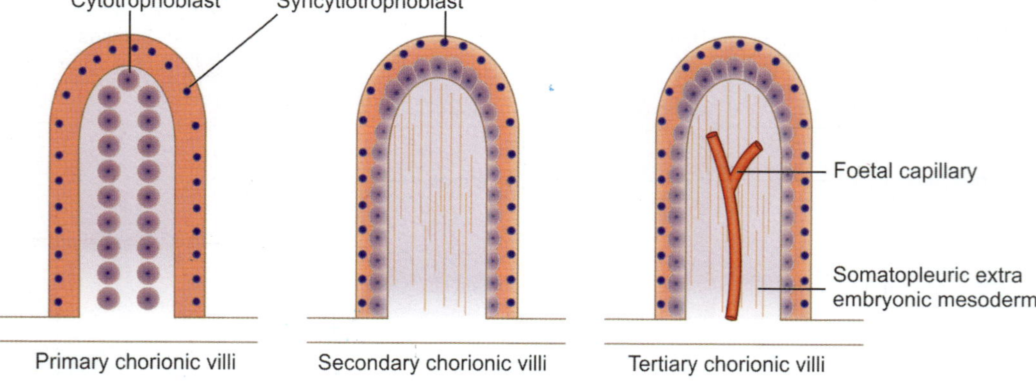

Fig. 44.14: Formation of various types of chorionic villi

Flowchart 44.5: Formation of placenta

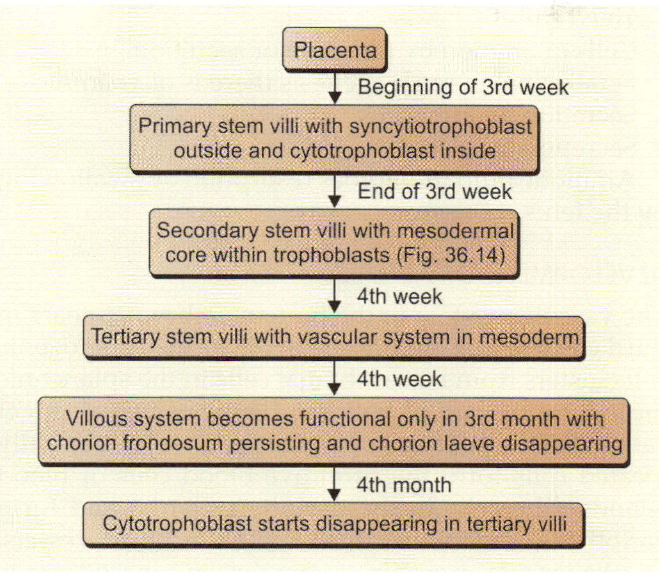

Thickness	:	2.5 cm
Weight	:	500 grams
Surfaces	:	2 surfaces, maternal and fetal

Fetal surface: This is smooth and covered with amnion. Umbilical cord is attached eccentrically on this surface. Umbilical vessels ramify under amnion.

Maternal surface: Rough and raw. It is divided into 15–20 cotyledons by decidual septa.

Type: Haemochorial

Microscopic structure at term: This shows cut sections of villi lying free in maternal blood. These sections, from without inwards, consist of:

1 Thinned out syncytiotrophoblast
2 Cytotrophoblast almost absent
3 Fused basement membranes of trophoblast and endothelium of fetal capillaries.
4 Thin core of mesoderm

Functions of Placenta

Placenta attaches the fetus to the mother and acting as membrane between maternal and fetal blood subserves the following functions for the fetus:

1 *Respiratory:* Functions as lungs and allows for free exchange of O_2 and CO_2.
2 *Nutritive:* Functions as gastrointestinal tract, absorbing products of carbohydrates, fats and proteins from maternal blood.
3 *Excretory:* Functions as kidney, excreting nitrogenous waste, plasma bilirubin, etc. into maternal blood.
4 *Dialysing membrane:* For exchange of water and electrolytes.
5 *Regulatory on metabolism:* (i) Converting glucose into glycogen and carbohydrates into fats. (ii) Concentrating iron selectively in fetal blood.
6 *Secretory:* Functions as an endocrine gland; secretes estrogen, progesterone, chorionic gonadotrophin and chorionic lactogen in the maternal blood. Levels of the human chorionic gonadotrophin hormone are used for pregnancy test.
7 Selectively absorbs maternal hormones like estrogen, progesterone, thyroxine, insulin and androgens administrated to mother.
8 Actively transport vitamins into fetus and also stores them.
9 Actively transports selective macromolecules like gamma globulin and lymphocytes from mother, conferring immunity against some diseases.
10 Though acts as a barrier to many bacteria and organisms, some of these or their toxins do manage to cross the barrier and cause fetal defects, e.g. rubella, syphilis, etc.

Yolk Sac

1 Initially transfers nutritive material from uterus through trophoblast and extraembryonic mesoderm and coelom to the developing embryo (Fig. 44.11).
2 Later dorsal part of it becomes incorporated in the embryo to form gut and allantoic diverticulum.
3 Vestigeal remnant (i.e. ventral part) is connected to mid-gut by vitello intestinal duct.
4 Vitelline vessels supplying yolk sac are later modified as coeliac axis, superior and inferior mesenteric vessels.

Umbilical Cord

1 Life line connecting fetus to mother through placenta.
2 Contents:
   a. Wharton's jelly
   b. Two umbilical arteries, right and left
   c. Left umbilical vein (Fig. 44.15)
   d. Remnant of yolk sac
   e. Remnant of allanto-enteric diverticulum.
3 Covered by amniotic membrane.
4 Length: 50–55 cm.
5 Attached eccentrically on the placenta.

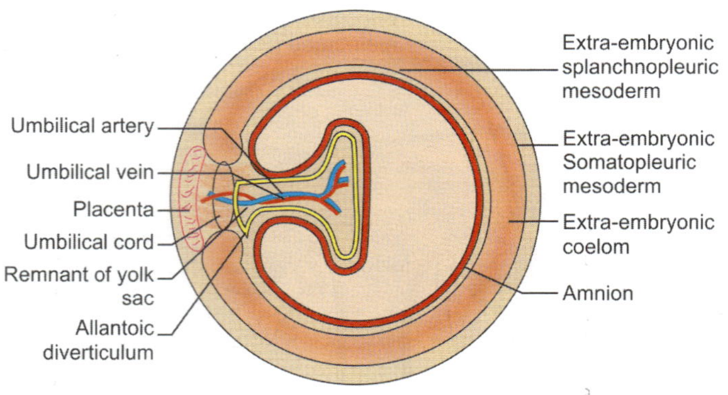

Fig. 44.15: Umbilical cord and allantoic diverticulum

Allantois

1 Diverticulum from caudal end of yolk sac.
2 Vascularised by allantoic vessels which later become umbilical vessels and get connected with placenta (Figs 44.16a and b).
3 Allantois gets incorporated into the apex of urinary bladder – urachus and the rest is fibrosed and forms median umbilical ligament.
4 Initially functions as dialyzing membrane.
5 May persist as urachal cyst, sinus or fistula.

Amnion

1 Derived from splitting up of ectodermal surface of inner cell mass from overlying trophoblast (7–12 days).
2 Completely surrounds the embryo and encloses a cavity filled with amniotic fluid (6 weeks).
3 Provides a watery cushion to absorb shock and protect the developing embryo and fetus. Promotes (a) symmetrical development (b) maintains constant temperature.
4 Metabolites and hormones (HCG, HPL) are excreted into it.
5 Allows for exchange of materials.
6 Helps dilate cervix at the beginning of labour.
7 Normal amount of fluid 1000 ml
Oligoamnios 400 ml or less
Polyhydramnios 2000 ml or more

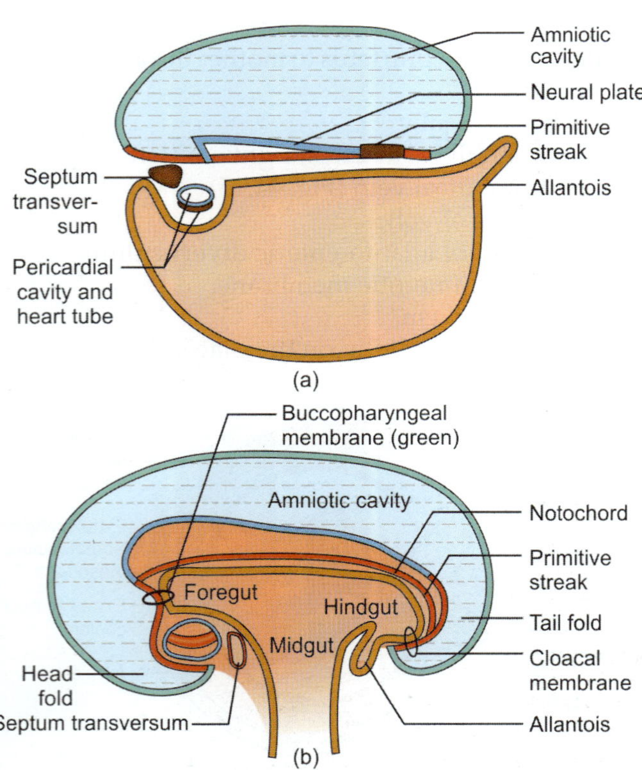

Figs 44.16a and b: Allantois: (a) Early stage, (b) later stage

Amniotic Fluid

Derived from
1 Cells of amnion by filtration or secretion.
2 Fetal urine. In renal agenesis there is oligoamnios.
3 Secretion by lung cells.
4 Secretion by placenta.

Amniotic fluid undergoes resorption by swallowing by the fetus.

DEVELOPMENT OF ARTERIES

The vascular system in the human embryo appears in third week of intrauterine life in the form of angiogenic cell clusters from mesenchymal cells in the splanchnic mesoderm of wall of yolk sac. These cell clusters get canalized by fusion of intercellular clefts. The centrally located cells form the primitive blood cells or blood islands. The cells in the periphery flatten and form endothelial cells which fuse and form blood vessels. Similar vessels appear in extraembryonic mesoderm as well as connecting stalk and thus a contact is established between the embryo and the placenta.

From the plexiform network to developing blood vessels following vessels are initially formed.

1 ***Extraembryonic***
  a. On yolk sac—vitelline vessels
  b. In allantois and chorion—umbilical vessels
2 ***Intraembryonic***
  a. 2 ventral aortae
  b. 2 dorsal aortae
  c. 2 heart tubes

Development of Intraembryonic Arteries

1 *Arch arteries:* The fused endocardial heart tubes form the ventral aorta which in turn forms the aortic sac. The aortic sac gets partitioned by a spiral septum into a dorsal part (pulmonary trunk) and ventral part, the aorta. This ventral part shows two horns—right and left—which are connected to the two dorsal aortae (right and left) by 6 pairs of arch arteries. The dorsal aortae fuse in their lower parts to form a single dorsal aorta (Fig. 44.17).

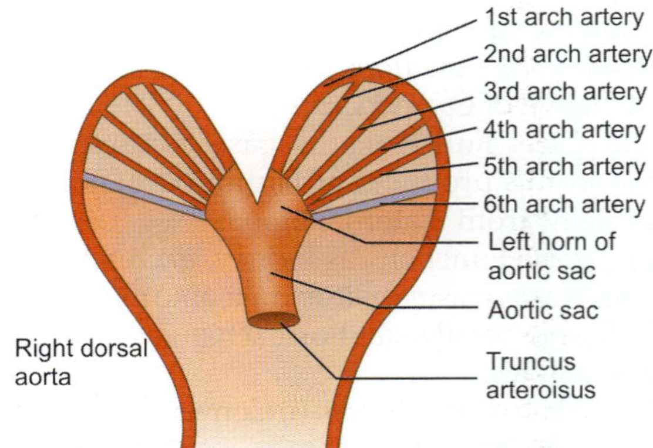

Fig. 44.17: Formation of aortic arches

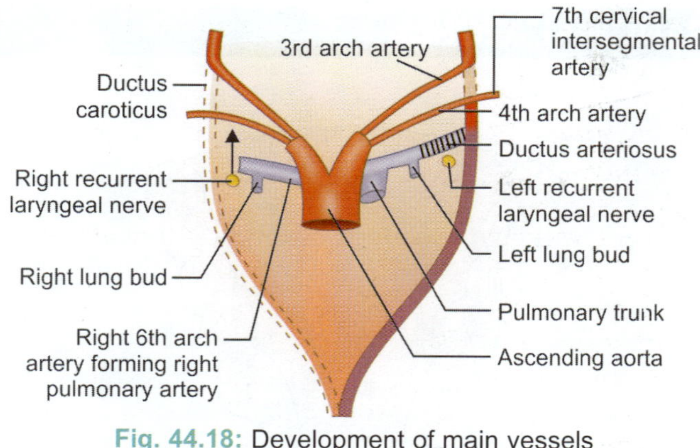

Fig. 44.18: Development of main vessels

Note: Neural crest cells get intermingled in the spiral septum. These cells are also incorporated in the processes forming the face. Thus abnormalities of face and heart appear simultaneously.

The final fate of arch arteries is depicted in Table 44.1 and Fig. 44.18.

Table 44.1: Fate of arch arteries

Arch artery	*Side*	*Part*	*Derivative*
I	Right and left	–	Major part disappears. Small part forms the maxillary artery.
II	Right and left	–	Major part disappears. Small part forms the stapedial artery.
III	Right and left	Proximal part	Common carotid artery
		Distal part	Internal carotid artery
		New sprout	External carotid artery
IV	Right	Entire	Right subclavian artery
	Left	Entire	Distal part of arch of aorta
V	Right and Left	Entirely	Disappear
VI	Right	Proximal part	Right pulmonary artery
		Distal part	Disappear
	Left	Proximal part	Left pulmonary artery
		Distal	Ductus arteriosus in the fetus and ligamentum arteriosum after birth.
Horns of aortic sac	Right	–	Brachiocephalic trunk
	Left	–	Proximal part of arch of aorta.
Blood vessels			**Development Components**
Ascending aorta			Truncus arteriosus
Arch of aorta (Fig. 44.18)			1. Ventral part of aortic sac and its left horn 2. Left 4th arch artery 3. Left dorsal aorta up to the 7th cervical intersegmental artery.
Descending aorta			1. Left dorsal aorta beyond 7th cervical intersegmental artery. 2. Fused dorsal aortae
Brachiocephalic artery			Right horn of aortic sac in which right 3rd and 4th arch arteries are opening.
Common carotid			Proximal half of 3rd arch artery.
Internal carotid artery			Distal half of 3rd arch artery and cranial parts of dorsal aorta.
External carotid artery			New off shoot from 3rd arch.
Subclavian artery	Right		1. Proximal part of right 4th arch artery 2. Part of right dorsal aorta 3. Distal part of right 7th cervical intersegmental artery.
	Left		Left 7th cervical intersegmental artery.

THE PHARYNGEAL OR BRANCHIAL ARCHES

INTRODUCTION

With the formation of head fold, the developing pericardial cavity lies on the ventral aspect of the embryo and developing forebrain forms a bulging above it on the ventral aspect. These two are separated by *stomatodaeum* (Fig. 44.19).

Stomatodeum is the future mouth. At this stage of embryonic period, the foregut is closed by buccopharyngeal membrane which is formed by ectoderm and endoderm without any intervening mesoderm.

The *buccopharyngeal membrane* ruptures by 3rd week of gestation and communicates with proximal part of foregut. The region between stomatodaeum and pericardial cavity elongates with descent of heart in the thoracic cavity forming the future neck.

The cranial most part of foregut forms the pharynx. This part shows mesodermal thickenings on the dorso-ventral side, covered outside by ectoderm and on the inner aspect lined by endoderm. This mesoderm gets arranged in six bars and grows ventrally in the floor of developing pharynx and fuses with the corresponding bar of the opposite side to form the pharyngeal arches (Fig. 44.20).

Initially, the arches consist of mesodermal tissue separated by deep clefts, in which ectoderm dips. These clefts are called *ectodermal clefts* or *pharyngeal clefts*. Simultaneously with the development of arches and clefts there are outpocketings in the form of pouches – *endodermal* or *pharyngeal pouches* to meet the ectoderm in pharyngeal cleft (Fig. 44.21).

Components of Each Arch

i. *Muscle (branchial):* Each branchial or pharyngeal arch is characterized by its own muscle component. The muscular component carries its nerve, spinal or cranial.

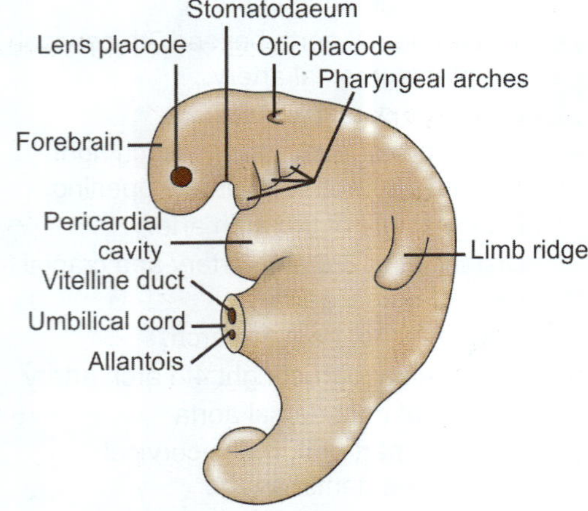

Fig. 44.19: Formation of the pharyngeal arches

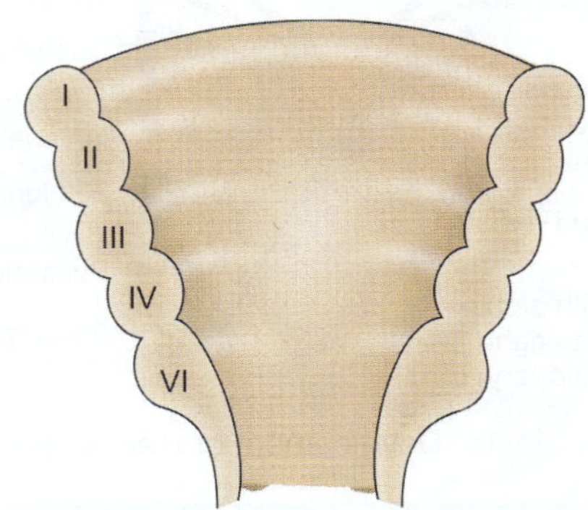

Fig. 44.20: I to VI pharyngeal arches, V arch has disappeared

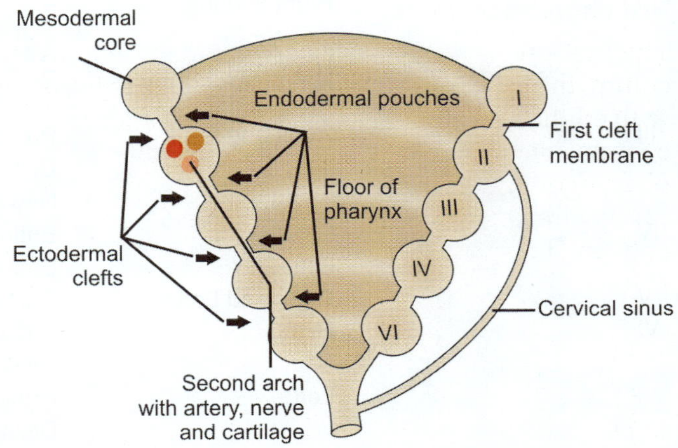

Fig. 44.21: Components of each pharyngeal arches

ii. *Skeletal element:* It may form cartilage to begin with, may develop into bone or may disappear (Fig. 44.21).

iii. *Nerve:* The formation of pharyngeal arches, clefts and pouches resemble formation of gills in fishes and amphibian; in the human embryo, real gills are never formed. In these animals, each arch is supplied by two nerves. The nerve which runs along the cranial border of arch is called post-tremetic nerve. Each arch also receives a branch from the nerve of next arch which runs along the caudal border of arch above it and is called pretremetic nerve. In the embryo of the human beings, *double nerve supply* of this type is seen only in the *first pharyngeal arch*.

iv. *Artery:* Each pharyngeal arch has its own artery arising from arterial arch which is formed by the arch between the branches of ventral and dorsal aortae in the embryo which becomes modified when the circulatory changes of the fetus takes place at birth. Mesodermal derivatives of Pharyngeal Arches are mentioned in Table 44.2.

Since the 5th arch disappears, early in embryonic stage, there are 5 arches left (Fig. 44.20).

Bones of face: Maxilla, mandible, zygomatic, palatine and part of temporal bone develop from 1st arch.

Some recent investigations suggest that mesenchyme giving rise to muscles of pharyngeal arches is derived from paraxial mesoderm, cranial to the occipital somites or preoccipital somites and its organization is influenced by neural crest cells.

PHARYNGEAL POUCHES

The epithelial endodermal lining of pouches gives rise to a number of important structures as listed below.

First Pharyngeal Pouch

The first pharyngeal pouch forms a stalk like diverticulum, the tubo-tympanic recess, that comes in contact with epithelial lining of first pharyngeal cleft, the future external auditory meatus. The proximal part forms the pharyngotympanic tube and distal part forms tympanic cavity, lining of tympanic membrane and mastoid antrum (Table 44.3).

Second Pharyngeal Pouch

Dorsal part of this pouch takes part in formation of tubo-tympanic recess. The ventral part of second pharyngeal pouch forms palatine tonsil. The epithelial lining of pouch proliferates and forms buds that penetrates the surrounding mesenchyme. During the 3rd and 5th months of fetal life it is infiltrated by lymphatic tissue. Part of the pouch remains and is found in the adult as tonsillar fossa.

Third Pharyngeal Pouch

In the 5th week of embryo, the epithelium of dorsal wing of the 3rd pouch differentiates into inferior parathyroid gland and ventral wing forms thymus.

Thymus: Both inferior parathyroid and thymus gland primordial lose their connection with pharyngeal wall. The thymus migrates in caudal and medial direction pulling the inferior parathyroid with it which finally rests on the posterior surface of thyroid gland. The main portion of thymus moves rapidly to its position in thorax, where it fuses with its counterpart of opposite side (Fig. 44.22).

Growth and development of thymus continue after birth until puberty. It lies behind sternum and anterior to pericardium and the vessels there.

Table 44.2: Mesodermal derivatives of pharyngeal/branchial arches

Arch	*Skeletal elements*	*Muscles*	*Nerve and artery*
I Arch			
(a) Maxillary swelling (palatopterygoquadrate cartilage) (b) Mandibular swelling (Meckel's cartilage)	Premaxilla, maxilla, zygomatic bone, part of temporal bone Incus Malleus, anterior ligament of malleus and sphenomandibular ligament Meckel's cartilage. Most of the mandible	Muscles of mastication, i.e. temporalis, masseter, lateral and medial pterygoid, tensor veli palatini, tensor tympani, mylohyoid and anterior belly of digastric	Mandibular division of V nerve is post-trematic, chorda tympani is pretrematic; maxillary artery
Note: By intramembranous ossification of mesenchyme of I arch, maxilla, zygomatic, squamous part of temporal are developed.			
II Arch Reichert's cartilage	Stapes, styloid process, stylohyoid ligament, lesser cornua and upper half of body of hyoid	Muscles of facial expression and occipitofrontalis, auricular muscles, platysma, stylohyoid and posterior belly of digastric	Facial nerve (VII) is post-trematic
III Arch	Greater cornua of hyoid and lower half of hyoid bone	Stylopharyngeus	Glossopharyngeal nerve is (IX nerve) post-trematic; Internal carotid artery
IV Arch	Thyroid, arytenoid, cuneiform and corniculate cartilages	Cricothyroid, muscles of palate except tensor veli palatini constrictors of pharynx	Sup. laryngeal nerve; Arch of aorta Right subclavian artery
VI Arch	Cricoid cartilage	Intrinsic muscles of larynx except cricothyroid	Recurrent laryngeal nerve, pulmonary arteries

Table 44.3: Derivatives of endodermal pouches

Pharyngeal pouch	*Derivatives*
Dorsal ends of I and II pouches form — Tubotympanic recess	Proximal part of tubotympanic recess gives rise to auditory tube. Distal part gives rise to tympanic cavity and mastoid antrum. Mastoid cells develop at about 2 years of age
Ventral part of II pharyngeal pouch	Epithelium covering the palatine tonsil and tonsillar crypts, lymphoid tissue is mesodermal in origin
III Pharyngeal pouch	Thymus and inferior parathyroid gland or parathyroid III. Thymic epithelial reticular cells and Hassall's corpuscles are endodermal. Lymphocytes are derived from haemopoietic stem cells during 12th week
IV Pharyngeal pouch	Superior parathyroid or parathyroid IV
V Pharyngeal pouch (ultimobranchial body)	Parafollicular or 'C' cells of the thyroid gland

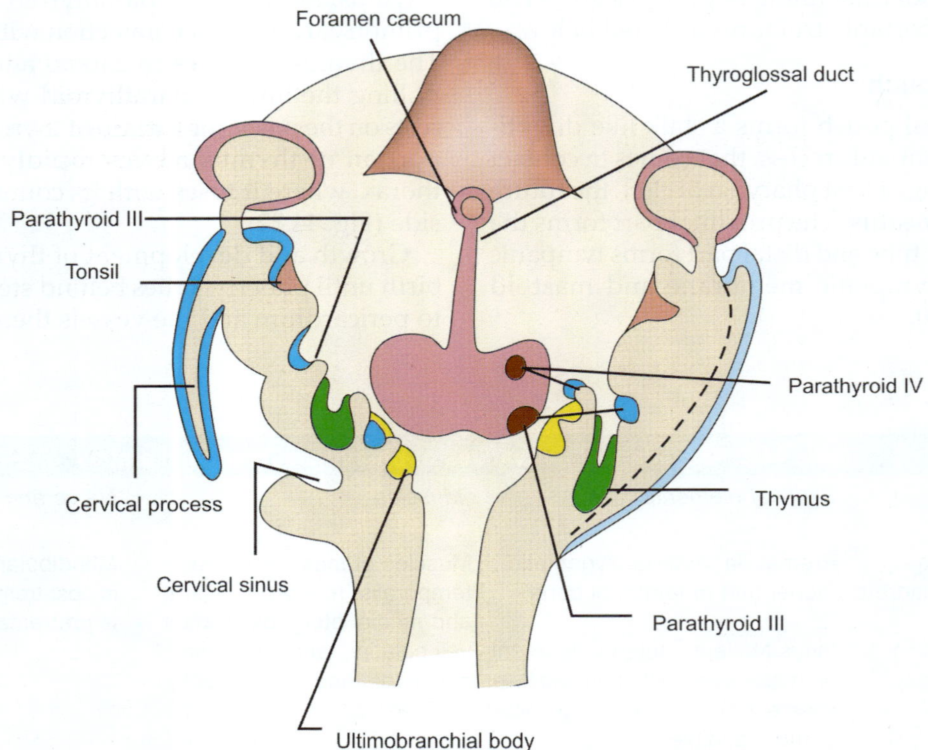

Fig. 44.22: Derivatives of various pharyngeal pouches, formation of cervical process and cervical sinus and development of thyroid and parathyroid glands

The endodermal cells of thymus are invaded by vascular mesoderm which contain numerous lymphoblasts. The mesoderm breaks thymic tissue into various masses giving it a lobulated appearance.

Soon after puberty, thymus atrophies and gets replaced by fatty tissue and it is difficult to identify it.

Fourth Pharyngeal Pouch

Epithelium of the dorsal wing of 4th pouch forms superior parathyroid gland. It migrates caudally and lies on the posterior surface of thyroid gland as superior parathyroid gland or parathyroid IV.

Fifth Pharyngeal Pouch

The fifth pouch is the last of the pharyngeal pouches to develop and is seen for a short period in the embryo. It gets incorporated in the 4th pouch. It forms ultimobranchial body in some species; which gives rise to Parafollicular or C′ cells of the thyroid gland. These cells secrete calcitonin, a hormone involved in calcium regulation in the blood.

It is believed that in human beings the fifth pouch gets incorporated into 4th pouch forming the caudal pharyngeal complex.

Table 44.4: Derivatives of ectodermal clefts	
Dorsal part of I ectodermal cleft	Epithelium of external auditory meatus and outer layer of tympanic membrane.
Auricle	Six auricular hillocks; three from I arch and three from II arch.
Rest of ectodermal clefts	Obliterated by the overgrowth of II pharyngeal arch over second and third pharyngeal clefts, it encloses space lined by ectoderm, called as cervical sinus. Overhanging second arch joins epicardial ridge, cervical sinus disappears.

ECTODERMAL CLEFTS

There are four pharyngeal clefts present in an embryo of about 5 weeks. Only one cleft contributes to the definitive structure of the embryo. The dorsal part of *first cleft* penetrates the underlying mesenchyme and gives rise to *external auditory meatus*. The ectodermal epithelium in addition to forming lining of meatus participates in the formation of tympanic membrane.

Pinna is formed from a number of swellings. These arise from first and second arches, where they adjoin the first cleft. The ventral part of this cleft is obliterated.

Active proliferation of the mesenchymal tissue in 2nd arch causes it to overlap 3rd, 4th and 6th arches. The space between overhanging 2nd arch and 3rd, 4th and 6th arches is called **cervical sinus** (Fig. 44.22). Finally the overhanging border of 2nd arch fuses with the tissues caudal to the arches, that is ectoderm overlying developing pericardium, thus obliterating ectodermal cleft and side of neck becomes smooth (Table 44.4).

Anomalies of Pharyngeal Pouches and Clefts

i. **Digeorge syndrome** or third and fourth pharyngeal pouch syndrome. Result from failure of development of third and fourth pouches. This syndrome is characterized by thymic hypoplasia which causes selective T cell deficiency and greatly reduced cell-mediated immunity. The absence of parathyroid glands result in hypocalcemia and tetany.

   If the above deficits are accompanied by cardiac defects, abnormalities of face and cleft palate, CATCH 22 syndrome occurs. Deletion of long arm of chromosome 22 is the likely cause of these multiple anomalies.

ii. **Nezelof's syndrome:** It results from failure of development of only the third pharyngeal pouch. In this case superior parathyroid glands are present but both inferior parathyroid glands and thymus are absent. Therefore, there is normal function of parathyroid glands. The symptoms due to absence of the thymus are present, these include absence of 'T' lymphocytes and absence of cell mediated immunity.

iii. Sometimes part of cervical sinus may persist and is known as **Branchial cyst**. These are most often located just below the angle of mandible along the anterior border of sternocleidomastoid (Fig. 44.23).

iv. **Internal branchial fistula:** These are rare. It occurs when cervical sinus is connected to lumen of pharynx by a small canal, which usually opens in tonsillar region. Such a fistula occurs from a rupture of membrane between 2nd pharyngeal cleft and pouch sometime during development.

DEVELOPMENT OF TONGUE

From development point of view, the tongue is divided into anterior 2/3rd, posterior 1/3rd and posterior most parts (Figs 44.24a to c).

Anterior Two-thirds

The anterior two-thirds of tongue is formed by

i. Two lateral mesodermal swellings.
ii. One median mesodermal swelling, called *Tuberculum impar*. These three swellings originate from first pharyngeal or mandibular arch. As the lateral swellings increase in size, they overgrow the tuberculum impar and merge with each other thus forming anterior two-thirds of tongue. The mucosa covering this part of tongue is supplied from lingual branch of mandibular division of

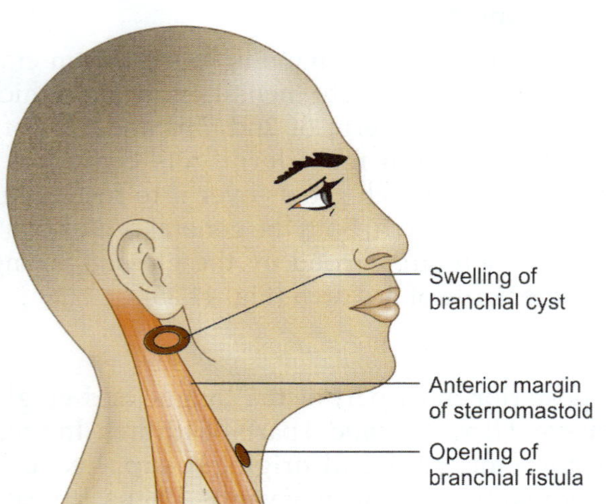

Fig. 44.23: Formation of branchial cyst

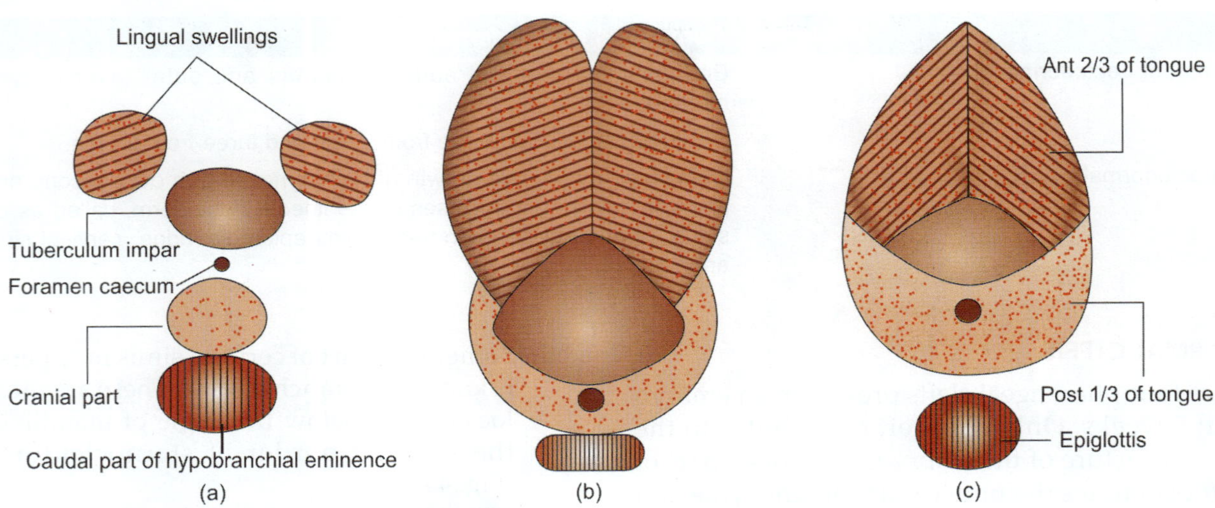

Figs 44.24a to c: Development of tongue

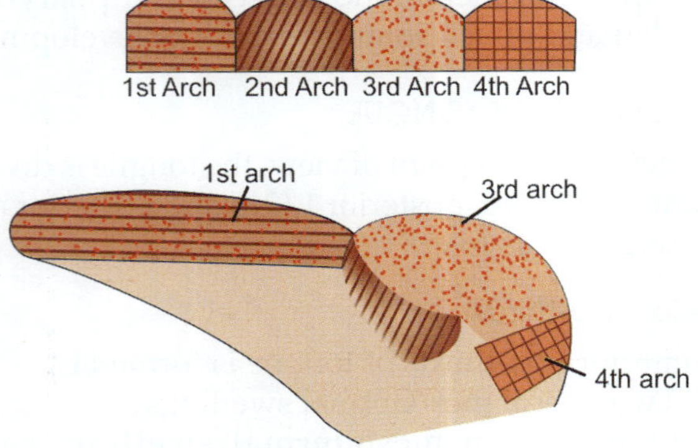

Fig. 44.25: Development of tongue

trigeminal nerve. Special sensory innervation, i.e. taste from most of the anterior two thirds is carried by chorda tympani branch of facial nerve which is pre-tremetic nerve of 2nd arch.

Posterior One-third

Posterior one-third of tongue is formed from cranial part of cupola or hypobranchial eminence which is derived from mesoderm of 2nd, 3rd and part of 4th arch. The 2nd arch mesoderm gets buried as the mesoderm of 3rd arch grows over it to fuse with the mesoderm of 1st arch. Both the general sensations and taste from here are carried by the glossopharyngeal nerve, the nerve of 3rd arch (Fig. 44.25).

Posterior Most Part

The posterior most part of the tongue and epiglottis are derived from the caudal parts of 4th arch. In keeping with the embryological origin. It supplied by the superior laryngeal branch of vagus. Vagus is the nerve of the 4th arch.

Muscles of the tongue migrate from *occipital myotomes* and are supplied by hypoglossal, the XII cranial nerve (Fig. 44.26).

Epithelium of tongue is made up of single layer. Later it gets stratified and forms papillae. The gustatory nerve cells of chorda tympani, glossopharyngeal and vagus nerves invade the epithelium to form taste buds.

Congenital Anomalies

a. *Macroglossia:* The tongue is large.
b. *Microglossia:* The tongue is small.
c. *Intralingual thyroid:* Thyroid tissue may be present in tongue.
d. Remnants of thyroglossal duct may form cysts at the base of the tongue.

DEVELOPMENT OF THYROID GLAND

The thyroid gland appears as on epithelial proliferation in the floor of the pharynx between tuberculum impar and cupola, approximately at 5th week of embryonic life, at a point later indicated by *foramen caecum*. The epithelial proliferation descends in front of the pharyngeal gut as a bilobed diverticulum. During this migration, the gland remains connected to the tongue by narrow duct, the *thyroglossal duct*. The duct later becomes solid and finally disappears (Fig. 44.27).

With further development, the thyroid gland descends in front of hyoid bone and laryngeal cartilages. It reaches the final position in front of trachea in 7th week of intrauterine life. By then, the two lobes are joined by well developed isthmus.

Parafollicular cells or 'C' cells are derived from the ultimobranchial body and according to some investigators by caudal pharyngeal complex in human (which is incorporated part of 5th with 4th pouches).

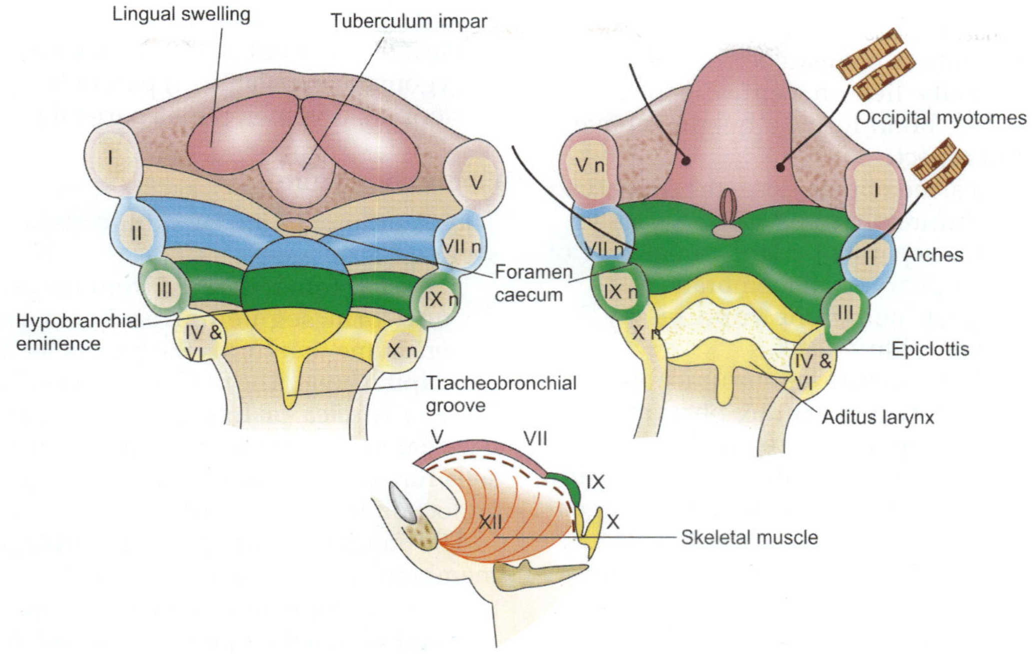

Fig. 44.26: Development of tongue

The gland begins to function approximately at the end of 3rd month of intrauterine life, when the first follicles containing colloid becomes visible. The 'C' cells serve as a source of calcitonin. Thyroid follicles first form at the periphery and later into the central part, i.e. follicular development is centripetal.

Anomalies of Thyroid Gland

A. Shape
   a. The pyramidal lobe as a normal structure may be present and it arises from isthmus
   b. Isthmus may be absent
   c. One of the lobes may be missing
   d. One of the lobes may be small
B. Position
   a. Lingual thyroid: Whole or part of the gland may be under the mucosa of dorsum of tongue to form a swelling, big enough to cause difficulty in swallowing (Fig. 44.27).
   b. The gland may be deep inside tongue, the intralingual thyroid.
   c. Gland is present above hyoid bone
   d. Gland descends just below hyoid bone, but above its normal position.
   e. Intrathoracic, retrosternal
C. Ectopic thyroid: Thyroid tissue has been observed in larynx, trachea, esophagus, pleura, pericardium and ovaries.
D. Remnants of thyroglossal duct
   a. Thyroglossal cyst
   b. Thyroglossal fistula
   c. Carcinoma of thyroglossal duct

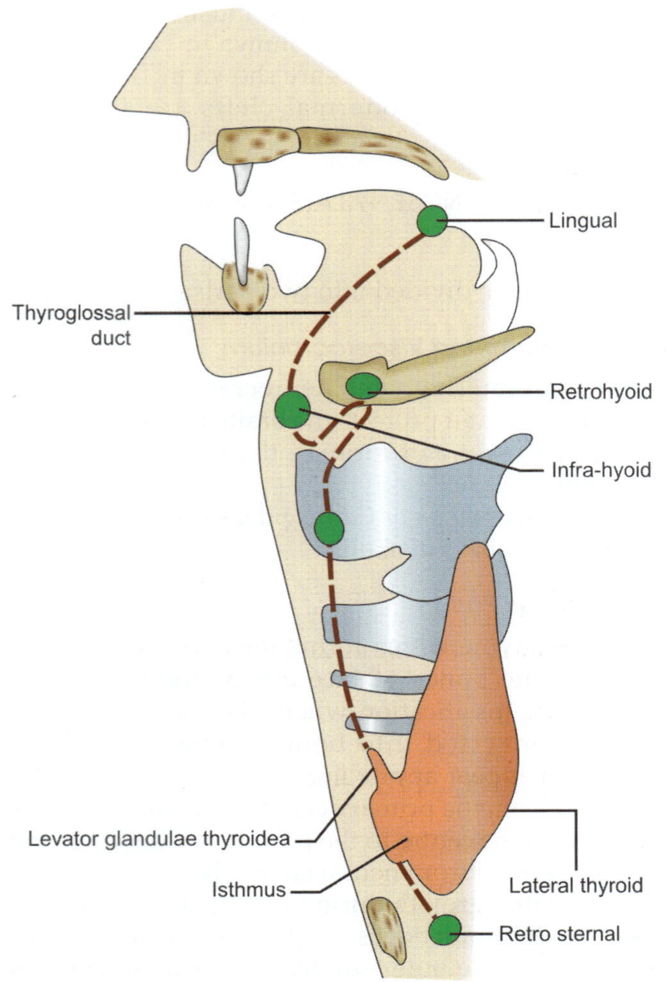

Fig. 44.27: Development of thyroid glands and its abnormal positions

SUMMARY

1 With the formation of head fold, developing pericardial cavity lies on ventral aspect and developing forebrain forms a bulging above it on the ventral aspect.
2 Buccopharyngeal membrane closes the cranial end of foregut, i.e. future pharynx.
3 Stomatodeum is separated from cranial part of foregut by buccopharyngeal membrane.
4 Buccopharyngeal membrane ruptures by 3rd week of embryonic life.
5 After its rupture, mouth communicates with proximal part of foregut or future pharynx.
6 Pharynx or cranial part of foregut shows mesodermal thickenings dorso-ventrally on either side and these thickenings are called Pharyngeal arches.
7 Pharyngeal or branchial arches are six in number, 5th disappears.
8 Each arch is covered on outside by ectoderm and lined on inside by endoderm, the lining of foregut.
9 Component of each arch is nerve, muscle (branchial), skeletal element and artery.
10 Derivatives of arches are shown in Table 44.2. Derivatives of pouches are shown in Table 44.3.

Derivatives of ectodermal clefts are shows in Table 44.4.

THE SKULL, FACE, NOSE, PALATE AND TEETH

The Skull

The skull can be divided into two parts:

Neurocranium and Viscerocranium

Neurocranium: The name neurocranium is derived from the fact that it protects the brain. It has two parts:

i. *Membranous part* forming the bones of vault of skull
ii. *Chondrocranium or Cartilaginous part* forming the bones of base of skull.

Membranous Part

The mesenchyme which forms the side and vault of skull and the bones of face are ossified by intramembranous ossification where the mesenchyme is directly converted into bone. Primary centre of ossification appear approximately in the centre of flat bones and from the primary centres, the bony spicules radiate from the centre to the periphery. Mesenchyme is partly derived from neural crest cells.

With further growth during fetal and postnatal life these membranous bones are formed by stacking of new layers on the outer surface and by simultaneous resorption of bone from the inside by osteoclastic activity.

Bones formed from membrane are:

a) Parietal, b) frontal, c) maxilla except premaxilla, d) zygomatic e) palatine, f) part of temporal, g) nasal, h) lacrimal, i) vomer, j) interparietal part of occipital.

Chondrocranium

The chondrocranium of skull consists of number of separate cartilages.

The sclerotomes derived from the occipital somites do not form segmentation but forms a mass of mesenchyme that forms the base of skull in the region of occipital bone. The notochord extends upto the level of sella turcica or hypophysis cerebri. The part of paraxial mesoderm that lies posterior to this limit i.e. sella turcica forms prechordal cartilage and ossifies by endochondral ossification.

The bones that form partly in cartilage and partly in membrane in the base of skull are:

a. *Temporal:* Squamous and tympanic parts ossify in membrane, while petrous and mastoid parts from ossification in cartilage of otic capsule.
b. *Occipital:* Interparietal part formed in membrane and rest of bone is from endochondral ossification from sclerotomes.
c. *Sphenoid:* Lateral parts of greater wing and pterygoid lamina in membrane, rest is in cartilage.

Bones completely formed in cartilage are ethmoid and inferior nasal concha. These are derived from cartilage of nasal capsule. *Septal and alar cartilage* do not ossify. These remain cartilages.

Viscerocranium

Viscerocranium consists of bones of face and are formed mainly form Ist and 2nd pharyngeal arches. The first arch gives rise to maxillary process which extends forwards beneath the region of eye and gives rise to maxilla and part of temporal bone. 1st arch also contains Meckel's cartilage. Mesenchyme around the Meckel's cartilage condenses and ossifies by membranous ossification to form most of the mandible and spheno-mandibular ligament. The dorsal part of Meckel's cartilage forms malleus and incus. Many investigators believe that mesenchyme formation of face is derived from neural crest cells.

Anomalies of Skull (Figs 44.28a to f)

Many investigators believe that most parts of facial skeleton and also most part of skull is formed from the neuroectoderm which originates from the neural crest cells.

These neuroectodermal cells are often targets for the teratogens during embryonic period i.e. 3rd to 8th week of intrauterine life, and these give rise to cranio-facial defects:

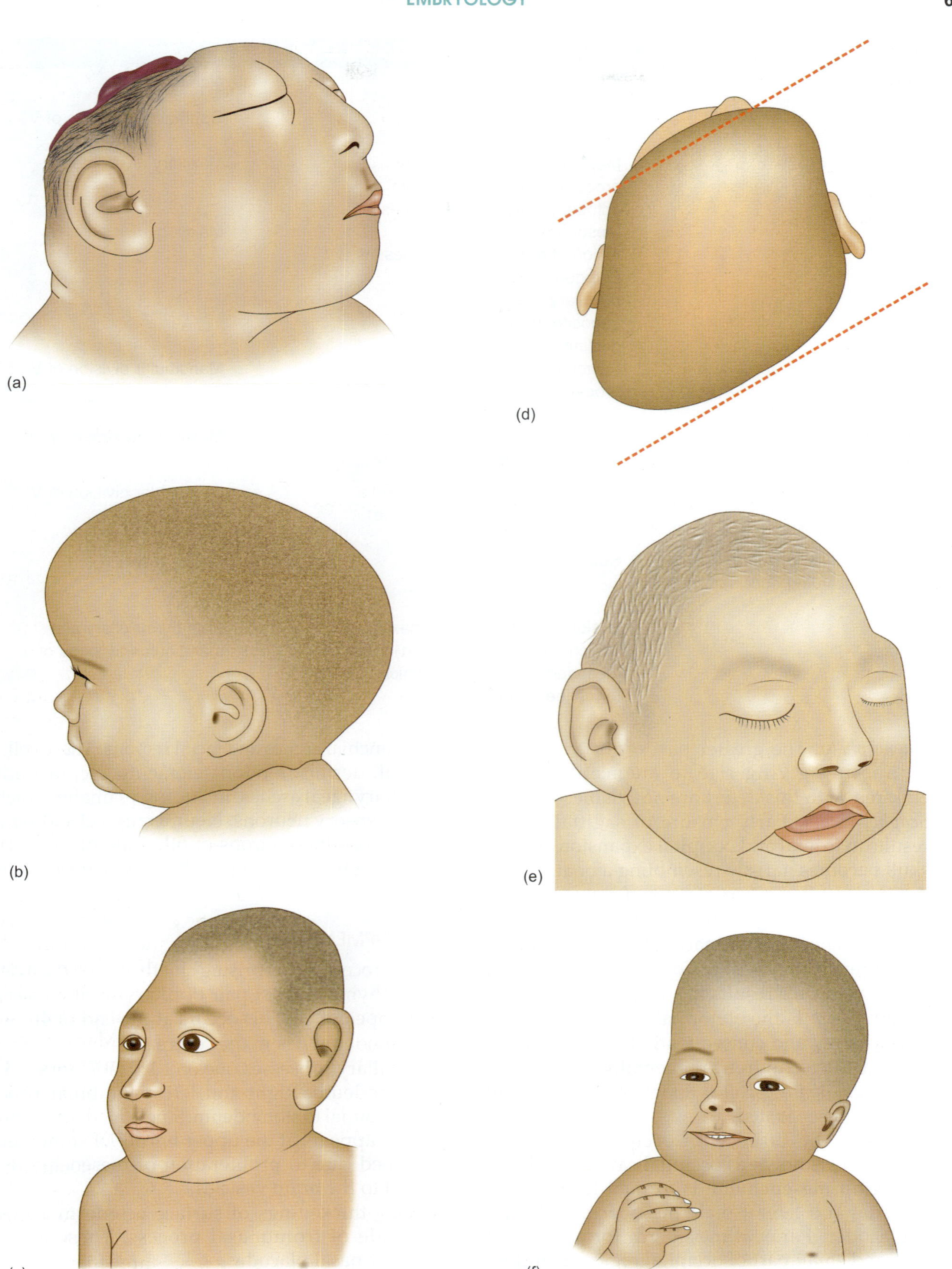

Figs 44.28a to f: Anomalies of skull (a) anencephaly, (b) scaphocephaly, (c) acrocephaly, (d) plagiocephaly, (e) microcephaly, (f) congenital hydrocephalus

Table 44.5: Developmental components of the face

Components	*Develop from*	*Nerves*
Forehead	Frontonasal process	Ophthalmic division of V
Upper lip:		
Lateral part	Mesodermal basis-maxillary process. Overlying skin from ectoderm covering the processes.	Maxillary division of V
Philtrum	Mesodermal part from fusion of medial nasal processes Ectoderm overgrows from maxillary process to meet opposite maxillary process in midline.	Maxillary division of V
Lower lip	Fusion of two mandibular processes.	Mandibular division of V
Upper jaw		
i) Premaxilla	Fused medial nasal processes	Maxillary division of V
ii) Maxilla	Mesoderm of maxillary process.	
Lower jaw	Mesoderm of first arch (Meckel's cartilage replaced by mandible)	Mandibular division of V
Muscles of facial expression, scalp, auricle including buccinator	Second arch	Facial nerve
Cheeks	Fusion of mesoderm on maxilla (which forms the upper part) with mesoderm on mandible which forms the lower part.	Both by maxillary and mandibular divisions of V

a. *Anencephaly:* The greater part of the vault may be missing giving rise to anencephaly and children with this defect are not viable.
b. *Scaphocephaly:* Early closure of sagittal suture results in frontal and occipital expansion and the skull becomes narrow resembling a boat.
c. *Acrocephaly:* Premature closure of coronal suture results in short high skull (tower skull).
d. *Plagiocephaly:* If the coronal and lambdoid sutures close prematurely on one side. This asymmetrical union of sutures results in a twisted skull.
e. *Microcephaly:* Is the abnormality in which brain fails to grow and consequently the skull fails to expand. Such children are mentally retarded.
f. *Congenital hydrocephalus:* Bones of vault of skull are widely separated.
g. Atlas may be fused with occipital bone. The condition is known as occipitalisation of atlas.

Head region mesenchyme is formed from neural crest, paraxial and lateral plate mesoderm and ectodermal placodes. Paraxial mesoderm forms floor of brain case and small part of occipital region including all skeletal muscles of head and neck.

Neural crest cells arise from neuroectoderm of forebrain, midbrain and hindbrain regions and migrate into branchial arches and facial regions. These cells form skeletal, dermis, tendons elements, etc. of midfacial and pharyngeal arches, including piamater, arachnoid mater, sensory neurons. Neural crest cells also participate in forming neurons of 5th, 7th, 9th, 10th cranial sensory ganglia along with cells from ectodermal placodes.

DEVELOPMENT OF FACE

Facial processes comprising chiefly neural crest derived mesenchyme and 1st pair of pharyngeal arches make their appearance. This occurs at the end of 4th week.

Stomodeum lies in the centre.

Maxillary processes one on each side appear lateral to stomodeum. Right and left mandibular processes appear caudal to stomodeum. Single median frontonasal process appears at the upper border of stomodeum. It is formed due to proliferation of mesenchyme lying ventral to the brain vesicles.

Local thickenings of surface ectoderm appear on each side of frontonasal process. These are called olfactory nasal placodes.

5th week: Nasal placodes invaginate to form nasal pits. Each nasal pit has lateral nasal process along lateral side and medial nasal process along its medial aspect.

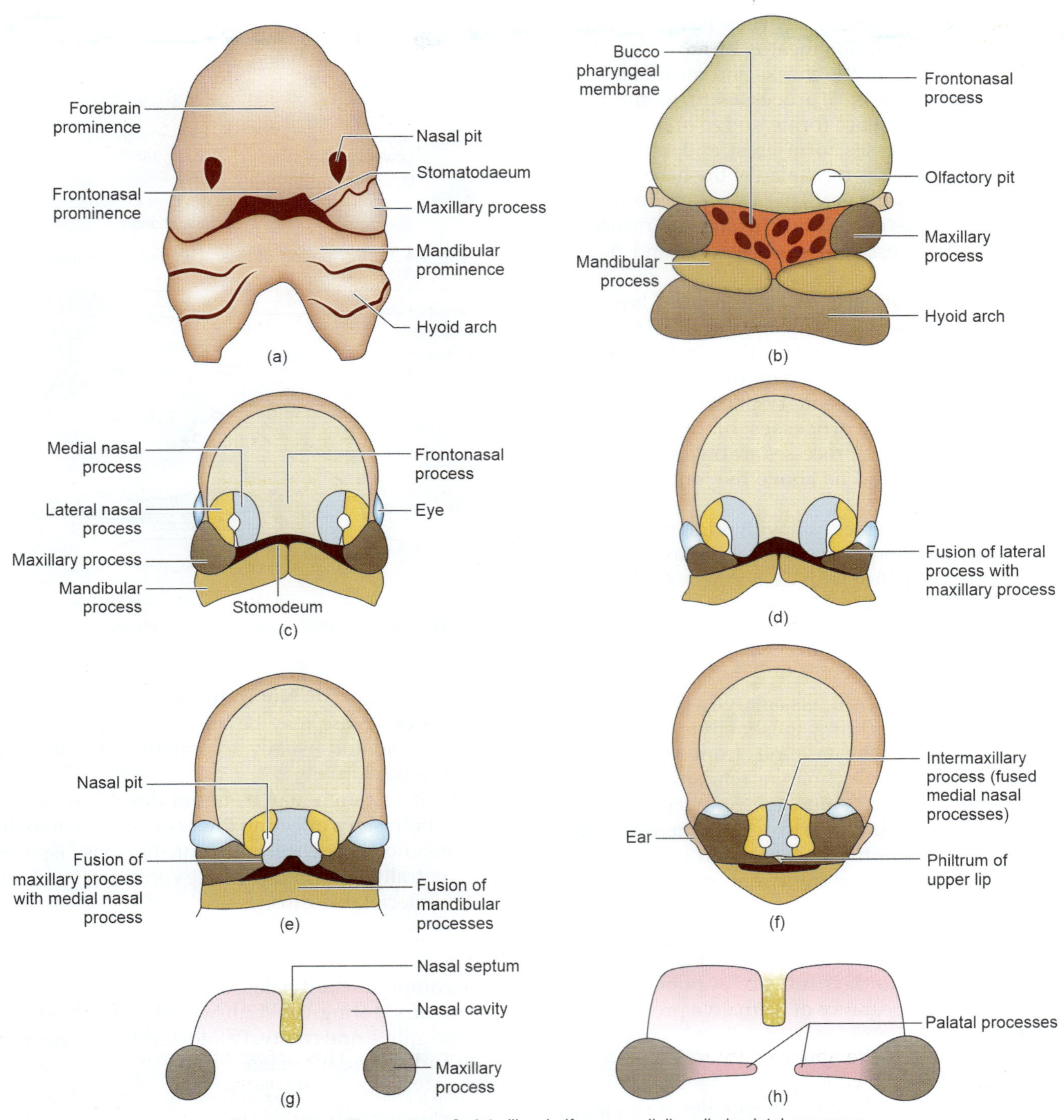

Figs 44.29a to h: Development of face and palate

6th and 7th week: Maxillary processes increase in size; grow medially to compress the medial nasal process. The cleft between the two processes is lost. Thus the upper lip develops from maxillary processes on lateral sides and only medial nasal processes in the central part. Upper lip does not take any contribution from lateral nasal process.

Nasolacrimal groove/cleft lies between maxillary process and lateral nasal process. Ectoderm in this, groove forms a solid cord. This cord after canalisation is known as nasolacrimal duct. The upper end of nasolacrimal duct dilates to form lacrimal sac. After detachment of the nasolacrimal duct, the maxillary prominence and lateral nasal prominence fuse with each other. Nasolacrimal duct runs between medial angle of eye and inferior meatus of nose. Maxillary processes form part of the cheeks and maxilla bones.

Formation of nose: 5 processes form the nose: Fronto-nasal prominence forms bridge of nose. Fused medial nasal processes form crest and tip of nose. Lateral nasal processes form alae of the nose.

Intermaxillary segment: This segment is formed by maxillary processes of each side fusing with respective medial nasal processes at surface level and deeper levels.

This intermaxillary segment thus formed has:

a. labial part forming philtrum of upper lip
b. upper jaw part which holds upper lip incisor teeth.
c. palate part which forms triangular primary palate.

6th and 7th week: Secondary palate: This palate is formed by palatine processes of the maxillary processes. At first these processes are oblique, later they become horizontal and lie above the tongue, to form secondary palate.

These palatal processes fuse with primary triangular palate. Their junction is marked by incisive foramen. The two processes fuse with each other as well. Even the nasal septum grows downwards to fuse with the palate.

Nasal Cavities

6th week: The small nasal pits enlarge a lot as these go deep into the underlying mesenchyme. Oronasal membrane separates the nasal pits from oral cavity by forming the primitive choanae (choana–singular). Primitive choanae lie behind the primary palate, on each side of the midline. Due to development of secondary palate the definitive choanae shift posteriorly to lie at the junction of nasal cavity and pharynx.

Paranasal air sinuses: These arise as diverticula from lateral nasal wall and invade into sphenoid, ethmoid, frontal and maxilla bones. These are very small in childhood and increase to their full size at puberty. These sinuses and the appearance of teeth give proper shape to the face.

Anomalies of Nose

i. Deflected septum: It is the commonest anomaly seen. The septum may not be in the midline. It may be deflected to one side.

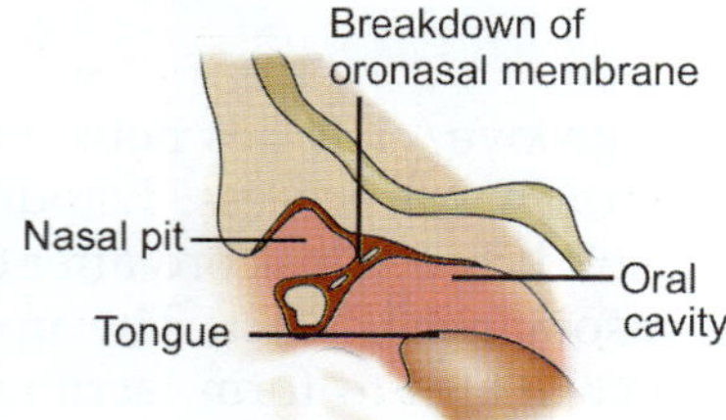

Fig. 44.30: Formation of nasal cavity

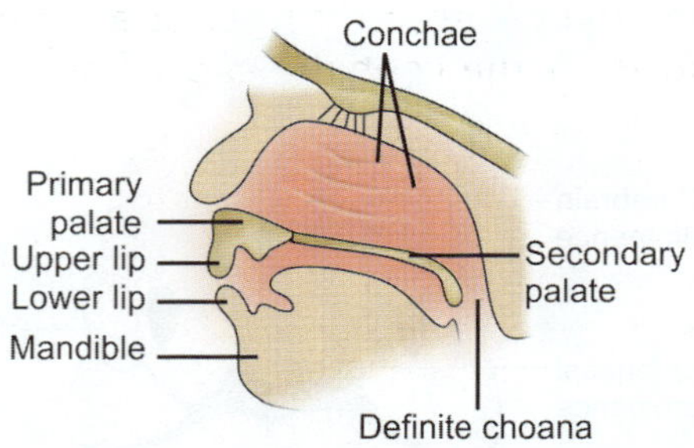

Fig. 44.31: Formation of lateral wall of nasal cavity

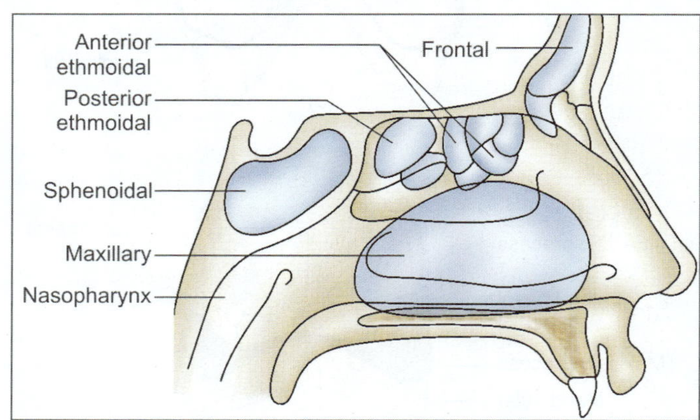

Fig. 44.32: Lateral wall of nasal cavity with location of paranasal sinuses.

ii. Absent septum: Not common.
iii. Process: Nose may be bifid jutting from below forehead and usually accompanied by fusion of eyes (cyclop).
iv. Entire 1st arch may be under developed on one or both sides affecting lower eyelid, the maxilla, mandible. The cheek is absent, the ear is displaced ventrally and caudally. The condition is mandibulofacial dysostosis.

PALATE

Palate comprises hard palate and soft palate. Development occurs during 6th–12th weeks from mesoderm in the primitive oral cavity. Palate develops as primary palate and secondary palate.

A. *Primary palate* is an area in front of incisive fossa and bears upper four incisor teeth. It is developed from fusion of medial nasal processes of frontonasal process with the maxillary process.

B. *Secondary palate* lies behind primary palate. It is developed by fusion of palatine processes of both maxillae. Fusion between primary and secondary palates takes place in 'y' shaped manner.

Soft Palate

The incisive foramen in midline marks junction between primary and secondary palate. At the same time as the palatine processes fuse, nasal septum grows down and joins the cephalic end of newly formed palate.

The mesoderm of anterior 3/4th palate undergoes intramembranous ossification. The ossification does not extend into the posterior 1/4th part which remains as soft palate and has components like epithelium, connective tissue and muscles. The posterior 1/4th part does not fuse with lower edge of nasal septum and hangs as soft palate.

ANOMALIES OF FACE AND PALATE

Hare lip: The upper lip of hare has a cleft. If there is a cleft in upper lip, it is called hare lip.

1 Lateral facial cleft: When the maxillary process does not fuse with lateral nasal process–it may give rise to a cleft running from medial angle of eye to mouth. The lacrimal duct is not formed (Fig. 44.33).

2 and 3 When one or both maxillary processes do not fuse with medial nasal process – may give rise to one or two clefts in the upper lip.

4 Defective development of lower part of frontonasal process may give rise to midline defect of upper lip.

5 If the two mandibular processes do not fuse with each other, it gives rise to defect in lower lip.

6 Incomplete or complete cleft palate including bilateral or unilateral cleft lip. These occur due to non fusion of palatine processes of maxilla with each other or with nasal septum and non fusion of maxillary process with medial nasal process. These give rise to:
   a. Bilateral complete cleft palate with bilateral hare lip
   b. Unilateral cleft palate and unilateral hare lip,
   c. Midline cleft extending into hard palate,
   d. Bifid uvula (Figs 44.34a to d).

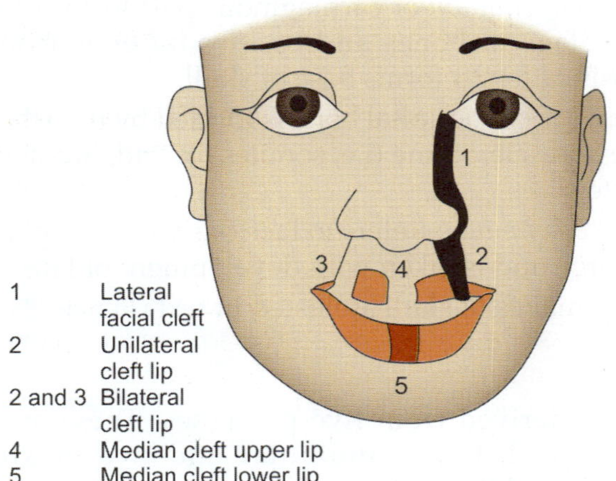

Fig. 44.33: Anomalies of face

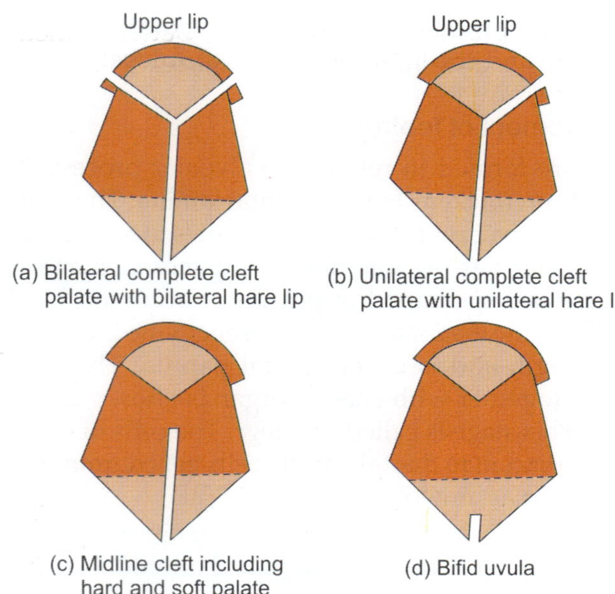

Figs 44.34a to d: Anomalies of palate

MOUTH

The mouth is derived from:
(a) Stomatodaeum, (b) from cranial part of foregut. The parts derived from these two parts are partly ectodermal and partly endodermal. After rupture of buccopharyngeal membrane, the junction between ectoderm and endoderm is difficult to define.

Structures derived from ectoderm lined stomatodaeum:

i. Lower part of nasal cavity.
ii. *Rathke's pouch:* It gives rise to anterior and intermediate lobes of hypophysis cerebri.
iii. *Vestibule of mouth:* The epithelium lining the inside of lips and cheeks.
iv. *Upper part of oral cavity:* The epithelium lining the palate.
v. *Dental ridges:* Give rise to maxillary and mandibular gums.
vi. Parotid gland.
vii. Anterior part of lower part of oral cavity up to linguogingival sulcus.

Structures Derived from Endoderm Lined Stomatodaeum

The epithelium of tongue is derived from endoderm. The tongue is separated laterally from the mandibular process by linguogingival sulcus.

Another sulcus forms between lip and gums and is called labiogingival sulcus which deepens rapidly and mesenchyme of mandibular arch lateral to it forms lower part of cheek. The tissue between the two sulci, i.e. labiogingival and linguogingival is raised and forms alveolar process of lower jaw.

Alveolar process of upper jaw is separated from the upper lip and cheek by labiogingival sulcus.

Development of Teeth

Teeth are formed in relation to alveolar process. The epithelium thickens to form dental lamina. The cells of dental lamina proliferate at various sites to form enamel organ, which grows into underlying mesenchyme and acquires a cup-shaped appearance, occupied by the mesenchyme (*bud stage*). This mesenchyme is of neural crest origin and is called dental papilla. The dental papilla together with enamel organ is known as tooth germ. This stage is called *cap stage*. The cells of enamel organ adjacent to dental papilla cells get columnar and are known as ameloblasts (Fig. 44.35).

The mesenchymal cells now arrange themselves along the ameloblasts and are called odontoblasts. The two cell layers are separated by a basement membrane. The rest of the mesenchymal cells form the "pulp of the tooth". This is the *bell stage*.

Now ameloblasts lay enamel on the outer aspect, while odontoblasts lay dentine on the inner aspect. Later ameloblasts disappear while odontoblasts remain.

The root of the tooth is formed by laying down of layers of dentine, narrowing the pulp space to a canal for the passage of nerve and blood vessels only (Fig. 44.35). The dentine in the root is covered by mesenchymal cells which differentiate into cementoblasts for laying down the cementum. Outside this is the periodontal ligament connecting root to the socket in the bone.

Permanent Teeth

The buds for permanent teeth are located on the medial or lingual aspect of milk teeth and are formed during third month of development. They give rise to permanent incisors, canines and premolars. The permanent molars are formed from buds that arise form the dental lamina posterior to last milk tooth.

These buds remain dormant till approximately 6 years of postnatal life, whereas the germs of premolars, 1st and 2nd molars are rudimentary for longer period of about 10–12 years. The germ of 3rd molar is formed after birth.

The buds for permanent teeth form teeth exactly like temporary teeth. When they begin to grow, they push against the underside of the corresponding milk tooth and end in their shedding. As a permanent tooth grows, the root of the overlying deciduous tooth gets resorbed by osteoclasts.

Permanent teeth erupt between 6 and 21 years.

Anomalies of Teeth

i. Teeth may be abnormal in number, shape and size.
ii. Two or more teeth may be fused called germination.
iii. The alignment of the upper and lower teeth may be incorrect—malocclusion.
iv. Sometimes lower incisors may be present at birth.
v. Eruption of teeth may be delayed.
vi. The teeth may be deficient in enamel, a condition caused by vitamin D deficiency.

SUMMARY

Skull

Two divisions

Neurocranium: Protects brain comprises two parts: (a) membranous, (b) cartilaginous

a. *Membranous:* Ossifies by intramembranous ossification. Membranous bones are:
   i. Vault of skull: Frontal, parietal, interparietal part of occipital, squamous and tympanic parts of temporal.
   ii. At birth the flat bones are separated by sutures: Main sutures are frontal or metopic, coronal, sagittal and lambdoid.
   iii. There are six fontanelles—anterior, posterior, two anterolateral and two posterolateral.
      1. Sutures and fontanelles allow growth bones of skull. These overlap each other during the time of vaginal delivery. The process is called as moulding; within few days, the membranous bones move back to their original position.
      2. Growth of bones of the vault continues after birth and is caused mainly by growth of brain.
b. *Chondrocranium* or cartilaginous part forms hyaline cartilage of bones and ossifies by endochondral ossification. It forms base of skull.

The base of occipital bone is formed by parachordal plate and sclerotome (i.e. somites) of 2nd, 3rd and 4th somites.

Viscerocranium: Refers to face derived from pharyngeal arch and is taken with development of face.

Anomalies of skull are listed in text (Fig. 44.28).

FACE

Face is derived from five processes. These are one frontonasal, two mandibular and two maxillary processes. All are derived from mesenchyme. This mesenchyme is of neural crest origin (*see* Table 44.5).

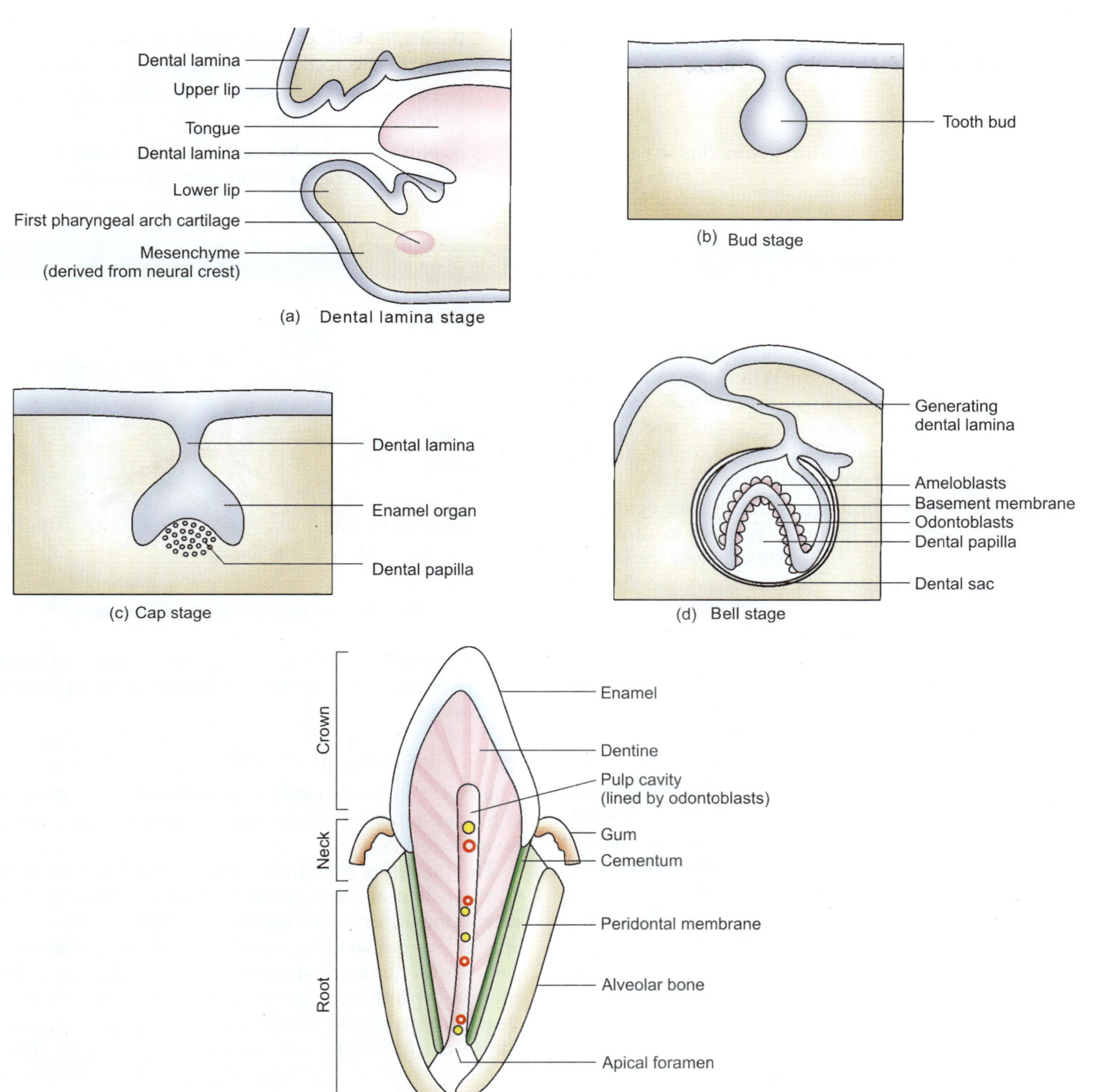

Figs 44.35a to e: Development of tooth

NOSE

i. Frontonasal process: On both side of nasal placodes.
ii. Nasal placodes invaginate raising nasal ridges on each side, called medial nasal process and lateral nasal process.
iii. Lateral nasal process forms ala of nose. The process fuses with maxillary process.
iv. Nasal pits deepen to form nasal sac or cavity. .
v. Nasal sacs separated by primitive nasal septum.
vi. Primitive nasal septum formed by frontonasal process.
vii. Nasal cavities initially communicate with oral cavity.
viii. Later, nasal cavity separated from oral cavity by primitive palate and oro-nasal membrane.

ix. Soon oro-nasal membrane ruptures in 2nd month—forms posterior nares which open in pharynx.

x. Nasal cavity
   a. Olfactory epithelium from nasal sac from olfactory placode.
   b. Respiratory epithelium from nasal sac from surface ectoderm.
   c. Paranasal sinuses arise as small diverticula from nasal cavity.
   d. Nasal septum formed by medial nasal process and deep part of frontonasal process.

DEVELOPMENT OF EYE

OPTIC VESICLE

In a 22 day embryo, a pair of shallow grooves appear, on each side of the forebrain. When the neural tube closes, these grooves form outpocketings from the diencephalon. These are known as *optic vesicles*. The proximal part of optic vesicles becomes constricted and elongated to form the optic stalk (Fig. 44.36a).

The optic vesicle approaches the surface ectoderm, comes in contact with it and induces it to form lens placode. The lens placode soon sinks below the surface and gets converted into lens vesicle. While the lens vesicle is forming, the optic vesicle forms a double layered optic cup due to differential growth of the wall of vesicle. The inner and outer layers of this cup are initially separated by a lumen, which is called inter-retinal space, but soon this lumen disappears and two layers get opposed to each other (Fig. 44.36b).

The invagination of inner layer into outer layer is not restricted to the central portion of the cup but also involves a part of inferior surface, as a result of which the wall of the cup shows deficiency on the inferior surface. This deficiency extends for some distance along the inferior surface of optic stalk and is known as choroid fissure or fetal fissure. Formation of this fissure allows the hyaloid artery to reach the posterior aspect of developing lens.

During the 5th week of development, lens vesicle loses contact with surface ectoderm and is then located in the mouth of optic cup and the margins of optic cup grow over the upper and lateral sides of lens to enclose it.

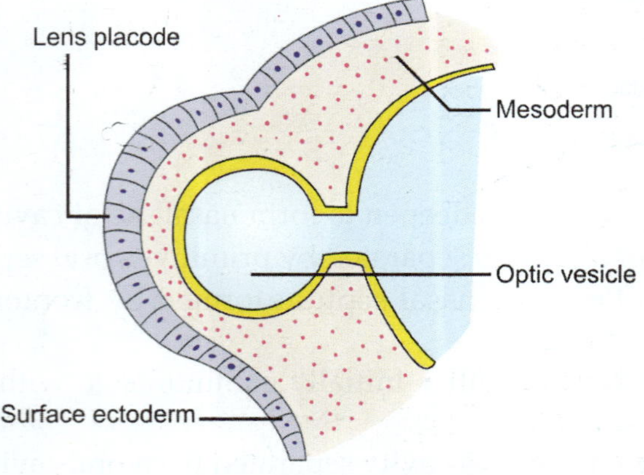

Fig. 44.36a: Formation of optic vesicle

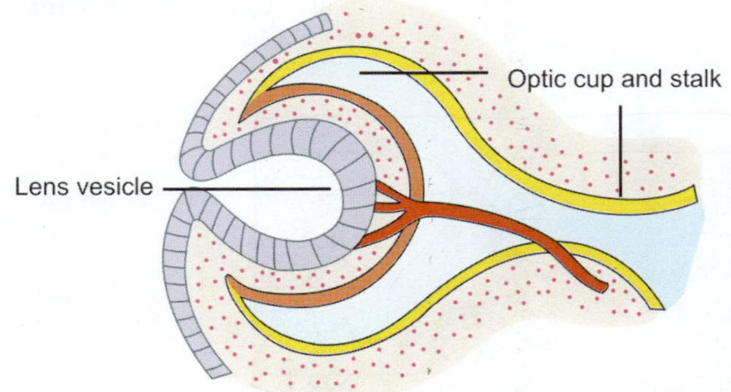

Fig. 44.36b: Formation of lens vesicle

RETINA, IRIS AND CILIARY BODY

The outer layer of optic cup remains thin, its cells contain pigment granules and is known as pigmented layer of retina.

The posterior four-fifths of the inner layer of optic cup is called as Pars optica retinae or optical part of retina and it contains cells bordering the inter-retinal space. This is also known as matrix cell layer and these cells differentiate into rods and cones. Adjacent to this photoreceptive layer is the mantle layer, which, as in the brain gives rise to neurons and supporting cells. These differentiate into outer nuclear layer, inner nuclear layer and ganglionic cell layer. Axons of ganglion cells migrate into marginal layer to form the layer of nerve fibres. These fibres grow into optic stalk through choroid fissure (Fig. 44.36c).

The anterior one-fifth forms ciliary and iridial parts of retina. Ciliary part of retina participates in formation of ciliary body. The anterior part of retina remains thin and forms an epithelial covering for the ciliary body and iris.

The region between the optic cup and overlying epithelium is filled with loose mesenchyme. In this tissue, sphincter and dilator pupillae muscles are formed. These muscles develop from neuroectoderm overlying the optic cup.

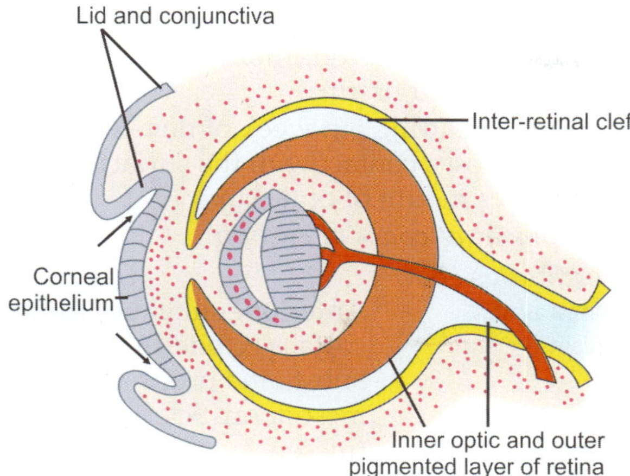

Fig. 44.36c: Formation of retina

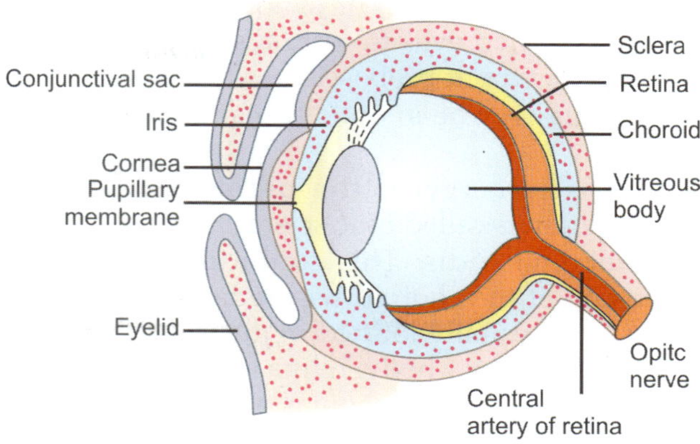

Fig. 44.36d: Formation of sclera, choroid and eyelids

The ciliary part of retina develops foldings, the ciliary processes. Externally, it is covered by layer of mesenchyme that forms ciliary muscle. It is connected to the lens by elastic fibres—the suspensory ligament. Contraction of ciliary muscle changes tension in the ligament and controls the curvature of lens.

LENS

Lens develops from lens vesicle. The cells of the anterior wall remain cubical. Cells of posterior layer begin to elongate in anterior direction and gradually fill the lumen of the lens vesicle during 7th week of development. These primary fibres reach the anterior wall of lens vesicle. They lose the nuclei and form lens fibres. However the new secondary fibres are continuously added to the central core (Fig. 44.36c).

Choroid, Sclera and Cornea

Approximately at the end of 1st month, the eye primordium gets surrounded by loose mesenchyme. The tissue differentiates into inner vascular layer, which forms choroid and an outer layer known as sclera. The choroid forms highly vascularised pigmented layer and the outer layer develops into sclera which is continuous with dura mater around optic nerve.

The substantia propria of cornea is formed from the same mesothelial layer that forms sclera. This mesoderm is in close contact with the surface ectoderm which forms epithelium covering superficial surface of cornea (Fig. 44.36d).

Anterior and posterior chambers of eye: These chambers are formed by splitting of the mesoderm in the region. The mesenchyme splits into an inner layer in front of lens, iris, the iridopupillary membrane and an outer layer on the inner aspect of the cornea. The pupillary membrane in front of lens disappears completely before birth thus providing communication between anterior and posterior chambers. Anterior chamber lies between cornea and iris. Posterior chamber lies between iris and lens.

Optic nerve: The optic stalk gets transformed into optic nerve with the closure of choroid fissure during 7th week of development. A narrow tunnel is formed inside the optic stalk by continuously increasing number of nerve fibres returning to the brain from retina.

It contains part of hyaloid artery, which is later called central artery of retina. On the outside, the optic nerve is surrounded by continuation of choroid and sclera, i.e. as pia-arachnoid and dura mater of brain.

ACCESSORY STRUCTURES OF EYEBALL

Eyelids

Eyelids are formed by reduplication of ectoderm above and below the cornea, and these folds contain mesoderm which forms muscles and tarsal plates. The margins of upper and lower lids fuse, thus cut off a space called conjunctival sac. The lids remain fused with each other till the 7th month of development (Fig. 44.36d).

Lacrimal Gland

The lacrimal gland arises as number of buds from upper angle of conjunctival sac. The lacrimal sac and naso-lacrimal duct are formed from the canalization of a strip of ectoderm buried in the naso-optic groove between the maxillary and lateral nasal processes. The upper part of this duct widens and forms lacrimal sac. The nasolacrimal duct then runs from the medial angle of eye to the inferior meatus of the nose.

Lacrimal canaliculi are formed by canalization of ectodermal buds that arise from the margin of each eyelid near the medial angles and join the lacrimal sac.

Anomalies of Eye

1 Enophthalmos: Entire eyeball may fail to develop.
2 Microphthalmos or microophthalmia: The eye remains very small.

3 Cyclops (single eye) or synophthalmia: There is fusion of two eyes to form a single midline eye, with or without proboscis.
4 Lens may not be in optic cup and may remain as cyst.
5 Thin sclera reveal the pigment of choroid. Condition is called blue sclera.
6 Coloboma iridis: This condition may occur if closure of the choroid fissure fails to occur. This fissure is usually located in the iris only but may extend to ciliary body, retina, choroid and even in the optic nerve. Colobomas of the eyelids may be due to underdevelopment of the nasal plate.
7 Persistent hyaloid artery: This artery may persist and form cyst or cord.
8 Persistent pupillary membrane: When the capsule persists on the anterior aspect of lens, it may completely occlude the pupil.
9 Congenital aphakia: Congenital absence of lens, due to disturbance in induction and formation of tissues responsible for formation of the lens.
10 Congenital cataract: A condition in which lens becomes opaque during intrauterine life. This is usually in children whose mothers suffered from German measles or rubella between 4th to 7th weeks of pregnancy.
11 Albinism: Various layer of eye show too little melanin pigment.
12 Palpebral fissure: May be abnormally wide or narrow and two eyelids may be partially or completely fused with each other.
13 Epicanthus: Abnormal folds in relation to the lids.
14 Entropian or ectropian: Lid may be inverted or everted.
15 Ptosis: Levator palpebrae superioris may fail to develop.
16 Atresia of nasolacrimal duct: May be partial or complete.
17 Non obliteration of naso-optic groove: It may be present as open groove on the face.

SUMMARY

- Optic vesicle develops from a shallow groove which appears on each side of forebrain in a 22-day embryo, when neural tube closes. The groove forms an outpocketing on each side known as optic vesicle.
- Lens placode develops from surface ectoderm after being inducted by optic vesicle. At first lens placode develops. Then it sinks below surface to forms lens vesicle.
- Optic cup is formed from optic vesicle. When lens is forming, the optic vesicle forms optic cup due to differential growth of walls of optic cup.
- Choroid fissure: As the optic cup is formed, wall of cup shows deficiency on inferior surface, which is known as choroid fissure.
- Lens vesicle: During 5th week of development, the lens vesicle loses contact with the surface ectoderm and occupies mouth of optic cup.
- ***Development of coats of eyeball:***

Outer fibrous coat

Cornea and sclera	Anterior epithelium from surface ectoderm Substantia propria from mesoderm. Sclera-mesoderm (mesenchyme around optic cup)

Middle coat and retina

a. Choroid, pigment cells and blood vessels	Mesoderm
b. Ciliary body, ciliary muscle and stroma	Mesoderm
c. Epithelium – iris, i.e. ciliary part of retina	Neuroectoderm
d. Pars iridis retina, i.e. Iridial part of retina	Neuroectoderm
e. Sphincter and dilator pupillae	Neuroectoderm
f. Mesothelial layer and stroma	Mesenchyme
g. Inner photo sensitive layer—Posterior 4/5th part of optic cup and 10 layers of retina	Neuroectoderm

- Optic nerve and central artery of retina: Develops from optic stalk. On the ventral surface there is a choroid fissure in which lie hyaloid vessels and nerve fibres returning to brain. Margins of choroid fissure fuse and hyaloid artery disappears. The part of hyaloid artery which lie in the centre of optic nerve forms central artery of retina.
- Development of contents of eyeball:
  - Anterior and posterior chambers from splitting of mesoderm in front of lens vesicle.
  - Lens from lens placode which develops from surface ectoderm.
  - Vitreous body from mesoderm inside the optic cup.
  - Pupil from rupture of irido-pupillary membrane or pupillary membrane.
- Accessory structures
  a. Eyelids from reduplication of surface ectoderm above and below the cornea with a core of mesoderm.
  b. Conjunctiva from surface ectoderm and mesoderm
  c. Lacrimal gland as buds from upper angle of the conjunctival sac.

d. Lacrimal sac and nasolacrimal duct from ectoderm of naso-optic furrow, upper dilated part forms lacrimal sac.

Anomalies

1 Enophthalmos
2 Microphthalmos
3 Cyclops or synophthalmos
4 Lens may not form, may be represented as a cyst
5 Blue sclera
6 Coloboma iris
7 Persistent hyaloid artery
8 Persistent pupillary membrane
9 Congenital aphakia
10 Congenital cataract
11 Albinism—Less pigment in the pigmented layer

DEVELOPMENT OF EAR

INTRODUCTION

In the adult, the ear forms one functional unit serving the functions of both hearing and equilibrium. Ear has three functional components:

a. External ear, which served as sound collecting organ in lower animals, but is almost vestigial in human, though it serves the purpose of supporting the spectacles, wearing the ear-rings and as an movable object for punishment. Lepra bacilli can be viewed from lobule of ear in infected cases. Y chromosome may manifest as "hairy pinna."
b. Middle ear which conducts sound waves from external to middle ear.
c. Internal ear which converts the sound waves into nerve impulses and identifies changes in the equilibrium.

The first indication of developing ear is seen in embryo approximately at 22 days. There is thickening of surface ectoderm on each side of hindbrain. These thickenings, otic placodes become depressed to form otic pits. The pits soon become rounded to form otic vesicles which get separated from surface ectoderm (Fig. 44.37).

Membranous labyrinth: Soon each otic vesicle divides into 2 parts:

i. Ventral part component that forms the *saccule and cochlear duct.*
ii. Dorsal component which gives rise to *utricle, semicircular canals* and *endolymphatic duct.*

i. By 6th week of development, the saccule forms a tubular shaped outpocketing at the lower end, which is known as cochlear duct, invading the surrounding mesenchyme in a spiral fashion and by 8th week, it has completed 2.5 turns. Its connection with the remaining part of saccule is confined through a narrow duct called ductus reunions.
ii. Simultaneously during 6th week of development, the semicircular canals appear as flattened outpocketings of utricular part of otic vesicle which give rise to superior, posterior and lateral semicircular ducts (Fig. 44.38).

Localised areas of epithelium of membranous labyrinth undergo differentiation to form *macula* of utricle and saccule; *organ of Corti* of cochlea and *cristae* of semicircular canals. These are sensory end organs of hearing and equilibrium.

The sensory end organs of hearing, i.e. macula of saccule and organ of Corti and of equilibrium, i.e. macula of utricle and cristae of semicircular ducts are innervated by peripheral processes of cochlear and vestibular ganglion. The ganglion are derived from neural crest. The cells remain bipolar throughout life.

Bony labyrinth: It is formed by the mesenchyme surrounding membranous labyrinth. The mesenchymal condensation soon gets converted into cartilage.

The layer of loose tissue known as *periotic tissue* around the saccule and utricle disappears to form a space called *vestibule*. The periotic tissue around the semicircular ducts also disappears to form semicircular canals which open into vestibule.

In the region of cochlea, two spaces are formed one on either side of the cochlear duct. These are *scala tympani* and *scala vestibuli*. The scala vestibuli

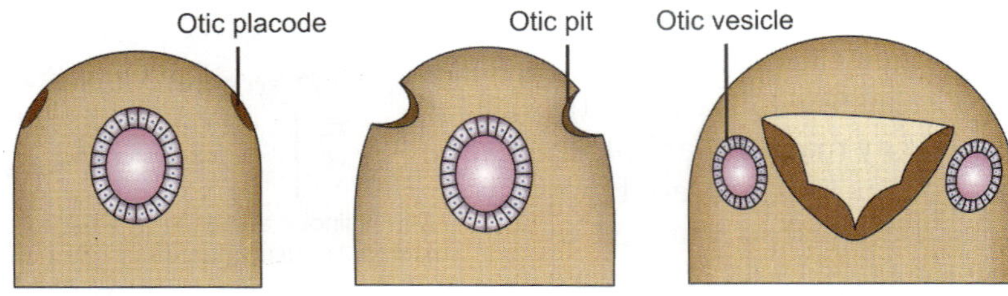

Fig. 44.37: Formation of otic placode, otic pit and otic vesicle

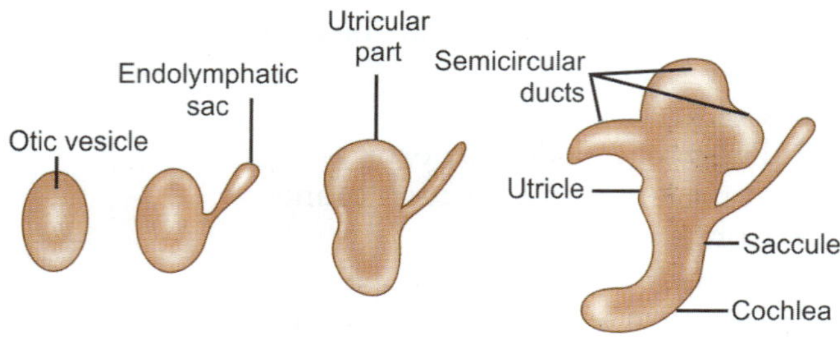

Fig. 44.38: Development of internal ear

communicates with the vestibule and scala tympani grows towards tympanic cavity from which it is separated by secondary tympanic membrane.

The cartilaginous labyrinth ossifies to form bony labyrinth. The membranous labyrinth is filled with endolymph. The periotic space between membranous and bony labyrinth is filled with perilymph.

MIDDLE EAR

The epithelial lining of middle ear and pharyngo-tympanic tube is of endodermal origin and both are derived from tubotympanic recess. The recess develops from the dorsal part of 1st pharyngeal pouch and it also receives contribution from the 2nd pouch. The distal part of the recess is wide and gives rise to primitive tympanic cavity, while the proximal part remains narrow and forms the pharyngotympanic or Eustachian tube. Through this channel tympanic cavity communicates with nasopharynx.

During fetal life, the tympanic cavity expands dorsally and forms tympanic antrum. After birth, bone of the developing mastoid process is invaded by the epithelium of tympanic cavity and epithelial lined air sacs are formed in the mastoid antrum.

Ossicles

Incus and malleus are derived form dorsal end of cartilage of 1st pharyngeal arch or Meckel's cartilage. Stapes is derived from dorsal end of 2nd pharyngeal arch.

The mucous membrane of the developing middle ear covers the ossicles after they invaginate it. The ossicles of the ear ossify during the 4th month of fetal life and these are the first bones in the body to do so.

Muscles

Tensor tympani develops from mesoderm of 1st pharyngeal arch and is supplied by mandibular branch of trigeminal nerve. Stapedius is derived from mesoderm of 2nd pharyngeal arch. It is attached to stapes and is innervated by the facial nerve, the nerve of 2nd pharyngeal arch.

EXTERNAL EAR

External auditory meatus is derived from dorsal part of 1st ectodermal cleft. Deeper part is formed by proliferation of cells which later get canalized.

Pinna or Auricle

Pinna develops from six mesenchymal proliferations located at dorsal ends of the 1st and 2nd pharyngeal arches around the opening of the dorsal part of 1st ectodermal cleft i.e. external auditory meatus. These six proliferations or hillocks fuse to form the pinna. Tragus is formed by 1st or mandibular arch. Rest of the auricle and muscles develop from 2nd or hyoid arch. The muscles of auricle are supplied by facial nerve, the nerve of 2nd arch.

Tympanic Membrane or Ear Drum

Tympanic membrane is formed by

a. The ectodermal lining of 1st ectodermal cleft, which forms the lining of external auditory meatus.
b. Endodermal epithelial lining of tympanic cavity.
c. Intermediate layer of connective tissue which forms the fibrous structure. Major part of the handle of malleus is firmly attached to the tympanic membrane (Fig. 44.39).

Congenital Anomalies

I *Pinna*

1. *Preauricular skin tags may be present:* These may be due to accessory hillocks.
2. *Preauricular pits and depression:* These represent abnormal development of auricular hillocks.
3. *Large pinna:* Occurs due to excessive development.
4. Fusion of auricle with head may occur.
5. Bat's ears: Abnormal lateral protrusion of auricle.
6. *Darwin's tubercle:* A small elevation on postero-superior part of helix-represents tip of the ear of lower mammals.

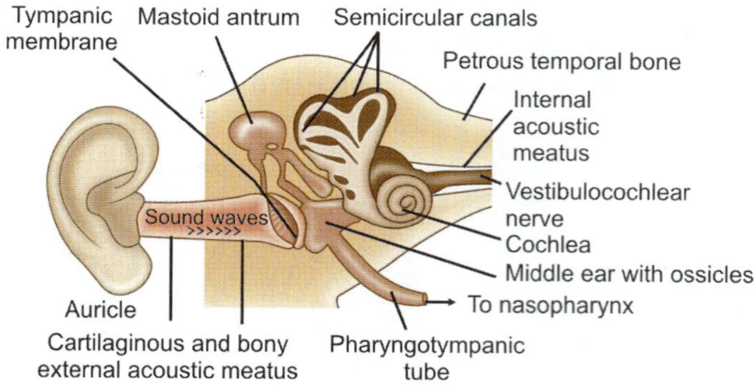

Fig. 44.39: Parts of external, middle and internal ear

II. *External Auditory Meatus*

1 Stenosis or atresia over the whole length of it or part of it.
2 The normal curvature may be accentuated as a result of which the tympanic membrane cannot be fully seen from outside.

III. *Middle Ear*

1 Ossicles may be malformed.
2 Stapedial artery may persist.

IV. *Internal Ear*

Rubella or Germal measles virus: During 7th or 8th week may cause severe damage to the organ of Corti. Poliomyelitis, diabetes and hypothyroidism during pregnancy may cause congenital deafness of the child. The various parts of membranous labyrinth may remain underdeveloped in the fetus.

SUMMARY

Components	*Develops from*
External Ear	
1 Pinna	From 6 auricular hillocks around dorsal part of 1st pharyngeal ectodermal cleft.
2 Tragus	1st arch
3 Rest of auricle and muscles	2nd arch
4 External auditory meatus	Dorsal part of 1st ectodermal cleft.
5 Tympanic membrane	Apposition of 1st ectodermal cleft with endoderm of tubotympanic recess with mesoderm in between.
Middle Ear	
1 Epithelial lining	Tubotympanic recess and (endoderm)
2 Malleus and incus	Dorsal end of 1st arch cartilage.
3 Stapes	Dorsal end of 2nd arch cartilage
4 Tensor tympani	Mesoderm of 1st pharyngeal arch
5 Stapedius	Mesoderm of 2nd pharyngeal arch

Internal Ear

1 Membranous labyrinth, i.e. cristae of semicircular canals, maculae of utricle and saccule and organ of Corti: Ectoderm overlying hindbrain forming otic placode and otic vesicle.
2 *Bony labyrinth:* Mesenchyme surrounding membranous labyrinth.

Chapter

45

Histology

"All that I am or hope to be, I owe to my angel mother."
—Anonymous

INTRODUCTION

Histology is the microscopic study of various tissues of the body. A tissue is made up of groups of cells performing the same function. The cell is the basic structural unit of the body (Fig. 45.1). The various tissues are:

- Epithelial tissue
- Connective tissue
- Muscular tissue
- Nervous tissue.
  Stain used is haematoxylin and eosin (H&E).

EPITHELIAL TISSUE

Functions of Epithelial Tissue/Epithelium

Epithelial tissue described below covers outer aspect of the body and lines various tubes and tracts.

a. *Protective*: The stratified squamous keratinised epithelium of skin offers mechanical protection including conservation of moisture.

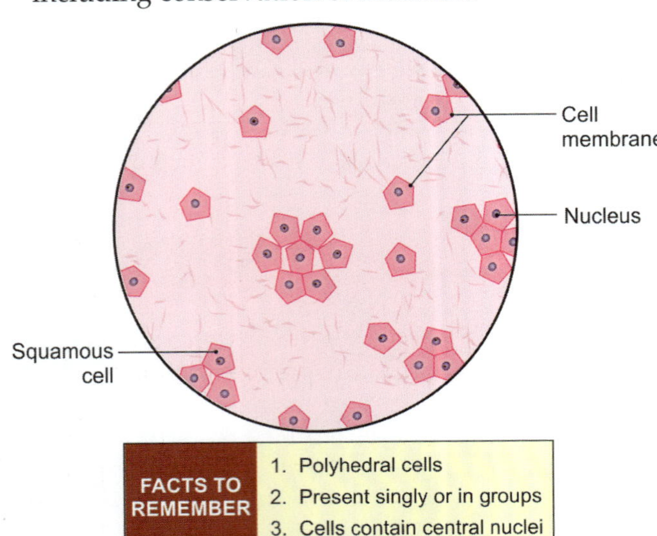

Fig. 45.1: Desquamated squamous cells: Cheek mucosa

b. *Secretory*: The glands which are derivatives of the epithelium secrete useful chemical substances.
c. *Absorptive*: Epithelia of small intestine and of proximal convoluted tubules of kidney are modified to specialise in absorptive functions.
d. *Excretory*: Epithelium of distal convoluted tubules and collecting ducts of kidney function as excretory organs.
e. *Sensory*: The rods and cones of retina and hair cells of olfactory mucous membrane are specialised sensory cells.

Characters of Epithelium

1. Epithelium may consist of one layer or many layers of cells.
2. The deepest layer of cells rest on a basement membrane.
3. There is minimal amount of intercellular substance.
4. Epithelium may develop from ectoderm, e.g. skin; from mesoderm, e.g. urinary system; from endoderm, e.g. gastrointestinal system.
5. Nutrition of epithelium is by diffusion from the underlying capillaries.
6. Epithelium covers the exterior of body surface and lines the interior of cavities/passages.

Classification of Epithelium

1. Simple epithelium
2. Pseudostratified epithelium
3. Compound epithelium

Simple Epithelium

It can be of the following types:

a. *Squamous (scale like) or pavement epithelium:* Seen in alveoli of lungs (Fig. 45.2), endothelium of blood vessels and mesothelium of serous membranes. The epithelium in sections is seen to consist of a single layer of thin cells with flattened nuclei.

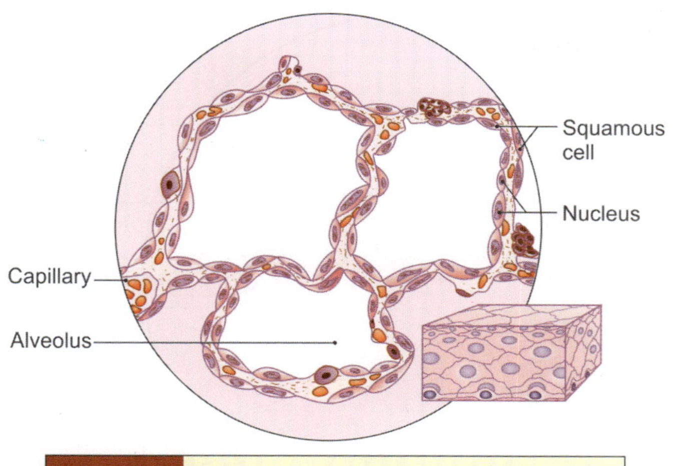

FACTS TO REMEMBER

1. Flattened cells lining the lung alveoli
2. Capillaries in between the alveoli
3. Squamous cells permit exchange of gases

Fig. 45.2: Squamous epithelium: Lung parenchyma

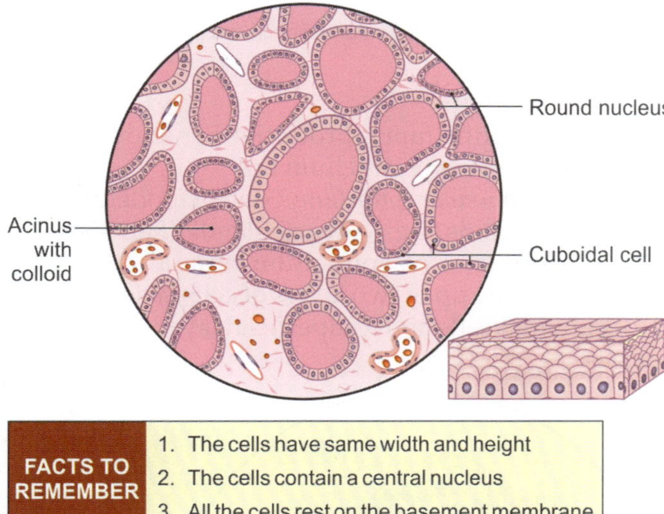

FACTS TO REMEMBER

1. The cells have same width and height
2. The cells contain a central nucleus
3. All the cells rest on the basement membrane

Fig. 45.3: Cuboidal epithelium: Thyroid gland

b. *Cuboidal epithelium*: Seen in thyroid gland acini during resting phase (Fig. 45.3), small ducts of the glands. The cells have equal width and height with the round central nuclei.

c. *Columnar epithelium*: The cells are almost three times taller than their width. Nucleus is basal and oval in shape. Its modifications are as follows:
   - *Simple columnar epithelium:* Lining of stomach (Fig. 45.4) and lining of cervical canal of uterus. This epithelium is secretory.
   - *Columnar cells with microvilli or brush border:* Seen in gall bladder (Fig. 45.5), lining of entire small intestine. The free margin of the cell shows bright red membrane.

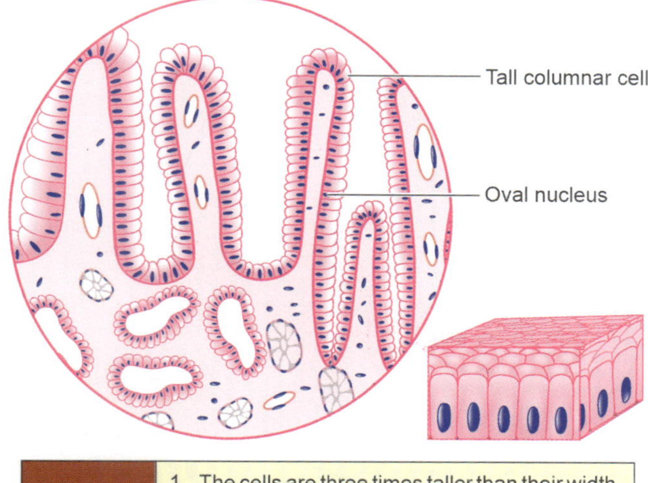

FACTS TO REMEMBER

1. The cells are three times taller than their width
2. Nucleus is basal and oval in shape
3. All the cells look alike

Fig. 45.4: Simple columnar epithelium stomach

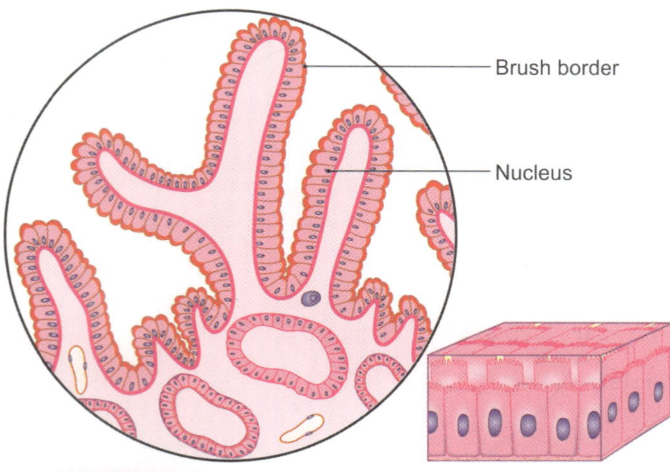

FACTS TO REMEMBER

1. The cells are columnar in shape
2. The free margin shows a bright red membrane called the brush border
3. The brush border is due to invaginations of the surface membrane

Fig. 45.5: Columnar epithelium with brush border: Gallbladder

   - *Ciliated columnar epithelium:* Seen in epithelium of fallopian tube (Fig. 45.6) and olfactory mucosa. Some of these columnar cells have hair-like processes projecting from their surfaces. The movement of the cilia propels the fluid.
   - *Goblet cells:* Plenty in large intestine (Fig. 45.7), small intestine, trachea, bronchi. These are unicellular glands and appear empty with haematoxylin and eosin staining, as the mucus contained in these cells gets dissolved during the staining procedure. The columnar cell assumes the

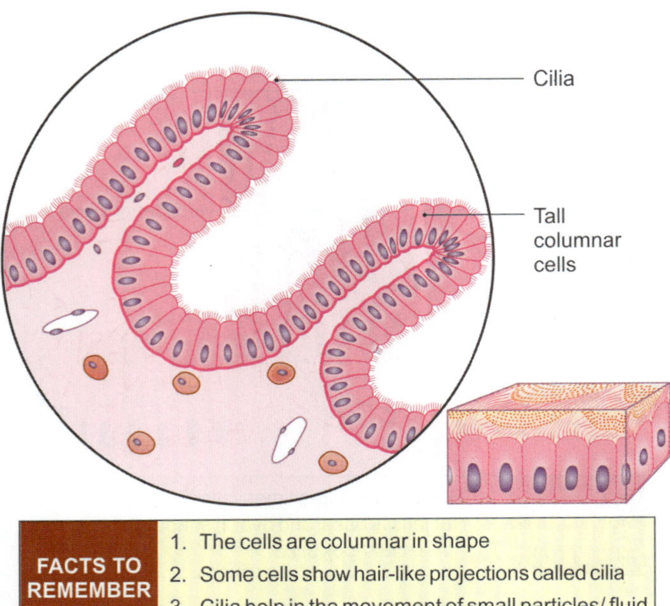

FACTS TO REMEMBER
1. The cells are columnar in shape
2. Some cells show hair-like projections called cilia
3. Cilia help in the movement of small particles/ fluid

Fig. 45.6: Ciliated columnar epithelium: Fallopian tube

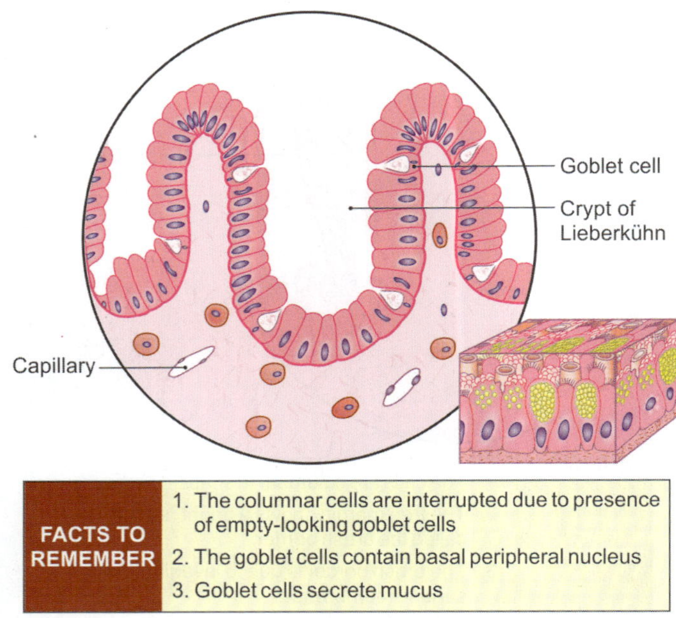

FACTS TO REMEMBER
1. The columnar cells are interrupted due to presence of empty-looking goblet cells
2. The goblet cells contain basal peripheral nucleus
3. Goblet cells secrete mucus

Fig. 45.7: Goblet cells: Large intestine

shape of a goblet. The cell full of mucus with flattened nucleus close to the base is seen with special stains.

Pseudostratified Epithelium

This type of epithelium is one cell thick, but cells are of varying heights. So it is a type of simple epithelium. Some cells are short, not reaching the surface, others are tall columnar and a few are goblet cells. Thus, the nuclei of these cells lie at different levels giving a false appearance of many layers. This epithelium is columnar and ciliated, e.g. trachea (Fig. 45.8).

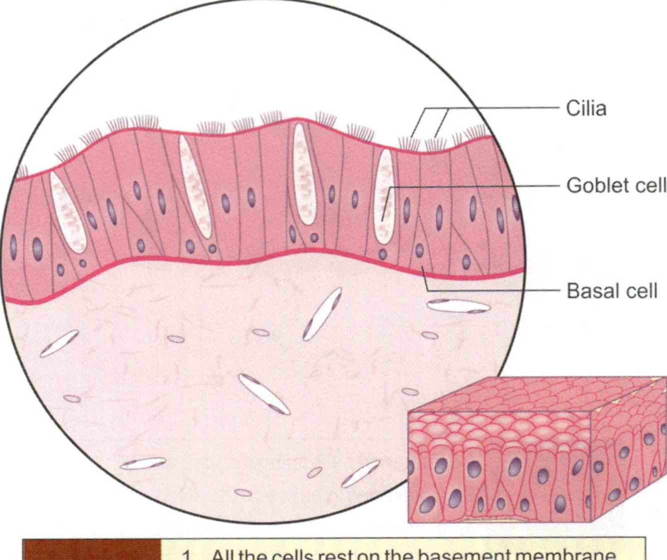

FACTS TO REMEMBER
1. All the cells rest on the basement membrane
2. Some cells are short and basal, others are tall ciliated columnar
3. A few empty-looking goblet cells are seen

Fig. 45.8: Pseudostratified columnar ciliated epithelium: Trachea

Compound Epithelium

This type of epithelium is protective in nature. Various types of compound epithelium are:

a. *Stratified columnar epithelium:* Seen in moderate sized ducts of glands, e.g. salivary glands (Fig. 45.9) and transition zone of epithelium of anal canal. It is usually made up of two layers of cells, a deeper layer of cuboidal cells and a superficial layer of columnar cells.

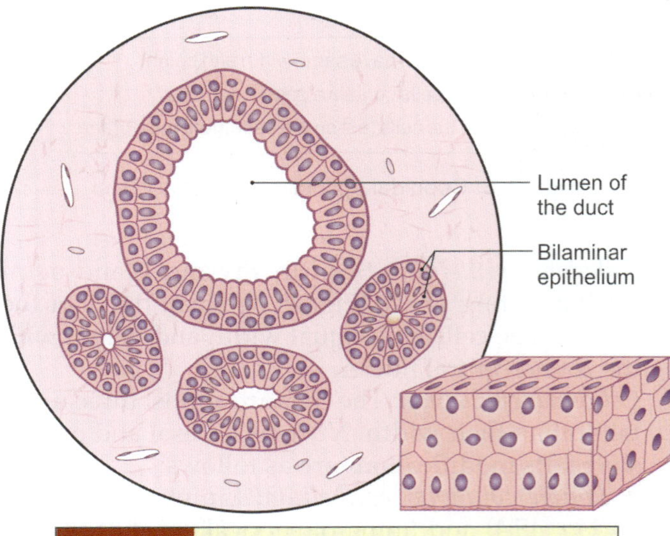

FACTS TO REMEMBER
1. Only the basal cells rest on the basement membrane
2. The basal cells are cuboidal
3. The luminal cells are columnar

Fig. 45.9: Stratified columnar epithelium: Large duct

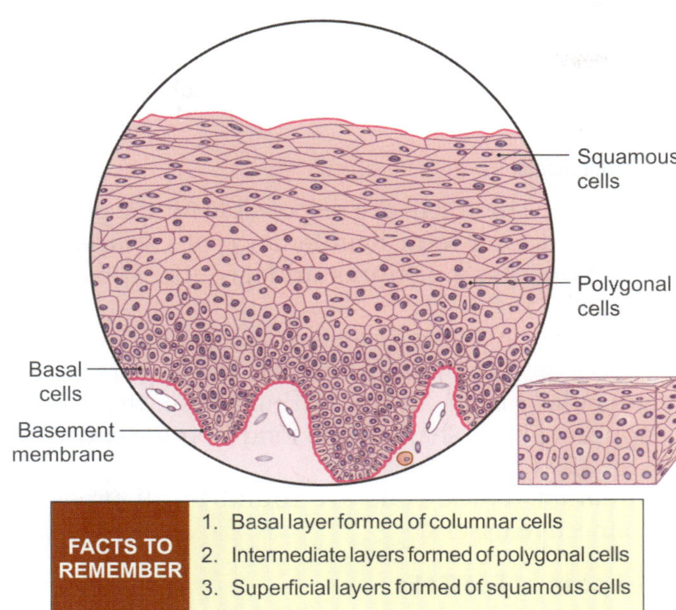

FACTS TO REMEMBER	1. Basal layer formed of columnar cells 2. Intermediate layers formed of polygonal cells 3. Superficial layers formed of squamous cells

Fig. 45.10: Stratified squamous non-keratinised epithelium: Oesophagus

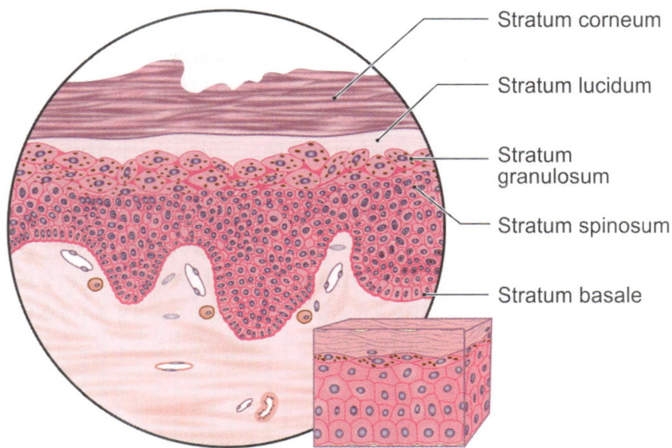

FACTS TO REMEMBER	1. Columnar cells of stratum basale rest on the basement membrane 2. Stratum spinosum, stratum granulosum, stratum lucidum and stratum corneum form the succeeding layers 3. Stratum corneum is the waterproof layer

Fig. 45.11: Stratified squamous keratinised epithelium: Skin

b. *Stratified squamous non-keratinised epithelium:* Example is oesophagus (Fig. 45.10); oral cavity and vagina. The cells occur in three layers or zones as follows:
- The deepest single layer of cells resting on the basement membrane is of columnar type and is called stratum basale.
- The intermediate zone is of 3–6 layers of polyhedral cells.
- The superficial zone is of 2–5 layers of flattened or squamous cells.

  The epithelium of oesophagus in lower animals shows keratinisation.

c. *Stratified squamous keratinised epithelium:* Seen in skin (Fig. 45.11). The layers or zones are as follows:
- *Stratum basale or stratum germinativum*: The cells are columnar, resting on the basement membrane. Varying number of pigment cells called melanocytes are also present here. These cells send dendritic processes amongst the next zone of cells. The melanocytes are derived from the neural crest.
- *Stratum spinosum*: The zone is made up of 3–7 rows of cells. The cells are polygonal in shape and are attached to each other by unstable desmosomes, giving it a prickly appearance. So this layer is known as *prickle cell layer*.
- *Stratum granulosum:* This zone consists of 2–3 layers of diamond shaped elongated cells which contain *keratohyalin granules*.
- *Stratum lucidum:* These cells lose their nuclei and form a zone of flattened ill-defined cells. These cells contain refractile *eleidin granules*. This layer looks unstained.

  v. *Stratum corneum:* The cells in this stratum are flat and cornified. The nucleus and cytoplasm get replaced by a protein called keratin. This zone is waterproof and protective in nature.

d. *Transitional epithelium:* It is a form of stratified epithelium capable of considerable distension. Examples are in the epithelium of ureter (Fig. 45.12); urinary bladder and proximal urethra.

The epithelium is made up of 4–6 layers of cells loosely applied to each other. The luminal cells are rounded or large cuboidal with a convex luminal border which stains more deeply than the cells of other layers.

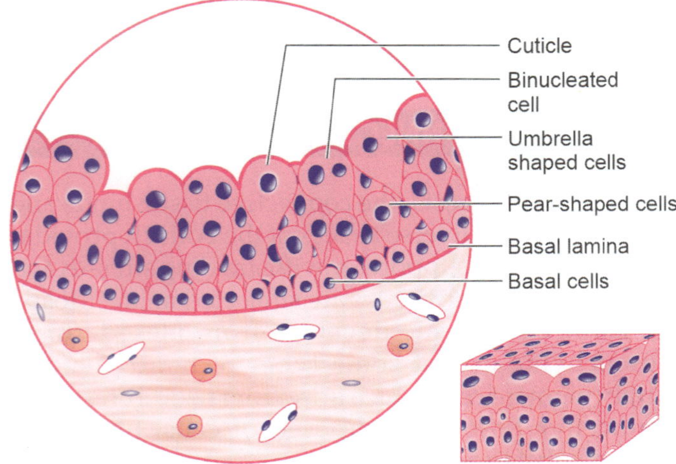

FACTS TO REMEMBER	1. The bright active luminal cells are umbrella shaped, some are binucleated 2. The pear-shaped cells form intermediate layer 3. The basal cells are cuboidal in shape

Fig. 45.12: Transitional epithelium: Ureter

These cells are also called *umbrella-shaped* cells. The surface membrane, called *cuticle* is seen as a thin eosinophilic band which makes the cells impermeable to urine present in the lumen. These cells may contain 2 nuclei and have depressions on their under surfaces to fit on the pear shaped cells of the underlying layer. The intermediate zone of cells of 2–4 rows are pear shaped or irregularly polyhedral in shape. The basal cells layer is made up of cuboidal cells. The number of cell layers decrease with distension of the organ and relatively increase when the organ is contracted or empty.

MEMBRANES

Membranes are sheets of epithelial tissue and their supporting connective tissue that lines/covers the cavities or internal structures. The membranes are of following types:

- *Mucous membrane/mucosa:* Lines the digestive tract, respiratory tract, genital tract. The epithelial cellsforming mucous membrane secrete mucus, which protects the underlying cells from mechanical or chemical injury.
- *Serous membrane/serosa:* Lines the outer aspects of the viscera. Serous membrane consists of a double layer of loose areolar tissue lined by simple squamous epithelium. Visceral layer surrounds the organ within the cavity while parietal layer lines the cavity. The two layers are separated by a thin layer of serous fluid. Serous membrane is seen in pleura, pericardium, peritoneum and tunica vaginalis of the testis. Small amount of serous fluid allows the organ free and frictionless gliding within the cavity.
- *Synovial membrane:* Lines the joint cavity. The synovial membrane secretes a clear sticky oily synovial fluid, which acts as a lubricant to the joint. The membrane consists of a thin flattened epithelial cells resting on a layer of connective tissue.

CONNECTIVE TISSUE

As the name suggests, the connective tissue binds and weaves through diverse tissues of the body. It provides them mechanical support for withstanding stresses and strains to which the tissues are subjected in life. Mostly the connective tissue develops from mesoderm or mesenchyme except some types of neuroglia and certain pigment cells which arise from neural crest cells. Connective tissue is composed of cells, fibres and ground substance.

CELLS

The cells may be

1 Fixed, e.g. fibroblasts, adipose cells, mesenchymal cells and pigment cells; or
2 Wandering, e.g. macrophages, plasma cells, mast cells and white blood cells.

FIXED CELLS

a. Fibroblasts

- *Function*: These cells are responsible for the production and long-term maintenance of extracellular components, e.g. fibres and ground substance (Fig. 45.13).
- *Morphology*: These are stem cells with multiple processes, basophilic cytoplasm, and large rounded vesicular nuclei. In the resting phase, these cells appear spindle shaped with long tapering ends and are called fibrocytes.
- *Situation:* These cells are found in all types of connective tissues.

b. Adipose or Fat Cells

- *Function*: Specialised cells for the synthesis and storage of fat (Fig. 45.13).
- *Morphology*: These cells are spherical/oval in shape. Each of the cells accumulate lipid to such an extent that the nucleus gets flattened and displaced to 'one side' and cytoplasm becomes so thinned that it is resolved only as a thin line around the rim of the single large droplet. The cells may appear singly or in groups, the resulting tissue is then called adipose tissue.

c. Mesenchymal Cells

Function: These cells have great potentialities and can change into any type of cell under a proper stimulus. Thus, mesenchymal cells are the precursors of all types of cells.

d. Pigment Cells

- *Function*: The pigment cells of skin and uveal tract protect these tissues against the harmful effects of ultraviolet light rays. Melanocytes produce the melanin and melanophores store it. Some pigment cells increase with age (Fig. 45.13).
- *Morphology*: These are stellate cells with branching processes. The cytoplasm contains dark brown/black pigment granules which are usually of melanin. These cells are of neural crest origin.

WANDERING CELLS

a. Macrophages/Histiocytes

- *Function*: Phagocytic (phage—to eat) in nature, i.e. they phagocytose and digest bacteria and foreign bodies, damaged and dead tissues.
- *Morphology*: These cells may be fusiform, stellate or spheroidal in shape. The nucleus tends to be smaller, darkly stained, usually indented and lies at one end

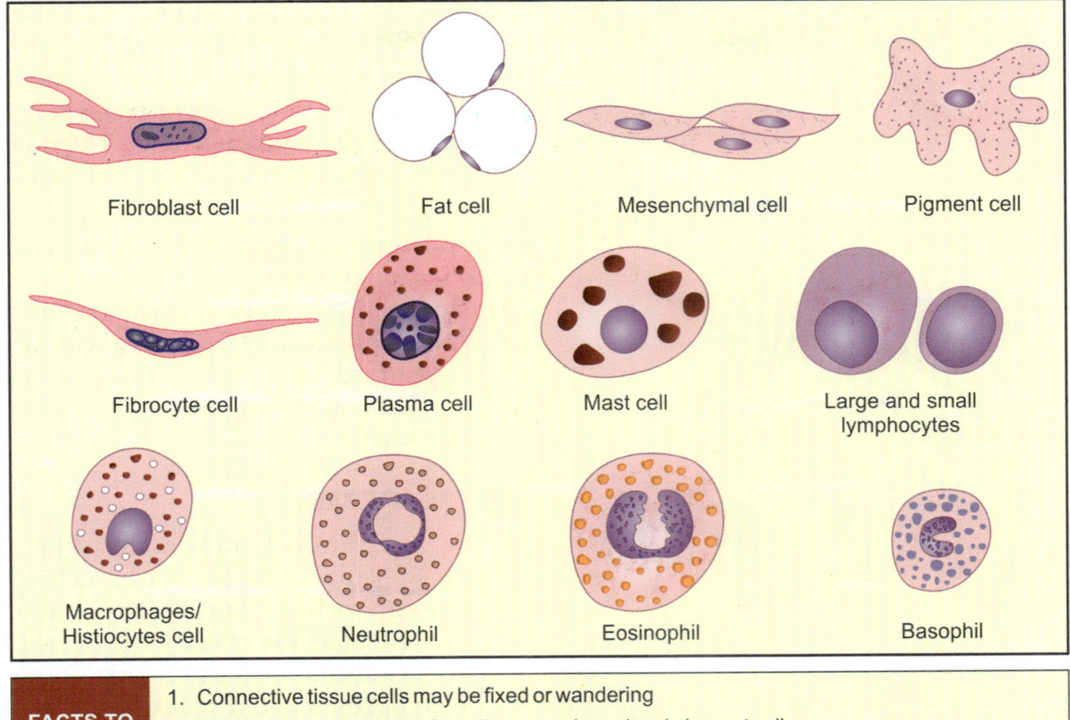

FACTS TO REMEMBER
1. Connective tissue cells may be fixed or wandering
2. Fixed cells are fibroblast, fat cell, mesenchymal and pigment cells
3. Wandering cells are macrophages, plasma cell, mast cell and white blood cells

Fig. 45.13: Various cells of connective tissue, 400X

of the cell. The cytoplasm often contains a variety of granules and vacuoles.

b. Plasma Cells

- *Function*: These are specialised for the manufacture of antibodies against antigens. Thus they impart resistance to the body against diseases (Fig. 45.13).
- *Morphology*: The cells are ovoid in shape, with a slightly eccentric, oval or round nucleus and intensely basophilic cytoplasm. The chromatin in the nucleus is arranged in a radial pattern, giving it a *cart wheel appearance*.

c. Mast Cells

- *Function*: These cells secrete
  a. Histamine responsible for producing allergic symptoms
  b. Heparin, the anticoagulant (Fig. 45.13)
  c. 5-hydroxytryptamine or serotonin which is vasoconstrictor.
- *Morphology*: These cells are large round or ovoid in shape. The nucleus is round and small, relative to the size of the cell. The cytoplasm is packed by intensely stained, coarse granules. The granules can be easily seen with methylene blue injection. The cytoplasmic coarse granules exhibit metachromasia, i.e. depict purple staining reaction when stained with either toluidine blue or alcian blue.
- *Situation*: Widely distributed in the connective tissues, serous membranes like peritoneum and pleura. These are also seen along the course of blood vessels.

d. White Blood Cells

For example, lymphocytes, neutrophils, eosinophil and basophil

- *Function*: These carry the antibodies and phagocytose bacteria, etc.
- *Morphology*: Lymphocytes are large or small according to the amount of contained cytoplasm. Neutrophils have usually three to five lobes of nuclei with small or fine eosinophilic granules. Eosinophils are associated with allergic reactions while small basophils are responsible for anaphylaxis.

FIBRES

Fibres are of three types (Fig. 45.14):

- Collagen fibres
- Elastic fibres
- Reticular fibres

COLLAGEN FIBRES

These are seen in all types of connective tissue (aponeurosis and superficial fascia). In unstained preparations of loose connective tissue, the collagen

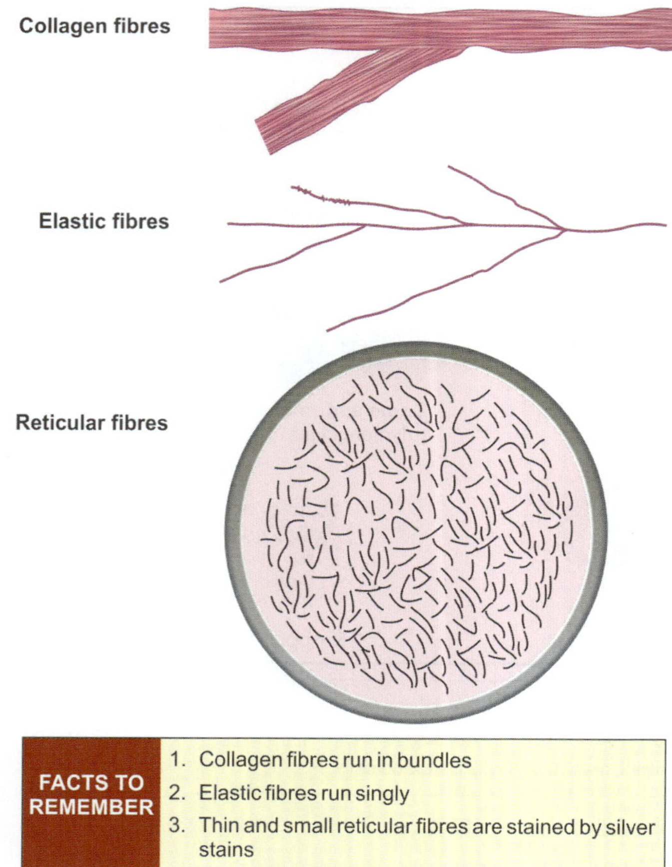

Fig. 45.14: Various fibres of connective tissue, 100X

fibres appear as colourless strands. These are made up of fibrils which run in various bundles and the bundles split into branches. The fibres are synthesised by the fibroblasts and are made up of a protein called collagen (Fig. 45.14).

a. ***Properties***
   - Fresh fibres appear colourless and run in bundles.
   - With haematoxylin and eosin the fibres are stained pink.
   - Van Gieson's stains them red.
   - If collagen fibres are treated with dilute acetic acid, they swell up. Acid digestion leads to the formation of gelatin.

b. According to the chemical composition, collagen fibres are classified into four grades. Grade I are the thickest fibres seen in bone and connective tissue.
   Grade II are visible in the hyaline cartilage.
   Grade III are in the walls of arteries.
   Grade IV are the thinnest fibres present in the basement membranes. Grade IV fibres are also termed as the reticular fibres.

ELASTIC FIBRES

These are found in the ligamentum nuchae, ligamentum flavum and in the walls of the large arteries. When in sufficient number, the fibres appear yellow in colour. These are made up of a protein called **Elastin**, which is highly resistant to boiling as well as dilute acids and alkalies. The fibres run singly, branch and anastomose with each other. When a fibre is broken, the ends retract or recoil (Figs 45.15 and 45.16).

Properties
- Fresh fibres appear colourless, run singly and branch to form network.
- With haemotoxylin and eosin the fibres appear pink.
- Elastic fibres stain dark brown with Verhoeff's stain.
- These fibres do not swell after treatment with acetic acid. They are synthesised by fibroblasts and smooth muscle cells.

RETICULAR FIBRES

These are seen in lymph nodes, liver, thymus and spleen. Reticular fibres are fine branching fibres, which form a supporting framework for the rich cellular lymphoreticular system and hepatocytes. The fibres are very delicate and form a network. These are Grade IV collagen fibres. *Staining properties*: These fibres cannot be seen with haematoxylin and eosin stain. Silver staining methods stain the reticular fibres black (Fig. 45.14).

GROUND SUBSTANCE

The formed elements of connective tissue, e.g. cells and fibres are embedded in the ground substance. Intercellular substance is the term used for combination of ground substance and fibres. Ground substance is comprised of water, carbohydrate and glycoproteins. The carbohydrates are in the form of polysaccharides, *sulphated* and *non-sulphated*. The former are comprised of *chondroitin sulphate* and keratosulphate, while the latter group belongs to hyaluronic acid.

Hyaluronic acid binds down water to the tissues and controls permeability of the ground substance. Hyaluronidase, an enzyme, dissolves the hyaluronic acid and increases tissue permeability. Thus, bacteria producing the enzyme hyaluronidase tend to spread the infection quickly.

Depending upon the relative proportion of cells, fibres and ground substance, the connective tissue is classified as follows:

CLASSIFICATION OF CONNECTIVE TISSUE

I. LOOSE CONNECTIVE TISSUE

1 *Areolar tissue,* e.g. superficial fascia (Fig. 45.15). It shows collagen fibres in bundles and elastic fibres dispersed singly. The nuclei seen belong to fibroblasts. Various other cell types may be seen scattered among the connective tissue fibres.

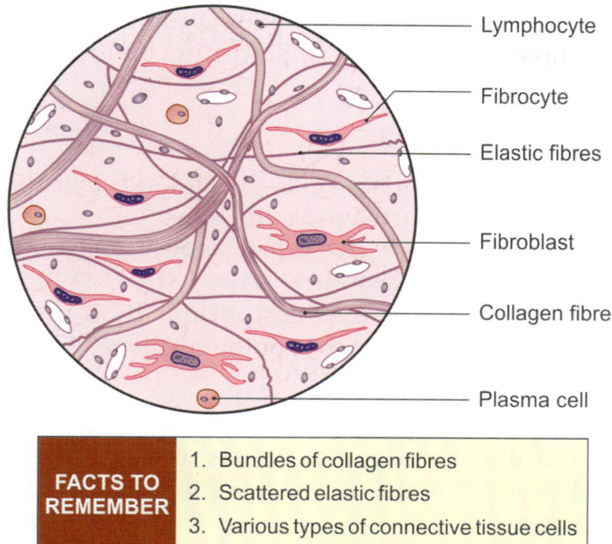

FACTS TO REMEMBER	
	1. Bundles of collagen fibres
	2. Scattered elastic fibres
	3. Various types of connective tissue cells

Fig. 45.15: Areolar tissue: Superficial fascia

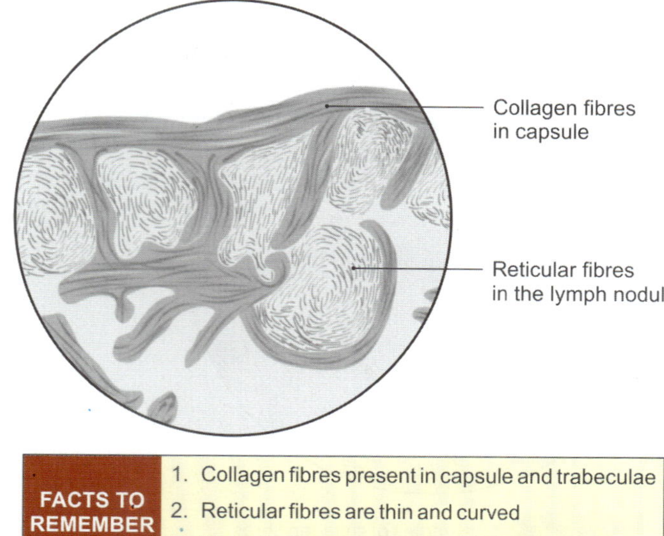

FACTS TO REMEMBER	
	1. Collagen fibres present in capsule and trabeculae
	2. Reticular fibres are thin and curved
	3. Reticular fibres support the cellular elements

Fig. 45.17: Reticular tissue: Spleen

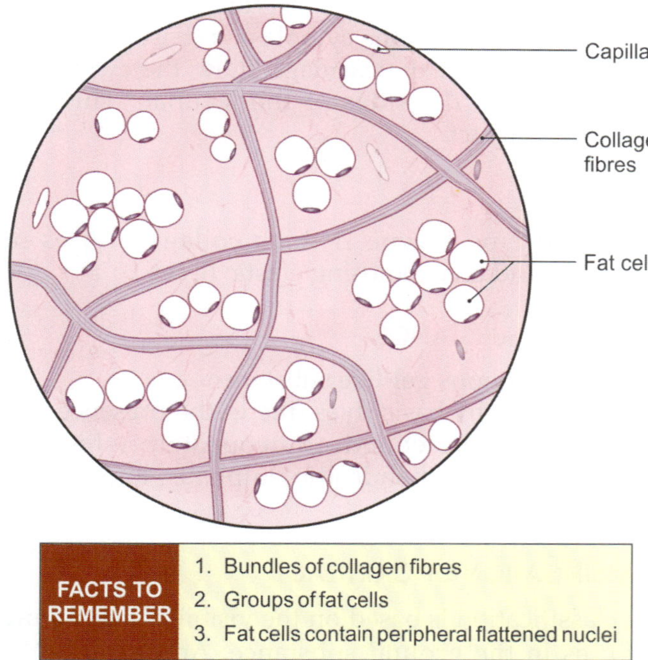

FACTS TO REMEMBER	
	1. Bundles of collagen fibres
	2. Groups of fat cells
	3. Fat cells contain peripheral flattened nuclei

Fig. 45.16: Adipose tissue: Mesentery

2 *Adipose tissue,* e.g. mesentery (Fig. 45.16). Adipose tissue contains fat cells (adipose cells). The fat cells synthesise and store large amounts of lipids.

The adipose tissue is also of two types:

- *White adipose tissue:* It contains unilocular fat cells. It is present in superficial fascia, in the mesentery, around eyeball and kidneys.
- *Brown adipose tissue:* It contains multilocular fat cells. The lipid is in form of small droplets and the round nucleus is pushed to one side. It is seen in newborn babies in some regions like the posterior triangle of neck and posterior abdominal wall. As the child grows the multiple fat droplets coalesce to form single fat droplet thus reducing the brown adipose tissue in adult. The brown adipose tissue is also seen in hibernating animals.

The brown colour of fat is because of presence of huge amounts of cytochrome oxidase present in mitochondria. This type of fat maintains the normal body temperature. The protein thermogenin of mitochondria regulates the temperature.

3 *Reticular tissue,* e.g. spleen, (Fig. 45.17), liver lymph node. Reticular tissue contains reticular fibres which get stained with silver stains.

4 *Myxomatous tissue,* e.g. umbilical cord (Fig. 45.18), vitreous humour of eye. This tissue shows fine collagen fibres with stellate-shaped cells and their nuclei. The matrix is mucoid in nature.

II. DENSE CONNECTIVE TISSUE

Dense connective tissue: The dense connective tissue is of following 2 types:

1 *Dense ordinary connective tissue*

- *Ordinary irregular dense connective tissue:* It is seen in the dermis of skin as papillary and reticular layers. The connective tissue is irregular in its disposition (Fig. 45.53).
- *Ordinary regular dense connective tissue:* The collagen fibres are arranged in a closely packed bundles in regular parallel manner with fibroblast nuclei which get pressed due to pressure of fibres. This type of tissue is seen in tendons of the muscles as these cross the joints. Tendons are easily visible on the dorsum of hands and feet (Fig. 45.19).

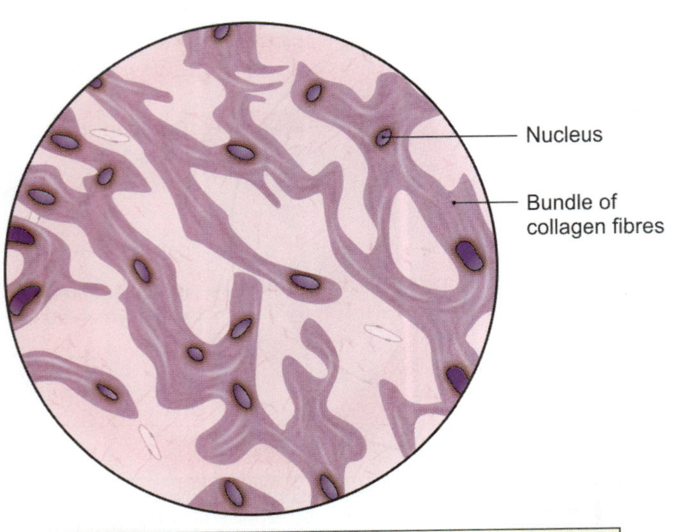

FACTS TO REMEMBER	1. Bundles of collagen fibres 2. Stellate-shaped cells 3. Seen in umbilical cord and vitreous humour

Fig. 45.18: Myxomatous tissue: Umbilical cord

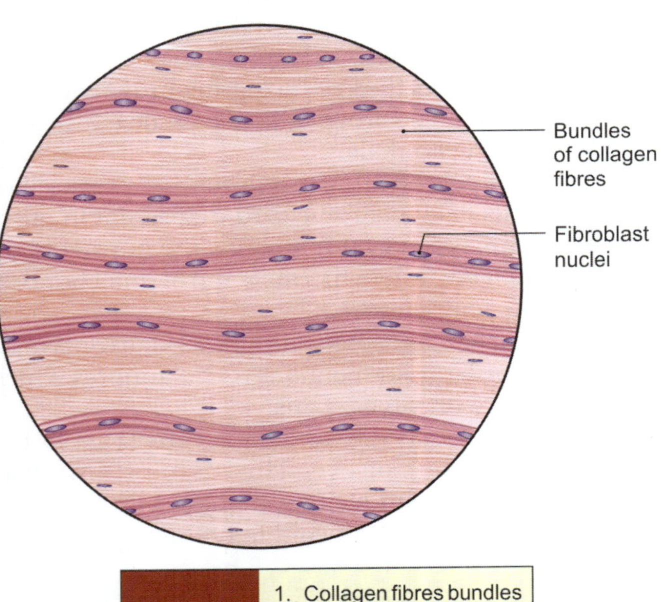

FACTS TO REMEMBER	1. Collagen fibres bundles 2. Fibroblast nuclei 3. Seen in tendons

Fig. 45.19: Dense connective tissue: Tendon

CARTILAGE

Cartilage is a specialised dense connective tissue. It is described in Chapter 2, Table 2.3 and Figs 2.6–2.7.

Functions

- It bears the weight of the body and plays an important role during the growth in length of long bones.
- Gives support to developing organs.
- Cartilage helps in withstanding bending and torsional forces.

Composition

The cartilage comprises cells, ground substance and fibres. Growth in cartilage occurs by:

a. *Appositional growth:* By surface deposition from the cells of inner perichondrial layer.
b. *Interstitial growth:* By the multiplication of cells situated within the matrix of the cartilage.

1. CELLS OF THE CARTILAGE

The mature cartilage consists of cells called chondrocytes, situated in spaces of the matrix known as lacunae.

Single cells are spherical in shape but the small groups of 2–4 cells are rounded with flat opposing surfaces (D-shaped). These group of cells are termed as 'cell nests'.

The nuclei of the cartilage cells are large and round with 1–2 nucleoli and the cytoplasm is basophilic. The stained sections of the cartilage show the cytoplasm shrunken from the sides of the lacunae. This is a shrinkage artefact.

2. FIBRES

Fibres are type I/type II thick collagen fibres or branching and anastomosing elastic fibres.

3. GROUND SUBSTANCE

It is an amorphous gel-like substance.

It is stained by basic dyes due to the presence of a glycoprotein, the chondromucoprotein which on hydrolysis yields chondroitin sulphates and kerato-sulphates.

CLASSIFICATION OF CARTILAGE

The classification is based on the visibility and nature of fibres in the ground substance. Accordingly the cartilage is classified as:

1 Hyaline cartilage containing thin (invisible) bundles of collagen fibres.
2 Elastic cartilage with branching elastic fibres.
3 Fibrocartilage containing thick bundles of collagen fibres.

HYALINE CARTILAGE

Features

- Cells are encapsulated in groups of 2–6 "Cell nests".
- The matrix appears homogeneous and has affinity for basic dyes (Fig. 45.20).

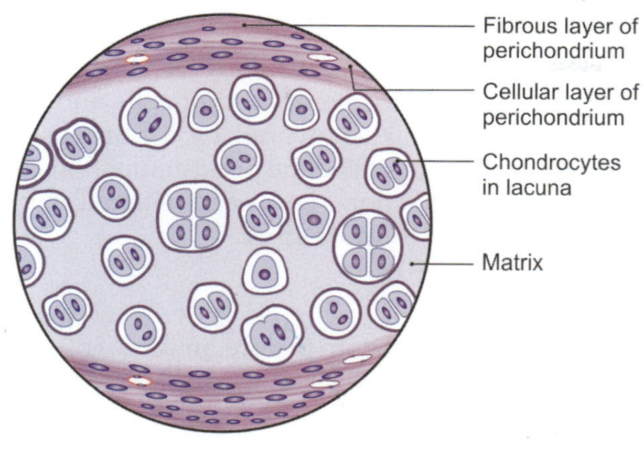

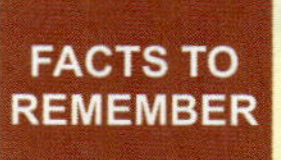
FACTS TO REMEMBER

1. Perichondrium seen all around
2. Ground substance appears homogeneous
3. Chondrocytes in lacuna lie in groups of 2–4 cells

Fig. 45.20: Hyaline cartilage: Trachea

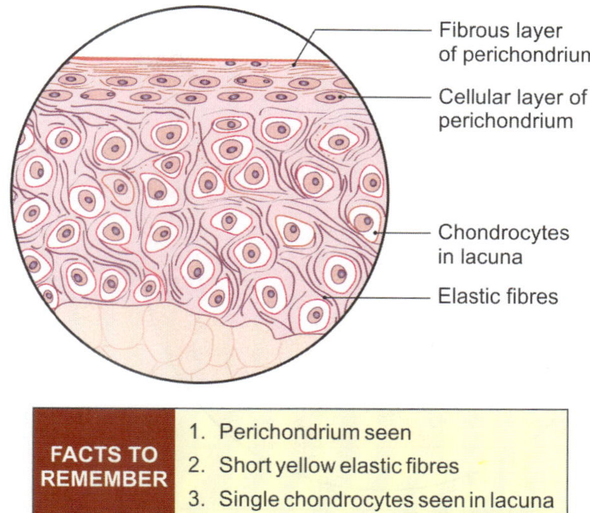

FACTS TO REMEMBER

1. Perichondrium seen
2. Short yellow elastic fibres
3. Single chondrocytes seen in lacuna

Fig. 45.21: Elastic cartilage: Epiglottis

- The type II collagen fibrils are not seen as a distinct entity in hyaline cartilage since the refractive index of fibres and ground substance is same.

ELASTIC CARTILAGE

This type of cartilage has elasticity, i.e. it comes back to its natural size after being stretched, i.e. it is highly flexible. It is present in pinna (external ear), epiglottis, external auditory meatus, part of arytenoid, corniculate and cuneiform cartilages. In fresh state this cartilage is yellowish in colour (Fig. 45.21).

Features

- Chondrocytes are larger than those of hyaline cartilage and are present singly or in small groups.
- The ground substance contains abundance of branching and anastomosing elastic fibres.
- Perichondrium is present and is comprised of an outer fibrous and an inner chondrogenic and vascular layer.

FIBROCARTILAGE

It is also termed as white fibrocartilage and is present in intervertebral discs, pubic symphysis, intra-articular discs (Fig. 45.22). It provides tensile strength, resists compression and bears weight.

Features

- Most of the chondrocytes lie singly and are in smaller numbers. These are squeezed and aligned in narrow rows between the thick parallel bundles of type I collagen fibres situated in the ground substance.
- Perichondrium is characteristically absent in the adult fibrocartilage (Table 45.1).

Table 45.1: Comparison of types of cartilages

	Hyaline cartilage	*Elastic cartilage*	*Fibrocartilage*
Perichondrium	Present, comprising of an outer fibrous layer and inner chondrogenic vascular layer	Present, comprising of an outer fibrous layer and inner chondrogenic vascular layer	Absent
Fibres	Thin collagen fibres	Elastic fibres branching and anastomosing	Thick bundles of collagen fibres
Cells	Chondroblasts and chondrocytes	Chondroblasts and chondrocytes	Fibroblasts and chondrocytes
Ground substance	Glycoprotein—the chondromucoprotein	Glycoprotein—the chondromucoprotein	Minimal ground substance
Calcification	Occurs in old age	Does not occur	Occurs only during bone repair
Sites	Most of the respiratory system, ossifying bones	External ear, epiglottis, cuneiform and corniculate cartilages of larynx	Intervertebral discs, menisci of knee joint and intra-articular discs of the joints

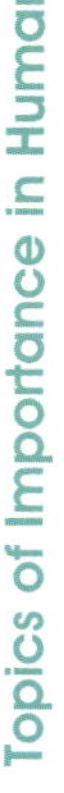

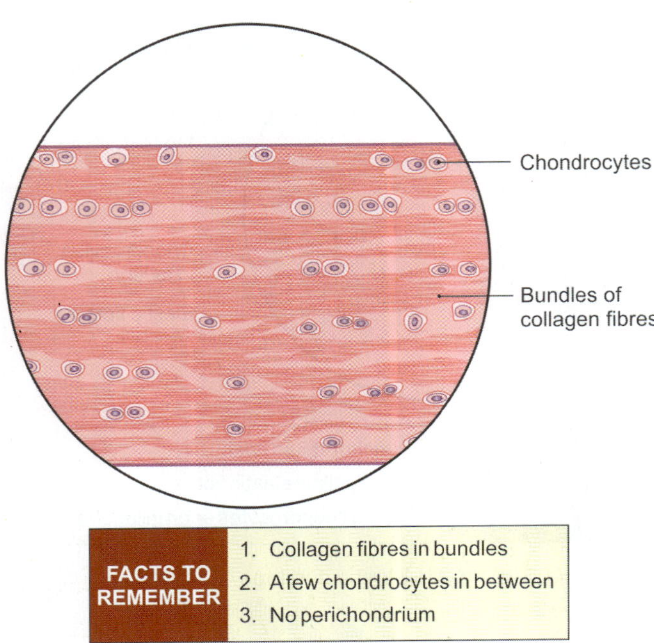

FACTS TO REMEMBER	1. Collagen fibres in bundles 2. A few chondrocytes in between 3. No perichondrium

Fig. 45.22: White fibrocartilage: Intervertebral disc

Nutrition of all cartilages: The nutrition of mature cartilage is derived by diffusion from capillaries in the adjoining connective tissue or by means of synovial fluid from joint cavities. Lack of nutrition affects the cartilage adversely. Lack of vitamins and proteins results in diminished thickness of epiphyseal plate. Deficiency of vitamin C causes improper matrix, while lack of vitamin D results in excessive proliferation of cartilage with diminished ossification, leading to deformity of bones.

BONE

Bone is another specialised dense connective tissue, where the matrix is impregnated with calcium salts making it hard and rigid. The calcium salts exist in the form of hydroxyapatite crystals $[Ca_{10}(PO_4)_6(OH)_2]$ in the form of 'plates or rods'. Matrix is the complex of organic and inorganic intercellular substances which surrounds the osteocytes in a bone.

FUNCTIONS

a. It is the storehouse of calcium and minerals
b. Bone marrow present in the bones manufacture RBC, granular WBC and platelets
c. Bones provide attachment to muscles and act as levers for movements
d. Bones form cavities for enclosing and protecting various viscera
e. Bones form supporting framework for whole body and transmit the body weight.

CHARACTERISTIC FEATURES

Bone has an organised canalicular mechanism and is highly vascular. Bone is composed of cells and intercellular substances. It is covered by a fibrovascular osteogenic membrane called the periosteum. Bone only grows by surface accretions, i.e. by appositional growth. It is a vascular tissue (Table 45.2).

CELLS OF BONE

a. *Osteogenic cells*: These are the precursors of other cell types and are found in the inner layer of the periosteum.
b. *Osteoblasts*: These are found where active bone is being formed. These are large basophilic cells with large rounded eccentric nuclei. These cells lay down fibres and matrix in the areas of bone formation.
c. *Osteocytes*: These are resting cells enclosed in the bony matrix. Osteocytes lie in spaces/lacunae in the matrix. Radiating in all directions from the lacunae are exceedingly slender branching tubular passages called the canaliculi. The canaliculi anastomose with similar canaliculi of the neighbouring lacunae. The processes of osteocytes occupy these canaliculi. The cytoplasm of osteocytes is less basophilic.
d. *Osteoclasts:* These are large/giant cells present where bony resorption is required. The cytoplasm is eosinophilic and nuclei are 5–15 in number. All the four types of bony cells work in harmony under normal circumstances.

INTERCELLULAR SUBSTANCES/MATRIX

a. *Inorganic matter*: It is comprised of calcium hydroxyapatite crystals $[Ca_{10}(PO_4)_6(OH)_2]$. The inorganic matter provides rigidity to the bone. If bone is put in strong acids, the salts get dissolved, and bone becomes flexible. Then it can be tied as a knot.
b. *Organic matter*: Formed by dense bundles of collagen fibres embedded in amorphous ground substance comprised of protein polysaccharides and hyaluronic acid. All these elements are secreted by osteoblasts. Organic matter can be destroyed by burning when the bone becomes brittle though its shape is retained.

HISTOLOGICAL CLASSIFICATION OF BONE

I. Compact or Dense

Bone is harder and denser, e.g. shaft of long bones.

II. Cancellous or Spongy

Bone has bigger marrow spaces and is relatively less hard, e.g. the ends of long bones.

MICROSCOPIC STRUCTURE OF COMPACT BONE

1 Bone is covered by the periosteum, consisting of an outer fibrous layer and an inner osteogenic and vascular layers. Collagen fibres from this layer penetrate into the outermost lamellae of bone nailing the two together. These are termed Sharpey's fibres.

2 Characteristic histologic feature of compact bone is haversian system or osteon. Each haversian system comprises the following:

a. A centrally situated haversian canal containing fine vessels, nerves and lymphatics. The haversian canal is surrounded by 6–12 concentric lamellae (Fig. 45.23).

b. Haversian lamella or matrix is composed of collagen fibres and the deposited calcium salts. The collagen bundles run spirally along the long diameter of the bone. The pitch and direction vary in the adjacent bundles. The variation in pitch and direction causes the lamellar appearance.

c. Between the lamellae or on the lamellae are small spaces/lacunae imprisoning the osteocytes. Canaliculi from the adjacent lacunae communicate with each other. These canaliculi are occupied by the processes of the osteocyte. Through these processes the nourishment reaches the distantly placed osteocytes.

d. Haversian canals are connected with one another and communicate with the marrow cavity via canals called Volkmann's canals.

e. Interstitial lamellae lie in the angles between the adjoining haversian lamellae. These lamellae belong to the relatively older bone. These lamellae also contain lacunae and canaliculi.

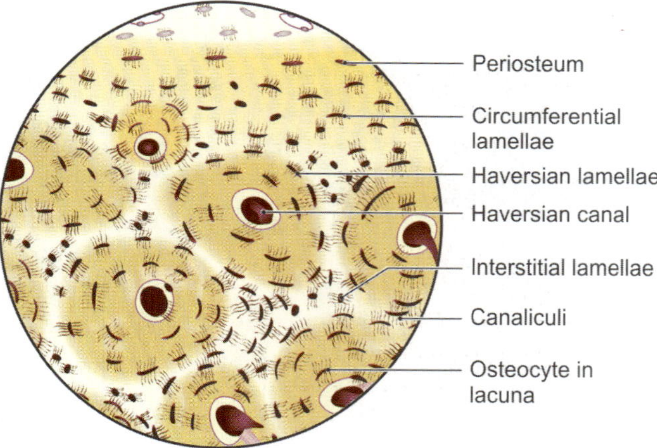

FACTS TO REMEMBER	
	1. Outer periosteum seen
	2. Three types of lamellae seen: haversian, interstitial and circumferential
	3. In between lamellae are osteocytes in the lacuna with canaliculi

Fig. 45.23: Shaft of a long bone

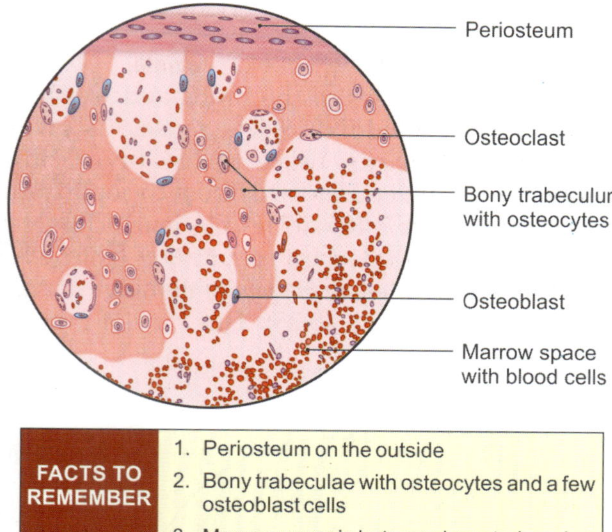

FACTS TO REMEMBER	
	1. Periosteum on the outside
	2. Bony trabeculae with osteocytes and a few osteoblast cells
	3. Marrow space in between bony trabeculae

Fig. 45.24: Cancellous bone

f. Subjacent to the periosteum are the outer circumferential lamellae.

g. Similarly next to the endosteum are the inner circumferential lamellae.

MICROSCOPIC STRUCTURE OF CANCELLOUS/SPONGY BONE

a. Haversian systems are absent in spongy bone.

b. Bone tissue is arranged as thin plates or trabeculae (Fig. 42.24).

c. Between the adjoining trabeculae are large irregular spaces containing red bone marrow.

d. At the margin of trabeculum are osteoblasts and osteoclasts and in the lacunae of trabeculum are present the osteocytes.

e. Cancellous bone is covered with the periosteum.

MUSCULAR TISSUE

Muscular tissue is responsible for movement of various parts of body with respect to one another. All muscles comprise elongated cells called fibres. The cytoplasm of muscle fibre is sarcoplasm, and the cell membrane is sarcolemma. The fibre contains myofibrils made of proteins myofilaments actin and myosin.

Types

1 Striated or skeletal or striped or voluntary.

2 Smooth or unstriated or unstriped or involuntary.

3 Cardiac or striated and involuntary.

See Chapter 4 for comparison of the muscle fibers.

SKELETAL MUSCLE

Skeletal or Striated Muscle

It is present in muscles of the limbs and trunk, e.g. deltoid and rectus abdominis. The muscle as a whole is enclosed in a connective tissue layer called *epimysium*. Septa extend inwards from the epimysium dividing the muscle into various fasciculi. Thus, each fasciculus is surrounded by *perimysium* from which extend fine septa called *endomysium* that invest individual muscle fibres (Fig. 45.25). This type of muscle is under conscious control.

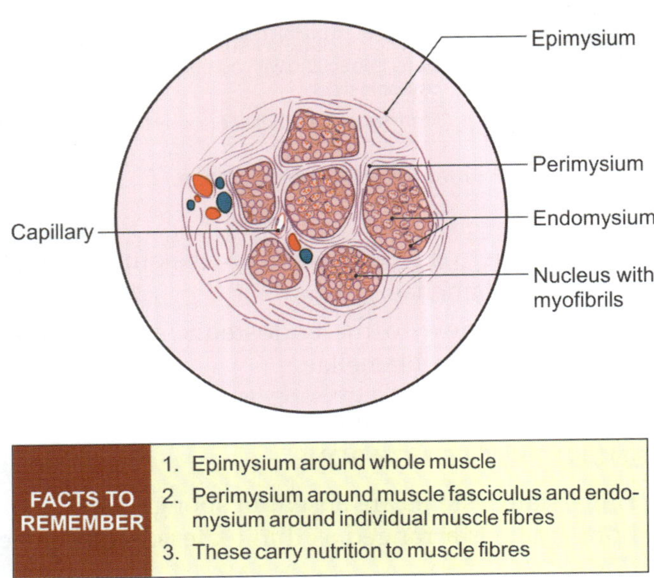

FACTS TO REMEMBER	
	1. Epimysium around whole muscle
	2. Perimysium around muscle fasciculus and endomysium around individual muscle fibres
	3. These carry nutrition to muscle fibres

Fig. 45.25: Deltoid muscle of a limb (transverse section)

Structure of Skeletal Muscle

With haemotoxylin and eosin stain, skeletal muscle fibres are seen as highly eosinophilic cylinders with multiple peripheral nuclei taking up a basic stain. Each fibre is surrounded by an outer limiting membrane called *sarcolemma* (Fig. 45.26).

The cytoplasm or sarcoplasm contains extensive sarcoplasmic reticulum, mitochondria and glycogen granules as well as large number of longitudinally running myofibrils. Under high power, the myofibrils depict alternate dark and light bands. These dark and light bands in all the myofibrils are "in register", providing a continuous cross striations in the muscle fibre. These well marked transverse/cross striations are a diagnostic and characteristic feature of the striated muscle (*see* Chapter 2).

These are mostly seen beneath the sarcolemma at the periphery of the fibre. Some nuclei appearing in the central part of the fibre belong to the connective tissue around the muscle fibres.

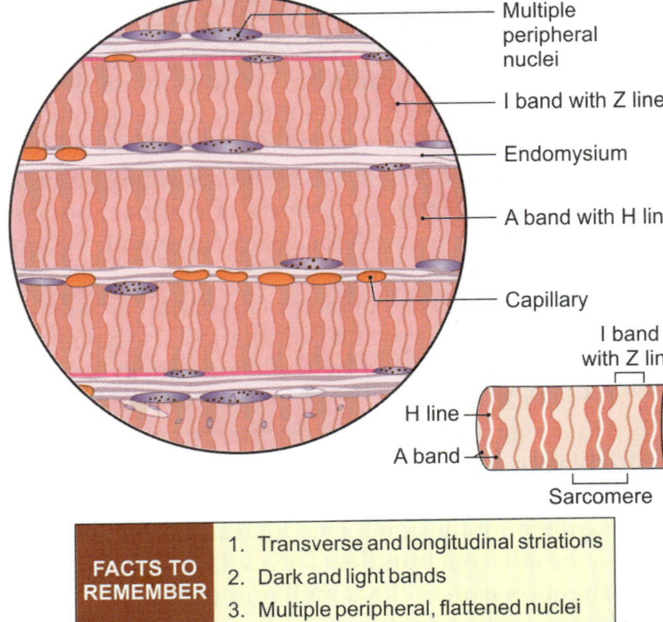

FACTS TO REMEMBER	
	1. Transverse and longitudinal striations
	2. Dark and light bands
	3. Multiple peripheral, flattened nuclei

Fig. 45.26: Striated muscle (longitudinal section): Tongue

SMOOTH MUSCLE

Smooth muscle is present in muscle of stomach, intestine, urinary and genital tracts, and in walls of blood vessels. A smooth muscle fibre or myocyte is an elongated spindle shaped or fusiform cell, which contains a single centrally placed nucleus (Fig. 45.27). The cell membrane is called the plasmalemma, and its cytoplasm is termed as the sarcoplasm. The sarcoplasm is eosinophilic and homogeneous. There are no transverse striations. However, longitudinal striations are visible.

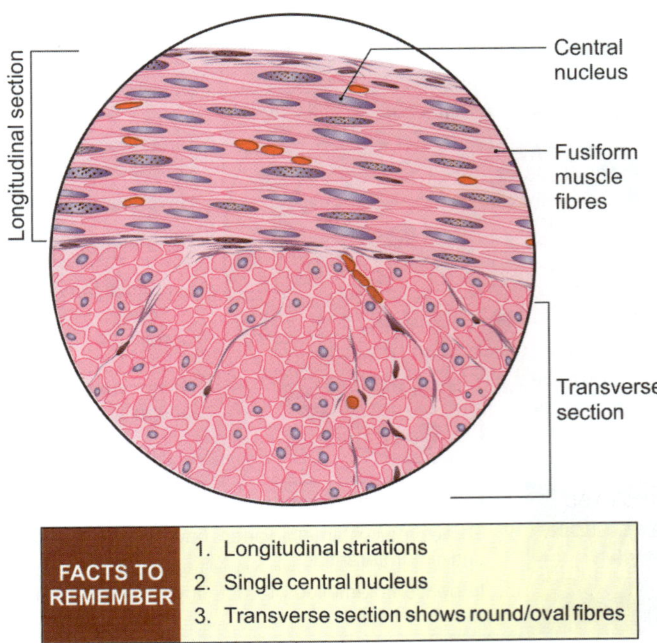

FACTS TO REMEMBER	
	1. Longitudinal striations
	2. Single central nucleus
	3. Transverse section shows round/oval fibres

Fig. 45.27: Smooth muscle: Stomach

Fibres in the smooth muscle are arranged in bundles. The thick segment of one fibre lies opposite the thin segment of the adjacent fibre and the nuclei are contained in the central thick segments only. The transverse section of the muscle would show fibres of varying sizes. Only the larger fibres have round central nuclei.

There is minimal connective tissue between the adjacent fibres. The smooth muscle fibres appear as sheets as these are connected to each other through nexus which is fusion of plasma membranes of adjacent myocytes (Fig. 45.27). Actin and myosin filaments are present, but lack regular arrangement or striations.

CARDIAC MUSCLE

Example of cardiac muscle is the muscle of the heart and large vessels attached to the heart. Cardiac muscle resembles skeletal muscle partially. Cross striations of actin and myosin filaments form A band, I band. It consists of short/cylindrical muscle fibres, which branch and anastomose with each other. Each fibre contains a single oval centrally placed large nucleus. Some cells show a perinuclear clear space. The transverse striations are present but are not as conspicuous as in skeletal muscle (Fig. 45.28).

The muscle fibres are joined together by surface specialisations known as intercalated discs which contain gap junctions. These intercalated/intercalary discs or junctional complexes appear as zigzag transverse lines and are caused by the apposed plasma membranes of the two fibres. These intercalated discs are better visible by silver stains. The spaces between the branchings of muscle fibres are occupied by fine connective tissue and blood capillaries. With increasing age, lipofuscin pigment is, deposited around the nuclei of the muscle fibres. Mitochondria are more abundant and larger in cardiac muscle.

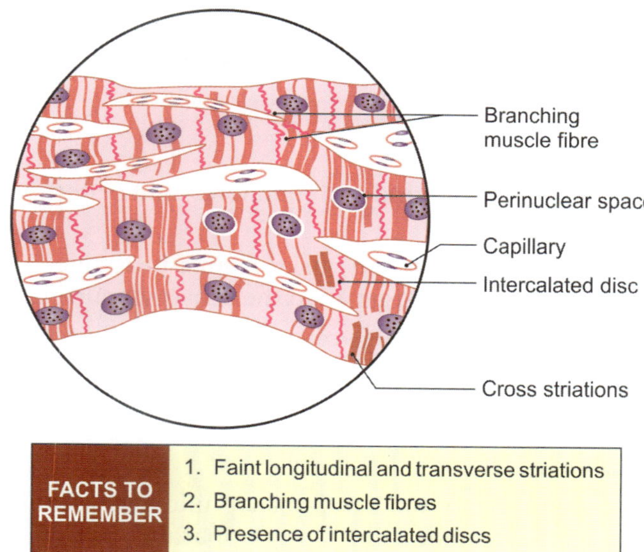

Fig. 45.28: Cardiac muscle

Table 45.2 shows comparison of these muscle fibers.

NERVOUS TISSUE

Nervous tissue is the specialised tissue responsible for excitability and conduction of impulses. Nervous tissue comprises:

Table 45.2: Comparing various types of muscles

Features	*Skeletal muscle*	*Smooth muscle*	*Cardiac muscle*
Location	Mostly in limbs, trunk	In wall of viscera, blood vessels	Heart
Connective tissue	Encloses the muscle as epimysium, perimysium and endomysium	Organised as only endomysium	Organised as only endomysium
Fibre:			
Length	Very long	Up to 15–200 mm	50–100 mm
Width	Wide fibre	Small	Small
Striations	Transverse striations prominent	Not seen	Faint transverse striations
Nucleus	Peripheral and multi-nucleated	Central and single	Central and single
Shape	Cylindrical	Spindle shaped	Short cylinders with branches
Junctional complexes	Nil	Gap junctions	Intercalated discs with desmosome
Nerve supply	Cranial and spinal nerves	Autonomic nervous system	Autonomic nervous system
Activity	Voluntary contraction strong, discontinuous quick voluntary contraction	Slow, weak involuntary contraction	Quick, strong continuous involuntary contraction

Neuron, i.e. nerve cells with its processes.

Neuroglia, the cellular connective tissue of the nervous system.

NEURON

Neuron is the structural and functional unit of nervous tissue.

Size: The size of a neuron varies from 4 to 20 microns. Motor neurons are larger than the sensory neurons.

Nucleus: It is large, pale, vesicular and usually central in position. It has a fine chromatin network and a large prominent nucleolus. The *sex chromatin* in the females is often visible as being attached to the nuclear membrane.

Cytoplasm: The cytoplasm is basophilic and contains usual cell organelles like Golgi apparatus and mitochondria. But the *centrosome* is conspicuously absent in mature neuron showing its inability to divide. The cytoplasm of neuron contains two specialised organelles, e.g. Nissl granules and neurofibrils (Fig. 45.29).

Nissl granules are chromophilic bodies which give a granular appearance to the neurons. These are easily stained by toluidine blue and cresyl violet. Nissl granules are the rough endoplasmic reticulum, responsible for synthesis of proteins. These are usually present around the nucleus and in the dendrites, but are absent from the axon hillock (the part of neuron which gives origin to the axon) and axon. Nissl granules degenerate due to fatigue/injury to the neuron and the process is called *chromatolysis*. Neurons synthesise neurotransmitters and neurohormones.

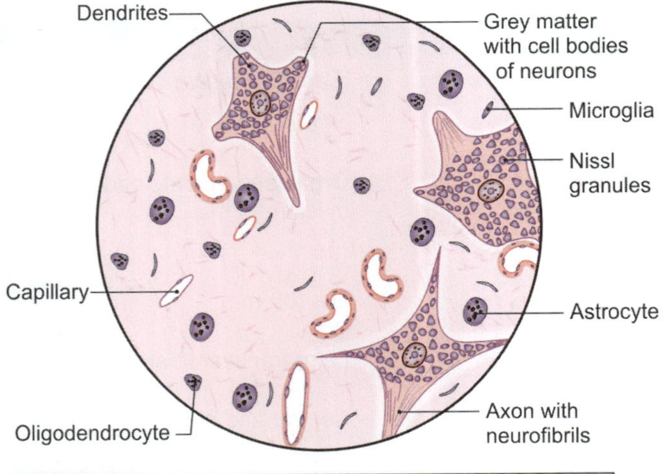

FACTS TO REMEMBER	1. Multipolar neuron is large irregular cell with central nucleus 2. Has multiple dendrites, single axon 3. Also seen are the astrocyte, oligodendrocyte, microglia, capillaries

Fig. 45.29: Grey matter of spinal cord

Neurofibrils are thread like structures easily stained with silver impregnation techniques. They form a plexiform pattern in the cell body and are arranged in parallel manner in both the dendrites and axon of the neuron. The neurofibrils give support to the body and processes of the neuron.

Pigments as inclusions are also present in the neuron in the form of lipofuscin and melanin. These increase with age.

Classification of neurons according to number of processes. Comparison of axon and dendrite, functions of neurologlical cells are given in Chapter 7.

NEUROGLIA

This is the cellular connective tissue of the nervous system. Various cells of neuroglia are:

Astrocytes: Protoplasmic and fibrous for nutrition of the neuron (Fig. 45.30).

Oligodendrocytes: For laying down myelin sheath in CNS.

Microglia: Phagocytose cellular debris.

Ependymal cells: Line the central canal of spinal cord and ventricles of brain.

Satellite or capsular cells: Surround the neurons of the ganglia.

Schwann cells: Lay down myelin sheath on peripheral nerves.

Astrocytes

These are star-shaped cells with multiple processes. These cells are small with large vesicular indented nuclei, and cytoplasm drawn into number of processes.

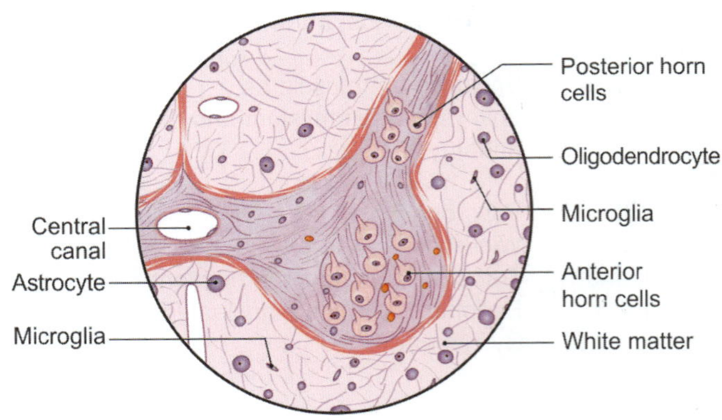

FACTS TO REMEMBER	1. Inner grey matter contains cell bodies of neurons 2. Outer white matter contains processes of neurons and neuroglial cells 3. Central canal lies in the grey commissure

Fig. 45.30: Neuron and neuroglia: Spinal cord

Oligodendrocytes

These cells have fewer and shorter processes, with no sucker feet. These make up three-fourth of the glial cells. These are smaller than astrocytes with deep basophilic round or oval nuclei, prominent nucleoli and abundant cytoplasm (Fig. 45.31).

Microglia

These are smallest of the neuroglia and are present both in the grey and white matter. The nuclei of microglial cells are small, comma shaped, deeply stained and surrounded by scanty cytoplasm.

Ependymal Cells

These are tall columnar ciliated cells. These cells line the ventricles of the brain and the central canal of spinal cord.

Satellite or Capsular Cells

These are flat cells with prominent nuclei. They surround the neurons of the spinal and autonomic ganglia, thus forming a multinucleated capsule for these irreparable cells.

Schwann Cells

These are derivatives of neural crest. The nucleus of a Schwann cell is flattened, surrounded by abundant cytoplasm.

It is responsible for laying down myelin sheath over a segment of a single axon after it indents into the Schwann cell. Myelin is stained with osmium tetroxide.

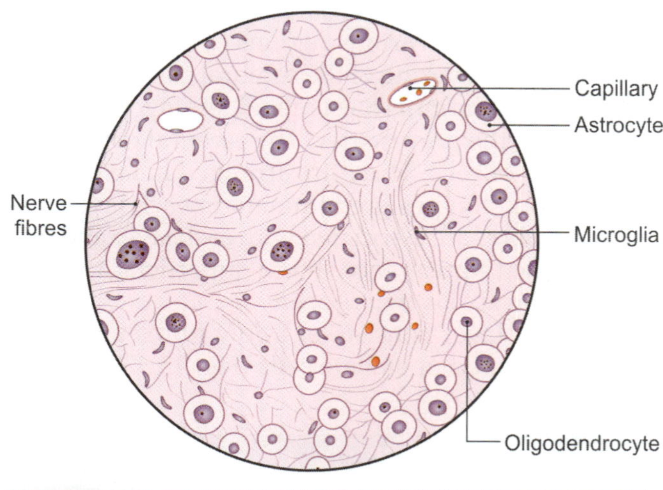

FACTS TO REMEMBER	
	1. Nerve fibres seen
	2. Neuroglial cells, i.e. astrocytes, oligodendrocyte and microglial cells seen
	3. Capillaries also seen

Fig. 45.31: White matter of spinal cord

NERVE FIBRES

A peripheral nerve fibre (Fig. 45.32) is an axon/dendron with its covering, i.e. myelin sheath and neurilemma.

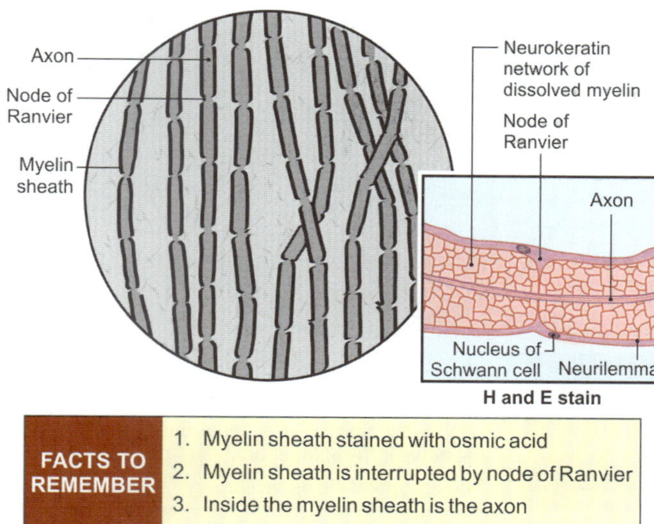

FACTS TO REMEMBER	
	1. Myelin sheath stained with osmic acid
	2. Myelin sheath is interrupted by node of Ranvier
	3. Inside the myelin sheath is the axon

Fig. 45.32: Longitudinal section of myelinated nerve fibres

These fibres are myelinated. Each fibre consists of:

- A central axon/axis cylinder with axoplasm and neurofibrils contained within the axolemma.
- Myelin sheath is composed of phospholipids, interrupted at intervals along with the length of the fibre. It is stained by osmic acid and not by H and E stain.
- Thin neurilemma sheath is present outside the myelin sheath. The cells of neurilemma are also known as Schwann cells, which are neuroectodermal in origin. At the points of interruption of myelin sheath the neurilemma comes into intimate contact with the axon and such areas are known as Nodes of Ranvier. The impulse jumps from one node to the next node.
- Endoneurium is a thin connective tissue layer of mesodermal origin. It supports the nerve fibres. The potential space between neurilemma and endoneurium contains tissue fluid for the nourishment of the nerve fibre.

NERVE TRUNK

Transverse section of nerve trunk shows that it is surrounded by connective tissue sheath called *epineurium*. It sends in septa dividing the nerve trunk into various fascicles, each of which is surrounded by a dense sheath, the *perineurium*. From the perineurium, numerous septa extend to form a sheath enclosing each nerve fibre. This sheath is known as *endoneurium*. This connective tissue skeleton supports the nerve fibres and carries capillaries with them.

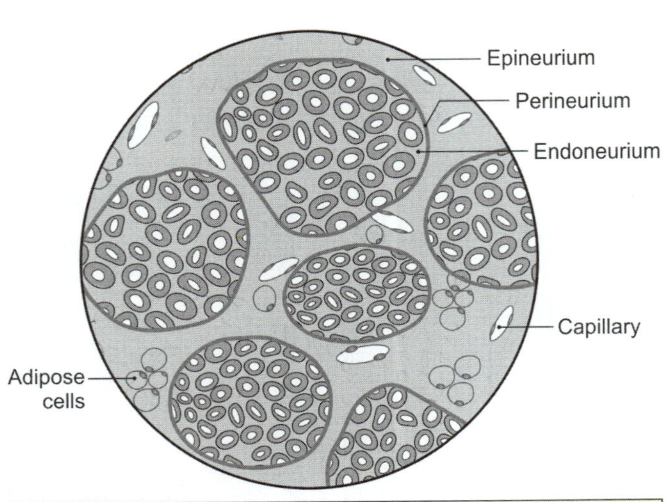

FACTS TO REMEMBER	
	1. Osmic acid preferentially stains the myelin sheath 2. Around each nerve fibre is endoneurium; around each nerve fasciculus is perineurium; and around the nerve is the epineurium 3. These support the nerve fibres

Fig. 45.33: Transverse section of nerve trunk (osmic acid stain)

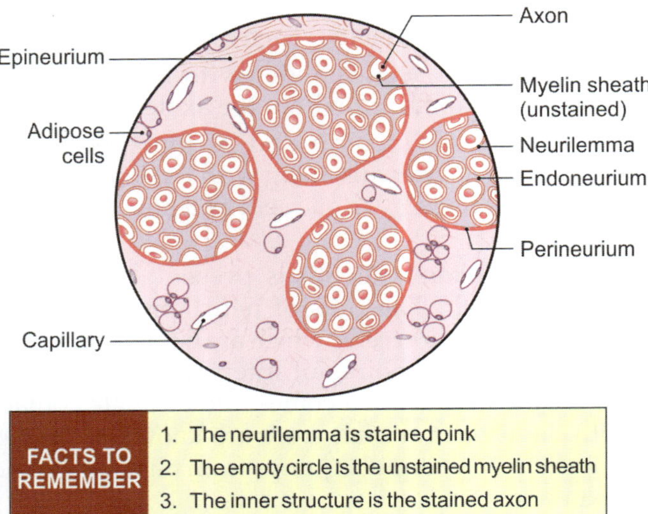

FACTS TO REMEMBER	
	1. The neurilemma is stained pink 2. The empty circle is the unstained myelin sheath 3. The inner structure is the stained axon

Fig. 45.34: Transverse section of nerve trunk

In transverse sections stained with osmic acid (Fig. 45.33) myelin sheath is stained black and neurilemma as well as axis cylinder (axon) remain unstained. With haematoxylin and eosin stain (Fig. 45.34), the neurilemma and the axis cylinder are stained pink, whereas the area occupied by myelin sheath is observed as halo or unstained space.

PARTS OF THE NERVOUS SYSTEM

SPINAL CORD

The spinal cord comprises a central canal surrounded by grey matter. Around this grey matter is the white matter (Fig. 45.30). Table 45.3 shows the comparison between the grey matter and white matter.

Transverse section of spinal cord stained with H & E stain (Fig. 45.30)

1. The central canal is seen as an oval cavity lined by columnar ciliated epithelium (Fig. 45.30).
2. The large cells in the anterior horn depict multiple angles/corners; the angles representing the origin of its processes.
   The grey matter reveals the neuroglial cells and lots of capillaries.
3. The peripheral white matter contains the fibres, neuroglia and fewer capillaries. In transverse sections the nerve fibres appear as hollow circles (myelin unstained) with central dots representing the axon (Fig. 45.34).

GANGLIA

Collection of neurons outside the central nervous system is called ganglion. There are two types of ganglia, spinal and autonomic. These are compared in Table 45.4 and shows in Figs 45.35 and 45.36.

CEREBRUM

It is characterised by *heterotypical cortex*, i.e. histological structure differs in various regions of cerebral cortex. The outermost covering of the cerebral cortex is the pia mater which is the innermost meningeal layer. It carries capillaries to the grey matter. The cerebral cortex contains variety of cells. These are arranged in layers with one or more cell types predominant in each layer. The horizontal fibres are associated with each layer and give it a laminated appearance. From superficial to deep, the following six layers are seen:

1. Molecular layer consists of a few fibres and some spindle-shaped or stellate cells (Fig. 45.37).

Table 45.3: Comparison of grey matter and white matter

Grey matter	*White matter*
1. Contains bodies of nerve cells	Bodies of nerve cells are absent
2. Has parts of dendrites and parts of the axon	Has most of the lengths of axon and dendrites
3. Contains protoplasmic astrocytes, oligodendroglia and microglia	Contains fibrous astrocytes, oligodendroglia and microglia
4. Has numerous capillaries	Has fewer capillaries

Table 45.4: Comparison of the ganglia

Dorsal root ganglion or sensory or spinal ganglion (Fig. 45.35)	*Sympathetic ganglion or autonomic ganglion* (Fig. 45.36)
1. Consists of pseudounipolar neurons	Consists of multipolar neurons
2. Has cell bodies of afferent neurons	Has cell bodies of efferent neurons
3. The cell body is large and rounded	The cell body is smaller and irregular
4. The nucleus is central with a prominent nucleolus	The nucleus is usually eccentric and has a prominent nucleolus
5. Around each neuron is a layer of flattened cells called capsular/satellite cells	Such capsular/satellite cells are a few in number
6. The neurons lie in groups separated by nerve fibres lying in groups	The neurons and nerve fibres lie scattered

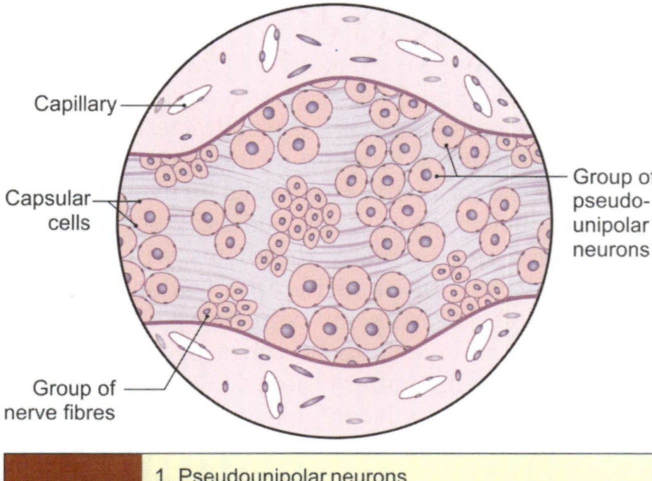

FACTS TO REMEMBER
1. Pseudounipolar neurons
2. Cell body is large and rounded
3. Neurons in groups separated by nerve fibres in groups

Fig. 45.35: Spinal/sensory/dorsal root ganglion

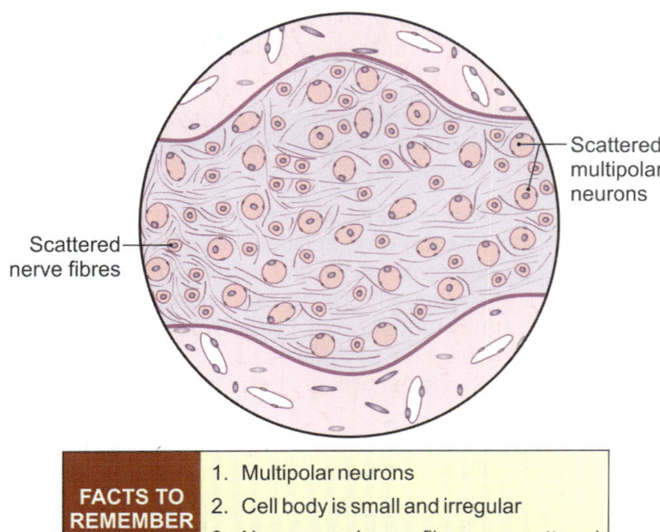

FACTS TO REMEMBER
1. Multipolar neurons
2. Cell body is small and irregular
3. Neurons and nerve fibres are scattered

Fig. 45.36: Autonomic ganglion

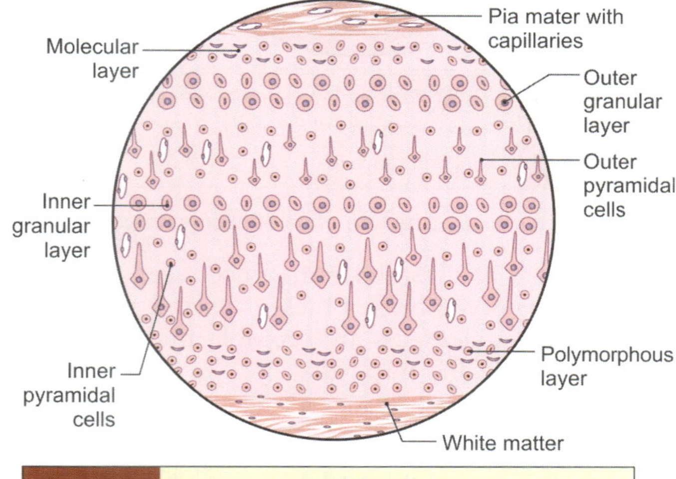

FACTS TO REMEMBER
1. Six layers of cells and fibres
2. Pyramidal cells more in motor cortex and granular cells more in sensory cortex
3. Numerous capillaries present

Fig. 45.37: Grey matter of cerebrum

2 Outer granular layer contains small cells, triangular in shape, with an apex directed peripherally and the base directed inwards. The axons leave from the basal part of the cell. A few stellate cells are also seen.
3 Outer pyramidal layer has similar cells as outer granular layer, but the cells are distinctly larger than those of the outer granular layer.
4 Inner granular layer contains cells which are larger than outer pyramidal cells, but have a large number of stellate cells between them.
5 Inner pyramidal layer contains cells which are triangular in shape and are the largest cells of the cerebral cortex, especially in the motor cortex where these are termed the Betz cells.
6 Fusiform layer or polymorphous layer contains mainly fusiform cells with a few stellate cells. No pyramidal cells are seen in this layer.

The *granular cell* layers are *afferent* in connection and the *pyramidal* cell layers are *efferent* in nature. The pyramidal cells are more pronounced in the motor areas, whereas the granular cells are more conspicuous

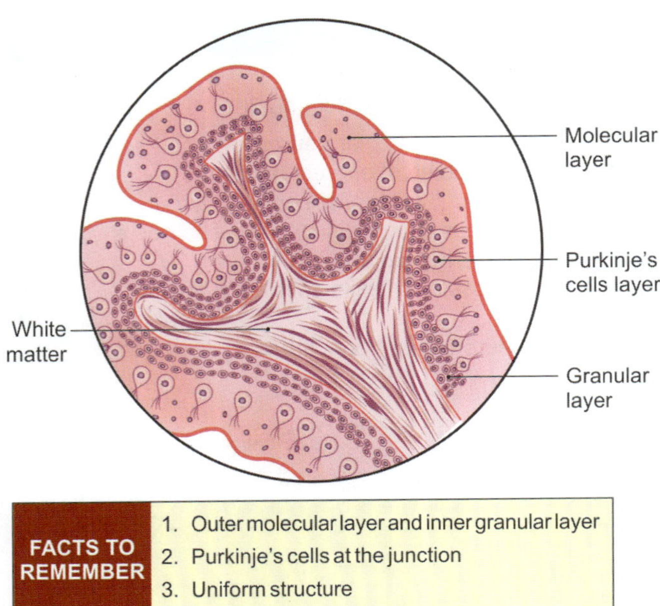

FACTS TO REMEMBER	
	1. Outer molecular layer and inner granular layer
	2. Purkinje's cells at the junction
	3. Uniform structure

Fig. 45.38: Structure of cerebellum cortex

in the sensory areas of the brain. In between the nerve cells are the nerve fibres of these cells and capillaries. The neuroglial elements are protoplasmic astrocytes, oligodendroglia and microglia.

CEREBELLUM

The histological structure of entire cerebellum is similar and is called **homotypical cortex**. The cerebellar cortex shows many deep folds called **cerebellar folia**, separated by fissures. The cerebellum consists of outer grey matter and inner white matter. The white matter is made up of myelinated fibres. The grey matter is greatly folded over the central core of white matter to increase the surface area. The appearance is known as the *arbor vitae* (Fig. 45.38). The white matter forms the core of each folium of cerebellum. It comprises myelinated fibres.

Layers of Grey Matter

It is composed of three layers:

1 *Outer molecular layer*: In this layer there are stellate cells, basket cells, axons and dendrites of both cell types, climbing fibres, axons of granule and Golgi cells (Table 45.5).
2 *Purkinje's cells*: These are the characteristic cells of cerebellum at the junction of outer molecular and inner granular layers. These cells lie in a single row and have flask-shaped cell bodies. The apex of the cell gives rise to many dendrites which branch repeatedly to form dendritic arborisations. From the base of the cell arises an axon that passes through the granular layer and becomes myelinated as it enters the white matter (Table 45.6).
3 *Inner granular layer*: It contains numerous small Golgi and granule cells with dark staining nuclei and scanty cytoplasm. There are also large stellate cells which have more cytoplasm.

Table 45.5: Types of neurons in cerebellum

Layers	*Neurons*	*Population*
Outer molecular layer	Stellate cells, basket cells	Sparse cells in this zone
Purkinje's cell layer	Purkinje's cells are characteristic cerebellar neurons	In single layer at the junction of molecular and granular layers
Granular cell layer	Granule cell, Golgi cell	Densely populated zone

Table 45.6: Depicting connections of various neurons

Neuron and its placement	*Course of dendrites*	*Course of axon*
Granule cells in deep part of granular layer	4–6 short dendrites which synapse with **mossy** fibres in granular	Axon passes upwards in the molecular layer (neuron lying upside down); divides into two subdivisions which run in opposite directions (T-shaped). These subdivisions of axon are termed parallel fibres and synapse with dendrites of Purkinje's cell
Outer stellate cell confined to the molecular layer	Synapse with parallel fibres (axons of granule cells)	Synapses with dendrites of Purkinje's cell
Basket cells in deeper part of molecular layer	Ramify in molecular layer synapsing with parallel fibres (axons of granule cells)	Form baskets around the cell bodies of Purkinje's cell
Golgi cells in superficial part of granular layer	Synapses with axons of granule cells (parallel fibres) in molecular layer	Ends in relation to dendrites of granule cells to form the glomeruli in granular layer

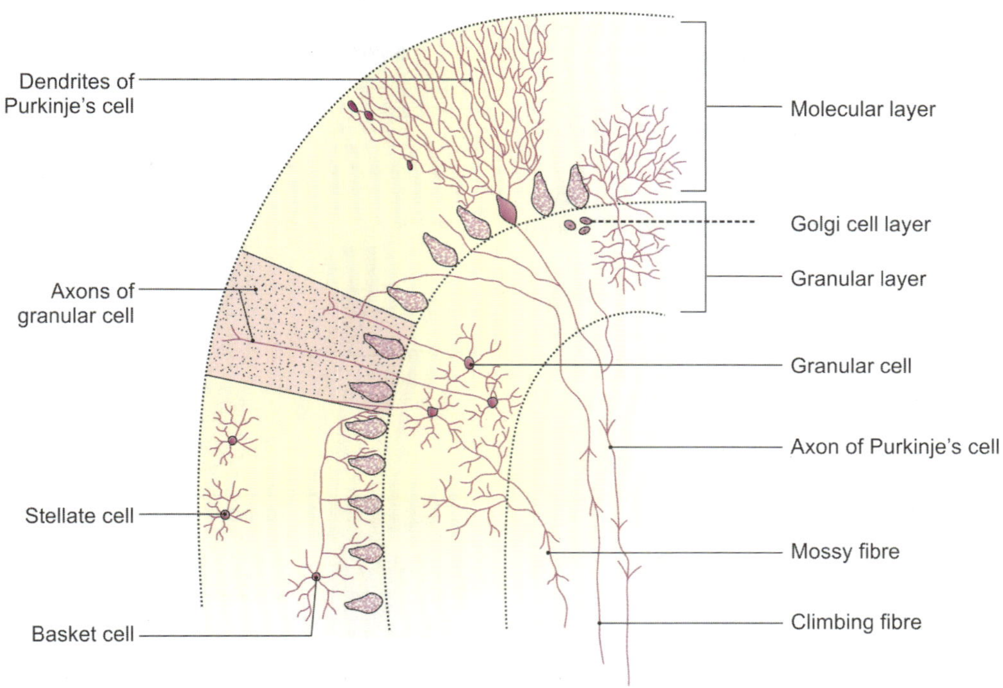

Fig. 45.39: Schematic figure to show layers and fibres of cerebellar cortex

White Matter

The core of white matter is formed by myelinated nerve fibres or axons. The axons are afferent and efferent fibres of the cerebellar cortex.

The afferent connections of cerebellum are through **mossy** and **climbing** fibres. Mossy fibres constitute all the afferents except those of olivo-cerebellar fibres. Mossy fibres synapse with granule and Golgi cells (Table 45.6). Olivo-cerebellar fibres climb up and make synaptic connections with dendrites of Purkinje's cells and are called climbing fibres (Fig. 45.39).

BLOOD VESSELS

All animals and human beings require a mechanism to distribute oxygen and nutritive materials to the tissues and to collect carbon dioxide and waste products of tissue metabolism and transmit these to excretory system. This mostly all done by the blood vessels. The various types of blood vessels are: (1) Arteries, (2) capillaries, (3) sinusoids, (4) veins. This chapter gives histology of arteries and veins.

ARTERIES

Arteries are classified as:

a. Elastic or large-sized arteries, e.g. aorta (Fig. 45.40)
b. Muscular or medium-sized arteries, e.g. brachial, radial, popliteal.
c. Arterioles—smallest divisions of arteries with a diameter of 100 micron.

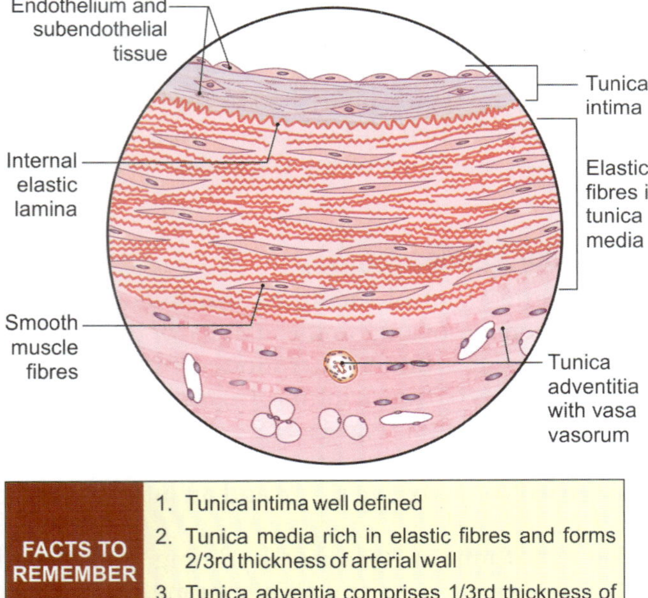

FACTS TO REMEMBER	
	1. Tunica intima well defined 2. Tunica media rich in elastic fibres and forms 2/3rd thickness of arterial wall 3. Tunica adventia comprises 1/3rd thickness of arterial wall

Fig. 45.40: Layers of elastic artery

a. Elastic Arteries

During systole, the elastic artery expands to accommodate increased amount of blood. During diastole of the heart, there is elastic recoil of the artery, so there is continuous blood flow to the peripheral parts of the body. Since these arteries have abundant elastic fibres in their walls, these are named elastic arteries. The lumen of the artery is surrounded by the three concentric coats (i) tunica intima, (ii) tunica media, and (iii) tunica adventitia.

- The tunica intima consists of an endothelium, subendothelial connective tissue and an internal elastic lamina.

  The **endothelium** is a thin layer, made up of flattened cells, lining the luminal surface of the artery. These cells rest on a basement membrane.

  Subendothelial connective tissue is a loose narrow layer containing elastic and collagen fibres along with nuclei of fibroblasts and macrophages.

  The **internal elastic lamina** is the limiting layer of tunica intima and is made up of fenestrated elastic fibres. The internal elastic lamina is not prominent as the elastic fibres merge with the elastic laminae of the tunica media.
- The tunica media or middle layer is the thickest and is dominated by concentric laminae of elastic fibres with smooth muscle fibres. It comprises two-thirds of the arterial wall. The outer layer of the tunica is the **external elastic lamina,** made up of elastic fibres, which is not so conspicuous.
- The tunica adventitia is a layer of collagen fibres, elastic fibres and fibroblasts. It contains a few arterioles called **vasa vasorum** which nourish the tunica adventitia and outer two-thirds of tunica media, the rest being nourished by the blood flowing through the lumen of the vessels. Tunica adventitia comprises one-third of the thickness of the arterial wall.

b. Muscular Arteries

These arteries control the amount of blood flowing through them according to the activity of the part.

It consists of a lumen surrounded by same three concentric coats (i) tunica intima, (ii) tunica media, and (iii) tunica adventitia (Fig. 45.41).

- The **tunica intima** consists of an endothelium, subendothelial connective tissue and an internal elastic lamina.

  The **endothelium** is formed by lining of flattened cells, resting on a basement membrane.

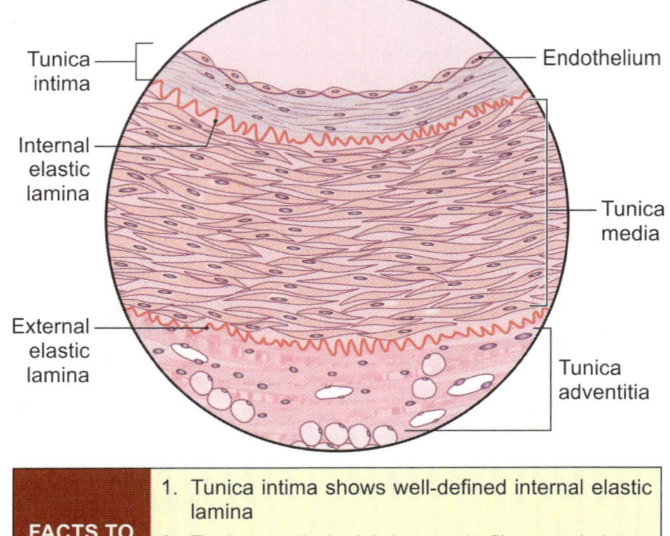

FACTS TO REMEMBER
1. Tunica intima shows well-defined internal elastic lamina
2. Tunica media is rich in muscle fibres and shows well-defined external elastic lamina
3. Tunica adventitia rich in collagen and elastic fibres

Fig. 45.41: Layers of muscular artery

  The **subendothelial connective tissue** consists of fine collagen and elastic fibres as well as fibroblasts.

  The **internal elastic lamina** is well defined. The lamina of elastic fibres stands out well as the media mainly consists of smooth muscle fibres.
- The **tunica media** forms two-thirds of the thickness of the arterial wall. It is made up of circularly or spirally running **smooth muscle fibres**. Among the muscle fibres are scattered elastic fibres.

  The **external elastic lamina** is made of elastic fibres and is better defined than in an elastic artery due to predominance of muscle fibres in the tunica media.
- The **tunica adventitia** is a well-defined layer comprising nearly **one-third** of the thickness of the arterial wall. It contains collagen and elastic fibres. Arterioles in the form of **vasa vasorum** are usually present in this layer.

Table 45.7 shows comparison of the three types of arteries.

Table 45.7: Comparison among elastic artery, muscular artery and arteriole

Layers	*Elastic artery*	*Muscular artery*	*Arteriole*
Tunica intima	Endothelium, subendothelial tissue and ill, defined internal elastic lamina	Endothelium, subendothelial tissue and prominent internal elastic lamina	Endothelium, subendothelial tissue and internal elastic lamina poorly developed
Tunica media	40–80 fenestrated elastic membranes with thin external elastic lamina	20–40 layers of smooth muscle cells, prominent external elastic lamina	Only 1–4 layers of smooth muscle cells
Tunica adventitia	Fibroelastic layer and prominent vasa vasorum	Fibroelastic layer, vasa vasorum not prominent	Loose connective tissue only

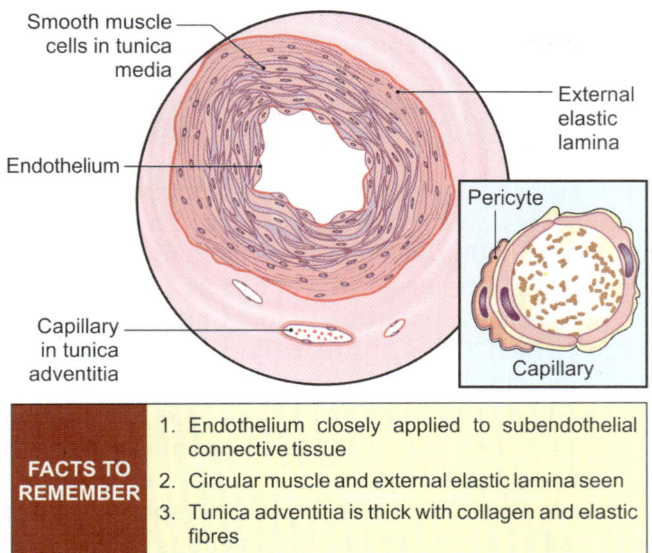

Fig. 45.42: Layers of arteriole. Insert shows a capillary

c. Arterioles

These are the smallest divisions of the arteries which have a diameter of **100 micron**. These act as resistance vessels to maintain peripheral blood pressure. Three concentric coats surrounding the lumen are (i) tunica intima, (ii) tunica media, and (iii) tunica adventitia.

- The **tunica intima** consists of endothelium closely applied to the **internal elastic** lamina with a mere trace of subendothelial connective tissue.
- The **tunica media** is made up of a layer of circularly arranged smooth muscle fibres and an outer elastic lamina (Table 45.7).
- The **tunica adventitia** is made of collagen as well as elastic fibres and is usually a thick layer (Fig. 45.42).

CAPILLARIES

Capillaries: Form a link between the arterioles (smallest division of an artery) and the venules (smallest tributary of a vein). The diameter of a capillary is about **8–10 micron**. Its lumen is slightly larger than the diameter of an erythrocyte. One to three endothelial cells with stretched out cytoplasm line the lumen and rest on the basement membrane. Outside the basement membrane is a fine layer of collagen and elastic fibres with **occasional perivascular cells** or **pericytes**. Usually the edges of endothelial cells fuse with those of adjacent cells, making the lining continuous. These capillaries are termed **"continuous capillaries"**. The exchange occurs through the cytoplasm by the formation of pinocytic vesicles.

In viscera like kidney, small intestine and endocrine glands the capillaries are **fenestrated**, i.e. have minute apertures/pores between the adjacent endothelial cells. These apertures may be closed by thin membrane either of the basal lamina or thinned out cytoplasm of the endothelial cell. The greater exchange in fenestrated capillaries occurs through these pores.

SHUNT VESSELS OR ARTERIOVENOUS ANASTOMOSES (AV ANASTOMOSES)

In many organs in the body, the arterioles and venules may also be connected to each other through a direct channels called AV anastomoses. Through these, most of the blood passes directly from arteriole to venule and bypasses the capillaries. These are present in skin of lips, nose, pinna, mucous membrane of GIT and are richly supplied by sympathetic nerves. These AV anastomoses help to maintain body temperature by decreasing the flow of blood through capillaries in cold weather and enhancing the flow in hot climate.

SINUSOIDS

Sinusoids are large irregular blood containing spaces lined by flattened **endothelial** as well as **reticulo-endothelial cells**. The latter type of cells are phagocytic in nature. In liver phagocytic cells are called Kupffer's cells. The lining of the sinusoids is **fenestrated**. These are seen in liver, spleen, endocrine glands and bone marrow. Table 45.8 shows differences between sinusoids and capillaries.

VEINS

These are vessels which collect and bring deoxygenated blood to the heart, exceptions being the umbilical, and pulmonary veins. Smallest veins are called venules with

Table 45.8: Differences between sinusoids and capillaries

Sinusoids	Capillaries
1. Wider, irregular spaces	Narrow regular spaces
2. Lined by endothelial as well as reticulo-endothelial cells, which may be interrupted, and fenestrated	Lined by a few continuous endothelial cells
3. Found in endocrine glands, lymphoid tissue, liver and bone marrow	Found in all the tissues of the body
4. Basal lamina is not continuous	Basal lamina is continuous

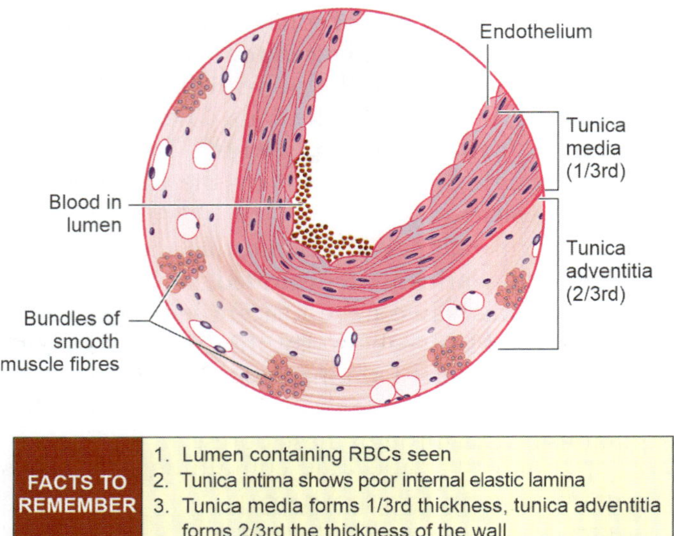

FACTS TO REMEMBER	
	1. Lumen containing RBCs seen 2. Tunica intima shows poor internal elastic lamina 3. Tunica media forms 1/3rd thickness, tunica adventitia forms 2/3rd the thickness of the wall

Fig. 45.43: Layers of large vein

extremely thin walls. These join to form medium sized and large veins (Fig. 45.43). The veins have relatively thin walls and large lumens. Many veins contain blood cells. The three concentric coats of the vein are (i) tunica intima, (ii) tunica media, and (iii) tunica adventitia.

- The tunica intima consists of an **endothelium** which rests directly on a poorly defined internal **elastic lamina** or is separated from it by a small amount of subendothelial connective tissue.
- The **tunica media** is thinner as compared to the tunica media of the arteries. It forms nearly one-third of the thickness of the wall of the vein. It contains smooth muscle fibres and collagen fibres (Fig. 45.43).
- The **tunica adventitia** forms two-thirds of the thickness of the wall of the vein. It consists of collagen fibres with a few elastic fibres. Large veins usually show longitudinally disposed smooth muscle fibres in this layer. The differences between arteries and veins have been tabulated in Table 45.9.

LYMPHATIC SYSTEM

The lymphatic system consists of lymphatic vessels, lymphocytes and lymphatic organs. The lymphatic capillaries are thin-walled tubes which form networks in most of the tissues of the body, except the central nervous system, epidermis, cornea and bone marrow. These collect tissue fluid called the lymph. The lymphatic capillaries unite to form larger vessels, the largest of these open into veins. The histological structure of large lymph vessels is identical to that of veins of corresponding size.

Lymphatic organs are: Lymph node, spleen, thymus and tonsil. Growth pattern and functions of lymphatic system are given in Chapter 6.

LYMPH NODE

It is a rounded or kidney-shaped structure. There is slight indentation, the hilum on one side of the node, where blood vessels enter and leave. Lymphatic vessels with valves enter the node at many places over the convex surface but only one vessel leaves it only at the hilum. Thus, it contains both afferent and efferent lymph vessels (Figs 45.44 and 45.45).

The lymph node surrounded by a pericapsular adipose tissue is covered by a capsule which consists of dense collagen fibres, fibroblasts and a few elastic fibres. **Trabeculae** of dense collagenous connective tissue arise from the capsule and penetrate the node. In the outer peripheral part of node the trabeculae divide the interior of the lymph node into roughly rounded areas. Features of lymph nodes can be studied from Chapter 6.

Table 45.9: Differences between arteries and veins

	Arteries	*Veins*
1. Lumen	Patent, RBC not seen	Lumen may be collapsed, RBC usually seen
2. Endothelial lining	Well defined	Not so well defined
3. Internal elastic lamina	Distinct	Poorly defined
4. Tunica media	Forms 2/3rd of the thickness of the wall	Forms 1/3rd of the thickness of the wall
5. External elastic lamina	Distinct	Not well defined
6. Tunica adventitia	Form 1/3rd of the thickness of the wall	Forms 2/3rd of the thickness of the wall
7. Extent of vasa vasorum	Supply extends up to outer 2/3rd of tunica media	Supply extends up to tunica intima

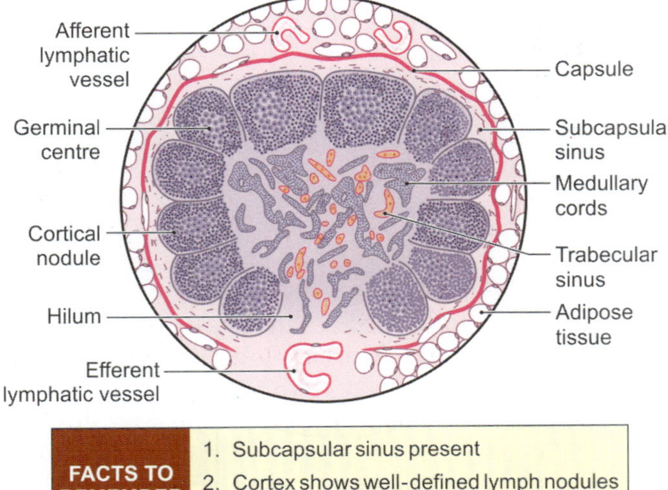

Fig. 45.44: Section of a lymph node

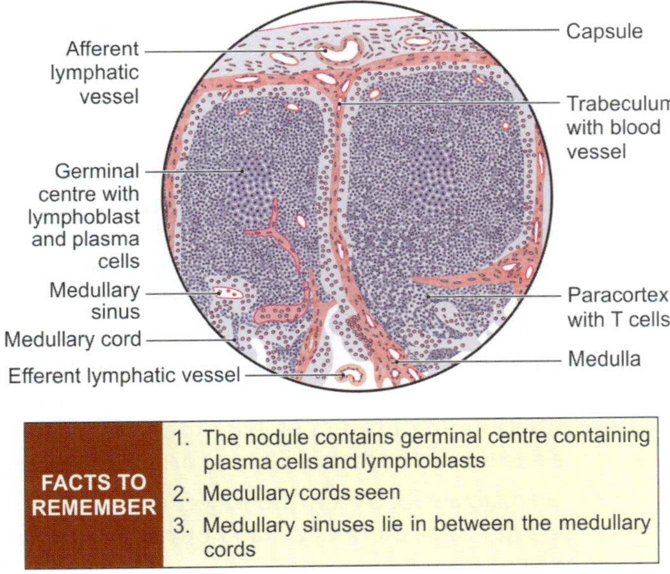

Fig. 45.45: Section of a lymph node

LYMPH FLOW

Beneath the capsule, the collagen fibres are loosely arranged to form the **subcapsular sinus**. From this sinus a number of radially directed cortical sinuses pass towards the medulla where these unite to form large medullary sinuses, which in turn join to form one efferent lymph vessel. Number of afferent lymphatics open into the peripheral subcapsular sinus. The lymph filters through the cortical and medullary sinuses and leaves the lymph node through the single efferent lymphatic channel (Fig. 45.45) at its hilum. The efferent lymphatic channel also has valves.

STRUCTURE OF LYMPH NODE

The cut surface of a lymph node is seen to be divided into an outer peripheral cortex and an inner medulla. The cellular components of these two zones are supported by a **reticular framework** which can be demonstrated by silver stain. The phagocytic reticular cells of mesodermal origin are present along the reticular fibres.

Cortex contains lymphatic nodules/primary nodules which are about 1 mm in diameter. These consist of peripheral darker area made up of mature lymphocytes and a lighter central zone called *germinal centre/ secondary centre* which contains lymphoblasts, medium-sized lymphocytes and plasma cells. Cortical nodules are separated by trabeculae containing capillaries (Fig. 45.45).

Medulla consists of lymphocytes arranged in cords called *medullary cords* which contain plasma cells, macrophages and small lymphocytes. Each cord consists of two or three rows of cells. The medullary sinuses, arterioles, venules occupy the area in between the medullary cords. The thymus derived "T lymphocytes" are confined in the deep cortical (**paracortical**) region. Rest of the lymphocytes belong to the bone marrow derived "B lymphocytes" (Fig. 45.45).

SPLEEN

Spleen contains a large amount of lymphatic tissues which **filters blood** instead of lymph. The spleen is surrounded by a connective tissue capsule which in lower animals contains smooth muscle fibres and elastic fibres. The outer surface of capsule is covered by a layer of flattened mesothelium. Trabeculae made up of reticular, elastic and collagenous fibres extend from the capsule and hilus into the **splenic pulp**. These run in various directions and become continuous with the reticular framework of the organ. There is no differentiation of tissue into cortex and medulla. Instead the spleen is comprised of **white pulp and red pulp** (Fig. 45.46).

White Pulp

Consists of lymphatic tissue which forms sheaths around the arterioles. In microscopic sections it is seen in the form of lymphatic nodules usually with an eccentric arteriole. These are known as splenic corpuscles or Malpighian corpuscles. Their peripheral part contains small lymphocytes while the central part/ *germinal centre* has large lymphocytes and plasma cells. Lymphocytes around the eccentric arteriole are T lymphocytes, whereas germinal centres contain B lymphocytes. These cells identify the antigens and bacteria. They interact with T cells resulting in immune responses.

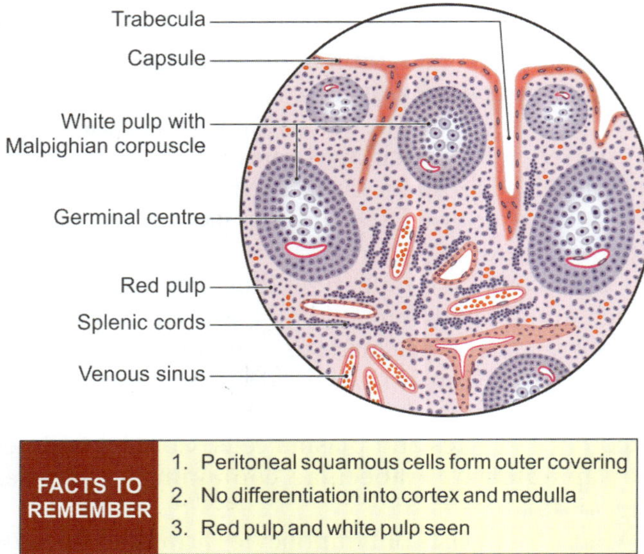

Fig. 45.46: Structure of spleen

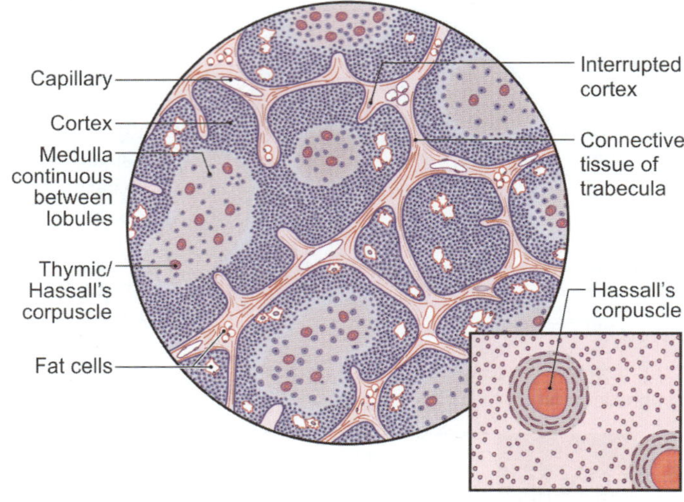

FACTS TO REMEMBER

1. Trabeculae only in cortical part with dark lymphocytes
2. Medulla of adjacent lobules continuous and contains lighter reticular cells
3. Hassall's corpuscles made up of concentric lamellae of epithelial cells surrounding a hyaline mass

Fig. 45.47: Structure of thymus of a child

Red Pulp

A loose framework of reticular fibres forms the foundation of red pulp. In the meshes of this framework are many lymphocytes, free macrophages and all the elements of circulating blood, i.e. red blood cells, neutrophils and monocytes. It also contains venous sinuses lined by the reticuloendothelial cells and splenic or Billroth's cords. Spleen contains only efferent lymph vessels. "T zone of lymphocytes" is around the perivascular sheath. For functions of spleen refer to Chapter 6.

THYMUS

Thymus is a lymphoepithelial lobulated organ that produces "T lymphocytes" and a lymphocyte stimulating hormone. Thymus involutes at puberty (Fig. 45.47). It is best developed in childhood. In adults it consists mainly of adipose tissue and Hassall's corpuscles.

STRUCTURE

It consists of a thin outer fibrous covering known as the capsule. From the capsule extend many thin connective tissue septa dividing it incompletely into various lobules. Each lobule has a peripheral darker cortex and a central lighter medulla. The interlobular septa are partial and do not extend into the medulla, so that there is continuity of the medullary tissue of the various lobules.

Chief cells present in thymus are:

a. *Thymic lymphocytes*: These are situated in the interstices of the thymic reticulum. These cells develop in thymus (their precursors migrated from bone marrow to thymus) and are immunologically competent but uncommitted cells.
b. *Epithelial reticular cells*: These are flattened cells with pale nuclei. Their processes branch and lie in apposition with the processes of the adjoining cells forming thin membrane. These reticular cells develop from the endoderm of third pharyngeal pouch. These cells secrete hormones, thymosin, thymopoietin, thymulin and thymic humoral factor. These hormones are required for proliferation, differentiation, maturation of T lymphocytes. They also are necessary for expression of surface markers.

Haemothymic barrier: Between the blood capillaries of thymus and its cells there is a haemothymic barrier. This comprises:

- Endothelial lining of the capillaries
- Minimal perivascular space
- Epithelial membrane constituted by the epithelial reticular cells.

The difference between cortex and medulla is due to the varying proportion of lymphocyte to reticular cells in each. The cortex consists mainly of densely packed small lymphocytes with their dark nuclei and between them are relatively a few reticular cells with pale staining nuclei.

In the medulla the reticular cells outnumber the lymphocytes. The medulla is more vascular than the cortex. It also contains Hassall's corpuscles which are made up of concentric lamellae of epithelial cells around a central degenerated hyaline mass. These stain with

Table 45.10: Comparison of the lymphatic organs

Features	*Lymph node*	*Spleen*	*Thymus*	*Palatine tonsil*
1. Outer covering	Connective tissue capsule with fat cells. Subcapsular sinus present	Connective tissue capsule covered with squamous epithelium of peritoneum	Thin connective tissue capsule	Connective tissue capsule on pharyngeal aspect is covered with stratified squamous non-keratinised epithelium, invaginating to form crypts
2. Lymph vessels	Both afferent and efferent lymph vessels	Only efferent lymph vessels	Only efferent lymph vessels	Only efferent lymph vessels
3. Trabeculae	Thin trabeculae all over	Abundant thick trabeculae with blood vessels	Trabeculae only in peripheral or cortical part	Occasional thin trabeculae from the capsule
4. Cortex	Contains well-defined lymph nodules with central germinal centre	Not differentiated into cortex and medulla. Instead there is white pulp with lymphatic nodules and red pulp	Contains collections of dark staining lymphocytes, and a few endodermal epithelial cells	Not differentiated into cortex and medulla Lymphocytes aggregated as small follicles along the sides of crypts. Germinal centre seen in a few follicles
5. Medulla	Lymphocytes are arranged in cords around lymph sinuses. These cords are known as medullary cords	Absent instead there is white pulp and red pulp	Medulla of one lobule is continuous with that of the adjoining lobules. Epithelial cells are arranged concentrically to form Hassall's corpuscles	Absent

acid dyes and increases with age. Thymus has only efferent lymphatics.

Functions of thymus can be studied from Chapter 6.

PALATINE TONSIL

It is a collection of paired lymphoid tissue at the oropharyngeal isthmus. Its oral aspect is covered by stratified squamous non-keratinised epithelium which dips into the underlying tissue to form crypts (Fig. 45.48). The lymphocytes lie beneath the epithelium and on the sides of the crypts. These are collected to form nodules. The germinal centre/secondary nodule may or may not be present. If present, these contain B large lymphocytes and plasma cells. "T lymphocytes" are present in the perifollicular area. The serous and mucous acini are seen on the deeper aspect of tonsil. Their ducts open on the sides of crypts. The outer aspect is covered by a capsule (hemicapsule). The deep aspect of tonsil contains serous and mucous acini and sections of skeletal muscle fibres. Table 45.10 shows

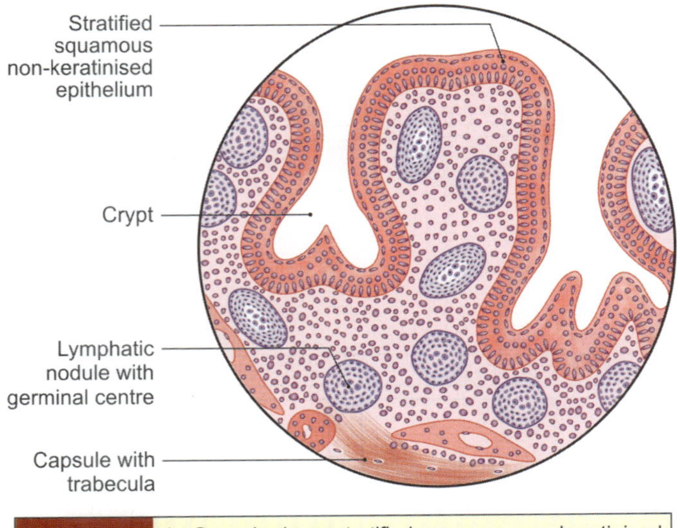

FACTS TO REMEMBER
1. Capsule shows stratified squamous non-keratinised epithelium on its oral aspect
2. The epithelium forms crypts
3. No differentiation into cortex and medulla

Fig. 45.48: Structure of palatine tonsil

the comparison of lymph node, spleen, thymus and palatine tonsil.

Functional Aspect

Palatine tonsils are one of the components of Waldeyer's ring of lymphoid tissue at the oropharyngeal isthmus. Others components are lingual, tubal and nasopharyngeal tonsils. All these try to prevent the entry of antigens and even attempt to destroy the antigens entering via nose and mouth.

THE GLANDS

The glands are epithelial invaginations of the surface epithelium, which are modified for the purpose of elaboration of secretion. These are classified as endocrine and exocrine glands.

Endocrine glands discharge their secretion directly into the blood or lymphatics and are called ductless glands, e.g. thyroid, suprarenal, hypophysis cerebri, etc.

Exocrine glands discharge their secretions onto a surface directly or by means of ducts and can be classified in five different ways as follows:

1 ***According to the branching of ducts:*** Simple and compound glands.
Simple: For example, gastric glands, pyloric glands, sweat glands. The secretion of these glands is conveyed to the surface by a single or unbranched duct (Fig. 45.49). The shape of gland may be coiled, simple branched tubular simple branched acinar.
Compound: For example, pancreas, parotid, Brunner's glands. The ducts of these glands divide into many branches. Shape of gland may be compound tubular, compound tubulo-acinar, compound acinar/alveolar.

2 ***According to the shape of the secretory unit***
Tubular racemose: For example, gastric glands, Brunner's glands of duodenum where the secretory unit is tubular in shape.
Acinar: For example, salivary glands, where the secretory unit is rounded or oval in shape.

3 ***According to the mode of elaboration of secretion:*** Holocrine, apocrine or merocrine also called epicrine.
Holocrine: For example, sebaceous glands. The secretory products first collect in the cytoplasm of the cell and then the cell disintegrates to form part of secretion.
Apocrine: For example, mammary glands. Only the apical part of the cell forms part of secretion. Some authorities believe it to be merocrine in type.
Merocrine or epicrine: For example, lacrimal and salivary glands. The secretion passes through the free surface of the cells into the lumen of the acinus. The wall of the secretory unit remains intact.

4 ***According to the type of secretion:*** Serous, mucous and mixed glands.

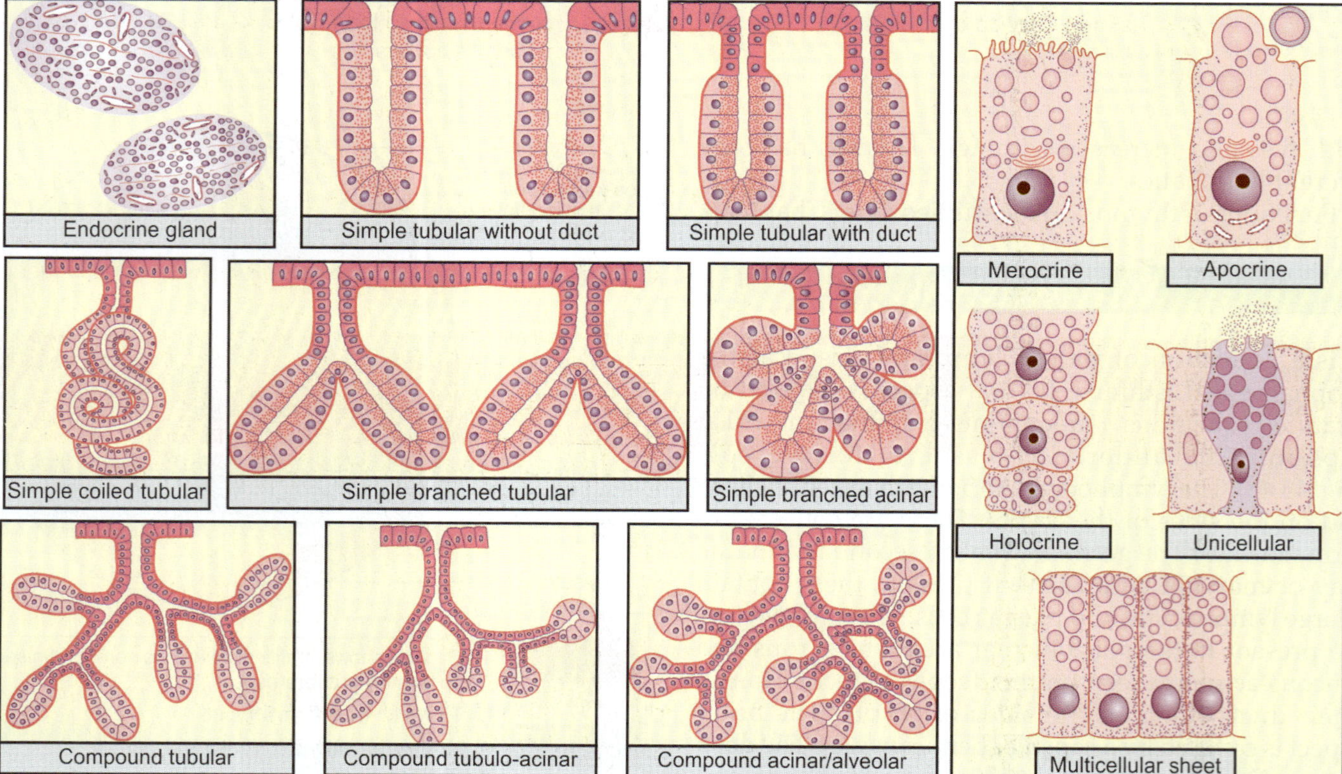

Fig. 45.49: Various types of glands (diagrammatic)

Serous: For example, parotid, exocrine part of pancreas. The secretion of these glands is a watery clear fluid. The cells have rounded nuclei close to the base of the cell with basal basophilia. Zymogen granules are in apical part of the cell.

Mucous: For example, sublingual gland. It is predominantly mucus in nature. The gland secretes mucin, which when mixed with water gets converted into mucous. These cells have flattened peripheral nuclei, lying against the bases of the cells. The cytoplasm is eosinophilic and vacuolated.

Mixed gland: For example, tracheal gland, submandibular gland. These have both serous and mucous type of acini.

5 ***According to number of cells:*** Unicellular and multicellular.

Unicellular: For example, goblet cells. These are unicellular glands situated in the epithelium of the trachea and intestines (Fig. 45.49).

Multicellular: For example, lacrimal, parotid gland. Most of the glands in the body are multicellular.

SALIVARY GLANDS

Three pairs of salivary glands secrete saliva which is poured into the oral cavity. These are:

- Parotid gland is chiefly serous.
- Submandibular gland is mixed, predominantly serous.
- Sublingual gland is mixed, predominantly mucous.

These glands are of the compound tubulo-alveolar variety. The connective tissue capsule and septa divide the gland into many lobes and lobules, carrying blood vessels, nerves and ducts. Various types of ducts are *intralobular*, *interlobar* and the *main duct*. These ducts are lined by cuboidal, columnar and stratified columnar epithelia respectively.

PAROTID GLAND

The acini of the gland secrete enzymes. The acinus is rounded and is lined by pyramidal cells surrounding a very small lumen. The cells show basal basophilia and lighter apical portion. The nuclei are rounded and basal in position. With higher magnification, the active cells show basal striations and apical eosinophilic zymogen granules (Fig. 45.50).

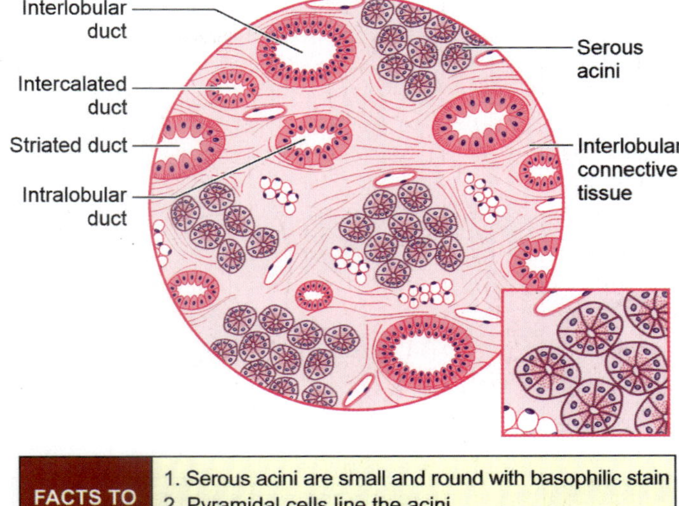

FACTS TO REMEMBER
1. Serous acini are small and round with basophilic stain
2. Pyramidal cells line the acini
3. Nuclei are round and basal

Fig. 45.50: Structure of serous gland: parotid gland

SUBMANDIBULAR GLAND AND TRACHEAL GLAND

These glands consist of both serous and mucous acini (Table 45.11). The mucous acinus is lined by truncated columnar cells. The size of the acinus is larger than the serous one and shows a bigger lumen. The nucleus is flattened against the basement membrane. Between mucous cells and the basement membrane are half-moon shaped polyhedral granular serous cells. These cells are known as **demilunes of Giannuzzi.** Fine canaliculi pass between mucous secreting cells from the demilunes to reach the lumen of the acinus. The secretions of the demilunes make mucous less viscid. A few **myoepithelial or basket cells** are present between the basement membrane and the acinar cells which help to squeeze the secretion from the acinus (Fig. 45.51).

Table 45.11: The differences between serous acini and mucous acini

Serous acini	*Mucous acini*
1. Smaller in size, rounded in shape	Larger in size, more variable in shape
2. Lumen hardly visible	Lumen mostly visible
3. Lining cells pyramidal in shape and relatively more in number	Lining cells truncated columnar in shape Cells relatively fewer in number
4. Nuclei are rounded and basal	Nuclei are flattened and peripheral
5. Cytoplasm depicts basal basophilia and apical eosinophilia	Cytoplasm is pale and vacuolated
6. Serous acinus may be present, as demilunes on one aspect of some mucous acini	Mucous acini only present as complete acini

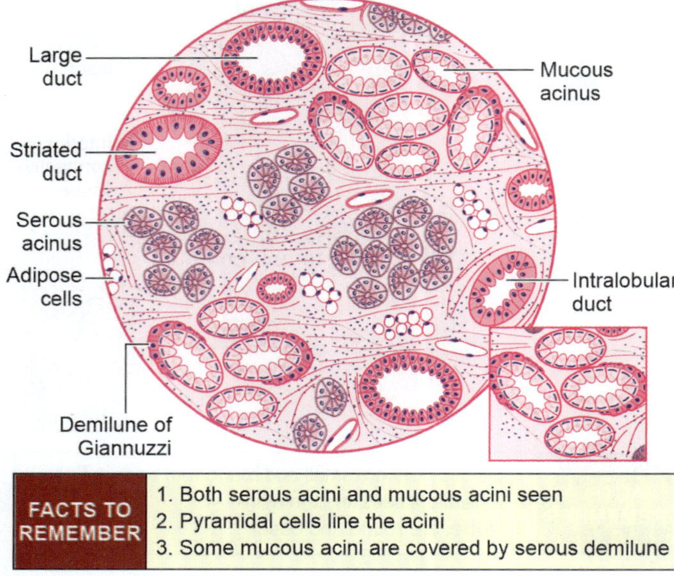

FACTS TO REMEMBER	
	1. Both serous acini and mucous acini seen 2. Pyramidal cells line the acini 3. Some mucous acini are covered by serous demilune

Fig. 45.51: Structure of submandibular salivary gland

SUBLINGUAL GLAND

Sublingual gland is predominantly mucus. These acini are lined by truncated columnar cells. The size of these acini and their lumen is bigger than the serous acini. The nuclei are flattened and rest against the basement membrane. With haematoxylin and eosin stain, the cytoplasm seems to be vacuolated and with periodic acid Schiff's (PAS) stain, the cytoplasm takes up magenta colour (Fig. 45.52). Demilunes of Giannuzzi are present here also. Table 45.11 compares the serous and mucous acini.

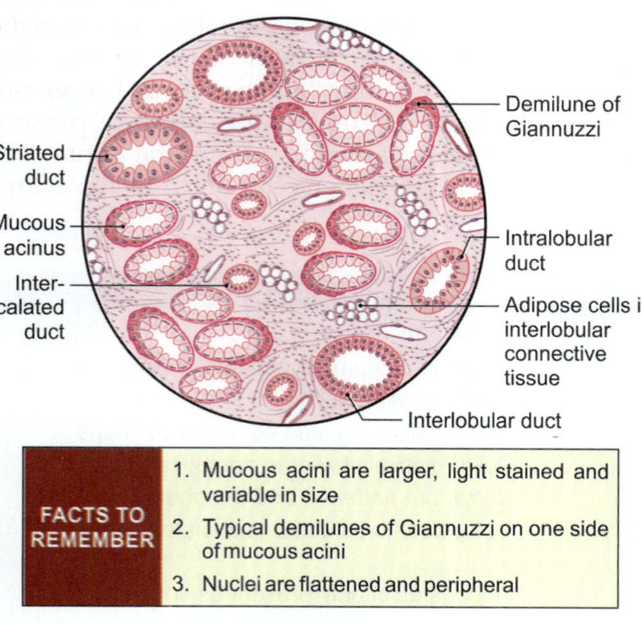

FACTS TO REMEMBER	
	1. Mucous acini are larger, light stained and variable in size 2. Typical demilunes of Giannuzzi on one side of mucous acini 3. Nuclei are flattened and peripheral

Fig. 45.52: Structure of biangugland

INTEGUMENTARY SYSTEM

Integumentary system consists of skin and its various appendages. Skin covers the surface of the body and consists of two main layers:

a. The surface epithelium or epidermis derived from ectoderm,
b. Subjacent deeper connective tissue layer or the dermis derived from mesoderm.

Thickness of skin varies from less than one millimeter to a few millimeters. The skin rests on a loose connective tissue layer called the superficial fascia.

SKIN

EPIDERMIS

Consists of stratified squamous keratinised epithelium nourished by diffusion from the capillaries of the dermis. It is primarily protective in nature. The epithelium is made up of the following.

- *Stratum basale*: It is the deepest single layer of columnar cells resting on the basement membrane with a few melanocytes in between, which produce melanin pigment. This pigment prevents the skin against ultraviolet rays of sun. In albinism (genetic disorder) the melanocytes are absent.
- *Stratum spinosum*: It is made up of 3–7 layers of polygonal cells which are attached to each other by unstable desmosomes, giving it a prickly appearance (Fig. 45.53).
- *Stratum granulosum*: Consists of 2–3 layers of diamond-shaped cells containing granules which stain deeply with basic dyes. These are keratohyalin granules.

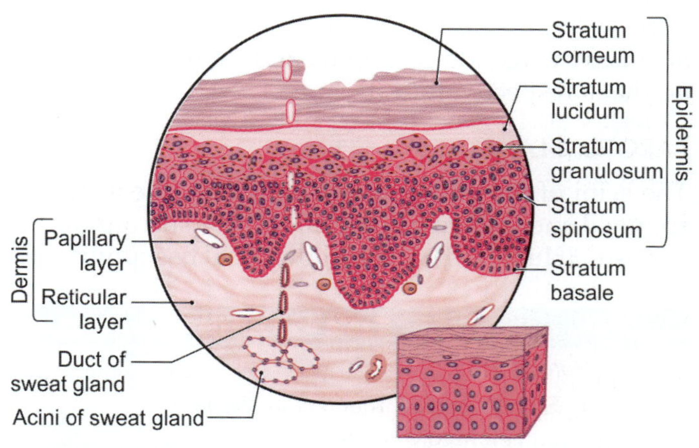

FACTS TO REMEMBER	
	1. Columnar cells of stratum basale rest on the basement membrane 2. Stratum spinosum, stratum granulosum, stratum lucidum and stratum corneum form the succeeding layers 3. Stratum corneum is the waterproof layer

Fig. 45.53: Layers of epidermis of thick skin

Table 45.12: Comparison between thick skin and thin skin

Features	*Thick skin (Fig. 45.53)*	*Thin skin (see Fig. 8.1)*
Epidermal layers	Comprises 5 layers: Stratum basale Stratum spinosum Stratum granulosum Stratum lucidum Stratum corneum	Comprises 4 layers Stratum basale Stratum spinosum Stratum granulosum Absent Thin stratum corneum
Epidermal ridges	Present	Absent
Sebaceous gland hair follicle and arrector pili muscle	Absent	Present
Sweat gland	Many	Few
Sensory receptors	Many	Few
Location	Palm and sole and palmar aspects of digits	All parts of body except palm, sole and palmar aspects of digits

- *Stratum lucidum*: These cells lose their nuclei and form a zone of flattened ill-defined cells. These cells contain refractile eleidin granules.
- *Stratum corneum*: The cells in this stratum are flat and cornified. The nucleus and cytoplasm are replaced by a protein called keratin. This zone is waterproof and protective in nature. The most superficial cells are constantly being desquamated.

A few Langhans' or clear cells may be seen in the stratum basale or stratum spinosum. These cells act as antigen—presenting cells to T lymphocytes. Langhans' cells recognise, phagocytose and process the antigens before presenting to T lymphocytes. A small number of Merkel's cells is seen in basal layer of epidermis. These act as mechanoreceptors to detect pressure in the finger tips.

DERMIS

Consists of an outer papillary and a deeper reticular layer. The outer **papillary layer**, in contact with the epidermis, is usually uneven and projects into papillae between the ridges on the deep surface of epidermis. These papillae, primary and secondary, bring about close contact between the capillaries of the dermis and cells of the epidermis. The papillary layer is thin and is made of fine collagen and elastic fibres with lymphocytes and plasma cells. It is very rich in capillaries and nerve endings. The deeper portion of the dermis is named the **reticular layer** and consists of dense irregular connective tissue with lymphocytes, fat cells, capillaries, lymphatics and nerve fibres.

TYPES OF SKIN—THICK AND THIN

Thick skin (Fig. 45.53), e.g. skin of palm and sole. The epidermis is very thick especially the stratum corneum. This skin contains numerous sweat glands.

Thin skin (*see* Fig. 8.1), e.g. skin over the rest of the body. Its characteristic features are the presence of hair follicles, sebaceous glands and arrector pili muscles. Table 45.12 shows the differences between thick skin and thin skin. Revise appendages of skin and functions of skin from Chapter 8.

UPPER RESPIRATORY SYSTEM

The respiratory system provides for the intake of oxygen and elimination of carbon dioxide, which are transported to and from the tissues of the body by the circulatory system.

Organs of respiration are nose comprising external nares, nasal cavity, posterior nares including the paranasal air sinuses.

- Nasopharynx
- Larynx
- Trachea
- Pleura, lungs including the bronchial tree.

Functionally the respiratory system is divided into:

- Conducting part which comprises nose, nasopharynx, larynx, trachea and bronchial tree till the level of terminal bronchioles. These are always patent for respiration.
- Respiratory part comprising of respiratory bronchioles, alveolar duct, atria, alveolar sac and alveoli. These are present in the spongy part of lung for exchange of gases.

HISTOLOGY OF NOSE, NASOPHARYNX AND LARYNX

NOSE

Comprises two nasal cavities separated by a nasal septum. Its functions are:

- Filtering, warming and moistening the inspired air
- Conducting air to and from the lungs
- As an organ for smell. The receptors for smell are placed in the upper one-third of nasal cavity and is lined by olfactory mucosa with special olfactory neurons. The lower two-thirds of nasal cavity is lined by respiratory mucosa, which is pseudostratified ciliated columnar epithelium with goblet cells. The lamina propria contains mucous and serous secreting glands, lymphocytes, plasma cells and large venous plexus.

NASOPHARYNX

It is situated between the posterior nares of nose and nasopharynx. It is lined by pseudo-stratified ciliated columnar epithelium with goblet cells.

LARYNX/VOICE BOX

It is made up of number of cartilages. It begins at root of tongue and ends at the trachea. Most of the larynx is lined by pseudostratified ciliated columnar epithelium interspersed with goblet cells.

Epiglottis is a very important elastic cartilage of larynx. There is lamina propria on both sides of the elastic cartilage. The anterior surface of epiglottis facing the tongue and upper part of posterior surface are lined with stratified squamous non-keratinised epithelium. The rest of the posterior surface is lined with respiratory epithelium, i.e. pseudostratified ciliated columnar epithelium.

TRACHEA AND CONDUCTING PART

Trachea is a thin-walled flexible tube. Its lumen is kept permanently patent by means of U-shaped hyaline cartilages. The trachea is lined by *pseudostratified ciliated columnar epithelium* with interspersed goblet cells resting on a basement membrane. The *lamina propria* consists of elastic fibres, lymphocytes both segregated and aggregated and short ducts of the glands (Fig. 45.54).

These ducts open on the free surface of the epithelium.

The deeper part of lamina propria is the *submucosa* which contains both mucous and serous acini that keep the epithelium moist. The mucus provided by mucous acini entangle the dust particles. Cilia move the mucous towards pharynx. Coughing also moves the mucus towards larynx and pharynx to be expelled from the respiratory system.

The most characteristic feature of trachea is its supporting framework of 16–20 U-shaped hyaline cartilages that encircle it on its ventral and lateral aspects. The posterior wall of the trachea adjacent to the oesophagus is devoid of cartilage. Its place is taken by transverse smooth muscle fibres, the *trachealis* muscle. The cartilage is covered by perichondrium on all sides which separates it from the neighbouring structures. The outermost layer is the adventitia which contains blood vessels and nerves.

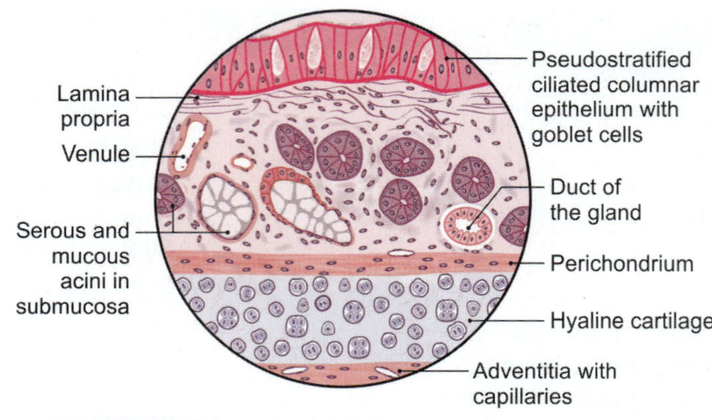

FACTS TO REMEMBER	
	1. Pseudostratified columnar ciliated epithelium
	2. Serous and mucous acini in between cartilage and epithelium
	3. C-shaped hyaline cartilage outside

Fig. 45.54: Various layers of wall of trachea

DIGESTIVE SYSTEM

The **digestive system** consists of digestive tract: (i) oral/ mouth cavity, oesophagus, stomach, small and large intestines, rectum and anal canal, and its associated glands and (ii) salivary glands, liver, gallbladder and pancreas.

Function

- Ingestion of food necessary for maintenance, development and growth.
- Absorption of broken down small molecules from lining of digestive tract.
- Its mucous membrane acts as a protective barrier to harmful substances.
- Expulsion of solid waste.

***Accessory organs and glands*:** These are teeth, tongue, salivary glands, liver, gallbladder and pancreas.

ORAL CAVITY

Digestive system comprises: Long gastrointestinal tract/ alimentary canal.

Canal: It starts at oral cavity, and continues as pharynx, oesophagus, small and large intestines to end at anus.

The oral cavity is divided into an outer smaller portion, the vestibule and an inner larger part the oral cavity proper. Vestibule of the mouth is narrow, bounded externally by the lips and cheeks and internally by the teeth and gums. The parotid duct opens into the vestibule. The vestibule communicates with the oral cavity when the mouth is open. The lining of vestibule is stratified squamous non-keratinised epithelium. The oral/mouth cavity proper contains teeth, openings of submandibular and sublingual salivary glands. Most of it is occupied by the tongue, described in Chapter 27. The opening of mouth cavity is guarded by the lips.

Lips: The lips are fleshy folds lined externally by skin and internally by mucous membrane. The mucocutaneous junction lines the edge or red margin of the lip, part of the mucosal surface is also normally seen. Each lip is composed of:

- Skin lined by stratified squamous keratinised epithelium with hair follicles, sweat and sebaceous glands in the dermis
- Superficial fascia
- Orbicularis oris muscle
- Submucosa, containing mucous labial glands and blood vessels
- Mucous membrane is lined by stratified squamous non-keratinised epithelium. The labial mucous glands are present in the lamina propria
- Mucocutaneous junction/red margin shows the transition from keratinised to non-keratinised epithelium, i.e. thick epithelium of skin changing to thin pink epithelium of mucous membrane, due to underlying blood vessels.

TEETH

Teeth form part of the masticatory apparatus and are fixed in the jaws. In man, the teeth are replaced only once (*diphyodont*) in contrast with non-mammalian vertebrates where teeth are constantly replaced throughout life (*polyphyodont*). The teeth of the first set (dentition) are known as *milk*, or *deciduous teeth*, and the second set, as *permanent teeth*.

The deciduous teeth are 20 in number. In each half of each jaw, there are two incisors, one canine, and two molars.

The permanent teeth are 32 in number, and consist of two incisors (Latin *to cut*) one canine (Latin *dog*) two premolars (Latin *millstone*) and three molars in each half of each jaw.

Parts of a Tooth

Each tooth has three parts:

1 A *crown*, projecting above the gum
2 A *root*, embedded in the jaw beneath the gum
3 A *neck*, between the crown and root and surrounded by the gum

Structure

Structurally, each tooth is composed of:

1 The pulp in the centre
2 The dentine surrounding the pulp
3 The enamel covering the projecting part of dentine, or crown
4 The cementum surrounding the embedded part of the dentine
5 The periodontal membrane.

The *pulp* is loose fibrous tissue containing vessels, nerves and lymphatics, all of which enter the pulp cavity through the apical foramen. The pulp is covered by a layer of tall columnar cells, known as *odontoblasts* which are capable of replacing dentine any time in life.

The *dentine* is a calcified material containing spiral tubules radiating from the pulp cavity. Each tubule is occupied by a protoplasmic process from one of the odontoblasts. The calcium and organic matter are in the same proportion as in bone.

The *enamel* is the hardest substance in the body. It is made up of crystalline prisms lying roughly at right angles to the surface of the tooth.

The *cementum* resembles bone in structure, but like enamel and dentine it has no blood supply, nor any nerve supply. Over the neck, the cementum commonly overlaps the cervical end of enamel; or, less commonly, it may just meet the enamel.

The *periodontal membrane (ligament)* holds the root in its socket. This membrane acts as a periosteum to both the cementum as well as the bony socket.

The pharynx contains the palatine tonsil, (Fig. 45.48).

The gastrointestinal tract from oesophagus to rectum follows a general plan.

General plan of gastrointestinal tract: The wall of the gastrointestinal tract (GIT) (Fig. 45.55) from oesophagus to anal canal is made up of the following four layers.

1 Mucous membrane consists of three layers:
   a. Epithelium resting on a basement membrane
   b. Lamina propria
   c. Muscularis mucosae
2 Submucosa
3 Muscularis externa
4 Serosa or adventitia

Mucous Membrane

a. *Epithelium*: It varies in different parts of GIT and is protective, absorptive and secretory. Its protective function against thermal, mechanical and chemical injury is clearly evident in oesophagus. This function is also seen in the distal part of the anal canal. Besides oesophagus and anal canal, the epithelium is single layered with various types of secretory cells. Its secretions are supplemented by the secretions of the glands which are present in different layers. The short ones are in the lamina propria, slightly longer ones in the submucosa and the other glands like liver, gall bladder and pancreas lie outside the gut.

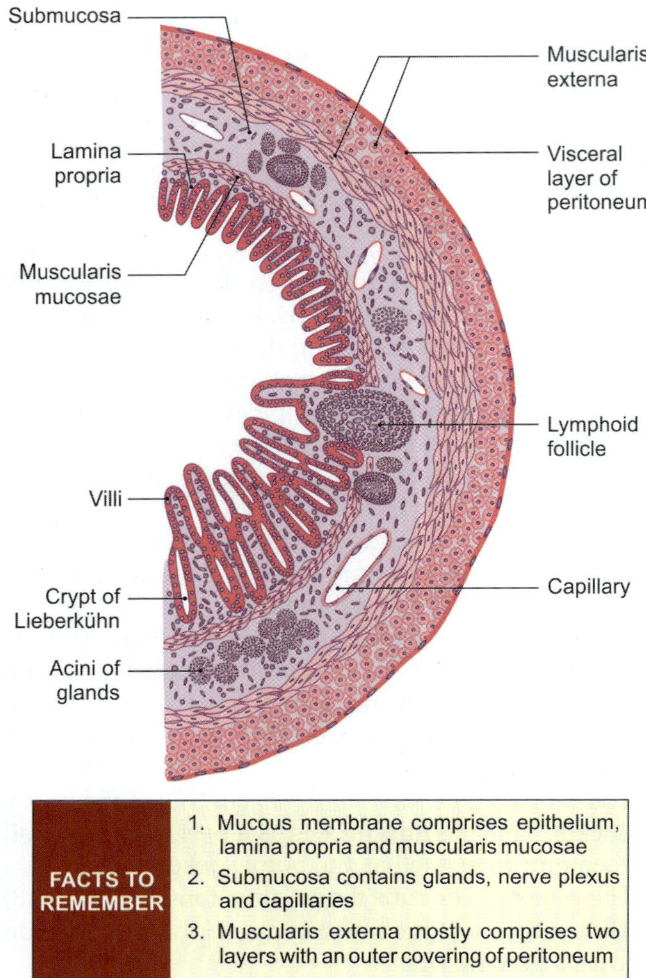

FACTS TO REMEMBER	
	1. Mucous membrane comprises epithelium, lamina propria and muscularis mucosae
	2. Submucosa contains glands, nerve plexus and capillaries
	3. Muscularis externa mostly comprises two layers with an outer covering of peritoneum

Fig. 45.55: General plan of gastrointestinal tract (diagrammatic)

b. *Lamina propria*: It consists of compact connective tissue with collagen, elastic and reticular fibres. It supports the epithelium. It contains capillaries, glands, fibroblasts, lymphocytes and sensory nerves which carry sensation of stretch and distension. This layer also contains extensions of muscularis mucosae. Lymphoid follicles are present in many regions like Peyer's patches in ileum. Cells in the lamina propria are also the source of growth factors which regulate the differentiation, turnover and repair of the epithelial cells.

c. *Muscularis mucosae*: It is made of an inner circular and an outer longitudinal layer of smooth muscle fibres. It is developed from oesophagus till distal part of rectum.
   - It causes localised movements of the mucous membrane helping in digestion and absorption.
   - The extensions of muscularis mucosae into the villus exert a milking effect on the lacteals of the villi of small intestine and promotes vascular exchange.
   - Its circular layer helps in emptying of the glands of lamina propria.

By its contraction, it modifies the shape of the local mucous membrane, permitting it to adapt to the altered shape due to its contents.

Submucosa

Submucosa consists of dense connective tissue, blood vessels and *Meissner's* or *submucous plexus* of nerves, ganglion cells, lymphatics and glands. It is a strong layer of the gut. It contains largest arterial network for supply of mucous membrane and muscularies externa. Submucosa enters into folds of oesophagus, stomach and intestine. Does not enter into the villus.

Muscularis Externa

Muscularis externa is comprised of an inner circular and an outer longitudinal layer of smooth muscle. The antagonistic activities of these two layers result in peristalsis. Circular layer is mostly thicker than the longitudinal layer. Only in colon the longitudinal layer is thicker, forming taenia. The contraction of this layer results in peristaltic movements along the intestines. Between the two layers of muscle fibres is the *Auerbach's* or *myenteric plexus* of autonomic nerves with a few ganglion cells. Parasympathetic system is (i) secretomotor to the glands, (ii) motor to the smooth muscle of the gut, and (iii) inhibitory to the sphincters of gut. Sympathetic system has the opposite effect.

Serosa or Adventitia

Serosa is the outermost protective layer which carries some blood vessels, nerves and lymphatics. A double layer of serosa forms the mesentery by which various organs are suspended from the abdominal wall.

OESOPHAGUS

The oesophagus is a muscular tube that rapidly propels the food from pharynx into the stomach. It is about 25 cm long. Its wall includes all the layers included in the general plan of GIT.

The **mucous membrane** is thrown into longitudinal folds when empty. These folds become smooth as the bolus of food passes through the oesophagus. The epithelium is *stratified squamous non-keratinised* in character and protective in function. The lamina propria sends papillae into the epithelium. The muscularis mucosae is indistinct at the beginning of oesophagus, but becomes distinct lower down. It is made up of longitudinal layer of smooth muscle fibres (Fig. 45.56).

The **submucosa** contains *oesophageal glands*. These are mucus secreting glands with acini which are round or oval in shape. The lining cells are truncated columnar with flattened peripheral nuclei. The cytoplasm is lightly stained and contains mucigen droplets.

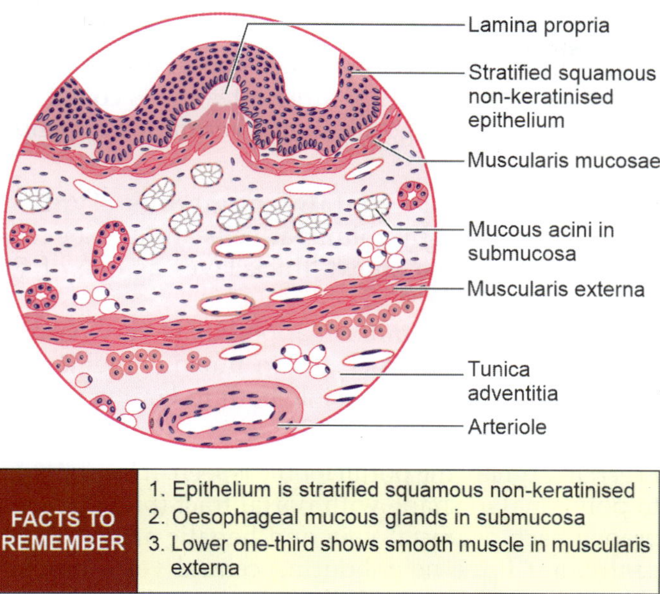

FACTS TO REMEMBER	1. Epithelium is stratified squamous non-keratinised 2. Oesophageal mucous glands in submucosa 3. Lower one-third shows smooth muscle in muscularis externa

Fig. 45.56: Oesophagus

The **muscularis externa** has striated muscle fibres in upper third, mixed, i.e. both striated and smooth muscle fibres in the middle third and smooth muscle fibres in the lower third of oesophagus.

The outermost layer is the **adventitia** which is made up of loose connective tissue with capillaries and nerves (Fig. 45.56).

Fundus and Body of Stomach

Epithelium of mucous membrane is tall columnar. All cells look alike. The free surface shows gastric pits, with 3–7 gastric glands opening into each pit. Deeper 2/3rd of gland is secretory and upper 1/3 is conducting part.

Chief cells and oxyntic cells line the gastric glands.

Muscularis externa shows 3 layers, inner oblique coat, middle circular coat and outer longitudinal coat. Rest is same (Fig. 45.57).

Small Intestine

Small intestine is characterised by the presence of evagination or villi of the mucous membrane for increasing suface area for absorption. In between villi are the crypts of Lieberkuln. Small intestien has 3 parts: Duodenum, jejunum and ileum. Duodenum contains mucous/Brunner's glands in submucosa. Rest is same as in general plan (Fig. 45.58).

Jejunum has neither Brunner's glands nor Peyer's patches. Rest is same as in general plan (Fig. 45.59).

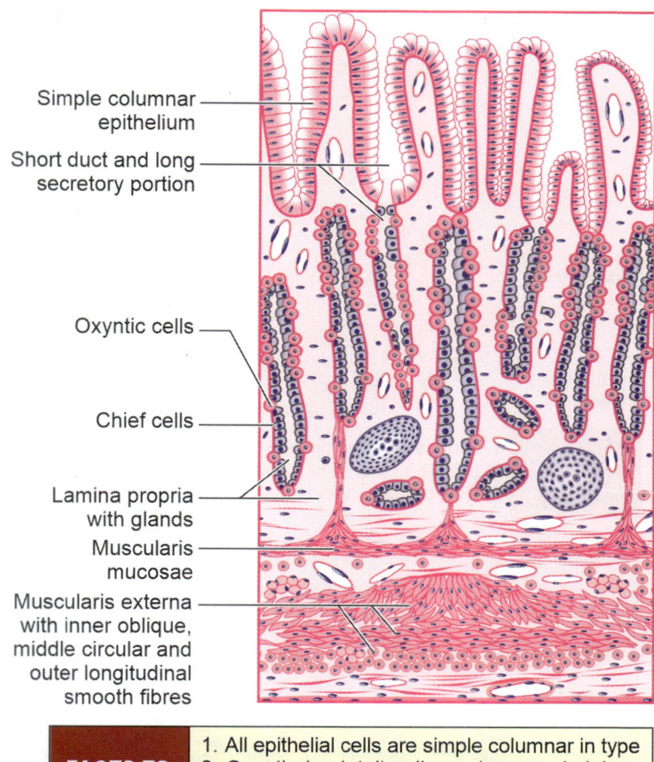

FACTS TO REMEMBER	1. All epithelial cells are simple columnar in type 2. Oxyntic (parietal) cells are large and pink, chief cells are small and blue 3. Duct is 1/3rd and secretory part is 2/3rd

Fig. 45.57: Fundus of stomach

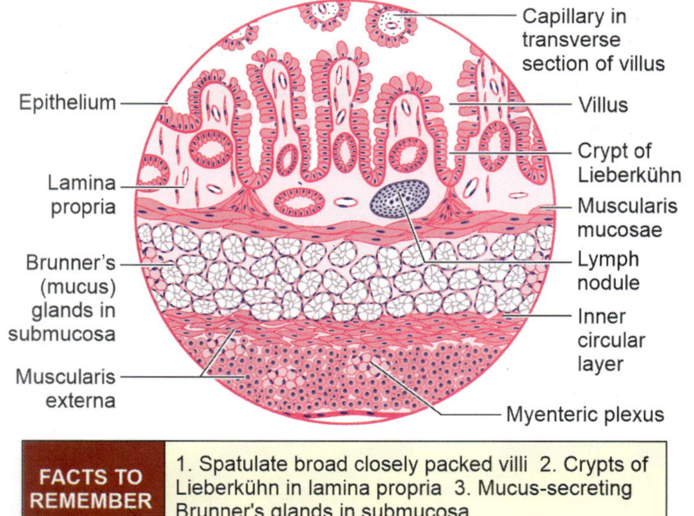

FACTS TO REMEMBER	1. Spatulate broad closely packed villi 2. Crypts of Lieberkühn in lamina propria 3. Mucus-secreting Brunner's glands in submucosa

Fig. 45.58: Duodenum

Ileum: Contains lots of lymph nodulus as Peyer's patches in lamina propria and submucosa. Rest is same as in general plan (Fig. 45.60).

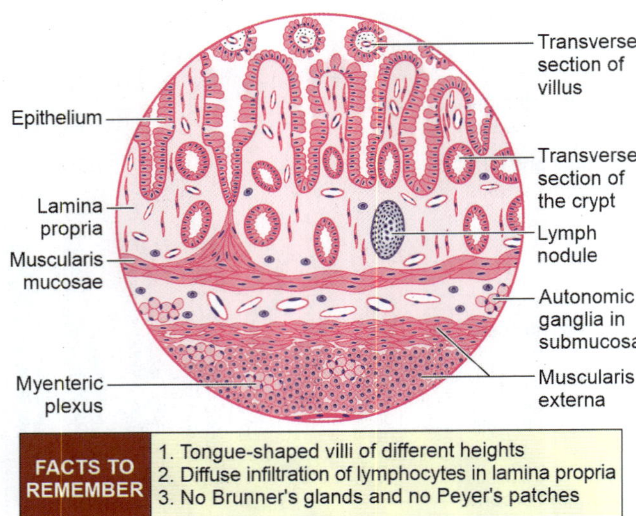

Fig. 45.59: Jejunum

Large Intestine

Large intestine extends from ileo-caecal orifice to anal orifice. Maximum part of large intestine is colon. The narrowest part of large intestine is vermiform appendix (Fig. 45.61).

Colon: Colon only contains numerous crypts of Lieberkühn, lined by columnar cells and goblet cells. Muscularis externa shows thick layer as one of the taenias (Fig. 45.61).

The lumen of vermiform appendix is very narrow. There are many deep crypts in mucous membrane. Lymphoid follicles are visible both in lamina propria and in submucosa (Fig. 45.62).

Liver: In human, the portal lobule is seen. It is triangular to polygonal in shape with portal tract (bile ductile, a branch each of portal vein and hepatic artery) in the centre and three neighbouring central veins on each side of it. Each liver cell/hepatocyte is hexagonal in

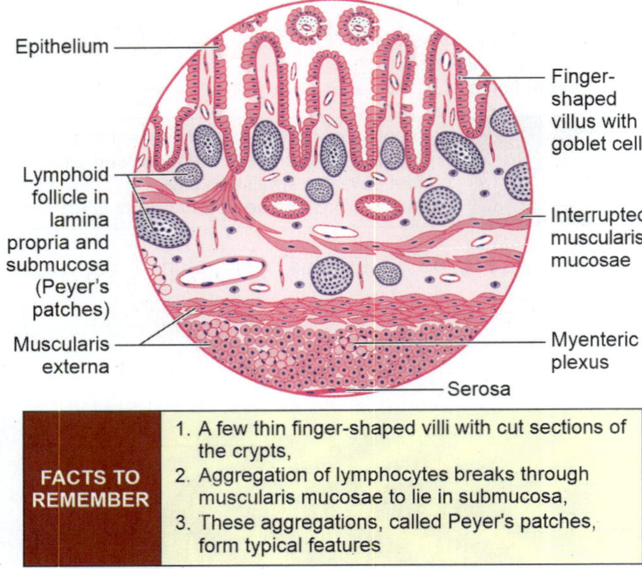

Fig. 45.60: Ileum

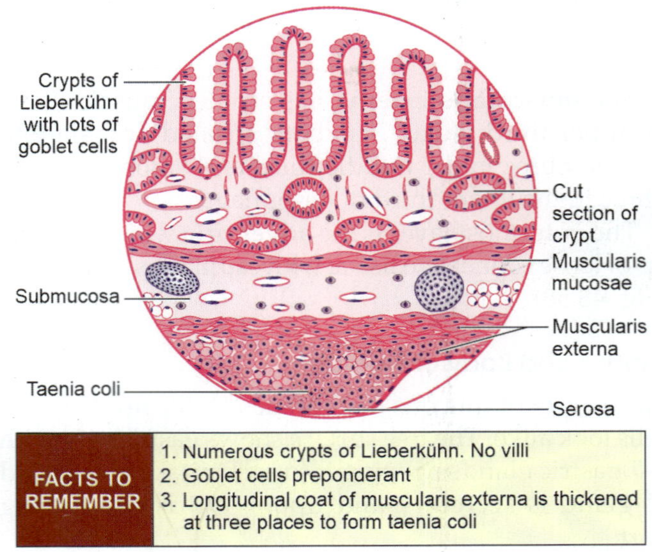

Fig. 45.61: Colon

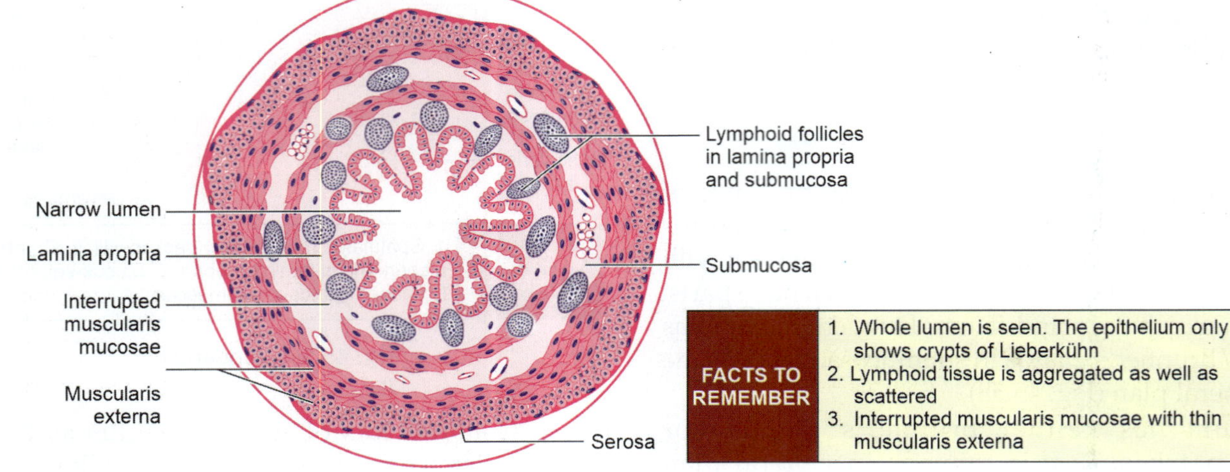

Fig. 45.62: Vermiform appendix

shape with around central nucleus. Liver cells run in laminae. Bile canaliculus lies in between adjacent cells of laminae. On one side of the cell is a bile canaliculus and on the other side is a sinusoid (Fig. 45.63).

Gallbladder: Epithelium consists of a single layer of tall columnar cells. Lamina propria shows cut sections of folds of mucous membrane. Deep to lamina propria is thin fibromuscular coat with subserous and serous coats (Fig. 45.64).

Pancreas: It is composed of an exocrine part, secreting pancreatic juice and an endocrine part called islets of Langerhans, secreting insulin from β cells and glucagon from α cells (Fig. 45.65).

Kidney: Comprises glomeruli made up of capillaries lined by endothelial cells; proximal and distal convoluted tubulus, loop of Henle and collecting ducts (Fig. 45.66).

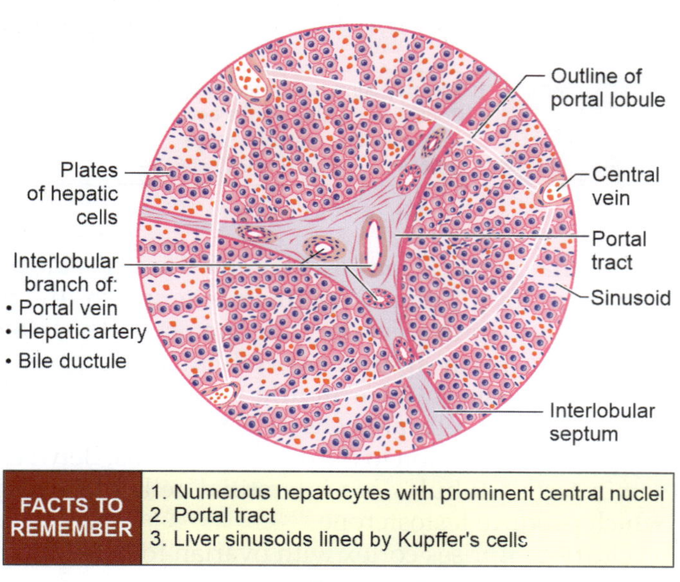

FACTS TO REMEMBER	1. Numerous hepatocytes with prominent central nuclei 2. Portal tract 3. Liver sinusoids lined by Kupffer's cells

Fig. 45.63: Liver

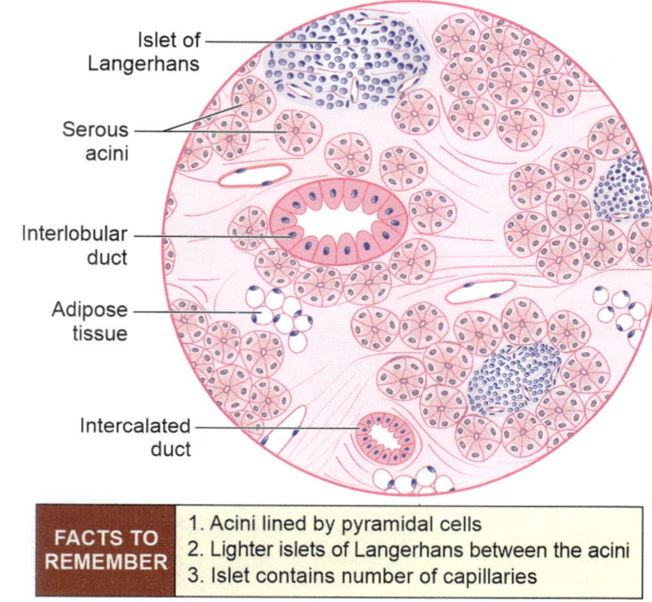

FACTS TO REMEMBER	1. Acini lined by pyramidal cells 2. Lighter islets of Langerhans between the acini 3. Islet contains number of capillaries

Fig. 45.65: Pancreas

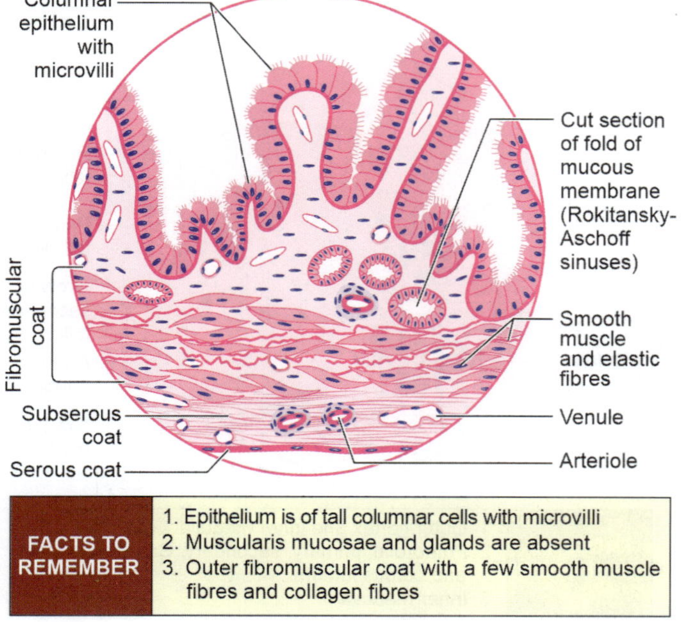

FACTS TO REMEMBER	1. Epithelium is of tall columnar cells with microvilli 2. Muscularis mucosae and glands are absent 3. Outer fibromuscular coat with a few smooth muscle fibres and collagen fibres

Fig. 45.64: Gallbladder

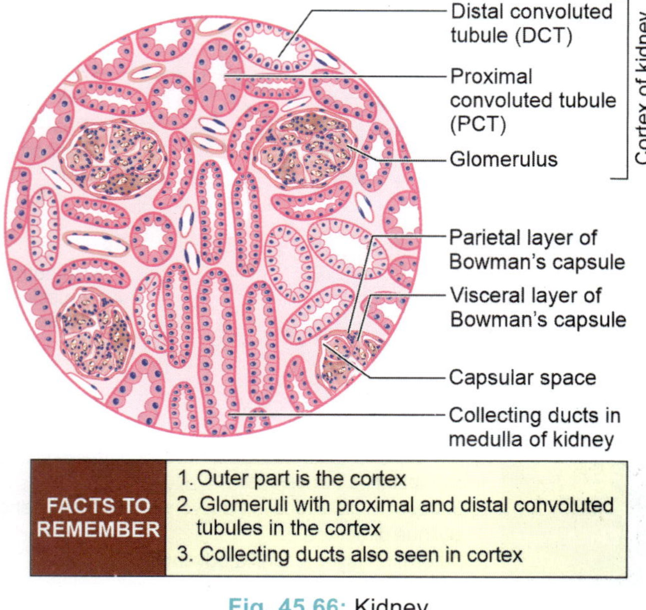

FACTS TO REMEMBER	1. Outer part is the cortex 2. Glomeruli with proximal and distal convoluted tubules in the cortex 3. Collecting ducts also seen in cortex

Fig. 45.66: Kidney

Ureter: Epithelial lining is of transitional variety. Lamina propria contains connective tissue. Muscular coat in upper 2/3rds has inner longitudinal and outer circular fibres. In lower 1/3rd, there is an additional outer longitudinal coat (Fig. 45.67).

Urinary bladder: The mucosa lined by transitional epithelium. Lamina propria is made up of connective tissue. Muscular coat is made up of smooth muscle fibres (Fig. 45.68).

Testis: Testis is made up of numerous lobules. Each lobule contains 1–4 seminiferous tubules. Each tubule is lined by stratified epithelium. The cell types are spermatogenic cells and supporting cells (Fig. 45.69).

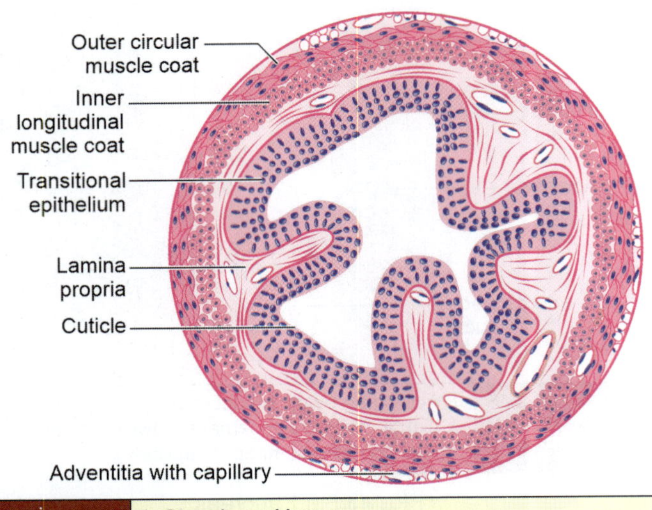

FACTS TO REMEMBER	1. Star-shaped lumen 2. Lining epithelium of transitional variety 3. Inner longitudinal and outer circular layer of smooth muscle fibres

Fig. 45.67: Ureter

FACTS TO REMEMBER	1. Epithelium is transitional 2. Detrusor muscle runs in transverse, longitudinal and oblique directions 3. Outermost layer is tunica adventitia

Fig. 45.68: Urinary bladder

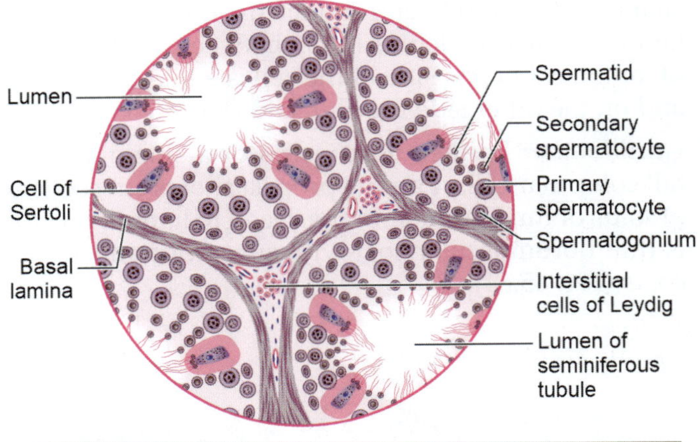

FACTS TO REMEMBER	1. Spermatogonia rest on the basal lamina 2. Reduction division occurs between primary and secondary spermatocyte stage 3. Cells of Leydig secrete testosterone

Fig. 45.69: Testis

Spermatogonia lie on basal lamina. These divide by mitosis to form primary spermatocyte, which divide by meiosis to form secondary spermatocyte. The latter divides to form spermatid, which undergoes a metamorphosis to form motile spermatozoa. With spermatogenic cells are cells of Sertoli for providing support and nutrition to the developing cells. Between seminiferous tubules are interstitial cells of Leydig which produce testosterone.

Ovary comprises cortex with ovarian follicles and a medulla with connective tissue and blood vessels. Ovary produces ova and secretes oestrogen and progesterone hormones.

Various follicles are primordial follicle, primary follicle, growing follicle, graafian follicle, atretic follicles and cellular corpus luteum (Fig. 45.70).

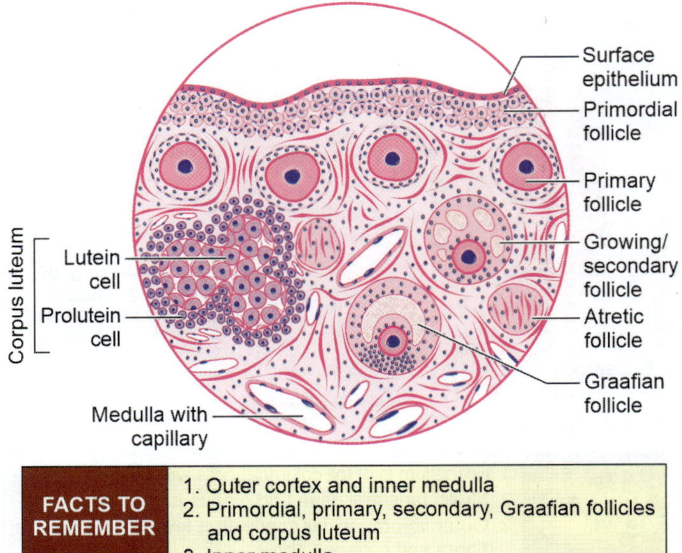

FACTS TO REMEMBER	1. Outer cortex and inner medulla 2. Primordial, primary, secondary, Graafian follicles and corpus luteum 3. Inner medulla

Fig. 45.70: Ovary

ENDOCRINE SYSTEM

The endocrine or ductless glands are situated in various regions of the body. They are devoid of ducts and the secretions are poured directly into the blood through the capillaries and numerous sinusoids draining and irrigating the gland. These have rich blood supply. Each of the gland secretes specific hormones with distinct functions. The principal endocrine glands are the hypophysis, thyroid, parathyroid, suprarenal, pineal glands and parts of pancreas, testis and ovary.

HYPOPHYSIS CEREBRI

The hypophysis cerebri lies in the cranial cavity and is attached to the base of the brain by the stalk or infundibulum. The hypophysis has two major divisions; the *neurohypophysis* which develops as a process growing downward from the floor of the diencephalon, and the *adenohypophysis* which originates in the embryo as a dorsal outpouching from the roof of the mouth. The neurohypophysis is also known as the posterior lobe.

There are three subdivisions of the adenohypophysis, the *pars distalis* or anterior lobe, *pars intermedia* and *pars tuberalis* (Fig. 45.71).

Pars Distalis

Pars distalis forms the largest subdivision of the hypophysis cerebri. It is composed of glandular cells arranged in irregular cords or clumps. These are intimately related to the extensive system of thin walled capillaries and sinusoids. The glandular cells are:

- Chromophobes which form 50 percent of the total cell population.
- Chromophils, forming the rest of the 50 percent of the cell population.

Chromophils are of two types: Acidophils or alpha cells and basophils or beta cells.

Chromophobes

Chromophobes are small cells, with homogeneous light staining cytoplasm. Nuclei are pale and lie in the centre of the cells. The cells are frequently arranged in groups or clumps. These cells are believed to give rise to chromophils or are fatigued secretory cells (Fig. 45.72).

Chromophils

Chromophils are larger than the chromophobes and contain granules in their cytoplasm. These cells are usually present at the periphery of the clump. Chromophils consist of *alpha* or acidophilic cells and *beta* or basophilic cells. Acidophilic cells can be further distinguished by differential histochemical stains into type A acidophil and type B acidophil. Type A acidophil secretes somatotropin hormone (STH) or growth hormone and type B acidophil secretes lactogenic/luteotropic hormone (LTH). Similarly basophils can be differentiated into beta basophils, responsible for the secretion of thyrotropic hormone (TSH) and adrenocorticotrophic hormone (ACTH) and delta basophils which elaborate gonadotropins (FSH, LH and ICSH).

Pars Intermedia

The pars distalis is separated from the neurohypophysis by a cleft lined on the juxtaneural side by a multilayered epithelium of basophilic cells

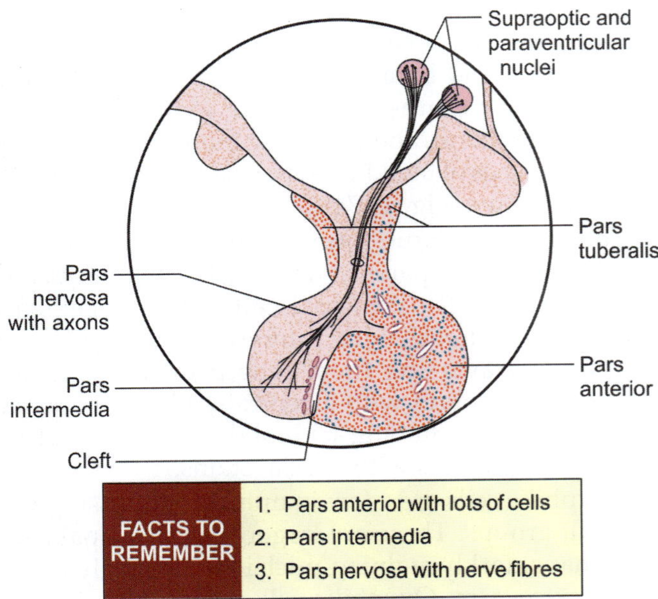

Fig. 45.71: Hypophysis cerebri

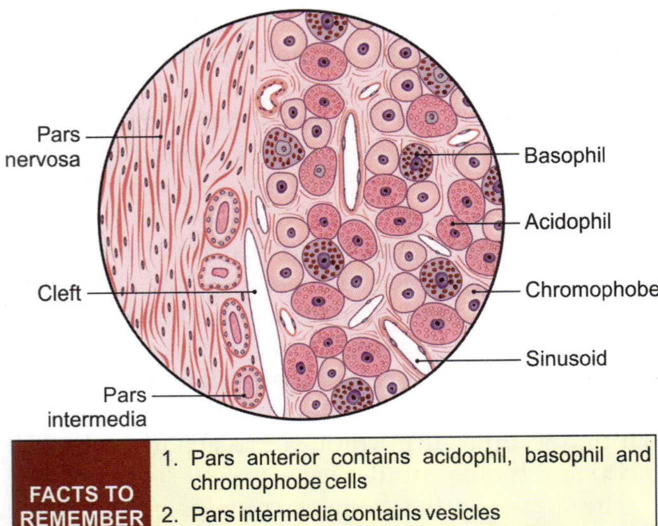

Fig. 45.72: Hypophysis cerebri

comprising the pars intermedia. The cells here are low columnar in shape and are basophilic in their staining properties. The cells are arranged in the form of vesicles which are lined by low columnar cells and contain colloid in their cytoplasm. The only hormone secreted by the pars intermedia is the *melanocyte stimulating hormone*.

Pars Nervosa

Pars nervosa consists of terminal portions of axons of extrinsic secretory neurons (supraoptic and paraventricular nuclei) whose cell bodies are located in the hypothalamus and an intrinsic population of modified neuroglial cells called the *pituicytes*. These cells are highly variable in size, shape and have cytoplasmic processes. Throughout the neurohypophysis are spherical masses that stain deeply with chrome-alum haematoxylin stain and are called *Herring bodies*. These are believed to be local accumulations of neurosecretory material in the axoplasm of the *hypothalamo-hypophyseal tract*, to be discharged into the sinusoids present therein. Hormones secreted by pars nervosa include *oxytocin, and antidiuretic hormone vasopressin*.

THYROID GLAND

Thyroid gland is responsible for maintaining the *basal metabolic rate* of the body by means of tetraiodothyronine (thyroxine) and tri-iodothyronine elaborated by the follicular cells. Another smaller number of cells called the *parafollicular cells* lower the calcium in the blood by means of *thyrocalcitonin*.

Thyroid gland is covered by the false capsule derived from pretracheal fascia. Its true capsule is comprised of collagen fibres. This capsule sends connective tissue septa into the gland to form lobes and lobules. These septa provide support to the abundant fenestrated capillaries present in the gland.

The structural and functional unit of thyroid gland is a *follicle*. Each follicle is an oval or round space lined by single layer of epithelial cells. The epithelial cells vary in size according to activity of the gland. The epithelium is cuboidal in normal functioning area, columnar in hyperactive stage and low cuboidal in resting phase. Different areas of gland show variance in height of cells (Fig. 45.73).

The epithelial cells rest on a basal lamina. The sparse connective tissue is rich in capillaries of blood and lymph, as thyroid hormones are absorbed both by blood and lymph capillaries.

The lumen of the follicles contains colloid which represents the stored product of the secretory activity of the gland and takes up acidophilic stain. Its main constituents are *thyroglobulin* and *iodothyroglobulin*.

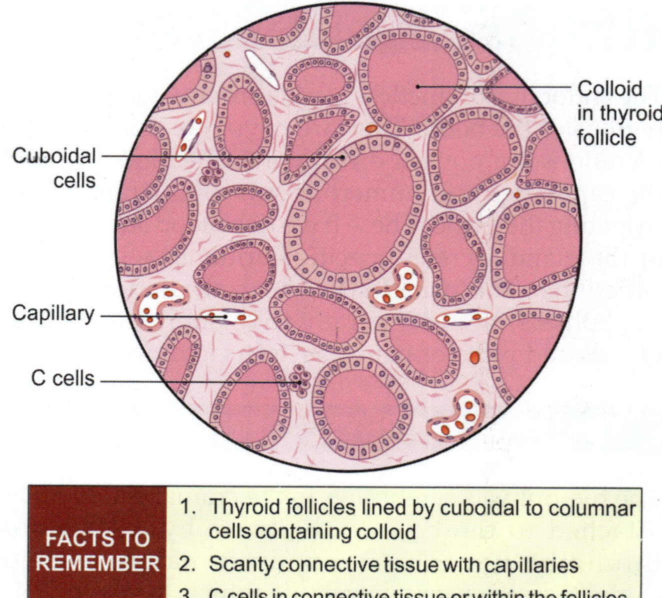

FACTS TO REMEMBER	
	1. Thyroid follicles lined by cuboidal to columnar cells containing colloid
	2. Scanty connective tissue with capillaries
	3. C cells in connective tissue or within the follicles

Fig. 45.73: Thyroid gland

In addition to the follicular cells, another smaller population of cells are seen. These are lighter in colour, bigger in size and are present amongst the follicular epithelium, situated between the basement membrane and the epithelial cells or between the follicles. These cells are termed *parafollicular* or *'C' cells*. These secrete a hormone named **thyrocalcitonin** or **calcitonin** responsible for lowering blood calcium level.

PARATHYROID GLAND

The parathyroid glands are two pairs of small, yellow brown bodies intimately connected with the posterior aspect of the thyroid gland. These glands are separated from the thyroid by a thin connective tissue capsule. The capsular connective tissue extends into the parathyroid gland, and it is along these trabeculae that larger branches of blood vessels, nerves and lymphatics enter and leave (Fig. 45.74).

The reticular tissue forms framework of the parathyroid gland. The parenchyma consists of *principal cells* and *oxyphilic cells*. Principal cells or chief cells are arranged in sheets with numerous sinusoids and capillaries traversing them. The principal cells are polygonal or round with a centrally placed vesicular nuclei and a pale staining acidophilic cytoplasm. These cells show granules with special stains.

Oxyphilic cells are a few in number, occur singly or in small groups. These are larger than principal cells. They have darkly staining nuclei and strongly acidophilic cytoplasm. Oxyphilic cells are seen to increase with age.

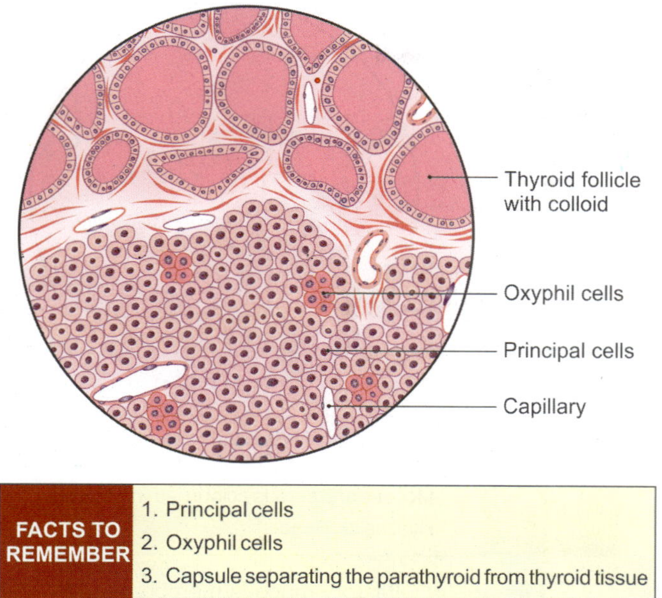

Fig. 45.74: Parathyroid gland

The principal or chief cells secrete *parathormone* responsible for maintaining the blood calcium level. In cases of hyperactivity of parathyroid gland, blood calcium level gets elevated by withdrawing it from the bones, thereby causing osteoporosis or fracture of bones. Increased calcium level also favours tendency for renal stone formation.

SUPRARENAL OR ADRENAL GLAND

The paired suprarenal or adrenal glands are roughly triangular or semilunar flattened glands, at the cranial pole of each kidney. It is surrounded by a thick capsule in which there are branches of main vessels, nerves and lymphatics. The septa penetrate from the capsule into the interior carrying blood vessels along them.

Each gland is comprised of outer yellow cortex surrounding the inner dark brown medulla. Medulla appears to be the "filling" of a sandwich formed by the cortex (Fig. 45.75).

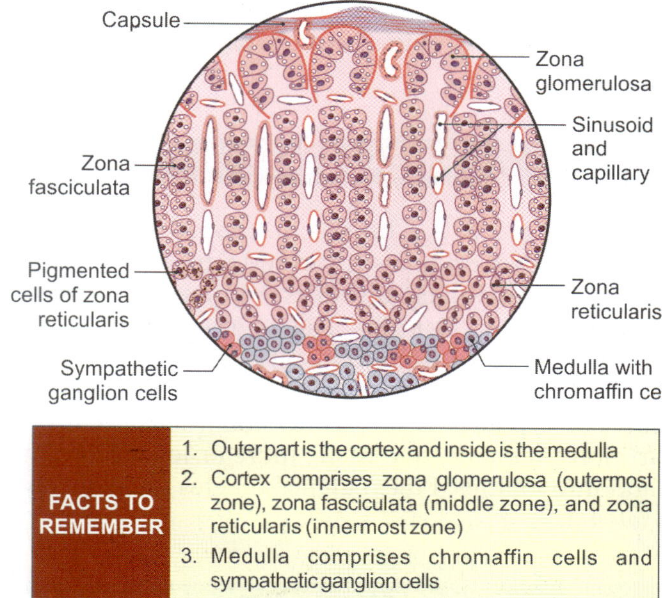

Fig. 45.75: Suprarenal gland

Cortex

The cortex shows three zones, outermost is the *zona glomerulosa*, a thick middle layer is the *zona fasciculata*, and moderately thick inner layer is the *zona reticularis* which is continuous with the medulla. The transition from one zone to the other is gradual and is not well demarcated.

The zona glomerulosa or outer zone consists of closely packed groups and **arches of columnar cells.** The nuclei are spherical and stain deeply. The cytoplasm shows vacuoles. Sinusoids are seen in between the groups of cells. The cells of the zona glomerulosa secrete *mineralocorticoids*.

In the middle zone or zona fasciculata the cells are arranged in vertical columns, with large number of vacuoles in their cytoplasm. These cells are also called **spongiocytes**. The cytoplasm is slightly basophilic and nuclei are central. The sinusoids follow a vertical course in this zone. The cells of the zona fasciculata secrete *glucocorticoids*.

In the inner zone or zona reticularis, the regular parallel arrangement of cords give way to an anastomosing network. The cytoplasm of cells contains fewer lipid droplets and is less vacuolated. Some of the cells contain yellow pigment. The intervening capillaries are irregularly arranged. These cells secrete *sex hormones*.

Another view about the functions of the cortex is that zona glomerulosa is the cell producing zone; zona fasciculata the hormone-producing zone and the zona reticularis the graveyard of the cells.

Medulla

Medulla is composed of chromaffin cells or pheochromocytes. These are arranged in irregular rounded groups or short cords isolated by fine septa. These are surrounded by blood capillaries and venules. The cytoplasm of the cells is basophilic. When the tissue is fixed in solution containing potassium bichromate, these cells are seen to be filled with fine brown granules and this is described as the *chromaffin reaction*. These granules are precursors of the hormone *epinephrine* or *adrenaline* and *norepinephrine* or *noradrenaline*. Norepinephrine producing cells are relatively more densely granulated. Interspersed between these cells are characteristic autonomic ganglion cells which are seen singly or in groups of two to four. The ganglion cells are large with big vesicular nuclei and nucleoli (Fig. 18.7).

PINEAL GLAND

The pineal gland is a little cone shaped body about 1 cm in length. It originates from and remains connected to third ventricle and lies dorsal to the midbrain. It contains two types of cells. The neuroectodermal cells give rise to parenchymal cells and are termed *pinealocytes*. The *mesenchymal cells* give rise to connective tissue of capsule of the gland and the incomplete partitions of connective tissue more or less divide the gland into lobules. Pineal gland secretes *serotonin* and *melatonin*.

PANCREAS

Islets of Langerhans of pancreas constitute the **endocrinal** part of the gland and have been described with the pancreas gland.

TESTIS AND OVARY

The hormones produced by these glands have been described with the respective reproductive systems.

ORGANS OF SPECIAL SENSES

Following are the organs of special senses:

1 Olfactory epithelium for sense of smell.
2 Taste buds of tongue for sense of taste (included with tongue).
3 Retina of the eye for sense of sight (included with eyeball).
4 Internal ear for sense of hearing and balance.
5 Skin for sense of touch (*see* Chapter 10).

OLFACTORY EPITHELIUM

The receptors of the sense of smell are located in the olfactory epithelium. The olfactory area extends from the middle of the roof of the nasal cavity, about 8 to 10 mm inferiorly on each side of the septum and on the upper surface of the superior nasal concha.

The epithelium is of tall *pseudostratified columnar* variety. It consists of three types—*basal cells, supporting or sustentacular cells* and *olfactory cells* (Fig. 45.76).

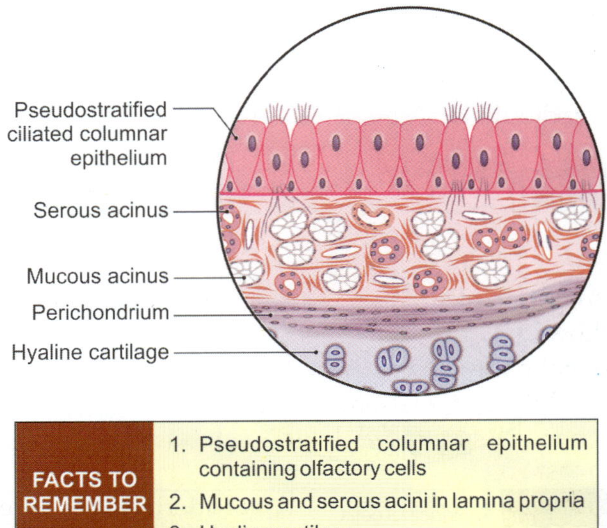

FACTS TO REMEMBER	
	1. Pseudostratified columnar epithelium containing olfactory cells
	2. Mucous and serous acini in lamina propria
	3. Hyaline cartilage

Fig. 45.76: Olfactory mucous membrane

BASAL CELLS

These cells form the deepest layer of the epithelium. They are triangular in shape with dark nuclei and branching processes. They have capability of regeneration.

SUPPORTING OR SUSTENTACULAR CELLS

These are tall cells, narrow at the basal end and wider at the free end. The nucleus is almost in the centre with light staining chromatin and nucleolus. A few gaps are present in between these cells through which olfactory cell processes pass.

OLFACTORY CELLS

These cells are evenly distributed between the supporting cells and are called the *bipolar neurons*. The nuclei of these cells lie towards the basement membrane between the basal cells and sustentacular cells. The apical portion of the bipolar cells is a modified dendron which passes through the gap between the sustentacular cells and reaches the surface of the epithelium. The proximal end tapers into a thin smooth filament, which is the axon, a fibre of the olfactory nerve. It passes into the connective tissue and with similar fibres forms small nerve bundles. Radiating from its apical surface there are six to eight olfactory cilia which are non-motile. These cilia are the components of the sense organ and are stimulated by contact with odorous substances.

The **lamina propria** contains a rich plexus of blood capillaries, large veins, lymphatics and elastic fibres. It also contains the branched tubuloalveolar olfactory *glands of Bowman*. The ducts of the glands assume a perpendicular course and open on the surface. The secretory part has mucous acini. The glands secrete a thin mucus secretion which bathes the cilia. The gases first get dissolved in this fluid before they can be smelt.

TASTE BUDS OF TONGUE

TONGUE

The tongue is a muscular organ and its functions are as follows.

- To move the bolus of food from side to side.
- To help in articulation of speech.
- To perceive the taste of various foodstuffs through the taste buds.

The tongue (Fig. 45.77) consists of interlacing bundles of striated muscles that run in different directions and cross one another. The musculature of the tongue is covered by *stratified squamous non-keratinised epithelium*. The epithelium on the ventral surface is thinner as compared to the epithelium on the dorsal surface which is much thicker.

In the anterior two-thirds on the dorsal surface of tongue, the underlying corium consists of collagen and elastic fibres which project upwards forming *papillae;* whereas in its posterior one-third or pharyngeal part, it presents only irregular bulges due to *lymphoid tissue*. The boundary between the two regions is inverted V-shaped. The principal gustatory region of the tongue is anterior to this line.

PAPILLAE

Three types of papillae are present: The *filiform*, the *fungiform* and the *circumvallate*.

- The *filiform papillae* are arranged in more or less distinct rows diverging to the right and left from the middle line.
- The *fungiform papillae* are a few in number. These have short, slightly constricted stalks and flattened hemispherical upper surfaces. The lamina propria core forms secondary papillae that project into the recesses on the undersurface of the epithelium. On some of the fungiform papillae the epithelium associated with secondary papillae contains taste buds.
- The *circumvallate papillae* (Fig. 45.78) are bigger than the other two types of papillae and lie just anterior to the junction of the anterior two-thirds and the posterior one-third of the tongue. The papillae are surrounded by deep circular furrows and **do not** project above the surface epithelium. The **lamina propria** core forms secondary papillae only on the upper surface. The epithelium is smooth on the lateral surface of papillae, and contains many taste buds.

Connected with the circumvallate papillae are glands of serous type, whose bodies are embedded in the underlying muscular tissue, ducts of which open at the bottom of the furrow. Mucous glands are present in

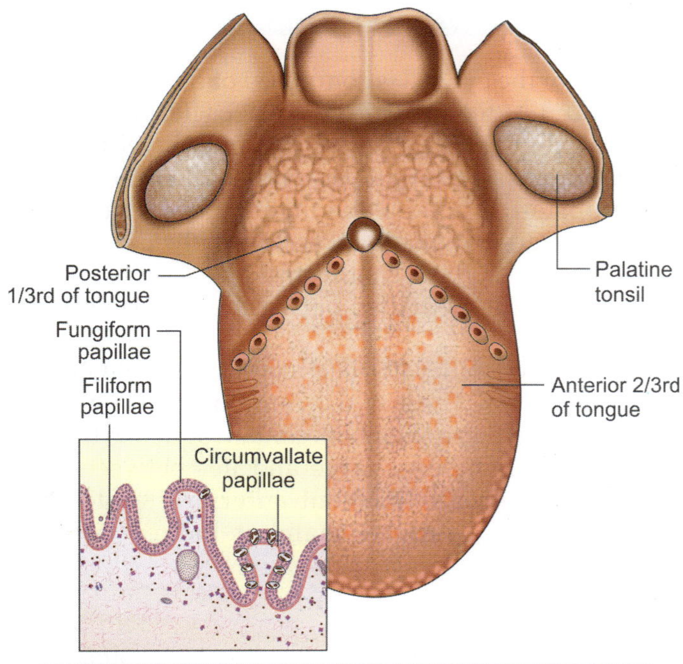

FACTS TO REMEMBER	
	1. Stratified squamous epithelium
	2. Filiform, fungiform and circumvallate papillae with taste buds
	3. Anterior 2/3rd contains papillae and posterior 1/3rd contains lymphoid follicles

Fig. 45.77: Tongue with its parts. The inset shows the various types of papillae

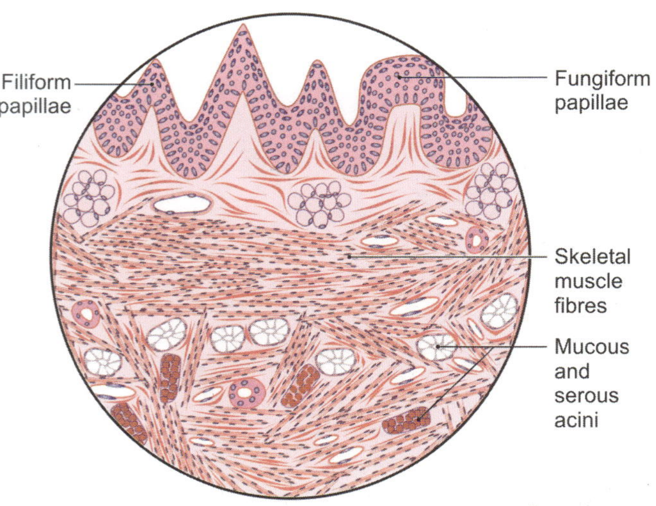

FACTS TO REMEMBER	
	1. Stratified squamous epithelium
	2. Filiform and fungiform papillae seen
	3. Striated muscle with mucous and serous acini

Fig. 45.78: Anterior part of tongue with papillae

relation to the pharyngeal part, tip and margins. Deep to the corium is striated muscle seen in all planes, i.e. longitudinal, transverse and oblique. The connective tissue in between muscle fasciculi contains blood vessels and nerves.

TASTE BUDS

The taste buds are seen on the lateral sides of the circumvallate papillae; some are also seen on the fungiform papillae. These are also present on the posterior part of the tongue, on the soft palate, on the posterior surface of epiglottis and on the posterior wall of the pharynx. Taste buds are barrel-shaped structures, narrower at the ends and broader in the middle. Two types of cells are distinguished in relation to the taste buds, the *supporting* or *sustentacular cells* and *neuroepithelial* or *gustatory cells.*

Sustentacular or Supporting Cells

These cells are arranged peripherally, have a curved course, narrow at each of its ends and broader in the centre, appearing almost spindle-shaped. At both ends the cells surround small openings known as the internal and external taste pores (Fig. 45.79).

Neuroepithelial or Gustatory Cells

These are distributed between the sustentacular cells and are long narrow cells having a slender rod-shaped form with a nucleus in the middle. On the free surface, these cells give rise to short hair which project into the lumen of the pit. The substances to be tasted first get dissolved in the saliva, stimulate the hair of neuroepithelial cells and then the impulse is conducted along the nerves. There are five fundamental taste sensations—sweet, bitter, sour, salty and umami. Last one is pleasant and gets triggered by amino acids, e.g. meat broth or old cheese (Fig. 45.80).

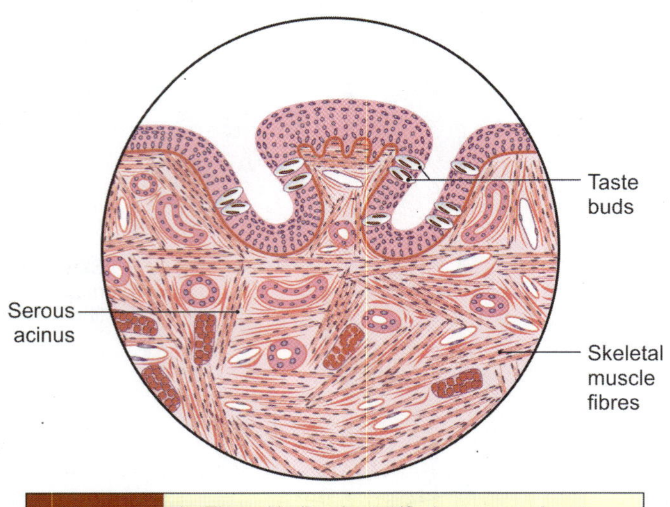

FACTS TO REMEMBER	
	1. The epithelium is stratified squamous in nature
	2. The side walls of the papilla contain numerous taste buds
	3. Taste buds comprise sustentacular and gustatory cells

Fig. 45.79: Circumvallate papilla

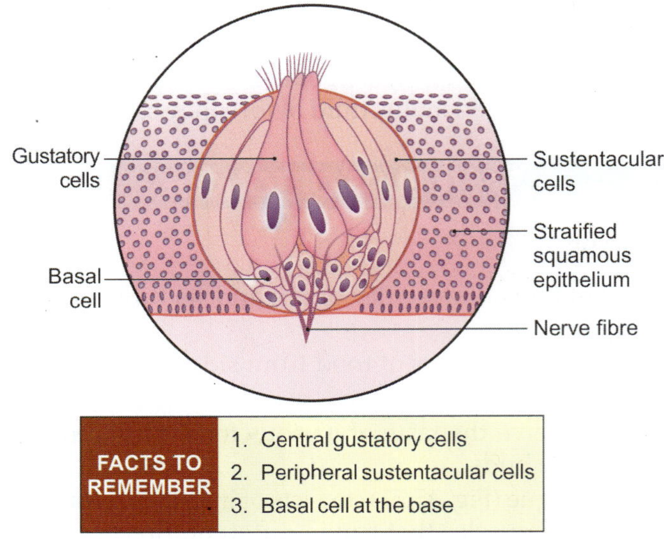

FACTS TO REMEMBER	
	1. Central gustatory cells
	2. Peripheral sustentacular cells
	3. Basal cell at the base

Fig. 45.80: Taste bud

STRUCTURE OF THE EYEBALL

The wall of the eyeball is composed of three concentric layers, the outer protective corneoscleral coat, the middle vascular coat, and the innermost layer which is the photosensitive retina. The corneoscleral coat has a large posterior opaque segment, the sclera, and a smaller anterior transparent segment, the cornea. The eyeball contains three chambers:

1 Anterior chamber lies between cornea, and iris (Fig. 45.81).
2 Posterior chamber lies between iris, anteriorly and ligament lens. These two communicate through the pupil. Both these chambers contain aqueous humor.
3 Vitreous chamber is large and lies between lens, with suspensory ligament anteriorly and retina posteriorly. Vitreous chamber lodges vitreous humor.

OUTER CORNEOSCLERAL COAT

Cornea

Cornea consists of five layers:

1 Corneal epithelium which is continuous at its margins with the conjunctiva.
2 The anterior limiting membrane or Bowman's membrane.
3 Substantia propria.

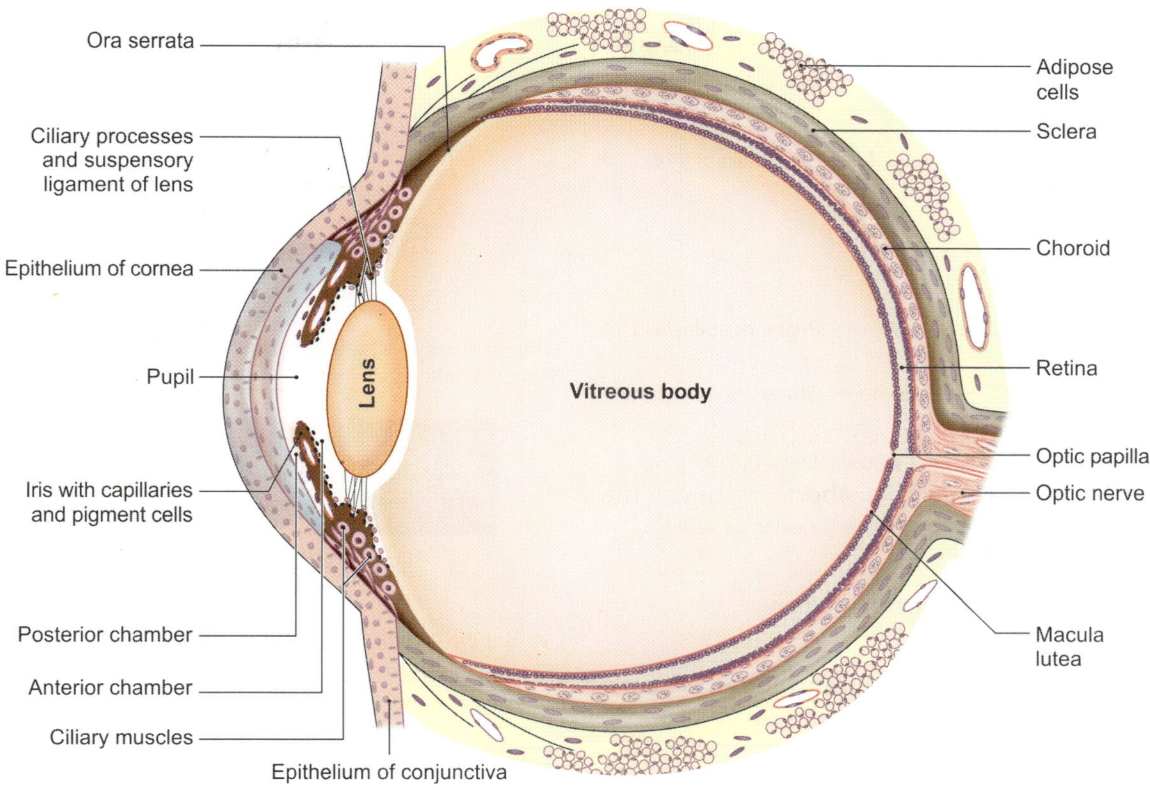

Fig. 45.81: Structure of the eyeball

4 The posterior limiting membrane or Descemet's membrane.
5 The posterior epithelium or mesenchymal epithelium of the anterior chamber.

Corneal Epithelium

It covers the front of the cornea and is stratified squamous, having four to five layers of cells. The deepest cells resting on the linear basement membrane are columnar with rod-shaped nuclei. In the superficial layers, the cells become progressively squamous. They contain flattened nuclei which do not become keratinised. The epithelium of the cornea is extremely sensitive and contains numerous free nerve endings.

Bowman's Membrane

The corneal epithelium rests on a structureless homogeneous membrane called the Bowman's membrane. It is formed by collagen fibres of substantia propria.

Substantia Propria

It is a transparent connective tissue whose bundles form thin lamellae arranged in many layers. Between the lamellae there is a metachromatic protein polysaccharide ground substance, the components of which are *chondroitin sulphate* and *keratosulphate*. The cells of the stroma are long slender fibroblasts lodged in narrow clefts among parallel bundles of collagen fibres.

Descemet's Membrane

It is homogeneous membrane deep to the substantia propria.

Posterior Epithelium or Mesenchymal Epithelium

The inner surface of Descemet's membrane is covered by a layer of low cuboidal cells.

SCLERA

Sclera consists of white fibrous tissue, the fibres of which run in bundles, parallel to the surface, between which are a few elastic and reticular fibres. The cells of the sclera are elongated fibroblasts.

CORNEOSCLERAL JUNCTION

The boundary between the opaque sclera and the transparent cornea is an oblique line. The outer edge of the sclera overlaps slightly the border of the cornea. The collagenous bundles of the sclera continue directly into those of the cornea where they become parallel with each other and the tissue becomes homogeneous as well as transparent. At the marginal zone or **limbus** of the cornea there is a gradual transition of its epithelium to

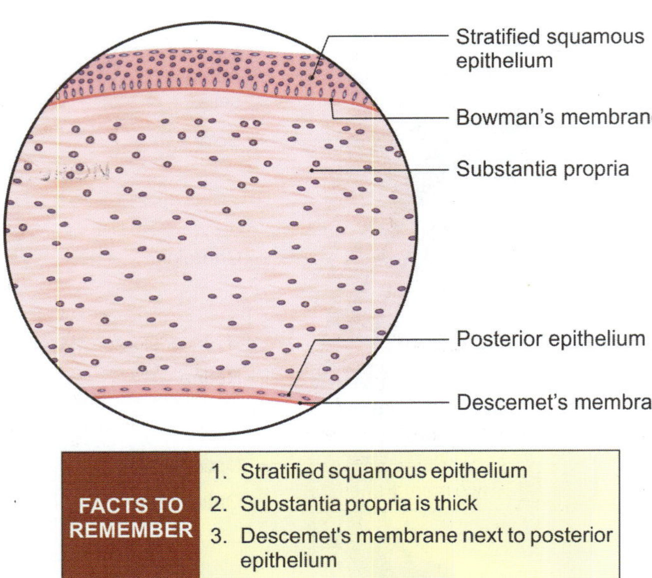

FACTS TO REMEMBER	1. Stratified squamous epithelium 2. Substantia propria is thick 3. Descemet's membrane next to posterior epithelium

Fig. 45.82: Structure of cornea

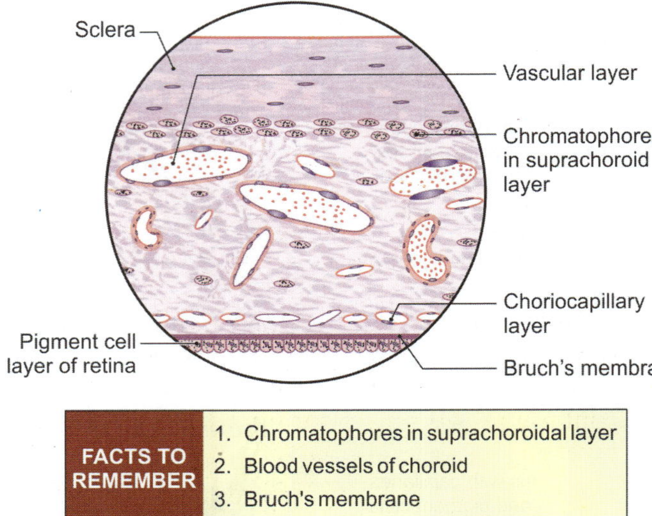

FACTS TO REMEMBER	1. Chromatophores in suprachoroidal layer 2. Blood vessels of choroid 3. Bruch's membrane

Fig. 45.83: Sclera and choroid

that of the conjunctiva. At this margin the Bowman's membrane ends and the subepithelial layer of loose connective tissue begins.

On its inner surface, the corneoscleral junction is marked by a shallow groove, the internal scleral furrow or sulcus. Its posterior lip forms a projecting ridge to which the ciliary body is fastened (Fig. 45.82). Just peripheral to the termination of Descemet's membrane is the trabecular meshwork enclosing small spaces known as *spaces of Fontana* which are lined by attenuated epithelium. These spaces communicate with the anterior chamber of the eye. There are also several small epithelial lined cavities, anterior and lateral to the trabecular meshwork near the bottom of the internal scleral furrow. These cavities are the cross-sections of a circular canal known as the *canal of Schlemm* which is parallel to the border of the cornea. This canal communicates with the venous system and is usually filled with clear **aqueous humor**.

MIDDLE VASCULAR COAT: CHOROID, CILIARY BODY AND IRIS CHOROID

From without inwards, choroid consists of the following four layers:

1 *Suprachoroid or epichoroid layer:* It is made up of fine collagenous fibres with elastic fibres and pigment cells called the *chromatophores* (Fig. 45.83).
2 *Vascular layer:* Contains large blood vessels. Between the vessels is fine connective tissue containing chromatophores.
3 *Choriocapillary layer:* Contains capillaries in a stroma of fine collagen and elastic fibres. These are the **widest capillaries in the body**. Through these capillaries the retina is constantly being nourished.
4 *Bruch's membrane:* It a thin glassy layer, which is made up of elastic fibres. It also acts as the basement membrane for the pigment cells of the retina.

Ciliary Body

It comprises a *ciliary ring*, the *ciliary muscles* which are made up of radial and circular fibres, and vascular *ciliary processes* which secrete the aqueous humor.

Iris

Iris is the anterior continuation of the ciliary body. The iris has an opening in its centre called the *pupil*. Between the iris and the cornea is the *anterior chamber* and between the iris and the lens is the *posterior chamber*. Both chambers are filled with **aqueous humor**.

Anteriorly the iris is lined by the mesothelial layer which is a continuation of the lining of the posterior surface of cornea. Posteriorly the iris is lined by two layers of cells which are the forward continuations of the two original layers of the retina. The stroma of the iris consists of fine connective tissue containing blood vessels, nerves, *sphincter and dilator pupillae muscles* as well as **chromatophores**. The number and distribution of chromatophores gives the appropriate colour to the iris.

INNER COAT—RETINA

Retina is the innermost of the three layers of the eyeball. In the retina ten parallel layers can be distinguished. Starting from the outer layers these are:

1 The pigment epithelium
2 Layer of rods and cones
3 Outer limiting membrane
4 Outer nuclear layer
5 Outer plexiform layer

6 Inner nuclear layer
7 Inner plexiform layer
8 Layer of ganglion cells
9 Layers of optic nerve fibre
10 Inner limiting membrane

1 *Pigment cell layer:* In this layer the cells have round nuclei. The apical cytoplasm is occupied by melanin granules.

2 *Layer of rods and cones:* This layer consists of dendritic cytoplasmic processes of the photoreceptors, i.e. rods and cones. Each rod or cone consists of an external or peripheral process, middle parts containing the nuclei forming the outer nuclear layer.

The internal or central processes or axons synapse with dendrites of bipolar cells and form outer plexiform layer. The peripheral processes of rods are cylindrical or rod shaped and are responsible for night vision. The peripheral processes of cones are conical in shape and are meant for **aquity, brightness of vision and for colour vision**. The *macula lutea* and *fovea centralis* contain only the **cones**.

3 *Outer limiting membrane:* It is made up of processes of neuroglial cells called *Müller's cells.*

4 *Outer nuclear layer:* The nuclei of rods and cones are present in this layer.

5 *Outer plexiform layer:* It is made up of synapses between the central processes of rods and cones along with the dendritic processes of the bipolar cells.

6 *Inner nuclear layer:* This layer contains nuclei of bipolar cells and Müller's cells.

7 *Inner plexiform layer:* It is formed by the synapses between the axons of bipolar cells and dendrites of the ganglion cells.

8 *Layer of ganglion cells:* The bodies of the ganglion cells are located in this layer.

9 *Layer of optic nerve fibres:* Axons of the ganglion cell layer form the layer of optic nerve fibres. These fibres acquire myelin only after piercing the sclera.

10 *Inner limiting membrane:* It is a thin homogeneous membrane formed by the termination of inner fibres of Müller's cells. It separates the rest of the layers of retina from the vitreous body (Fig. 45.84).

LENS

The lens is biconvex with anterior and posterior poles and an equator. Outermost is the lens capsule. Anteriorly the lens is lined by the *anterior epithelium* which is cuboidal in type. The rest of the lens is made up of *lens fibres* which are transparent (Fig. 45.81).

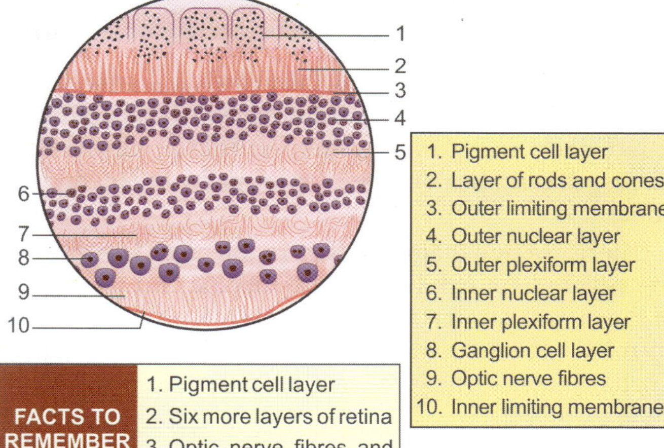

FACTS TO REMEMBER

1. Pigment cell layer
2. Six more layers of retina
3. Optic nerve fibres and two membranes

Fig. 45.84: Structure of retina

LACRIMAL GLAND

Lacrimal gland is a serous gland situated chiefly in the lacrimal fossa on the anterolateral part of the roof of the bony orbit and partly in the upper eyelid. It secretes lacrimal fluid for friction free movements of eyelids. When lacrimal fluid is produced in excess, it is called tears.

STRUCTURE OF EYELID

Each lid is made up of the following layers from without inwards:

1 The *skin* is thin, loose and easily distensible by oedema fluid or blood.

2 The *superficial fascia* is without any fat. It contains the palpebral part of the orbicularis oculi muscle.

3 The *palpebral fascia* of the two lids forms the orbital septum. Its thickenings form tarsal plates or *tarsi* in the lids and the *palpebral ligaments* at the angles. Tarsi are thin plates of condensed fibrous tissue located near the lid margins. They give stiffness to the lids.

4 The *conjunctiva* lines the posterior surface of the tarsus.

Apart from the usual glands of the skin and mucous glands in the conjunctiva, the larger glands found in the lids are:

a. Large sebaceous glands also called *Zeis' glands* at the lid margin associated with cilia.

b. Modified sweat glands or *Moll's glands* at the lid margin closely associated with Zeis' glands and cilia.

c. *Tarsal glands* or meibomian glands are embedded in the posterior surface of the tarsi; their ducts open in a row behind the cilia.

INTERNAL EAR

The internal ear is called labyrinth because of its complex structure. It is composed of a series of fluid-filled sacs and tubules suspended in cavities of corresponding form in the petrous part of the temporal bone.

There are two major cavities in the bony labyrinth—the vestibule which houses the saccule and the utricle of the membranous labyrinth. Anteromedial to it is the spirally coiled cochlea which contains the organ of Corti.

COCHLEA

Cochlea consists of a complex bony canal that makes two and three quarter spiral turns around a central axis formed by a conical pillar of the spongy bone called the *modiolus*. The *spiral ganglion* which receives the nerve fibres from the cochlear division of the statoacoustic (eighth cranial) nerve lies within the modiolus along the inner wall of the cochlear canal. Cell bodies in the spiral ganglion are *bipolar* afferent neurons (Fig. 45.85).

The lumen of the canal of the osseous cochlea is divided along its whole course into upper and lower sections by a *spiral lamina*. The lamina is divided into two zones, the inner zone containing bone (the osseous spiral lamina), and a fibrous outer zone (the membranous spiral lamina); the latter is also called the *basilar membrane*. At the attachment of the basilar membrane to the outer wall of cochlea, the periosteum is thickened and forms a distinct structure, the *spiral ligament*. The cochlear membrane (*Reissner's membrane*), extends obliquely from spiral lamina to the outer wall of the bony cochlea.

Thus a cross-section of the bony cochlea shows three compartments: An upper cavity the *scala vestibuli*; a lower cavity, the *scala tympani*; and an intermediate cavity the *scala media*. The latter is the cochlear duct, a portion of the endolymphatic system. The scala vestibuli and scala tympani are perilymphatic spaces.

SCALA MEDIA OR COCHLEAR DUCT

The roof of the scala media is formed by the vestibular or Reissner's membrane separating the scala vestibuli from the cochlear duct. The outer wall of the cochlear duct is formed by a vascular layer of the stratified columnar epithelium, under which lies the collagenous spiral ligament. The vestibular membrane is attached to the upper end of this spiral ligament. The medial end of the membrane is continuous with the periosteum of the *osseous spiral lamina*. The osseous spiral lamina bulges into the medial end of the scala media. The spiral limbus is thickened connective tissue continued from

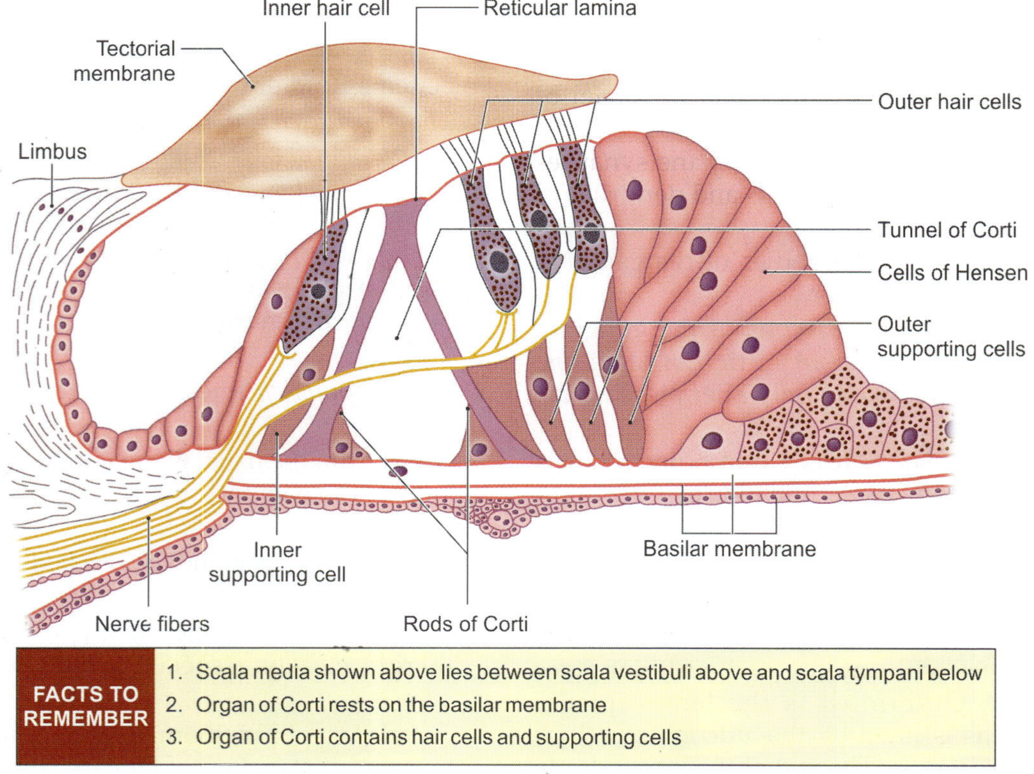

FACTS TO REMEMBER

1. Scala media shown above lies between scala vestibuli above and scala tympani below
2. Organ of Corti rests on the basilar membrane
3. Organ of Corti contains hair cells and supporting cells

Fig. 45.85: Structure of scala media (diagrammatic)

the periosteum of the osseous spiral lamina and it forms the floor of the cochlear duct. The spiral limbus is covered by columnar epithelium which is continuous at its lateral extension with *tectorial membrane* overlying the spiral organ of Corti. The *basilar membrane* lies between the lateral end of the osseous spiral lamina and the lower end of the spiral ligament. The *organ of Corti* rests on the basilar membrane.

Organ of Corti

Organ of Corti is composed of hair cells (the receptors of stimuli produced by sound) and various supporting cells. These are tall, slender cells extending from the basilar membrane to the free surface of the organ of Corti. The supporting cells include the **inner and outer pillar cells, inner and outer phalangeal cells** and **Dieter's cells**. The *inner pillar cells* have broad bases that rest on the basilar membrane and conical cell bodies with their apices extending upwards. The cytoplasm contains a nucleus at its inner end. The most distinctive feature of the cells is the darkly staining tonofibril that courses from the cell base through the body to end in the junctional complexes of the other cells at the apex. The *outer pillar cells* are longer than the inner but cell bodies are similar to those of the inner pillar cells. *Inner phalangeal cells* are arranged in a row on the inner surface of the inner pillar cells and completely surround the inner hair cells.

Hair Cells

Two types of hair cells are present. The inner hair cells are arranged in a single row along the whole length of the cochlea. The outer hair cells form three rows and are lodged between the outer pillar and outer phalangeal cells. In the second coil of the cochlea, a fourth, and in the upper coil, a fifth row of outer hair cells are present. The peripheral processes of bipolar neurons end in the hair cells of the spiral organ of Corti.

COMPONENTS OF VARIOUS LAYERS OF GI TRACT

Histological sections of oesophagus fundus, pylorus of stomach, duodenum, jejunum, ileum, vermiform appendix, colon and anal canal are shown in Fig. 45.86.

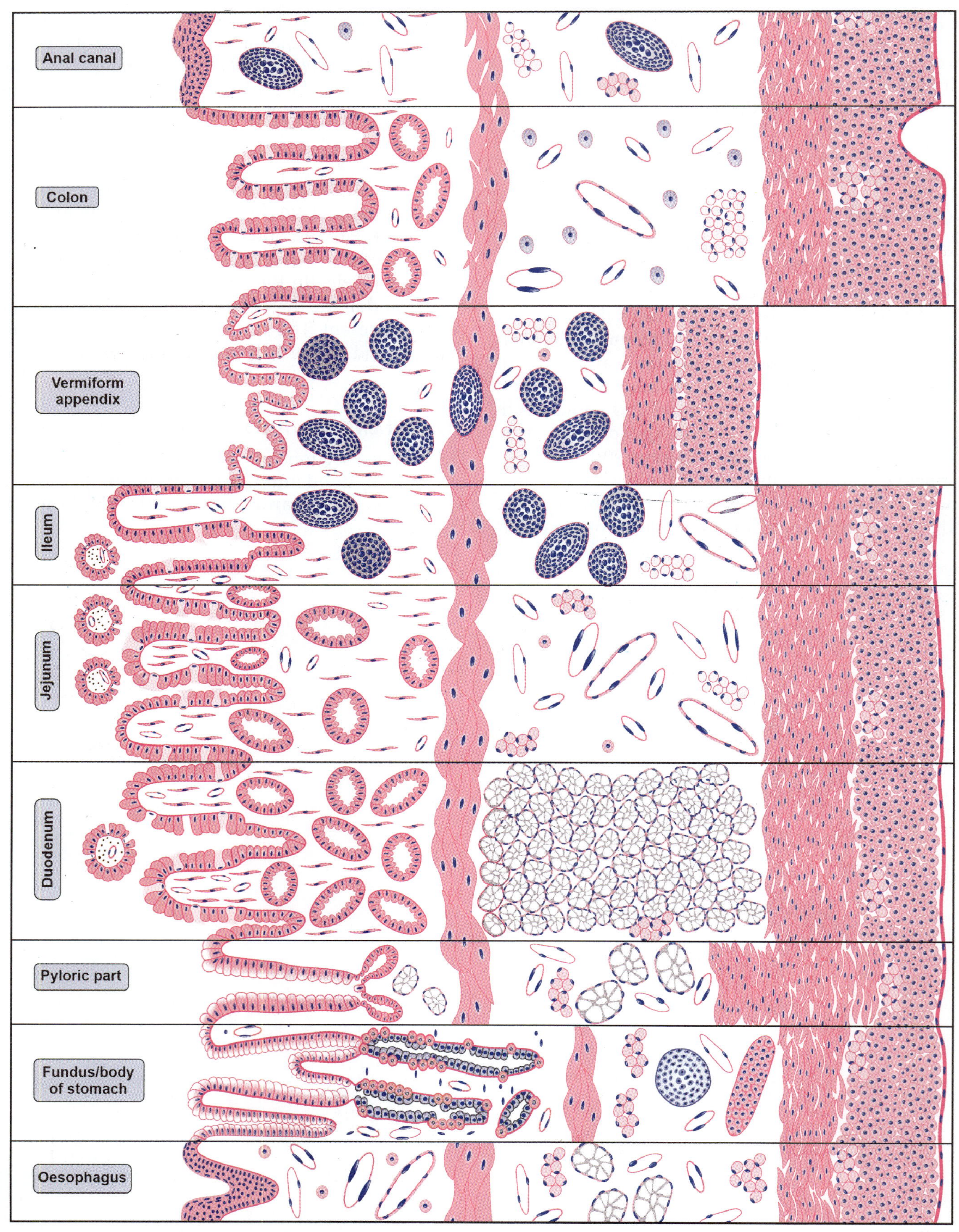

Fig. 45.86: Components of various layers of gastrointestinal tract

Index